NHS Staff Library at the L.G.I.

This book must be returned by the date shown below or a fine will be
charged. To renew this book please phone **0113 39 26445 or e-mail
stafflibraries@leedsth.nhs.uk.** You can also renew this book online
using the NHS Library Catalogue. Please ask library staff for details.

Leeds Teaching Hospitals NHS Trust

D1357524

Basic Orthopaedic Biomechanics & Mechano-Biology

Third Edition

Basic Orthopaedic Biomechanics & Mechano-Biology

Third Edition

Editors

Van C. Mow, PhD

Stanley Dicker Professor of Biomedical Engineering
Department of Biomedical Engineering
Director, Shelley Liu Ping Laboratory for Functional Tissue Engineering Research
Fu Foundation School of Engineering and Applied Science
Columbia University
New York, New York

Rik Huiskes, PhD

Professor of Biomedical Engineering
Department of Biomedical Engineering
Eindhoven University of Technology
Eindhoven, The Netherlands

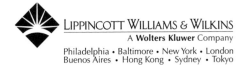

LIPPINCOTT WILLIAMS & WILKINS
A **Wolters Kluwer** Company
Philadelphia • Baltimore • New York • London
Buenos Aires • Hong Kong • Sydney • Tokyo

Acquisitions Editor: Robert Hurley
Developmental Editor: Jenny Kim
Project Manager: Alicia Jackson
Senior Manufacturing Manager: Benjamin Rivera
Marketing Manager: Sharon Zinner
Designer: Melissa Walter
Production Service: TechBooks
Printer: Maple Press

© 2005 by LIPPINCOTT WILLIAMS & WILKINS
530 Walnut Street
Philadelphia, PA 19106 USA
LWW.com

Printed in the USA

Library of Congress Cataloging-in-Publication Data

Basic orthopaedic biomechanics & mechano-biology / editors, Van C. Mow, Rik Huiskes.–
3rd ed.
    p.   ; cm.
Rev. ed. of: Basic orthopaedic biomechanics / editors, Van C. Mow, Wilson C. Hayes.
2nd ed. c1997.
Includes bibliographical references and index.
ISBN 0-7817-3933-0
1. Orthopedics.   2. Human mechanics.   I. Title: Basic orthopaedic biomechanics and
mechano-biology.   II. Mow, Van C.   III. Huiskes, Rik.   IV. Basic orthopaedic
biomechanics.
    [DNLM: 1. Biomechanics.   2. Orthopedics. WE 103 2005]
RD732.B353 2005
616.7–dc22   2004026755

---

10 9 8 7 6 5 4 3 2

To my many brilliant and creative graduate students, and postdoctoral fellows, to whom I owe much of my academic success.
&
To my wife, Barbara, for all her loving support over the years and for her unfailing encouragement throughout my long hours pursuit of excellence year after year.
—Van C. Mow, Columbia University

To my graduate students, who taught me more than I taught them.
—Rik Huiskes, Eindhoven University of Technology

CONTENTS

CONTRIBUTING AUTHORS

Steven D. Abramowitch, PhD
Research Assistant Professor, Department of
  Bioengineering
Musculoskeletal Research Center
University of Pittsburgh
Pittsburgh, Pennsylvania

Thomas P. Andriacchi, PhD
Professor, Departments of Mechanical
  Engineering and Orthopedic Surgery
Biomechanical Engineering
Stanford University
Stanford, California

Gerard A. Ateshian, PhD
Director, Musculoskeletal Biomechanics
  Laboratory
Professor of Mechanical Engineering and
  Biomedical Engineering
Columbia University
New York, New York

Faye Hui Chen, PhD
Staff Scientist
Cartilage Biology and Orthopaedics Branch
National Institute of Arthritis and
  Musculoskeletal and Skin Diseases
National Institutes of Health
Bethesda, Maryland

Lutz E. Claes, PhD
Director, Institute of Orthopaedic Research
  and Biomechanics
University of Ulm
Ulm, Germany

Paul Ducheyne, PhD
Professor of Bioengineering and Orthopaedic
  Surgery Research
Director, Center for Bioactive Materials and
  Tissue Engineering
Department of Bioengineering, School of
  Engineering and Applied Science
University of Pennsylvania
Philadelphia, Pennsylvania

Georg N. Duda, PhD
Professor of Biomechanics
Center of Musculoskeletal Surgery
Charité University of Medicine Berlin
Free & Humboldt University Berlin
Berlin, Germany

Felix Eckstein, MD
Director, Institute of Anatomy and
  Musculoskeletal Research
Professor of Anatomy
Paracelsus Private Medical University
Salzburg, Austria

Ahmed El-Ghannam, PhD
Assistant Professor of Biomedical Engineering
Center for Biomedical Engineering
University of Kentucky
Lexington, Kentucky

Thomas W. Gilbert
Graduate Student Researcher
Department of Bioengineering
McGowan Institute for Regenerative Medicine
University of Pittsburgh
Pittsburgh, Pennsylvania

Steven A. Goldstein, PhD
Henry Ruppenthal Family Professor of
  Orthopaedic Surgery and Bioengineering
Associate Chair for Research
University of Michigan
Ann Arbor, Michigan

Farshid Guilak, PhD
Professor, Departments of Surgery and
   Biomedical Engineering
Director of Orthopaedic Research
Duke University Medical Center
Durham, North Carolina

Wei Yong Gu, PhD
Associate Professor of Biomedical Engineering
Director, Tissue Biomechanics Laboratory
Department of Biomedical Engineering
College of Engineering
University of Miami
Miami, Florida

Frans C. T. van der Helm, PhD
Adjunct Professor of Biomechanical
   Engineering
Twente University of Technology,
   The Netherlands
Associate Professor of Mechanical Engineering
Department, Mechanical Engineering
   & Marine Technology
Man Machine Systems Laboratory
Delft University of Technology
Delft, The Netherlands

Rik Huiskes, PhD
Adjunct Professor of Orthopaedic Research
University of Maastricht, The Netherlands
Professor of Biomedical Engineering
Section 'Bone and Orthopaedic Biomechanics'
Department, Biomedical Engineering
Eindhoven University of Technology
Eindhoven, The Netherlands

Clark T. Hung, PhD
Associate Professor, Department of Biomedical
   Engineering
Director, Cellular Engineering Laboratory
Columbia University
New York, New York

Debra E. Hurwitz
Department of Orthopedic Surgery
Rush–Presbyterian–St. Luke's Medical Center
Chicago, Illinois

James C. Iatridis, PhD
Assistant Professor, Department of Mechanical
   Engineering
Director, Spine Bioengineering Laboratory
University of Vermont
Burlington, Vermont

Keita Ito, MD, ScD
Department of Biomedical Engineering
Eindhoven University of Technology
Eindhoven, The Netherlands
AO Research Institute
Davos Platz, Switzerland

Thay Q. Lee, PhD
Research Career Scientist, VA Long Beach
   Healthcare System
Professor and Vice Chairman for Research,
   Department of Orthopaedic Surgery
Professor, Department of Biomedical
   Engineering
University of California, Irvine
Irvine, California

Van C. Mow, PhD
Stanley Dicker Professor of Biomedical
   Engineering
Department of Biomedical Engineering
Director, Shelley Liu Ping Laboratory for
   Functional Tissue Engineering Research
Fu Foundation School of Engineering and
   Applied Science
Columbia University
New York, New York

Raghu N. Natarajan
Department of Orthopedic Surgery
Rush–Presbyterian–St. Luke's Medical Center
Chicago, Illinois

Patrick J. Prendergast, PhD
Associate Professor, Mechanical and
   Manufacturing Engineering
Director, TCBE
Department of Mechanical Engineering
Trinity College
Dublin, Ireland

Bert van Rietbergen, PhD
Associate Professor of Biomedical Engineering
Section 'Bone and Orthopaedic Biomechanics'
Department, Biomedical Engineering
Eindhoven University of Technology
Eindhoven, The Netherlands

Ian A. F. Stokes, PhD
Research Professor
Departments of Orthopaedics and
    Rehabilitation and Mechanical Engineering
University of Vermont
Burlington, Vermont

Jan Stolk, PhD
Department of Orthopaedics
University Medical Center Maastricht
Maastricht, The Netherlands

Frans C. T. van der Helm, PhD
Adjunct Professor of Biomechanical
    Engineering
Twente University of Technology,
    The Netherlands
Associate Professor of Mechanical Engineering
Department, Mechanical Engineering
    & Marine Technology
Man Machine Systems Laboratory

Delft University of Technology
Delft, The Netherlands

Gordana Vunjak-Novakovic, PhD
Principal Research Scientist
Harvard–MIT Division of Health Sciences
    and Technology
Massachusetts Institute of Technology
Cambridge, Massachussetts
Adjunct Professor
Tufts University
Boston, Massachusetts

Peter S. Walker, PhD
Research Professor
Department of Orthopaedics
Laboratory for Minimally-Invasive Surgery
New York University School of Medicine
VA Medical Center
New York, New York

Savio L-Y. Woo, PhD, DSc
Whiteford Professor and
    Director
Musculoskeletal Research Center
Department of Bioengineering
University of Pittsburgh
Pittsburgh, Pennsylvania

FROM THE FIRST THROUGH THE SECOND TOWARD THE THIRD EDITION

The first edition of *Basic Orthopaedic Biomechanics*, published in 1991, grew from a conversation I had with Wilson C. (Toby) Hayes in his office at Harvard Medical School in early 1986, out of our perceived need for a good book that captured the essence of the then-burgeoning field of orthopaedic biomechanics. This need was sensed by the establishment of the *Journal of Orthopaedic Research* in 1982 (with W. C. Hayes as Co-Editor-in-Chief and V. C. Mow as Chairman of the Editorial Advisory Board), by the large number of manuscript submissions, and by the high percentage of the ever-increasing number of orthopaedic biomechanics abstracts submitted to the annual meetings of the Orthopaedic Research Society. Graduate students and orthopaedic resident fellows were desperately in need of a good source of information that covered orthopaedic biomechanics. On the occasion of the Inaugural Symposium of the Orthopaedic Research Laboratory at Columbia University, April 20–21, 1987, a list of stellar speakers was invited and asked to write a chapter summarizing their assessment of their specialties within the field. The invited speakers, and the chapter co-authors, were judged by Hayes and I to be the leaders of their subspecialties. As with all edited books of this type, it took awhile to receive the contributed chapters, and awhile to edit all the chapters so as to put some coherence and continuity into the first edition. The first edition finally appeared in 1991 and soon became one of the leading authoritative sources for students interested in orthopaedic and musculoskeletal biomechanics.

The second edition appeared in 1997 shortly after the first edition was sold out. This second edition contained a new chapter that was inexplicably omitted in the first volume, i.e., total

knee prostheses. Toby and I were pleased to have Peter Walker write this chapter. Peter is one of the world's foremost experts on the design and performance of total knee replacements. During the early 1990s, quantitative anatomy came into its own; thus a separate chapter by Gerard Ateshian and Louis Soslowsky was added in the second volume to cover the topic of quantitative anatomy of human joints. As subfields sprout in any field, new topics were added. In January 1988, the first conference on tissue engineering was held at Squaw Valley, California. At the end of the conference, the organizers wrote the broad definition for tissue engineering that was adopted shortly thereafter by the U.S. National Science Foundation (NSF). An NSF funding program was soon established. The proceedings of this first tissue engineering conference were published in a 1991 volume of the *ASME Journal of Biomechanical Engineering*. To the surprise of many, these efforts launched a feverish pace of tissue engineering activities in the go-go decade of the 1990s. Indeed, many tissue engineering programs were established in universities and research laboratories, and new business ventures worth billions of dollars were created worldwide. Thus, in the 1997 second edition, Hayes and I included a chapter on the "physical regulation of cartilage metabolism" by Farsh Guilak and co-workers. Guilak is now, along with Rik Huiskes, Co-Editor-in-Chief of the *Journal of Biomechanics*.

Many things have changed since 1991, when the first edition of *Basic Orthopaedic Biomechanics* was published, with modest ambitions, and since 1997, when the second edition appeared. The editors of these editions were Van C. Mow and Wilson C. (Toby) Hayes. First and foremost among the changes for the third edition was a new choice for the second editor. A few years ago, Toby decided to retire from his faculty position at Harvard Medical School to pursue other, perhaps more enjoyable endeavors. Toby moved from Boston, Massachusetts, to Eugene, Oregon, and away from basic orthopaedic research, an area of intellectual endeavor in which he spent more than 30 years of his life. I wish Toby good luck in his future endeavors.

I am indeed pleased that Professor Rik Huiskes from the Department of Biomedical Engineering, Eindhoven University of Technology, The Netherlands, agreed to take the responsibility as my coeditor for this third edition. Rik was already principal author for a chapter on hip prostheses in the first and second editions, and he brings a world of experience in orthopaedic biomechanics, particularly from the European side. This is in fact timely. European orthopaedic biomechanics has been blooming for many years, and Rik brings many of the best Europeans to this third edition as contributors. Moreover, Rik has served since 1980, and continues to serve, as Co-Editor-in-Chief of the *Journal of Biomechanics*. This is one of the flagship journals in the field. Rik has his fingers on the pulse not only of European biomechanics activities, but also of those throughout the world. Hence, this third edition has a more ecumenical flavor and appeal.

Over the years, during my travels around the world delivering lectures on various topics covered in *Basic Orthopaedic Biomechanics*, more often than not I have spied a copy of either the first or the second edition of the book on the desks or bookshelves of my hosts. Indeed, it has been very gratifying to see the wide acceptance of *Basic Orthopaedic Biomechanics* over time, around the world.

Van C. Mow, PhD
Columbia University

PREFACE TO THE THIRD EDITION

In any human endeavor it is difficult to perceive the scope and importance of events in a contemporaneous manner. However, 50 years after the creation of the American Orthopaedic Research Society (perhaps the first of its kind in the world), nearly 50 years after the clinically important, successful development of joint prostheses, after more than 50 years of advances in orthopaedic biomechanics and the more recent developments in the fields of orthopaedic biochemistry, tissue engineering, molecular biology, genomics, and a profuse array of subspecialties, perhaps an attempt at a chapter sketching a brief history of orthopaedic biomechanics is not untimely. We undertook the task of writing such a chapter with a certain amount of trepidation. Any attempts at writing a brief history of any subject will undoubtedly have omissions and a certain amount of incorrect interpretation of the underlying historical events. Thus, we took a long perspective going all the way back to Aristotle, as perhaps the first to have tried his hand at doing biomechanics. In this way, the topics covered must necessarily be superficial. Nevertheless, the reader can gain a broad philosophical understanding of the grand sweep of how knowledge is gained, and how knowledge can block progress. Advancements in knowledge of orthopaedic biomechanics followed the same conceptual milestones, the same progression of ideas and thoughts. We have attempted to take the reader from the ancient philosopher Aristotle, the classical physician Galen, the renaissance scientist Galileo, the age of enlightenment with mathematician/physicist Newton and the physician/physiologist Harvey, to the contemporary orthopaedic engineers and scientists.

History is not the only new addition to this third edition. Chapter 2, "Analysis of Muscle and Joint Loads," found new authors in Patrick J. Prendergast, Frans C. T. van der Helm, and Georg N. Duda, a European team, who deepened and widened the subject. Chapter 3, "Musculoskeletal Dynamics, Locomotion, and Clinical Applications," whose principal author is again Thomas P. Andriacchi, has an additional co-author, Todd S. Johnson. Chapter 4, "Biomechanics of Bone," was taken over from Toby Hayes by Rik Huiskes and his colleague Bert van Rietbergen, although it must be said that some of Toby's original text remained intact. Chapter 5, "Structure and Function of Articular Cartilage and Meniscus," by Van C. Mow, comes with the alternative co-authors Wei Yong Gu and Faye Hui Chen. Chapter 6, "Physical Regulation of Cartilage Metabolism," was again authored by Farshid Guilak, but with a new co-author, Clark T. Hung, a young biomedical engineering professor at Columbia University, specializing in tissue engineering. Chapter 7, "Structure and Function of Ligaments and Tendons," by Savio L-Y. Woo, was updated, with the assistance of co-authors Thay Q. Lee, Steven D. Abramowitch, and Thomas W. Gilbert. Because of the importance of bone and cartilage tissue engineering, mechanosignal transduction, and mechanisms of controlling tissue growth and regulation, there is a new Chapter 8, entitled "Biomechanical Principles of Cartilage and Bone Tissue Engineering," by the two world-renowned authors Gordona Vunjak-Novakovic and Steven A. Goldstein. In fact, because of its importance, the title of this third edition was changed to *Basic Orthopaedic Biomechanics and Mechano-biology*, reflecting current trends in the field. Chapter 9, "Quantitative Anatomy and Imaging of Diarthrodial Joint Articular Layers," by Gerard A. Ateshian, was updated, with the assistance of new co-author Felix Eckstein from Austria, a specialist in novel imaging methods. Chapter 10, "Friction, Lubrication, and Wear of Articular Cartilage and Diarthrodial Joints," was updated and enlarged, with Gerard A. Ateshian now as first and Van C. Mow as second author. A new addition is Chapter 11, "Biomaterials," by Ahmed El-Ghannam and Paul Ducheyne, which, in our opinion, completes the full set of relevant basic sciences for this book. "Biomechanics of the Spine," Chapter 12, found new authors in Ian A. F. Stokes and James C. Iatridis. "Biomechanics of Fracture Fixation and Fracture Healing," Chapter 13, is new, authored by Lutz E. Claes and Keita Ito from Ulm, Germany, and Davos, Switzerland, respectively; this is also an addition that completes orthopaedic sciences, with a clinical flavor. Chapter 14, "Biomechanics and Preclinical Testing of Artificial Joints: The Hip," by Rik Huiskes, has a new co-author in Jan Stolk. Finally, Chapter 15, "Biomechanics of Total Knee Replacement Designs," by Peter S. Walker, is the only chapter with both title and author unchanged from the second edition. The text, however, was seriously updated, as can be expected from a creative innovator such as Peter. Altogether, *Basic Orthopaedic Biomechanics and Mechano-biology* can be seen as a new book, with a new title, reflecting progress.

This third edition has taken a number of years to complete because of various professional and personal adversities and unexpected turns of events in our lives, including relocations of jobs and health problems. We wish to thank the people at Lippincott Williams & Wilkins Publishers for their patience, which we are sure we have stretched to the breaking point. Their supportive attitude and constant offers of help were very encouraging for us. In particular, Mr. Robert Hurley and Ms. Jenny Kim of LW&W are to be mentioned and thanked. We hope this third edition will be worthwhile for the readers and the publisher alike. The book has grown tremendously in size, perhaps reflecting the enormous growth of the field. As a rough measure, by attendance of the annual meeting of the Orthopaedic Research Society, the field has grown by a factor of four from approximately 900 attendees in 1991 to 3,600 in 2004. This does not include all those interested in many foreign lands who cannot attend the ORS meeting in America. It is certain that the field will keep growing, with no end in sight yet.

Van C. Mow, PhD
Columbia University

Rik Huiskes, PhD
Eindhoven University of Technology

A BRIEF HISTORY OF SCIENCE AND ORTHOPAEDIC BIOMECHANICS

VAN C. MOW
RIK HUISKES

1 INTRODUCTION

An insight into how knowledge is gained, how "knowledge" can block new discoveries, and how new knowledge is advanced to form a new and higher level of understanding of any field is a crucial step in our current understanding of the state of knowledge in *basic orthopaedic biomechanics and mechanobiology* of the 21st century. Going from prior knowledge to a new level of knowledge often requires a paradigm shift (37,59). For the beginner, it is important to know that there are several necessary but basic steps in the acquisition and accumulation of knowledge and the establishment of a new paradigm. Indeed, the great Roman physician Galen in the 2nd century AD wrote that all knowledge is accumulative (6). It was true then, and it is true now, that there will always be prior knowledge and there will always be new discoveries.

First, to gain new knowledge, one must start from a domain of generally accepted and ac-cumulated or prior knowledge, i.e., that which we learned when we were young (the common everyday information), and the more advanced knowledge (also now part of the commonly accepted everyday knowledge), i.e., that which we learned or might have learned as an undergraduate or a graduate student in science, mathematics, and engineering. Indeed, this accumulated domain of knowledge determines the way we think, the way we behave, and the way we work, whatever our profession may be (15). Most of the accumulated knowledge in science and engineering is obtained by routine experiments and analyzed by well-accepted theories, working within accepted paradigms that frame our understanding. However, with the accretion of knowledge, conflicts and inconsistencies will arise, and theories will fail to explain or to predict. Clever new experiments or tools need to be crafted (e.g., Galileo's telescope or Hooke's microscope), perhaps to measure the data or to improve their coherence so as to resolve conflicts, or shed new light on a particular phenomenon. Perhaps a new theory needs to be developed to explain the phenomenon. Throughout the ages, with the accumulation of data and conflicts within a given framework of understanding (or paradigm), new hypotheses have arisen. Although most have not been successful, a few have been spectacularly so (e.g., Newtonian mechanics, Darwin's theory of evolution, Einstein's relativity theory, Planck's quantum theory). Even today Darwin's theory of evolution (1809–1882) is still not generally accepted as a scientific truth (7).

Each new hypothesis needs to be validated, and each new paradigm needs to overcome an existing theory or paradigm in logical and rational ways before it can be accepted and generally used by scientists and engineers, and by the public. Thus there is an endless cycle of creating, validating, or confuting existing theories, accumulating knowledge, developing a new working paradigm, proposing new hypotheses, developing new theories, inventing new instruments, devising new experimental methods for the acquisition of data, and finally forging a paradigm shift (37,49). Indeed, the domain of knowledge is, and must be, a dynamic one. It must also be the fertile ground from which all new ideas are created, no matter what the field of endeavor, and it is independent of the time of discovery. In this process, conflicts will almost always occur (scientific, political, religious, or personal), and in a constructive way they become the catalysts and the fuel needed for creativity and advancement of knowledge (15). In a destructive way, conflicts can block progress and create serious personal tragedies (5). Thus, all new ideas must be put in the context of the domain of prior knowledge from which they sprang, and tested in that domain as well. In other words, the history of science has taught that prior "knowledge" can and does block the advancement of knowledge (6). Since the beginning of time, this cycle is one of the most intellectually absorbing aspects of the history of human civilization, and this theme is repeated over and over in this book. This monograph is about the advancement of knowledge in orthopaedic biomechanics that mainly took place over the past 50 years, and the creation of, and advancements made

in, the newly developing field of mechanobiology.

In subsequent sections of this chapter, we give a brief account of a few examples of the monumental and famous historical struggles for advancements in science and of paradigm shifts. In a very small way, these same ideas and struggles (for the most part, sans religious overtones) have led to the theme of this book: *basic orthopaedic biomechanics and mechanobiology*. Obviously, it is not possible today to comprehensively cover this now-large domain of knowledge in a single monograph. Selection of topics to be covered in the various chapters of this book and selection of the senior authors were entirely at the discretion of the editors. These senior authors have all achieved a certain level of credibility in their fields of specialization and have contributed significantly to their specialties. In most cases, the senior authors had total freedom in their choice of coauthors.

2 EARLY HISTORY OF SCIENCE

It is impossible to trace back to the beginning of the scientific discipline that we know today as biomechanics. From ancient times, though, it is a safe bet to attribute to Aristotle (384–322 BC; Fig. 1-1) as the first who might have studied and written extensively on physiology and animal motions (6,25). Aristotle also wrote on many aspects of the natural sciences including physics,[1] astronomy, meteorology, zoology, metaphysics, and other areas encompassing such topics as logic, theology, psychology, politics, economics, ethics, rhetoric, and poetics. Many of Aristotle's ideas on animals, physics, and other broad scientific topics laid the broad foundations of the biological and physical sciences, and they were not to be superseded for nearly 2,000 years, until the Renaissance beginning in the 15th century. Indeed, it was his

---

[1] Mechanics and physics in Aristotle's time were not the same as those we know today. Obviously, Newton and Newtonian mechanics did not appear onto the scene for another 2,000 years.

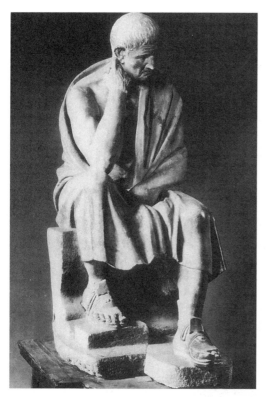

FIGURE 1-1. A Roman copy of a statue of Aristotle (384–322 BC). From Lyons and Petrucelli (40), plate 326.

aim to write on the totality of human knowledge. Yet, Aristotle himself was a kindly and affectionate man with little to indicate his self-importance; his major goal appeared to be to teach and to transmit his accumulated knowledge and thoughts to his pupils. However, much of his ideas were flawed in the context of today's science (6).

During the middle ages Aristotelian knowledge blocked progress. In fact one of Galileo's (1564–1642) major preoccupations was to overcome both the accepted but antiquated domain of Aristotelian knowledge and the dogmas of Christian-sanctified science (51). Nevertheless, even in the context of our time, some of Aristotle's ideas, observations, and principles have proven to be true (e.g., he believed that the earth is round because he observed that the masts of tall ships disappear at great distances as a result of the curvature of the earth). Teaching and transmitting knowledge, and the spirit of dis-

covery of new knowledge, are also the goals of this book.

Aristotle's geocentric system of the stars, sun, earth, and planets was later reinforced by Claudius Ptolemy (Alexandria, Egypt; ca. 150 AD). This schema was further reinforced when it was incorporated into the Christian belief that the earth was flat, and that the earth is at the center of the universe. By the time of the Renaissance, the Aristotelian–Ptolemaic views of the universe and sciences became rigidified. To overcome this idea was nearly impossible. Indeed, classical "knowledge" that had been so self-evident and common sense became a formidable barrier for the discovery of new knowledge . . . a paradigm shift was clearly in the making (37). Despite strong doctrinal religious teachings, many doubts on the validity of the geocentric schema for the universe did arise; these doubts were steadily reinforced by the ever-increasing problems with the calendar in calculating holy days, and with the inability to predict astronomical observations or even provide a simple explanation for planetary motion.

Into this rigidified schema of science and religious beliefs, and into the cauldron of intellectually fomenting society, Nicolaus Copernicus was born (1473–1543; Fig. 1-2). He was a bright, precocious lad: At the age of 9, while a student in Krakow, he purchased and studied Euclid's 13 mathematics books[2] on *The Elements* (Fig. 1-3). At that time, these books constituted the authority on mathematics and geometry (Euclid, Alexandria, Egypt, 325–265 BC). Indeed, these books represent some of the crowning intellectual achievements by ancient scholars. With his father urging him to study medicine, and his uncle urging for him to have a career in the Church, and with a sinecure arranged by his uncle as canon of the Frauenberg Cathedral, Copernicus went to the University of Bologna, and later to Padua, ostensibly to study medicine and law. Instead he actually studied mathematics and astronomy! Eventually his astronomical studies gave rise to his seven axioms on planetary

---

[2] Amazingly, the books that Copernicus purchased, inscribed with his name, still exist today.

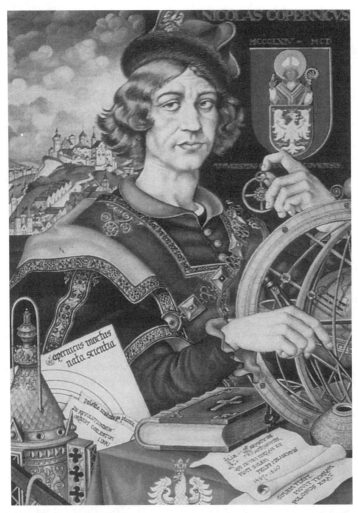

FIGURE 1-2. Nicholas Copernicus (1743–1543), Krakow, Poland, depicting astronomical observations. From Glenn (25), p. 22.

motions that led inexorably to the hypothesis of a heliocentric solar system.

This new theory can more simply and elegantly explain most of the orbital characteristics of the known planets, with the sun being at the center and planets moving in *circular* orbits. Because the Catholic Church was under great pressure from the Protestant movement in the mid-1500s, and the heliocentric *hypothesis* was thought to be heretical, the publication of his hypothesis in the book *De Revolutionibus Orbium Colestium* was postponed and did not occur until 1543, near the time of his death. Many scientists of the day also eschewed the idea of a heliocentric solar system for fear of religious persecution. Indeed, more than a few heretics were burned at the stake for unsanctified religious beliefs. Fortunately, the publication of *De Revolutionibus* was soon followed by the *careful observational data* of Tycho Brahe (1546–1601), a Danish astronomer who observed and catalogued the motion of more than 1,000 stars, the known planets, and comets. These astronomical *data* did much to reinforce Copernicus' heliocentric hypothesis. To further understand these observations, Brahe solicited the mathematician Johannes Kepler to help him explain the motions of these heavenly bodies.

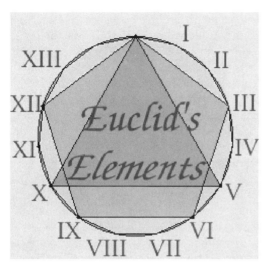

FIGURE 1-3. A diagram figuratively illustrating Euclid's 13 elements of mathematics by Jaume Domenech Larraz (2005; www.euclides.org/). *The Elements* has been studied for nearly 2,500 years throughout the world.

Johannes Kepler (1571–1630), a brilliant mathematician, is now mainly remembered for his three famous laws of planetary motion that we all learned in a high school or college physics course (Fig. 1-4). Of these laws, Kepler's concept

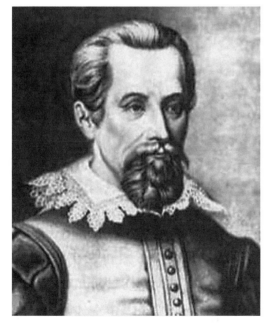

FIGURE 1-4. Johannes Kepler (1571–1630). Steven J. Dick (2005); webmaster@euler.ciens.ucv.ve.

of *elliptical* planetary orbits was the most revolutionary, and helped explain simply and consistently the known planetary motions when the theory of circular orbits could not (6). These laws would become one of the cornerstones for Newton's law of universal gravitation and the consequent movement of planets in an attractive central force field.

Kepler was a profoundly religious man and a mystic (Fig. 1-4). He received his education at the University of Tübingen in Germany, where he learned Aristotelian–Ptolemaic astronomy (geocentric system). Even with his religious beliefs, and the "knowledge" he gained at the university, he became skeptical of the geocentric theory. His skepticism led to his excommunication from the Church in 1612; this ban was to remain in force for the rest of his life. His mother was also charged with witchcraft by the Church, but prosecution was not carried out because of legal complications. Such were the times. The combination of the geocentric flat-earth universe, an idea that had lasted for more than a millennium, and Christian beliefs made a paradigm shift incredibly difficult. Nevertheless, with the Copernican *hypothesis*, reinforced by Brahe's astronomical *data* and Kepler's *theory*, the stage was set for the *paradigm shift* necessary to understand planetary motions (37).

Galileo Galilei (1564–1642; Fig. 1-5), a contemporary of Kepler, was born 21 years after Copernicus' death. During his studies of planetary motion, Galileo had corresponded with Kepler (51). In his personal letters, Galileo secretly stated that he was a "Copernican." There were many personal parallels between Galileo and Copernicus. As with Copernicus, Galileo's father wanted him to study medicine, which he did for a little while, since even at that time doctors made a better living than mathematicians. In his late teens, like Copernicus, he learned much of his mathematics from Euclid's 13 texts *The Elements,* and also from Archimedes' writings. Galileo was inquisitive and a free thinker. Being inquisitive, at the age of 19 while sitting in the Cathedral of Pisa, he noted that the period of a pendulum was not dependent on the amplitude of swing, no matter how large (we now know that there is a limit before nonlinear effects

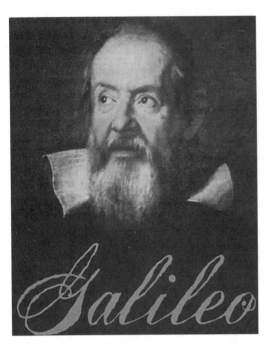

FIGURE 1-5. Galileo Galilei (1564–1462). From Reston (51).

well, could perfect his own telescope before Lippershey could sell his in Italy. Indeed, in 1623, Galileo wrote that "we are certain [that] the first inventor of the telescope was a simple spectacle-maker [Han Lippershey] from the Netherlands" (6). This event shows that Galileo was not above skullduggery to achieve his ends.

Once this *new instrument* was perfected, Galileo was able to obtain nearly a tenfold magnification. When he turned the telescope to the heavens, he saw the mountains of the moon, the moons of Jupiter,[3] the rings of Saturn, the sun spots, that Venus has phases like the moon, and the star clusters in the Milky Way. These observations further reinforced his belief in the correctness of the heliocentric view of the solar system; these observations were published in the *Starry Messenger* (*Sidereus Nuncius*, Venice, 1610).

Twenty-two years later, Galileo wrote, with his undaunted and perhaps foolhardy spirit, a small pamphlet on planetary motion (*Dialogue Concerning the Two Chief Systems of the World— Ptolemaic and Copernican*, Florence, February 1632). This pamphlet depicts a dialogue mainly between individuals (Salviati, a Florentine nobleman in support of the Copernican system, and Simplico, a supporter of the Aristotelian–Ptolemaic system, for the benefit of the third listener). Galileo had already been admonished in 1616 by Pope Paul V never to publish or speak about the Copernican heliocentric system. Now, under Pope Urban VIII, he published the *Dialogue*, which fortified the Copernican theory with *new data*—and in quite obvious terms, it was evident that Galileo's Simplico was a caricature of Urban VIII! Subsequently, Galileo was hulled to Rome from Florence to face the Inquisition in February 1633 (6). At the end of the Inquisition, Galileo was condemned for heresy and was forced to abjure the Copernican theory: "I, Galileo of Florence, must altogether abandon the false opinion that the sun is at the center of the world and immobile, and that the earth is not the center of the world and moves. . . ."

become important). He timed the period of the swing by his own pulse. This simple physical phenomenon led him to even greater curiosity about physics and mathematics. Free thinking is rare in any era, but during the early Renaissance it was downright dangerous. Galileo's free-spirited and arrogant nature eventually led the Pope to put him under house arrest for the last 9 years of his life.

By 1600, Hans Lippershey, a Dutch spectacle maker, had chanced upon a method to make a telescope by using more than one lens. In 1608, the Dutch government received a request from Lippershey for patent rights. He contended that such a telescope would give great advantage to the Dutch government during the wars then raging in Europe. However, because of charges and countercharges by "retroactive inventors," the Dutch government never agreed to Lippershey's petition. Thus, Lippershey decided to journey to Italy to sell his invention to the rich and powerful duchies of Florence and Venice and other vying city-states. Upon hearing of this, Galileo somehow had Lippershey "detained" in Europe so that he, being an excellent instrument maker as

---

[3] To curry favor, he named the moons of Jupiter after the Grand Duke of Tuscany, Cosimo de Medici; today these moons are known as the Medician satellites of Jupiter. De Medici was a patron of Galileo.

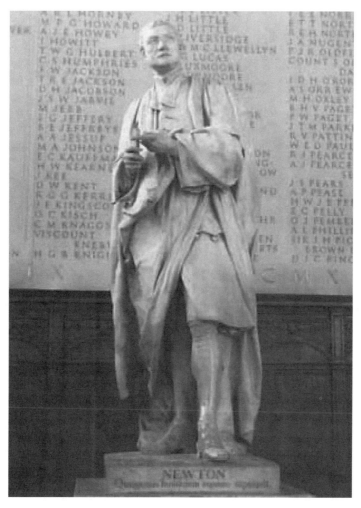

FIGURE 1-6. Statue of Sir Isaac Newton at Cambridge University.

Following this condemnation, Galileo was kept under house arrest, first in Siena, and then at his home in Arcetri near Florence, until his death 9 years later. He was also not allowed to see anyone except with the approval of officers of the Inquisition. Nevertheless, during this period, nearly blind, Galileo managed to write his *Discourses and Mathematical Demonstrations Concerning Two New Sciences*. These were smuggled out of Italy to Leyden, Holland, for publication. These manuscripts dealt with the new sciences now known as statics, strength of materials, and dynamics. For example, he wrote that "the distance that a body moves from rest under uniform acceleration is proportional to the square of the time taken." Today, every physics and engineering student knows this from studies of falling bodies under the influence of constant gravitational force on the surface of the earth. Thus the stage is set within the Aristotelian domain for a paradigm shift to Newtonian mechanics.

Isaac Newton (1642–1727) was born on Christmas Day, 1642, in Lincolnshire (Fig. 1-6), England, in the year Galileo died. Isaac never knew his father, who had passed away the previous October. His mother remarried when he was 2 years old. She moved to a nearby town with her new husband and left Isaac to the care of his grandmother. In his later years, he would claim that he was treated like an orphan by his mother and stepfather. During his growing years, he did not demonstrate academic promise. Teachers' reports indicated inattentiveness and poor performance (6). Nevertheless, a maternal uncle did see some talent in young Isaac. He *mentored* the boy and encouraged his mother (by then a widow again) to allow Isaac to return to grammar school to prepare for university entrance. In his academic preparations, Isaac learned mathematics and geometry by reading Euclid's 13 books on *The Elements*; Newton was also encouraged to further develop his ample mechanical skills, which would become very useful later in life at Cambridge University. In 1661, he entered Trinity College to study law. However, like others before him, young Isaac did not study law but rather studied the writings of Euclid, Descartes, Boyle, Kepler, Galileo, and other great thinkers. At that time Isaac Barrow (1630–1677), the Lucasian chair professor of mathematics at Cambridge, mentored him.

Because of the 1665 plague, Newton returned to Lincolnshire, taking a 2-year of leave of absence from Cambridge. During these 2 years, he made astounding progress in mathematics, physics, optics, and astronomy. Barrow, recognizing Newton's talents and the novelty of his work, sent his manuscript on mathematics to colleagues at the Royal Society to make sure that Newton's contributions were recognized. Shortly thereafter, Barrow resigned from his Lucasian chair to pursue religious studies. Thus at the age of 28, Newton was appointed his successor as the Lucasian chair professor of mathematics. With the domain of knowledge filled with the scholarly contributions from the giants before him, Newton developed theories on calculus, law of universal gravitation, mechanics, optics, celestial mechanics, fluids, solids, and gases, and chemistry (particularly as it relates to alchemy). His theory on calculus and his law of universal gravitation remain today high points of intellectual achievement. These in turn provided the tools necessary to study celestial mechanics that eventually put a mathematical unity on Kepler's three laws on planetary motion. In 1672, Newton was elected to the Royal Society at the age of 30. However, much of Newton's work remained contested and controversial. He maintained animosity toward Robert Hooke on the priority of discovery of results in optics and toward the German mathematician Gottfried Leibnitz on the development of calculus, as well as toward a number of other prominent European scientists and mathematicians.

As we have seen, creation of new knowledge and scientific advancements can be quite hazardous. It requires from scientists courage (or foolhardiness), imagination, strength, and perseverance. It also requires domains of prior knowledge, hypothesis generation, new tools and instruments for better data collection or mathematical calculations, resolution of conflicts and inconsistencies of theories, and data. For multidisciplinary work, although each of the domains is stocked with vastly different set of tools and knowledge, they must also intersect and communicate. The knowledge within this book, *Orthopaedic Biomechanics and Mechanobiology*, occurs at the intersections of the domains of mechanics, engineering, mathematics, computer science, biology, biochemistry, musculoskeletal science, and orthopaedic surgery.

3 BIOLOGICAL AND BIOMEDICAL RESEARCH DURING THE RENAISSANCE

The gladiatorial games were major public attractions during the time of Emperor Marcus Aurelius (121–180 AD) and his son Commodus (161–192 AD), who succeeded as co-Augustus at the age of 19. Both father and son were fond of gladiatorial games. In these games, the Emperor Commodus was often involved in mortal combat with gladiators and beasts alike. (It was these contests that were recently depicted in the Russell Crowe movie *Gladiator*.) Galen (Fig. 1-7), a famous physician of his time, was appointed by Emperor Marcus Aurelius as physician to the gladiators (25).

During his earlier years, Galen learned his medical and anatomical knowledge from the writings of Hippocrates. He was also trained in Aristotelian physics and philosophy and Euclidean mathematics. He learned anatomy of the upper and lower extremities (bone, joints, and

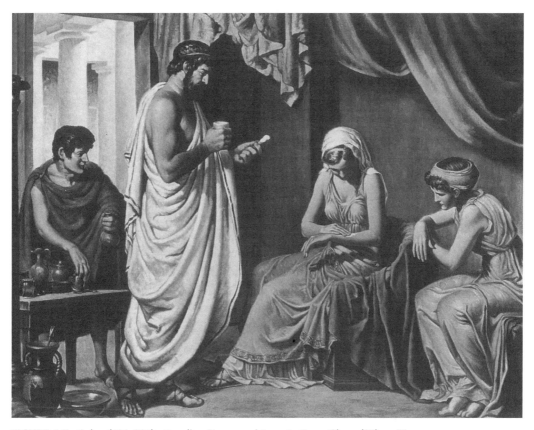

FIGURE 1-7. Galen (131–201) attending Roman aristocrats. From Glenn (25), p. 36.

muscles) from the numerous injured gladiators. However, since Roman laws prohibited human dissections, much of his knowledge of the vital organs, e.g., the heart, was obtained from dissections of Barbary apes available in northern Africa, and these apes only have two-chambered hearts (Fig. 1-8). More than 500 articles on medicine and healing are attributed to Galen, and much of the "knowledge" they contained is incorrect. Nevertheless, Galen's teaching was, for more than 1,400 years, the paradigm for medieval European physicians. This knowledge, along with all its erroneous concepts, became what was known as the "tyranny of Galen." This revered "knowledge" also became the obstacle to progress in medical science.

As with other great thinkers of the Renaissance, many physicians and anatomists began to challenge Galen's dogma. One such genius was Leonardo da Vinci (1452–1519), and another was anatomist Andreas Vesalius (1514–1564). Da Vinci was an artist and an engineer, much like Archimedes. In recent times, H. R. Lissner (4), at the dawn of modern American biomechanics in the last century (1966), would quote da Vinci: "Mechanical science is the noblest and above all others the most useful, seeing that by means of it all animated bodies which have movements perform their interactions. . . . "

Although da Vinci's sketches of human anatomy from dissections are remarkable (43), they did not create the scientific revolution that Vesalius's anatomic studies produced (6). Unlike Da Vinci's time, during Vesalius's time there was no taboo against dissection of the human body, thus allowing him to handle human bodies and dissect human organs. He discovered much about human anatomy, and found numerous errors in Galen's anatomical depictions. He could not, for example, confirm Galen's

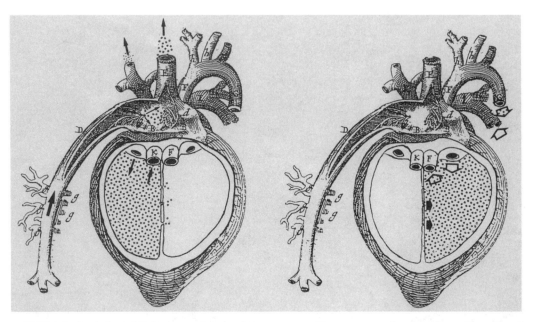

FIGURE 1-8. Depiction of Galen's two-chamber heart separated by a perorated septum from dissection of Barbary apes. From Glenn (25), p. 32.

two-chamber heart with perforations in the septum between the two chambers (Fig. 1-8). He published the finding in exquisite drawings (artists unknown) in his magnum opus *De Humani Corporis Fabrica* in 1543. The *Fabrica* quickly revolutionized not only the understanding of human anatomy but also scientific teaching. Thus, to Vesalius goes the credit of making the first major scientific challenge to Galen's dogma, and the beginnings of a release from Galen's tyrannical grip on medical science. *Fabrica* was published in Basel, Switzerland, and the printing was overseen by Vesalius. Within a mere half-century, this work had become the standard reference for human anatomy; indeed, a paradigm shift had occurred (37). An example of Vesalius's magnificent work is the illustration of the venous system of the human body (Fig. 1-9). A number of copies of the magnum opus still exist in rare book libraries around the world and at the U.S. Library of Congress.

Another paradigm shift away from the Galen tyranny during the Renaissance was the understanding of the blood circulation system. William Harvey (1578–1657), physician to King James I and King Charles I of England,

proposed the concept of continuous circulation of blood—blood leaving the heart, going through the arterial system, and coming back to the heart via the venous system. Also, Harvey's hypothesis of circulation is based on a four-chambered heart, whereas Galen's was based on a two-chambered heart with a perforated septum (Fig. 1-8). Harvey, despite his association with royalty, was nevertheless under severe attack from the numerous Galenists of his time. From a simple calculation of the sheer volume of blood that is pumped by the heart in a day, 234 kg (40), logic would seem to dictate that blood must circulate in the body. However, there was no proof that the venous system (Fig. 1-9) was actually connected to the arterial system in a closed system. As with Galileo's telescopic observations of the heavens that brought new data concerning motions of the planets and eventually brought about a paradigm shift away from the Aristotelian–Ptolemaic view of the geocentric universe, the microscope of Robert Hooke (1635–1703), along with the works of Antonie van Leeuwenhoek (1632–1723) and his reported examinations of the microscopic world existing in droplets of pond water, would

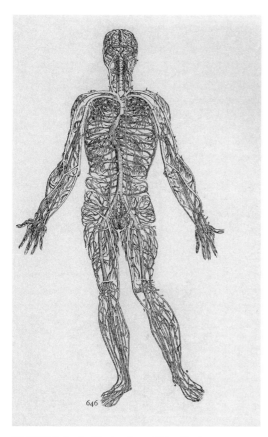

FIGURE 1-9. An illustration of Vesalius's venous system. From Lyons and Petrucelli (40), plate 646, p. 417.

eventually lead to the defeat of the Galenists' view of blood circulation.

The hero of this story is Marcello Malpighi (1628–1694), who is widely regarded today as one of the first true microscopists (6,40). Malpighi was guided by his mentor Giovanni Alfonso Borelli (1608–1679), who not only earned a degree in medicine, but also studied physics and mathematics at the University of Naples. Borelli founded the field of "iatrophysics," which is the study of application of physics to the study of human motion . . . a predecessor of modern biomechanics. In 1680, Borelli published *De Motu Animalium* (*On the Motion of Animals*; Fig. 1-10), where it can be seen that he used the concepts of physics and mathematics to understand human motion, much like some of the concepts proposed by da Vinci. Borelli encouraged Malpighi to delve into the microscopic

world using the new instruments of Hooke, the experimental techniques of Leeuwenhoek, and Harvey's theory on circulation; thus, Malpighi began to tackle the problem of validating the theory of a continuous circulation system. To do this, he needed to find the connections between the arterial and the venous system. Until then, Harvey's hypothesis could not convince many influential Galenists. In 1661, Malpighi announced to his mentor Borelli that he had discovered the capillary system that connects the arterial and venous systems, thus proving Harvey's hypothesis. These studies were quickly published. However, this was not the end of the story.

History has recorded that this discovery of the capillary system did not settle the raging debate on continuous circulation. Much to his sadness, Malpighi had to defend himself against attacks even from a few of his own students, who claimed that his conclusions were rash, and defend his priority against his mentor Borelli. After his death, in 1697, a professor of anatomy in Rome published an article in the *Transactions of the Royal Society* supporting all of Malpighi's conclusions and claims of priority.

Throughout all this, we see the concepts of mechanics at work, where forces and motions are essential for the understanding of a physiological system. It was more than a century later that D'Arcy W. Thompson (1860–1948), in his celebrated publication *On Growth and Form,* argued cogently and elegantly that zoologists, morphologists, and physiologists should eagerly enlist the aid of the physical and mathematical scientists for their studies (59). The subjects embodied in the current book are excellent examples of the thesis put forth by Thompson.

Such titanic paradigm shifts have launched new studies in the domains of physics, biology, medicine, mechanics, engineering, and so on. In recent times, there have also been some equally titanic paradigm shifts, e.g., relativity theory and quantum mechanics; discovery of the double helix; new theories on cosmology; development of large-scale supercomputers; "complete" discovery of the human genome; and many other engineering science endeavors that may include, broadly speaking, biomechanics and

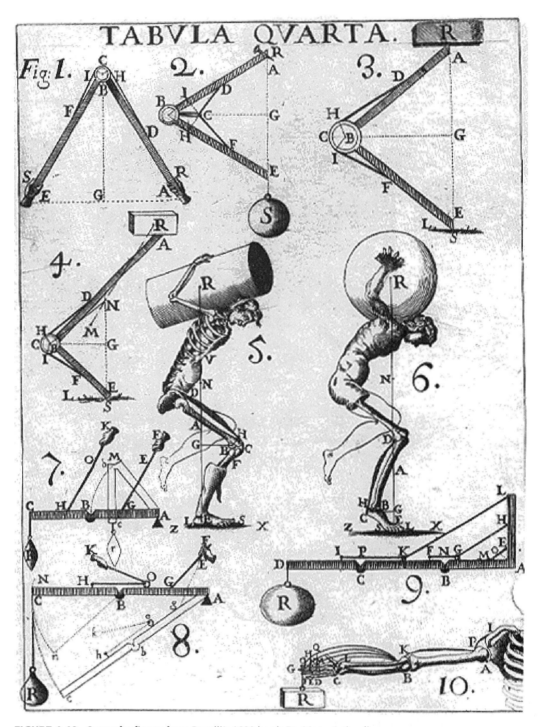

FIGURE 1-10. Copy of a figure from Borelli's 1680 book *De Motu Animalium*.

bioengineering. We repeat again the necessary ingredients for the search for new knowledge: (1) a domain of prior knowledge based on some paradigms; (2) conflicts of the specific data within the paradigm(s); (3) proposed new hypotheses to bridge and resolve the conflicts; (4) creation of new experiments, and better or new instruments for data collection; (5) development of new theories to analyze and to predict; (6) validation of the theories with experimental data; and (7) establishment of a new paradigm. In the subsequent chapters, this theme repeats itself.

4 ORTHOPAEDICS AND BIOMECHANICS

Hippocrates (460–370 BC) preceded Galen by nearly 500 years and wrote on many pragmatic treatments of common ailments. There were many other physicians at his time, and because of Hippocrates' fame, it is likely that many of these physicians attributed their authorships to Hippocrates. Consequently, a legend was created, often with embellished facts and stories told (40). In time, more than 171 books and treatises on medicine and surgery were attributed to Hippocrates. Among these writings, much was devoted to bone fractures and joint dislocation and the observation that damaged cartilage does not heal. Hippocrates also promoted the application of biomechanics for reducing dislocated knee and straightening a dislocated spinal column (Fig. 1-11—Lyons plate 316 and 317). Germane to this book, the observation of Hippocrates on cartilage was reaffirmed by the great British anatomist William Hunter (1718–1783), i.e., that articular cartilage, when it is injured or possesses pathology, does not heal (33). Tissue engineers to this day are attempting to find new ways to cause articular cartilage to heal (see Chapters 5, 6, and 8).

The word *orthopaedics* was coined by the French doctor Nicolas André in 1741: *ortho,* "to straighten," and *paideia*, "children" (40). From Fig. 1-11, we see that even during the times of Hippocrates, mechanics (force and motion) were

part of orthopaedics. Until the 20th century, orthopaedists were mainly involved in straightening the spine in scoliosis,[4] performing fracture fixation with braces and plaster casts, treating infections of the bone and joints, and other nonoperative procedures. It was the advent of the development of modern orthopaedic surgical techniques, and the development of durable total joint replacements that was achieved by mid-20th century, that brought orthopaedics to the realm of orthopaedic surgery. With the desire to continually improve the outcome of total joint replacement, orthopaedic surgeons joined hands with biomechanists (e.g.,11,17,19), which led to the present-day field of orthopaedic biomechanics. Indeed, today orthopaedic biomechanics constitutes a major part of orthopaedic research worldwide.

The historical record shows that John Barton of Great Britain surgically performed a subtrochanteric osteotomy to create a pseudoarthrosis at the hip in 1827 (50). In 1894, Themistocles Gluck surgically replaced the femoral head with an ivory ball and secured it with a mixture of resin, powdered pumice, and plaster of Paris. This procedure was later adopted by a number of orthopaedic surgeons of the day. Obviously many of these procedures failed. In the 1940s, the Judet brothers in France developed prosthetic femoral head replacements made of an acrylic hemisphere cap and a short metal stem inserted in the osteotomized femur; this was inserted in more than 600 patients. Most of these endoprostheses quickly failed, due to improper biomechanical design, poor-quality acrylic used for the femoral head, and overuse by the patient. However, advances in the mid-20th century in the development of biocompatible materials such as poly(methyl methacrylate) (PMMA or Plexiglas), vitallium (a cobalt, chrome, and molybdenum alloy), ultrahigh-molecular-weight polyethylene (UHMWP),

---

[4] In the early 20th century, major advances in scoliosis treatment were made by Russell Hibbs of New York Orthopaedic Hospital (NYOH) in 1911; later NYOH would become the Department of Orthopaedic Surgery at Columbia University.

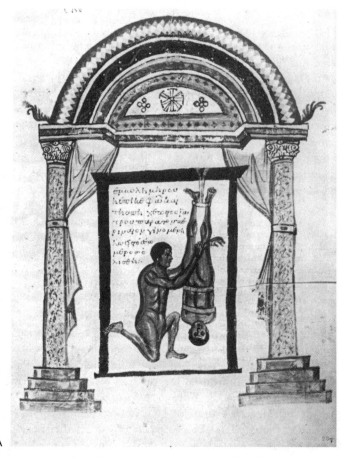

A

FIGURE 1-11. Eleventh-century Byzantine copy of 9th-century Greek "orthopaedic biomechanics." **(A)** Reducing a dislocated knee; **(B)** reducing a dislocated spine. Both figures are from the teaching of Hippocrates. From Lyons and Petrucelli (40), pp. 212–213, plates 316 and 317.

stainless steel, and titanium made longer-lasting prosthetic designs possible for the hip and the knee (8,17). To increase the longevity of hip prostheses, G. K. McKee, in the United Kingdom, developed a device with metal-on-metal articulation. Eventually, in patients, metal-on-metal articulation caused high frictional torque that led to loosening and produced unacceptable metallic wear debris. Today wear from UHMWP and metal articulation is a major problem arising from long-term use of total joint replacements in patients. To counter the loosening problem, McKee incorporated the stem design of an American orthopaedic surgeon (F. R. Thompson) into

his hip replacement design in the late 1950s and early 1960s. Later, in collaboration with J. Farrar, McKee made further improvements in stem designs for the femoral head endoprosthesis with improved surgical outcomes. The system they developed is still in use today and is known as the McKee-Farrar prosthesis. Chapter 14, by R. Huiskes and co-workers, provides a modern treatment of biomechanical analysis of hip prostheses designs, and Chapter 15, by P. S. Walker, provides the same for knee prostheses.

No discussion of total joint replacements, however brief, can be credible without mentioning the contributions of Sir John Charnley

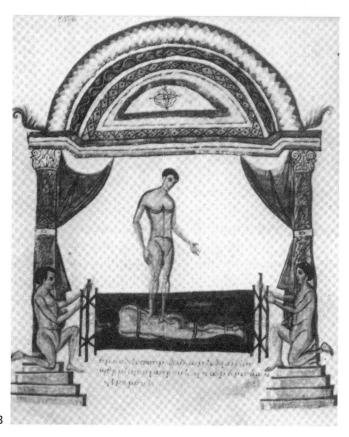

B

FIGURE 1-11. (Cont.)

(1911–1982) (Fig. 1-12). Motivated by his observation that cartilage is more slippery than ice, he began to study various phenomena related to friction, lubrication, and wear of cartilage and joints, in the mid-1950s and 1960s (11); this is now a field known as biotribology[5] (17). Using UHMWP for the acetabular cup, vitallium for the femoral replacement component, and PMMA for cement, Charnley successfully developed and promoted the concept of low-friction arthroplasty for total hip replacements. The first successful such prosthesis was surgically implanted in 1961, and its continued high de-

gree of success led to the worldwide acceptance of total hip joint replacement. For this achievement, John Charnley was knighted.

During the mid-1960s, there was a crescendo of bioengineering and biomechanics efforts throughout the UK as represented by the newly formed Bioengineering Unit at the University of Strathclyde in Glasgow, Scotland, led by R. M. Kenedi (35,36), and in the Bio-engineering Group at the University of Leeds, led by D. Dowson and V. Wright (17). Whereas the efforts at Strathclyde were more varied, covering many topic areas in bioengineering, including studies on the cardiovascular system, hemodynamics, biomaterial, prostheses, biotribology, bone biomechanics, physicochemical and biomechanical properties of cartilage, and gait analysis (36), the studies by the Leeds group were more focused, concentrating on bone, cartilage, joints, and soft tissues (17). The Strathclyde

---

[5] Biotribology is a term popularized by Duncan Dowson: Tribology derives from the Greek word *tribo* (to rub) and thus tribology is the science of friction lubrication and wear. Biotribology is the study of friction, lubrication, and wear of biological materials, e.g., articular cartilage and joints–see Chapter 10 by Ateshian and Mow.

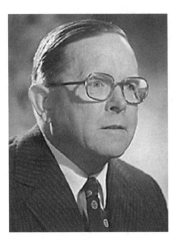

FIGURE 1-12. Portrait of Sir John Charnley. The latter half of the 20th century witnessed the development of successful total hip replacements for arthritic patients. This success served as a catalyst for orthopaedic biomechanics research that is ongoing today. One of the pioneers and innovators in this field was Sir John Charnley, an English orthopaedic surgeon. (2004, H. D. Huddleston, www.hipsandknees.com/hip/charnley.htm)

group's efforts have now largely dissipated in orthopaedic biomechanics on the international scene; the group at Leeds continues to be active in research on biotribology of both natural and artificial joints. The third active group in the UK during that time was led by M. A. R. Freeman, a well-known orthopaedic surgeon in London. Under his leadership, the Biomechanics Unit of the Imperial College of Science and Technology promoted many of the new concepts on the basic biological, biochemical, biomechanical, and morphological studies on articular cartilage and osteoarthritis (20,34). Notable among these studies were those led by Alice Maroudas, who advanced and used some of the concepts from physicochemistry, particularly ion exchange through cartilage, Donnan theory for equilibrium ion distribution, and osmotic pressure for studies on articular cartilage. Two editions of an influential monograph came from this Imperial College group in 1973 and 1979 (20).

On the European continent, a notable publication became available in 1944 by Carl Hirsch, then of the Nobel Institute, Stockholm, Sweden (30). This work was one of the first attempts to correlate the characteristics of the indentation viscoelastic creep behaviors of normal and arthritic articular cartilage with the details of tissue composition (water and chondroitin-sulfuric acid contents) and its histomorphological appearance.[6] However, as with any early studies in a field, Hirsch's work contained numerous fundamental experimental and theoretical errors in the context of today's engineering standards. These errors may be summarized as incorrect stress–strain law, oversimplification of the geometric form, mathematical errors, poor precision in experimental procedure, and lack of statistical analysis. Some of these errors would later be committed by the bioengineers at all three UK groups on the determination of articular cartilage biomechanical properties and subsequently by various orthopaedic bioengineering groups around the world (see detailed discussion in Chapter 5 by Mow and co-workers). Nevertheless, Hirsch's studies on cartilage and his other orthopaedic biomechanics studies (35) captured the imagination of many orthopaedists and budding bioengineers. Indeed, a number of future leaders in American orthopaedic surgery (including Victor Frankel, then of Case Western Reserve University, Cleveland, OH; Jorge Galante of Chicago's Rush Presbyterian Hospital; Augustus White, then of Yale University Medical School; and others) and American biomechanists (Wilson C. Hayes, then of Stanford University; Albert B. Schultz, then of the University of Illinois, Chicago; and others) spent sabbaticals or did postdoctoral fellowships with Hirsch, first at Stockholm, and later at Gothenburg, Sweden, during the 1960s and early 1970s.

Hirsch was not by any stretch of imagination the only one to have performed biomechanics studies on articular cartilage, nor was he the first. German researchers such as E. Bär (1926; ref. 1) and C. Göcke (1927; ref. 26) long preceded Hirsch in biomechanical studies, and German microscopists such as J. W. Hultkrantz (1898; ref. 32) and A. Benninghoff (1925; ref. 2) performed morphological studies of cartilage fine structures. What was novel was Hirsch's attempt

---

[6] Chondroitin-sulfuric acid is now known as proteoglycan.

to correlate the biomechanical results with the details of biochemical composition and morphological appearance, under light microscopy, of normal and osteoarthritic human cartilage. This is an approach much like that encouraged by D'Arcy Thompson (59). Indeed, for research on articular cartilage, Hirsch's work ushered in the modern era of structure–function relationship studies that is currently ongoing in a multitude of robust ways and in many laboratories around the world (see discussions in Chapter 5 by Mow and co-workers).

On this side of the Atlantic, investigators such as L. Sokoloff, a pathologist who was Chief of the Section on Rheumatic Diseases of the Laboratory on Experimental Pathology at the National Institutes of Health, have also been pursuing cartilage indentation studies (58). Sokoloff's studies added new dimensions to cartilage biomechanics studies. During the early and mid-1960s, Sokoloff and co-workers showed that the indentation viscoelastic creep behavior of cartilage depended not only on the health of the tissue (normal or diseased), but also on its water content. In addition these indentation viscoelastic creep behaviors strongly depended on the electrolyte concentrations in the bathing solution, and the type of salt (e.g., Na^+, Ca^{2+}) used in the solution. These results were consistent with, and preceded, the inchoate results from the Biomechanics Unit at the Imperial College in London, and thus set the stage for most of the later work, and current research, on cartilage biomechanics research (see Chapter 5 by Mow and co-workers). However, the engineering errors committed by Hirsch were also propagated into Sokoloff's otherwise careful studies. In his book, *The Biology of Degenerative Joint Diseases,* University of Chicago Press, 1969, Sokoloff wrote an important motivation for many latter-day bioengineers:

> The morphological characteristics of the lesions allow no serious question that mechanical factors are instrumental in causing the abrasion and reshaping of the joint characteristics of osteoarthritis. From the mechanical view, this requires an analysis of the stresses acting on the joints, and the material properties of the tissue and lubrication.

In fact, many studies on cartilage biomechanics that are ongoing today, and forming a large part of orthopaedic biomechanics studies in this century, have specifically addressed the issues raised by Sokoloff in 1969. Indeed, the history of paradigm shift has been repeated again.

5 BIOMECHANICS AND ORTHOPAEDIC BIOMECHANICS

In the mid-1960s several events took place in America that greatly promoted the development of biomechanics in general, and orthopaedic biomechanics in particular. First, the American Society of Mechanical Engineers (ASME) published a collection of papers in a monograph edited by Y. C. Fung (22). The proceedings included studies by Richard Skalak of Columbia University on wave propagation in blood flow and flows through porous tapered elastic tubes; by Benjamin Zweifach of the University of California, San Diego, on transport phenomena in capillary walls; by Y. C. Fung of California Institute of Technology on microscopic blood flow in the rabbit mesentery (i.e., Zweifach and Fung addressed the problem started by Harvey and Malpighi); by Y. K. Liu of the University of Michigan on the impact of human torso; and by T. Y. Wu of California Institute of Technology on the mechanics of swimming of microorganisms. Others who have studied locomotion of microscopic organisms are Sir G. I. Taylor, 1952, and Sir M. J. Lighthill, 1952. Both Taylor and Lighthill in their time held the Lucasian chair professorship at Cambridge University, the same chair held by I. Barrow and Sir I. Newton in the 17th century.

In 1967, Byars, Contini, and Roberts edited an ASME monograph (4), with an introduction by H. R. Lissner of Wayne State University with a provocative title: "Biomechanics—What Is It?" Naturally, these individuals emphasized topics that related more to orthopaedic and musculoskeletal biomechanics as we know it today. Topics such as human gait analysis, anisotropic elastic properties of lamellar bone, dynamic response of musculoskeletal tissues (bone and soft tissues), mechanics of the arm and back, response of the human body due to impact loading, and tensile properties of collagenous tissue were covered.

Other influential orthopaedic biomechanics contributors of that period who deserve honorable mention are Frankel and Burstein on bone properties and general orthopaedic biomechanics (19); Evans on stresses and strains in bone (18); Paul on transmission of forces in human joints (44); Chaffin on modeling of body segment motion (10); Charnley, Dowson, and Wright on biotribology studies (11,17,66); Frankel and Burstein on orthopaedic biomechanics (19); Freeman and Maroudas on cartilage biochemistry, biology, and physicochemical studies (20); Greenwald and O'Connor on hip joint articulation studies (27); Hayes et al. on cartilage biomechanics studies (29); Currey and Pauwels on form and function of bone relationships (14,46–48); Schultz and Galante on spine biomechanics (57); and Viidiik on rheological properties of collagenous tissues (62). By the beginning of the 1970s, these and others made a major impact on accelerating the growth of the field. Consequently, orthopaedic biomechanics today is a basic scientific and engineering discipline that is robust, vital, and dynamic.

To Y. C. Fung (Fig. 1-13), in our opinion, rightly goes the honor of the title "father of modern biomechanics." His greatest influence over the latter half of the 20th century on the development of biomechanics as a scientific discipline is his massive contributions to the literature (22–24). His archival publications and his textbooks on biomechanics have defined and shaped a broad range of its development. His second greatest contribution is his untiring efforts to the development of biomechanics on both the national and international scenes. His efforts have fostered numerous biomechanics journals, agendas, organizations, meetings, and symposia worldwide. Every element of the critical events leading up to a paradigm shift can be found in his contributions. What has attracted such worldwide acceptance is the rigor of his work, both theoretical and experimental, on studying biological materials and systems. Perhaps this is best summed up by a quotation from his 1968 paper "Biomechanics: Its Scope, History, and Some

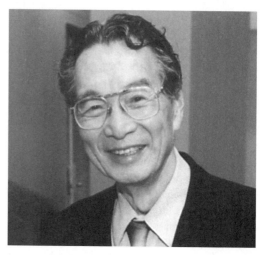

FIGURE 1-13. Portrait of Y. C. Fung, October 30, 2000, taken at the Inaugural Symposium of the Biomechanical Engineering Department of Columbia University. Professor Fung is widely regarded as the "father of modern biomechanics."

Problems of Continuum Mechanics in Physiology" (23):

> What contributions can be expected from [engineers]? I am sure that there are many answers to these questions, but the main thing that engineers have to offer is clear: a set of new tools. It appears that much of the serious application of theoretical and experimental mechanics is new to biology [then and now]. Since every scientific advance in history is heralded by a new tool, it is hoped that the analytical tool of mechanics [and mathematics] may open up a new chapter in medicine and biology, as did in engineering.

6 APPLICATION OF MODERN MECHANICS THEORIES: MATHEMATICAL AND COMPUTATIONAL TOOLS FOR THE STUDY OF ARTICULAR CARTILAGE

Throughout the ages, many anatomists, biologists, biochemists, engineers, physicians, and scientists have reported on anecdotal observations and studies on articular cartilage. The fact that the degeneration of articular cartilage often leads to degenerative joint disease [i.e., osteoarthritis (OA)] has presaged a major effort today on OA and articular cartilage research worldwide (3). Modern biomechanics studies on articular cartilage have been built up on the previous works of Bär, Göcke, Hirsch, Kempson, Sokoloff, Hayes, and others. Prior to 1980, the predominant assumption of biomechanics studies on this tissue was an isotropic, homogeneous, linearly elastic solid. A few authors used viscoelastic laws to model the deformational behavior of such tissue. In general, the disparate theoretical and experimental studies using *ad hoc* constitutive assumptions and experimental methods have led to confusion and controversy along the way. Today, studies based on such elementary (and inaccurate) constitutive assumptions and poor experimental techniques are rare. However, they still do exist.

The major breakthrough in cartilage biomechanics research began with the publication of a paper by Mow and co-workers in 1980 (41). The hypothesis of this paper is based on the well-known fact that soft biological tissues such as articular cartilage contain large amounts of water, and that the frictional drag of flow through the interstices of the tissue is a dominant factor in controlling frictional dissipation within the tissue and hence its viscoelastic behaviors. This paper immediately won the ASME Melville Medal (1982) for best archival literature of that year and it rapidly became the most frequently quoted paper ever published in the *Journal of Biomechanical Engineering*. It has led to a paradigm shift not only for cartilage research, but also for other biological tissues, both hard and soft. This theory, based on a continuum mechanics approach, allowed a theoretically sound and rational approach to ever-increasing sophistication in the modeling of articular cartilage deformational behaviors, e.g., incorporating the some of the details of cartilage collagen–proteoglycan microstructural information into the theory. Detailed description of cartilage biomechanics research and its evolution over time is provided in Chapter 5 by Mow and co-workers.

Though the biphasic theory has been successful in providing a detailed accounting of the major influence of water on the compressive viscoelastic behaviors of cartilage, the theory lacked an accounting of the effects of charges that are fixed on the proteoglycans within the organic matrix, and dissolved ions (e.g., Na^+ and Ca^{2+}) in the interstitial fluid. Earlier osmotic pressure and ion equilibria theories were developed by F. G. Donnan (16) for charged electrolyte solutions (i.e., a liquid) and were adopted by Maroudas to describe the swelling behavior of cartilage. The Donnan theory for electrolyte solutions obviously cannot be correctly used for a charged solid (i.e., the proteoglycan–solid matrix). Ten years after the publication of the biphasic paper, Mow and co-workers (42) published a paper that included a treatment of ions in the interstitial liquid and charges fixed to the porous–permeable solid matrix. This paper received the best paper award of the Bioengineering Division of ASME in 1991 and appears to be changing the paradigm on the theory for soft–hydrated–charged tissues. The biphasic and triphasic theories, their varying assumptions on tissue inhomogeneities and anisotropies, and the adoption of various finite deformation theories seem to satisfy the needs of most theoretical and experimental researchers on studying cartilage and other multiphasic biological materials. It remains to be seen if these two fundamental mixture theories developed for biological tissues, in particular for articular cartilage, will withstand the test of time.

7 APPLICATION OF MODERN MECHANICS THEORIES: MATHEMATICAL AND COMPUTATIONAL TOOLS FOR THE STUDY OF BONE

Throughout the centuries, bones have been studied by mankind because they lasted and were supposed to reveal hidden meaning. In ancient times, they were often studied for prediction of the future, in a generic sense. We now view these ancient "witch-doctor" studies with some amusement, at best, but in fact the goals were not so different from what we are after today: to predict the future. Not in a generic sense, but rather to predict whether a broken bone will heal when applying a particular fixation method, or whether osteoporosis will be prevented by a

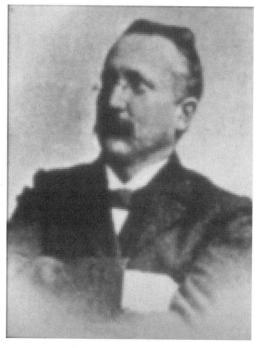

FIGURE 1-14. Wilhelm Roux (ca. 1895) developed theories about cells, bone modeling, and tissue differentiation. No experimental validation studies were performed, thus leaving it up to others to test his hypotheses.

of bone biomechanics that find their roots in the 19th century. This will show that the theories we address are based in history, while the progress we make we owe to modern tools.

The first example is that of *tissue differentiation* in bone. Bones start their constitution in the embryo as cartilaginous anlagen that originate from the differentiation of mesenchymal tissues. These cartilaginous anlagen mineralize in the course of time, starting in the middle of the bone and progressing in both directions toward the epiphyses. Mineralization lingers there, for a while, in the form of cartilaginous growth plates, which eventually mineralize in adulthood—providing in fact the definition of maturity. How and why cartilaginous tissues are mineralized is not entirely clear, but the influence of mechanical loading was already

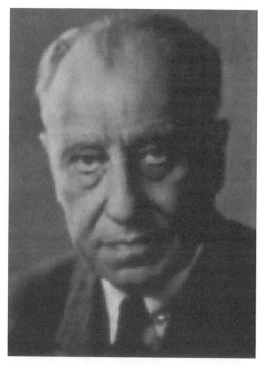

FIGURE 1-15. Friedrich Pauwels (ca. 1970), an MD/PhD, used photoelasticity as a "new tool" to measure the strain field within anatomically shaped models of bones, such as the proximal femur and femoral head. His hypothesis that deviatoric stress stimulates the formation of fibrous connective tissue and that hydrostatic pressure stimulates cartilage formation was the foundation of many latter 20th-century studies on bone morphogenesis.

particular drug or a particular lifestyle, for example. Indeed, our offspring will look at our contemporary efforts with some amusement as well. Or will they? "Amused" is certainly not our state of mind when we look at the bone drawings of Andreas Vesalius (56), or when we study a text of Wilhelm Roux (Fig. 1-14) from 1895 (54). It is respect, not amusement, that we feel. Vesalius applied a new tool to depict the anatomy of bones in detail, thereby allowing theoreticians to ponder about meaning. Roux developed theories about cells, bone modeling, and tissue differentiation, leaving it up to others to validate them. The research for this chapter on the history of biomechanics made us feel humble. The point is, theories and tools are the vehicles of true science, one inspiring the other and vice versa. As to tools, we are certainly much better equipped than our ancestors. However, as to theories in the area of biomechanics, our ancestors were surprisingly modern. Next we present two examples of contemporary research in the area suggested by Wilhelm Roux in 1895 (53,54) in his theory of "functional adaptation" in fracture healing, where fibrous repair tissue differentiates to cartilage, which is later mineralized to bone. Roux was far ahead of his contemporaries, so it is not so strange that it took some time before his hypotheses were taken up in orthopaedics. It was only in the 1920s that his work was seriously considered again in relation to fracture healing. Roux had proposed, for instance, that particularly shear stress on mesenchymal tissues would produce cartilage. Several orthopaedic scientists in prewar Germany took this up and wrote about it, such as Benninghof in 1925 (2) and F. Pauwels in 1940 (45–48). Pauwels (Fig. 1-15) was an orthopaedic surgeon and a professor (PhD in both medicine and engineering), working in Aachen, who actually performed laboratory experiments, measuring strain transfer in bone models with photoelasticity equipment. His work was first collected in a German book (46), then translated into English in 1980—he was 95 years old then—so it did not perish (48). His success as a

scientist was largely based on experimental tools: photoelasticity measurements of strain in laboratory models of bones, in addition to the use of "strength of materials" theory. He hypothesized that deviatoric stress stimulates the formation of fibrous connective tissue and that hydrostatic, compressive stress stimulates cartilage to be formed. The tissue-differentiation theory he developed from these studies is depicted in Fig. 1-16 (47).

It is no wonder that this hypothesis of bone formation was again taken up when new tools emerged in our time—such as the use of finite-element analysis (FEA)—by D. R. Carter (9). Carter and his students made FEA computer models of bones and cartilaginous anlagen, to which they applied the appropriate external loads. They calculated the local stress values in the models, and from those calculations they predicted the kinds of tissues that would locally emerge. Of course, to accomplish that, one needs a theory about what stress (or strain) type produces what tissue. That is exactly the same

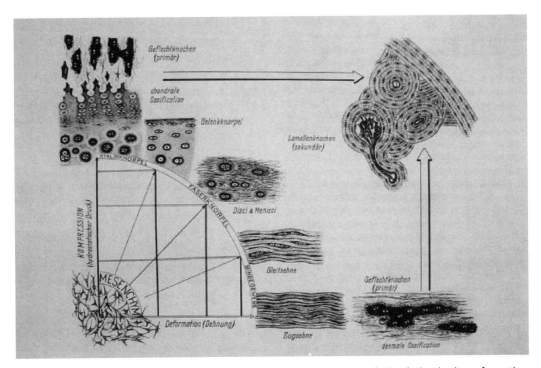

FIGURE 1-16. Diagram depicting Friedrich Pauwels' theory on mechanical stimulation in tissue formation and differentiation from cartilage to bone (47).

question the late 19th- and early 20th-century scientists quibbled over. Carter proposed a combination of octahedral shear stress and hydrostatic stress for his ossification formula, which indeed predicted realistic mineralization patterns in his FEA models. Originally, his computer models were made for FEA *analysis* only, in the sense that the tissue types were predicted directly from the stress patterns computed. Later, they became FEA *simulations* in which the differentiation processes of tissues were included in the computer algorithm. Others followed in his path, considering tissue differentiation patterns in fracture healing and implant interface incorporation, using FEA simulation to predict the courses of the differentiation pathways (12,39). Although the differentiation formulas used were different, and also algorithms for mesenchymal cell migration were included, all used a combination of deviatoric and hydrostatic stress or strain values to regulate the differentiation process, and all provided reasonable predictions.

So after more than a century of research on the relationship between mechanical loading and tissue differentiation (from visual contemplation of tissues to theoretical closed-form solid mechanics, to photoelasticity studies, to FEA analyses and FEA simulations), no paradigm shift had occurred. The theory of Wilhelm Roux still stands, but now we can actually use it for predictions of tissue differentiation patterns, owing to better tools, such as computer simulation using large and incredibly fast computers. That is a great achievement of modern biomechanics. However, although tissue differentiation is obviously related to mechanical stimulation, it is definitely executed by cells, whose biological sensing and signaling activities are implicitly assumed, but not actually considered, in most of these simulation studies. So, in *concept*, the modern computational analyses are not so different from those performed by our ancestors. Fortunately, several mechanobiologists are now studying these relationships between mechanical signals and cell expressions (60).

Other examples of how contemporary theories are based in history are the late 19th-century works of the anatomist Hermann von Meyer (63), the engineer Karl Culmann, and

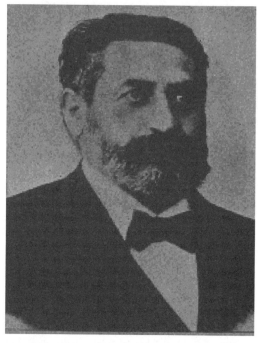

FIGURE 1-17. Julius Wolff (1892), an orthopaedist in Berlin, adopted Karl Culmann's engineering idea that bone may be a mechanically optimal structure of maximal strength and minimal weight. This idea was later to become known as "Wolff's law" of bone remodeling.

the orthopaedic surgeon Julius Wolff (Fig. 1-17; ca. 1892). Culmann, inspired by von Meyer, discovered a remarkable similarity between the trabecular architecture of the proximal femur and the patterns of stress trajectories, calculated in a mathematical model, using the new method of "graphic statics" he had developed.[7] From its results grew the paradigm that bone may be a mechanically optimal structure of maximal strength and minimal weight. This idea was adopted by Wolff, who, an orthopaedic surgeon in Berlin, had collected numerous postmortem bones. Studying the morphologies of the internal trabecular structures of normal and postfracture bones, he visually confirmed this idea and

---

[7] Culmann was a world-renowned mechanical engineer owing to his invention of graphic statics, used for, among other things, stress analyses of the Brooklyn Bridge and the Eiffel Tower.

wrote a book about it (64,65). This hypothesis—for it was no more than that—became known as "Wolff's law." The work of Culmann is a good example of how new tools—scientific methodology—can inspire new paradigms.

This begs the question of how bone can actually organize its structure in such an efficient way. In fact, it was Roux who had suggested in 1881 (53) that trabecular bone architecture is formed, maintained, and adapted by mechanical loads, in a local self-organizing process, regulated by cells. Although Wolff invited Roux as a coauthor for his book (64), he refused because of the shallowness he perceived in Wolff (52). Be that as it may, the question is still with us: There is an obvious relationship between bone mass and morphology, on the one hand, and its mechanical usage on the other, so how does this "self-organizing process" work? A scientist who wrote and taught extensively about these issues was, again, Friedrich Pauwels. In the 1980 English translation of his collected work (48), we find that he applied theoretical and photoelastic stress analyses to models of bones, and found that

> The analysis thus leads to the surprising [sic!] finding that the trajectorial arrangement of cancellous bone (Roux, 1895) and its reorientation when the stressing is altered (Wolff, 1892) appear as a forceful consequence of the principle of construction of the bone (Pauwels, 1973). Neither Roux nor several anatomists could find a satisfactory basic explanation of this phenomenon during the last hundred years.

Today this sounds a little naive because there was not really a "basic explanation" in the work presented. The consequence that he mentioned, "of the principle of construction of the bone," refers to the hypothetical reactions of bone morphology to stresses. Pauwels believed that tensile stresses produce bone resorption and compressive stresses produce bone formation (48). In fetal development and growth, the skeleton would be structurally optimized by muscle contractions, in such a way that in the end all bone stresses are compressive (Fig. 1-18). We no longer believe that, so here we detect the beginnings of a paradigm shift. However, more

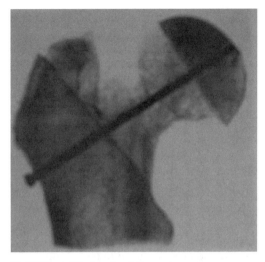

FIGURE 1-18. Proximal-femoral roentgenogram of a postmortem specimen taken from a hipreplacement patient. The superior side of the femoral neck shows bone resorption, the inferior side bone conservation. According to Pauwels, this was caused by tensile versus compressive stresses (48).

important is that the "basic explanation" must be found in the reactions of bone cells to stresses, not in the stresses themselves.

Yet, still, Pauwels can be seen as pivotal for modern bone biomechanics research, picking up the flag from Wilhelm Roux and delivering it to—well, history will tell. In any case, around the same time as Pauwels' conclusion just cited, S. C. Cowin and D. H. Hegedus (1976) published a closed-form mathematical solution for their "theory of adaptive elasticity" to predict mass and shape adaptations as effects of external loading (13). Analytically speaking, this was a totally different ball game, which now allowed analysts to incrementally compute mass and shape adaptations from stresses, strains, or other force-related variables in the bone concerned, based on a phenomenological *feedback* remodeling rule. This would, in the late 1980s and early1990s—note how slowly science progresses, even in our time and age—inspire many an orthopaedic biomechanician. Cowin also presented analytical proof that in these mechanical adaptation analyses the principle of conservation of mass is not violated. This is almost neglected, but still vital, information for those who perform these stress- and strain-related bone modeling and re-modeling studies.

This fundamental question now actually begged for the use of FEA, and it was only a matter of time before this method was applied to link stresses in bone to its morphology and morphological adaptations in so-called "FEA remodeling models"(28) (see also Chapter 4). Initially, FEA theories and models were developed to simulate the regulation of—cortical and trabecular—bone density, or shape, as effects of loading permutations. In principle, however, these studies did not more than confirm what Pauwels had already heuristically concluded: that there was a relationship between bone density morphology and the stresses applied to it. Of course, the new tools made the theory manageable for orthopaedic questions, such as how particular implants would influence bone density postoperatively (see also Chapter 14).

The computer-simulation models predicting bone shape and density of bones based on external loads were later augmented with algorithms to predict trabecular structure (see Chapter 4). This development eventually culminated in a "unified computational theory" for modeling (change of bone shape) and remodeling (coupled osteoclast resorption and osteoblast formation) for both trabecular and cortical bone, as effects of dynamic mechanical loading (31) (see also Chapter 4). It includes mathematical descriptions of osteocyte mechanosensing and signaling for osteoblast bone formation in modeling, osteoclast resorption as effects of bone microcracks, and osteoclast–osteoblast coupling in remodeling. This theory predicts disuse osteoporosis as an effect of reduced loads, and postmenopausal osteoporosis as an effect of estrogen deficiency, making it a suitable research tool for questions related to mechanical stimuli in bone metabolism.

So, finally, the bone cells were included in the computational models, at least by explicit specification of their assumed metabolic expressions as effects of mechanical stimuli. These developments were greatly inspired, or enabled, by the biological theories of Harold Frost (21) and Lance Lanyon (38). Frost proposed the roles of osteoclasts and osteoblasts in the processes of bone modeling and remodeling in his "mechanostat" theory, relative to mechanically induced cell signaling. Lanyon and associates, based on numerous *in vivo* strain-gauge and cell-signaling experiments, proposed the roles of osteocytes in bone as "strain gauges" and signal transducers. Equally important for these developments was the contemporary availability of large-scale computers for testing the theory in simulation studies. Without those the theory would have been useless—that is, not testable. Thus, all the ingredients necessary for a paradigm shift are now in place, and the future bodes well for major advances in understanding bone mechanobiology.

A development that affected biomechanical bone research in a major way was the invention of microcomputed tomography or μCT scanning (55). This enabled 3D visualization and measurements of trabecular structure, which greatly enhanced research and clinical testing in osteoporosis. Using the feasibilities of this measuring tool, μFEA models of trabecular structure could be developed to compute trabecular stresses and strains. Initially, these studies were limited to small bone cubes, but eventually trabecular stresses and strains in whole bones could be evaluated (61). Potentially, these μFEA models could also be used to analyze bone modeling and remodeling, as discussed previously. However, the feedback loops required to simulate these cell-driven processes in an entire bone require computer capacities presently not available. No doubt, a time for this will come!

The examples just discussed suggest that the questions posed, the hypotheses analyzed, and the theories investigated in 20th-century biomechanics were largely derived from 19th-century scientific culture. Nothing can illustrate this better than a quote from an article by H. Roesler, one of Pauwels' students, which he wrote for the special *Journal of Biomechanics* "F. Gaynor Evans Anniversary Issue on Bone Biomechanics"(52):

> Wolff's doctrine... became nearly inextricably involved with Roux's principle of functional adaptation because Roux, searching for impressive examples of his new principle, tried to interpret Wolff's trajectorial structures as a result of functional adaptation. This again was thankfully accepted by Wolff... as further support of his

doctrine, although he apparently did not realize that Roux's "quantitative self-regulating mechanism" was just what he a few years ago had violently rejected as a "theory of permanent structural upheaval."

A computational theory from our time, mentioned earlier (31), can indeed be characterized as such a "theory of permanent structural upheaval." It is fascinating that more than 100 years ago, Roux already saw bone development and maintenance as "principles of functional adaptation," which is now commonly referred to as "Wolff's law," but that Julius Wolff himself rejected the consequences of that proposal. This information should make us humble: We are not smarter than our ancestors; we just have better tools.

The 21st century, however, brought us "mechanobiology" and the associated paradigms and tools to study cell function in the context of mechanical loading. Citing from "Why Mechanobiology?" (60):

> So why mechanobiology? While the term is the inverse of biomechanics, the definition of biomechanics clearly encompasses the experimental and computational models described here: "The science that studies the effects of forces on biological tissues, organs and organisms, in relation to biological and medical problems" [ESB 1978]. As a word, however, mechanobiology moves the emphasis from mechanics to biology and to determining the mechanisms behind "form follows function." But then what does "function" follow? In an evolutionary sense, one could consider function to follow form, a strategy that has enabled vertebrates to successfully breed and survive. This then produces ". . . form follows function follows form. . . ." Considering this cycle of repetition, one can now distinguish between the two terms: biomechanics focuses on the latter part, whether function follows form, whereas mechanobiology emphasizes the former, whether function determines form.

To put it bluntly: To measure stresses in a bone to check whether it would break during a particular musculoskeletal task is biomechanics. To measure stresses in a bone to explain its morphology from its musculoskeletal task is mechanobiology. Having said that, although it is clear from the definition that both examples discussed in this section are mechanobiological in purpose, in both cases the actual treatment was a biomechanical one. Because whereas mechanical signals were determined in those studies, their effects on biology were just inherently assumed, but not explicitly considered. In the first example of tissue differentiation studies, computational models determined strains in tissues, which determined pathways of differentiation. However, how that works in terms of cell functionality was not considered. In the second example of bone modeling and remodeling, stresses were assumed to produce microcracks in bone that block osteocytic signaling, so that osteoclasts are free to resorb bone. Yet, the nature of the osteocytic signal, and how its absence provokes osteoclasts to be formed, was not specified. Seen in that light, "mechanobiology" seems to be a promise rather than an occupation. However, this century has seen the emergence of many new university departments in "Biomedical Engineering," in the United States and in Europe. Visiting those, one will find bioengineers and students involved in actual laboratory studies on, for instance, cell signaling. Many examples are discussed in this book. Musculoskeletal mechanobiology may be a promise, but it will be fulfilled. This is going to be a very interesting century, we predict, full of shifting paradigms.

8 SUMMARY

We have provided a brief synopsis of how scientific advances took place throughout history, and of the often titanic struggles that were involved in making a paradigm shift (i.e., when scientific revolutions occur). Some specific examples have been described from the time of Aristotle down to our present time. We must appreciate that the examples we provided are just a few of the vast numbers of such endeavors and struggles that have that taken place along the way. However, there are certain fundamental elements that are common to all such scientific and engineering endeavors, and these elements must exist for real scientific advances to take place. We repeat again the ingredients that are necessary for the search for new knowledge: (1) a domain of prior knowledge based on some paradigms, (2) conflicts of the specific data within the paradigm(s), (3) proposed new hypotheses to bridge and resolve the conflicts, (4) creation of new experiments and better or new instruments for data collection, (5) development of new theories to analyze and to predict, (6) validation of the theories with experimental data, and (7) establishment of a new paradigm. This scheme is illustrated by the struggles of Galileo for the study of our planetary system, Harvey's struggles on his hypothesis on blood circulation, and, pertaining to the topic of this book, on the advancement of our knowledge of the biomechanics and mechanobiology for the elements of the skeletal system, i.e., bone, cartilage, intervertebral disc, ligament, meniscus, and tendon.

9   ACKNOWLEDGMENT

This work was supported in part by the Stanley Dicker Endowed Chair for Biomedical Engineering, the Liu Ping Functional Tissue Engineering Laboratory funds, and the Whitaker Foundation Special Development Award (Columbia University). Special thanks are due to Ms. Diana Arnold for her excellent assistance in the final editing of this chapter.

REFERENCES

1. Bär E. Elastizitätsprüfungen der Gelenkknorpel. *Arch Entwicklungsmech Organ* 1926;108:739–760.
2. Benninghoff A. Form und Bau der Gelenkknorpel in ihren Beziehungen zur Funktion. *2. Der Aufbau des Gelenkknorpels in seinen Beziehungen zur Funktion. Z Zellforsch* 1925;2:783–862.
3. Brandt KD, Doherty M, Lohmander LS. *Osteoarthritis,* 2nd ed. Oxford: Oxford University Press, 2003:511.
4. Byars EF, Contini R, Roberts VL. *Biomechanics monograph.* New York: The American Society of Mechanical Engineers, 1967:245.
5. de Boer R. Highlights in the historical development of porous media theory: toward a consistent macroscopic theory. *Appl Mech Rev* 1996;49:201–262.
6. Boorstin DJ. *The discoverers: a history of man's search to know his world and himself.* New York: Vintage Books, 1983:745.
7. Browne J. *Charles Darwin: voyaging—a biography.* New York: Alfred A. Knopf, 1995:605.
8. Callaghan JJ, Rosenberg AG, Rubash HE. *The adult hip.* Philadelphia: Lippincott-Raven, 1998:826.
9. Carter DR, Beaupré GS. *Skeletal function and form.* Cambridge, UK: Cambridge University Press, 2001:318.
10. Chaffin DB. A computerized biomechanical model development of and use in the study of gross body action. *J Biomech* 1969;2:418–428.
11. Charnley J. The lubrication of animal joints. In: *Proc. Symp. Biomechanics.* London: Inst Mech Engng, 1959.
12. Claes LE, Hegele CA. Magnitudes of local stress and strain along bony surfaces predict the course and type of fracture healing. *J Biomech* 1999;32:255–266.
13. Cowin SC, Hegedus DH. Bone remodeling I: theory of adaptive elasticity. *J Elasticity* 1976;6:313–326.
14. Currey J. *The mechanical adaptations of bones.* Princeton, NJ: Princeton University Press, 1984:293.
15. Csikszentmihalyi M. *Creativity: flow and the psychology of discovery and invention.* New York: Harper Perennial, 1996:456.
16. Donnan FG. The theory of membrane equilibria. *Chem Rev* 1924;1:73–90.
17. Dowson D, Wright V. *Introduction to the biomechanics of joints and joint replacements.* London: Mechanical Engineering Publications, 1981:254.
18. Evans FG. *Stresses and strains in bone.* Charles C Thomas, 1956:185.
19. Frankel VH, Burstein AH. *Orthopaedic biomechanics.* Philadelphia: Lea & Feabiger, 1970:188.
20. Freeman MAR. *Adult articular cartilage,* 2nd ed. Kent, UK: Pitman Medical Publishing, 1979:560.
21. Frost HM. *Intermediary organization of the skeleton.* Boca Raton, FL: CRC Press, 1986.
22. Fung YC. Biomechanics. *Trans Am Soc Mech Eng* 1966;204.
23. Fung YC. Biomechanics: its scope, history, and some problems of continuum mechanics in physiology. *Appl Mech Rev* 1968;21(1):1–20.
24. Fung YC. *Biomechanics: mechanical properties of living tissues.* New York: Springer-Verlag, 1981:433.
25. Glenn J. *Scientific genius: the twenty greatest minds.* New York: Crescent Books, 1996:160.
26. Göcke C. Elastizitätsstudien am jungen und alten Gelenkknorpel. *Verhandl Deutsch Orthop Ges* 1927;22:130–147.
27. Greenwald AS, O'Connor JJ. The transmission of forces through the human hip joint. *J Biomech* 1971;4:507–528.
28. Hart RT, Fritton SP. Introduction to finite element based simulation of functional adaptation of cancellous bone. *Forma* 1997;12:277–299.

29. Hayes WC, Keer LM, Herrman G, et al. A mathematical analysis of indentation tests of articular cartilage. *J Biomech* 1972;5:541–551.
30. Hirsch C. The pathogenesis of chondromalacia of the patella. *Acta Chir Scand Suppl* 1944;83:1–107.
31. Huiskes R, Ruimerman R, van Lenthe GH, et al. Effects of mechanical forces on maintenance and adaptation of form in trabecular bone. *Nature* 2000;405:704–706.
32. Hultkrantz JW. Über die Spaltrichtungen der Gelenkknorpel. *Verhandl d anat Gesellsch Kiel* 1898;12:248–256.
33. Hunter W. Of the structure and diseases of articulating cartilage. *Phil Trans* 1743;42:514–521.
34. Kempson GE, Spivey CJ, Swanson SAV, et al. Patterns of cartilage stiffness on normal and degenerate human femoral heads. *J Biomech* 1971;4:597–609.
35. Kenedi RM. Biomechanics and related bioengineering topics. *Proc Symp Glasgow.* 1965;493.
36. Kenedi RM. *Perspectives in biomedical engineering.* London: Macmillan, 1973:314.
37. Kuhn TS. *The structure of scientific revolutions,* 3rd ed. Chicago: University of Chicago, 1996:210.
38. Lanyon LE. Functional strain in bone as an objective and controlling stimulus for adaptive bone remodelling. *J Biomech* 1987;20:1083–1093.
39. Lacroix D, Prendergast PJ. A mechano-regulation model for tissue differentiation during fracture healing: analysis of gap size and loading. *J Biomech* 2002;35:1163–1171.
40. Lyons AS, Petrucelli RJ. *Medicine: an illustrated history.* Harry N. Abrams, 1978:616.
41. Mow VC, Kuei SC, Lai WM, et al. Biphasic creep and stress relaxation of articular cartilage in compression: theory and experiments. *J Biomech Eng* 1980;102:73–84.
42. Mow VC, Lai WM, Hou JS. A triphasic theory for the swelling properties of hydrated charged soft biological tissues. *Appl Mech Rev* 1990;43(2):134–141.
43. O'Malley CD, Saunders JB. *Leonardo da Vinci on the human body.* Avenel, NJ: Wing Books, 1982:506.
44. Paul JP. Force actions transmitted by joints in the human body. *Proc R Soc Lond B* 1976;192:163–172.
45. Pauwels F. Biomechanik der Frakturheilung. Proc. 34th Congress, German Orthop Assoc, 1940.
46. Pauwels F. *Gesammelte Abhandlungen zur funktionellen Anatomie des Bewegungsapparates.* Berlin: Springer-Verlag, 1965;543.
47. Pauwels F. *Atlas zur Biomechanik der gesunden und kranken Hüfte.* Berlin: Springer, 1973:276.
48. Pauwels F. *Biomechanics of the locomotor apparatus [translation of Pauwels, 1973].* Berlin: Springer-Verlag, 1980:518.
49. Popper K. *The logic of scientific discovery,* 7th ed. Guildford, UK: Routledge Classics, 2002:513.
50. Rang M. *The story of orthopaedics.* Philadelphia: WB Saunders, 2000:587.
51. Reston J Jr. *Galileo: a life.* New York: HarperCollins, 1994:319.
52. Roesler H. The history of some fundamental concepts in bone biomechanics. *J Biomech* 1987;20:1025–1034.
53. Roux W. *Der züchtende Kampf der Teile, oder die 'Teilauslese' im Organismus (Theorie der funktionellen Anpassung').* Leipzig: Wilhelm Engelman, 1881.
54. Roux W. *Gesammelte Abhandelungen über die Entwicklungsmechanik der Organismus.* Leipzig: Wilhelm Engelmann, 1895.
55. Rüegsegger P, Koller B, Müller R. A microtomographic system for the nondestructive evaluation of bone architecture. *Calcif Tissue Int* 1996;58:24–29.
56. Saunders JB deCM, O'Malley C. *The anatomical drawings of Andreas Vesalius.* New York: Bonanca Books, 1982:248.
57. Schultz AB, Galante JO. A mathematical model of the study of the mechanics of the human spine. *J Biomech* 1970;3:405–416.
58. Sokoloff L. *The biology of degenerate joint disease.* Chicago: University of Chicago Press, 1969:162.
59. Thompson, DW. *On growth and form.* Cambridge, UK: Cambridge University Press, 1942:1116. Revised edition: Dover Publications, 1992.
60. Van der Meulen MCH, Huiskes R. Why mechanobiology? *J Biomech* 2002;35:401–414.
61. Van Rietbergen B, Huiskes R, Eckstein F, et al. Trabecular bone strains in the healthy and osteoporotic human femur. *J Bone Miner Res* 2003;18:1781–1788.
62. Viidiik A. A rheological model for uncalcified parallel-fibred collagenous tissue. *J Biomech* 1968;1:3–11.
63. von Meyer H. Die Architectur der Spongiosa. *Arch Anat Physiol* 1867;615–628.
64. Wolff J. *Das Gesetz der Transformation der Knochen.* Berlin: Hirschwald, 1892.
65. Wolff J. *The law of bone remodeling [translation of Wolff, 1892].* Berlin: Springer-Verlag, 1986:126.
66. Wright V. *Lubrication and wear in joints.* Philadelphia: Lippincott, 1969:152.

2

ANALYSIS OF MUSCLE AND JOINT LOADS

PATRICK J. PRENDERGAST
FRANS C. T. VAN DER HELM
GEORG N. DUDA

1 INTRODUCTION

Almost all animals possess the ability to move. It has often been said that the success of *Homo sapiens* as a species is due to their ability to combine movements that are precise, accurate, and controlled with movements that require strength, flexibility, and endurance. Generating movement from muscle forces is performed by the musculoskeletal system. It is a direct result of the arrangement of the individual muscles and connective tissues, and of the control given to them by the central nervous system. Degeneration of the musculoskeletal system with age and disease affects mobility and can seriously reduce a person's quality of life. The challenge of orthopaedics is to ensure that each individual maintains mobility—a mobility that is as pain-free as possible—throughout his or her lifetime.

Biomechanical knowledge forms the scientific basis for understanding how the musculoskeletal system works, and of how repair and reconstruction strategies for the skeleton may be developed. Investigations of the musculoskeletal system, like those of any system, usually require the development of a *model*. A model is used to answer some question about the behavior of a system. Models may be constructed as a physical apparatus, or alternatively models may be theoretical or computational. The ability to devise the best model to answer a research question is one of the hallmarks of excellence in scientific investigation. The model should not be so complex that the inputs cannot be measured or the outputs related to the question at hand, but neither should it be so simplified that the predictions are obvious. Creating a model that balances these two aspects requires knowledge of modeling tools and how they may be applied—but it also requires judgment and experience.

Biomechanical models of varying levels of complexity have been developed for the musculoskeletal system—from simple static models to computer models that integrate complex control mechanisms. Simple models are usually employed to illustrate a fundamental principle, whereas more elaborate complex models are used for quantitative predictions. The complex output of large-scale models sometimes makes it difficult to use them to discover the fundamental behaviors of the system; oftentimes fundamental knowledge can be obtained using relatively simple models. Therefore, simple models are always important in scientific investigation. However, if a large-scale musculoskeletal model can be successfully validated, it can be used for quantitative analysis of musculoskeletal performance and of the effect of surgical interventions, and

can therefore provide much valuable information.

In writing this chapter, we aimed to show how representative models of the musculoskeletal system can be developed. The reader is encouraged to learn how to analyze forces and motion in articulating joints. First of all, the reader should review some concepts of basic mechanics. Next, these concepts are extended to consider modeling of the musculoskeletal system under the control of the central nervous system (CNS)—this will be the basis for creating large-scale models. Experimental assessment of musculoskeletal performance required for 'validation' or evaluation of models is described in Section 6. In the final two sections of the chapter, analysis of joint and muscle loading applied to the upper and lower extremities is presented.

2 BASIC CONCEPTS OF MECHANICS

Some preliminaries relating to basic mechanics are:

- *Scalars and vectors:* a scalar quantity is described by a single number—its magnitude, e.g., mass, volume, density. A vector quantity also needs specification of direction, e.g., velocity, acceleration, force, moment.
- *Units:* all quantities are measured in units; for mass the unit is kilogram denoted as kg; for volume, m^3; for density, kg/m^3; for force, newtons (N). Capital letters are used to symbolize units named after a person.
- *Notation:* a special notation is used for vector quantities; often an arrow is used so that a force is written as $\vec{F}$. Alternatively, it may be denoted thus $\underline{F}$ or $\mathbf{F}$. The special notation is often omitted if the context makes it clear that the quantity is a vector. An elementary introduction to mechanics is given in Özkaya and Nordin (104).

2.1 Velocity and Acceleration

The velocity v is the rate of change of position with respect to time. If the position is denoted x, then $v = \frac{dx}{dt}$ or $v = \dot{x}$. Integral calculus is used to express the inverse relationship, i.e., $x = \int_{t_1}^{t_2} v \, dt$. The $\int$ symbol may be thought of as an elongated S indicating *sum of* so that $\int_{t_1}^{t_2} v \, dt$ represents the sum of $v.dt$ over the time interval t_1 to t_2. Because the unit of displacement is the meter, velocity is given in meters per second (denoted m/s or ms^{-1}). Acceleration a is the rate of change of velocity, i.e., $a = \dot{v} = \ddot{x}$, where the "double dot" denotes the second derivative, i.e., it denotes $\frac{d^2}{dt^2}$. The units of acceleration are m/s^2 or ms^{-2}. If a mass falls freely under gravity, experiments have shown that it accelerates toward the ground at approximately 9.81 ms^{-2}. This value of acceleration is denoted g and is called the "acceleration due to gravity".

2.2 Angular Velocity and Acceleration

If an object rotates, it turns through an angle in a certain time interval. If the angle is measured in radians, then the angular velocity is given in radians per second (denoted rad/s). Note that 2π radians ≈ 6.236 radians = 360 degrees. The angular acceleration is the rate of change of angular velocity, given in rad/s^2. Because muscles create rotations about joints, the concepts of angular velocity and angular acceleration appear frequently in biomechanics. If the angle is denoted θ then the angular acceleration, usually denoted by α, is given by $\alpha = \frac{d^2\theta}{dt^2} = \ddot{\theta}$. Integral calculus can be used to calculate the angle of rotation if the angular acceleration is known, i.e., $\theta = \iint \ddot{\theta}.dt$, where the $\iint$ symbol denotes double integration.

2.3 Forces

A force can be described as an action between two bodies, such as when one pushes or pulls the other, or a force causes, or tends to cause, motion. However, we cannot rely on simple definitions to give a good understanding of the concept of force—force is a quantity best appreciated by example. If you rise from your chair, your quadriceps muscles will cause knee extension by the generation of a muscle force; in this case the force causes motion. As you sit in your chair, the downward force of your weight is balanced by

an upward force from the chair; in this case the forces are balanced and there is no motion.

Objects do not have to be physically connected to exert a force on each other. Any mass in the earth's gravitational field will have the force of gravity acting on it, pulling it toward the center of the earth; in this case the action occurs between the object and the earth. If you throw a ball in the air, its velocity changes because of a gravitational force acting on it. The magnitude of the gravitational force acting on an object is calculated as its weight multiplied by the acceleration due to gravity. Hence, an object that weighs, say, 20 kg will have a force acting on it of 20 kg × 9.81 ms^{-2} = 19.62 N.

2.4 Moments

A moment rotates, or tends to rotate, an object. A moment is equal to the force multiplied by the perpendicular distance between the force and the axis of rotation, stated as $\vec{M} = \vec{d} \times \vec{F}$, where $\vec{d}$ is the moment arm vector from the center of rotation to the line of application of the force, see Fig. 2-1A. This multiplication is called the cross product of two vectors; consult a mathematics textbook for further explanation. Moments have the units of newton-meter (symbolized by Nm). Moments are vector quantities, and the direction of a moment can be determined using the 'right-hand rule' as follows: imagine the fingers of your right hand curling in the direction of rotation, then your thumb is pointing in

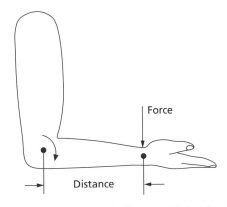

FIGURE 2-1A. Moment is force multiplied by distance.

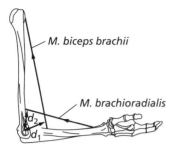

FIGURE 2-1B. Both muscles create moments around the elbow joint.

the direction of the moment vector $\vec{M}$. For the situation depicted in Fig. 2-1A, the moment vector points downward into the plane of the paper.

Motion of a limb is caused by moments generated by muscle contractions acting at a distance from the joint. Consider the simple case of the muscles acting as flexors in the forearm. If *m. biceps brachii* generates a force of F_1 and *m. brachioradialis* a force of F_2, and the perpendicular distances between the lines of action of the forces and the center of rotation at the elbow are d_1 and d_2 respectively (Fig. 2-1B), then the moment generated is

$$\vec{M} = \vec{d_1} \times \vec{F_1} + \vec{d_2} \times \vec{F_2}.$$

The further the line of action of the force from the center of rotation of the joint (i.e., the greater the lever arm), the greater will be the moment of the force.

2.5 Newton's Laws

Isaac Newton (1642–1727) was a genius who discovered the fundamental laws of mechanics that now take his name. Newton's laws relate force to motion, and they relate moment to angular velocity and angular acceleration.

■ Newton's First Law: *A body will remain at rest, or continue in uniform motion in a straight line, unless it is acted on by an external force.* An external force is one that originates outside the object, whereas an internal force originates inside it. As an example of an internal force:

if you sit in your stationary automobile and push against the dashboard, no matter how hard you push the car will remain at rest because your force is balanced by an equal and opposite internal force (the reaction of the dashboard) leading to zero net force. Internal forces do not cause accelerations because they are balanced within the body itself.

■ Newton's Second Law: *An external force will cause a body to accelerate in the direction of the force with an acceleration directly proportional to the magnitude of the force and inversely proportional to the mass of the body.* Newton's Second Law can be written as $\vec{F} = m\vec{a}$, where m is the mass and $\vec{a}$ is the acceleration vector. Because acceleration is the second derivative of the displacement, this may be written as $\vec{F} = m\ddot{x}$. This law also relates moment to angular acceleration. If the moment acts about the instantaneous rotation axis then $\vec{M} = I\vec{\alpha}$, where I is moment of inertia and $\vec{\alpha}$ is the angular acceleration. In this case, the angular acceleration can also be written as the second derivative of the angle to give $\vec{M} = I\ddot{\theta}$. A more complex expression is required for three-dimensional (3D) rotation, see (103) for further information.

■ Newton's Third Law: *To every force, there is an equal and opposite reaction force.* This means that when two objects exert a force on each other then the forces are equal in magnitude and opposite in direction. This law can be used to develop free-body diagrams. A free-body diagram is the first step toward modeling mechanical systems. A mechanical system can be isolated from its environment by replacing this environment by the forces exerted on it. Consider the forearm holding a weight (Fig. 2-2). A free-body diagram can be constructed by replacement of the humerus by the reaction force it exerts; the reaction force is given the symbol R in Fig. 2-2. Likewise, *m. biceps brachii* is replaced by the upward force it generates B_1, *m. brachioradialis* is replaced by B_2, the weight of the ball is replaced by its force W, and the weight of the forearm itself is represented by G. In this way we have isolated the forearm from its environment by

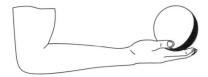

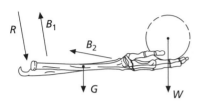

FIGURE 2-2. Free-body diagram of the forearm. Note that the *internal forces* (such as between the wrist bones) are not represented.

substitution of the forces created by that environment.

These three laws are the basis of Newtonian mechanics. Other concepts in mechanics derive from these laws. One of the most important is the concept of static equilibrium. An object is in static equilibrium when the forces acting on it sum to zero and the moments acting on it sum to zero. Letting the $\sum$ symbol denote "sum of", an object is in static equilibrium when:

$$\sum \vec{F} = 0 \qquad (1)$$

$$\sum \vec{M} = 0 \qquad (2)$$

If the forces and moments did not add up to zero, then the object would not be in static equilibrium and motion would occur because the object would accelerate according to Newton's second law. Illustration of static equilibrium in two dimensions requires that the forces balance in *any* two perpendicular directions (say *x* and *y*). Eq. (1) gives two separate equations as follows:

$$\sum F_x = 0, \qquad \sum F_y = 0, \qquad (3)$$

and Eq. (2) requires moments created by forces in the x-y plane to balance. Because the forces lie in the x-y plane, the moment created points in the *z*-direction (right-hand rule), and so

we have

$$\sum M_z = 0 \qquad (4)$$

Notice the subscript *z* in Eq. (4). In two-dimensional (2D) models, having co-planar forces, these three equations can be used to determine up to three unknown variables in the model. However, in reality musculoskeletal loading is not planar and static equilibrium in three dimensions must be considered. In that case, three orthogonal directions are taken (say *x*, *y*, and *z*), and Eqs. (1) and (2) are expanded to give six equations of equilibrium: the three equations of translational equilibrium,

$$\sum F_x = 0, \qquad \sum F_y = 0, \qquad \sum F_z = 0 \quad (5)$$

and the three equations of rotational equilibrium,

$$\sum M_x = 0, \quad \sum M_y = 0, \quad \sum M_z = 0 \quad (6)$$

In 3D static equilibrium we can solve for six unknowns because there are six equations of equilibrium.

2.6 Static versus Dynamic Analysis

If an object is not in static equilibrium, it moves. Problems involving moving objects are called dynamic problems. If a body accelerates, then the inertial forces are calculated according to Newton's second law. Sometimes dynamic problems can be analyzed as quasi-static problems; in that case a static analysis is performed for every time step. In the next section, the solution of problems using static equilibrium will be addressed. In later sections, dynamic models of the musculoskeletal system will be addressed.

The solution of dynamic problems allows computation of motions in a musculoskeletal system. There are two classes of solution methods: (i) forward dynamic models where the forces are known and the motion is calculated by integrating once with respect to time to obtain the velocity and twice to obtain the acceleration, and (ii) inverse dynamic models where the motions are known and differentiation is performed to obtain displacements/rotations, see Fig. 2-3.

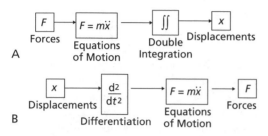

A

B

FIGURE 2-3. Solution schemes for (A) a forward dynamics problem and (B) an inverse dynamics problem.

3   STATIC EQUILIBRIUM

The classical text, *De Motu Anamalium* (10) by G.A. Borelli, first applied static mechanics to analysis of the musculoskeletal system. At the time it was a radical text because it viewed the human body as a machine. The kind of analysis performed by Borelli is still relevant today because it is the basis of fundamental musculoskeletal analysis.

3.1   Calculations with Force Vectors

Any force $\vec{F}$ may be split or *resolved* in two components. If we define the x and y as orthogonal directions as shown in Fig. 2-4, where θ is the angle between force vector and x direction, then $F_x = F \cos \theta$ and $F_y = F \sin \theta$. This process is called "the resolution of vectors." If $\vec{i}$ and $\vec{j}$ denote unit vectors in the x and y directions, then we can write $\vec{F} = F_x \vec{i} + F_y \vec{j}$. We can add two vectors by first resolving them into the same coordinate system and adding their components, so that if θ_1 and θ_2 denote the angles of $\vec{F}_a$ and

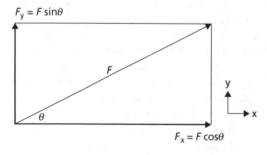

FIGURE 2-4. Trigonometric resolution of vectors.

$\vec{F}_b$ with respect to the x axis, then

$$\vec{F}_a + \vec{F}_b = (F_a \cos \theta_1 + F_b \cos \theta_2)\vec{i}$$
$$+ (F_a \sin \theta_1 + F_b \sin \theta_2)\vec{j}.$$

The vectors can also be added graphically by drawing the diagonal of the parallelogram made by the force vectors. The graphical method is a useful visualization tool: consider for example the resolution of the resultant force from the quadriceps tendon force $\vec{F}_Q$ and the patellar tendon force $\vec{F}_P$ exerted on the patella by the femur. The parallelogram of forces can then be used as shown in Fig. 2-5. Note, however, that we have assumed a 2D problem whereas we know that the patella contacts on the femoral condyles so that the force $\vec{R}$ in Fig. 2-5 is actually the sum of two forces acting at both condylar surfaces.

In a 3D analysis the forces must be resolved in the x, y, and z directions as $F_x = F \cos \alpha$, $F_y = F \cos \beta$, $F_z = F \cos \gamma$, as shown in Fig. 2-6, and the force may be represented as $\vec{F} = F_x \vec{i} + F_y \vec{j} + F_y \vec{k}$. If we wish to add two forces $\vec{F}^1$ and $\vec{F}^2$ in 3D space then

$$\vec{F}^1 + \vec{F}^2 = (F_x^1 + F_x^2)\vec{i} + (F_y^1 + F_y^2)\vec{j}$$
$$+ (F_z^1 + F_z^2)\vec{k}.$$

3.1.1   Static Equilibrium of Two-dimensional Force Systems

In this section, some applications using static equilibrium to analyze musculoskeletal systems are presented. The most important assumption for the solution is that all forces act in one plane, i.e., they are co-planar.

Example 1: A weight 10 kg is held at 90 degrees of abduction, as shown in Fig. 2-7A. The weight of the arm is 3 kg. The perpendicular distance from the glenohumeral (GH) joint to the center of the hand is 60 cm, and the distance to the center of gravity of the arm is 35 cm. Assume that the deltoid muscle is the only muscle acting to support the arm. Anatomical measurements have estimated that the perpendicular distance from the center of the head of the humerus to the line of action of the deltoid muscle is 5 cm and

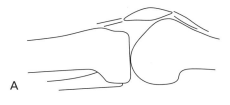

A

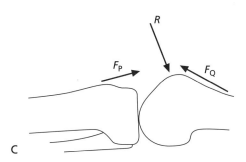

B

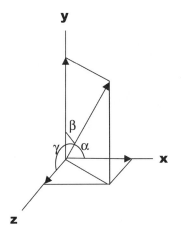

C

FIGURE 2-5. (A) A schematic illustration of the knee joint. **(B)** A free-body diagram of the patella. F_P represents the force in the patellofemoral tendon, F_Q represents the force in the quadriceps tendon, and R is the reaction force at the patellofemoral joint. **(C)** Forces acting on the femur.

that the deltoid muscle connects to the humerus at a point 9 cm distal to the GH joint.

(i) Write the three equations of static equilibrium, and hence

(ii) Calculate the deltoid muscle force and the joint reaction force.

(iii) How much is the magnitude of the joint reaction force reduced if the weight is dropped but the arm still remains at 90 degrees abduction?

Solution: Use symbols to denote the length and force quantities, and use the SI units of kg, N, and m as follows:

F_{GH} = glenohumeral joint reaction force
  α = angle between F_{GH} and the arm
  F_D = deltoid muscle force
  β = angle of F_D and the arm. From Fig. 2-7B, $\sin \beta = 5/9$ giving $\beta = 33.7°$
  W_A = weight of the arm = 3 kg × 9.81 ms^{-2}
    = 29.43 N
  W_B = weight in the hand = 10 kg × 9.81 ms^{-2}
    = 98.1 N
  a = distance of center of gravity of arm to GH joint = 0.35 m
  b = distance from weight to GH joint = 60 cm
    = 0.6 m
  c = 9 cm = 0.09 m
  d = 5 cm = 0.05 m

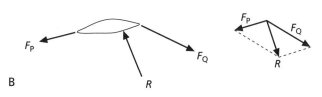

FIGURE 2-6. Resolution of vectors in 3D.

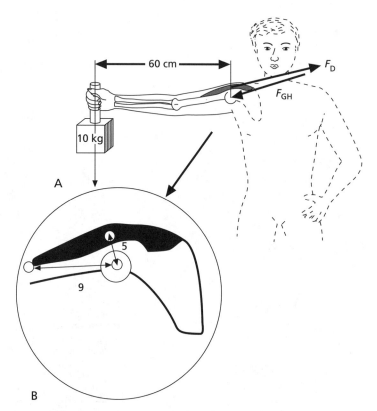

FIGURE 2-7. Analysis of the shoulder joint from Example 1. **(A)** Suggest: "Arm extended showing deltoid muscle and glenohumeral joint reaction force with weight held perpendicular." **(B)** Suggest: "Angle of deltoid muscle force."

There are three unknowns in this problem (F_{GH}, α, and F_D). Using the equations of static equilibrium all of these unknowns can be calculated.

(i) Write the three equations of static equilibrium.

The three equations of static equilibrium are those given in Eqs. (3), (4), and (5) above. Take the x-direction as being along the length of the arm and the y-direction as perpendicular to that. First the F_{GH} and F_D must be resolved into the x and y directions using the trigonometric rule described in Fig. 2-2. Then we can write

...... for the x direction

$$F_{GH} \cos \alpha = F_D \cos \beta \qquad \text{(a)}$$

...... for the y direction

$$F_{GH} \sin \alpha + W_A + W_B = F_D \sin \beta \qquad \text{(b)}$$

...... and taking moments about the GH joint gives

$$W_A \cdot a + W_B \cdot b = F_D d \qquad \text{(c)}$$

(Note that moments could be taken around any point but it is convenient to take them about the GH center of rotation because it eliminates from the algebraic equations those forces that go through the point, i.e., in this case F_{GH}).

(ii) Calculate the deltoid muscle force and the joint reaction force.

If we substitute the known values into Eq. (c) we get

$$29.43 \times 0.35 + 98.1 \times 0.6 = F_D \times 0.05.$$

This gives a value for the deltoid muscle force as

$$F_D = 1383 \text{ N.}$$

Substituting the known values into Eq. (b) we get

$$F_{GH} \sin \alpha + 29.43 + 98.1 = 1383 \times \sin 33.7°$$
$$F_{GH} \sin \alpha = 540.19. \qquad (d)$$

and

$$F_{GH} \sin \alpha = 639.8$$

Using Eq. (a) gives

$$F_{GH} \cos \alpha = 1383 \times \cos 33.7° = 1150.6 \qquad (e)$$

If we divide Eqs. (d) and (e), because $\sin \alpha / \cos \alpha = \tan \alpha$ we get

$$\tan \alpha = 0.556$$

and

$$\alpha = 29°$$

giving

$$F_{GH} = 1315.54$$

(iii) How much is the magnitude of the joint reaction force reduced as the weight is let go but the arm still remains at 90 degrees abduction?

In this case, W_B is set to zero and using Eq. (c) we get

$$F_D = 206.01$$

Using Eq. (b) gives

$$F_{GH} \sin \alpha = 85.02$$

Using Eq. (a) gives

$$F_{GH} \cos \alpha = 206.01 \times \cos 33.7° = 171.39$$

giving

$$\tan \alpha = 0.496$$

and

$$\alpha = 26.38°$$

therefore

$F_{GH} = 191.34 \, \text{N} \ldots$ a reduction of many times what it is when the weight is held. The solution of this problem leads to an important conclusion about joint reaction forces first noted by Borelli in 1680—the joint reaction forces are rather large. As the problem above demonstrates, holding a 10-kg weight at arm's length generates a reaction force at the glenohumeral joint of approximately 1.3 kN. This is approximately twice body weight (say that a weight of a person is typically 70 kg, then 70 times 9.81 equals 686.7 N). You could use what you have learned here to calculate what the effect is of varying the insertion site of the deltoid muscle (*c* in this example). Using a computer package (such as Microsoft Excel, or Matlab) will make this easy. If the insertion site is moved 2 cm proximally to 6 cm (i.e., let c = 0.06 m) then the joint reaction force doubles to 2.5 kN. It is also instructive to apply your anatomical knowledge to criticize this model. What are the assumptions and how may they affect the result? Some assumptions are (i) constant center of rotation and therefore constant moment arm for the glenohumeral joint, (ii) only one muscle acts at the joint, which is clearly a very great simplification, (iii) a unique insertion point for the muscle, whereas the muscle inserts over an area, (iv) a straight line of action for the muscle whereas, in reality, it wraps over other anatomical structures.

Example 2: An arm is flexed to 90 degrees, as shown in the diagram of Fig. 2-1A. A weight of 2 kg is held in the hand as shown in Fig. 2-2. The weight of the forearm is 1.5 kg. Anatomical measurements have given the following dimensions:

$a =$ distance of *m. biceps brachii* attachment to elbow joint = 3 cm = 0.03 m
$b =$ distance of *m. brachioradialis* attachment to elbow joint = 20 cm = 0.2 m
$c =$ distance from center of gravity of forearm to elbow joint = 15 cm = 0.15 m
$d =$ distance from weight to elbow joint = 35 cm = 0.35 m
$\beta =$ angle of B_1 and the arm = 75°
$\gamma =$ angle of B_2 and the arm = 20°

(i) Ascribe symbols to each of the variables in the problem, and hence, write the equations of static equilibrium, and show that there are four unknowns. Explain why there is no unique solution to this problem.

(ii) By assuming that the force in *m. brachioradialis* is equal to zero,

a. Calculate the force in the *m. biceps brachii* and the force (direction and magnitude) acting at the elbow.

b. If the arm is extended a further 30 degrees the angle of the *m. biceps brachii* with the forearm is reduced to 45 degrees. Does the magnitude of the joint reaction force increase or decrease?

Solution: Use symbols to denote the length and force quantities, and use the SI units of kg, N, and m as follows:

G = weight of the forearm = 1.5 kg × 9.81 ms^{-2}
  = 14.72 N
W = weight in hand = 2 kg × 9.81 ms^{-2}
  = 19.62 N
R = elbow joint reaction force
α = angle between R and the forearm
B_1 = *m. biceps brachii* force
B_2 = *m. brachioradialis* force

There are four unknowns, R, α, B_1, and B_2, and only three equations of static equilibrium. Therefore, there is no unique solution. They can be solved by optimization methods (see Section 3.2 below), or by assuming a value for one of the unknowns.

(i) *Write the three equations of static equilibrium*

Referring to Fig. 2-2, and noting the definitions of α, β, a, b, c, and d as above:
... ... for the horizontal direction

$$R \cos\alpha = B_1 \cos\beta + B_2 \cos\gamma \qquad (a)$$

... ... for the vertical direction

$$R \sin\alpha + G + W = B_1 \sin\beta + B_2 \sin\gamma \qquad (b)$$

... ... and taking moments about the elbow joint gives

$$B_1 \sin\beta.a + B_2 \sin\gamma.b = G.c + W.d \qquad (c)$$

(ii) *By assuming that the force in* m. brachioradialis *is equal to zero*,

a. *Calculate the force in the m. biceps brachii and the force (direction and magnitude) acting at the elbow.*

Letting $B_2 = 0$, and using Eq. (c) to obtain an expression for B_1 as:

$$B_1 = \frac{G.c + W.d}{\sin\beta.a} = 313.3\,\text{N}.$$

Eq. (a) gives

$$R \cos\alpha = B_1 \cos\beta + B_2 \cos\gamma = 81.05\,\text{N}.$$

Eq. (b) gives

$$R \sin\alpha = B_1 \sin\beta + B_2 \sin\gamma - G - W$$
$$= 268.2\,\text{N}$$

which gives tan $\alpha = 3.08$, and $\alpha = 73.2°$ and using Eq. (a) allows R to be calculated as

$$R = 280.3\ \text{N}$$

b. *If the arm is extended a further 30 degrees the angle of the* m. biceps brachii *with the forearm is reduced to 45 degrees. Does the magnitude of the joint reaction force increase or decrease?*

The free-body diagram of this problem is shown in Fig. 2-8. To solve this problem, the equations of static equilibrium must first be written, as before. However, it will be seen that the solution can be most easily obtained if the forces are resolved parallel and perpendicular to the humerus, rather than vertically and horizontally.

The following symbol is introduced:

δ = angle of further arm extension = 30°, and now
β = angle of B_1 and the arm = 45°

... ... for the forces parallel to the forearm,

$$R \cos(\alpha - \delta) + G \sin\delta + W \sin\delta = B_1 \cos\beta \qquad (d)$$

... ... for the forces perpendicular to the forearm,

$$R \sin(\alpha - \delta) + G \cos\delta + W \cos\delta = B_1 \sin\beta \qquad (e)$$

... ... and taking moments about the elbow joint gives

$$B_1 \sin\beta.a = G \cos\delta.c + W \cos\delta.d \qquad (f)$$

Using Eq. (f) allows B_1 to be computed as:

$$B_1 = 370.5\,\text{N}.$$

Next Eq. (d) can be used to get

$$R \cos(\alpha - \delta) = 202.6 \qquad (g)$$

and Eq. (e) can be used to get

$$R \sin(\alpha - \delta) = 232.2 \qquad (h)$$

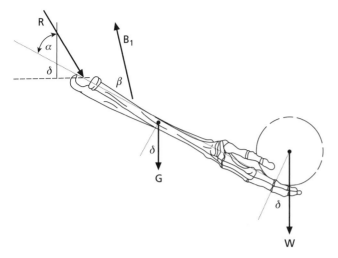

FIGURE 2-8. Free-body diagram for Example 2, part (b).

Dividing Eq. (h) by Eq. (g) gives:

$$\tan(\alpha - \delta) = 0.9485$$

and therefore

$$\alpha - \delta = 43.5°$$

and

$$\alpha = 73.5°$$

Taking either Eq. (g) or Eq. (h) allows the elbow joint reaction force R to be determined as

$$R = 337.4\,\text{N}$$

3.1.2 Static Equilibrium of Three-dimensional Force Systems

In some situations it cannot be assumed that the forces are co-planar. Consider the situation of a weightlifter at a bench press. If we assume that the weight, denoted P, is divided equally between both arms, and if the weight of the arms themselves is neglected, then we can calculate the translational forces and rotational moments that must be resisted by the shoulder joint. Assuming the weightlifter to be lying on his or her back, and defining a coordinate system with an origin at the center of rotation of the joint with x pointing distally in the horizontal direction, y pointing vertically, and z pointing laterally, then we can describe the load vector at the hand as $(0, -P/2, 0)$. If the position of the hand relative to the center of rotation of the joint is given by the coordinates (d_x, d_y, d_z), i.e., the hand grips the bar at a distance d_z lateral to the shoulder and d_x distal to the shoulder, assume $d_y = 0$ so that the grip and the shoulder are on the same vertical level, then the moment to be resisted is given as

$$\vec{M} = (d_x, 0, d_z) \times \left(0, -\frac{P}{2}, 0\right)$$

The cross product[1] of the vectors in terms of the components gives that the moment to be resisted at the joint (by the bones and restraining soft tissues) is

$$\vec{M} = -\frac{P}{2}d_z\vec{i} + \frac{P}{2}d_x\vec{k}$$

therefore, increasing d_x creates an increased moment about the z axis, there is no moment about the y axis, and increasing d_z creates a larger moment about the x axis.

3.2 Indeterminate Force Systems

In the examples described above it was possible to calculate the unknown muscle forces because the number of unknowns was equal to the

---

[1] The cross product of (a_1, a_2, a_3) and (b_1, b_2, b_3) is $(a_2 b_3 - a_3 b_2)\vec{i} + (a_3 b_1 - a_1 b_3)\vec{j} + (a_1 b_2 - a_2 b_1)\vec{k}$.

number of equations. Such problems are said to be statically determinate problems. In general, there are many more muscles present than *degrees of freedom* $(\mathrm{Df})^2$ at the joint, and multiple combinations of muscle forces can result in the same net moments around the joint. However, electromyogram (EMG) recordings show that the muscle activation patterns are very reproducible for the same motion. Hence, it is likely that an optimal pattern is being used to generate the motion. It is currently unknown what optimization criterion is being used in the body, but generally it is assumed that energy consumption is one of the factors.

In statically *indeterminate* problems the number of unknowns is greater than the number of equations. If the force due to *m. brachioradialis* given in Example 2 above were not known (taken to be zero in this model) then the problem would be statically indeterminate, as there would be more unknown forces than equations available. Any number of combinations of the muscle forces from *m. brachialis* and *m. brachioradialis* could counterbalance the weight. If the antagonistic (extensor) muscle were also included, even more combinations of muscle forces producing in the same net moment could result. By applying the appropriate optimization criterion, the muscle forces in statically indeterminate systems can be calculated.

3.2.1   The Optimization Procedure

Optimization procedures allow solutions to be found if there are more unknown variables than equations. In optimization, the equations can be solved exactly with multiple combinations of the variables. If there are *m* equations and *n* variables:

- $m < n$: optimization procedures can be used to solve the problem,
- $m = n$: one unique solution. Paul (107) and Ghista et al. (58) reduce the unknown forces

by grouping muscles, until the equations form a determinate system with one unique solution. This is called the "reduction method" for solving indeterminate systems,

- $m > n$: parameter estimation ('fitting of parameters'). In this case there are more equations than unknowns and it is usually not possible to solve each equation exactly. Instead a solution is found by "fitting the parameters" to minimize the error.

3.2.2   Inverse and Forward Dynamic Optimization

As described in Section 2.5, dynamical systems can be simulated as forward dynamic problems or inverse dynamic problems. When optimization is used, equations are written for an inverse dynamic optimization problem. Because the accelerations and velocities are known in an inverse dynamic model (Fig. 2-3), the differential equations of motion reduce to algebraic equations. The advantage of algebraic equations is that the optimization problem is independent for each time sample. For each time sample the optimization criterion can be calculated, and the muscle forces can be estimated; e.g., if a motion is recorded for 5 seconds with a sampling frequency of 100 Hz, the optimization procedure must be repeated 500 times, but each repetition is independent from the other optimizations. In a forward dynamic optimization problem, the muscle force at one time sample affects the motion of the mechanism, and hence the force at the next time sample is likely to result in another moment. The whole motion will be different. Therefore, the forward dynamic optimization problem becomes much more complex than the inverse dynamic optimization problem because the variables are not independent from each other in time. The whole motion must be optimized in one large optimization procedure.

3.2.3   Optimization Criterion

If *A* is a matrix with the moment arms of *n* muscles with respect to *m* Df at the joints, $\underline{F}(F_1 . . F_n)$ is a vector with the muscle forces, and *M* is a vector with net joint moments, then a general

---

[2]The number of independent translations and rotations that can occur at a joint determines the number of degrees of freedom.

description of the problem is given by:

$$M = A.\underline{F} \qquad (7)$$

If the number of muscles equals the number of degrees of freedom at a joint ($n = m$), one unique solution would exist (determinate problem). This is never the case in the human body, where at least two antagonistic muscles must be present to move a joint in one direction and back. Therefore, in any musculoskeletal model, $m < n$ and no unique solution can be found for muscle force vector $\underline{F}$. In case of a simple one Df musculoskeletal model with two antagonistic muscles, both muscles could co-contract, resulting in high muscle forces but no net muscle moment. Additional requirements (equations) are needed in order to arrive at a unique solution. Such requirements are implemented in an *optimization criterion*. For example, we may decide to find the set of muscle forces that minimizes the total stress generated in all muscles; in that case the optimization seeks to minimize J, where

$$J = \sum_i \left(\frac{F_i}{PCSA_i} \right)$$

F_i denotes the force of the *i*th muscle, and $PCSA_i$ is the physiological cross-sectional area of the muscle, i.e., the area of the cross section perpendicular to the muscle fibers. The muscle force divided by the PCSA is the muscle stress (σ), and muscle stress is related to the energy consumption of the muscle. The higher the muscle stress, the more energy will be used by the muscle. Hence, minimizing this criterion will minimize the sum of squared muscle stresses in the musculoskeletal model, and a unique solution for the variables F_i will be found.

Both linear and non-linear optimization criteria exist. Examples of linear optimization are:

 (i) minimizing the sum of forces (113,114),
(ii) minimizing the sum of moments (131,132),

or a combination of these criteria (131,134). New optimization criteria could guarantee that muscles that were reported inactive from electromyographic measurements are excluded from the calculation. Physiological-based criteria include, for example,

 (i) minimizing the summation of stress (3,32,33),
 (ii) minimizing work done (22),
(iii) minimizing fatigue damage (44),
(iv) minimizing mechanico-chemical energy (105,106).

The above-mentioned criteria can also be applied in a non-linear form, e.g., the sum of forces squared or the sum of stresses squared is to be minimized (3,14,32,33,45,113,132). While linear criteria lead, commonly, to large but few muscle recruitments, non-linear criteria simulate synergistic activity and tend to have more muscles with lower muscle forces. Multiple studies have been performed to compare the linear and non-linear approaches, as well as additional optimization criteria (45,59–61,122,150). Calculations from such studies indicated that the muscle force data was more dependent on the exact determination of the joint angles and the resultant joint moments (a factor of 3 to 4) than on the use of a particular optimization criterion (a factor of 2 according to Patriarco et al. (106)).

3.2.4 Constraints

In addition to the optimization criterion, there are also a number of constraints that should be fulfilled by the variables F_i, otherwise a very trivial solution to the minimization problem would be that all muscle forces would be zero (indeed a very energy efficient solution!). The first set of constraints to be fulfilled are the moment equations $A.\underline{F} = M$, which are a set of linear equality constraints.

An example of a constraint is that a joint should not rotate beyond the restraints of the ligaments. The force in the ligament is a function of the muscle forces loading the ligaments. A loaded ligament will act as a constraint in an inverse dynamic analysis. The constraint is expressed by the equation $A_{lig}.\underline{F} = C_{lig}$ in which the $k \times n$ matrix A_{lig} describes the sensitivity of k ligaments for a linear combination of specific muscle forces, and C_{lig} ($k \times 1$ vector) describes offset terms. Because no compression forces can exist in a ligament, the combination should be constrained to zero or larger than zero. This unidirectional constraint can be represented by a linear inequality equation:

$$A_{lig}.\underline{F} - C_{lig} \geq 0, \qquad (8)$$

or

$$A_{lig}.\underline{F} \geq C_{lig}$$

Another set of linear inequality constraints is formed by the restrictions on muscle forces themselves; muscle forces can only be tensile and they are limited to a maximal value. The maximal value can be calculated as $F_{max} = \sigma_{max} \cdot PCSA$. However, most musculoskeletal models underestimate the maximal joint moment if this value would be used because most data for musculoskeletal models have been acquired from cadavers of old persons. Especially the PCSA values (or the σ_{max}) should be scaled up to be representative for younger persons. Hence, the following linear inequality constraints are added:

$$F_i \geq 0,$$
$$F_i \leq PCSA_i.\sigma_{max} \qquad (9)$$

Another constraint might be that the coordination between muscles is such that dislocation of the joints is prevented, even without stressing the ligaments. This happens when the two articular surfaces of the joint are compressed onto each other, and hence, the joint reaction vector intersects both articular surfaces. If this would not be the case, no equilibrium between 'action forces' from the one bone on the other and 'reaction forces' of the other bone on the first one could occur (Newton's third law), and the bones would move (dislocate) with respect to each other. The joint reaction force vector is a linear summation of the muscle forces (and other forces acting on the bone). Because only the direction of the joint reaction vector is constrained, and not the magnitude, this imposes a non-linear inequality constraint:

$$f(\underline{F}) \leq C_{joint,} \qquad (10)$$

in which $f(\underline{F})$ represent the non-linear function of muscle force vector $\underline{F}$, and C_{joint} is the constraint.

Summarizing, in an optimization procedure, an optimization criterion is minimized with the restriction that the calculated muscle forces must obey linear equality constraints (motion equations), linear inequality constraints (ligament constraints and minimal and maximal muscle forces), and non-linear inequality constraints.

4 MUSCULOSKELETAL SYSTEMS

4.1 Introduction

The wide variety of movements carried out by the human musculoskeletal system are all performed by the same elements: muscles, bones, joints, sensors, and the CNS. Control of the musculoskeletal system is very important in order to understand the resulting behavior. One would never build a robot without a controller, and similarly the musculoskeletal system has a controller in the form of the CNS. The CNS and the sensors cannot be neglected in determining the performance and pathology of the musculoskeletal system.

The dynamic properties of the musculoskeletal system are determined by the inertia of the segments, the visco-elastic, activation, and contraction properties of the muscles, and the proprioceptive feedback loops, in which especially the time delays caused by transportation and processing of the neural signals dominate the behavior. In order to analyze the effect of pathology of one of the components, the function and interaction of the whole system must be considered.

4.2 A Control System Approach

In this section, a theory for modeling the musculoskeletal system as a control system is described. When using a systems theory approach, we do not limit ourselves to the musculoskeletal system, but also incorporate the properties of the CNS and analyze a neuro-musculoskeletal system. We represent each element (skeletal link, joint, muscle, etc.) as a block where each block describes the (static or dynamic) behavior of a sub-system. Each block has certain input signals and output signals. In a block scheme, the signals (or variables) are depicted as arrows, and the relation between (input and output) signals is depicted as blocks. The flow of signals goes

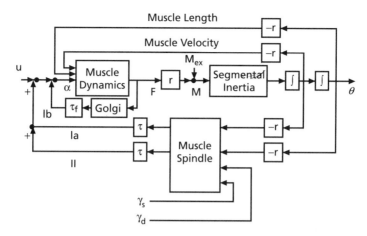

FIGURE 2-9. Block scheme of a neuro-musculoskeletal system. The flow of signals goes from left to right, feedback pathways go from right to left. Input signal is a supraspinal signal from the brain to the spinal cord, output signal is joint angle θ. An α-motor neuron sends an efferent nerve signal to a muscle. The muscle generates force, which also depends on the two other input signals of the muscle, i.e., muscle length and muscle velocity. The force is transferred to a moment through the moment arm r. The muscle moment acts on the skeletal system, which will be accelerated. Also perturbation moments M_{ex} affect the skeletal system, and are added to the effect of the muscle forces. One time integration of the angular acceleration signal will result in the angular velocity of the skeletal system, a second integration results in the joint angle θ. The anatomy of the musculoskeletal system is represented by the segmental inertia (i.e., joint rotation center, center of gravity, mass distribution) and by the moment arms (i.e., the distance between the muscle line of action and the joint rotation center).

The feedback pathways can be distinguished into the intrinsic feedback due to the visco-elastic properties of the muscle, and the reflexive pathways through the muscle spindles and Golgi tendon organs. For the intrinsic feedback the muscle length and velocity can be calculated from the joint angle θ and joint angle velocity $\dot{\theta}$, respectively, by multiplying with the negative moment arm –r. Muscle length and velocity are fed back to the muscle dynamics model, and affect the resulting force through the force-length and force-velocity relationship. For the reflexive feedback the muscle spindles are sensitive to muscle length and velocity. The γ_d and γ_s- motor neurons innervate the intrafusal muscle fibers of the muscle spindle, in order to maintain the sensitivity of the spindle for large length excursions. The Golgi tendon organ is sensitive to the muscle force. The output of the muscle spindles (Ia and II afferent nerve signals) and the Golgi tendon organ (II afferent nerve signals) are fed back as input to the α-motor neuron.

from left to right, and starts from input signals (supraspinal signals originating from the brain) into the whole system and ends with the output signals (the joint angle θ). The supraspinal signals activate the α-motor neuron and result in efferent nerve signals to the muscles. The muscle generates force, which is transferred to a muscle moment through the moment arm r. The muscle moment M acts on the segment with inertia I and results in an angular acceleration: $\ddot{\theta} = M/I$, as described in Section 2.5. The angular acceleration is twice integrated in order to obtain the joint angle θ. The block diagram describing the neuro-musculoskeletal system is given in Fig. 2-9, where a detailed description is given in the caption.

4.3 Muscle Biomechanics

4.3.1 Morphology

Muscles are the actuators of the skeletal system. They transfer efferent neural signals into forces

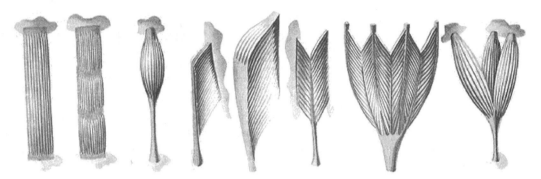

FIGURE 2-10. Variety of muscle architectures. Adapted from *Gray's Anatomy* (Warwic and Willems, 1973).

that will cause motion (or forces exerted on the environment). The basic morphology of a muscle is a muscle belly with the muscle fibers and a tendon. Often muscle fibers attach to a tendinous sheet inside the muscle belly. These tendinous sheets are called the aponeurosis. The tendons are made of connective tissue, mostly collagen fibers, just like ligaments. They tend to be very strong and stiff, elongating only about 5% to 7% of their rest length. Sometimes the tendon is very short, and the muscle appears to be directly attached to the bone. The muscle belly consists of muscle bundles, which are subdivided into muscle fibers in parallel. The more muscle fibers are in parallel, the higher the force a muscle can exert. The area perpendicular to the muscle fiber direction is called the PCSA. Often the PCSA is approximated by

$$PCSA = \frac{V_m}{l_{fiber}} \qquad (11)$$

in which V_m is the muscle volume (equivalent to the muscle mass because the muscle density is about one and l_{fiber} is the optimum muscle length), see Weber (146). The maximal muscle stress (= maximal muscle force per unit area) along the fiber direction is about 37 N/cm^2 (147), as has been measured in animal experiments. The maximal muscle stress can be used to calculate the maximal force that a muscle can exert. For instance, if a muscle has a PCSA of 7 cm^2, the maximal muscle force is 7 [cm^2] × 37 [N/cm^2] = 259 N. Usually in musculoskeletal models, higher values for the maximal muscle stress are used to match with

young and healthy subjects, e.g., ranging from 60–100 N/cm^2 to account for the muscle atrophy in elder cadavers and, presumably, for the non-physiological stimulation using electrodes in the animal experiments, e.g. Winters and Stark (152).

There is a wide variety of muscle architectures, see Fig. 2-10. The proximal attachment of the muscle is called the origin, the distal attachment is called the insertion. Muscles with parallel fibers running straight from origin to insertion exert forces in line with the fiber direction. There are also unipennate, bipennate, and multipennate muscles, in which the fibers are attached with a (pennation) angle α to the tendon (Fig. 2-9). The forces exerted in the muscle fibers are not in line with the muscle force, which should be corrected for the pennation angle:

$$F_{muscle} = F_{fibers} \cdot \cos \alpha \qquad (12)$$

The muscle architecture has an effect on the function of the muscle. The force exerted in a fiber should be maintained over the whole fiber, which costs energy. Therefore, muscles with short muscle fibers and long tendons (to cover for the distance between origin and insertion) are more suitable for static tasks, whereas muscles with longer fibers are more suitable for motion tasks. Within the same muscle volume (= fiber length × PCSA), there can be more fibers in parallel (= higher PCSA and thus higher force) with smaller fiber length. Usually this configuration would be seen in combination with a certain pennation angle. The pennation angle results in a lower muscle force (see Eq. (12)), but this is compensated because more muscle fibers are in parallel. For example, in a pennated muscle the fiber length could be one quarter of the fiber length of a parallel fibered muscle, but then also four times as many fibers are in parallel (in the same muscle volume). The muscle force is four times higher, multiplied by the cosine of the pennation angle α. The cosine of $30°$ (which is a high pennation angle) is 0.866, hence the resulting muscle force in the pennated muscle is $0.866 \times 4 = 3.46$ times higher than in the parallel fibered muscle.

4.3.2 Muscle Contraction

The smallest contractile unit in a muscle is the sarcomere (see Fig. 2-11). In a sarcomere the actin and myosin filaments slide over each other, and the muscle can shorten. The areas where the filaments overlap and the areas where they do not overlap result in the typical pattern of striated muscles, which can be observed by light microscopy.

Muscles exert force when activated by stimuli from a nerve (or artificially by an electrode, a technique called functional electrical stimulation (FES)). These stimuli start a chain reaction of chemical processes that results in a connection between the actin filament and the opposite myosin filament. When a neural signal arrives at the neuromuscular junction (the 'motor end-plate'), the signal is transferred into action potentials that travel over the muscle fibers. These action potentials, in the order of milli-volts (mV), can be recorded as EMG through wire or surface electrodes. Through a system of small tubuli, the action potentials can penetrate deep into the muscle fiber (Fig. 2-12). Inside the muscle cell, Ca^{2+}-ions are stored in high concentrations in the sarcoplasmic reticulum (SR). Through the action potentials the permeability of the SR increases and the Ca^{2+}-ions are released into the cellular medium.

The connection between the actin and myosin filaments is made by the so-called cross-bridges (also called 'myosin heads'). The cross-bridges are firmly connected to the myosin filament, and can be regarded as a prestretched spring with elastic energy stored inside. With calcium (Ca^{2+}) as a catalyst, the cross-bridges attach to the actin filament, the 'clamp' is released from the prestretched spring, and the cross-bridge exerts a force between the two filaments. While Ca^{2+}-ions are present in the cellular medium, there is a constant turnover (attachment–release cycles) of the cross-bridges. Shortening of a muscle is the result of the cross-bridge turnover. The cross-bridges can be regarded as galley slaves rowing the myosin ship along the actin sea. The Ca^{2+} concentration in the cellular medium follows with some delay (in the order of 10–50 ms) the muscle excitation by the α-motor neuron. The number of attached cross-bridges is directly related to the Ca^{2+} concentration. The Ca^{2+}-ions are continuously 'pumped back' into the SR. This is one of the major energy-consuming processes in the muscle, and accounts for roughly one-third of the energy consumption of the muscle. One should consider that the Ca^{2+}-ions are stored ready for action in the SR, and that the Ca^{2+}

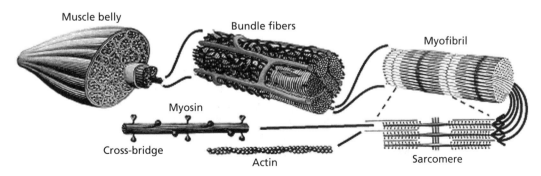

FIGURE 2-11. Muscle anatomy. Adapted from *Gray's Anatomy* (Warwic and Willems, 1973).

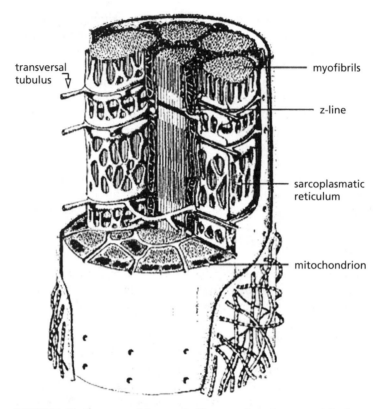

transversal tubulus

myofibrils

z-line

sarcoplasmatic reticulum

mitochondrion

FIGURE 2-12. Structure of the muscle fiber or cell. Action potentials along the cell membrane are transported deep inside the muscle cell through the transversal tubuli. Adapted from Ganong (1981).

release is a very fast process (in the order of 10 ms). The active Ca^{2+}-pump to restore the Ca^{2+} concentration in the SR is a slow process (in the order of 50 ms). Human (and most other mammals) are sacrificing a large amount of energy for the ability to initiate very fast movements, which might be very beneficial from an evolutionary point of view. If the Ca^{2+} concentration in the cellular medium is decreased through the calcium pump, the number of attached cross-bridges will decrease, and the muscle force decreases (92).

4.3.3 Force-length Relation

At the point of maximal overlap between the actin and myosin filaments, most cross-bridges can be attached, and maximal force can be exerted. This is called the optimum muscle length. If the muscle is stretched above the optimum length, a smaller population of cross-bridges have the opportunity to attach and the force will drop, even with the same activation and the same Ca^{2+} concentration. When the muscle is stretched to about 140% of the optimum length, no active force can be generated through the cross-bridges.

If the muscle is shortened below the optimum length, a similar mechanism occurs. One should consider a 3D structure of actin and myosin filaments. When shortening, the actin filaments slide over each other, and the number of troponin molecules to which the myosin heads can potentially bind diminishes. As a result, less cross-bridges will be formed and the force will drop. At about 60% of the optimum length, no active force can be generated through the cross-bridges.

The length-dependency of the sarcomere is shown in Fig. 2-13. Figure 2-14 shows that the

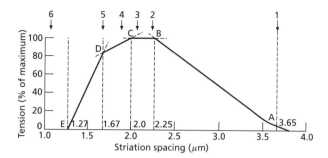

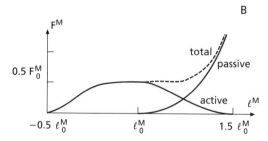

FIGURE 2-13. The sarcomere force-length relation results from the overlap between actin and myosin filaments.

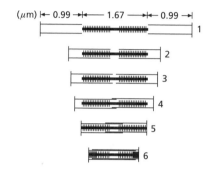

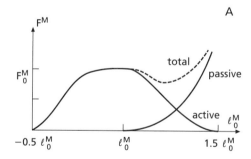

FIGURE 2-14. The active and passive force-length relationship of a muscle. **(A)** Representation of maximal muscle activation is shown here. **(B)** Representation of sub-maximal (50%) muscle activation is shown here.

single sarcomere behavior is reflected in the force-length relation of a whole muscle. In addition to the active force-length relation resulting from the actin-myosin overlap, there is also the passive force-length relationship. If the passive muscle is stretched above the rest length (muscle length where the passive forces start to increase, not necessarily equal to the optimum length), passive force will result. The passive force-length relation is approximately an exponential relation, and also shown in Fig. 2-14. The active and passive force-length relations are additive mechanisms.

When a muscle insertion is transferred, one should consider if the muscle will be able to exert forces in the new position. The optimum muscle length will adapt to the length at which the muscle is exerting the highest forces (62,63). But the adaptation mechanism only happens when the muscle is above the optimum length, and the sarcomeres are stretched. Then, additional sarcomeres will be formed in series with the existing sarcomeres. If the muscle is way below optimum length (attached in too short a position), no adaptation will take place, and the muscle will not be functional (53).

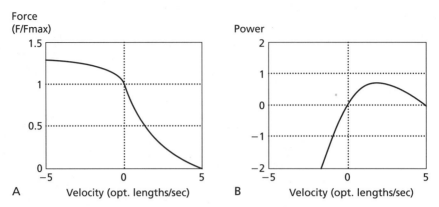

FIGURE 2-15. **(A)** The force-velocity relation. **(B)** The velocity-power curve.

4.3.4   Force-velocity Relation

The muscle force depends also on the contraction velocity (Fig. 2-15). The maximal isometric force is recorded at zero velocity, i.e., in isometric contractions the muscle remains at the same length. If the muscle is contracting and shortening (concentric contractions), the force drops. Two mechanisms are thought to be responsible for this. On the one hand, attached cross-bridges cannot be released in time, and are drawn beyond their shortest length in the opposite direction, where they exert a force in the opposite direction. On the other hand, the cross-bridge attachment rate drops due to the velocity of the moving filaments. If the muscle is lengthened (eccentric contractions), up to 30% higher forces than the maximal isometric force can be exerted, because the cross-bridges are further stretched and therefore exert higher forces.

The maximal contraction velocity v_{max} depends on the fiber type of the muscle. For slow twitch muscles like the *m. soleus* in the lower leg, v_{max} is about two times muscle length per second: $v_{max} = 2\, l_0/s$, in which the muscle length is defined as optimal at l_0. For fast twitch muscles like the *m. gastrocnemius* (also in the lower leg), v_{max} is about 8 l_0/s. Most other muscles, e.g., in the upper extremity, are intermediate, and have about 50/50 distribution of slow twitch and fast twitch fibers, and hence a v_{max} of about 5 l_0/s.

The power output is the amount of external energy per second (Nm/s or J/s or Watt) that is generated by the muscle. The muscle power P_{mus} is the product of the muscle force F_{mus} and muscle velocity v_{mus}: P_{mus} [Watt] $= F_{mus}$ [N] $\times v_{mus}$ [m/s]. At maximal velocity v_{max} the muscle force F_{mus} is about zero, and hence the power output is also about zero (Fig. 2-15). At zero contraction velocity (isometric conditions: $v_{mus} = 0$), the power output is also zero. The maximal power output of a muscle is around 30% of its maximal contraction velocity v_{max} (Fig. 2-15). During eccentric contraction (muscle lengthening), the power output is negative, and the muscles are actually dissipating energy. Energy dissipation is very important to stop a motion, e.g., when throwing, or absorbing an impact, e.g., when landing with feet on the ground during running.

Generating muscle force costs energy, whether power output is produced or not. If no mechanical power output is generated, the energy is transferred into heat. The muscle is most efficient at the maximal power output, i.e., at 30% of the maximal contraction velocity. The contraction efficiency (defined as the muscle power output P_{mus} divided by the energy consumption of the muscle) is then about 35%, meaning that still 65% of the energy is 'wasted' into heat. Heat accumulation can be a problem, e.g., for marathon runners, whose body temperature can increase to $40°C$.

4.3.5   Muscle Stiffness and Viscosity

Muscles have elastic and viscous properties. Elastic properties ($\sim$ stiffness) mean that the muscle force increases as the muscle is stretched, just as a spring. With a constant stiffness K, the resisting force F_{muscle} increases linearly with the relative displacement between the muscle endpoints, denoted Δx. The force acts in the opposite direction to displacement in order to restore the initial situation:

$$F_{muscle} = -K.\Delta x \qquad (13)$$

Viscous properties make the muscle forces increase with the speed of muscle stretching. Viscous properties are less intuitive than stiffness properties. A well-known viscous effect is if you stir a pot with honey; the faster you stir the greater the force against you. A viscous force is proportional to the speed of movement, and always in the opposite direction:

$$F_{muscle} = -B.\dot{x} \qquad (14)$$

If movement stops the viscous force disappears. If a muscle is stretched with a certain velocity, the force will increase. If the muscle is shortened with a certain velocity, the force will decrease.

It is tempting to take the slope of the force-length curve (Fig. 2-14) to estimate the muscle stiffness, and the derivative of the force-velocity curve (Fig. 2-15A) to estimate the muscle viscosity. However, the force-length curve is obtained by drawing a line through a sequence of isometric conditions, which is not the same as moving a muscle through this sequence of lengths. Similarly, the force-velocity curve is obtained through measurements in a number of separate isokinetic (constant velocity) conditions. The visco-elastic properties of the muscle are the result of biochemical processes, for instance the dynamics of cross-bridge turnover. These are highly nonlinear dynamic properties, which will change with the velocity and the magnitude of the perturbating force. Typically, muscle stiffness and viscosity are a factor 2 to 3 higher than the derivative of the force-length or force-velocity curves. Moreover, above muscle optimum length the derivative of the force-length curve is negative, meaning a decrease in force when the muscle is stretched. Actually, the force will increase when the muscle is stretched above optimum length (47,70,137).

4.3.6 EMG and Muscle Force

The electrical action potentials traveling over the muscle fibers can be picked up by wire or surface electrodes. Wire electrodes are inserted by a hollow needle. After inserting the needle with the wire inside, the needle is retracted and the wire electrode remains in place because of a little barb, which hooks in the muscle. The wire electrode consists of two threads, which register the difference in electrical potential. Wire electrodes register typically a volume of a few cm^3. Surface electrodes are glued to the skin, after thoroughly removing hairs and dead cells by sanding and cleaning with alcohol. Two surface electrodes are used, which are placed along the fiber direction. Surface electrodes pick up the difference in electrical potential, in a registration volume of a few tenths of cm^3.

A *motor unit* consists of all muscle fibers (typically between 10 and 100) that are innervated by one α-motor neuron. The action potentials have positive and negative peaks. When many motor units are activated, the action potentials are superimposed and show a chaotic pattern in the EMG.

The EMG signal is low-pass filtered, sampled, rectified, and integrated, and the IEMG signal (integrated rectified EMG) is obtained.[3] IEMG is related to the generation of muscle force. As a result of the electrical potentials, the

---

[3] The recorded EMG signal is high-pass filtered (only frequencies above, e.g., 15 Hz are passed) in order to remove movement artifacts (surface electrodes moving with respect to the muscle). The EMG is also low-pass filtered (only frequencies below half the sample frequency are passed: If the sample frequency is 500 Hz, the low-pass filter frequency should be below 250 Hz), in order to prevent aliasing ('leakage' of high-frequency signal power into the low frequencies). Filtering is done by analogous filters in the EMG equipment, before the sampling by an A/D (analog/digital) converter. After sampling, the EMG is rectified: all negative peaks are mirrored to positive peaks. Rectifying again introduces low frequencies in the signal, representative for instance. For slowly activating and deactivating the muscle. Usually the high-frequency content of the EMG can be neglected because muscle activation and deactivation takes place at low frequencies (up to 10 Hz). The frequency content of the EMG is reduced by averaging, low-pass filtering, or integration. Integrating the EMG signal results in the low-frequent IEMG.

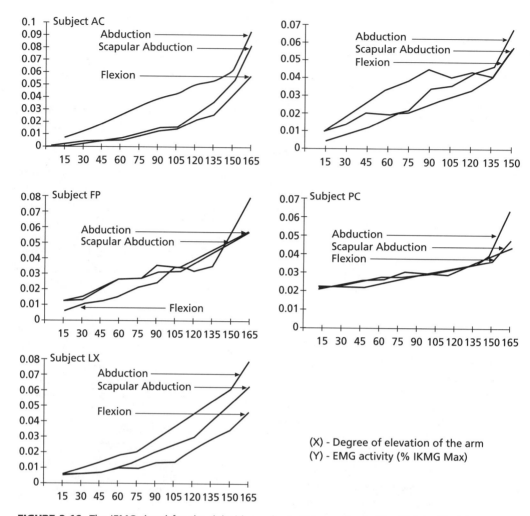

FIGURE 2-16. The IEMG signal for the deltoid muscles in three patients. The highest EMG is recorded near maximal elevation, while the highest force output is around 90° humerus elevation. The discrepancy between the maximal EMG output and maximal muscle output can be explained by the effect of the force-length curve.

Ca^{2+} concentration will increase, cross-bridges will attach and muscle force will result. After a burst of IEMG, it takes about 60–100 ms before the peak in force is present. (The exact time difference is a result of all dynamic processes inbetween, and depends on the rise time of the IEMG.) The amplitude of the EMG signal and the amplitude of the force are related by the force-length and force-velocity relationships. Maximal EMG (~ maximal activation) results in maximal isometric force near the optimum of the muscle force-length curve, but in almost zero muscle force near 60% of optimum muscle length. In Fig. 2-16 the EMG and force of the deltoid muscle is shown during abduction of the arm. The peak in the muscle force is around 90° elevation of the arm, when the external moment is maximal. The peak in EMG is near maximal elevation, when the deltoid muscle is at its shortest length! Similarly, at higher contraction velocities the EMG is not very representative for the resulting muscle force, since the force-velocity relationship would predict much lower muscle forces.

Summarizing, one should be very cautious to use EMG as representative for muscle force or muscular effort. It would be better to consider EMG as representative for the neural activation of the muscle, and take the dynamic effects (Ca^{2+} flow) and force-length and force-velocity relationships explicitly into account. However, the necessary parameters for these relationships (e.g., the optimum muscle length is seldom known) are lacking and therefore the force-length and force-velocity relationships are (erroneously!) neglected. The timing patterns of the EMG signal, i.e., when the EMG is increasing or decreasing, can be compared with the rise and fall of the muscle force. Very often, a fixed time delay (the EMD: electromechanical delay) of about 70 ms is taken into account to relate the EMG to muscle force.

4.4 Muscle Models

Biochemical processes in muscle fibers and nerves result in the generation of force that depends on muscle length and contraction velocity, as described above. A number of computer models have been developed in order to analyze the mechanical behavior of the muscle. Muscle models have three input signals (neural activation, length, and contraction velocity) and one output signal (force)—is depicted in the block diagram of Fig. 2-9. Muscle models can be divided into Hill-type models and cross-bridge models. In Hill-type models, the active muscle fibers are represented by a contractile element (CE) in series with a series-elastic (SE) element representing visco-elastic tendon and cross-bridge properties (Fig. 2-17). The passive muscle properties are modeled by a parallel elastic element (PE).

A Hill-type model contains activation dynamics and contraction dynamics (72). The activation dynamics represent the dynamic process of calcium release from the SR, with a fast outflow and a slow inflow. Neural activation (in arbitrary units between 0 and 1) is the input signal, and Ca^{2+} concentration (also called active state) is output signal. In the contraction dynamics, the mechanical properties of the muscle fibers and tendon are represented, with active state, length, and contraction velocity as input, and force as output. The force-length $f(l_{ce})$ and force-velocity $f(v_{ce})$ relations are incorporated

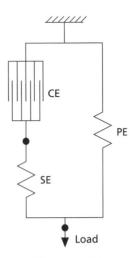

FIGURE 2-17. In Hill-type models: the active muscle fibers are represented by a contractile element (CE) in series with a series-elastic (SE) element representing visco-elastic tendon and cross-bridge properties. Passive muscle properties are represented in the parallel elastic element (PE).

in a descriptive way into the CE, without referring to the underlying cross-bridge dynamic behavior. The resulting force is calculated in a multiplicative way:

$$F_m = a . f(l_{ce}) . f(v_{ce}) . F_{max} \qquad (15)$$

The advantage of Hill-type models is that only a few parameters are required, which could be derived from gross morphological parameters of the muscle, such as tendon length, mass, and fiber type. The muscle optimum length is the most difficult parameter to acquire because it must be reconstructed from the sarcomere length (85). Disadvantage of Hill-type models is that the not very detailed model description only allows for a rough approximation of the energy consumption of the muscle because the active state and cross-bridge turnover are not modeled.

Cross-bridge models include the partial differential equations, which describe the cross-bridge attachment and deattachment (79). This results in a model that can explain the resulting force-velocity relation, instead of only describing it. Cross-bridge models are generally too difficult to solve to be useful in musculoskeletal modeling. The advantage of the cross-bridge models is that precise estimates are made of the energy consumption of the muscle. Disadvantages are the large number of (unknown) parameters and the computational complexity.

Muscle models are mainly used in forward dynamic simulations (with activation as input and force as output), in which the non-linear differential equations are numerically solved. Muscle models are seldom used in inverse dynamic models, in which the recorded motions are input and the muscle forces and neural activation are output. However, most calculations in musculoskeletal models are done inverse-dynamically, which generally means that in these calculations the muscle dynamic properties are not included. The disadvantage of inverse dynamic calculations without muscle dynamics is that the muscle force can vary instantaneously from zero to maximal, while in reality muscle dynamics prevents these very fast changes in force.

4.5   Joints

Diarthrodial joints and artificial hip and knee joint replacements are described in other chapters of this book. Of relevance here is to summarize that the shapes of the articular surfaces determine the possible motions between the bones. The articular surfaces restrict the freedom of the bones to move with respect to each other, and ligaments restrict the freedom of movement even further by keeping the articulating surfaces together, and stabilizing the joints. Some joints allow only rotational degrees of freedom and may be sufficiently described as ball-and-socket joints.

A ball-and-socket joint has three degrees of freedom, i.e., three rotations and no translations. More complex-shaped articular surfaces result in more complex motions, in which the rotation axis is more difficult to predict. For instance, saddle joints have two rotation axes, which do not necessarily intersect each other. However, in many musculoskeletal models only the hinge and ball joints are represented.

4.6   Bones and Segments

In the joints the bones articulate with respect to each other. Together with the bones, the attached

muscles, but also fat, skin, blood vessels, nerves, etc., will move. This whole ensemble of morphological structures is seen as a segment.

One of the most important properties of segments for the neuro-musculoskeletal model is that they have mass and rotational inertia. Referring to Section 2.5 we have then,

$$\ddot{x} = \frac{1}{m} F \qquad (16)$$

which is Newton's second law written in order to maintain causality, i.e., that a motion results from forces, and not the other way around. In a similar fashion the relation between joint torque T and angular acceleration can be written as,

$$\ddot{\theta} = \frac{1}{J} T \qquad (17)$$

In which J is the angular momentum (in kgm^2). Usually the segments are considered as rigid bodies, which means that it is assumed that the mass particles inside the rigid body do not move with respect to each other. For the trunk this is a very approximative assumption because the internal organs do move quite a lot during fast motions. For most other segments the assumption is very reasonable.

In earlier days, the segment masses and rotational inertias were measured at cadavers. The cadavers were disarticulated; for some segments it is quite arbitrary which part of the body is attributed to the one segment or to the other. The segments are weighed to assess the mass. The centers of gravity are usually determined by a pendulum test.

4.7   Sensors

Sensors are required to enable a controller (the CNS) to adjust the motions. There is an abundance of sensor types in the human body, which provide, in part, redundant information about the state of the body. The redundancy can be used to improve the accuracy of the recordings (because the individual sensors are sensitive to noise and threshold effects), to compensate for sensory conflicts, and to be able to function when some sensors are blocked out (e.g., in the dark without information of the visual system).

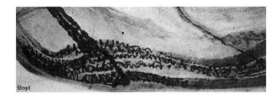

FIGURE 2-18. Photo of the sensory part of the muscle spindle, in which the nerve ending is wrapped around the nuclear chain and nuclear bag fibers. In addition, the emergence of the sensory nerve toward the CNS can be seen at the left side.

For the neuro-musculoskeletal system, the following sensors are important:

- The muscle spindle provides information about the muscle length and contraction velocity
- Golgi tendon organs provide information about muscle force
- Capsule receptors provide information about the joint orientation.
- The tactile system provides information about external forces acting on the body
- The visual system provides information about the environment, and is used to assess motion of the body with respect to the environment.
- The vestibulary system consists of two parts. The otoliths are sensitive to translational accelerations and to the direction of the gravitational field. The semicircular canals are sensitive to angular accelerations (though for most frequencies the sensitivity is effectively for angular velocities).

These are described in detail below.

4.7.1 Muscle Spindles

A muscle spindle is a complex sensory unit consisting of about 3–5 nuclear chain fibers, and 1–2 nuclear bag fibers. A muscle spindle has a length of about 8 mm and is located parallel to the muscle fibers. The muscle spindle endings are attached to the muscle fibers, and hence the spindles are lengthened and shortened together with the muscle fibers. Hence, the length and velocity of a muscle spindle are always proportional to the length and contraction velocity of the muscle fibers (64).

Both the nuclear chain and nuclear bag fibers consist of two small muscles at the endings, and a sensory part in the middle. A nerve ending is wrapped around the sensory part, and essentially is sensitive to the stretch of the sensory part

(Fig. 2-18). The small muscles inside the muscle spindle are called 'intrafusal' muscles. The intrafusal muscle spindles are innervated by a separate motor neuron, the γ-motor neuron, which is an *efferent* innervation to the muscle spindle (carrying signals from the CNS to the periphery).

The nuclear bag fibers are sensitive to the stretch velocity, and the nuclear chain fibers are sensitive to the stretch length. There are two types of *afferent* nerves, Ia and II sensory nerves. The Ia sensory nerve receives branches from the sensors of both the nuclear bag and nuclear chain fibers, and thus contains length and velocity information. The II sensory nerve receives only branches from the nuclear chain fibers, and contains only length information. According to the specific sensitivity of the nuclear bag and nuclear chain fibers, the innervating γ-motor neurons are called γ_d (dynamic) and γ_s (static) motor neurons, respectively (Fig. 2-19). Their input into the block diagram is shown in Fig. 2-9.

The muscle spindle is sensitive to length and contraction velocity. The resulting spike trains in the Ia and II afferent nerves are shown in Fig. 2-20, indicating that the muscle spindle is primarily sensitive to muscle *stretch* and *stretching velocity* (note that the stretch of the muscle spindle is proportional to the stretch of the extrafusal muscle fibers). During shortening, the spike trains almost disappear, especially in the Ia afferent fibers. The II afferent fibers are mainly length dependent, and show their highest activity at the length peaks. The Ia afferent fibers have their highest activity at the highest lengthening velocity (81).

The visco-elastic properties of the intrafusal muscle fibers, as well as the neural output, are changed when the muscle fibers are activated by the γ-motor neurons. As a direct effect, when the intrafusal muscle force increases, the sensory part is stretched. As a secondary effect the stiffness and viscosity increase, and the sensor becomes

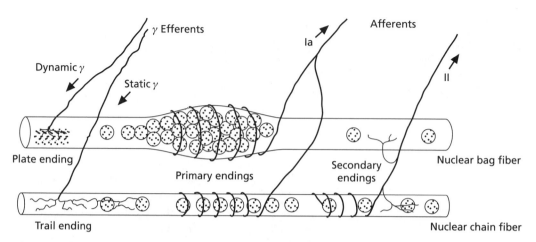

FIGURE 2-19. A muscle spindle has two efferent nerve inputs (γ_d to the nuclear bag muscle fiber and γ_s to the nuclear chain muscle fiber) and two afferent nerve outputs (Ia from both the nuclear bag and nuclear chain sensory parts, and II mainly from the nuclear chain sensory part). After Matthews (1984).

more sensitive: A relatively more compliant sensory part means that more of the stretch is taken up by the sensory part. Here, an important role of the γ-motor neurons arises: They can keep the muscle spindle in the most sensitive region even for the extreme range of lengthening and shortening of the muscle. However, it also implies that for the correct interpretation of the afferent output in terms of length and velocity, the efferent input to the muscle spindle must also be known.

It is assumed that the γ-motor neuron activation has a two-fold function: maintaining the muscle spindle in the most sensitive region, and adjusting the gain of the muscle spindle and thereby affecting the loop gain of the length and velocity feedback. The gain of the muscle spindle is the magnitude of sensory output compared with the length or velocity input. In that respect, increasing the spindle sensitivity and the spindle gain is the same action, though functionally interpreted in a different way.

The transmission speed of the sensory nerves depends on the thickness of the myelin sheaths (77). In Table 2-1, it can be seen that the tactile sensors and free nerve endings have a very slow transmission. The fastest transmission speeds are found for the Ia and Ib afferents. These sensory nerves are part of the inner loop of a feedback system. A pure time delay causes a phase lag in the open-loop transfer function, which limits the bandwidth of the system. Especially the inner loops (force and velocity) need to be very fast, in order to enable higher feedback gains in the outer loop (position feedback). For a position-controlled system, a higher loop gain will result in a higher admittance, i.e., less sensitivity to force perturbations.

4.7.2 Golgi Tendon Organs

The Golgi tendon organs (GTOs) are located in the muscle tendons; they provide information about muscle force. About 50 GTOs are

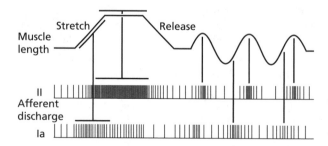

FIGURE 2-20. Response of the muscle spindle to a regime of stretch and release. From the spike trains in the afferent nerves it can be seen that the II afferent nerve is mainly sensitive to length, and the Ia afferent nerve is sensitive to lengthening velocity. During release, the Ia afferent nerve is almost silent.

TABLE 2-1. DIAMETER AND TRANSMISSION SPEED OF SOME OF THE PROPRIOCEPTIVE SENSORS IN THE BODY, I.E., SENSORS THAT PROVIDE INFORMATION ABOUT THE 'INNER STATE' OF THE BODY

	Diameter (μm)	Transmission Speed (m/s)	Type of Sensor	Stimulus
Ia	12–20	70–100	Muscle spindle	Length & velocity
Ib	12–20	70–100	GTO	Force
II	6–12	35–70	Muscle spindle	Length
	2–5	12–30	Pacini corpuscle	Pressure
	0.5–2	3–12	Free nerve ending	Nociceptive

located in a major tendon. The GTOs consist of nerve endings that are intertwined with the collagen fibers of the tendon (Fig. 2-21). When the tendon is stretched, the nerve endings are 'squeezed'. The deformation of these nerve endings results in a spike train along the afferent nerve to the CNS. This afferent nerve is called the Ib afferent nerve fiber. Inside the GTO, there are no dynamic effects, i.e., the Ib afferent nerve output is always proportional to the muscle force. Hence, there is a static (no

time-history) and linear relation between the muscle force and the afferent nerve (28).

In the earlier days, experiments in which the whole muscle was stretched resulted in little activity of the GTO. Therefore, it was thought that the function of the GTO was not in the fine motor control, but merely to detect large forces in the tendons and protect the tendon against damage. This theory was also in accordance with the fact that the GTO is connected to the α-motor neuron through an inhibitory

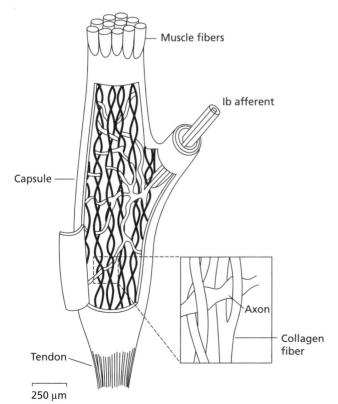

Muscle fibers

Ib afferent

Capsule

Axon

Collagen fiber

Tendon

250 μm

FIGURE 2-21. The Golgi tendon organ (GTO) is sensitive to the muscle force exerted through the tendon.

interneuron, i.e., when the tendon was stretched, the GTO caused the α-motor neuron to cease firing. However, this theory has been abandoned for two reasons. In the first place, if the α-motor neurons cease firing while the large external force is still stretching the muscle, the muscle will be stretched rapidly, and presumably the muscle fibers will be damaged. More recent experiments showed that the GTOs are especially sensitive to the forces exerted by the *active* muscle fibers, more than to the passive forces transmitted through endomysium and perimysium (the connective tissue around the muscle fibers), see Guyton (66).

4.7.3 Joint Capsule

The range of motion of a joint is determined by the capsule and ligaments, in which stretch and pressure sensors are located. The ligaments are strings of connective tissue, strengthening the joint capsule. Often, only at the end of the range of motion the ligaments are stretched. Hence, these sensors are not firing at the mid-range of motion; therefore, it is not likely that they play a major role in the control of movement. On the other hand, information about the boundaries of the joint motion is necessary to learn to move within these boundaries, in order to prevent damage.

4.7.4 Tactile Sensors

The skin is the boundary between the outside world and the inside body. One important function is the information exchange between the inside body and the direct environment. In the skin, sensory organs are sensitive for touching (mechanoreceptors), heat and cold (thermoreceptors), and pain (nociceptors).

Tactile sensors in the skin provide information about the external forces, i.e., normal and shear forces at the skin. Humans are capable of sensing the forces under their feet, which is an important cue for postural control while standing. In addition, there are pressure sensors and temperature sensors. The shape of the sensor cells determines if they are more sensitive to certain deformations, and result in pressure or stretch sensors, for instance.

Tactile sensors are only sensitive to *changes* in the stimuli. For example, after sitting for a long time one is no longer aware of the pressure at the seat. Only after some movements, the pressure is felt again. Tactile information is very important for use in daily life, for the upper extremities as well as for the lower extremities. For example, information about slip when holding a cup provides feedback for muscle co-contraction necessary to hold the cup. The importance of tactile information can be appreciated if a patient with a hand prosthesis is observed. These patients have many difficulties in holding delicate objects like a plastic cup, an egg, or a banana. They have to rely completely on the visual system that only provides position information and no force information!

4.7.5 Vestibulary System

The vestibulary system consists of three perpendicular semicircular canals and an otolith system in each of the inner ears (Fig. 2-22). The semicircular canals are sensitive to rotational accelerations of the head. Because there are three perpendicular rotational sensors, any rotational movement of the head will be detected. The semicircular canals are filled with fluid, and sealed off by a membrane (cupula) that prevents the fluid flow. The excursion of the cupula is sensed and transmitted to the CNS. Through the mass-spring-damper properties of the fluids and the cupula, the semicircular canals act as rotational velocity sensors for an important range of frequencies, i.e., between 0.1 and 10 Hz (142). The orientation of the head can only be reconstructed through time integration of the rotational acceleration. This will result in an integration offset that can be experienced when rotating with the eyes closed. After several turns, it is difficult to know one's orientation in the room.

Translational accelerations are being detected by the otolith system in the inner ear. The otolith system consists of small bony parts on little hairs. The amount of bending of the hairs gives an indication of the acceleration and weight of the bone parts. The otolith system gives information about the translational accelerations of the head, but is also sensitive to gravity (50). The

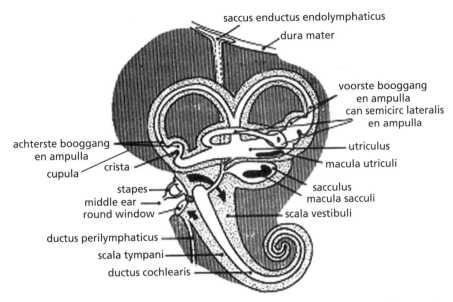

FIGURE 2-22. The three semicircular canals in the vestibulary organ are sensitive to rotational accelerations. The otolith near the center of the semicircular canals is sensitive for translational accelerations and for gravitational forces.

perceived integration offset directly points to the role of the visual system, which provides direct position and orientation information of the head. Humans are capable of deriving velocity information from the visual system (how fast an object is moving), but no acceleration information (changes in the speed of the object). The combination of the visual and vestibulary system provides position, velocity and acceleration information of the head. It is obvious that for the position of the rest of the body in space, the relative position of the head, with respect to the trunk, must be detected by sensors in the neck musculature.

4.8 The Central Nervous System

From a control systems perspective, the CNS is the controller of the neuro-musculoskeletal system. The CNS has been praised for its capabilities, for instance in comparison to control systems of robots. Robots usually have a very limited set of sensors and actuators, and a controller reconstructs the exact position of the whole linkage system, before it updates the control signal to the actuator. In the human body, there are many muscles active in controlling the joints,

and there is an abundance of sensors present, as described above. These provide different modalities of information (many different types of sensors), but also provide the same information simultaneously by multiple identical sensors (e.g., by the large number of muscle spindles and Golgi tendon organs in one muscle). The CNS is a distributed control system, receiving sensory information through many channels, and sending control signals to the actuators, also over many channels. A distributed control system means that at different locations in the CNS the information is processed and an adequate response is generated. If one of these locations is damaged, then part of the information is lost, but much of the information might still be accessible.

The CNS is unique in its capacity to control a wide variety of tasks, ranging from standing, walking, and jumping to fine motor tasks such as grasping and manipulating. Instantaneously, the human can switch from accurate positioning tasks to contact tasks. The neuromusculoskeletal system consists of many nonlinear components, which have nicely distributed properties enabling these difficult control tasks. Many scientists have focused on the separate components of the system, while others study the interactions of the components and their relative importance.

The CNS consists of four major parts, the cerebrum, the cerebellum, the brainstem, and the spinal cord. The CNS is a massive parallel information processing system, with the interneurons as relatively simple building stones, merely subtracting and adding incoming information. The 'programs' of the CNS are an interesting mixture of software and hardware. The information storage depends on the strength of the synapses, i.e., the strength of the connections between the interneurons. The strength of a synapse increases when it is frequently used, and decreases when it is not used. The stronger a synapse, the more likely it is that the next neuron will also be excited (or inhibited) and start firing (or be prevented from firing). About 80% of the interneurons are excitatory neurons (increase the potential of the next neuron), and the remaining 20% are inhibitory interneurons (decrease the potential of the next neuron).

In many tasks humans have to deal with all types of perturbations. For example, while walking with a cup of coffee, the perturbations of the trunk must be neutralized by very compliant behavior of the arm. On the contrary, while using a drill, the drill must be kept from slipping, while exerting a force in the drilling direction. Two strategies are used by humans to resist perturbations. On the one hand, by co-contraction of antagonistic muscles the joints are stiffened. This strategy works against all sorts of perturbations, though it is highly energy consuming. On the other hand, by using proprioceptive feedback the perturbations are detected and the muscles will generate a restoring force. This strategy is energy efficient because muscles are only activated when perturbations are present. Due to the time delays in the feedback caused by neural transportation and processing, this strategy will only be effective against low-frequency perturbations.

5 MUSCULOSKELETAL ANALYSIS

The mechanical interactions of bone, muscle, and soft tissue structures must be considered to fully understand how loads are transmitted within the body. Load transmission determines whether or not implants fail mechanically (78), and how the tissues react around artificial joint prostheses or during reconstruction of fractured bones (23,89) because adaptation processes are triggered by mechanical stimuli (27). Many studies have been performed to examine the mechanical conditions in the musculoskeletal system of the upper and lower limbs. Only seldom have these investigations incorporated the relationship between the bones and the muscular and ligamentous structures.

In the first part of this section, calculation methods for the load transfer in the long bones of the lower limb are explained. The unknowns associated with these calculations are the muscle, ligament, and joint contact forces; in addition, the precise anatomy is seldom known. Joint contact and ligament forces may be determined from *in vivo* and *in vitro* experiments. Muscle forces can be estimated by mathematical models and by direct measurements requiring the monitoring of electromyographic activity. The literature on these measurements and calculations is also reviewed.

5.1 Historical Review of Musculoskeletal Analysis

The load transfer within a bone has been the subject of research for many years (123). As early as 1638, Galileo studied the mechanics of long bones and analyzed the gross anatomical structure of the thigh. The basis of his work, and further descriptive analysis, assumed a relationship between mechanical principles and the anatomical shape of the femur. Surprisingly, the inner structure, not the macroscopic anatomy, was the main focus in these early biomechanical analyses of bone. Based on Meyers' 1867 description of the trabecular architecture in the proximal femur (100), Wolff postulated that bone structure corresponds to the load transfer (Fig. 2-23). The trabecular structures were not found to be irregular in orientation, but aligned to form a pattern. Wolff postulated that form follows function (154) and quoted the work of the Swiss engineer Gustav Culmann in which

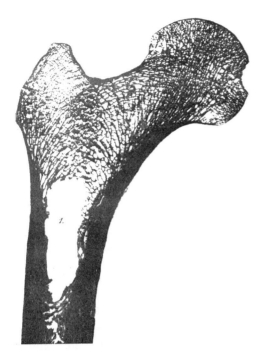

FIGURE 2-23A. Trabecular orientation within the proximal femur. (After Wolff J. *Das Gesetz der Transformation der Knochen.* Berlin: A. Hirschwald, 1892, with permission.)

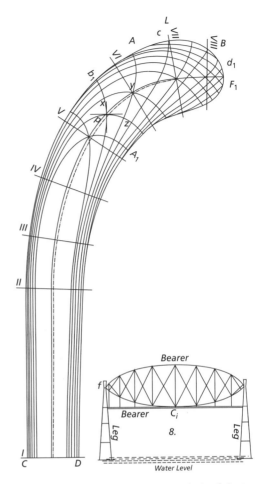

FIGURE 2-23B. "Graphic static" analysis of the trabecular structure of the proximal femur.

the advantages offered by the orientation of the trabecular structure could be demonstrated with "graphic static" analysis. Agreeing that bone was an optimum structure, it was obvious to suggest that the bony architecture resulted from the mechanical influences that occurred during evolution. In addition, Wolff found that fully healed misaligned fractures also obeyed mechanical rules. In his work from 1892, Wolff stated explicitly that bony structures were not only predetermined by genetics but also by adaptation to mechanical load transfer ("law of bone remodeling" or Wolff's law (153)).

Although Wolff proposed the adaptation of bone to mechanical load, it was Koch (86) who first tried to quantify mechanical load transfer within a bone by calculating stresses and strains. In his publication, Koch thoroughly analyzed the anatomy of the femur by calculating the cross-sectional area and moment of inertia at seventy-five locations (Fig. 2-24). The cross sections were aligned perpendicular to a line between the centers of knee and femoral head.

Using the geometry of the bone and an assumed set of material properties, Koch was able to calculate the internal forces acting in the long axis of the bone (axial forces) and the ones acting perpendicular to the long axis (shear forces), as well as the bending moments and principal stress lines within the femur. For his calculation, Koch used "beam theory" (see Chapter 14 or Gere and Timoshenko (56)). Koch assumed a hip-joint contact force of 445 N ($\approx$0.7 BW) during walking and running. For this load, the axial force in the femur increased from 177 N at the hip to 445 N distal of the lesser trochanter. A maximal shear force of 409 N was present at the femoral head, which decreased toward the lesser trochanter. The maximal bending moments occurred at the

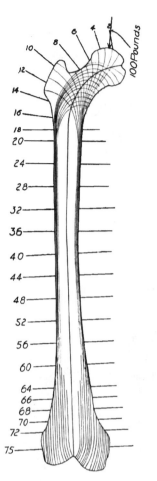

FIGURE 2-24. Cross-sectional description of the femur (86).

level of the lesser trochanter, with values of up to 18 Nm (≈0.03 body weight meters, BWm). Rather surprisingly perhaps, the direction of his computed principal stresses agreed well with the descriptions of trabecular architecture made by Wolff in 1892 (Fig. 2-23). Koch's analysis only represented femoral curvatures in the frontal plane and did not include muscle activities. The latter produced an underestimation of the joint contact force and, consequently, femoral loads in general. Nevertheless, his work is considered as the classical approach to femoral stress calculation that opened the door for many similar studies. Shortly afterward, Grunewald (65) and Marique (97) published similar works on mechanical load transfer within the femur. Evans

and Lissner (49), and later Frankel (52), used brittle stress coatings to experimentally investigate the stress at the surfaces of the loaded bones. Evans and Lissner found, in good agreement to Koch's calculations, stress peaks in the femoral head and knee-condylar regions. Stresses in the diaphyseal region were found to be reasonably constant; no muscle forces were considered.

Pauwels was one of the first scientists to include the effects of muscles on femoral loading in his analysis (110) and experiments (109). Due to the experimental conditions used in his photoelastic investigations, the 3D characteristics of the long bones were ignored. Nevertheless, Pauwels stated that a bone is loaded in bending, superimposed onto compression (108). He was able to detect tensile (lateral) and compressive (medial) patterns in the femoral neck and shaft regions. Furthermore, he showed that tension in a collagenous band between the greater trochanter and the femoral condyles significantly reduced the bending moments in the bone shaft.

Torodis (139) reported a method to calculate the femoral stresses using beam theory. In contradiction to Pauwels, he assumed that the effects of muscle loads on the mechanical behavior of a bone was not as important as that of body weight. However, Torodis included muscle forces in his mechanical description for those situations in which the muscles were thought to have a "more pronounced effect." Unfortunately, no force, moment, or stress data were reported in this article. A mathematical approach to quantify the muscular influence on femoral stresses was published by Rybicki et al. (124). They used the anatomical description of the femur from Koch to analyze femoral stresses in the one-legged stance phase of gait. They included the joint contact force (2,318 N ≈ 3.6 BW), the hip abductors (*m. gluteus medius* and *m. gluteus minimus*, 1,592 N) and the iliotibial band. The latter was modeled as a tension band between the tibial epicondyles and the iliac crest, gliding on, but not connected to, the greater trochanter. The muscle forces were taken from calculations by Inman (80) and the joint forces from studies conducted by Bresler and Frankel (15). The effects associated with a wide range of forces in the iliotibial band (0... 1,557 N) were investigated using both beam theory and 2D finite element modeling (see Chapters 4 and 14 for thorough descriptions of finite element modeling). Similar to Pauwels, Rybicki's results indicate a reduction of the maximal stresses (70–77% of the original values) within the bone due to iliotibial activity. The author argued that including more muscles would most likely result in further reduction of bending moments, and hence, the stresses acting in the bone. Although Rybicki considered the *mm. abductores* and the iliotibial band, no other muscular influences were analyzed (*mm. adductores, mm. vasti*). His model was basically 2D, representing only one load situation and single-legged stance. No distinctions were made among the six load components or between the resulting stress directions.

Ghista et al. (58) published a mathematical description of the internal stresses in a bone during gait. The muscle forces were determined by application of an inverse dynamic calculation of the resultant loads at the instantaneous joint centers. To satisfy the equilibrium conditions for a limb segment, Ghista simplified the model such that only three muscles and three joint contact forces were active at a time (Fig. 2-25). The method allowed computation of the internal stresses of the bone using the force data and geometric properties of the femur. Unfortunately, calculated values for the forces, moments, and internal stresses were not reported.

Raftopoulos and Qassem (120) published a method for calculating the stresses in a femur including its 3D curvature and composite nature. Similar to the approach of Carter and Vasu (19), Raftopoulos and Qassem transformed the composite beam into a homogeneous beam by changing the cross-sectional geometry (area and moments of inertia) of the stiffer material. Thereafter, the composite beam could be treated as a simple beam in which the stress and strain calculations were based on Hooke's law. Calculated values for the internal loads or stresses were not reported.

Salathe et al. (127) applied beam theory to determine the stresses and deformations in long

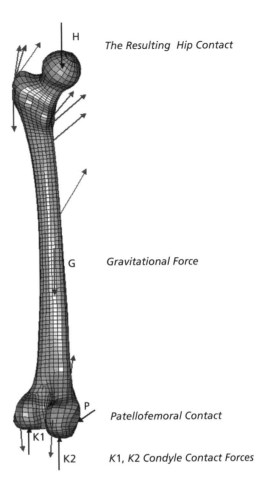

The Resulting Hip Contact

Gravitational Force

Patellofemoral Contact

K1, K2 Condyle Contact Forces

FIGURE 2-25. Finite element model of a femur subjected to complex musculo-skeletal loading conditions. Illustrated are the muscle forces, the gravitational force (G), the resulting hip contact (H), patellofemoral contact (P), and condyle contact forces (K1, K2).

bones. Cross-sectional properties were calculated for the fifth metatarsal along the curved centroid line of the bone. Assuming a distributed load along the long axis of the bone, the internal forces and moments were calculated. Using the axial, bending, torsion, and shear components and assuming elastic properties, the stresses and deformations were computed.

In conclusion, mechanical analyses of bones have been frequently performed. It is important that the loading conditions of the bones concerned are known if research questions requiring more detailed analysis of local stress patterns are to be answered. In addition to beam theory, finite element analyses (see Prendergast (116) for a review) and experimental testing techniques (see Cristofolini (30) for a review) may be used to quantify stresses in the femur and other bones with and without prostheses implanted (78,91, 116).

5.2 Factors Influencing Musculoskeletal Loading of the Femur

Forces are exerted on the femur by those muscles with insertions or origins on the femur, by the joint contact forces at the hip and knee, and by the adjacent soft tissue structures. The forces on the bone must be in equilibrium. If the bone moves, there is the additional load due to the acceleration of the bone. To fulfill the equilibrium conditions at any instant, the parameters that describe these loads must be known. A first step in an analysis is to determine the anatomical information relating the orientation of the forces relative to the bone position. Second, the muscle, ligament and joint force values must be computed in such a way that, for a given anatomical configuration, a certain movement can be performed. Finally, the elastic properties of the materials need to be included if the force orientations change with the deformation of the bone.

5.2.1 Muscle Anatomy

Muscle anatomy, particularly the locations of origin and insertion, must be known to calculate the effects of muscle activity. Multiple studies have been conducted to determine muscle attachment locations. Seireg and Arvikar (132) measured lower limb muscle attachment coordinates from anatomical textbook descriptions. Crowninshield et al. (34) and Dostal and Andrews (40) located the origin and insertion coordinates of the leg musculature on dry bone specimens. Brand et al. (12) marked the muscle origins and insertions on three pairs of lower limb specimens and calculated the attachment coordinates using biplanar x-ray images. Pierrynowski and Morrison (115) digitized the

bony landmarks on disarticulated dry bones; no information was given on how the muscle attachment locations were determined. White et al. (149) located the sites of muscle origin and insertion on six pelvises and nine lower limbs using dry bones. Muscle anatomy may be derived from magnetic resonance imaging (MRI) data (135). Even though these data are more complex and allow representation of the 3D configuration of muscles, they are seldom used to gain representative data on anatomical variations.

5.2.2 Muscle Activity

To calculate the internal loads of the lower limb, knowledge of the muscle force values is essential. Approaches to quantify the relation between electromyographic signals and muscle forces are mentioned in the previous section. Muscle forces may also be determined using analytical methods. It is possible to record the relative motions of body segments and the force between a subject and the ground during, for example, a gait cycle (4,15,21). The forces and moments acting at the joints between the segments may then be calculated by implementation of an inverse dynamic approach. This approach uses data describing the motion of a body to calculate the forces that must be acting upon it to produce the observed motion.

However, these forces between body segments are in reality produced by a combination of the reaction forces at the joint surfaces and the actions of the muscles crossing each joint. From a mechanical point of view, there are an infinite number of muscle force combinations that can produce the required force between the body segments. This type of mechanical problem is described as indeterminate and can be approached using 'optimization' procedures, together with a specific optimization criterion or cost function to solve for muscle and joint contact forces. These techniques have been described in more detail in Section 3.2. The optimization criteria have been found to produce muscle forces that correlate with electromyographic data (121,138) though this is more than just inverse dynamics and muscle optimization. Although a more general solution to these mechanically indeterminate problems has yet to be developed, a more complex approach that applies an EMG-based optimization criterion could aid in the calculation of realistic muscle force data in the lower extremity. An optimization approach used in conjunction with instrumented devices (14) may allow the governing equations for various muscle activities to be determined.

5.2.3 Other Soft Tissue Structures

In addition to the forces exerted by the muscles, the force contributions of ligaments and fascial structures can also be considered. Forces that are exerted by these soft tissue structures give a direct contribution to the state of load equilibrium. *In vivo* knee ligament forces have been reported by France et al. (51). The joint stabilizing effects of the knee ligaments have also been investigated by a number of other researchers (9,25,76,98,155).

The anatomy of the fasciae has been described by, for example, Gerlach and Lierse (57). Investigations of the magnitudes and directions of the fascial forces are, however, unknown. The fascial structures of the thigh combine to form three large compartments. The pressure differences that exist between these compartments directly contribute to the shear forces produced by muscles and ligaments. Compartment pressures have been measured by Heckman et al. (68), Schwartz et al. (130), Mannarino and Sexson (96), and Jerosch et al. (83).

6 MUSCULOSKELETAL MEASUREMENTS

In the previous sections of this chapter, we have considered how both static equilibrium and control system theory may be used to create a musculoskeletal model to determine joint and muscle loadings. When these loads are determined, they may be used together with data on the constitutive behavior of the tissues to analyze the deformation of musculoskeletal elements—as outlined in Section 5 above. Such analysis may be done using physical *in vitro* models or using

computational models based on finite element analysis. Often the *in vitro* or *in vivo* measurements are used for what has been termed "validation" of the model. Obviously the data used for validation of the model must be independent of that used to construct the model. For example *in vitro* surface strain measurements of the femur have been recorded for various applied loads, for which, together with bone geometry and material property information, one can calculate the internal forces and moments. If these calculated forces and moments are similar to those used in the model this is considered a "validation." Some researchers eschew the word validation because it has connotations of "proving the model to be true" whereas, by definition, a model is a simplification of the real system and will only be "valid," or need to be valid, in a limited sense relevant to the question under investigation. It might be better to say that a similarity between a prediction of the model and an independent experimental measurement "confirms" the model, or provides a corroboration of the model. In any case, such similarity will give the investigator greater confidence that the model is an acceptable representation of the real system. Another issue is that, for some models, corroboration with experimental data is difficult if not impossible; obviously models that can be tested against experimental data of the kind presented below are usually preferred (117).

6.1 Strain on Bone Surfaces

Cristofolini et al. (31) measured the strains in the proximal portion of the femur to show the influence of muscle groups on the loading of the bone. The experimental setup included contributions from the *m. adductor longus, m. adductor magnus, mm. glutei, mm. vasti, m. rectus femoris,* and *m. biceps femoris.* A single gait phase was used to show the influence of the muscles on the strain distribution within the proximal portion of the femur; it was shown that proximal femoral strains of up to ten times higher when the influence of muscles was considered. According to Cristofolini, the *mm. glutei* account for 50 to 100% of the strain changes induced by muscles within the proximal femoral third. However, strain gauge measurements can only provide surface information; material and geometric properties must be known to compute the internal loads. Furthermore, evaluation of the load situation at a selected position during gait (as used by Cristofolini) provides limited information about the internal femoral loads that occur during daily activities.

If muscles are to be included in experiments or calculations, it is difficult to use "correct" muscle force values. Cristofolini et al. used a combination of muscle forces from Patriarco et al. (106) and Crowninshield (32). Each of these data sets represented, in itself, a state of equilibrium. A combination of the forces from different data sets applied to a particular anatomical position, as performed by Cristofolini, results in a totally new load situation that may not be in equilibrium. Furthermore, due to the manner in which the forces were calculated, the *mm. glutei* and *m. biceps femoris* have rather large force values, whereas the iliotibial band has none. Other muscle force calculation methods and electromyographic measurements have reported different levels of muscle activity (14,151).

The influence of the *mm. abductores* on femoral surface strain patterns has been extensively discussed in both experimental and finite element models. But the vector pair of *mm. abductor* and hip contact forces can by no means completely represent the complex loading that occurs in the femur during normal daily activities. Sharar et al. (133) calculated stress distributions in the canine femur using full muscle loads. They showed that the magnitude of the bone stresses is lower when all muscle forces are included. Despite the differences in anatomy and size, the same principle may operate in the human femur. Further investigations, which determine the role that each of the different muscle groups play in femoral loading, seem to be necessary (see also Chapter 14).

Although the method of *in vivo* strain measurement in animals has been used since at least 1969 [90], limited information exists about the strains in human femora. This is an important issue because the results obtained from *in vitro* experiments cannot be validated without *in vivo* knowledge. According to Cordey et al. (26), the

possibility of conducting accurate *in vivo* surface strain measurements could be greatly enhanced by appropriate telemetric devices. Such devices have been previously discussed by Bergmann et al. (7).

Weinans and Blankevoort (148) measured the *in vivo* loads in goat tibiae using strain gauges. Directly after sacrifice, the strain gauges were calibrated using externally applied forces. A transformation matrix was later used to calculate the corresponding forces from the measured strains. Similar to the method described previously, the load equilibrium in the goat tibia was assumed to be incomparable to that of the human femur. Nevertheless, the study shows that *in vivo* measurements are invaluable in determining unknown musculoskeletal forces.

6.2 Tendon Forces

An et al. (1) presented a method for direct *in vivo* tendon force measurement using buckle transducers. Komi (87) described a similar method to conduct transcutaneous *in vivo* ligament force measurements of the Achilles tendon. He reported tendon forces of up to 3,885 N ($\approx$6 BW) during sprinting. According to Komi, *in vivo* ligament force measurements represent a viable method to verify mathematical calculations of muscle forces (optimization, reduction, etc.). Such analytical distribution type solutions, with the exception of electromyographic measurements, lack validation. The use of *in vivo* ligament force measurements as a method of verifying complex mathematical calculations raises many questions. First, ethical issues have to be considered prior to *in vivo* measurements. Second, a number of unknowns must be determined to perform muscle force calculations. In contrast, direct measurements provide actual force information that can be used to validate analytical approaches. The limitations shared with other techniques of *in vivo* measurement (few patients, selected activities) remains a concern.

6.3 Joint Contact Forces at the Hip

Hip contact forces have also been determined using *in vivo* measurements. The first measurements were reported by Rydell (125, 126). Telemetric devices were developed by many others (6,18,37,48,95). A review of telemetric devices was published by Bergmann et al. (6). Bergmann et al. (8) published the hip joint contact forces for two patients with telemetrized hip prostheses at different walking speeds. The force maxima observed in this study were between 2.9 BW (2 km/h) and 4.7 BW (6 km/h) for the endoprostheses. On one occasion, a maximal resultant force at the hip of 8.7 BW was reported during stumbling. The existence of such data provides verification for calculated hip contact forces (contact force maximal, e.g., Brand et al. (13): 4–5 BW; Crowninshield et al. (34): 3.6–5.6 BW; Seireg and Arvikar (131): 5.3 BW). Important for a comparison of calculated and measured forces is, however, not only the maximum value but also the force distribution during a gait cycle. Bergmann found this type of hip contact force pattern for both of his patients walking at various speeds; most calculations report a socalled "double peak" (5). The "double peak" pattern may therefore be a convention rather than the real pattern occurring *in vivo*. One possible explanation for the differences existing between the experimental and computational approaches may be directly related to muscle activity. The true muscle activity pattern is measured by experimentation, whereas an assumed pattern of activity is used for calculation.

6.4 Internal Loads of the Femur

Schneider et al. (128) presented *in vivo* measurements of the internal loads on an intramedullary nail that was implanted in a 33-year-old male. The patient had suffered a comminuted midshaft fracture of his left femur that was treated with a telemetric nail, similar to the AO/ASIF universal nail. Loads within the nail were monitored in supine, sitting, and standing positions. According to Schneider et al. the implant loads decreased during partial weight bearing after the seventh post-operative week by about 50%. However, during the healing process, training of the quadriceps produced an increase in the axial force ($\approx$40%). The authors concluded from their measurements that, even after the frac-

ture had completely healed, approximately 50% of the loads were transmitted through the nail. Throughout the healing process, the torsional moments remained relatively small (2–5 Nm $\approx$ 0.003–0.008 BWm). The bending moments reached values of 18–22 Nm before and 4 Nm after fracture healing. The axial force had peaks of up to 300 N and shear forces of 60–80 N during post-operative measurement (standing position, partial weight bearing). In addition, the study showed that even in static patient positions, significant axial loads (130 N $\approx$ 0.2 BW) could be produced by isometric muscular activity.

The forces and moments measured in the nail may not completely represent the load situation that exists in a healthy individual. However, they do provide information about the relative magnitude of the loads acting within the femur. The measured forces and moments were relatively small in magnitude. Therefore, it may be necessary to validate the load information associated with other dynamic activities in addition to those investigated in this study. It may also be interesting to determine to what degree the forces and moments are transferred through the fracture fragments, instead of passing through the nail.

6.5 Muscle Activity

One of the greatest obstacles encountered in biomechanics concerns the ability to quantify muscle force values. *In vivo* measurements can be made using EMG, as described in Section 4.2.6 above. Unfortunately, not all muscles are accessible for the application of surface or needle electrodes. Also, the errors associated with signal cross talk from the electrodes cannot always be eliminated. Approaches for transferring EMG measurement data to muscle force values have been developed by a number of researchers. For example, van Ruijven and Weijs (143) measured the activity in the jaw muscles in cats. Hof and van den Berg (73,74) performed measurements on the human triceps surae and various calf muscles. Herzog and ter Keurs (71) introduced a technique in which the force-length relation was first calculated and then measured *in vivo*. With this approach, the changes in muscle force for a group of muscles (*m. rectus femoris*) may be calculated.

6.6 Concluding Remarks

The literature regarding joint contact forces (e.g., Bergmann et al. (5)), femoral loads (e.g., Schneider et al. (128)), and muscle (e.g., Herzog and ter Keurs (71)), as well as ligament forces (e.g., Komi (87)), is somewhat limited. These measurements were established using a very small population performing a standard set of activities. In addition, these measurement devices were directly applied to the musculoskeletal system. It is unknown to what degree the measurement devices themselves may have modified the internal load situation. Therefore, the use of analytical models, which attempt to calculate the internal thigh loads, remain useful and viable approaches. In parametric studies, they allow the determination of the load conditions and their influencing factors. Nevertheless, *in vivo* measurements play a key role in analytical modeling by forming the gold standard necessary to evaluate the accuracy of the various theoretical approaches.

7 APPLICATIONS TO UPPER EXTREMITY

The upper extremity incorporates the bones from the thorax to the hand. In this section, the emphasis will be on shoulder and elbow joints. The relevant bones are the thorax as a base, and the clavicle, scapula, humerus, ulna, and radius. For most of the arm motions the medial border of the scapula slides over the thorax in the so-called 'scapulothoracic gliding plane'. The shoulder girdle (thorax-clavicle—scapula-thorax) is a closed-chain mechanism. The rotations in the sternoclavicular (SC) and acromioclavicular (AC) joints are restricted, and depend on the shape of the thorax, length of the clavicle, and the triangular shape of the scapula. Whenever a muscle exerts a moment about one of these joints, the scapula is also pressed against the thorax, and scapulothoracic reaction forces will be present. Due to these reaction forces, the muscle

actions around the SC or AC joint will also affect the moment equilibrium about the other joints.

Most of the muscles in the shoulder girdle insert at the scapula. The scapula is the 'driven bone', whereas the clavicle merely keeps the acromion at a distance, and provides a good lever arm to the *m. serratus anterior*. There are two scapulohumeral muscles present: the *m. latissimus dorsi* and the *m. pectoralis major*. These muscles exert moments about the SC, AC, as well as the glenohumeral (GH) joint. Seven monoarticular muscles cross the GH joint and, in addition, there are two biarticular shoulder-elbow muscles. One pure flexion/extension monoarticular muscle pair exists at the elbow, which consists of the *m. brachialis* and the *m. triceps*, with pars medialis and lateralis. The other elbow muscles also have an effect on the pro/supination motion in addition to the flexion/extension moment.

Muscles in the shoulder have unusually large attachment sites, and the fiber orientation can change throughout the muscle. Different parts of the muscle can contract independently from other parts, as has been shown in EMG studies of the *m. trapezius*, *m. deltoideus*, and *m. pectoralis major*. It is appropriate to represent one muscle by multiple muscle lines of action, as is shown in Fig. 2-26.

7.1 Biomechanical Model of the Shoulder Joint

The Delft shoulder and elbow model (DSEM) is presented as an example of a large-scale musculoskeletal model (van der Helm (140)). In such large-scale models the muscle moment arms cannot be derived using the methods described in Section 2 of this chapter, and instead numerical methods appropriate for computers are used. However, the same mechanical principles apply for the simple as well as for the more elaborate large-scale models.

The DSEM is based on a finite element approach, in which each morphological structure is represented by an appropriate element of which the mechanical properties are known. By connecting the elements to each other at the common nodes, the mechanical properties of the

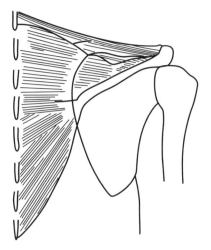 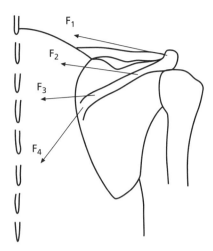

FIGURE 2-26. The *m. trapezius* has a large attachment site at the origin as well as at the insertion. The muscle fibers of the m. trapezius run directly from origin to insertion, without a tendon. It is appropriate to represent this muscle by multiple muscle lines of action (F_1, F_2, F_3, F_4), along which the muscle force vectors act.

whole mechanism can be calculated. The elements of the model are represented as follows:

- Bones are represented as 'rigid body elements', which do not deform and provide attachment nodes for other elements.
- Joints are represented as 'hinge elements'. One hinge element can represent a single axis joint as the elbow or the pro/supination joint. Three perpendicular hinge elements can represent a ball-and-socket joint as the GH joint with three rotational degrees-of-freedom (df). Also the SC and AC joints are represented with ball-and-socket joints. The use of a hinge joint assumes a fixed rotation center, and the small joint translations can be neglected.
- Muscles are represented by 'truss' elements, which can exert forces at their attachment sites in the direction of the truss (i.e., the muscle line of action). Truss elements can be straight between origin and insertion, but also curved around intervening bony contours. In the latter case, the line between the tangential point at the bony contour and the attachment site at the other bone determines the effective moment arm (see Fig. 2-27). Multiple muscle lines of action can represent one muscle (Fig. 2-26).

- Ligaments are represented similarly as the muscles, though in dynamic analysis they are restricted to exerting passive forces only depending on loading and stretch. The scapulothoracic connection is modeled with a special 'surface' element, which restricts a point at the medial border of the scapula to follow the surface of the thorax (approximated by an ellipsoid). The reaction forces between thorax and scapula act perpendicular to the surface of the ellipsoid.

In Fig. 2-28, the DSEM model with a few of its elements is shown. In total, 31 muscles and muscle parts are represented by 139 muscle elements, accounting for the broad muscles with independent parts. The bony contour of the thorax is modeled as an ellipsoid, forcing the *m. serratus anterior* to follow the surface. The *tuberculum majus* and the *caput humeri* are each represented by a sphere, with the *m. deltoid* and the rotator cuff muscles wrapping around, respectively. The *collum humeri* is represented by a cylinder, forcing the *m. latissimus dorsi* and *m. pectoralis major* to wrap around. Also the pro/supination muscles are wrapping around the ulna and radius, if applicable. In each position of the upper extremity, the shortest path of the muscle around the bony contour is calculated, thereby

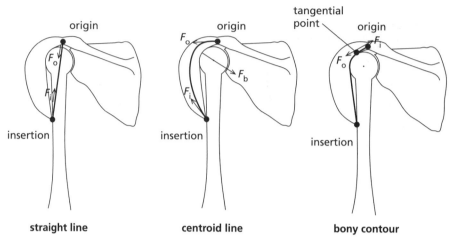

straight line   **centroid line**   **bony contour**

FIGURE 2-27. Three methods to model the muscle line of action. In the straight line method, the muscle line of action connects origin and insertion, but can intersect the bony contour in between. The moment arm is obviously underestimated. In the centroid line method, it is assumed that the muscle line of action is in the middle of the muscle contours. However, because a full free-body diagram of the muscle is not usually made, all forces acting on the muscle (e.g., from the underlying bone) are not taken into account. It is not straightforward to derive the moment arm from the centroid line. In the bony contour method, the shortest line (in three-dimensional space) around the bony contour between the origin and insertion is calculated. The effective moment arm is derived from the part between the tangential point and the origin. The thickness of the muscle is neglected in this approach. F_o denotes the force at the origin and F_i denotes the force at the insertion.

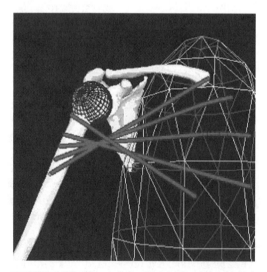

FIGURE 2-28. View of the Dutch shoulder and elbow model (DSEM). The muscle lines of action of the *m. pectoralis* major are shown, as well as the sphere representing the bony contour of the tuberculum majus (used for the wrapping of the *m. deltoideus*). The thorax is modeled by an ellipsoid (shown as a wire frame), on which the medial border of the scapula slides.

changing the moment arm of the muscle continuously.

The SC and AC joints are represented as spherical with three rotational df, neglecting the small translations in the joints. However, since the medial border of the scapula is connected to the thorax, there are two constraints (i.e., two points on a line determine the position of the line). So the number of df will diminish by two. An additional problem is that the conoid ligament is very short and very stiff. If the length were predicted from the bony motions of the scapula and clavicle, it would be very inaccurate. It is better to impose a fixed length on the conoid ligament, which will determine the axial rotation of the clavicle (rather than using the inaccurately recorded axial rotation of the clavicle to determine the length of the conoid ligament). The fixed length of the conoid ligament will diminish the number of df by one, so three df remain at the shoulder girdle. Additional df in the upper extremity are in the GH joint (three rotations), humeroulnar joint (1 df), ulnoradial joint (1 df), and the wrist (2 df). Assuming a free-moving thorax as a base, with 6 df (three rotations and three translations), the total number of df is 16.

7.2 Model Parameters

Cadaver measurements are performed to obtain a complete and accurate data set. The following data are important for a large-scale musculoskeletal model:

- Inertia parameters of the segments (mass, rotational inertia, center of mass). Inertia parameters are difficult to record directly from humans, but also on cadavers. The parameters are derived using regression equations based on anthropometric measures, such as segment length and overall weight;
- Geometric parameters (joint rotation centers, muscle attachment positions, muscle architecture: multiple muscle lines of action per muscle, position and shape of the bony contours, ligament attachment positions); geometric parameters have been measured using a specially built spatial linkage device, ready to point at and record the 3D coordinates. Some of these geometric data can be obtained using MRI measurements. However, it is difficult to make out whether a muscle is attached to a bone, or just wrapping around it. Hence, the accuracy of such measurements using MRI might be low. Some data, such as muscle fiber direction, are not available on normal MRI images.
- Muscle parameters (mass, physiological cross-sectional area, force-length, force-velocity relationships, architecture, pennation); muscle volume can be assessed using MRI. Physiological cross-sectional areas are more difficult because the fiber direction cannot be seen. For the force-length curve the optimal muscle length must be derived. In cadaver measurements this is done by measuring the sarcomere length, using laser diffraction. In living humans this will be very difficult. The muscle architecture and pennation depend on the fiber direction.

7.3 Inverse Dynamic Analysis

An inverse dynamic analysis is employed in almost all applications of large-scale musculoskeletal models. In an inverse dynamic analysis, the recorded position, its derivatives (velocity and acceleration), and the external forces like gravity and hand forces applied to the environment are input variables to the model (see Fig. 2-29). Using the biomechanical model, the muscle forces, which are in (static or dynamic) equilibrium with the external forces and inertial forces can be calculated. From these muscle forces, all other forces in the musculoskeletal system, such as joint reaction forces and ligament forces, can be calculated using optimization procedures.

7.4 Motion Recording

The position, velocity, and acceleration of the bones must be recorded to be used as input for the biomechanical model (Fig. 2-30). Few 3D motion recording techniques have been

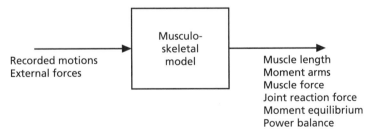

FIGURE 2-29. In an inverse dynamic model, the recorded motions and external forces are input, and the muscle forces are calculated through optimization. Many other relevant variables are also calculated, such as muscle length, muscle moment arms, joint reaction forces, muscle power, and moment equilibrium.

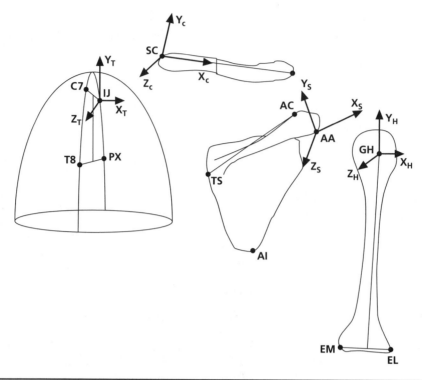

Bone Segment	Bony Landmark	Description
Thorax	IJ	Incisura jugularis (suprasternal notch)
	PX	Processus xlphoideus, most caudal point on sternum
	C7	Processus spinosus of 7th cervical vertebra
	T8	Processus spinosus of 8th cervical vertebra
Clavicle	SC	Most ventral point on sternoclavicular joint
	AC	Most dorsal point on acromioclavicular joint
Scapula	AC	Most dorsal point on acromioclavicular joint
	TS	Trigonum spinae, point on medial border in line with the scapular spine
	AI	Angulus inferior, most caudal point of scapula
	AA	Angulus acromialis, most laterodorsal point of scapula
	PC	Most ventral point of processus coracoideus
Humerus	GH	Glenohumeral rotation center, estimated by regression
	EM	Most caudal point on medial epicondyle
	EL	Most caudal point on lateral epicondyle

FIGURE 2-30. Local coordinate systems of the thorax, clavicle, scapula, and humerus are defined with bony landmarks.

published. Högfors et al. (75) used a 3D roentgen technique with two roentgen cameras and implanted markers. Apparent problems are the difficult localization of the markers with respect to bony landmarks, the small field of view and low sample frequency. Advantage is the high accuracy and capacity to record dynamic motions. Other authors used a palpation technique in which bony landmarks were retrieved and subsequently digitized using a palpator (119,141) or electromagnetic devices, such as 3-Space or Flock-of-Birds (84). Advantages are the noninvasive methodology and the direct retrieval of the bony landmarks. However, it is a static method: Only positions can be measured, no motions. 3D video recordings (VICON, Optotrack, etc.) of the thorax and humerus are widely used. However, due to the large bone-to-skin displacements, no clavicular or scapular motions can be recorded using external markers. Advantages of the method are the fully dynamic capacity and high sampling frequency.

Motions recorded in the various studies are difficult to compare because the local coordinate systems and rotation orders are different. A standardized protocol for motion description is lacking, and due to the recording methodology some data sets are incomplete, i.e., in video techniques scapular and clavicular motions are missing, and bony landmarks have been missing in the roentgen technique. A standardized protocol for 3D motion description has been published by Van der Helm and Pronk (141). The following steps are described below: (i) definition of global and local coordinate systems with respect to *bony landmarks,* (ii) the choice of

tracking markers, and (iii) motion description by choice of *reference frame* and *order of rotation.*

7.4.1 Definition of Coordinate Systems with Respect to Bony Landmarks

Because the shape of bones and joints are different between individuals, it must be acknowledged that an absolute reference frame for comparing motions does not exist. Bony landmarks are well-retrievable references in a bone, and are preferred above bony ridges, like the scapular spine or humeral shaft. Bony ridges require additional definition because a straight line must be fitted through them. Bony landmarks are used to define local coordinate systems of the bones for the shoulder girdle as shown in Fig. 2-31. For comparison of motions between studies, at least the same bony landmarks must be used; otherwise, the results cannot even be calculated in another coordinate system. In the definition of

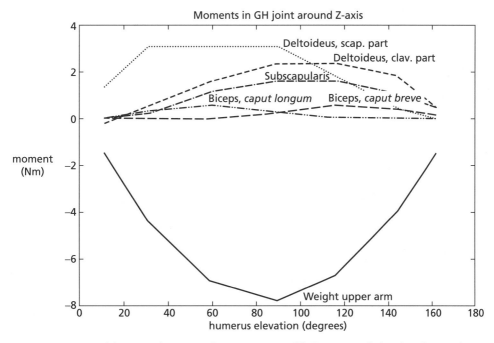

FIGURE 2-31. Model output browser: The moment equilibrium around the dorsal-ventral axis through the glenohumeral joint is shown during humeral abduction. At one side of the equilibrium is the weight of the upper arm, counterbalanced by the muscle moments due to the scapular and clavicular part of the *m. deltoideus, m. subscapularis,* and some smaller contributions of the *m. biceps, caput longum,* and *caput breve.*

coordinate systems the following principles are considered:

- The global coordinate system and the local coordinate systems of the bones are as much aligned as possible in the initial (resting) position.
- Rotations about intuitively recognizable axes are more easily interpreted.
- Gimbal lock orientations anywhere in the range of motion must be avoided. Gimbal lock is described in Section 7.4.3 below.

Definition of global coordinate system. $\underline{X}_g$: horizontal, pointing from left to right; $\underline{Y}_g$: vertical, pointing upward; $\underline{Z}_g$: horizontal, pointing backward. The global coordinate system is more or less aligned with the body. However, this is task dependent. Sitting and standing tasks do not pose a big problem, but in discus throwing, for example, the throwing direction can be used as the forward-backward direction. If motions of the left side of the body are recorded, it is advised to *start* data processing with mirroring the *raw* data in the *measurement coordinate system* (X = −X), in order to avoid left-handed coordinate systems or changes of definition.

Definition of local coordinate systems in the shoulder. A special notation is required (Craig (29)). The local coordinate system, e.g., for the thorax, with respect to the global coordinate system is denoted ^GT where the post-fix G stands for global. Similarly we have ^GC for the clavicle, ^GS for the scapula, and ^GH for the humerus.

Thorax: Bony landmarks of the thorax are shown in Fig. 2-30. The local coordinate system ^GT is defined as $[^G\underline{x}_t, {}^G\underline{y}_t, {}^G\underline{z}_t]$ where, e.g., $^G\underline{y}_t$ represents the y-axis of the thorax with respect to the global coordinate system. It is defined as:

$$^G\underline{y}_t \, \{(^G\underline{IJ} + {}^G\underline{C7})/2 - (^G\underline{PX} + {}^G\underline{T8})/2\}$$

$$\| \, \{(^G\underline{IJ} + {}^G\underline{C7})/2 - (^G\underline{PX} + {}^G\underline{T8})/2\} \|$$

(vector from the midpoint between PX and T8 to the midpoint between IJ and C7, approximately vertical in the initial position)

$^G\underline{x}_t$: Perpendicular to the plane fitted to the points $^G\underline{IJ}$, $^G\underline{C7}$, and $(^G\underline{PX} + {}^G\underline{T8})/2$, pointing to the right.

$^G\underline{z}_t$: Perpendicular to $^G\underline{x}_t$ and $^G\underline{y}_t$.
Origin: $^G\underline{IJ}$

and $^GT = [^G\underline{x}_t \, {}^G\underline{y}_t \, {}^G\underline{z}_t]$. $^G\underline{IJ}$ is the position vector of bony landmark IJ (incisura jugularis), etc. The thorax coordinate system is defined such that in the initial resting position it is approximately aligned with the global coordinate system G.

Clavicle: Bony landmarks of the clavicle are shown in Fig. 2-30. The local coordinate system ^GC is defined as:

$^G\underline{x}_c$: $(^G\underline{AC} - {}^G\underline{SC}) \| (^G\underline{AC} - {}^G\underline{SC}) \|$

$^G\underline{z}_c$: Perpendicular to $^G\underline{x}_c$ and $^G\underline{y}_t$, pointing backward.

$^G\underline{y}_c$: Perpendicular to $^G\underline{z}_c$ and $^G\underline{x}_c$.
Origin: $^G\underline{SC}$.

and $^GC = [^G\underline{x}_c \, {}^G\underline{y}_c \, {}^G\underline{z}_c]$. Nota bene, only two bony landmarks can be identified on the clavicle. Therefore, the thorax $^G\underline{y}_t$ axis is used for definition of the initial orientation of the clavicle. Once the orientation of the initial position of the clavicle has been defined, subsequent rotations can be found by the displacement of tracking markers (75) or, e.g., by minimizing AC joint rotations (141). Pronk (119) and Johnson et al. (84) used the bony landmark AA instead of bony landmark AC. Here, AC is preferred because it is a common point with the clavicle, and the rotation between the clavicular and scapular local coordinate systems closely approximates the AC joint rotations.

Scapula: Bony landmarks of the scapula are shown in Fig. 2-30. The local coordinate system ^GS is defined as:

$^G\underline{x}_s$ $(^G\underline{AC} - {}^G\underline{TS}) \| (^G\underline{AC} - {}^G\underline{TS}) \|$

$^G\underline{z}_s$: Perpendicular to $(^G\underline{AI} - {}^G\underline{AC})$ and $^G\underline{x}_s$, pointing backward, i.e., perpendicular to the scapular plane.

$^G\underline{y}_s$: Perpendicular to $^G\underline{z}_s$ and $^G\underline{x}_s$.
Origin: $^G\underline{AC}$.
and $^GS = [^G\underline{x}_s \, {}^G\underline{y}_s \, {}^G\underline{z}_s]$.
Humerus

$^G\underline{y}_h$: $(^G\underline{GH} - {}^G\underline{E}) \| (^G\underline{GH} - {}^G\underline{E}) \|$

$^G\underline{z}_h$: Perpendicular to $^G\underline{y}_h$ and $(^G\underline{EL} - {}^G\underline{EM})$, pointing backward.

$^G\underline{x}_h$: Perpendicular to $^G\underline{y}_h$ and $^G\underline{z}_h$.
Origin: $^G\underline{GH}$.

and $^GH = [^G\underline{x}_h\ ^G\underline{y}_h\ ^G\underline{z}_h]$. GH is *not* a bony landmark. It can be obtained by a regression equation using the bony landmarks AC, AA, TS, AI, and PC (Meskers et al. (99): standard deviation of the residual error between 2 and 5 mm per coordinate). GH provides a useful operationalization of the longitudinal axis of the humerus. It can also be operationalized in another way, e.g., by a cuff mounted to the upper arm.

7.4.2 Choice of Tracking Markers

Tracking markers are those that can be retrieved during the motion under study. The tracking markers can be used to calculate the position and orientation of the local coordinate system in each recorded position. For the various recording methods different tracking markers are used. In a 3D roentgen study tantalum balls implanted to the bones are used. In a palpation study the bony landmarks serve both for the definition of the local coordinate systems, but also as tracking markers because they are recorded in each position. A Flock-of-Bird system provides a direct recording of the position and orientation of the local coordinate system; the sensor replaces the set of tracking markers. In a 3D video recording, marker trees mounted to the segments are used as tracking markers.

The calculation procedure contains the following steps:

1. Before the start of the experiment, the position of the tracking markers (or sensor) are recorded with respect to the local coordinate system, i.e., the bony landmarks are recorded simultaneously: recording of initial position.
2. The position of the marker tree is recorded during the experiment.
3. The rotations of the marker tree with respect to that in the initial position can be calculated using an algorithm provided by Veldpaus et al. (144).
4. The orientation of the local coordinate system during the experiment can be calculated

using the rotation of the marker tree and the initial position of the local coordinate system.

Step 1 is especially important for 3D roentgen recordings. It must be attempted to record the position of the bony landmarks together with the position of the tantalum balls; otherwise, the results cannot be generalized to non-invasive situations. If no tracking markers can be used for clavicle and scapula (i.e., in 3D video measurements), the orientation of these bones can be calculated by a regression equation using the humeral orientation, a marker at AC, and the initial position of the scapula as regressors (71). De Groot (38) found that there were no major effects of movement velocity and external forces of the scapulohumeral rhythm. This allows for extrapolation of static (palpation) measurements to dynamic situations (3D video).

7.4.3 Motion Description by Choice of Reference Frame and Order of Rotation[4]

An important distinction in the definition of rotation is the difference between rotations with respect to the *global* coordinate system and with respect to a *local* coordinate system. A general description of rotations with respect to the global coordinate system is given by:

$$^GA \cdot {}^A_BR = {}^GB \Rightarrow {}^A_BR = {}^GA^T \cdot {}^GB$$

where R denotes the rotation from local coordinate system ^GA to local coordinate system ^GB and is defined as a rotation about the axes of the global coordinate system. Postfix ^{T} means the transposed matrix. Premultiplying with a rotation matrix means rotations about the axes of the global coordinate system. Postmultiplying with a rotation matrix means rotations about the axes of the (first) local coordinate system as is usually the case in biomechanical definitions.

Choice of reference frame: There are two ways to describe the orientation of a bone, with respect

---

[4]The two prefixes of rotation matrices define the first and second coordinate system between which the rotation is defined, e.g., $A \cdot {}^A_BR = B$

TABLE 2-2. CALCULATION OF ROTATION MATRICES FOR JOINT ROTATIONS[a]

	Joint	Rotation Matrix
Clavicle w.r.t. Thorax	Sternoclavicular joint	$^{G}T.Rc_i = {}^{G}C \Rightarrow Rc_i = {}^{G}T^{T}.{}^{G}C$
Scapula w.r.t. Clavicle	Acromioclavicular joint	$^{G}C.Rs_i = {}^{G}S \Rightarrow Rs_i = {}^{G}C^{T}.{}^{G}S$
Humerus w.r.t. Scapula	Glenohumeral joint	$^{G}S.Rh_i = {}^{G}H \Rightarrow Rh_i = {}^{G}S^{T}.{}^{G}H$

[a] The i refers to the with realization of Rt, Rc, etc., i.e., the time frame.

to the proximal bone (*joint rotations*) and a 'global' orientation (*bone rotations*). A global orientation would mean the orientation with respect to the global coordinate system. However, if, for example, the motion of a discus thrower is considered, the orientation of the clavicle with respect to the track does not make much sense. Therefore, for the 'global' orientation the thorax is chosen as a reference. It is very common to describe the humerus orientation with respect to the thorax (the virtual 'thoracohumeral' joint, often referred to as shoulder joint!). The thorax is also very useful as a reference frame for the interpretation of the scapular motions over the scapulothoracic gliding plane.

Joint rotations: Joint rotations are defined in Table 2-2. The thorax is defined with respect to the global coordinate system (GCS) because there is no proximal bone. Next, the SC joint rotations are defined as rotations of the clavicle with respect to the thorax, AC joint rotations of the scapula with respect to the clavicle, and GH joint rotations of the humerus with respect to the scapula. It is important to note that these rotations are calculated using the rotations of local coordinate systems based on bony landmarks. For true joint rotations the location of the (sometimes moving) joint rotation center with respect to the local coordinate system is needed. However, because the bony landmarks SC and AC are close to the joint rotation centers, and GH is

actually an approximation of the joint rotation center, the deviations will be small.

Bone rotations: Bone rotations are defined in Table 2-3. The thorax is defined with respect to the GCS, similar to the definition of joint rotations. The clavicle, scapula, and humerus are defined with respect to the thorax. For the clavicle the rotations are also similar to the joint rotations because the thorax is the proximal bone.

Euler angles: A rotation matrix is a 3×3 matrix consisting of the cosines between the axes of the first and second local coordinate system between which the rotation is defined. These nine numbers contain only three independent variables. One way to decompose the three independent variables is the choice of Euler angles. Euler angles can be interpreted as subsequent rotations around axes of the (local or global) coordinate system.

$$R_x = \begin{bmatrix} 1 & 0 & 0 \\ 0 & \cos\alpha & -\sin\alpha \\ 0 & \sin\alpha & \cos\alpha \end{bmatrix}$$

$$R_y = \begin{bmatrix} \cos\beta & 0 & \sin\beta \\ 0 & 1 & 0 \\ -\sin\beta & 0 & \cos\beta \end{bmatrix}$$

$$R_z = \begin{bmatrix} \cos\gamma & -\sin\gamma & 0 \\ \sin\gamma & \cos\gamma & 0 \\ 0 & 0 & 1 \end{bmatrix}$$

TABLE 2-3. CALCULATION OF ROTATION MATRICES FOR BONE ROTATIONS

	Rotation Matrix
Thorax w.r.t. Global C.S.	$G.Rt_i = {}^{G}T \Rightarrow Rt_i = G^{T}.{}^{G}T$
Clavicle w.r.t. Thorax	$^{G}T.Rc_i = {}^{G}C \Rightarrow Rc_i = {}^{G}T^{T}.{}^{G}C$
Scapula w.r.t. Thorax	$^{G}T.Rs_i = {}^{G}S \Rightarrow Rs_i = {}^{G}T^{T}.{}^{G}S$
Humerus w.r.t. Thorax	$^{G}T.Rh_i = {}^{G}H \Rightarrow Rh_i = {}^{G}T^{T}.{}^{G}H$

for rotations α, β, and γ about the x-, y-, and z-axis, respectively. Successive rotations (α, β, and γ) result in

$$R = R_x(\alpha) \cdot R_y(\beta) \cdot R_z(\gamma)$$

Note that the second and third rotations occur about rotated axes redirected by one (R_x) or two ($R_x.R_y$) previous rotations. The rotation order is very important: x-y-z result in different angles than y-z-x, for instance. The following was considered in the choice of rotation order:

- The definitions are more or less according to medical terminology, though the latter only refers to the anatomical position and often misplaces rotations by translations.
- The last rotation is about the 'longitudinal' axis. The advantage is that the first two rotations determine the orientation of this axis.

Because in the initial (resting) position the local coordinate systems of the bones are not aligned, the rotations do not start with zero-zero-zero. Often, the zero-zero-zero position cannot even be obtained (e.g., alignment of the clavicular and scapular coordinate systems is physically impossible). Gimbal lock orientations should be avoided. The gimbal lock orientation occurs if the second rotation is $+/- 90°$ (when three different axes are used, like x-y-z, etc.) or if the second orientation is $0°$ or $180°$ (when two different axes are used, like y-z-y, etc.). Then in the gimbal lock position the first and third rotation axis coincide, and no solution can be found for the decomposition into Euler angles. Close to the gimbal lock position the rotations become very sensitive to measurement errors, resulting in large intra- and interindividual standard deviations.

Choice of order of rotations: Because the order of rotations is important, as described above, an order of rotations at the joints (Table 2-4) and at the bones (Table 2-5) must be defined. In Tables 2-4 and 2-5 the proposed order of rotations using Euler angle decomposition is shown. The rotation axes are shown in Fig. 2-30. Euler angles are defined about axes of the first coordinate system (where it should be kept in mind that the second and third rotations are about displaced axes). The description of the rotations in anatomical terms is also given. The rotations should be interpreted as follows. To start, imagine that the second local coordinate system (e.g., the scapula) is aligned with the first local coordinate system (e.g., the thorax: ^GT). The first rotation occurs about the common axis, e.g., the $^G\underline{y}_t$ (and thus $^G\underline{y}_s$ axis). After this first rotation the x- and z-axis are not aligned any more. Then the second rotation occurs about the displaced $\underline{z}_s$ axis, and the third rotation about the twice-displaced $\underline{x}_s$ axis. Then the resulting scapular

TABLE 2-4. DEFINITION OF ROTATION ORDER OF THE SC, AC, AND GH JOINT ROTATIONS[a]

	Rotation Order	Description
Sternoclavicular joint	Y	Pro/retraction about the *thoracic* $^G\underline{y}_t$ axis
	Z′	elevation/depression about the local $\underline{z}_c$ axis
	X″	axial rotation about the local $\underline{x}_c$ (longitudinal axis)
Acromioclavicular joint	Y	Pro/retraction about the *clavicular* $^G\underline{y}_c$ axis
	Z′	lateral/medial rotation about the local $\underline{z}_s$ axis perpendicular to the scapular plane
	X″	tipping forward/backward about the local $\underline{x}_s$ axis through the scapular spine
Glenohumeral joint	Y	Plane of elevation with respect to the *scapular* $^G\underline{y}_s$ axis
	Z′	Elevation/depression about the local $\underline{y}_h$ axis
	Y″	axial rotation about the local $\underline{y}_h$ axis

[a] Axes denoted with single and double quotes are rotated with respect to the initial aligned orientation of the local coordinate systems.

TABLE 2-5. DEFINITION OF ROTATION ORDER OF THE THORAX, CLAVICLE, SCAPULA, AND HUMERUS ROTATIONS[a]

	Rotation Order	Description
Thorax	X	Forward/backward rotation about the *global* $\underline{Y}_G$ axis
	Z'	Lateral flexion about the local $^G\underline{z}_t$ axis
	Y"	Torsion about the local $^G\underline{y}_t$ axis
Clavicle	Y	Pro/retraction about the *thoracic* $^G\underline{y}_t$ axis
	Z'	Elevation/depression about the local $\underline{z}_c$ axis
	X"	Axial rotation about the local $\underline{x}_c$ (longitudinal axis)
Scapula	Y	Pro/retraction about the *thoracic* $^G\underline{y}_t$ axis
	Z'	Lateral/medial rotation about the local $\underline{z}_s$ axis perpendicular to the scapular plane
	X"	Tipping forward/backward about the local $\underline{x}_s$ axis through the scapular spine
Humerus	Y	Plane of elevation with respect to the *thoracic* $^G\underline{y}_s$ axis
	Z'	Elevation/depression about the local $\underline{y}_h$ axis
	Y"	Axial rotation about the local $\underline{y}_h$ axis

[a] Axes denoted with single and double quotes are rotated with respect to the initial aligned orientation of the local coordinate systems.

orientation is equal to the recorded position ^{G}S. The magnitude of the first, second, and third rotations can be uniquely solved from the rotation matrix R[5].

7.5 Model Output

The above system is solved using the optimization procedures described in Section 3.2 above. All kinematic (motion-related) and dynamic (force-related) data can be calculated in inverse dynamic applications. For large-scale models it is always attempted to build a user-friendly interface, such that the user can easily surf through all the data, and generate and check his/her own hypothesis. For instance, you might be interested in the function of a muscle during the motion that has been simulated. Using a model browser, it will be possible to look at the muscle force during the motion. If the muscle is generating force, it is likely that there is a good reason for it. First, it is logical to assume that the muscle has a good location, and will act as an agonist. However, it is

also possible that the muscle is active to compensate for another muscle. When you look closer to the model output, in this case to the muscle moment arms, it is possible to derive which of these options is most likely.

In Fig. 2-31 an example of such model output is shown. In this case, the moment equilibrium around the ventral-dorsal axis during abduction is shown. In the moment equilibrium, the moment contributions of all forces around the joint, i.e., M = r x f, are added. The resulting moment should be zero because the muscle and ligament forces should cancel the weight of the segments and external forces. It can be seen in the figure that the scapular and clavicular parts of the *m. deltoideus*, *m. subscapularis*, and *m. biceps, caput breve* and *c. longum* are the main muscles counterbalancing the weight of the arm. From the figure it can be concluded that *m. supraspinatus*, often indicated as the second glenohumeral abductor, is not large enough to generate a significant moment contribution.

The moment equilibrium around the SC joint is shown in Fig. 2-32. In this figure it can be seen that the most important abducting moment around the SC joint is due to the reaction force acting from the thorax on the angulus inferior at the scapula. Apparently, the *m. serratus anterior* latero-rotates the scapula in such a position that

---

[5]In fact, there are two solutions to determine the Euler angles from a rotation matrix. However, if the second rotation is constrained between −90° and 90° (x-y-z, etc.) or between 0° and 180° (y-z-y, etc.), the best interpretable solution remains.

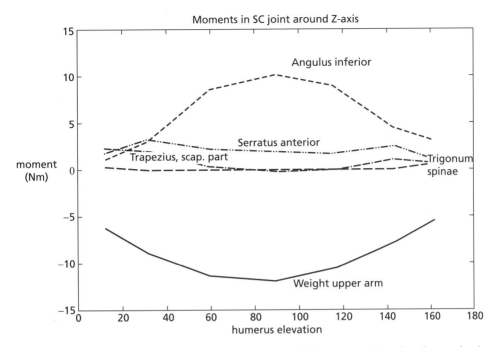

FIGURE 2-32. Model output browser: The moment equilibrium around the dorsal-ventral axis through the sternoclavicular joint is shown during humeral abduction. At one side of the equilibrium is the weight of the upper arm, counterbalanced mainly by the reaction force between angulus inferior and thorax, and also by *m. serratus anterior, m. trapezius,* scapular part. The position of the scapula lateral to the thorax at 90° seems to be very favorable to use the passive scapulothoracic reaction forces instead of active (energy-consuming) muscle forces.

hardly any muscle force is necessary to resist the segment weights!

7.6 Data for Clinical Applications

Musculoskeletal models are very helpful in answering what-if questions: "What would happen if. . . ?". In this case, the new situation can be implemented in the model and the consequences can be checked. For clinical applications, this will mean that the first task is to record the motions of the patients, and then the model can be applied. The model must in general be adapted to the specific dysfunction of the patients, e.g., some paralyzed muscles, alternative rotation center, fixated joints, etc. It is often also interesting to test why the patients are not able to generate specific motions. Joint reaction force and muscle loading information can also be used to generate finite element models of, for example, implanted scapulae under adduction and flexion loading,

and these can be use to assess glenoid component designs (88,102).

8 APPLICATIONS TO LOWER EXTREMITY

8.1 Musculoskeletal Loading of the Lower Limb

Musculoskeletal loading plays an important role in the biological processes of fracture healing (23,89), bone modeling and remodeling (67), and primary stability of implants (145). Nevertheless, current knowledge of musculoskeletal loading of the lower limb is still limited. Whereas there is strong evidence that muscles are major contributors to femoral loading (41,43), and that some of the muscles are also required to model failure of joint prostheses in the femur (136), the actual forces occurring *in vivo* remain largely unknown.

To date, noninvasive measurement of *in vivo* muscle forces is still impossible, whereas ethical considerations discourage the use of invasive methods to determine muscle forces in humans. Therefore, the only opportunity to estimate the complex distribution of muscle forces is offered by computer analysis. Optimization algorithms have been employed to solve the distribution problem and simulate loading conditions at the hip in a large number of studies (14,24,35,54,69,111,112,131,132). A common approach to validating these models has been to compare muscle activation patterns obtained from simulation with measured muscle activities as determined by EMG. However, this method does not allow quantitative validation of the musculoskeletal loading conditions. Instrumented implants, as discussed in Section 5.2, provide hip contact forces for different activities for individual patients *in vivo*. A method of validating predicted musculoskeletal loading conditions is to compare the calculated hip contact forces with these *in vivo* measured forces. This comparison makes it possible to determine whether the calculated results are within the range of those found from *in vivo* studies. The study of Lu et al. (93) presented a model of the lower limb in the sagittal plane that was validated by a cycle-to-cycle comparison of predicted axial forces in the femur to *in vivo* forces measured by a massive femoral prosthesis. However, they did not investigate the loading conditions at the hip. To our knowledge, computed hip contact forces and those measured *in vivo* in the same patient have only been compared in one study (11). In this study, hip contact forces were measured 58 days post-operatively, while gait analysis was performed 90 days post-operatively. Hence, a cycle-to-cycle comparison of measured and calculated hip contact forces was not possible.

8.2   Loading and Load History: An Example of How to Obtain Loading Information

Patients: Four total hip arthroplasty (THA) patients were included in the study. In all patients, an instrumented femoral prosthesis was used to measure the *in vivo* hip contact forces (8). All subjects gave informed consent to participate in the experiments and to the publication of their images and names. In two patients the prosthesis was implanted in the left hip, in the others in the right hip. At the time of surgery, the mean age of the patients was 61 years, ranging from 51 to 76 years. The mean time between surgery and measurements was 17 months, ranging from 11 to 31 months. For each patient, extensive anthropometric data were collected to determine bone dimensions, segment masses, center of gravity positions, and inertia parameters (39).

8.2.1   Gait Analysis and Inverse Dynamics

Clinical gait analysis was conducted for a number of different activities of everyday life (5). The present study concentrates on activities with the highest frequencies during daily living (101), such as walking and stair climbing. Each patient performed several trials of each activity. The average speed during walking was 3.9 km/h. The stair climbing exercise was performed on custom-made stairs composed of three single steps without handrail support. The patients selected an average stride length of 45 cm. Three patients climbed all steps (HSR, PFL, KWR), while patient IBL climbed only the first one. All measurements were taken during climbing of the first step. Start and end of the walking and stair climbing exercises were determined by instants of heel contact. The beginning of the exercise was defined as the moment of heel strike (0% stride). The end of the exercise was marked by the next heel strike of the same leg (100% stride). During all activities, time-dependent kinematic and kinetic data were gathered: two Kistler force plates measured ground reaction forces. The *in vivo* hip contact force with magnitude F and components $-F_x$, $-F_y$, $-F_z$ were measured in the femur system x, y, z during all activities. The x-axis of the femur system was parallel to the dorsal contour of the femoral condyles in the transverse plane and the z-axis was parallel to an idealized midline of the femur (8). An optical system (Oxford Metrics, UK), consisting of a set of six infrared cameras and 24 reflective markers attached to the patients' skin, was used to determine movement of the lower limbs.

Positional information given by the skin markers and the anthropometric data were combined to derive the locations of bony landmarks. From these landmarks, the segment coordinate systems (origins and orientations) were computed with respect to the fixed gait laboratory system. The resultant intersegmental forces and moments at ankle, knee, and hip joint were computed from the kinematic and kinetic gait analysis data with respect to the local coordinate systems using an inverse dynamics approach.

Peak values of the vertical force during a gait cycle were used to define interindividual variability. The mean vertical peak force was computed as the arithmetic mean of the peak vertical forces of all trials performed by a single patient. The relative variability was defined as the maximal difference between the peak force of a single trial.

Similarly, interindividual variability of the flexion-extension moment at the hip was defined. The mean peak moment was computed as the arithmetic mean of the peak flexion-extension moments of all trials performed by a single patient. Relative variability was defined as the maximal difference between the peak moments of a single trial.

To allow interindividual comparison, the data were mirrored for those patients with a prosthesis on the right side. Thus, all data were available for a prosthesis on the left side.

8.2.2 Musculoskeletal Model

Based on computed tomography (CT) data from the visible human (NLM, Bethesda, MD, USA), a musculoskeletal model of the human lower extremity was developed. The visible human data set was chosen because it is the most complete official data set available that describes the human anatomy. The CT scans were available at a spacing of 1 mm with a slice thickness of 1 mm (in plane scan resolution: 0.9375 mm/pixel) and thus allowed an accurate description of bony anatomy to be obtained. From the CT scans, surface contour data of all hip bones (left and

right iliac bone, sacrum, and vertebra S1) and all the bones of the left leg (femur, patella, tibia, fibula, and all the bones of the foot) were determined. This was achieved by thresholding methods available in the "Medical Image Editor" software by courtesy of the German Heart Center, Berlin. The bony surfaces were reconstructed from the contours (55). To remove noise, the surfaces were filtered by a polygonal mesh filter available in the Visualization Tool Kit (129).

Muscles were represented as straight lines spanning from origin to insertion based on descriptions from the literature (Fig. 2-33) (42). Muscles with large attachment areas, such as the glutei, were modeled by more than one line of action. Some muscles were wrapped around the bones to approximate their real curved path. This was necessary to gain an adequate representation of their lever arms at the joints. In total, the muscle model included 95 lines of action.

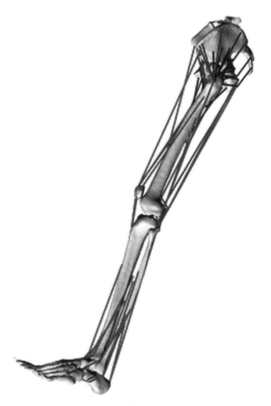

FIGURE 2-33. Musculoskeletal analysis of lower limb loading.

Data on the PCSA of the individual muscles was taken from the literature (43).

8.2.3 Joint Kinematics

The hip and ankle were modeled as joints with three rotational df. At the knee, the femorotibial joint was modeled as a joint with three rotational df, while the patellofemoral joint was modeled as a joint with one rotational df around the medio-lateral axis, and two translational df in the sagittal plane.

The tracking of the patella during gait analysis proved impossible. An *in vitro* experiment was conducted to determine the kinematics of the patellofemoral joint. A human knee specimen was mounted in a knee joint simulator allowing unconstrained knee motion and loading (46). The motion of the patella in the sagittal plane was derived for a complete flexion-extension cycle of the knee. In order to adapt the data obtained from the knee specimen to the patients, anterior-posterior and axial translations were scaled based on the patella position in full extension of the knee.

8.2.4 Adaptation to the Individual Patient

Adaptation of the visible human to the individual patient anatomy was accomplished by a scaling process. The procedure employed bony landmarks between which bone dimensions were defined. These landmarks were determined for the visible human and the patients. Scaling factors were calculated as the ratio of patients to visible human bone dimensions. Linear scaling was applied individually to each bone and all attached muscle origins, insertions, or wrapping points in order to obtain individual patient musculoskeletal models.

Mediolateral scaling of the pelvis was based on the distance between the left and right hip joint centers. The thigh was scaled to match the length between the transition point of the prosthesis neck and shaft and the knee joint center. The same scaling factor was applied to the patella. The distance between knee and ankle

joint center was used to compute the scaling parameter for the shank. The foot was scaled based on the distance between calcaneal tuberosity and the phalanx of the fifth digit. The PCSA of each muscle was scaled according to the patients' body weight.

The head and neck of the visible human femur were resected to simulate THA surgery. In a first step, the proximal part of the femoral prosthesis (neck modeled as a cylinder, prosthesis head modeled as a sphere) was scaled based on the patient's neck length and head diameter. In a second step, neck and head were positioned and oriented toward the resected femur according to femoral anteversion, caput collum, and diaphyseal and neck-stem angle to match the individual implantation.

8.2.5 Computation of Muscle and Joint Contact Forces

Muscle force distribution was computed using a linear optimization algorithm, minimizing the sum of muscle forces (34). Inequality constraints were imposed on the maximal muscle forces (20). Maximal muscle activation during the everyday activities under investigation was unlikely to occur. Therefore, the muscle forces were restricted to below 85% of the physiological muscle force. This force was calculated as the product of each muscle's PCSA and a physiological muscle stress of 1.0 MPa (2).

A distribution of muscle forces was required to fulfill the resultant intersegmental moments at the ankle (flexion-extension moment), knee (flexion-extension and ab-adduction moments), and hip joint (all moments). From the individual muscle and the resultant intersegmental forces, joint contact forces were calculated for ankle, knee, and hip joints for all patients and activities. The calculated hip contact forces and those measured *in vivo* were compared for all trials.

8.2.6 Ground Reaction Forces

The general patterns and the magnitudes of the ground reaction forces were similar for all trials involving one individual patient during walking. The ground reaction forces were characterized by a dominant, vertically directed component. The relative variability of the vertical peak forces for a single patient ranged from 2% to 5% with an average of 4% for the patients (IBL: 2%, HSR: 4%, PFL: 5%, KWR: 5%). Findings for stair climbing were similar. Again, vertical forces dominated. Relative variability of vertical peak forces for a single patient ranged from 1% to 6% with an average of 4% for all patients (IBL: 5%, HSR: 4%, PFL: 1%, KWR: 6%).

8.2.7 Resultant Intersegmental Moments at the Hip

For both walking and stair climbing, the general characteristics of the resultant intersegmental moments at the hip were similar for the different trials for each patient. The largest moment was always the flexion-extension moment. The average relative variability in the flexion extension moment for all patients was 19% during walking (IBL: 11%, HSR: 27%, PFL: 27%, KWR: 11%) and 11% during stair climbing (IBL: 21%, HSR: 5%, PFL: 4%, KWR: 15%)

8.2.8 Measured versus Calculated Hip Contact Forces

Calculated hip contact forces and those measured *in vivo* were compared in all investigated trials. Graphical representation is restricted to one trial per patient. The cycle-to-cycle comparison revealed good agreement in patterns and magnitudes of computed and measured hip contact forces for walking in all four patients. Relative deviation was defined as the difference between measured and calculated hip contact forces divided by the measured force and evaluated for each moment during the gait cycle. During the stance phase, where absolute forces were much larger than during the swing phase, relative deviations in absolute hip contact force magnitudes were smallest (Fig. 2-34). The smallest relative deviation of all three force components was found for the axially directed component F_z. The smaller, mediolateral and anterior-posterior directed contact forces F_x and F_y showed larger relative deviations, both under or overestimating the *in vivo* measured forces. At the moment of maximal measured hip contact force, the

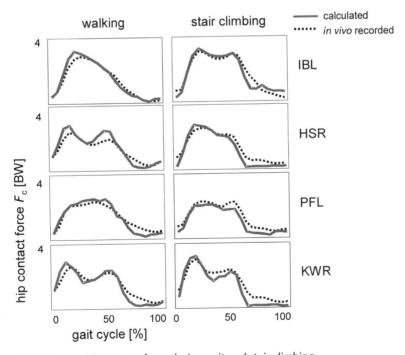

FIGURE 2-34. Hip contact force during gait and stair climbing.

minimal relative deviation between measured and calculated hip contact forces for all trials was 0.3% (patient KWR). In the trial with the largest deviation, the calculation overestimated the hip contact force by 33% (patient HSR). The arithmetic mean of the relative deviation of absolute measured and calculated force magnitudes during walking was 12% for all patients (mean values determined from all trials for the individual patients: IBL: 13%, HSR: 23%, PFL: 10%, KWR: 2%).

The findings for stair climbing were similar. General pattern and magnitudes of the calculated hip contact forces agreed well with the *in vivo* measured data (Fig. 2-34), especially during the stance phases. The smallest relative deviation was found for the axially directed contact force component F_z, while the mediolateral and anterior-posterior forces F_x and F_y showed larger relative deviations. For a single trial of an individual patient, the smallest relative deviation between measured and calculated absolute force magnitudes at the moment of maximum measured hip contact force was 3%, the largest 37%. Relative deviation of the absolute force magnitudes during stair climbing showed a mean of 14% for all patients (mean values determined from all trials for the individual patients: IBL: 8%, HSR: 15%, PFL: 21%, KWR: 13%).

8.3 Simplification of the Derived Muscles

The stability of joint endoprostheses depends on the loading conditions to which the implant-bone complex is exposed. Due to a lack of muscle force data, however, it is only possible to consider simplified loading conditions *in vitro*.

The complete set of muscle forces across the hip joint only becomes of practical value if it can be applied to improve implants or surgical techniques. The complete derived muscle set is not only complex, but also consists of variations for every patient, activity, and time point of measurement. The application of these loads to, for instance, implant testing machines is made more difficult due to size and space constraints (118). To avoid oversimplified loading conditions, a load profile has been developed that resembles the *in vivo* loading conditions of a "typical" total hip replacement patient, considering the interdependence of muscle and joint forces, and is achievable in an *in vitro* test. It has been implemented experimentally where it is shown that muscle loading affects migration of a femoral prosthesis (16,17,94,145).

The development of the load profile was based on a computer model of the lower extremities that was validated against *in vivo* data. This model was then simplified by grouping functionally similar hip muscles. Muscle and joint contact forces were computed for an average data set of up to four patients, throughout walking and stair climbing. The calculated hip contact forces were compared with the average of the *in vivo* measured forces.

The developed load profile was then simplified to include the forces of up to four muscles at the instances of maximum *in vivo* hip joint loading during both walking and stair climbing (Fig. 2-35). The resulting muscle configuration showed hip contact forces that differed by less than 10% from the peak *in vivo* value for a "typical" patient.

The simplified load profile presented (Fig. 2-35) is one that is based on validated musculoskeletal analysis and yet seems achievable in an *in vitro* test setup. It could form the basis for further standardization of preclinical testing by providing a more realistic approximation of physiological loading conditions (14).

8.4 Summary

In this section it has been shown how to determine the musculoskeletal loading conditions of the proximal femur during walking and stair climbing. Addressing the limitations, it is well known that skin movement errors can affect location of bony landmarks derived from the marker positions. Therefore, special care was taken to minimize skin movements and other artifacts. Furthermore, because the inverse dynamics calculation is an iterative process starting from the ankle joint, the largest errors due to error propagation and error accumulation were most likely to occur at the most proximal joint in

Walking (BW = 836N)

Force	x	y	z	Acts at Point
hip contact	−54.0	−32.8	−229.2	P0
intersegmental resultant	−8.1	−12.8	−78.2	P0
abductor (1)	58.0	4.3	86.5	P1
tensor fascia latae, proximal part (3a)	7.2	11.6	13.2	P1
tensor fascia latae, distal part (3b)	−0.5	−0.7	−19.0	P1
vastus lateralis (4)	−0.9	18.5	−92.9	P2

Stair Climbing (BW = 847N)

Force	x	y	z	Acts at Point
hip contact	−59.3	−60.6	−236.3	P0
intersegmental resultant	−13.0	−28.0	−70.1	P0
abductor (1)	70.1	28.8	84.9	P1
ilio-tibial tract, proximal part (2a)	10.5	3.0	12.8	P1
ilio-tibial tract, distal part (2b)	−0.5	−0.8	−16.8	P1
tensor fascia latae, proximal part (3a)	3.1	4.9	2.9	P1
tensor fascia latae, distal part (3b)	−0.2	−0.3	−6.5	P1
vastus lateralis (4)	−2.2	22.4	−135.1	P2
vastus medialis (5)	−8.8	39.6	−267.1	P3

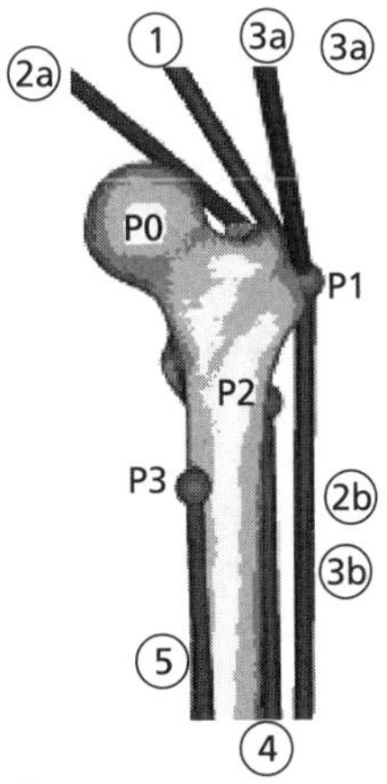

Coordinates

Point	x	y	z
P0	0.00	0.00	0.00
P1	−67.83	−12.04	−35.45
P2	−49.40	−5.01	−79.52
P3	−18.79	8.82	−106.23

FIGURE 2-35. Simplification of the hip joint muscle set.

the model, the hip joint. While the ground reaction forces showed an intraindividual variation of 4%, the flexion-extension moments at the hip varied by as much as 19%. The impact of error propagation or actual intraindividual variations on the observed findings remains to be clarified.

In order to predict musculoskeletal loading conditions, an accurate model of bones and muscles was mandatory. Muscles were modeled as straight lines. Wrapping of muscles was used to simulate their real force distribution and lever arms relative to the joints. Nevertheless, the actual 3D volumetric structures and curved pathways of the muscles had to be simplified. This might explain why the correlation between hip contact forces measured *in vivo* and calculated hip contact force components in the transverse plane was not as good as for the axial component (82).

The optimization approach used to estimate muscle forces was similar to that previously used in other studies. Consequently, all limitations discussed therein also apply to the present study, e.g., the dependency of individual muscle forces on PCSA (11) or the dependency of individual

muscle forces on the objective function employed in the optimization calculation (111).

The musculoskeletal model of the lower extremity presented in this study allowed prediction of proximal femoral loading for walking and stair climbing in four THA patients. Although the patients were of different ages and the implantation varied considerably in the anteversion angle, the musculoskeletal loading conditions were characterized by similar patterns and magnitudes.

The calculated hip contact forces and those measured *in vivo* during walking and stair climbing were similar. However, a varying degree of conformity between the individual force components was found. The component acting along an idealized femoral midline showed best agreement, while the results for the significantly smaller forces in the transverse plane were less accurate. For the first time, a direct cycle-to-cycle validation of proximal femoral loading was possible. The cycle-to-cycle validation revealed that absolute peak loads differed by an average of only 12% during walking and 14% during stair climbing.

Two general principles seem important when predicting musculoskeletal loading conditions. First, a suitable measuring procedure to validate the prediction should be accessible. In this study, the *in vivo* measured hip contact forces can be used for cycle-to-cycle validation of the predicted hip contact forces. Second, patient-specific models should be used to approximate the loading conditions in each individual case. The biomechanical model used in the present study was adapted to the individual anatomy and prosthesis configuration.

9 CONCLUSION

Analysis of joint and muscle loading is fundamental to advancing the science of orthopaedic biomechanics. A wide range of research has been done on the subject, and the knowledge has been applied to the etiology of musculoskeletal disorders and to the design of improved joint replacements. This chapter introduces the fundamental principles and demonstrates how large-scale musculoskeletal models are being developed.

Fundamental principles involve the application of mechanics and optimization methods; using these methods allows the solution of many musculoskeletal loading problems. A potentially powerful methodology is offered by control systems theory, which models the musculoskeletal system under CNS control. Whatever theory is used for modeling of joint and muscle loading, the predictions should be supported by measurements of strain, forces, or muscle activity. Our review shows how these measurements have been performed in previous studies. Examples of analyzing joint and muscle loading in the upper and lower extremities show how modeling methods have been developed in practice, and how they can be used to give fundamental information about the performance of the musculoskeletal system.

REFERENCES

1. An KN, Berglund L, Cooney WP, et al. Direct in vivo tendon force measurement system. *J Biomech* 1990;23:1269–1271.

2. An KN, Kaufman KR, Chao EYS. Physiological considerations of muscle force through the elbow joint. *J Biomech* 1989;22:1249–1256.
3. An KN, Takahasi K, Harrigan TP, et al. Determination of muscle orientations and moment arms. *J Biomech Eng* 1984;106:280–282.
4. Andrews JG. Biomechanical analysis of human motion. *Kinesiology* 1974;4:32–42.
5. Bergmann G, Deuretzbacher G, Heller M, et al. Hip contact forces and gait patterns from routine activities. *J Biomech* 2001;34:859–871.
6. Bergmann G, Graichen F, Rohlmann A. *Implantable telemetry in orthopaedics*. Berlin: Freie Universität Berlin, 1990.
7. Bergmann G, Graichen F, Rohlmann A. Instrumentation of a hip joint prosthesis. In: Bergmann G, Graichen F, Rohlmann A, eds. *Implantable telemetry in orthopaedics*. Berlin: Freie Universität Berlin, 1990:35–63.
8. Bergmann G, Graichen F, Rohlmann A. Hip joint loading during walking and running, measured in two patients. *J Biomech* 1993;26:969–990.
9. Blankevoort L, Kuiper JH, Huiskes R, et al. Articular contact in a 3-dimensional model of the knee. *J Biomech* 1991;24:1019–1031.
10. Borelli GA. *De motu animalium*. Rome: Anglei Bernabò, 1681. [*On the movement of animals*. Berlin: Springer-Verlag, 1989]. Maquet P, translator.
11. Brand RA, Pedersen DR, Davy DT, et al. Comparison of hip force calculations and measurements in the same patient. *J Arthroplasty* 1994;9:45–51.
12. Brand RA, Crowninshield RD, Wittstock CE, et al. A model of lower extremity muscular anatomy. *J Biomech Eng* 1982;104:304–310.
13. Brand RA, Pedersen DR, Davy DT, et al. Comparison of hip force calculations and measurements in the same patient. *Trans Orthop Res Soc* 1989;1:96.
14. Brand RA, Pedersen DR, Friederich JA. The sensitivity of muscle force predictions to changes in physiological cross-sectional area. *J Biomech* 1986;19:589–596.
15. Bresler B, Frankel JP. The forces and moments in the leg during level walking. *J Biomech Eng* 1950;A-62:27–36.
16. Britton JR, Walsh LA, Prendergast PJ. Mechanical simulation of muscle loading on the proximal femur: analysis of cemented femoral component migration with and without muscle loading. *Clin Biomech* 2003;18:637–646.
17. Britton JR, Prendergast PJ. Detection of differences in migration between cemented femoral component designs under long term cyclic loading in vitro. *Trans Orthop Res Soc* San Francisco, 2003 (*in press*).
18. Carlson CE, Mann RW, Harris WH. A radio telemetry device for monitoring cartilage surface

pressures in the human hip. *IEEE Transon Biomed Eng* 1974;21:257–264.

19. Carter DR, Vasu R. Plate and bone stresses for single and double-plated femoral fractures. *J Biomech* 1981;14:55–62.

20. Challis JH. A procedure for determining rigid body transformation parameters. *J Biomech* 1995;28:733–737.

21. Chao EYS, Rim K. Application of optimization principles in determining the applied moments in human leg joints during gait. *J Biomech* 1973;6:497–510.

22. Chow CK, Jacobson DH. Study of human locomotion via optimal programming. *Math Biosci* 1971;10:239–307.

23. Claes LE, Heigele CA, Neidlinger-Wilke C, et al. Effects of mechanical factors on the fracture healing process. *Clin Orthop* 1998;355[Suppl]:S132–S147.

24. Collins JJ. The redundant nature of locomotor optimization laws. *J Biomech* 1995;28:251–267.

25. Collins JJ, O'Connor JJ. Muscle-ligament interactions at the knee during walking. *Proc Inst Mech Eng: Part [H]* 1991;205:11–18.

26. Cordey J, Gautier E, Sumner-Smith G, et al. 'In-vivo' strain gauge technique in biomechanics. In: Bergmann G, Graichen F, Rohlmann A, eds. *Implantable telemetry in orthopaedics.* Berlin: Freie Universität Berlin, 1990:3–10.

27. Cowin SC, ed. *Bone mechanics handbook.* Boca Raton: CRC Press, 2001.

28. Crago PE, Houk JC, Rymer WZ. Sampling of total muscle force by tendon organs. *J Neurophysiol* 1982;47:1069–1083.

29. Craig JJ. *Introduction to robotics, mechanics and control.* Addison Wesley, 1989.

30. Cristofolini L. A critical analysis of stress shielding evaluation of hip prostheses. *Crit Rev Biomed Eng* 1997;25:409–483.

31. Cristofolini L, Viceconti M, Toni A, et al. Influence of thigh muscles on the axial strain in a proximal femur during early stance in gait. *J Biomech* 1995;28:617–624.

32. Crowninshield RD. Use of optimization techniques to predict muscle forces. *J Biomech Eng* 1978;100:88–92.

33. Crowninshield RD, Brand RA. A physiologically based criterion of muscle force prediction in locomotion. *J Biomech* 1981;14:793–801.

34. Crowninshield RD, Johnston RC, Andrews JG, et al. A biomechanical investigation of the human hip. *J Biomech* 1978;11:75–85.

35. Davy DT, Audu ML. A dynamic optimization technique for predicting muscle forces in the swing phase of gait. *J Biomech* 1987;20:187–201.

36. Davy DT, Kotzar GM, Berilla J, et al. Telemetrized orthopaedic implant work at Case Western Reserve University. In: Bergmann G, Graichen F, Rohlmann A, eds. *Implantable telemetry in orthopaedics.* Berlin: Freie Universität Berlin, 1990:205–219.

37. Davy DT, Kotzar GM, Brown RH, et al. Telemetric force measurement across the hip after total hip arthroplasty. *J Bone Joint Surg [Am]* 1988;70-A:45–50.

38. De Groot JH. The variability of shoulder motions recorded by means of palpation. *Clin Biomech* 1997;12:416–492.

39. Deuretzbacher G, Rehder U. A CAE (computer aided engineering) approach to dynamic whole body modeling—the forces in the lumbar spine in asymmetrical lifting. *Biomed Tech (Berl)* 1995;40:93–98.

40. Dostal WF, Andrews JG. A three-dimensional biomechanical model of hip musculature. *J Biomech* 1981;14:803–812.

41. Duda GN. Influence of muscle forces on the internal loading in the femur during gait. *PhD Thesis, Arbeitsbereich Biomechanik Tu Hamburg–Hamburg,* 1996.

42. Duda GN, Brand RA, Freitag S, et al. Variability of femoral muscle attachments. *J Biomech* 1996;29:1183–1190.

43. Duda GN, Heller M, Albinger J, et al. Influence of muscle forces on femoral strain distribution. *J Biomech* 1998;31:841–846.

44. Dul J, Johnson GE, Shiavi R, et al. Muscular synergism—II. A minimal-fatigue criterion for load sharing between synergistic muscles. *J Biomech* 1984;17:675–684.

45. Dul J, Shiavi R, Green NE. Simulation of tendon transfer surgery. *Eng Med* 1985;14:31–38.

46. Dürselen L, Claes L, Kiefer H. The influence of muscle forces and external loads on cruciate ligament strain. *Am J Sports Med* 1995;23:129–136.

47. Edman KAP. Force enhancement by stretch. *J Appl Biomech* 1997;13:432–436.

48. English TA, Kilvington M. In vivo records of hip loads using a femoral implant with telemetric output (a preliminary report). *J Biomed Eng* 1979;1:111–115.

49. Evans FG, Lissner HR. Stresscoat deformation studies of the femur under static vertical loading. *Anat Rec* 1948;100:159–190.

50. Fernandez C, Goldberg JM. Physiology of peripheral neurons innervating otolith organs of the squirrel monkey. II Directional selectivity and force-response relations. *J Neurophysiol* 1976;39:996–1008.

51. France EP, Daniels AU, Goble EM, et al. Simultaneous quantitation of knee ligament forces. *J Biomech* 1983;16:553–564.

52. Frankel V. *The femoral neck.* Uppsala: Almquist and Wiksells, 1960.

53. Friden J, Lieber RL. Tendon transfer surgery: clinical implications of experimental studies. *Clin Orthop* 2002;403[Suppl]:S162–S170.

54. Fuller JJ, Winters JM. Assessment of 3-D

joint contact load predictions during postural/stretching exercises in aged females. *Ann Biomed Eng* 1993;21:277–288.

55. Geiger B. Three dimensional modeling of human organs and its application to diagnosis and surgical planning. *PhD Thesis Institut National de Recherche en Informatique et Automatique* 1993.

56. Gere JM, Timoshenko SP. *Mechanics of materials.* Boston: PWS Engineering, 1984.

57. Gerlach UJ, Lierse W. Functional construction of the superficial and deep fascia system of the lower limb in man. *Acta Anat (Basel)* 1990;139:11–25.

58. Ghista DN, Toridis TG, Srinivasan TM. Human gait analysis: determination of instantaneous joint reaction forces, muscle forces and the stress distribution in bone segments part II. *Biomed Tech (Berl)* 1976;21:66–74.

59. Glitsch U. Comparison of different optimization approaches for the evaluation of internal loads of the lower limb. *Proceedings of the International Society of Biomechanics,* Paris, 1993;1:492–493.

60. Glitsch U, Baumann W. The three-dimensional determination of internal loads in the lower extremity. *J Biomech* 1997;30:1123–1131.

61. Glitsch U, Farkas R. Applications of a multi-body simulation model in human movement studies. *Proceedings of the International Society of Biomechanics,* Paris, 1993;1:490–491.

62. Goldspink G, Scutt A, Loughna PT, et al. Gene expression skeletal muscle in response to stretch and force generation. *Am J Physiol* 1992;262:R356–R363.

63. Goldspink G, Williams P. Muscle fibre and connective tissue changes associated with use and disuse. In: Ada L, Canning C, eds. *Key issues in neurological physiotherapy.* Oxford: Butterworth-Heinemann, 1990:197–218.

64. Gordon J, Ghez C. Muscle receptors and spinal reflexes. The stretch reflex. In: Kandel ER, Schwarttz JH, Jessell TM, eds. *Principles of neuroscience.* Englewood Cliffs, NJ: Prentice-Hall, 1991.

65. Grunewald J. Die Beanspruchung der langen Röhrenknochen des Menschen. *Z Orthop Chir* 1920;39:27–49.

66. Guyton AC. *Textbook of medical physiology.* Philadelphia: WB Saunders, 1991.

67. Hart RT. Bone modelling and remodelling: theories and computation. In: Cowin SC, ed. *Bone mechanics handbook.* Boca Raton: CRC Press, 2001.

68. Heckman MM, Whitesides Jr TE, Grewe SR, et al. Compartment pressure in association with closed tibial fractures. The relationship between tissue pressure, compartment, and the distance from the site of the fracture. *J Bone Joint Surg [Am]* 1994;76:1285–1292.

69. Herzog W. Individual muscle force estimations using a non-linear optimal design. *J Neurosci Methods* 1987;21:167–179.

70. Herzog W, Leonard TR. Force enhancement following stretching of skeletal muscle: a new mechanism. *J Exp Biol* 2002;205:1275–1283.

71. Herzog W, ter Keurs Hedj. A method for the determination of the force-length relation of selected in-vivo human skeletal muscles. *Pflügers Arch* 1988;411:637–641.

72. Hill AV. The heat of shortening and the dynamic constants of muscle. *Proc R Soc Lond B Biol Sci* 1938;126:136–195.

73. Hof AL, van den Berg JW. EMG to force processing I: an electrical analogue of the Hill muscle model. *J Biomech* 1981;14:747–758.

74. Hof AL, van den Berg JW. Linearity between the weighted sum of the EMGs of the human triceps surae and the total torque. *J Biomech* 1977;10:529–539.

75. Hogfors C, Peterson B, Sigholm G, et al. Biomechanical model of the human shoulder joint. 2. The shoulder rhythm. *J Biomech* 1991;24:699–709.

76. Holden JP, Grood ES, Korvick DL, et al. In vivo forces in the anterior cruciate ligament: direct measurements during walking and trotting in a quadruped. *J Biomech* 1994;27:517–526.

77. Houk J, Henneman E. Responses of Golgi tendon organs to active contractions of the soleus muscle of cat. *J Neurophysiol* 1967;30:466–481.

78. Huiskes R. Failed innovation in total hip-replacement: diagnosis and proposals for a cure. *Acta Orthop Scand* 1993;64:699–716.

79. Huxley AF. Muscle contraction and theories of contraction. *Prog Biophys Biochem* 1957;7:225–318.

80. Inman VT. Functional aspects of the abductor muscles of the hip. *J Bone Joint Surg [Am]* 1947;29:607–619.

81. Jankowska E. Interneuronal relay in spinal pathways from proprioceptors. *Prog Neurobiol* 1992;38:335–378.

82. Jensen RH, Davy DT. An investigation of muscle lines of action about the hip: a centroid line approach vs the straight line approach. *J Biomech* 1975;8:103–110.

83. Jerosch J, Castro WH, Geske B. Intracompartmental pressure in the lower extremity after arthroscopic surgery. *Acta Orthop Belg* 1991;57:97–101.

84. Johnson GR, Stuart PR, Mitchell S. A method for the measurement of three-dimensional scapular movement. *Clin Biomech* 1993;5:123–128.

85. Klein Breteler MD, Spoor CW, Van der Helm FCT. Measuring muscle and joint geometry parameters of a shoulder for modeling purposes. *J Biomech* 1999;32:1191–1197.

86. Koch JC. The law of bone architecture. *Am J Anat* 1917;21:177–298.

87. Komi PV. Relevance of in vivo force measurements to human biomechanics. *J Biomech* 1990;23[Suppl 1]:23–34.

88. Lacroix D, Murphy LA, Prendergast PJ. Three dimensional finite element analysis of glenoid replacement prostheses: a comparison of pegged and keeled anchorage systems. *J Biomech Eng* 2000;112:430–436.

89. Lacroix D, Prendergast PJ. A mechanoregulation model for tissue differentiation during fracture healing: analysis of gap size and loading. *J Biomech* 2002;35:1163–1171.

90. Lanyon LE, Smith RN. Measurements of bone strain in the walking animal. *Res Vet Sci* 1969;10:93–94.

91. Lennon AB, Prendergast PJ. Evaluation of cement stresses in finite element analyses of cemented orthopaedic implants. *J Biomech Eng* 2001;123:623–628.

92. Lieber RL. *Skeletal muscle: structure and function.* Baltimore: Williams & Wilkins, 1992.

93. Lu TW, O'Connor JJ, Taylor SJG, et al. Validation of a lower limb model with in vivo femoral forces telemetrized from two subjects. *J Biomech* 1998;31:63–69.

94. Maher SA, Prendergast PJ. Discriminating the loosening behaviour of cemented hip prostheses using measurements of migration and inducible displacement. *J Biomech* 2002;35:257–265.

95. Mann RW, Hodge WA. In vivo pressures on acetabular cartilage following endoprosthesis surgery, during recovery and rehabilitation, and in the activities of daily living. In: Bergmann G, Graichen F, Rohlmann A, eds. *Implantable telemetry in orthopaedics.* Berlin: Freie Universität Berlin, 1990:181–204.

96. Mannarino F, Sexson S. The significance of intracompartmental pressures in the diagnosis of chronic exertional compartment syndrome. *Orthopaedics* 1989;12:1415–1418.

97. Marique P. Etudes sur le femur, *Libr Sci Bruxelles* 1945;1–180.

98. Markolf KL, Amstutz HC. The clinical relevance of instrumented testing for ACL insufficiency. Experience with the UCLA clinical knee testing apparatus. *Clin Orthop* 1987;223:198–207.

99. Meskers CGM, Fraterman H, van der Helm FCT, et al. Calibration of the "Flock of Birds" electromagnetic tracking device and its application in shoulder motion studies. *J Biomech* 1999;32:629–633.

100. Meyer H. Die Architectur der Spongiosa. *Archiv fur Anat Phys und Wissensch Medizin* 1867;34:615–628.

101. Morlock M, Schneider E, Bluhm A, et al. Duration and frequency of every day activities in total hip patients. *J Biomech* 2001;34:873–881.

102. Murphy LA, Prendergast PJ, Resch H. Structural analysis of an offset-keel design glenoid component compared with a center-keel design. *J Shoulder Elbow Surg* 2001;10:568–579.

103. Nigg BM, Herzog W, eds. *Biomechanics of the musculo-skeletal system,* 2nd ed. Chichester: John Wiley and Sons, 1999.

104. Özkaya N, Nordin M. *Fundamentals of biomechanics. equilibrium, motion, and deformation.* New York: Van Nostrand Reinhold, 1991.

105. Patriarco AG. *The prediction of individual muscle forces during human movement.* [dissertation]. Cambridge, MA: Harvard University, 1982.

106. Patriarco AG, Mann RW, Simon SR, et al. An evaluation of the approaches of optimization models in the prediction of muscle forces during human gait. *J Biomech* 1981;14:513–525.

107. Paul JP. The biomechanics of the hip joint. *Proc R Soc Med* 1966;59:943–951.

108. Pauwels F. *Atlas zur Biomechanik der gesunden und kranken Hüfte.* Berlin: Springer-Verlag, 1973.

109. Pauwels F. Über die Bedeutung der Bauprinzipien des Stütz- und Bewegungsapparates für die Beanspruchung des Röhrenknochens. *Acta Anat (Basel)* 1951;12:207–227.

110. Pauwels F. Über die mechanische Bedeutung der gröberen Kortikalisstruktur beim normalen und pathologisch verbogenen Röhrenknochen. *Anat Nachr* 1950;1:53–57.

111. Pedersen DR, Brand RA, Cheng C, et al. Direct comparison of muscle force predictions using linear and nonlinear programming. *J Biomech Eng* 1987;109:192–199.

112. Pedersen DR, Brand RA, Davy DT. Pelvic muscle and acetabular contact forces during gait. *J Biomech* 1997;30:959–965.

113. Pedotti A, Krishnan VV, Stark L. Optimization of muscle-force sequencing in human locomotion. *Math Biosci* 1978;38:57–76.

114. Penrod DD, Davy DT, Singh DP. An optimization approach to tendon force analysis. *J Biomech* 1974;7:123–129.

115. Pierrynowski MR, Morrison JB. Estimating the muscle forces generated in the human lower extremity when walking: a physiological solution. *Math Biosci* 1985;75:43–68.

116. Prendergast PJ. Finite element models in tissue mechanics and orthopaedic implant design. *Clin Biomech* 1997;12:343–366.

117. Prendergast PJ. An analysis of theories in biomechanics. *Eng Trans (Warsaw)* 2001;49:117–133.

118. Prendergast PJ. Bone prostheses and implants. In: Cowin SC, ed. *Bone mechanics handbook* Boca Raton: CRC Press, 2001:35.1–35.39.

119. Pronk GM. Three-dimensional determination of the motion of the shoulder girdle during humerus elevation. *Proceedings of the 11th International Society of Biomechanics Congress,* Biomechanics XI B, Eds. De Groot G, Hollander AP, Huijing PA,

Ingen Schenau GJ van. Amsterdam: Free University Press, 1987:1070–1076.

120. Raftopoulos DD, Qassem W. Three-dimensional curved beam stress analysis of the human femur. *J Biomed Eng* 1987;9:356–366.

121. Raikova RT, Prilutsky BI. Sensitivity of predicted muscle forces to parameters of the optimization-based human leg model revealed by analytical and numerical analysis. *J Biomech* 2001;34:1243–1255.

122. Raikova R. A general approach for modelling and mathematical investigation of the human upper limb. *J Biomech* 1992;25:857–867.

123. Roesler H. The history of some fundamental concepts in bone biomechanics. *J Biomech* 1987;20:1025–1034.

124. Rybicki EF, Simonen FA, Weis EB. On the mathematical analysis of stress in the human femur. *J Biomech* 1972;5:203–215.

125. Rydell NW. Forces acting in the femoral head-prosthesis. *Acta Orthop Scand* 1966;37[Suppl. 88]:1–132.

126. Rydell NW. Intravital measurements of forces acting on the hip joint. In: Evans FG, ed. *Intravital measurements of forces acting on the hip joint.* Berlin: Springer-Verlag, 1966:52–68.

127. Salathe Jr EP, Arangio GA, Salathe EP. An application of beam theory to determine the stress and deformation of long bones. *J Biomech* 1989;22:189–199.

128. Schneider E, Michel MC, Genge M, et al. Loads acting in an intramedullary nail during fracture healing in the human femur. *J Biomech* 2001;34:849–857.

129. Schroeder W, Martin K, Lorensen B. *The visualization toolkit,* Vol. 1, 2nd ed. Englewood Cliffs, NJ: Prentice-Hall, 1998.

130. Schwartz Jr JT, Brumback RJ, Lakatos R, et al. Acute compartment syndrome of the thigh. A spectrum of injury. *J Bone Joint Surg [Am]* 1989;71:392–400.

131. Seireg A, Arvikar RJ. The prediction of muscular load sharing and joint forces in the lower extremities during walking. *J Biomech* 1975;8:89–102.

132. Seireg A, Arvikar RJ. A mathematical model for evaluation of forces in lower extremities of the musculo-skeletal system. *J Biomech* 1973;6:313–326.

133. Sharar R, Banks-Sills L, Elisay R. Stress and strain distributions in the canine femur: finite element analysis. *Med Eng Phys* 2003;25:387–395.

134. Siebertz K, Baumann W. Biomechanische Belastungsanalyse der unteren Extremität. *Biomed Tech (Berl)* 1994;39:216–221.

135. Spitzer V, Ackerman MJ, Scherzinger AL, et al. The visible human male: a technical report. *J Am Med Inform Assoc* 1996;3:118–130.

136. Stolk J, Verdonschot N, Huiskes R. Hip-joint and abductor-muscle forces adequately represent in vivo loading of a cemented total hip reconstruction. *J Biomech* 2001;34:917–926.

137. Sugi H, Tsuchiay T. Stiffness changes during enhancement and deficit of isometric force by slow length changes in frog skeletal muscle fibers. *J Physiol* 1988;407:215–229.

138. Thelen DG, Anderson FC, Delp SL. Generating dynamic simulations of movement using computed muscle control. *J Biomech* 2003:36:321–328.

139. Torodis TG. Stress analysis of the femur. *J Biomech* 1969;2:163–174.

140. Van der Helm FCT. Analysis of the kinematic and dynamic behaviour of the shoulder mechanism. *J Biomech* 1994;27:527–550.

141. Van der Helm FCT, Pronk GM. 3-Dimensional recording and description of motions of the shoulder mechanism. *J Biomech Eng* 1995;117:27–40.

142. Van Egmond AAJ, Groen JJ, Jongkees LBW. The mechanics of the semicircular canals. *J Physiol* 1949;110:1–17.

143. Van Ruijven LJ, Weijs WA. A new model for calculating muscle forces from electromyograms. *Eur J Appl Physiol* 1990;61:479–485.

144. Veldpaus FE, Woltring HJ, Dortmans LJMG. A least squares algorithm for equiform transformation from spatial marker coordinates. *J Biomech* 1988;21:45–54.

145. Verdonschot N, Bergmann G, Britton JR, et al. A European proposal for pre-clinical testing methods of cemented femoral THA implants. *J Arthroplasty* 2003 (*in press*).

146. Weber EF. Ueber die Langenverhaltnisse der Fleischfasern der Muskeln im *Algemeinen. Berichte u.d. Verh. D. Konigl. Sachs. Ges. D. Wiss. Math.-Phys. Cl.* 1851;5–86.

147. Weijs WA, Hillen B. Cross-sectional areas and estimated intrinsic strength of the human jaw muscles. *Acta Morphol Neerl Scand* 1984;23:267–274.

148. Weinans H, Blankevoort L. Reconstruction of bone loading conditions from in vivo strain measurements. *J Biomech* 1995;28:739–744.

149. White SC, Yack HJ, Winter DA. A three-dimensional musculoskeletal model for gait analysis. Anatomical variability estimates. *J Biomech* 1989;22:885–893.

150. Willinger R, Renault D. Determination of muscular and articular forces through physiological optimization. *Biomed Sci Instrum* 1987;23:15–22.

151. Winter DA. *The biomechanics and motor control of human gait: normal, elderly and pathological.* Waterloo, Ontario, Canada: University of Waterloo Press, 1991.

152. Winters JM, Stark L. Estimated mechanical-properties of synergistic muscles involved in

movements of a variety of human joints. *J Biomech* 1988;21:1027–1041.

153. Wolff J. *Das Gesetz der Transformation der Knochen.* Berlin: A. Hirschwald, 1892.

154. Wolff J. Über die innere Architectur der Knochen und ihre Bedeutung für die Frage vom Knochenwachsthum. *Virchow's Archiv* 1870;50:389–450.

155. Zavatsky AB, Beard DJ, O'Connor JJ. Cruciate ligament loading during isometric muscle contractions. A theoretical basis for rehabilitation. *Am J Sports Med* 1994;22:418–423.

MUSCULOSKELETAL DYNAMICS, LOCOMOTION, AND CLINICAL APPLICATIONS

THOMAS P. ANDRIACCHI
TODD S. JOHNSON
DEBRA E. HURWITZ
RAGHU N. NATARAJAN

An analysis of the biomechanics of human locomotion is fundamental to understanding normal and pathological function. Although many parameters can be used to describe the biomechanics of human movement, there are several kinematic (study of motion) and kinetic (study of the relationship between motion and force) parameters that are particularly relevant to the understanding of the pathomechanics of human movement. This chapter will focus on the description of these kinematic and kinetic parameters, as well as identify specific applications where they have been clinically relevant.

1 KINEMATICS OF LOCOMOTION

Kinematic measurements of human locomotion are usually based on the assumption that the limb segments can be idealized as rigid bodies. Relative segmental angular motions have been a frequently used kinematic measure of locomotion. The temporal patterns of segmental angles have been well described (26,27,32,49) in studies of walking and other activities of daily living. It has been shown that temporal characteristics of these segmental angles are quite reproducible during normal gait. The common features of

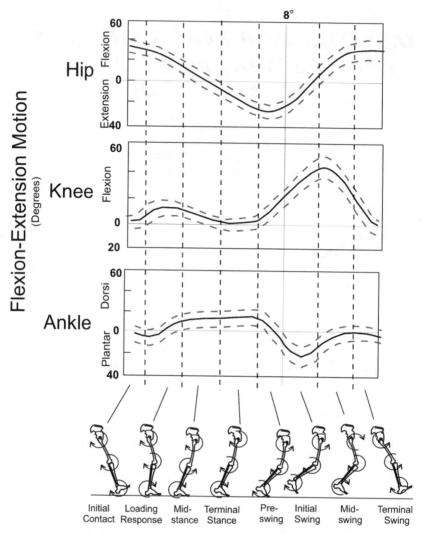

FIGURE 3-1. The position of the hip, knee, and ankle during gait. The stance phase is divided into five segments, and the swing phase is divided into three segments. The curves represent the normal patterns of motion for the hip, knee, and ankle. The position of the limb below the curves illustrates the position of the pelvis, thigh, and shank segments as they would be observed during each of these phases of the gait cycle. The normal sequence of events is quite regular and reproducible, as indicated by the relatively narrow bandline segments around the solid bars, which represent the average of the normal motion patterns.

the sagittal plane motion of the hip, knee, and ankle during the stance and swing phases of gait can be divided into eight segments. During the stance phase, the events are described as initial contact, loading response, midstance, terminal stance, and preswing. The swing phase is described in terms of initial swing, midswing, and terminal swing (Fig. 3-1). It is important to note that the narrow band around each of the motion curves (Fig. 3-1) at the hip, knee, and ankle suggests that the characteristics of these patterns do not vary substantially during normal gait (49). However, care must be taken in measuring certain peak amplitudes because it has been shown that these values are related to walking speed (7,9).

Although the planar segmental angles described above are very useful for many clinical applications (46) where the primary movement is flexion, there are a number of applications that require a more rigorous analysis of the 6 degree of freedom (Df) movement of limb segments. This is particularly true at the knee where secondary translations (e.g., anterior-posterior) and rotations (e.g., internal-external rotation) are important to the normal function of the joint. This section provides some basic kinematic definitions and indicates general applications to locomotion studies.

1.1 Motion Relative to a Global Coordinate System

Consider the motion of the knee joint. Typically, video-based measurements during locomotion describe the motion of limb segments with respect to a global coordinate system G fixed in the laboratory. For example, the translation of the femur can be represented by the vector **d**, which locates the moving or local coordinate system origin in the fixed or global coordinate system G (Fig. 3-2). Three normalized unit vectors can represent the orientation of the local coordinate system embedded in the femur relative to the fixed coordinate system. If x, y, and z and X, Y, and Z are used to describe the orthogonal moving and fixed coordinate systems, respectively, then the x-axis orientation relative to the global coordinate system is represented by the unit column vector

$$\hat{e}_x = \{\hat{e}_{xX}, \hat{e}_{xY}, \hat{e}_{xZ}\}^T,$$

where $\hat{e}_x = \dfrac{e_x}{\|e_x\|} = \dfrac{V_x - d}{\|V_x - d\|}.$

Similarly, the local y- and z-axis orientation can be expressed as the unit vector quantities

$$\hat{e}_y = \{\hat{e}_{yX}, \hat{e}_{yY}, \hat{e}_{yZ}\}^T$$

and $\hat{e}_z = \{\hat{e}_{zX}, \hat{e}_{zY}, \hat{e}_{zZ}\}^T$

with respect to the fixed coordinate system. The three column vectors can be combined into a 3 × 3 rotation matrix $[R]$, which will completely describe the rotational orientation or attitude of the

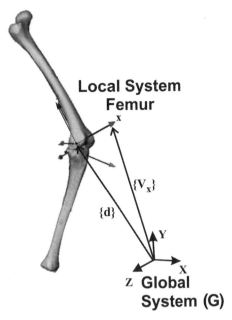

FIGURE 3-2. An illustration of the position of the local coordinate system in the femur relative to the fixed global system **G**. The vector **d** located the origin of the femoral system. The vector **V$_X$** is used to locate the direction **e$_X$** of the local femoral x axis relative to the global system **G**. Each of the local femoral axes can be located in a similar manner.

moving coordinate system relative to the fixed coordinate system where

$$[R] = \left[\{\hat{e}_x\}\{\hat{e}_y\}\{\hat{e}_z\}\right].$$

The 6-Df rotations and translations between a fixed and moving coordinate system in three-dimensional (3D) space can be conveniently represented in a single matrix by utilizing a 4 × 4 square matrix known as a homogeneous transformation matrix. A 4 × 4 homogeneous transformation matrix $[T]$ is composed of the 3 × 3 rotation matrix $[R]$, the displacement vector $\{d\}$, and an additional row as represented in the equation below:

$$[T] = \begin{bmatrix} [R] & \{d\} \\ 0\,0\,0 & 1 \end{bmatrix}$$

where $[R]$ and $\{d\}$ represent the previously described rotational orientation and distance between coordinate system origins, respectively. The last row of $[T]$ uses a scaling factor of 1 so that the transformed homogeneous coordinates are the same as transformed ordinary coordinates (54). The main benefit of utilizing homogeneous coordinates in rigid-body kinematics analysis is that the transformation matrix can be inverted because it is square.

The global positions of the femur and tibia at any instant in time relative to the fixed laboratory coordinate system **G** is given by the 4×4 homogeneous transformation matrices $[T]_{f,G}$ and $[T]_{t,G}$ using the method previously described.

1.2 Relative Motion Between Moving Segments

The method described above can be used to independently describe the motion of the femur and the tibia relative to a fixed global coordinate system (47). However, relative segmental motion is often more useful for physical and clinical interpretations of kinematic measurements. Thus, the relative motion of the femur with respect to a fixed axis in the tibia provides a more meaningful description of knee motion than the global motion of each segment.

The position of the femur relative to the tibia $[T]_{f,t}$ can be obtained by employing a method known as a forward transformation utilizing the following equation,

$$[T]_{f,t} = [T]_{t,G}^{-1}[T]_{f,G}.$$

The femoral transformation $[T]_{f,G}$ is premultiplied by the inverse of the tibial to the global transformation. The transformations employed in a forward transformation proceed from right to left and are performed with respect to the global reference frame.

1.3 Definition of a Joint Coordinate System

The appropriate interpretation of kinematic measurements requires a precise and physically meaningful definition of anatomical references (13,23,48,64). As a general rule, caution needs to be employed when one attempts to compare results between various researchers and techniques because the choice of coordinate systems does influence the magnitudes of rotations and displacements. In fact, equivalent knee motions can be described quite differently based on the orientation and displacement technique used as well as the choice of reference coordinate systems (13,48).

A joint coordinate system (JCS) described by Grood and Sontay (36) has been proposed to define a standard by the International Society of Biomechanics (82). The proposed benefit of using this coordinate system is that it provides a temporally independent method for describing the motion with an attempt to relate the rotations and translations to clinically used terms. Some ambiguity still exists in this coordinate system in that there remains flexibility in choosing the anatomic reference points that define the body's fixed axes.

The JCS described above can be reduced to a convenient and conceptually simple method of defining coordinate systems and relative motions for knee kinematics (13). The approach utilizes bony landmarks and projection angles of the motion of the femur relative to the tibia. The origin of the femoral coordinate system is located at the midpoint of the transepicondylar line of the distal femur (Fig. 3-3). The

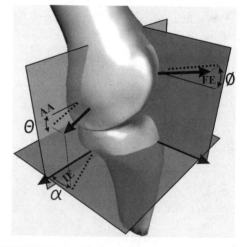

FIGURE 3-3. An illustration of the projection angles used to define anatomical position of the femur in a fixed tibial system. Abduction-adduction (AA), flexion-extension (FE), and internal-external rotation are calculated by projecting the axis embedded in the femur onto planes fixed in the tibia. The definitions remain anatomically consistent at all flexion angles.

origin of the tibial coordinate system is set at the midpoint of a line connecting the medial and lateral points of the tibial plateau. Anatomically relevant projection angles can be extracted from the 3×3 rotation submatrix of $[T]_{f,t}$, where flexion-extension (FE), internal-external (IE), and abduction-adduction (AA) rotations are represented by ϕ, α, and θ, respectively.

The rotation submatrix $[R]$ of the transformation matrix is represented by the following premultiplied concatenation of the individual rotations (34), which were assumed to be performed in the following order about their respective axes: (a) $\phi(x)$, (b) $\alpha(y)$, and (c) $\theta(z)$.

$$[R] = \begin{bmatrix} \cos\theta & -\sin\theta & 0 \\ \sin\theta & \cos\theta & 0 \\ 0 & 0 & 1 \end{bmatrix}$$

$$\times \begin{bmatrix} \cos\alpha & 0 & \sin\alpha \\ 0 & 1 & 0 \\ -\sin\alpha & 0 & \cos\alpha \end{bmatrix} \begin{bmatrix} 1 & 0 & 0 \\ 0 & \cos\phi & -\sin\phi \\ 0 & \sin\phi & \cos\phi \end{bmatrix}$$

$$= \begin{bmatrix} \cos\alpha\cos\theta & -\sin\theta\cos\phi + \sin\alpha\cos\theta\sin\phi \\ \cos\alpha\sin\theta & \cos\theta\cos\phi + \sin\alpha\sin\theta\sin\phi \\ -\sin\alpha & \cos\alpha\sin\phi \end{bmatrix}$$

$$\left. \begin{matrix} \sin\theta\sin\phi + \sin\alpha\cos\theta\cos\phi \\ -\cos\theta\sin\phi + \sin\alpha\sin\theta\cos\phi \\ \cos\alpha\cos\phi \end{matrix} \right]$$

At each time step, the projection angle rotations representing the orientation of the femoral component with respect to the tibia can be calculated from the rotation matrix representation using the following series of equations.

$$\alpha = -\arcsin[R]_{3,1}$$

$$\phi = \arctan\left(\frac{[R]_{3,2}}{[R]_{3,3}}\right)$$

$$\theta = \arctan\left(\frac{[R]_{2,1}}{[R]_{1,1}}\right)$$

The displacement vector $\{\mathbf{d}\}$ between the origins of the two coordinate systems is also extracted from $[T]_{f,t}$ at each time step to position the femur relative to the tibia. When the assumed

sequence-dependent projection angle rotations (a) $\phi(x)$, (b) $\alpha(y)$, and (c) $\theta(z)$ are extracted from the rotation submatrix, of the experimentally determined transformation with respect to the fixed tibial system x, y, and z axes, respectively, the magnitudes of the rotations and displacements are equivalent to the JCS.

Translations can be expressed as the displacement of the origin of the femoral coordinate system relative to the tibial system. Anterior-posterior (AP) motion is the femoral displacement projected on the AP (z) axis of the tibia. Similarly, medial-lateral (ML) and inferior-superior motion are determined from the projection on the corresponding tibial (x) and (y) axes, respectively. Note that locating the position of the femoral reference along the transepicondylar axis minimizes the amount of translation caused by pure rotation because this axis is close to the instantaneous axis of motion. The rotation angles of α and θ are expressed as projection angles of the femoral axis projected onto planes defined by the axis of the tibia. IE rotations are measured by projecting the ML femoral axis onto a plane created by two reference axes in the tibia, the AP and ML axes. AA angles are also calculated by projecting the ML femoral axis onto a plane created by the ML and superior-inferior tibial axes.

1.4 Knee Kinematics During Walking

The application of this technique can be illustrated in a study of knee kinematics during walking (13). This example describes some of the common features of FE, IE rotation, and AP displacement. At heel strike the knee is near full extension and the femoral component is located posteriorly and internally rotated relative to the tibia. During the period from midstance, the femur displaces anteriorly and externally rotates while flexing and extending to terminal extension during stance phase (Fig. 3-4). The offset on the AP translation between heel strike and terminal extension is consistent with the knee operating within an envelope of motion during normal function (21). Note AP translation was determined by calculating the temporal change

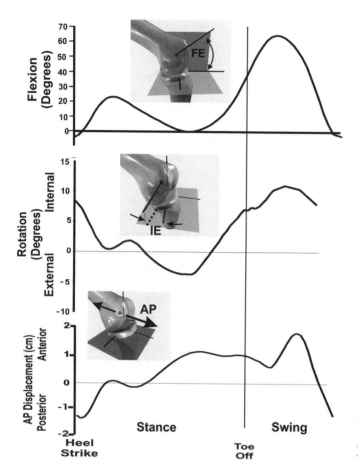

FIGURE 3-4. An illustration of the flexion-extension (FE), internal-extension (IE), and anterior-posterior (AP) motion of the knee during walking. The IE motion was based on the projection angle definition (Fig. 3-3.) and the AP motion of the knee was based on the displacement of a point (midpoint of transepicondylar axis) on the femur relative to a fixed tibial axis.

in distance between the origins of the femoral and tibial coordinate systems in the sagittal plane. The projection angles can be related to the anatomical function of the joint. For example, consider internal rotation of the femur with respect to the tibia with the knee at full extension. IE rotation of the femur will stress the anterior portion of the lateral meniscus and the posterior portion of the medial. Using the projection angle definition, similar stress is applied to the menisci during internal rotation with the knee at 90 degrees of flexion. The projection angle approach is particularly important when studying rotation of the knee in deep flexion because the projected rotations on the tibial planes are anatomically consistent at all flexion angles.

Obtaining meaningful six-Df motion of the knee during unencumbered movement remains challenging. Markers placed on the skin will move relative to the underlying bone and limit the resolution of detailed joint movement (68). In most cases only large motions such as FE have acceptable error limits with most skin-based marker systems. Skeletal movement has been measured using alternative approaches to a skin-based marker system including stereoradiography (45,74,83), bone pins (48,68), external fixation devices, and single-plane fluoroscopic techniques (15,77). All of these methods are invasive or expose the test subject to radiation. Therefore, the widespread applicability of these methods is limited. The results described above use a point cluster technique (PCT) that permits direct *in vivo* measurement of the complete 6-Df motion of the femur on the tibia while performing activities of daily living. The technique uses a cluster of points placed on the thigh and shank to measure the motion of the knee. The method minimizes the error associated with skin movement and permits *in vivo* kinematic measurements of the knee with sufficient resolution to analyze the complete 6-Df motion of the joint. A complete description of the method can be found elsewhere (3,13).

2 KINETICS: EXTERNAL FORCES ON LIMB SEGMENTS, MASS, AND INERTIA

An understanding of the kinetics of human movement is fundamental to the understanding of the musculoskeletal system. The motion of the musculoskeletal system is the result of a balance between those forces and moments that act external to the body, and the forces and moments that act internally.

Before one can begin to analyze the forces acting at different joints in the human body during human movement, some basic definitions and assumptions must be made. In most studies of locomotion, as noted before, the limb segments are assumed to be rigid bodies. This simplifies the analysis because the structure is assumed not to deform under load. Forces acting on the rigid body may be classified as either external forces or internal forces. External forces represent the action of other bodies on the rigid body under consideration. In gait analysis, ground reaction forces, gravitational forces, and inertial forces are taken as external forces. Internal forces are responsible for holding together the component parts that make up the rigid body. For example, the forces that hold together the shank and thigh are called internal forces. Force will be expressed in units of Newtons (N). The moment of a force about an axis measures the tendency of the force to impart to the body a rotational motion about this axis. A moment of a force will be expressed in units of Newton-meters (Nm).

Inertia is a body's resistance to acceleration. Inertial resistance to linear acceleration depends on mass, whereas resistance to angular acceleration depends on geometry and mass distribution

(and is generally referred to as mass moment of inertia). The mass moment of inertia must be referenced to a coordinate system. The analysis of forces and associated motion is a branch of mathematics called dynamics. Newton's second law of motion links the kinematics of a body to its kinetics. This law may be stated as follows: "If the resultant force acting on a body is not zero, the body will have an acceleration proportional to the magnitude of the resultant and in the direction of this resultant force."

2.1 Calculation of Intersegmental Forces and Moments

2.1.1 General Approach

Newton's second law makes it possible to solve for intersegmental forces and moments. The foot-ground reaction forces are usually measured using a force plate. The weight and inertial forces are often approximated by modeling the leg as a collection of rigid segments representing the thigh, shank, and foot (22,24). Limb motion is measured using various types of optoelectronic or electromagnetic methods. The following is a description of how Newton's second law of motion is used in calculating external intersegmental forces and moments at different joints during human locomotion. The first step in this process involves the establishment of a model. The model we are describing here is a link model (Fig. 3-5A) in which inertial properties for each rigid segment are lumped at its mass center (a lumped mass approximation). It is also assumed that each segment is symmetric about its principal axes and that the angular velocity and acceleration about the longitudinal axis of the segment are negligible. The second step in the process involves the measurement of the external ground reaction forces, some method for approximating limb segment inertial properties, and a method of locating the 3D position of the joint centers in space and time.

Once these data are obtained, the analysis begins with a free-body diagram for each of the segments (Fig. 3-5B). The free-body diagram

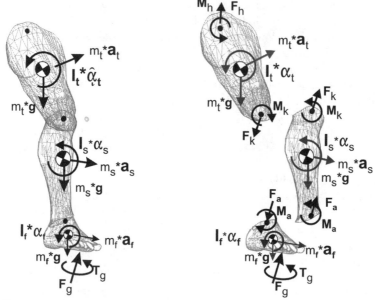

(A) External Loads Acting on Leg   **(B) Intersegmental Forces and Moments**

FIGURE 3-5. A: The lower extremity model consists of three rigid-body segments: foot, shank, and thigh. The known forces and moments are the ground reaction force and moment, inertial forces and moments, as well as gravitational forces on the three rigid bodies. **B:** Free-body diagram. Free-body diagrams for the three rigid links are shown here. The calculations proceed from the distal to proximal end and start at the foot. With the help of rigid-body equilibrium equations, the force and moment at the ankle ($\mathbf{F_a}$, $\mathbf{M_a}$) are calculated. The force and moment at the distal end of the shank are equal and opposite to the force and moment at the ankle ($-\mathbf{F_a}$, $-\mathbf{M_a}$). With the distal force and moment of the shank known, the proximal shank force and moment are then calculated ($\mathbf{F_k}$, $\mathbf{M_k}$).

includes the intersegmental forces and moments at the joint centers, and the inertial forces and moments and gravitational forces acting at the center of mass of the segment. The calculations start at the foot because the only unknown force and moment is at the ankle and then proceeds from distal to proximal. Segmental equilibrium equations are written at the mass center using Newton's second law of motion. Unknown intersegmental forces and moments at the proximal end of the segment are obtained from the solution of these equilibrium equations. Once the intersegmental forces and moments are calculated at the ankle, they are applied to the next segment as an equal and opposite force and moment at the distal end of the segment (shank). The process continues with solving for the unknown intersegmental forces and moments at the proximal end of the segment.

2.1.2   Details of the Calculation

The free-body diagram for each of the rigid segments is shown in Fig. 3-5B. The governing equations for the ankle can be expressed as two vector equations representing six scalar equations. The first vector equation represents the equilibrium of the rigid body under external forces. The second vector equation represents the moment equilibrium equation. Bold letters indicate vector quantities. Each of these vector equations has three components, one along each of the global axes: x, y, and z.

The two vector equations of equilibrium for the foot (subscript f) are given as

$$\sum \mathbf{F} = m_f \mathbf{a}_f \qquad (1)$$

(force equilibrium equations) and

$$\sum \mathbf{M} = \mathbf{I}_f\, \alpha_f \qquad (2)$$

(moment equilibrium equations, in which moments are taken about the center of mass of the rigid body), where m_f is the mass, $\mathbf{I}_f$ the moment of inertia, $\mathbf{a}_f$ the linear acceleration of the mass center, and α_f the angular acceleration of the foot.

The forces and moments at the distal end ($\mathbf{F}_g$ and $\mathbf{T}_g$) of the foot are the ground reaction forces and moment measured by the force plate. The intersegmental forces and moments at the ankle ($\mathbf{F}_a$ and $\mathbf{M}_a$) are unknowns. The mass center is located at a distance of $\mathbf{r}_{cm,p}$ and $\mathbf{r}_{cm,d}$, respectively, from the proximal and distal ends of the rigid body.

To solve for the intersegmental force ($\mathbf{F}_a$) at the ankle, apply the force equilibrium equation as follows:

$$\mathbf{F}_a + \mathbf{F}_g + m_f\mathbf{g} = m_f\mathbf{a}_f \qquad (3)$$

where $\mathbf{g}$ is the acceleration due to gravity. Thus, the intersegmental force at the ankle is given by

$$\mathbf{F}_a = m_f\mathbf{a}_f - \mathbf{F}_g - m_f\mathbf{g} \qquad (4)$$

To solve for the intersegmental moment at the ankle, the moment equilibrium equation for the rigid body is written as

$$\mathbf{M}_a + \mathbf{T}_g + (\mathbf{r}_{cm,p} \times \mathbf{F}_a) + (\mathbf{r}_{cm,d} \times \mathbf{F}_g) = \mathbf{I}_f\alpha_f \qquad (5)$$

Thus, the intersegmental moment at the ankle is given by

$$\mathbf{M}_a = -\mathbf{T}_g - (\mathbf{r}_{cm,p} \times \mathbf{F}_a) - (\mathbf{r}_{cm,d} \times \mathbf{F}_g) + \mathbf{I}_f\alpha_f \qquad (6)$$

The above method of calculating the intersegmental forces and moments at the ankle joint can be extended to calculate intersegmental forces and moments at the knee joint. For the next rigid body, the shank, the forces, and moments at the distal end ($\mathbf{F}_a$ and $\mathbf{M}_a$) are known from the previous calculations (Eqs. 4 and 6). The forces and moments at the proximal end ($\mathbf{F}_k$ and $\mathbf{M}_k$) are assumed to be unknown. The shank has a mass of m_s, the mass center is located at a distance of $\mathbf{r}_{cm,p}$ and $\mathbf{r}_{cm,d}$, respectively, from the proximal and distal ends of the rigid body. The shank is assumed to move with an acceleration of $\mathbf{a}_s$. The subscript s in the following equations

(Eqs. 7–10) indicates that the segment under consideration is the shank.

The force equilibrium equation for the rigid body is

$$\mathbf{F}_k + \mathbf{F}_a + m_s\mathbf{g} = m_s\mathbf{a}_s \qquad (7)$$

Thus, the intersegmental force at the knee is given by

$$\mathbf{F}_k = m_s\mathbf{a}_s - \mathbf{F}_a - m_s\mathbf{g} \qquad (8)$$

where $\mathbf{F}_a$ is given in Eq. 4.

The moment equilibrium equation for the rigid body is written as:

$$\mathbf{M}_k + \mathbf{M}_a + (\mathbf{r}_{cm,p} \times \mathbf{F}_k) + (\mathbf{r}_{cm,d} \times \mathbf{F}_a) = \mathbf{I}_s\alpha_s \qquad (9)$$

Thus, the intersegmental moment at the knee is given by:

$$\mathbf{M}_k = -\mathbf{M}_a - (\mathbf{r}_{cm,p} \times \mathbf{F}_k) - (\mathbf{r}_{cm,d} \times \mathbf{F}_a) + \mathbf{I}_s\alpha_s \qquad (10)$$

The above method of calculation of forces and moments at the knee joint can also be extended to calculate intersegmental forces and moments at the hip. The equations remain the same except that the subscript s in the equations is replaced by t (thigh). Further, because we now know the forces and moments at the knee joint, subscripts a and k are to be replaced by k and h, respectively. Thus, the force at the hip is given by:

$$\mathbf{F}_h = m_t\mathbf{a}_t - \mathbf{F}_k - m_t\mathbf{g} \qquad (11)$$

Similarly, the moment at the hip joint is given by:

$$\mathbf{M}_h = -\mathbf{M}_k - (\mathbf{r}_{cm,p} \times \mathbf{F}_h) - (\mathbf{r}_{cm,d} \times \mathbf{F}_k) + \mathbf{I}_t\alpha_t \qquad (12)$$

The preceding 3D example is an application of the rigid-body equations to solve for the intersegmental forces and moments at any joint. The analysis is done from distal to proximal. The unknown intersegmental loads are solved sequentially at the ankle, knee, and hip. The intersegmental load at the distal segment is applied with equal magnitude and opposite direction to the distal joint of the next segment up the limb. This leaves one unknown force, the proximal intersegmental load. In the next section, we will

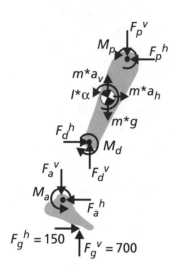

FIGURE 3-6. Sagittal plane intersegmental forces and moments at ankle and knee joints. Intersegmental forces at the ankle and knee joints, as well as the ground reaction force, are resolved in the horizontal and vertical directions. Note that the inertia forces and moments of the foot are neglected.

see how the intersegmental forces and moments at the joints can be used to calculate the internal forces, i.e., muscle and internal joint reaction forces.

Example 1: Application of kinetics in gait analysis to estimate external forces and moments. This example illustrates the basic steps used to calculate the intersegmental forces and moments at the ankle and knee joints from measurements of limb segment displacements, body mass, and ground reaction forces during gait (Fig. 3-6). For this example, the forces and moments acting on the segments in the sagittal plane alone will be considered. The foot is assumed to be of negligible mass compared with the mass of the shank. The ground reaction forces, inertial forces of the shank (both linear and angular), distance of ankle from floor, and length of shank are known. Because the current example deals with forces in only one plane (the sagittal plane), the forces are expressed in horizontal and vertical components. The vertical component of force is denoted by a superscript of v, and the horizontal component is denoted by a superscript of h. The numerical values for this example are given in Table 3-1.

Thus, the force equilibrium equation for the foot segment can be rewritten as

$$-F_a^h + F_g^h = 0$$

$$-F_a^v + F_g^v = 0$$

Substituting the known values of F_g^h and F_g^v into the above equations, the external forces at the ankle along horizontal and vertical directions can be obtained. The numerical solution is given in Table 3-1.

The moment equilibrium equation for the foot is reduced to

$$M_a + F_g^h \cdot v_1 + F_g^v \cdot h_1 = 0$$

where h_1 and v_1 are the horizontal and vertical distances of the ankle joint from the position of the ground reaction force. Table 3-1 contains the numerical value of this moment.

In regard to the analysis of the forces and moments in the shank, at the distal end the forces will be equal and opposite in nature to those acting at the ankle. Thus, $F_d^h = - F_a^h$, and $F_d^v = - F_a^v$. Now, if we write the force equilibrium equations for the shank along horizontal and vertical directions, respectively,

$$F_d^h - F_p^h = ma_h$$

from which the unknown force F_p^h is calculated, and

$$F_d^v - F_p^v = ma_v - mg$$

from which the unknown force F_p^v is calculated.

The moment equilibrium equation is written about the center of mass of the shank and given as

$$F_d^h \cdot v_2' - F_d^v \cdot h_2' + F_p^h \cdot v_2'' - F_p^v \cdot h_2'' \\ - M_d + M_p = I\alpha$$

where h_2' and v_2' are the horizontal and vertical distances, respectively, of the center of mass of the shank from the ankle joint. The corresponding horizontal and vertical distances, respectively, of the center of mass of the shank from the knee joint are h_2'' and v_2''. In the above equation, all quantities are known except M_p. The results are shown in Table 3-1.

TABLE 3-1. NUMERICAL VALUES FOR EXAMPLE 1: APPLICATION OF KINETICS IN GAIT ANALYSIS

Description	Symbol	Value
Knowns		
Ground reaction force		
Vertical	F_g^v	700 N
Horizontal	F_g^h	150 N
Lever arms		
Floor to ankle		
Horizontal	h_1	0.13 m
Vertical	v_1	0.10 m
Ankle to center of mass of the shank		
Horizontal	h_2'	0.06 m
Vertical	v_2'	0.16 m
Knee center to center of mass of the shank		
Horizontal	h_2''	0.09 m
Vertical	v_2''	0.12 m
Shank weight	mg	28 N
Inertial forces		
Shank mass (m) ×		
horizontal acceleration (a_h)	ma_h	0.7 N
Shank mass (m) × vertical acceleration (a_v)	ma_v	3.3 N
Shank inertia (I) × angular acceleration (α)	$I\alpha$	0.06 Nm
Unknowns		
Force at ankle		
Horizontal	F_a^h	150 N
Vertical	F_a^v	700 N
Moment at ankle	M_a	106 Nm
Force and moment at shank		
Distal end		
Horizontal force	F_d^h	150 N
Vertical force	F_d^v	700 N
Moment	M_d	106 Nm
Proximal end		
Horizontal force	F_d^h	149.3 N
Vertical force	F_p^v	696.7 N
Moment	M_p	43.16 Nm

2.2 Equilibrium Between External and Internal Forces

Equilibrium requires a balance between intersegmental forces and internal forces such that there is no change in the state of rest or motion of the body. For locomotion studies, the state of equilibrium at the joint is of relevance. The intersegmental forces and moments calculated by the methods described in Example 1 must be balanced by a set of forces and moments acting internally to maintain equilibrium. These internal forces are generated primarily by muscle contraction, passive soft tissue stretch, and articular reaction forces. Equations of equilib-

rium can be resolved into a total of six equations (three forces and three moments). Thus, in three dimensions, it is only possible to solve for six unknowns. In general, there are more internal forces (unknowns) than equations, thereby rendering the problem statically indeterminate. Thus, a unique solution for individual muscle forces is not possible without further assumptions. However, it is possible to reduce the problem, with appropriate assumptions, to a case in which there are an equal number of unknowns and equations. The problem thus becomes statically determinate and can be solved. Important insight into the forces sustained by internal

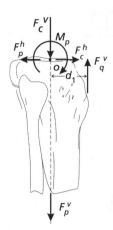

FIGURE 3-7. Free-body diagram of external and internal forces acting at the center of the knee on the tibial plateau. This problem is statistically determinate because there are three unknowns, which can be determined from the three equilibrium equations of the rigid body.

structures has been gained using this approach (44,56,57,71).

Example 2. Statically determinate analysis for estimating internal forces. To illustrate how a statically determinate analysis can be used to calculate internal forces, let us consider a two-dimensional statically determinate example. The external as well as internal forces are treated as scalar quantities as opposed to being considered vectors. The free-body diagram in Fig. 3-7 contains the external forces (known) and the internal forces (unknown) acting on the knee joint. The external vertical and horizontal components of the forces, F_p^v and F_p^h, have been explicitly calculated in the previous example. The external moment, M_p, acting at the knee has also been calculated explicitly and is tending to flex the knee. The internal forces acting at the knee include the vertical and horizontal components of the tibial-femoral contact force, F_c^v and F_c^h, and the vertical and horizontal components of the quadriceps muscle force, F_q^v and F_q^h, which are all unknown.

For the purpose of this example, we will not consider the horizontal component of the quadriceps force.

The external moment for this example tends to flex the joint. One approach to simplifying the

problem would be to assume that the antagonist muscles (hamstring muscles) are inactive. The quadriceps muscle would then generate a moment equal and opposite to this external flexion moment. This solution would provide a conservative estimate of the tibiofemoral contact force and quadriceps muscle force. The problem then becomes statically determinate because there are three unknowns, horizontal and vertical contact forces and the vertical quadriceps force, and three independent equations of equilibrium. The contact point between the tibia and femur is assumed to be at the center of the tibial plateau.

Summing forces in a vertical direction gives:

$$-F_c^v + F_q^v - F_p^v = 0$$

Summing forces in a horizontal direction gives:

$$F_c^h - F_p^h = 0$$

Summing moments at the center of contact on the tibial plateau to eliminate the unknown contact force, we obtain:

$$F_q^v * d_1 - M_p = 0$$

where d_1 is the distance from the vertical component of the contact force F_c^v to the vertical component of the quadriceps force F_q^v.

The equations of equilibrium contain three unknown forces, which are the vertical components of the quadriceps, F_q^v; the contact force, F_c^v; and the horizontal component of the contact force, F_c^h. Mathematically, the system consists of three linearly independent equations with three unknowns and is therefore statically determinate. Numerical values are provided in Table 3-2.

The external moment that tends to flex the knee is balanced by the vertical component of the quadriceps force, F_q^v, acting at a distance d_1 from the tibial-femoral contact point, 0. In general, this situation, in which the external moment acting at the joint is balanced by internal moments generated by muscle forces, occurs with most joints. Muscles are in mechanically efficient positions to balance external moments at the joints and usually provide the largest portion of the internal joint moment. As a result,

TABLE 3-2. NUMERICAL VALUES FOR EXAMPLE 2: STATICALLY DETERMINATE ANALYSIS

Description	Symbol	Value
Knowns		
External reaction force and moment		
Vertical force	F_p^v	697 N
Horizontal force	F_p^h	149 N
Moment	M_p	43.2 Nm
Unknowns		
Quadriceps force (vertical)	F_q^v	1080 N
Tibiofemoral contact force		
Vertical force	F_c^v	382 N
Horizontal force	F_c^h	149 N

large joint reaction forces are generated primarily from muscle contraction.

For the case in which antagonistic muscle activity is present, the problem again becomes statically indeterminate (the equations of equilibrium cannot be solved explicitly) because the number of unknowns exceeds the number of equations. Sophisticated mathematical models incorporating additional information have been used to solve these problems.

2.3 Techniques for Solving the Indeterminate Problem

The techniques illustrated in Examples 1 and 2 have been used to predict muscle forces at the joints. As with most biological systems, there is a redundancy of muscle (synergistically and antagonistically) that can equilibrate the external joint moments and forces generated during locomotion. Thus, the problem of predicting muscle forces is indeterminate because there are many feasible muscle force distributions that satisfy equilibrium. In general two approaches have been used to solve the indeterminate problem. The first is a "reduction" method that groups muscles into functional units reducing the indeterminate problem to a determinate one as illustrated in Example 2. The second approach uses optimization methods that assume the force distribution among the muscles must also satisfy some physical condition such as mechanical efficiency.

Early attempts to use optimization methods (29,72,73) solved for muscle force distributions

that were based on laboratory measurements. More recent approaches can predict patterns of motion to achieve a particular objective (4,60). The selection of an appropriate physiologically based optimization criteria is a major limitation of optimization methods (28), especially when antagonistic muscle activity is present. Optimization criteria are usually based on the assumption of an energy efficient gait (29,63) and have predicted reasonable estimates of muscle activity (1) for normal locomotion. Meaningful optimization solutions are also dependent on an accurate estimate of muscle moment arms (61). These moment arms can substantially change during movement. For example, at the knee the moving contact point changes the effective length of the lever arm of the forces generated by the muscles crossing the joint (8). Also the maximum force-generating capacity of each muscle is related to the length and velocity of muscular contraction using Hill's equation (2,31,38). The ultimate challenges for optimization models include selecting appropriate assumptions for the physiological function of muscle and the selection of appropriate global optimization criteria. The selection of appropriate optimization criteria is further complicated for pathological gait.

In spite of the complexity of predicting individual forces, there is amazing similarity between the measurements of the predicted contact forces at the hip joint during gait (12). In general, the force at the hip joint reaches an initial peak in early stance phase and a second peak in late stance phase. This pattern was described in the initial work of Paul and McGrouther (62) using a reduction method and subsequent studies, using optimization methods (29,70,76), as well as studies of direct force measurement using an instrumented total hip replacement (17).

An alternative approach to the reduction and optimization approaches is to determine all possible combinations of muscle forces that balance the external moments. Although there are an infinite number of combinations of muscle forces that will equilibrate the external forces, the magnitude of these forces are constrained by the physiological limits of the muscle. Mikosz et al. (55) used a stochastic approach to select potential solutions for muscle forces at the knee with physiological constraints. Hurwitz et al. (41) applied a parametric approach to estimate the full range of physiologically feasible muscle forces that balance the external moments at the hip. The parametric approach permits direct evaluation of the effect of agonist and antagonist muscle force distributions on the resulting contact force and can predict a maximum and minimum range based on the assumed level of antagonistic muscle activity.

The above discussion illustrates the complexity of predicting muscle force during locomotion. Thus, these techniques must be applied with care. Yet, meaningful estimates of joint contact forces can be derived from external measurements of joint reaction moments because joint contact force prediction is relatively insensitive to the modeling approach.

Example 3: Prediction of joint and muscle forces. This example illustrates the application of a reduction model to predict the joint reaction forces, muscle forces, and soft tissue forces at the knee during walking.

Model description. The model (71) is similar to Morrison's (56). Input to the model consists of knee flexion angle, intersegmental moments, and forces (Table 3-3). The model differs from that of Morrison's in that the point of contact changes with knee flexion, the cruciate ligaments resist only AP shear forces, and collateral ligaments resist only abducting-adducting moments. The movement of the tibial-femoral contact and the resulting changes in muscle mo-

ment arms are modeled by a third-order polynomial relating the angle of knee flexion to the tibial-femoral contact point (33). The medio-lateral location of the tibial-femoral contact remains fixed at 25% of the tibial width from the knee joint center on each plateau, while the AP contact changes with flexion (33,52). The average width of the tibia is taken as 80 mm. A linear relationship is assumed to exist between the knee flexion angle and the inclination of the patellar ligament with the long axis of the tibia (52). In common with Morrison's model, the three muscle groups in this model consist of the quadriceps, hamstrings, and gastrocnemius.

The activity of the flexor-extensor muscle groups was assumed to be dependent on the direction of the external moment. For example, the quadriceps muscles were active to balance the intersegmental flexion moment, and the hamstring and gastrocnemius resist the intersegmental extension moment. The external adduction moment (M_{ad} is balanced by the muscle group forces (F_m) plus the axial load (F_A) acting about the medial contact (Fig. 3-8). If the moment generated by the muscle force and axial load does not balance the external adduction moment about a pivot on the medial surface, then lateral soft tissue (F_s) tension (active or passive) was used to balance the remaining adduction moment. The force in the iliotibial band resulting from contraction of the tensor fascia latae and *m. gluteus maximus*, along with the tensile forces in the

TABLE 3-3. EXTERNAL MEASUREMENTS AND INTERNAL PREDICTIONS

		Normal Group
Adduction moment	(input)	3.30 ± 0.67% (bw × ht)
Flexion moment	(input)	1.81 ± 0.65% (bw × ht)
Extension moment	(input)	2.86 ± 0.82% (bw × ht)
Axial load	(input)	1.01 ± 0.08 bw
Extensor muscle force	(output)	0.75 ± 0.26 bw
Flexor muscle force	(output)	1.65 ± 0.46 bw
Medial joint reaction	(output)	2.25 ± 0.39 bw
Lateral joint reaction	(output)	0.91 ± 0.24 bw
Lateral pretension	(output)	0.50 ± 0.18 bw

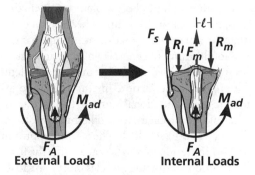

FIGURE 3-8. The external adducting moment was resisted by the summed muscle force(F_m) and axial load acting over a lever arm (l). Pretension in the lateral soft tissues would maintain equilibrium if the muscle force were insufficient (71).

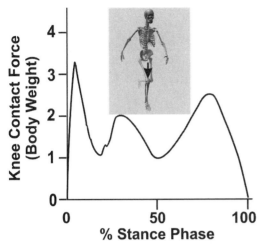

FIGURE 3-9. The total joint reaction for a normal subject during walking consisted of three peaks. The first peak is a result of the hamstrings, the second the quadriceps, and the third the gastrocnemius (71).

lateral collateral ligament and capsular forces, are grouped together and referred to as lateral soft tissue pretension.

Model results. The model was used to predict the contact forces, extensor and flexor muscle force, and lateral soft tissue tension for an average normal subject walking. The predicted total contact force during normal level walking (1.2 m/sec) consisted of three peaks (Fig. 3-9). The first peak just following heel strike was approximately three times body weight. The first peak in the contact force was produced primarily from force generated by the hamstring muscles. The second contact force peak was the result of the quadriceps muscles, and the third contact force peak was produced by the gastrocnemius muscles. It should be noted that the joint reaction force described here was predicted without antagonistic muscle activity, and therefore represents a lower bound to the contact force at the knee. The muscle forces, medial and lateral contact force predicted when the contact force (1st peak, Fig. 3-9) was greatest, are given in Table 3-3. It should be noted that the minimum muscle force (no antagonist) to maintain equilibrium was insufficient to balance the adduction moment and keep the knee joint closed laterally in this example. Co-contraction of antagonistic muscle action and/or pretension in the passive

soft tissue was needed for dynamic joint stability during walking. These observations suggest a possible explanation for the presence of antagonistic muscle action during normal walking. A high adduction moment in a patient with severe lateral laxity could lead to a condition in which the joint opens laterally and transfers the entire joint reaction through the medial compartment.

3 JOINT MOMENTS IN LOCOMOTION

An analysis of the temporal characteristics of the moments acting at the joints of the lower extremity during walking and other activities of daily living demonstrates characteristic patterns. These patterns include predictable phasic changes in the magnitude and direction of the joint moment during the walking cycle (Figs. 3-10 and 3-11). To differentiate variations detected in gait among individuals from variations in individual body sizes, the moment magnitudes shown are reported as a percentage of body weight times height [%(bw × ht)]. This normalization assumes that the moments, typically measured in Newton-meters (Nm), are proportional to the height and weight of an individual. Thus, differences detected among individuals would be associated with differences in gait rather than body size.

3.1 Flexion-extension Moment Patterns During Walking

The appropriate application of the joint moment to the study of normal and abnormal function requires characterizing the patterns that can be expected in a normal population. Shown in Fig. 3-10 are the FE moment patterns at the hip, knee, and ankle throughout the stance and swing phases of gait. The hip has the most reproducible characteristics of FE moments of the three major joints (11). At heel strike, the external moment tends to flex the hip joint, reaching a maximum value just before midstance. The pattern reverses direction after midstance to a moment tending to extend the joint. This

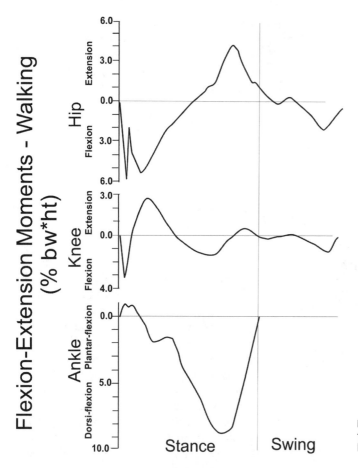

FIGURE 3-10. The patterns of flexion-extension moments at the hip, knee, and ankle.

sinusoidal pattern was found at all walking speeds and among both male and female subjects. The maximum magnitude of moments at the hip was greatest in the direction tending to flex the joint.

The most frequently occurring pattern of FE moment at the knee is biphasic, tending to produce extension at heel strike, flexion through midstance, extension in late stance, and flexion just prior to toe-off. Deviation from the biphasic pattern has been reported at slow walking speeds (11). At slow walking speeds, the external moment at the knee tends to extend the knee during the entire portion of middle stance phase. At faster walking speeds, there was less variability in the FE pattern. The patterns of the FE moment at the ankle was also reported to be reproducible for normal gait.

The external moment tends to dorsiflex the ankle throughout the entire portion of stance phase.

3.2 Adduction-abduction Moment Patterns During Walking

The patterns of AA moments at the hip, knee, and ankle are quite reproducible, with only one pattern present for all subjects at all walking speeds (Fig. 3-11). There is an abduction moment at the hip at heel strike, which reverses immediately to adduction throughout the entire period of stance phase. A similar pattern is observed at the knee. The pattern of the plantar-dorsiflexion moment at the ankle was more variable than the patterns at the hip or knee (11).

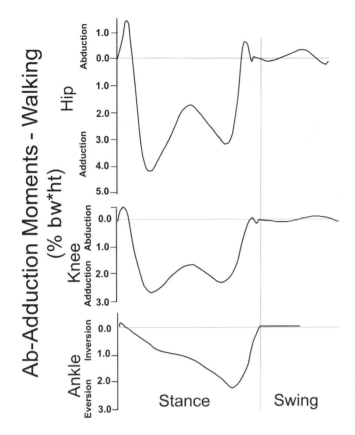

FIGURE 3-11. The patterns of abduction-adduction moment at the hip, knee, and ankle during level walking (11).

3.3 Amplitudes of Moment Patterns as a Function of Walking Speed

As previously illustrated, the magnitude of the moment pattern can be related to the magnitudes of the net muscle force and internal joint reaction forces. Using this relationship, the relative magnitudes of the moments during various activities can be used as an indicator of forces acting on the joint. For example, the magnitude of the FE moments has been shown to be dependent on walking speed. Because the internal forces are related to the joint moments, the internal forces acting on the joints can also be expected to vary with walking speed.

This speed dependency is present at the hip, knee, and ankle joint (Fig. 3-12). The flexion moment has the greatest dependency on speed, exhibiting a nearly threefold increase as

the walking speed approximately doubles. The only moment component that does not substantially change with walking speed in the sagittal plane is the moment tending to plantarflex the ankle. The other components of the moments, for AA and IE rotation, do not substantially change with walking speed.

To provide estimates of the actual moments that occur during walking, the normalized values of the moments (Fig. 3-10) can be converted to actual values. For example, the average product bw × ht for the male portion of the population represented in Figs. 3-10 through 3-12 is 1,370 Nm, whereas the average bw × ht for the female population is 990 Nm. Thus, if one were to take the magnitude of the hip flexion moment at a normal walking speed as 6%(bw × ht), this represents an average flexion moment magnitude at the hip of 82.2 Nm for a man of average size and 59.4 Nm for a woman of average size.

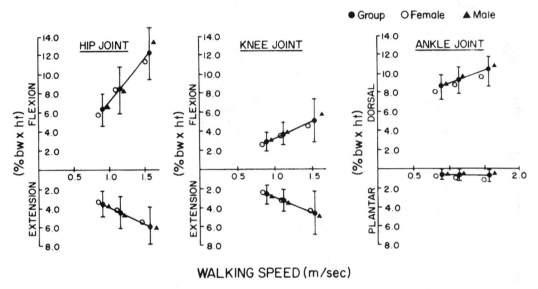

FIGURE 3-12. An illustration of the walking speed dependence of the flexion-extension moments at the hip, knee, and ankle (11).

It should be noted that the normalized data shown in Fig. 3-10 show no statistical difference between the moment magnitudes for the male and female population for the FE components (11). The only differences that appear in the moment magnitudes after normalization between the men and women are in the moments tending to adduct the hip and knee joints. The moment is approximately 8% greater at the knee and 4% greater at the hip for the female subjects. These differences are present during all walking speeds and seem to reflect differences in pelvic structure between men and women. The women with relatively larger pelvises probably have a relatively higher moment tending to adduct the hip and the knee. Clearly, normalization that accounts only for height differences does not account for other types of structural differences.

3.4 Moment Magnitudes During Level Walking

The largest moments in the joints of the lower extremities occur in directions tending to flex the hip and dorsiflex the ankle. These flexion moments at the hip and ankle are more than twice the magnitude of the flexion moment that occurs at the knee for a walking speed of 1.2 m/sec (Fig. 3-13). Assuming equal muscle lever arms at the hip, knee, and ankle, these differences suggest that the extensor musculature at the hip and the muscles involved in plantarflexion at the ankle sustain greater forces than the knee extensor musculature for normal walking. Again, it should be noted that the patterns described during level walking are measured external to the joint and use the fundamental principles of mechanical equilibrium to determine a lower boundary for the muscle forces.

The dorsiflexion moment at the ankle joint is sustained through nearly the entire portion of stance phase (Fig. 3-10). Thus, in addition to having the largest magnitude, it is sustained for the greatest duration. Hence, the endurance of the calf muscles is important because they sustain a large force for a relatively long time during the gait cycle. The knee in contrast to the ankle has a FE moment that oscillates about the zero axis and sustains relatively low maximum moments during walking. In addition the peak FE moments at the knee are sustained for only short periods during a normal gait cycle. It appears that the normal biphasic FE moment at the knee minimizes demands on the quadriceps and

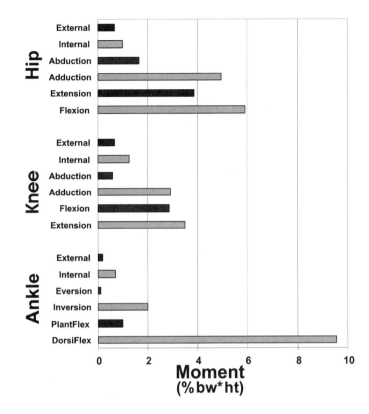

FIGURE 3-13. A comparison of the relative peak moment magnitudes at the hip, knee, and ankle during level walking.

knee flexors during walking. It will be shown in the following section that this efficient biphasic pattern at the knee changes when an abnormal gait is present.

The relative magnitudes of the FE, AA, and IE rotation moments are also illustrated in Fig. 3-13. As can be seen, with the exception of the ankle, the moment tending to adduct each joint is of comparable magnitude to the flexion or extension moments. At the knee, the magnitude of the adduction moment is comparable with the FE moments and probably represents one of the major factors influencing the loads at the knee joint. The adduction moment in Fig. 3-13 results primarily from the medial offset of the body's center of mass, and the medial and lateral acceleration and deceleration of the center of mass during walking. An adduction moment on the limb tends to force the ankle medially and, without internal resistance, would thrust the knee into increasing varus. Thus, it is this moment component that causes the medial compartment of the knee to bear a higher

load than the lateral compartment (46). Approximately 60% to 80% of the total compressive load transmitted across the knee is on the medial compartment.

3.5 Moments During Activities of Daily Living

The largest moments during most activities of daily living are in directions tending to flex the joints. This type of limb motion places demands on the extensor antigravity muscles. A comparison of the maximum flexion moments during walking, ascending stairs, descending stairs, rising from a seated position, and jogging indicates a substantial variation in the peak values at each of the joints (Fig. 3-14). At the hip and knee, walking produces the lowest flexion moment, whereas the lowest flexion moment at the ankle occurs when rising from a seated position. Using the magnitude of the moment during walking as a basis, comparison of the relative muscular efforts can be made. For example, the flexion

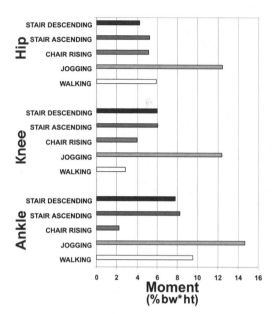

FIGURE 3-14. A comparison of the magnitude of the flexion moments during various activities of daily living.

moment at the hip during walking is approximately 6%(bw × ht). This magnitude increases to approximately 12%(bw × ht) during jogging. Thus, the range of joint loadings is relatively uniform during a variety of activities of daily living, with an approximately 30% increase in joint loads experienced during jogging over the base level for straight walking. The knee joint, with a relatively small flexion moment during level walking, sustains substantial increases during several activities including descending stairs and jogging. The large increases in the flexion moment at the knee joint for descending stairs and jogging are likely associated with the high incidence of patellofemoral problems in individuals involved in middle- and long-distance running as well as the difficulty in descending stairs for those with patellofemoral problems. It is likely that the relative increase (by approximately a factor of five) in flexion moment during jogging over the nominal level of walking values is more important on a comparative basis than the absolute magnitude. For example, the ankle dorsiflexion moment during jogging is higher than the flexion moment at the knee. However, the relative increase in the dorsiflexion moment sustained during jogging as compared with level

walking is only by a factor of two as compared with the fivefold increase seen in the knee flexion moment.

4 CLINICAL APPLICATIONS

The quantitative analysis of human locomotion can be a useful method for improving our understanding of various musculoskeletal diseases and injuries. In many cases, the functional changes associated with an injury or disease result from an adaptation to the condition rather than as a direct result of the mechanical change associated with the pathologic or anatomic change. For example, in patients with knee ligament injuries, such as an anterior cruciate ligament rupture, walking may not produce an abnormal anterior drawer on the tibia because the subject can stabilize the knee using muscular substitution. Thus, the gait adaptation would be associated with a compensatory mechanism that provides muscular stabilization. These types of dynamic adaptations appear during locomotion and, in most cases, represent the manifestation of the pathologic condition and thus require an interpretation of the adaptation. Pathologic stimuli such as pain, instability, or muscle weakness can cause dynamic adaptations. Often, a biomechanical analysis of the adaptation reflects the nature of the underlying pathology. Another example is the case of the Trendelenburg gait. The adaptation in this situation is the avoidance of stress in the abductor muscles of the hip by shifting the body weight over the center of the hip joint, thereby eliminating the need for the abductors to balance the moment because of the offset of bodyweight.

An understanding of the cause and effect of functional adaptations is extremely important for the development of methods for training, rehabilitation, and treatment of functionally impaired individuals (66). The purpose of this section is to illustrate some aspects of our current knowledge of biomechanical functional adaptations and to discuss the clinical implications of these adaptations.

Total knee replacements. An analysis of level walking in patients following total knee replacement provides an excellent example of the use of several types of parameters for the evaluation and analysis of function (74). There are a large number of parameters that can be measured during walking. These gait measures range from fundamental measures of time and distance to motion (kinematics) and forces (kinetics). The choice of which gait measurements to use depends on the intended application. These three general classes of gait measurements (time-distance, kinematics, and kinetics) can be applied to an evaluation of patients with total knee replacement. Time-distance measurements include measures of stride length, walking speed, and cadence. These are important measures of normal and abnormal walking (65). Stride length (distance between consecutive unilateral heel strikes) is one of the simplest and most sensitive indicators of walking abnormalities. It is important to note that stride length is dependent on walking speed (7,35); thus, in comparing measurements among normals and individuals with walking disabilities, it is important to account for differences in walking speed. For example, the relationship between stride length and walking speed for normal individuals is relatively linear and reproducible. It has also been shown that recovery of function from surgical reconstruc-

tions, such as total knee replacement, can be evaluated by comparing the overall stride length-walking speed relationship over a range of walking speeds. An improvement in walking ability is indicated by the stride length-walking speed relationship approaching normal between the 3- and 6-month postoperative gait evaluations (Fig. 3-15). The range of speeds selected by the patients are substantially less than normal, and without examining the relationship of stride length to speed, it would be extremely difficult to make comparisons between patients and normals or between the patients' observation at 3 and 6 months.

Time-distance parameters, although extremely efficient in evaluating quantitative changes in the overall characteristics of walking, do not provide specific information that can be related to the cause of the walking abnormality. For example, it has been shown (7) that the stride length-walking speed relationship does not fully return to normal following total knee replacement (Fig. 3-15). Patients continue to walk with shorter than normal stride lengths when differences in walking speed are taken into account. This observation suggests that patients with total knee replacement, in spite of a successful clinical result, do not completely recover

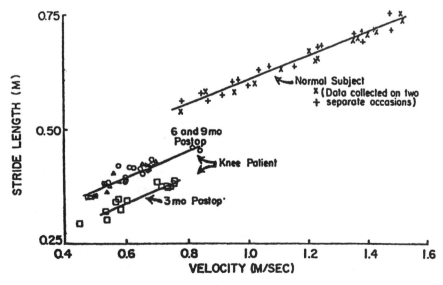

FIGURE 3-15. An illustration of the normal stride length-walking speed relationship in comparison to the measurements taken from a postoperative patient with total knee replacement (7).

normal function during level walking. The cause of these functional differences cannot, however, be obtained from simple stride length measurements.

Measurement of joint kinematics can be used to quantify specific joint involvements in walking disabilities (69). In particular, relative segmental angles are joint specific and have been used to quantify changes in patterns of motion related to specific joints. Consider again the example of the gait of patients with total knee replacements. In addition to the shorter than normal stride lengths, these patients have reduced knee flexion (9,69) during the midportion of stance phase (Fig. 3-16). The normal midstance knee flexion is approximately 20 degrees at an average speed, whereas patients, in spite of a pain-free clinical result, tend to walk with less than 10 degrees of midstance knee flexion. Thus, it appears that the adaptation to knee reconstruction is associated with a subtle inhibition in knee flexion. This type of kinematic analysis permits the localization of the adaptation to the knee joint and to the specific phase of the gait cycle, but at present it does not provide an explanation for the mechanism of this adaptation.

Joint moments during locomotion can also be used to identify the nature and cause of functional abnormalities in total knee replacement. As indicated previously, the magnitude and direction of the FE moment can be related to muscular function (50) and to joint loading. In patients with total knee replacements, it has been reported (7,52) that the moment at the knee joint is an important measure to identify functional changes.

A study of patients during stair climbing (6,8) following total knee arthroplasty illustrates the contribution of the posterior cruciate ligament (PCL) to normal knee function. Examination of the stair-climbing differences between the cruciate-substituting and cruciate-retaining designs indicates that the functional abnormality in patients with the cruciate-sacrificing designs is associated with a forward lean of the body (Fig. 3-17) in such a way that the moment tending to flex the knee during stair climbing is substantially reduced. This reduction in the moment tending to flex the knee reflects either a weakness or avoidance of the quadriceps during stair climbing. This change in function has been described as an adaptation to a knee in which the normal posterior movement of the femur on the tibia (rollback) with flexion is inhibited in designs where the PCL is removed (Fig. 3-17). This normal posterior movement of the tibiofemoral contact provides a larger lever arm for the quadriceps mechanism as the knee flexes. If this mechanism is lost through either constraint of the articulating surface or removal of the PCL, the normal rollback is inhibited. The normal interaction between tibiofemoral contact motion has also been demonstrated in cadaver studies (8,33). The passive kinematics of the knee influence the efficiency of active muscle function by changing the moment arm of various muscles as the knee is flexed.

Functional evaluation in high tibial osteotomy. Gait analysis has been used to evaluate patients with varus gonarthrosis prior to and following

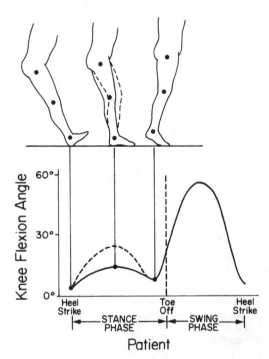

FIGURE 3-16. An illustration of the change in midstance knee flexion angle following total knee replacement.

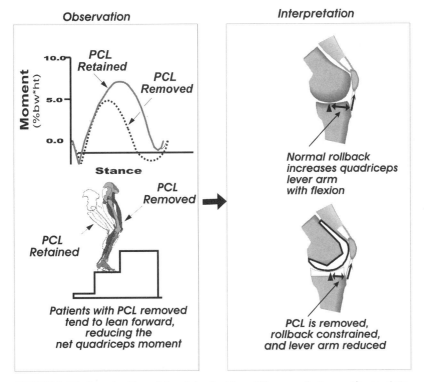

FIGURE 3-17. Examination of the stair-climbing differences between the cruciate-substituting and cruciate-retaining designs.

treatment with high tibial osteotomy. The fundamental premise of this procedure (51) has been that the varus deformity places an increased stress on the medial compartment of the knee and that this stress is, in part, responsible for the symptoms of the degenerative process as well as for accelerating the degeneration. The rationale for the treatment of medial compartment arthritis with high tibial osteotomy is, therefore, to reduce the stress on the medial compartment of the knee. The procedure is particularly suitable for the younger patient because it is more conservative than other treatment modalities such as total joint arthroplasty. The results, however, have been somewhat variable and unpredictable (42). It has been assumed that the amount of stress on the medial compartment is proportional to the degree of varus deformity measured by standing x-rays (51). However, the dynamic loads that occur during walking may play a more important role than do the static loads resulting from varus malalignment (67).

This observation is based on a study of patients tested in the gait laboratory before a high tibial osteotomy and at yearly intervals following treatment (67,80). The investigation focused on the dynamic peak adduction moment at the knee, with the analysis based on the relationship described earlier relating the adduction moment to the stress on the medial side of the knee. One might predict that patients with a large varus deformity would have a higher than normal adduction moment. However, a preoperative gait analysis indicated that only about one-half of the patients had a higher than normal adduction moment ("high adduction moment" group) in spite of the varus deformity at the knee joint.

The clinical outcome of the treatment of patients with varus gonarthrosis with high tibial osteotomy has been related to the magnitude of the adduction moment measured in the gait laboratory before surgery (67,80). Patients were grouped on the basis of the magnitude of their preoperative adduction moment; they were considered to have "high" adduction moments if the adduction moment exceeded 4%(bw × ht). All other patients were classified as having a "low" adduction moment. Approximately one-half of the patients in the original study group had an adduction moment lower than 4%(bw × ht). Thus, it was possible for approximately one-half of the patients to adapt their gait dynamically to reduce the loading across the knee joint.

Following surgery, the adduction moment was reduced in both groups. However, the average postoperative adduction moment in the "low" adduction moment group was still significantly lower than the average adduction moment in the "high" adduction moment group (Fig. 3-18). The two groups were indistinguishable based on preoperative knee score, initial varus deformity, immediate postoperative correction, age, and weight. In a follow-up of between 3 and 8.9 years after surgery, the patients in the "low" adduction moment group had significantly better clinical outcome (Fig. 3-18). The passage of time caused a decline in the clinical results in both the "high" and "low" adduction moment groups. However, the patients who had a low preoperative adduction moment maintained a better clinical result than did patients in the "high" adduction moment group at an average of 6 years. Further, 79% of the knees in the "low" adduction moment group had maintained valgus correction, whereas only 20% of the knees in the "high" adduction moment group remained in valgus alignment.

The adaptive mechanism used by some patients to reduce the adduction moment has been related to a shorter stride length and an increased external rotation (toe-out) of the foot during stance phase. The adaptation using the toe-out mechanism altered the adduction moment during gait. The mechanics of this technique simply involved moving the ground reaction vector closer to the center of the knee joint and, thus, reducing the lever arm of the external ground reaction force.

It is possible for patients to reduce the dynamic loading on the medial compartment of the knee. Preoperative gait analysis provides a means of detecting which patients develop these adaptive mechanisms. Gait analysis can be used as an additional means of selecting patients who have a higher probability of a good result with a high tibial osteotomy. It also provides a basis for training patients to lower the loads at the knee joint and slow the progression of degenerative changes or increase the probability of a better result with a high tibial osteotomy.

It is well accepted that mechanical loading influences the mass and architecture of bone. Previous studies have shown that bone mineral density or content is correlated with the peak external moments during gait (1,40,79). In particular, the knee adduction moment has been correlated with the distribution of bone between

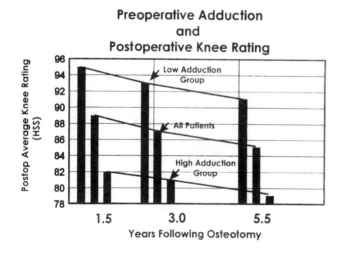

FIGURE 3-18. Postoperative knee adduction moments and postoperative knee rating.

the medial and lateral sides of the knee joint in both young normal subjects and subjects with knee osteoarthritis (40,79). These studies provide additional evidence that the external moments are good measures of the internal joint loads.

Function following anterior cruciate ligament injury. An analysis of the patterns of locomotion (16,78) in patients following rupture of the anterior cruciate ligament (ACL) provides an example of the importance of applying biomechanical principles when interpreting functional measurements. The ACL is one of the four major ligaments of the knee. It provides primary restraint to anterior displacement of the tibia as well as rotational stability. Rupture of the ACL of the knee is a common sports injury. Clinical studies have shown that more than two-thirds of patients with chronic ACL deficiency discontinue athletic activity or reduce their participation in more vigorous activities (37,58,59). The development of cartilage degradation in chronic ACL deficiency has also been reported even in some patients that reduce activity levels (30). The observation (58) that some patients develop degenerative changes while others do not develop symptoms suggest that some patients can adapt their patterns of locomotion to accommodate for the loss of the ACL.

A study of the changes in patterns of locomotion with respect to the time past the index injury (81) has demonstrated that patients with ACL deficiency adapt their patterns of locomotion over time. Patients that had an ACL-deficient knee for greater than 7.5 years demonstrated a change in the net moments sustained by the knee flexors and extensors relative to patients that were less than 2.5 years past index injury as well as relative to normal subjects. The pattern of the FE moment during stance phase was interpreted in terms of the net quadriceps muscle force or net knee flexor muscle force (hamstrings and/or gastrocnemius) during stance phase. Typically among the normal subjects, at heel strike, there was an external moment tending to extend the knee joint (demanding net knee flexor force) as the knee moved into midstance, the external moment reversed its direction (demanding net quadriceps

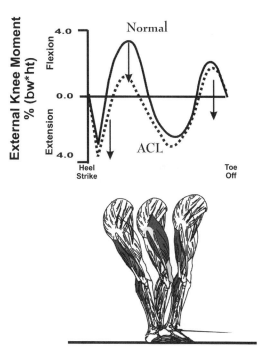

FIGURE 3-19. Knee flexion-extension moment pattern for the patients with ACL-deficient knees.

force), as the knee passed midstance the moment again reversed its direction (demanding net knee flexor muscle force), and finally, in the preswing phase, the moment tended to flex the knee (demanding net quadriceps muscle force) (Fig. 3-19). In contrast, the subjects with ACL deficiencies over 7.5 years had a different moment pattern.

An analysis of the biomechanics of knee anatomy assists in interpreting the adaptive changes in locomotion following ACL injury. The shift in the moment pattern showing a reduced external flexion moment and increased extension moment could indicate a reduction/avoidance of the force generated by the quadriceps muscles or an increase in the force generated by the knee flexors muscles. The potential for antagonistic muscle activity prohibits the exact prediction of muscle force solely on the basis of the moment magnitude. However, the biomechanics of the knee supports the interpretation that the reduction of the external flexion moment during walking is consistent with a reduction in quadriceps activity rather than an increase in hamstring activity. From an anatomic viewpoint the hamstrings do not serve as effective synergists to the ACL when the knee is near full extension (the situation during walking). Their ability to compensate for the loss of the ACL during the loading response and early midstance phases of gait would be limited. However, quadriceps contraction during these phases of the gait cycle would induce an anterior drawer, causing the quadriceps to act as an antagonist to the ACL (14,18,19). A decrease in quadriceps activity would appear to be a more effective mechanism for reducing anterior drawer during this portion of the gait cycle. Strength deficits of the quadriceps muscle reported among patients with ACL deficiency (19,53,78) is also consistent with a reduction in quadriceps activity during walking rather than with an increase in hamstring activity.

The time-dependent changes in the patterns of locomotion in patients following ACL rupture suggest that these adaptations are the result of repetitive experiences following the loss of the ACL. It is possible that reprogramming (5) of the locomotor process occurs such that the adaptations occur before instability and excessive anterior displacement results. This can be accomplished by altering the pattern of muscle contracture as part of an adaptive locomotor program. Thus, the adaptations anticipate the instability and avoid the abnormal displacement. This general locomotor reprogramming could be part of a learning process that takes place during the early stages following an ACL injury. It would be necessary for the locomotor system to be reprogrammed in a manner such that it anticipates instability prior to the occurrence of the episode producing the instability because the latency time for muscle contraction would be too slow to instantaneously respond to such a rapid stimulus.

This example illustrates a process that can be used to interpret functional measurements. There are numerous potential causes for a particular change in the patterns of locomotion. The adaptive change can have a positive or negative influence on long-term clinical outcome. Thus, the integration of functional measurements with appropriate biomechanical analysis

and clinical experience can provide a useful approach to the clinical interpretation of functional measurements.

Running injuries and joint moment magnitudes. An analysis of the joint loading during jogging can be used to evaluate some of the mechanisms of the overuse injury occurring in middle- and long-distance runners (10,25). Overuse injury results from cyclic loading of the joint with sufficient magnitude to produce injuries when applied over a large number of cycles. This overuse pattern differs from a traumatic injury in which the load is substantially higher and is of sufficient magnitude to cause injury during a single occurrence.

The knee—in particular, the patellofemoral joint—is a frequent site of overuse injury patterns in middle- and long-distance runners (43). Other frequent sites of overuse injury in runners are the iliotibial band, Achilles tendon, and metatarsal heads (10). Shown in Fig. 3-20

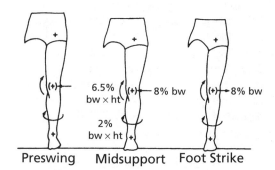

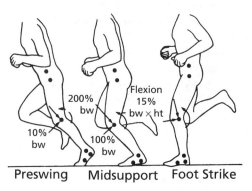

FIGURE 3-20. An illustration of the limb configuration during running.

are three portions of the running cycle including the foot strike, midsupport, and preswing configurations of the limbs and torso. At foot strike, the hip and knee are slightly flexed, and the foot contacts the ground dorsiflexed. During running, the body has a more vertical posture at heel strike with slightly more hip and knee flexion than during level walking. Landing in this flexed position provides a potential for absorbing the higher impact that occurs during running. An analysis of the intrinsic loading at the knee at foot strike indicates compressive and posteriorly directed force components and a moment that tends to flex the joint. As the body moves forward to the midsupport phase, the axial force reaches a maximum of two times body weight, the posterior shear reaches body weight, and the moment tending to flex the knee approaches 12%(bw × ht). Again, it should be noted that this maximum knee flexion moment is greater than five times the moment that normally occurs during level walking. As the limb moves to the preswing position, the hip and knee joints extend and the ankle plantar flexes.

Also shown in Fig. 3-20 is the configuration of the limb in the frontal plane during the three phases of the support phase of running. At foot strike, there is a medially directed shear of 8% body weight as well as a moment tending to abduct the knee and internally rotate the joint. At midsupport, the shear reverses direction to a maximum of 8% body weight directed laterally, the internal rotation reaches a maximum of 2%(bw × ht), and the moment tending to adduct the knee reaches a maximum of 6.5% (bw × ht). As the body moves toward preswing, internal rotation, AA, and the medially directed force continue in the same direction but reduce in magnitude before the foot leaves the ground.

A comparison of the maximum loads at the knee that occur during running (3 m/sec) and walking (1.2 m/sec) indicates that the moment tending to flex the knee increases the most. This increase in flexion moment can be related to an increase in quadriceps force, patellofemoral contact force, and joint compressive force. Therefore, there appears to be a correspondence between the frequency of running injuries to the knee joint and the increase in magnitude of the flexion moment during level walking. Similarly, the large adduction moment at the hip increases the iliotibial band stress, and the dorsiflexion moment at the ankle stresses the Achilles tendon. Clearly, structures that are more highly stressed during running are operating in a range where any perturbation (such as change in distance, speed, or shoe style) may be sufficient to alter the delicate balance between healing and repair mechanisms associated with the overuse injury. Thus, it is important to first describe, and then evaluate, any adaptations to these perturbations, because they may cause increased loading to already high loads.

It is hoped that the examples above provide a broad although by no means inclusive overview of the types of clinical orthopedic problems where the application of biomechanical principles, as briefly described in this chapter, may aid in the understanding of the body's response to such abnormal or disease states.

5 PROBLEMS

1. A person at the gym is going to strengthen his or her quadriceps muscles by doing a series of leg extension exercises.

   Case 1: Assume that the femur is at a right angle to the tibia and that the weight exerts an external force, F, which acts perpendicular to the tibia through the ankle joint at a distance, d_1, to the center of the tibial plateau. Calculate the external moment generated at the knee in response to the force, F, at the ankle and the mass of the shank, m. The distance from the ankle to the center of the knee joint is $d_1 = 0.4$ m, the weight lifted is $F = 400$ N, and the mass of the shank is $m = 2.89$ kg.

   Case 2: Assume that the leg is fully extended. Use the same values given for Case 1. The distance from the mass center to the tibial plateau is $d_2 = 0.1$ m.

2. Using the result for the external reaction moment at the knee obtained from Problem 1, calculate the internal force in the quadriceps muscle necessary to balance the external

reaction moment when the knee joint is flexed at 90° and when it is at full extension. Assume that the quadriceps is the only muscle acting and that the distance from the quadriceps muscle force to the tibiofemoral contact point is $d = 0.02$ m. Calculate the force in the quadriceps muscle if the distance from the quadriceps force, F_q^v, to the tibiofemoral contact point, 0, is $d = 0.04$ m. Refer to Fig. 3-7 in the text.

3. Consider the left leg of a person walking in the gait laboratory with a cluster of points located on the thigh and shank (13). The cluster coordinates used to locate the orientation and location of coordinate systems embedded in the femoral and tibial bones with respect to a global coordinate system centered on the force plate are represented by the 4 × 4 homogeneous transformation matrices of $[T]_{f,G}$ and $[T]_{t,G}$ respectively, where

$$[T]_{f,G} =$$
$$\begin{bmatrix} 0.257006 & -0.442300 & 0.859256 & 5.35 \\ 0.385660 & -0.768320 & -0.510840 & 22.04 \\ 0.886123 & 0.462670 & -0.026890 & 72.76 \\ 0 & 0 & 0 & 1 \end{bmatrix}$$

and

$$[T]_{t,G} =$$
$$\begin{bmatrix} 0.116158 & 0.650180 & -0.750850 & -1.46 \\ -0.078970 & 0.759618 & 0.645557 & 16.04 \\ 0.990087 & -0.015700 & 0.139578 & 32.21 \\ 0 & 0 & 0 & 1 \end{bmatrix}$$

with the origin locations given in units of cm. Utilizing the forward transformation technique presented in this chapter, determine the three rotation angles and displacements for the total joint replacement femoral component moving with respect to a fixed tibial component coordinate system. The total joint femoral and tibial components are oriented and located relative to the respective bone coordinate systems with the following rigid-body fixed 4×4 homogeneous transformations of:

$$[T]_{fc,f} =$$
$$\begin{bmatrix} 0.049061 & 0.998508 & -0.023926 & -26.37 \\ -0.570085 & 0.04766 & 0.820200 & -2.08 \\ 0.820115 & -0.026609 & 0.571573 & -4.34 \\ 0 & 0 & 0 & 1 \end{bmatrix}$$

and

$$[T]_{tc,t} =$$
$$\begin{bmatrix} -0.095664 & 0.973703 & 0.205821 & 13.98 \\ 0.678769 & 0.215064 & -0.702154 & -2.57 \\ -0.728095 & -0.072534 & -0.681628 & -3.88 \\ 0 & 0 & 0 & 1 \end{bmatrix}$$

where $[T]_{fc,f}$ locates the femoral component to the femoral bone and $[T]_{tc,t}$ locates the tibial component to the tibia bone. Assume that the rotations are performed in the following order about their respective axes: (a) $\phi(x)$, (b) $\alpha(y)$, and (c) $\theta(z)$ in order to calculate the femoral projection angles and translations along the tibial component axes where FE rotation occurs about the x axis (positive lateral), IE rotation occurs about the y axis (positive superior), and AA rotation occurs about the z axis (positive anterior).

REFERENCES

1. Advisory Committee on Artificial Limbs, National Research Council. *The pattern of muscular activity in the lower extremity during walking*. Prosthetic Devices Research Project, Institute of Engineering Research. Berkeley: University of California, Series II, Issue 25,1953.
2. Abbot BC, Wilkie DR. The relation between velocity of shortening and the tension length curve of skeletal muscle. *J Physiol* 1953;120:214–223.
3. Alexander EJ, Andriacchi TP. Correcting for deformation in skin based marker systems. *J Biomech* 2001;34(3):355–362.
4. Anderson FC, Pandy MG. Static and dynamic optimization solutions for gait are practically equivalent. *J Biomech* 2001;34:153–61.
5. Andriacchi TP. Dynamics of pathological motion: applied to the anterior cruciate deficient knee. *J Biomech* 1990;23[Suppl]:99–105.
6. Andriacchi TP, Galante JO. Retention of the posterior cruciate ligament in total knee arthroplasty. *J Arthroplasty* 1988;3:513–519.
7. Andriacchi TP, Ogle JA, Galante JO. Walking speed as a basis for normal and abnormal gait measurements. *J Biomech* 1977;10:261–268.
8. Andriacchi TP, Galante JO, Draganich, LE. Relationship between knee extensor mechanics and function following total knee replacement. In: Dorr L, ed. *Proceedings 1st annual meeting of the Knee*

Society. Baltimore: University Park Press, 1985:83–94.

9. Andriacchi TP, Galante JO, Fermier RW. The influence of total knee replacement design on walking and stairclimbing. *J Bone Joint Surg* 1982;64A:1328–1335.

10. Andriacchi TP, Kramer GM, Landon GC. The biomechanics of running and knee injuries. In: Finerman G, ed. *American Academy of Orthopaedic Surgeons, symposium on sport medicine, the knee.* St. Louis: Mosby, 1985:23–32.

11. Andriacchi TP, Strickland AB. Lower limb kinetics applied to the study of normal and abnormal walking. In: Berme N, Engin AE, Correia Da Silva KM, eds. *KM Biomechanics of normal and pathological human articulating joints, NATO ASI series, series E: No. 93.* Dordrecht: Martinus Nijhoff 1985;83–102.

12. Andriacchi TP, Hurwitz DE. Gait biomechanics and the evolution of total joint replacement. *Gait Posture* 1997;5:256–264.

13. Andriacchi TP, Alexander EJ, Toney MK, et al. A point cluster method for *in vivo* motion analysis: applied to a study of knee kinematics. *J Biomech Eng* 1998;120(12):743–749.

14. Arms SW, Pope MH, Johnson RJ, et al. The biomechanics of anterior cruciate ligament rehabilitation and reconstruction. *Am J Sports Med* 1984;12:8–18.

15. Banks SA, Hodge WA. Accurate measurement of three-dimensional knee replacement kinematics using single-plane fluoroscopy. *IEEE Trans Biomed Eng* 1996;43(6):638–649.

16. Berchuck M, Andriacchi TP, Bach BR Jr, et al. Gait adaptations by patients who have a deficient ACL. *J Bone Joint Surg* 1990;72A:871–877.

17. Bergmann G, Deuretzbacher G, Heller M, et al. Hip contact forces and gait patterns from routine activities. *J Biomech* 2001;34:859–71.

18. Beynnon BD, Howe JG, Pope MH, et al. The measurement of anterior cruciate ligament strain in vivo. *Int Orthop* 1992;16(1):1–12.

19. Beynnon BD, Johnson RJ, Fleming BC, et al. The effect of functional knee bracing on the anterior cruciate ligament in the weight bearing and non-weight bearing knee. *Am J Sports Med* 1997;25:353–359.

20. Branch TP, Hunter R, Donath M. Dynamic EMG analysis of anterior cruciate deficient legs with and without bracing during cutting. *Am J Sports Med* 1989;17:35–41.

21. Blankevoort L, Huiskes R, de Lange A. The envelope of passive knee joint motion. *J Biomech* 1988;21(9):705–720.

22. Bresler B, Frankel JP. The forces and moments in the leg during level walking. *Trans Am Soc Mech Eng* 1953;48A:62.

23. Cappello A, Cappozzo A, La Palombara PF, et al.

Multiple anatomical landmark calibration for optimal bone pose estimation. *Hum Mov Sci* 1997;16(2–3):259–274.

24. Cappozzo A, Figura E, Marchetti M. The interplay of muscular and external forces in human angulation. *J Biomech* 1976;9:35–43.

25. Cavanaugh PR, Pollock ML, Landa J. A biomechanical comparison of elite and good distance runners. *Ann N Y Acad Sci* 1977;301:328–345.

26. Chao EYS. Justification of triaxial goniometer for the measurement of joint rotation. *J Biomech* 1980;13:989–1006.

27. Chao EY, Laughman RK, Stauffer RN. Biomechanical gait evaluation of pre- and postoperative total knee replacement patients. *Arch Orthop Trauma Surg* 1980;97:309–317.

28. Crowninshield RD. Use of optimization techniques to predict muscle forces. *J Biomech Eng* 1978;100:88–92.

29. Crowninshield RD, Brand RA. A physiologically based criteria of muscle force prediction in locomotion. *J Biomech* 1981;14:793–801.

30. Daniel DM, Stone ML, Dobson BE, et al. Fate of the ACL-injured patient: a prospective outcome study. *Am J Sports Med* 1994;22:632–644.

31. Delp SL, Loan JP, Hoy MG, et al. An interactive graphics-based model of the lower extremity to study orthopaedic surgical procedures. *IEEE Trans Biomed Eng* 1990;37:757–767.

32. Dillman CJ. Kinematic analyses of running. In: Wilmore JH, ed. *Exercise and sport sciences review,* Vol. 3. New York: Academic Press, 1975:193–218.

33. Dragnich LF, Andriacchi TP, Anderssoln GBJ. Interaction between intrinsic knee mechanics and the knee extensor mechanism. *J Orthop Res* 1987;5:539–547.

34. Goldstein H. *Classical mechanics,* 1st ed. Reading, MA: Addison Wesley, 1950.

35. Grieve DW. Gait patterns and the speed of walking. *J Biomed Eng* 1968;3:119–122.

36. Grood ES, Sontay WJ. A joint coordinate system for the clinical description of three-dimensional motions: application to the knee. *J Biomech Eng* 1983;105:136–144.

37. Hawkins RJ, Misamore GW, Mewitt TR. Followup of the acute nonoperated isolated anterior cruciate ligament tear. *Am J Sports Med* 1986;14:205–210.

38. Hill AV. The mechanics of active muscle. *Proc R Soc Lond B Biol Sci* 1953;38:57–76.

39. Hurwitz DE, Foucher KC, Sumner DR, et al. Hip motion and moment during gait relate directly to proximal femoral bone mineral density in patients with hip osteoarthritis. *J Biomech* 1998;31(10):919–926.

40. Hurwitz DE, Sumner DR, Andriacchi TP, et al. Dynamic knee loads during gait predict proximal tibial bone distribution. *J Biomech* 1998;31:423–430.

41. Hurwitz DE, Foucher KC, Andriacchi TP. A new parametric approach for modeling hip forces during gait: a technical note. *J Biomech (submitted 2001)*.

42. Insall, JN, Joseph DM, Msika C. High tibial osteotomy for varus gonarthrosis. *J Bone Joint Surg* 1984;66A(7):1040–1048.

43. James SL, Bates BT, Osternig LR. Injuries to runners. *Am J Sports Med* 1978;6(2):40–50.

44. Johnson E, Scarrow P, Waugh W. Assessment of loads in the knee joint. *Med Biol Eng Comput* 1991;19:237–243.

45. Jonsson H, Karrholm J. 3-Dimensional knee-joint movements during a step-up: valuation after anterior cruciate ligament rupture. *J Orthop Res* 1994;12(6):769–779.

46. Kettelkamp DB, Johnson RJ, Smidt GL, et al. An electrogoniometric study of knee motion in normal gait. *J Bone Joint Surg* 1970;52A(4):775–790.

47. Kinzel GL, Hall AS, Hillberry BM. Measurement of the total motion between two body segments 1: analytical development. *J Biomech* 1972;5:93–105.

48. Lafortune MA, Cavanagh PR, Sommer HJ, et al. Three-dimensional kinematics of the human knee during walking. *J Biomech* 1992;25:347–357.

49. Lamoreux L. Kinematic measurements in the study of human walking. *Bull Prosthet Res* 1971;10–15:3–84.

50. Lindahl O, Movin A. The mechanics of extension of the knee joint. *Acta Orthop Scand* 1967;38:226–234.

51. Maquet P. The biomechanics of the knee and surgical possibilities of healing osteoarthritic knee joints. *Clin Orthop* 1980;146:102–110.

52. Mathews LS, Sonstegard DA, Henke JA. Load bearing characteristics of the patellofemoral joint. *Acta Orthop Scand* 1977;48:511–516.

53. McHugh MP, Spitz AL, Lorei MP, et al. Effect of anterior cruciate ligament deficiency on economy of walking and jogging. *J Orthop Res* 1994;12:592–597.

54. McKerrow PJ. *Introduction to robotics,* 1st ed. Reading, MA: Addison Wesley, 1991.

55. Mikosz RP, Andriacchi TP, Andersson GBJ. Model analyses of factors influencing the prediction of muscle forces at the knee. *J Orthop Res* 1987;6:205–214.

56. Morrison JB. Bioengineering analysis of force actions transmitted by the knee joint. *Biomed Eng* 1968;3:164–170.

57. Morrison JB. The mechanics of the knee joint in relation to normal walking. *J Biomech* 1970;3:51–61.

58. Noyes FR, Bassett RW, Grood ES, et al. Arthroscopy in acute traumatic hemarthrosis of the knee: incidence of anterior cruciate tears and other injuries. *J Bone Joint Surg Am* 1980;62:687–695.

59. Noyes FR, Matthews DS, Mooar PA, et al. The symptomatic anterior cruciate deficient knee. Part II: the results of rehabilitation, activity modification, and counseling on functional disability. *J Bone Joint Surg* 1983;65A:163–174.

60. Pandy MG, Anderson FC. Dynamic simulation of human movement using large-scale models of the body. *Phonetica* 2000;57(2–4):219–228.

61. Patriarco AG, Mann RW, Simon SR, et al. An evaluation of the approaches of optimization models in the prediction of muscle forces during human gait. *J Biomech* 1981;14:513–525.

62. Paul JP, McGrouther DA. Forces transmitted at the hip and knee joint of normal and disabled persons during a range of activities. *Acta Orthop Belg* 1975;41[Suppl]:78–88.

63. Pedotti A, Krishner VV, Stark L. Optimization of muscle-force sequencing in human locomotion. *Math Biosci* 1978;38:57–76.

64. Pennock GR, Clark KJ. An anatomy-based co-ordinate system for the description of the kinematic displacements in the human knee. *J Biomech* 1990;23(12):1209–1218.

65. Perry J. Clinical gait analyzer. *Bull Prosthet Res* 1974;10–22:188–192.

66. Perry J, Hoffer MM, Giovan P, et al. Gait analysis of the triceps surae in cerebral palsy: a preoperative and postoperative clinical and electromyographic study. *J Bone Joint Surg* 1974;56A(3):511–520.

67. Prodromos CC, Andriacchi TE, Galante JO. A relationship between gait and clinical changes following high tibial osteotomy. *J Bone Joint Surg* 1985;67A(8):1188–1194.

68. Reinschmidt C, van den Bogert AJ, Nigg BM, et al. Effect of skin movement on the analysis of skeletal knee joint motion during running. *J Biomech* 1997;30:729–732.

69. Rittman N, Kettlekamp DB, Pryor P, et al. Analysis of patterns of knee motion walking for four types of total knee implants. *Clin Orthop* 1981;155:111–117.

70. Rohrle H, Scholten R, Sigolotto C, et al. Joint forces in the human pelvis-leg skeleton during walking. *J Biomech* 1984;17:409–424.

71. Schipplein OD, Andriacchi TP. Interaction between active and passive knee stabilizers during level walking. *J Orthop Res* 1991;9:113–119.

72. Seireg A, Arvikar RJ. A mathematical model for evaluating forces in lower extremities of the musculo-skeletal system. *J Biomech* 1973;6:313–326.

73. Seireg A, Arvikar RJ. The prediction of muscular load sharing and joint forces in the lower extremities during walking. *J Biomech* 1975;3:51–61.

74. Selvik G. *A roentgen stereophotogrammetic method for the study of the kinematics of the skeletal*

system (dissertation), University of Lund, Sweden, 1974.

75. Simon SR, Trieshmann HW, Burdett RG, et al. Quantitative gait analysis after total knee arthroplasty for monarticular degenerative arthritis. *J Bone Joint Surg* 1983;65A(5):605–613.

76. Simonsen B, Dyhre-Poulsen, Voight, et al. Bone on bone forces during loaded and unloaded walking. *Acta Anat (Basel)* 1995;152:133–142.

77. Stiehl JB, Dennis DA, Komistek RD, et al. *In vivo* kinematic analysis of a mobile bearing total knee prosthesis. *Clin Orthop* 1997;345:60–66.

78. Tibone JE, Antich TJ, Fanton GS, et al. Functional analysis of anterior cruciate ligament instability. *Am J Sports Med* 1986;14(4):276–284.

79. Wada M, Maezawa Y, Baba H, et al. Relationships among bone mineral densities, static alignment and dynamic load in patients with medical compartment knee osteoarthritis. *Rheumatology* 2001;40:499–505.

80. Wang JW, Kuo, KN, Andriacchi TP, et al. The influence of walking mechanics and time on the results of proximal tibial osteotomy. *J Bone Joint Surg* 1990;72A:905–909.

81. Wexler G, Hurwitz DE, Bush-Joseph CA, et al. Functional gait adaptations in patients with ACL deficiency over time. *Clin Orthop* 1998;348:166–75.

82. Wu G, Cavanagh PR. ISB recommendation for standardization in the reporting of kinematic data. *J Biomech* 1995;28(10):1257–1260.

83. You BM, Siy P, Anderst W, et al. In vivo measurement of 3-D skeletal kinematics from sequences of biplane radiographs: application to knee kinematics. *IEEE Trans Med Imag* 2001;20(6):514–525.

BIOMECHANICS OF BONE

RIK HUISKES
BERT VAN RIETBERGEN[*]

1 INTRODUCTION

1.1 Scope of This Chapter

Orthopaedic surgeons are frequently nicknamed "bone doctors." Although they are often engaged in surgical procedures treating cartilage, ligament, tendon, and muscle affections as well, bone is seen as their central concern, in patient care and research. Hence, the title of this chapter is by nature overly ambitious; the material treated must be limited. Examples of bone affections and diseases are congenital deformities (e.g., scoliosis) and osteopetrosis (a bone disease creating overly dense, but brittle bones) in children, fractures due to trauma in all ages, and osteoporosis in the elderly. Osteoarthrosis and arthritis, requiring artificial joint replacement, is a main issue in orthopaedics.

To fulfill their protective and locomotory functions, bones must be stiff and strong. Both are properties determined by their architectures (shape, dimensions), on the one hand, and the mechanical quality of the bone material itself on the other. These properties are not static during life. Bone mass and structure change considerably in growth, remain more-or-less constant in adulthood, and deteriorate in the elder. When structural deterioration in the elderly is particularly pronounced we call it "osteoporotic." Osteoporosis is a severe condition in older ages, leading to a significant increase in bone fracture risk. It also affects the effectiveness of orthopaedic restorative procedures, such as articular joint replacement. One—biomechanical—emphasis of this chapter is the question whether and how we can estimate bone strength and stiffness more precisely.

The second main emphasis is a mechanobiological one: Can we do something about osteoporosis? This question may seem misplaced here, as orthopaedic surgeons do not normally treat osteoporosis; this is a subject for internal medicine (endocrinology). However, the history of orthopaedic research is deplete with

---

[*] With contributions from Marjolein van der Meulen, Ronald Ruimerman, and Esther Tanck

indications that bone mass and structure are affected—indeed depend on—mechanical loading. Bone is an adaptive structure in which cells sense mechanical loads and adapt bone mass and structure accordingly. The questions are how this—literally mechanobiological—tprocess works, and whether we can use it to prevent and cure osteoporosis. In other words how, precisely, do loads on bone produce increased bone mass and strength? Conversely, how does lack of loads reduce it?

These two questions relative to mechanical bone quality and load-induced bone metabolism, one diagnostic and one therapeutic, are emphases of this chapter. The literature on these issues is reviewed. There is an emphasis on scientific methodology in biomechanics and mechanobiology, relative to experimental, but particularly computational tools. However, they should be seen as scientific flagpoles at the end of the course. Along the way the purpose of the text is to teach the basics and inform the student about what is known and what is done, and what not.

1.2 Composition of Bone

Bone tissue consists of cells embedded in a fibrous organic matrix (in this case, osteoid), which is primarily collagen (90%) and 10% amorphous ground substance (primarily glycosaminoglycans and glycoproteins). Osteoid comprises approximately 50% of bone by volume and 25% by weight. The characteristic rigidity and strength of bone derive from the presence of mineral salts that permeate the organic matrix. The mineral phase comprises approximately 50% of bone by volume and 75% by weight. The principal constituents of bone mineral are calcium phosphate and calcium carbonate, with lesser quantities of sodium, magnesium, and fluoride. The mineral components consist mainly of hydroxyapatite $[Ca_{10}(PO_4)_6(OH)_2]$ crystals and amorphous calcium phosphate. Bone apatite crystals are approximately 50 to 100 angstroms (Å) long and are arranged in an orderly pattern within the collagen network. Bone collagen is the same type I collagen as found in dermis, tendon, and fascia.

Because of the presence of stable intermolecular cross links, bone collagen is extremely insoluble in the solvents commonly used to extract collagen from connective tissues.

The cells of bone include osteoblasts (bone-forming cells), osteoclasts (bone-resorbing cells), osteocytes (bone-maintaining cells), and bone-lining cells. Osteoblasts and osteoclasts are cells that reach the bone for metabolic purposes only. Osteocytes and lining cells reside permanently in (respectively on) the bone, interconnected by a system of canaliculi. Osteocytes represent osteoblasts trapped by secretion of the extracellular matrix. During bone formation, uncalcified osteoid is secreted by osteoblasts. Hydroxyapatite crystals then precipitate in an orderly fashion around collagen fibers present in the osteoid. Although the osteoid rapidly becomes about 70% calcified within a few days, maximal calcification occurs only after several months.

Whole bones are composed of two types of bony tissue (Fig. 4-1). Cortical bone comprises the diaphysis of long bones and the thin shells that surround the metaphyses. Trabecular bone in the metaphyses and epiphyses is continuous with the inner surface of the metaphyseal shell and exists as a three-dimensional, interconnected network of trabecular rods and plates. The trabeculae divide the interior into intercommunicating pores of varying dimensions, thereby resulting in a structure of variable porosity and density (Fig. 4-2). A network of rods produces low-density, open cells, while a network of plates can result in higher density, nearly closed cells (77). The classification of bone tissue as cortical or trabecular is based on relative density; i.e., the ratio of specimen density to that of fully dense cortical bone (usually assumed to have a density of 1.8 g/cc). The relative density of trabecular bone varies from 0.7 to about 0.05, corresponding to porosities that range from about 30% to more than 90%. The relative density of cortical bone ranges from about 0.7 to about 0.95. Obviously, the distinction between low-density cortical bone and high-density trabecular bone is somewhat arbitrary.

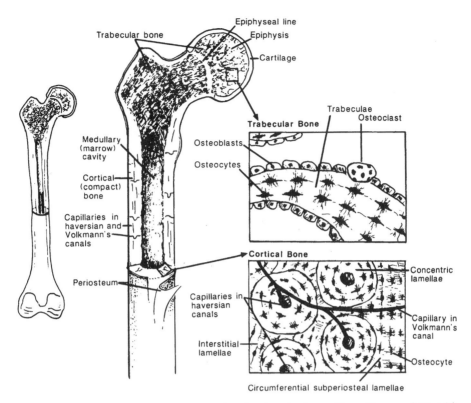

FIGURE 4-1. Schematic diagram of cortical and trabecular bone. (From Hayes, ref. 95, with permission.)

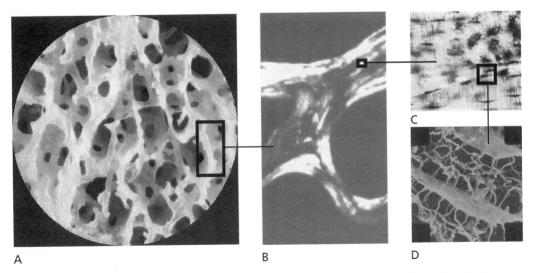

A   B   D

FIGURE 4-2. Morphological levels of trabecular bone: **A:** Bone trabecular structure. **B:** Polarized-light picture of a trabecula; the microstructural inhomogeneity of the bony material is evident. **C:** A detailed histological slice shows the osteocyte cells and the canalicular network that connects them. **D:** Two osteocytes with canaliculi.

1.3 Gestation and Development of Bone

During growth and throughout life, there is a continuous and highly regulated process of bone resorption by osteoclasts followed by osteoblast deposition of new bone. All bone formed by this process is called secondary bone, to distinguish it from the first bone (primary bone) formed through endochondral ossification—mineralization of cartilage—or direct subperiosteal deposition. Three types of primary bone are found in humans: (a) circumferential lamellar bone, (b) woven-fibered bone, and (c) primary osteons. At birth, cortical bone consists largely of woven-fibered bone with randomly arranged collagen bundles and large, irregularly shaped vascular spaces lined with osteoblasts. The osteoblasts deposit successive layers (lamellae) of new bone and thus progressively reduce the volume of the vascular spaces. The resulting convoluted areas, occupying what were previously vascular channels, are called primary osteons. These primary osteons are generally (but not always) parallel to the long bone axis and may contain one to several vascular canals. On the periosteal surface, the diameter of long bone is increased during growth by the deposition of new primary lamellar bone consisting of an orderly arrangement of collagen fibers.

In the adult cortical bone, remodeling continually changes the internal architecture. The process is initiated by osteoclast resorption to create longitudinally oriented tubular channels. Osteoblasts on the surfaces of these channels then deposit successive layers of lamellar bone until the diameter of the cavity is reduced to a small, singular vascular canal. The newly formed, layered lamellar cylinders surrounding a longitudinally oriented vascular canal are called secondary osteons or haversian systems. Unlike primary osteons, secondary osteons are always bounded by cement lines formed where osteoclast activity ceases and osteoblast bone formation begins. Such cement lines are strongly basophilic, contain little or no collagen, and exhibit a high content of inorganic matrix. The irregular areas of bone between secondary osteons are referred to as "interstitial" bone and consist of the remnants of woven-fibered bone, circumferential lamellar bone, or primary and secondary osteons that previously occupied the area.

Normal cortical bone in the adult human consists of regions of secondary osteons bounded on the endosteal and periosteal surface by circumferential lamellar bone. Woven-fibered bone is found only during rapid bone formation such as with fracture healing, hyperparathyroidism, and Paget's disease. Lamellar bone consists of alternating sheets (each with a characteristic collagen fiber orientation) of about 7 μm thickness, separated by thin interlamellar cement layers of about 0.1 μm thickness. Thus, at both the microstructural level (where osteons and circumferential lamellae are formed from layers of fibers with alternating orientations) and at the whole bone level (where the diaphysis is formed by longitudinally oriented secondary osteons), cortical bone exhibits a number of the features of fiber-reinforced engineering composites.

The microstructural features of trabecular bone are more involved, and also more important, as they are mostly affected by osteoporotic loss of bone mass and strength. Individual trabecular plates and rods are composed primarily from interstitial bone of varying composition, although on occasion lamellar trabecular plates and osteonal trabecular rods are found. The architectural features of trabecular bone are remarkably similar to porous engineering foams, and indeed, many of the features of its mechanical behavior can be described using techniques first developed for characterizing the mechanical behavior of porous foams (28,229). It has also long been suspected that the morphology and density of trabecular bone are related to the stresses imposed during the activities of daily living (55, 258,296). Although the laws by which form follows function have not been comprehensively described, the general assumption is that the direction of trabecular orientation is related to the directions in which the imposed stresses reach maximum and minimum values (principal directions). If the loads are about equal in all directions, trabecular bone tends to form approximately equiaxed cells. If one load is much larger then the others, the trabecular cell walls tend to align and thicken in the directions that will best support the load (77). It is also generally accepted that the density of trabecular bone depends on the magnitude of the imposed load. In regions where trabecular loading is low, trabeculae tend to form a rod-like network of open cells. As the loads increase, the cell walls thicken and spread so that they resemble perforated plates (77). However, there is considerable uncertainty as to which of the many time-varying loads the bone experiences most influences trabecular architecture. It was also suggested that mechanisms exist for integrating loading information, so that trabecular architecture and density are influenced by both the number and magnitude of loading cycles (9,31).

1.4 Osteoporosis—Development and Definitions

During growth, bone mass continuously increases until it reaches a peak at about the age of 30 years (Fig. 4-3). Afterward, bone mass gradually decreases. For some individuals, however, there is a much steeper decrease in bone mass. This is found in particular for women after menopause, in which case this is due to hormonal changes—particularly loss of estrogen—that disturb the normal bone turnover process

(postmenopausal osteoporosis). Dramatic decreases in bone mass are found as well after loss of activity (disuse osteoporosis), for example, after long bed rest or space flights. In these cases, bone loss is due to a normal, though undesired, bone turnover mechanism that adapts the skeleton to a situation of reduced mechanical loading. As a result of the reduction in bone mass, the strength of bones is reduced and, consequently, the chances that a bone will fracture in a fall are increased. Predominant sites for these fractures are hip, spine, and wrist. In particular for the elderly, bone fractures are catastrophic events. The 1-year mortality rate for hip fractures is 25%, and the probability of an older patient regaining the previous level of function after a hip fracture is less than 30% (46,49,170). With the increase in average age, the number of fractures will become an increasing problem. It is estimated that the number of hip fractures will increase to over 6.2 million worldwide in 2050 (50). An improved and accurate diagnosis is of great value to recognize those patients at risk of fractures. In order to diagnose osteoporosis, however, an accurate definition is required.

Osteoporosis was defined as "a condition characterized by low bone mass and microarchitectural deterioration, leading to enhanced

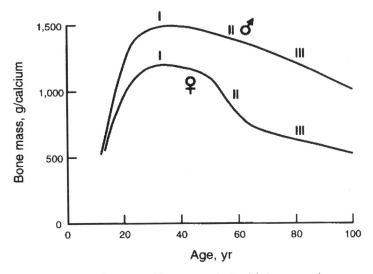

FIGURE 4-3. Development of bone mass during life in men and women. (From Riggs BL, Melton LJ III. Evidence for two distinct syndromes of involutional osteoporosis. *Am J Med* 1983;75:899–901, with permission.)

bone fragility and a consequent increase in fracture risk" (75). Hence, in order to assess osteoporosis one needs parameters quantifying "bone mass," "bone micro-architecture," and "bone fragility." However, to measure "bone fragility" one must test the bone's strength, and that can only be done destructively; not a pleasant perspective for a patient. For practical purposes the World Health Organization (WHO) established other criteria for making the diagnosis of osteoporosis. These criteria are based on comparing bone density in a particular patient with the average bone density for a 25-year-old female. Patient bone-density values that are 2.5 standard deviations below the average are diagnosed as "osteoporotic." If a patient has a value less than the normal 25-year-old female, but not 2.5 standard deviations below the average, the bone is said to be "osteopenic." This implies that, rather than strength, one now needs to measure bone density to diagnose osteoporosis. How this can be done is discussed below.

As we will see later in this chapter, osteoporosis is a trabecular affection predominantly, although in its later stages also cortical thickness can severely be reduced. It is not considered a "disease," but rather a "condition," because there are no symptoms that the subjects suffer from. There is only the increased risk of fracture in the case of a fall (i.e., hip and wrist fractures) or in cases of repetitive functional loads (i.e., vertebral body fractures).

1.5 Introduction to Bone Biomechanics

According to the definitions of osteoporosis, as quoted above, its diagnosis involves the assessment of mechanical and structural properties. In this section, the most important mechanical and morphological parameters used for this are introduced.

To understand the complex relationships between failure of bone tissue and fracture of the whole bone requires a critical analytical step involving calculation of the internal stresses (force intensities) in the whole bone. This step in turn requires knowledge of the material properties of the involved tissues, of the geometric features of the whole bone and of the loads being applied. Once the internal stresses are known, they can be compared with the strength properties of bone tissue to provide an assessment of fracture risk. Thus, the process of failure (or fracture) prediction involves (a) characterization of tissue-level material properties, (b) information on bone geometry, (c) knowledge of the loads being applied, (d) an analysis (which incorporates geometric and loading information) of the internal stresses, and (e) a comparison of the predicted stresses against the known strength properties at the tissue level. If the predicted stresses exceed the known strengths, the bone is at risk of fracture under the assumed loading conditions.

In the next sections we define some of the biomechanical concepts required to predict bone fracture and assess fracture risk. We use a simple case of axial loading to define stress, strain, modulus, and strength and to contrast the material behavior of bone as a tissue with the structural behavior of whole bones. More complex loading modes, such as bending and torsional loading, are discussed in the appendix to this chapter.

1.5.1 Stiffness and Strength

When forces are applied to any solid object, the object is deformed from its original dimensions. At the same time, internal forces are produced within the object. The relative deformations created at any point are referred to as the *strains* at that point. The internal force intensities (force/area) are referred to as the *stresses* at that point. When a bone is subjected to forces, these stresses and strains are introduced throughout the structure and can vary in a complex manner. To avoid some of these complexities and demonstrate some important mechanical concepts, it is useful to focus on a regular structure loaded under well-defined conditions (Fig. 4-4A). Similar specimens of regular geometry are used to determine the material properties of bone tissue.

In Fig. 4-4A, a cylindrical bar of length L and a constant cross-sectional area (A) is shown subjected to pure tensile force (F). As load is applied,

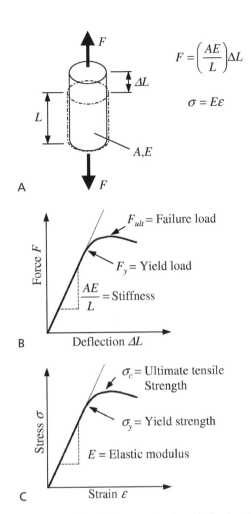

$$F = \left(\frac{AE}{L}\right)\Delta L$$

$$\sigma = E\varepsilon$$

A

F_{ult} = Failure load

F_y = Yield load

$\dfrac{AE}{L}$ = Stiffness

Force F

Deflection ΔL

B

σ_c = Ultimate tensile Strength

σ_y = Yield strength

E = Elastic modulus

Stress σ

Strain ε

C

FIGURE 4-4. Material versus structural behavior: **A:** Compressive loading of a cylinder of trabecular bone (with length *L* and cross-sectional area *A*) results in a deflection Δ*L*. **B:** Plot of force versus deflection defines structural behavior because specimen geometry influences the stiffness *AE/L* and the ultimate load *F*ᵤₗₜ. **C:** Plot of stress versus strain defines material (or tissue-level) behavior because the effects of geometry have been eliminated. (From Hayes et al. (95), with permission.)

the cylinder begins to stretch. This situation can be described by analogy to the simple equation that describes stretching of a spring

$$F = kx \qquad (1)$$

where *F* is the applied force, *x* is the change in length or elongation of the spring, and *k* is the spring constant or stiffness of the spring. Invert-

ing this simple relationship ($x = F/k$) demonstrates that with a very stiff spring (high *k*), the elongation *x* is small for a given applied force. The analogous relation for stretching of the cylinder is

$$\Delta L = \frac{FL}{AE} \qquad (2)$$

where (ΔL) is the elongation of the cylinder, *L* is the original unstretched length, *A* is the cross-sectional area, *F* is the force, and *E* is a factor (which we will subsequently define as the modulus) that describes whether the material is rigid (such as with steel) or flexible (as with rubber). According to the simple relationship shown in Eq. 2, the elongation (ΔL) is directly proportional to the applied force and to the original length and inversely proportional to the cross-sectional area and to factor *E*. Note also from Fig. 4-4A and Eq. 2 that the total elongation (ΔL) depends both on the original length and on the cross-sectional area of the bar.

We can plot a force-deflection curve to represent the structural behavior of the cylindrical bar (Fig. 4-4B). A cylinder of bone tested in tension would yield a linear region (also known as the elastic region) followed by a nonlinear region where "yielding" occurs and there is an internal rearrangement of the structure, often involving damage accumulation. After yielding, nonelastic deformation occurs until finally fracture results in the loss of load-bearing capacity of the bar. The load at which yielding occurs is referred to as the yield load, F_y. The load at which failure occurs is called the ultimate or failure load, F_{ult}. It is particularly important to note that a force-deflection curve describes the behavior of the structure because the curve would differ for a cylindrical bar of different cross-sectional area or different length (Eq. 2).

To provide a standardized representation of the mechanical behavior of the material (as opposed to the behavior of the structure), we plot a normalized curve known as a stress-strain curve (Fig. 4-4C). This normalizes the force-deformation relationship (i.e., eliminates the influence of the geometry of the cylinder) by dividing the applied force (*F*) by the cross-sectional area (A) and the deformation (ΔL) by the original length (L). We define this internal force intensity as stress (s). The units of stress are Newtons per square meter (N/m^2) or Pascals (Pa). [1 N = 0.225 lb force; 1 Pa = 145.04 × 10^{-6} lb per square inch (psi).] We often express stress in terms of megapascals (MPa) (1 MPa = 1 × 10^6 Pa) or gigapascals (GPa) (1 GPa = 1 × 10^9 Pa).

The ratio of the elongation to the original length is defined as the strain (ε). Note that strain is a nondimensional quantity. We can rewrite Eq. 2 in terms of stress and strain as

$$\sigma = E\varepsilon \tag{3}$$

In a stress-strain curve (Fig. 4-4C), the slope of the linear elastic region is referred to as the modulus (E). Because the modulus is defined as the slope of the stress-strain curve in the elastic region, and because the units of stress are megapascals and strain is nondimensional, the units of modulus are the same as those of stress (MPa or GPa). In the stress-strain curve, the material yields at a stress level known as the yield strength (again with units of megapascals). Ultimately, the material fractures at a stress level known as the fracture strength or ultimate tensile strength (units of megapascals). Note that the stress-strain representation allows us to compare different materials in terms of both the slope of the stress-strain curve and these strength parameters. From such stress-strain curves, the modulus of steel is shown to be approximately ten times that of cortical bone. The ultimate tensile strength of steel is approximately five times that of cortical bone.

Example 1: Axial stiffness. The results of a nondestructive (i.e., fully elastic) tensile test of a small circular cylinder of bone removed from the femoral diaphysis of an adult man yields the force-deformation curve shown in Fig. 4-4B. Assume that the cylinder is of cross-sectional area A, length L, and modulus E.

What happens to the force-deformation curve when we cut the specimen in half (so that L becomes $\frac{1}{2}L$) and repeat the test? Derive an expression for the ratio of the new to the old slopes of the two force-deformation curves.

Solution: Rewriting Eq. 2 in the form ($y = mx$) where m is the slope, we have

$$F = \frac{AE}{L}\Delta L$$

The slope $\frac{AE}{L}$ of the force-deformation curve is known as the *axial stiffness*. Written this way, it is immediately apparent that the slope increases directly with increasing A and E and decreases with increasing L. Thus, the ratio of the new to the old axial stiffness is

$$\frac{m'}{m} = \frac{\frac{AE}{\frac{1}{2}L}}{\frac{AE}{L}} = 2$$

As becomes clear from this example, the axial stiffness of the cylinder is dependent on its length. It is therefore immediately apparent that different force-deformation curves result from cylinders of different geometries even though the material (as reflected by the modulus E) remains the same. Thus, a force-deformation curve describes structural behavior since it reflects not only the material, but also the geometry of the specimen. By contrast, a stress-strain curve describes only the material behavior because the geometric influences were eliminated by the normalization process. Note that for the case of compression instead of tension the solution can be found in a similar way, by just acknowledging the negative sign for this case.

The calculations performed in this way can be validated with the use of "strain gauges," electrical filaments glued to the bone surface (see also Chapter 14) that measure local strains, which can be calculated to stresses, using Hooke's law. For the femoral cortex, for example, it was shown that the stresses found in this way approximated those computed with closed-form bar theory (as discussed above) and beam theory (discussed in the chapter 14 appendix) quite well (112,113).

The mechanical properties of trabecular bone are traditionally determined with compression tests on excised specimens. In order to obtain meaningful results, such specimens must meet certain size restrictions. It has been stated that the specimen must be at least five intertrabecular widths in size (approximately 5 mm) in order to meet the continuum assumption required for the determination of its mechanical properties (90). Even if this condition is met, however, results of compression tests on trabecular bone specimens can be seriously influenced by several factors, among which are alignment errors, specimen geometry, test protocols, and random and systematic errors (129,134,165,210). The most important source of errors are the end-artifacts that emerge when a specimen is extracted from its surrounding. Trabeculae near the boundaries of the specimen which were connected to the neighboring bone, are cut off after extraction. As a result, the specimen is less stiff than it was in situ. This effect is inherent to the extraction of the specimen and would occur even if the extraction process causes no damage. The underestimation of the stiffness due to end-artifacts is in the range of 20% to 40% (129,134). This error is less severe in a test protocol that uses waisted specimens glued in end-caps (118,130). In that case all test measurements are done on a subvolume of the specimen, which is then still connected to its environment.

Although it is possible to measure bone stiffness and strength from bone biopsies, this procedure is limited to certain non–load-bearing sites (typically the ilia crest) from where biopsies can be taken without jeopardizing the bone as a whole and clearly is unsuitable for follow-up or screening studies. Hence, a direct measurement of bone mechanical properties *in vivo* is not feasible in most cases. The only noninvasive techniques that can provide some information about bone stiffness are acoustic tests. With these tests, a high frequency ($\sim$200 kHz–2 MHz) signal is transmitted through the bone by a transducer and received on the other side. By measuring the speed of the acoustic waves, the stiffness E can be calculated from density ρ and acoustic velocity v, as

$$E = \rho v^2 \qquad (4)$$

The application of this technique *in vivo*, however, is complicated by the existence of soft tissues around the bone. In this chapter, this technique will not be further discussed and the interested reader is referred to the literature (158,273,277).

1.5.2 The Finite Element Analysis Method for Structural Mechanics Analysis

As is demonstrated in the previous section, and is extended upon in the appendix to this chapter, it is possible to calculate the axial or bending stiffness and strength of a bone by measuring its tissue properties (e.g., modulus, strength) and some geometric parameters (e.g,. length, area, second moment of inertia). However, this is possible only if the bone geometry can be largely simplified (e.g., as a hollow tube). Whereas this may be reasonable for the diaphysis of long bones, it is not in most other cases.

To derive mechanical properties of complex geometry, a computational technique called the method of finite element analysis (FEA) was developed. With this technique, the complex geometry ("domain") is divided in a large number of subdomains with a simple geometry, called elements (Fig. 4-5). The geometry of the domain can be two-dimensional, in which case the elements are usually triangles of quadrilaterals, or three-dimensional, in which case the elements are usually tetrahedrons or hexahedrons.

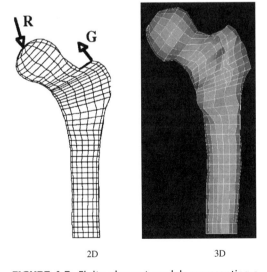

2D   3D

FIGURE 4-5. Finite element models representing a human femur. The left model is a two-dimensional one built of four-node and triangular elements. The right model is a three-dimensional one, built of eight-node brick and tetrahedral elements.

After subdividing the object in relatively simply shaped elements, a computer model ("mesh") of the object can be made that describes its geometry by the nodes of the elements and their connectivity. Based on this information, finite element computer programs can calculate what the deformation of the object is for a set of so-called boundary conditions. Boundary conditions represent the loading conditions (e.g., forces acting on the object) and kinematic constraints (e.g., locations where the object is fixed). Based on the deformation field calculated and the material properties, such programs can also calculate the stresses and strains within the object. The accuracy of the technique depends, among other factors, on the number of elements used. By increasing the number of elements, a better representation of the actual geometry is obtained and a more detailed stress/strain/deformation field results. There is a trade-off, though: The computer resources needed to solve large FEA problems rapidly increase with the number of elements. A detailed description of the FEA method and references to classical textbooks on this method are given in the appendix of Chapter 14.

The FEA method is widely used in the field of orthopaedic research to calculate stresses and strains in bones for specific loading configurations. Based on two- or three-dimensional measurements of their geometry, computer models of bones can be generated as input for the finite element program. When loaded by physiological forces, such models reveal the stresses and strains in the bone tissue. Hence, when the strength of the bone tissue is known, these analyses can be used to predict the whole-bone failure load in a similar way as described in the previous section, but without the limitation to simple geometry. Moreover, the method also enables, for example, calculating the effects of implants on the stresses and strains in the bone (see Chapter 14 for an overview).

In most FEA studies done so far, trabecular bone was represented as a continuum material (see appendix of Chapter 14) whereby the porosity of the bone was spread out over an element. The bone porosity is then accounted for by adjusting the material properties of the element. Recently, however, it became possible as well

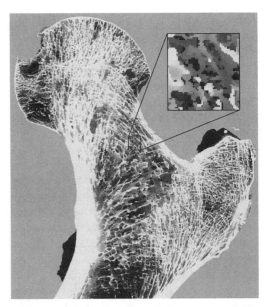

FIGURE 4-6. A microfinite element model of a human femur. The model is generated by stacking high-resolution sequential micro-CT images in a computer to create a 3D voxel (= 3D pixel) model. By converting voxels representing bone tissue to equally shaped eight-node brick elements, a micro-FEA model is obtained that represents the actual trabecular architecture with a very large number of elements (~ 97 million). (From van Rietbergen B, et al. Trabecular bone tissue strains in the healthy and osteoporotic human femur. *J Bone Miner Res* 2003;18:1781–1788, with permission.)

to create FEA models that represent trabecular bone architecture in detail (104,202,280,284). With such analyses, a very large number of equally shaped brick elements are used to represent the complex trabecular architecture in a similar way like a Lego model (Fig. 4-6). Such analyses, often referred to as "micro-FEA" or "large-scale" FEA—referring to the large number of brick elements—enable the calculation of stresses and strains at the level of trabeculae as well as the calculation of bone mechanical properties as they relate to its microarchitecture. Results of such studies are summarized in the following sections.

In this chapter, only FEA in structural mechanics is discussed. It should be noted, however, that the technique could also be used to analyze fluid flow or temperature distributions. For example, FEA was applied in an orthopaedic setting to calculate increases in bone temperatures due to acrylic-cement polymerization during joint replacement, both at the continuum (113) and the microlevel (250). It was also applied to evaluate the effects of frictional heating in hip replacement on thermal damage of bone (12).

1.5.3 Bone Density

Given the WHO definition of osteoporosis, bone density is the parameter that should be measured to diagnose osteoporosis. It should be noted though, that the popularity of bone density for this purpose is largely based on it being the only parameter that could be accurately measured *in vivo*. Bone density is bone mass per volume of bone (kg.m^{-1}). With this definition, the volume is taken as the total volume of a bone specimen, hence, including any holes. Bone density calculated in this way is also called "structural density" or "apparent density" because it measures the density of an "apparent" continuum material. A similar scalar value is the bone "volume fraction," which is the dimensionless volume of bone per tissue unit of volume. Bone volume fraction is often represented by *BV/TV* (bone volume over total volume) or V_V. Under the assumption that the trabecular bone tissue itself is homogeneous and of constant density ρ_{tissue}, the relationship between the different parameters becomes

$$\rho_{apparent} = (BV/TV)\rho_{tissue}, \qquad (5)$$

indicating that each of the density parameters mentioned above can be used as a measure of bone density. For excised specimens, bone density can be measured in a straightforward manner from measurements of its weight and volume. Bone volume fraction can be measured using Archimedes' principle (136) or from two-dimensional slices using stereology techniques (206).

The most common technique for measuring bone density *in vivo* is dual energy x-ray absorptiometry (DEXA). With this technique, a calibrated digitized radiograph of the bone is made in which the gray level of the pixels corresponds to the amount of bone passed by the x-rays. Two common parameters measured with this technique are the bone mineral content (BMC) and

bone mineral density (BMD). BMC gives the total amount of bone mass (unit: g) for a two-dimensional region of interest (e.g., the femoral neck) selected in the radiograph. For calculating BMD, the BMC value is divided by the area of the selected region (unit: g.cm^{-2}). DEXA measurements are commonly used to diagnose osteoporosis by comparing the measured BMD and BMC values of a patient with those of a population. According to the definition proposed by the WHO, the diagnosis "osteoporosis" results if the patient bone density is more than two-and-a-half standard deviations below the average of the young healthy female population (75). Major advantages of DEXA measurements are the reasonable accuracy, its simplicity, and the fact that the equipment required is widely available. A serious shortcoming of DEXA measurements is the fact that they are dependent on the size of a bone. BMD is not a real density in the sense as discussed above, but a two-dimensional estimate of it. As a result, the BMC and BMD values for a bone of a large patient will be higher than those of a smaller patient, even if the real bone density of the bone in these patients is the same. Consequently, the chance to be incorrectly diagnosed as osteoporotic are higher for smaller patients whereas the chances that severe loss of bone mass is overseen is higher for larger patients.

A more accurate measurement of bone apparent density is possible with quantitative computed tomography (QCT) scanning. With this technique, a cross-sectional image of the bone is obtained in which the gray level of the pixels corresponds to the bone density at that point. This technique enables a very sensitive determination of local changes in density (60). The QCT method also permits a distinction to be made between trabecular and cortical bone, which offers an advantage in terms of treatment choice, because cortical and trabecular bone densities do not necessarily change in the same way in osteoporosis. It was found that QCT measurements of vertebrae could better separate groups with and without prevalent fractures than DEXA measurements, suggesting that QCT is a superior predictor for bone fracture risk (13,61,305). For the distal radius, however, the predictive value of

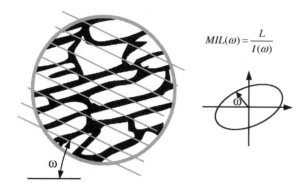

$$MIL(\omega) = \frac{L}{I(\omega)}$$

FIGURE 4-7. Mean intercept length (MIL) measurement. A grid of parallel lines is projected over a trabecular cross section and the total number of bone marrow intercepts is counted. The MIL value for line orientation angle ω is then calculated as the total line length within the image over the number of intercepts. By repeating this procedure for a large number of line orientation angles ω, a polar plot can be generated, representing the MIL value as a function of the orientation angle ω.

QCT and DEXA measurements for bone failure load was found to be very similar (167).

1.5.4 Morphological Parameters

Because neither trabecular bone density, nor volume fraction, provide any information about the actual structure of the bone (other than its density), other parameters were introduced. Among these are scalar parameters that quantify the average geometry of the trabeculae, such as average trabecular thickness (Tb.Th), average trabecular spacing (Tb.Sp), and the average number of trabeculae per unit of length ("trabecular number": Tb.N). Another commonly used parameter is the connectivity density (Conn.D), which characterizes the number of redundant connections between two points in the bone per unit of volume (205,206). If this number is high, the bone structure is well connected, which is generally considered as advantageous. A large number of other scalar parameters to define its trabecular architecture appeared in the literature. Although some of these may be useful for specific purposes, their interpretation is often difficult and outside the scope of this chapter.

To quantify directionality and anisotropy of trabecular structures, so-called "fabric parameters" were introduced. To quantify "fabric" of a structure, a single scalar is not enough. Instead, second- or higher-order tensorial parameters are needed to quantify a direction-dependent value (59,91,123–125). The one most commonly used fabric tensor is the mean intercept length (MIL) (295). It can be graphically represented by an ellipse-shaped figure, with its largest principal

axis indicating the principal or axial direction of the material (Fig. 4-7). The ratio between the lengths of the principal axes is an indication of the anisotropy of the structure. It should be emphasized, however, that no unique definition exists for the structural anisotropy of bone; other tensor measures were developed as well (209).

Measurements of structural parameters require imaging methods to visualize trabecular structure. Traditionally, these parameters were determined from thin slices of bone, overlaid by a grid of points or lines and viewed through a microscope (290). For example, to measure MIL, a grid of parallel lines was projected over a thin slice of bone. The number of bone-marrow interfaces was then counted for a large number of grid angles. When representing the number of bone marrow interfaces in a polar plot, an ellipse-shaped figure results (a three-dimensional ellipsoid) (Fig. 4-7). A shortcoming of the traditional determination of parameters from measurements on a single bone slice is that they do not provide information about architecture in the third dimension. It is usually assumed that the trabeculae are either rod-like or plate-like (212), and morphometric parameters such as Tb.N and Tb.Sp are determined based on this assumption, which can cause inaccuracies (205,206).

A more accurate and convenient way to measure bone structural parameters is by using digitized sets of cross-sectional images and computer algorithms. To accurately measure the trabecular structure, the resolution of the images should be 50 μm or better. Presently, three techniques are available for this task. The first is a serial sectioning method using a digital camera mounted on top of a microtome to generate sequential images of a bone specimen while it is sliced (11,207,208). The second is a microcomputed tomography (micro-CT) technique—a small version of a CT scanner—that creates sequential cross-sectional images at a very high resolution (89,149,237). The third is a micromagnetic resonance imaging (micro-MRI) method that uses the distribution of protons (hence, water) in a cross section to quantify nuclear spin. Because there is more water in bone marrow than in bone tissue, this technique provides the contrast between bone tissue and marrow, needed to visualize the trabecular microstructure. All three techniques can provide images with similar resolutions of up to 10 μm, depending on the field of view and measurement time. Until recently, such high-resolution images could be made only for very small specimens ($\sim$1 cm^3), but recent developments in CT and MRI now enable imaging larger bones and even bone *in vivo* (17,63,151,154, 166,171,172,194,195,205,222,289). Presently, however, applications to bone *in vivo* are limited to the peripheral skeleton because adequate resolutions can be obtained for these sites only.

By stacking a large number of sequential images in a computer, the three-dimensional trabecular structure can be represented in a rectangular grid in which some voxels (i.e., three-dimensional pixels) represent bone tissue and other voids. Using computational algorithms, it then is relatively easy to determine structural parameters in a real three-dimensional manner. Measurements based on such three-dimensional reconstructions are more accurate since the full three-dimensional structure is accounted for; hence, no assumptions about the geometry of the structure in the third dimension (e.g., plate or rod model) are required. The availability of such three-dimensional reconstructions also created possibilities for the measurement of new structural parameters that could not be measured with the classical approach. Examples of these are structural model index (SMI) (101) that characterizes the trabecular structure as either rod-like (SMI = 3) or plate-like (SMI = 0). Another

one is ridge number density (RND), a measure for the trabecular number that can be extracted directly from high-resolution three-dimensional images of patients (152).

2 STRUCTURAL AND MECHANICAL PROPERTIES OF BONE

The relationships between the mechanical behavior of bone tissue as a material and the structural behavior of whole bones suggest that the properties of bone should be approached at three levels (96,97,131). At the smallest level of the mineralized osteoid the mechanical properties of the local tissue are of interest. Specimen representative for the apparent structural organization of bone tissue in complex geometric arrangements—trabecular or cortical—represent the second level. The structural behavior of whole bones, or their sub-regions, forms the third level. In the first part of this section, mechanical properties at the first level, the bone tissue level, are described. The mechanical properties of trabecular bone, however, are largely determined by its structural organization, i.e., the second level. This is discussed in the second part of this section. The last section summarizes recent insights into the mechanical behavior of bone as obtained with novel imaging and computational analysis techniques.

2.1 The Mechanical Properties of Bone Tissue

Mineralized bone tissue forms the basic building material of bones. Both cortical and cancellous bone have very similar compositions. There are, however, differences in their structural organization. In cortical bone, haversian canals are present, containing blood vessels or nerves (Fig. 4-1). Bone tissue is deposited in cylindrical layers around these canals. In trabecular bone no haversian canals exist, but bone tissue is deposited in longitudinal layers. It was long assumed that this difference in microstructural composition, in combination with the small sizes of the trabeculae, would result in lower stiffness and strength for trabecular bone tissue. As discussed below, however, recent studies have demonstrated that, in fact, the mechanical properties might be very similar.

2.1.1 Cortical Bone Tissue

To determine the mechanical properties of bone tissue, small uniform specimens are loaded under well-defined conditions. As shown in Fig. 4-4, such testing conditions produce uniform stresses throughout the specimen. Specimen deformation can then be measured and the strains calculated using the relationships between stress and strain. With this, and other modes of loading, this general approach to materials testing allowed documentation of cortical bone material properties in tension, compression, bending, and torsion (27,29,39,56,57,86,226,227,229,242).

Several factors influence the material properties of cortical bone. One is the rate at which the bone tissue is loaded. Specimens of cortical bone loaded very rapidly exhibit increased elastic moduli and ultimate strengths as compared

with specimens loaded more slowly. To quantify the rate of deformation, one can refer to the strain rate (units: s^{-1}) to which the tissue is exposed. In normal activities, bone is subjected to strain rates generally below $0.01\ s^{-1}$. Materials such as bone, for which stress-strain characteristics and strength properties depend on the applied strain rate, are said to be *viscoelastic* (or time-dependent) materials. However, this rate dependency is relatively weak (68). The elastic modulus and ultimate strength of bone are approximately proportional to the strain rate raised to the 0.06 power (Fig. 4-8). Hence, over a very wide range of strain rates, the ultimate tensile strength increases by a factor of three, and the modulus increases by a factor of about two (68).

The stress-strain behavior of cortical bone is also strongly dependent on the orientation of the bone microstructure with respect to the direction of loading. Several investigators have demonstrated that cortical bone is stronger and stiffer in the longitudinal direction (direction of osteon orientation) than in the transverse direction. In

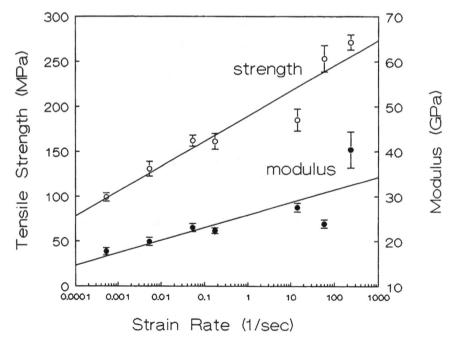

FIGURE 4-8. The influence of loading rate on the tensile strength and modulus of cortical bone. The ultimate tensile strength increases by about a factor of 3, and the modulus by a factor of 2. (From Wright TM, Hayes WC. Tensile testing of bone over a wide range of strain rates: effects of strain rate, microstructure and density. *Med Biol Eng* 1976;14:671–680, with permission.)

addition, bone specimens loaded in a direction perpendicular to the osteons tend to fail in a more brittle manner, with little non-elastic deformation after yielding. Long bones are therefore better able to resist stresses along their axes than across their axes. Materials such as bone, for which elastic and strength properties are dependent on the direction of applied loading, are said to be anisotropic materials. A consequence of anisotropic behavior is that measurements of mechanical properties are direction dependent and more parameters need to be measured to fully characterize their mechanical behavior. The viscoelastic and anisotropic nature of cortical bone distinguishes it as a complex material. Because of these characteristics, one must specify the strain rate and the direction of applied loading when describing material behavior.

Ultimate strength values of adult femoral cortical bone under various modes of loading, in both the longitudinal and transverse directions, are summarized in Table 4.1 (39,86, 226,228). These indicate that the material strength of bone tissue depends on the type of loading as well as on the loading direction. The compressive strength is greater than the tensile strength in both longitudinal and transverse directions. Transverse specimens are weaker than longitudinal specimens in both tension and compression. The shear strength (determined by torsion tests about the longitudinal axis and

TABLE 4-1. STRENGTH OF FEMORAL CORTICAL BONE[a]

Loading Mode	Ultimate Strength (MPa)
Longitudinal	
Tension	133
Compression	193
Shear	68
Transverse	
Tension	51
Compression	133

[a] Age span of population 19–80 years. From Hayes WC, Gerhart TN. Biomechanics of bone: applications for assessment of bone strength. In: Peck WA, ed. *Bone and mineral research.* Amsterdam: Elsevier Science, 1985:259–294, with permission. Mean values from Reilly DT, Burstein AH. The elastic and ultimate properties of compact bone tissue. *J Biomech* 1975;8:393–405, with permission.

TABLE 4-2. MODULAS OF FEMORAL CORTICAL BONE[a]

Longitudinal	17.0 GPa
Transverse	11.5 GPa
Shear	3.3 GPa

[a] Age span of population 19–80 years. 1 GPa (gigapascal) = 1,000 MPa. From Hayes WC, Gerhart TN. Biomechanics of bone: applications for assessment of bone strength. In: Peck WA, ed. *Bone and mineral research.* Amsterdam: Elsevier Science, 1985:259–294, with permission. Mean values from Reilly DT, Burstein AH. The elastic and ultimate properties of compact bone tissue. *J Biomech* 1975;8:393–405, with permission.

reflecting shear stresses along transverse and longitudinal planes) is about one-third of the compressive strength. The modulus values for adult femoral cortical bone are shown in Table 4.2 (39,86,226,228). The longitudinal elastic modulus is about 50% greater than the transverse elastic modulus. The shear modulus for torsion about the longitudinal axis is about one-fifth the longitudinal modulus.

The material properties of cortical bone also decline with age (28) (Fig. 4-9). Both tensile strength and modulus decrease at about 2% per decade for the age range from 20 years to 90 years. Thus, the ultimate tensile strength declines from 140 MPa in the third decade to 120 MPa in the ninth decade. Over the same period, the elastic modulus decreases from 17 to 15.6 GPa (28).

2.1.2 Trabecular Bone Tissue

Trabecular bone tissue elastic properties and strength were also measured, using standard engineering test methods—tensile, three- or four-point bending and buckling[2]—on excised trabeculae. Values found for the tissue moduli range from 0.76 to 10 GPa in tensile, from 3.2 to 5.4 GPa in three- or four-point bending, and from 8.7 to 14 GPa in buckling tests (for an

---

[2] Buckling is a mode of failure occurring in slender bars when these are loaded in axial compression. This mode of failure does not directly depend on material strength, but rather on elastic modulus, in combination with bar width and force value. It is in fact an instability problem related to slenderness.

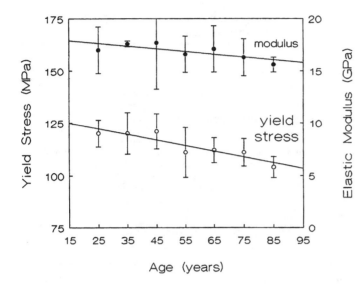

FIGURE 4-9. Ultimate tensile strength and modulus versus age for human femoral cortical bone. (From Burstein AH, Reilly DT, Martens M. Aging of bone tissue: mechanical properties. *J Bone Joint Surg Am* 1976;58:82–86, with permission.)

overview see Rho et al. (229)). Although Young's moduli of trabecular tissue were determined experimentally in many studies, its strength was rarely reported. In one of the few experimental studies in which trabecular tissue strength was measured, using four-point bending tests, a static strength of about 160 MPa was reported (44). This value is about 15% lower than values measured for similar cortical bone specimens. A major problem with using standard engineering tests for the determination of bone tissue properties is the relatively small size of trabeculae (thickness: 100–200 μm, length 1–2 mm), resulting in inaccuracies in displacement measurements, hence in the calculation of moduli. Another problem is the irregular shape of trabeculae, where standard engineering tests require standardized specimen geometry. To overcome this problem, some authors used machined specimens (44,45), but it is unclear to what extent machining artifacts can affect their stiffness. In other studies ultrasound was used to measure tissue elastic properties. Values found with this method are generally higher than those obtained from standard tests: 11 to 15 GPa (3,229), approaching the stiffness measured for cortical bone.

A new approach for the determination of bone tissue elastic properties and strength uses micro-FEA models. With this approach, the stiffness or strength of a cancellous bone cube is calculated using micro-FEA models for which certain assumptions are made concerning stiffness and strength of the tissue. The results of the calculations are then compared with results of laboratory compression tests in which stiffness or strength of the specimens were measured. By comparing the results, it is possible to calculate what tissue material properties would provide the best agreement with the experimental results (118,121,150,277,284). A major advantage of this approach (and the ultrasound approach) is that the stiffness of trabeculae is determined in situ. Hence, errors due to machining, the excision of trabeculae or other experimental artifacts related to experimental tests can be excluded. The values found in these studies for the stiffness of trabecular bone tissue are generally higher than those obtained from bending or other mechanical tests on excised specimens, but they were still considerably less than values found for cortical bone tissue. However, in most of these studies standard compression tests were used to measure the bone apparent stiffness, and such tests are bound to underestimate it (129,134,165,210). As a result, values found for the tissue stiffness are underestimated as well. This was confirmed by recent studies, in which more accurate experimental tests were used to determine the apparent stiffness of trabecular bone specimens. By comparing micro-FEA and accurate experimental results, considerably higher values were obtained for the trabecular bone tissue stiffness, at only 10% less than the stiffness of cortical bone tissue (7,201). This difference, however, cannot be explained by differences in mineralization, suggesting that it originates from differences in the ultrastructure (86).

Using a similar set-up, and comparing experimental to micro-FEA results, it was possible to determine trabecular bone tissue yield strain. These studies indicated that micro-FEA analyses that include cortical-like strength asymmetry at the tissue level with a yield strain of 0.60% in tension and 1.01% in compression, can predict apparent level failure of trabecular bone for multiple loading modes to an outstanding level of accuracy (200,201). It was concluded that, although the elastic moduli and yield strains for trabecular tissue are just slightly lower than those of cortical tissue, tissue strength is about 25% higher for cortical bone.

Based on its micro-structural composition, it is generally assumed that trabecular tissue material behaves transversally isotropic with its symmetry axis in the longitudinal trabecular direction, but little quantitative information about anisotropy at this level is available. However, for the common loading modes of trabeculae, compression, tension, or bending, only the longitudinal and shear moduli of the bone tissue are relevant. Hence, the value found for the tissue stiffness with a micro-FEA approach in fact represents the longitudinal stiffness of the bone tissue material.

2.1.3 Microcracks and Damage in Bone Tissue

Healthy bone tissue contains a considerable amount of microcracks. Their number was quantified as ranging from zero in young people to 5 cracks/mm^2 in the elderly (243,294, 307,309). Their number increases with age and is greater for females than males at a comparable age (66,243,307). These cracks are due to material fatigue of the bone tissue under repetitive loading. In bone tissue, however, such cracks are repaired in the process of bone remodeling. Hence, crack formation rate, on the one hand,

and the remodeling rate on the other determine the number of microcracks in bone tissue at any time. Normally, this process reaches some equilibrium status. If the mechanical loading of bone is increased, however, microcracks can accumulate, leading to damage of the tissue and, eventually, fracture of the bone ("stress fracture"). There are two different scenarios that can lead to this type of bone failure. According to the first scenario, the magnitudes of the forces acting on the bone are strongly increased (e.g., due to a fall). In this situation, damage in the bone rapidly accumulates, leading to almost instantaneous bone fracture, leaving no time for repair. According to the second scenario, the magnitude of the force is still in its physiological range, but the cycle frequency is much increased. A typical example of the latter condition is the formation of stress fractures in new army recruits and athletes (117,159,218). In this case, the crack formation rate far exceeds the repair rate, leading to crack accumulation and eventually bone fatigue fractures.

Both instantaneous and fatigue fractures of bone tissue were studied using classical engineering strength and fatigue tests (18,30,34, 58,98,178,204,244). Obviously, in such laboratory tests on excised specimens, microcrack repair cannot take place. However, given that this repair process hardly plays a role in the two scenarios mentioned above, the results can be considered representative for the *in vivo* situation. It was found that repetitive loading gradually reduces both stiffness and strength of bone tissue (32,34,215,308). In fact, with an increasing number of microcracks, the load-bearing cross-sectional area is reduced. Hence, the stresses in the remaining tissue are increased and the bone tissue ultimate stress is reached earlier.

It was suggested that microcracks might play a role in the regulation of the bone remodeling process (see further in this chapter). Because the number of cracks increases with increased loading, the actual number of cracks in the bone could be an indicator for its loading history. Osteocyte cells within the bone tissue could detect cracks either because they act as stress risers or because cracks would cut the canaliculi, thus inhibiting fluid flow (22,224). Based on such hypotheses, damage and repair theories were developed and tested with computer simulation (225,257).

2.2 Trabecular Bone Strength and Stiffness

The major physical difference of trabecular bone in comparison with cortical bone is its increased porosity. This is reflected by measurements of the apparent density (i.e., the mass of bone tissue divided by the bulk volume of the test specimen, including mineralized bone and bone marrow spaces). In the human skeleton, the apparent density of trabecular bone ranges from approximately 0.1 to 1.0 g/cm^3. The apparent density of cortical bone is about 1.8 g/cm^3. A trabecular specimen with an apparent density of 0.2 g/cm^3 has a porosity of approximately 90%.

Bone apparent density has a profound influence on the compressive stress-strain behavior of trabecular bone (33,35,76–78,115,131,230, 248) (Fig. 4-10). These stress-strain properties are markedly different from those of cortical bone and are similar to the compressive behavior of many porous engineering materials that are used to absorb energy on impact (77). The stress-strain curve for trabecular bone exhibits an

initial elastic region followed by yield. Yielding occurs as the trabeculae begin to fracture. Yield is then followed by a long plateau region, which is created as progressively more and more trabeculae fracture. The fractured trabeculae begin to fill the marrow spaces. At a strain of approximately 0.50, most of the marrow spaces have filled with the debris of these fractured trabeculae. Further loading of trabecular bone after pore closure is associated with a marked increase in specimen modulus. Figure 4-11 shows compressive strength data for trabecular bone from a wide variety of studies, plotted against apparent density (77,99). These curves clearly show that both strength and stiffness of trabecular bone can vary over a wide range, spanning at least three orders of magnitude, and that these properties are largely dependent on apparent density. Because the bone density varies only from about 0.1 to about 1.0 g/cm^{-3}, i.e., over one order of magnitude, it is clear that even a small variation in density can have a large influence on trabecular bone mechanical properties. This also explains why diseases affecting bone mass and structure, such as osteoporosis, have such a dramatic effect on bone mechanical properties and fracture risk. The strong dependency on bone density led to the development of stochastic relationships

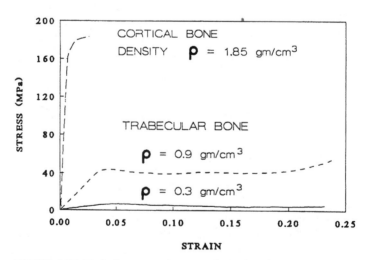

FIGURE 4-10. Typical stress-strain curves for trabecular bone of different apparent densities. (From Hayes WC, Gerhart TN. Biomechanics of bone: applications for assessment of bone strength. In: Peck WA, ed. *Bone and mineral research.* Amsterdam: Elsevier Science, 1985:259–294, with permission.)

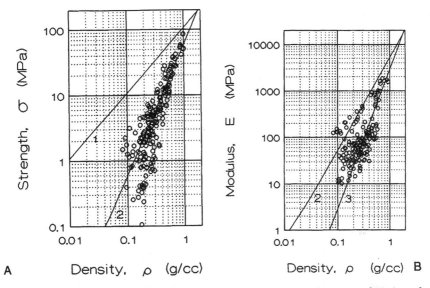

FIGURE 4-11. Compressive strength and modulus of trabecular bone as a function of apparent density: **(A)** compressive strength varies as a power-law function of apparent density with an exponent of approximately 2; **(B)** compressive modulus also varies as a power-law function of apparent density with an exponent ranging between 2 and 3. (From Hayes WC, Piazza SJ, Zysset PK. Biomechanics of fracture risk prediction of the hip and spine by quantitative computed tomography. *Radiol Clin North Am* 1991;29:1–18, with permission.)

for the prediction of bone strength and stiffness, based on measurements of bone density. These relationships are discussed later.

The results presented in Fig. 4-11 also demonstrate that bone density alone is not a perfect predictor for trabecular bone strength or modulus. For example, for a density value of 0.3, the strength can vary from approximately 0.8 to 11 MPa and the modulus from 12 to 140 MPa. This implies that the mechanical properties are not determined by bone density alone, but also by other factors, in particular the structural organization of the bone tissue. Hence, including parameters that describe bone morphology in stochastic relationships could potentially improve the prediction of trabecular bone strength and modulus. However, which parameters should be measured is still not clear and the subject of many studies, the results of which are summarized later.

It is commonly accepted now that the large variation in trabecular bone mechanical properties enables trabecular bone to adapt itself to local loading conditions, in the sense that stiffer/stronger bone is formed at highly loaded

locations and weaker bone in low-loaded regions. It is also known that trabecular bone manages to do so primarily by varying its structure, such that it is somehow optimal for its load-carrying task (see the section on bone modeling and remodeling for more details). However, it is still not known what, exactly, bones are optimized for. Huiskes (109) phrased this enigma as: "If bone is the answer, then what is the question?" Some recent insights with regard to this question are presented later in this chapter.

2.2.1 Compressive Versus Tensile Properties

Because compression seems the more physiological loading mode, most studies focused on the determination of the compressive properties of trabecular bone. The elastic constants of trabecular bone for tensile loading, however, were determined as well (4,38,234) and the conclusion of these studies was that there are no differences between tensile and compressive stiffness of trabecular bone. The tensile strength of bone, however, is not the same as its compressive strength.

There are some conflicting data in the literature, with some authors reporting that trabecular bone tensile strength is at least as high as its compressive strength (38,234), while others reported the opposite (126,251). Based on accurate experiments with bovine bone, Keaveny et al. (135) later concluded that the compressive strength is higher, but that the difference is dependent on the bone stiffness. This view was later confirmed for human bone (147).

2.3 Stochastic Relationships for the Prediction of Trabecular Bone Mechanical Properties

The protocol used to derive stochastic relationships between bone structural and mechanical parameters was largely similar for most authors who published on this issue. A large number of cancellous bone specimens are obtained and their mechanical properties are measured from compression or ultrasound tests. For the same set of specimen, the density is measured using Archimedes' principle. In some cases, the structural anisotropy—or other morphometric parameters of the specimens—are measured. Mechanical and structural parameters are then correlated with each other and statistical analysis is used to identify the predictive value of structural parameters for the mechanical behavior of bone.

2.3.1 Relationships Based on Bone Apparent Density

In the past, the relationships were usually limited to the prediction of the cancellous bone axial properties (the properties of the bone in its load-bearing direction) from measurements of bone volume fraction or density. In an often-cited study by Carter and Hayes (35), a cubic relationship was found between the axial modulus and the apparent density for a set of human and bovine cancellous and cortical bone specimens, as

$$E_{longitudinal} = 3790\dot{\varepsilon}^{0.06}\rho^3 \qquad (6)$$

with ρ the apparent density of cancellous bone in g/cm^3 and $\dot{\varepsilon}$ the strain rate (s^{-1}). This rela-

tionship was developed to describe the stiffness of both cortical and trabecular bone and is valid for the full range of densities. Rice et al. (230) later found that a square relationship yields more accurate results for bone stiffness when human cancellous bone alone is considered. In more recent studies, the power p in the general relationship $E = a\rho^p$ was not limited to integer values. These studies have indicated that the power is somewhere between two and three (80,102). In some of these studies, very high coefficients of determination were reported between the mean elastic modulus of cancellous bone and its density. However, such highly predictive relationships based on volume fraction (or density) alone are found only if the set of bone specimens covers a wide range of densities. Ulrich et al. (267) demonstrated that although more than 86% of the variation in the elastic properties of a set of specimens could be explained by bone volume fraction, differences in moduli between samples with the same volume fraction could be as large as 53%. In this study, it was demonstrated that the inclusion of other structural parameters (Tb.Sp, anisotropy ratio, Tb.N) could improve the predictive value of the relationship. However, the most effective indices were not the same for different anatomical sites. This site dependency of such relationships was also confirmed in another recent study (181).

Similar relationships were developed for the prediction of bone strength from bone density. In the study by Carter and Hayes (35), cited earlier, a relationship between ultimate stress σ_{ult} and apparent density was found as

$$\sigma_{ult} = 68\dot{\varepsilon}^{0.06}\rho^2. \qquad (7)$$

In later work, general power-law relationships of the form $\sigma_{ult} = a\rho^p$ were developed for trabecular bone only and for different sites (for an overview, see Keaveny (128)). Although different relationships were reported for different sites, the values predicted do not vary tremendously across sites. The predictive value of these relationships was generally very good, with coefficients of determination ranging from 0.76 for the lumbar spine (88) up to 0.93 for the proximal femur (168). Interestingly, the yield strain of trabecular bone is almost independent of its density

(135,147,234,260). Human vertebral bone starts yielding for strains of about 0.008.

Example 2. Trabecular bone properties: Effects of density. Consider Eqs. 6 and 7. Assuming that the initial apparent density of vertebral trabecular bone is 0.20 g/cc, what is the effect on compressive strength and modulus when the density decreases (as with aging) to 0.15 g/cc for a physiological strain rate of 1,000 microstrain.s^{-1}?

Solution. For a strain rate of 1,000 microstrain/sec (0.001 s^{-1}) and a $\rho = 0.20$ g/cc, the compressive strength is $\sigma = 1.8$ MPa, and the compressive modulus is 20 MPa. A 25% reduction in apparent density to $\rho = 0.15$ g/cc results in a compressive strength of 1.0 MPa and a compressive modulus of 8.5 MPa. Thus, a 25% reduction in density is associated with a 44% reduction in strength and a 58% reduction in modulus. Note that these density values correspond to those measured in elderly cadaveric vertebrae (99,176,184). It is thus not surprising that vertebral compression fractures are common among the elderly and often occur before there is clear radiographic evidence of density reductions. Also note that doubling the strain rate will have little effect on the results.

be included in the relationships (107). This is not a trivial task because stiffness is represented by a fourth rank tensor, fabric by a second rank tensor, and bone density by a scalar. Hence, some sort of mathematical framework is needed for a stochastic relationship. A general form for such relationships was derived by Cowin et al. (51). Using this form, Turner et al. (262) derived a relationship to predict the three Young's and three shear moduli from measurements of density and normalized MIL. The coefficients of determination (R^2) were 0.70 and 0.80 for the Young's and shear moduli, respectively.

With the development of high-resolution microstructural imaging methods described in the previous section, it became possible to calculate structural parameters in a real three-dimensional manner. With the micro-FEA technique, it became possible to derive all engineering constants—three Young's, three shear moduli, and three Poisson's ratios—for cancellous bone specimens. Based on the same mathematical basis formulated by Cowin (51), Kabel et al. (122) quantified a relationship that predicted the full stiffness tensor from measurements of bone volume fraction and normalized mean intercept length, as

$$
\begin{cases}
S_{iiii} = E_{tissue}\left\{0.0291 + 0.8650\,V_V^{1.6} + \left(0.1332 - 5.506\,V_V^{1.6}\right)II + \left(-0.5109 + 5.1440\,V_V^{1.6}\right)H_i \right. \\
\qquad \left. + \left(0.8208 - 0.0754\,V_V^{1.6}\right)H_i^2\right\}(R^2 = 0.946) \\[6pt]
S_{iijj} = E_{tissue}\left\{-0.0065 + 0.6238\,V_V^{1.6} + \left(0.2758 + 11.570\,V_V^{1.6}\right)II + \left(-0.2631 - 13.4430\,V_V^{1.6}\right)(H_i + H_j) \right. \\
\qquad \left. + \left(0.2629 + 11.590\,V_V^{1.6}\right)\left(H_i^2 + H_j^2\right) + \left(0.2739 + 18.790\,V_V^{1.6}\right)H_i\,H_j\right\}(R^2 = 0.852) \\[6pt]
S_{ijij} = E_{tissue}\left\{0.0178 + 0.1206\,V_V^{1.6} + \left(-0.0713 - 8.5380\,V_V^{1.6}\right)II + \left(0.0038 + 8.0010\,V_V^{1.6}\right)(H_i + H_j) \right. \\
\qquad \left. + \left(0.0053 - 10.510\,V_V^{1.6}\right)\left(H_i^2 + H_j^2\right)\right\}(R^2 = 0.929) \\
i, j = 1, 2, 3; i = j
\end{cases}
\tag{8}
$$

2.3.2 Relationships for the Prediction of Trabecular Bone Anisotropic Properties

Because bone volume fraction, density, and the morphometric parameters mentioned above are all scalar parameters, they cannot predict the anisotropic behavior of bone. To predict cancellous bone mechanical anisotropy, structural parameters such as MIL, which describe the average orientation of the trabeculae, must

with S_{ijkl} the components of the stiffness tensor, E_{tissue} the isotropic tissue Young's modulus, and H_i the eigenvalues of the MIL fabric tensor. The coefficient of determination for the pooled data was 0.97. After calculating the Young's and shear moduli from the predicted stiffness matrix, it was found that these engineering constants were accurately predicted as well ($R^2 > 0.93$).

Using the same data, Yang et al. (302) demonstrated that all nine elastic engineering constants could be well predicted from the cancellous bone volume fraction alone. They used a spectral decomposition method to align the micro-FE calculated stiffness matrices in the same coordinate system in which the first coordinate corresponds to the stiffest direction and the third coordinate to the weakest direction. In this common coordinate system, the engineering constants could be written as a function of volume fraction V_V alone, as

$$E_{11} = E_{\text{tissue}} \left(1240 \, V_V^{1.8}\right), \; E_{22} = E_{\text{tissue}} \left(885 \, V_V^{1.89}\right),$$
$$E_{33} = E_{\text{tissue}} \left(529 \, V_V^{1.92}\right), \, (R^2 = 0.924)$$
$$G_{23} = E_{\text{tissue}} \left(533.3 \, V_V^{2.04}\right), \; G_{13} = E_{\text{tissue}} \left(633.3 \, V_V^{1.97}\right),$$
$$G_{12} = E_{\text{tissue}} \left(972.6 \, V_V^{1.98}\right) \, (R^2 = 0.884) \qquad (9)$$

$$\nu_{23} = E_{\text{tissue}} \left(0.256 V_V^{-0.086}\right), \nu_{13} = E_{\text{tissue}} \left(0.316 V_V^{-0.191}\right),$$
$$\nu_{12} = E_{\text{tissue}} \left(0.176 V_V^{-0.248}\right) (R^2 = 0.755) \qquad (10)$$

In these relationships, the bone volume fraction alone could explain more than 92% of the variation in the Young's moduli. Clearly, no information about the directionality can be derived from bone volume fraction, which is a scalar. It was suggested, however, that information about the directionality can be derived from the anatomical site from which the sample originates. The results obtained by Yang et al. (303) suggest that bone density and anisotropy are coupled in the sense that trabecular bone anisotropy increases with decreasing density. This becomes clear if the anisotropy of the sample is written as

$$\frac{E_{11}}{E_{33}} = \frac{1240 \, V_V^{1.8}}{529 \, V_V^{1.92}} = 2.3 \, V_V^{-0.12} \qquad (11)$$

i.e., a negative exponent evolves. For a bone sample with a volume fraction of 5%, the anisotropy ratio would be 3.35, whereas for a bone sample with a volume fraction of 50% it would be 2.54.

Similar to the stiffness, the yield and ultimate stress of trabecular bone is dependent on the loading direction as well as on bone density. The yield strain of trabecular bone, however, is almost independent of loading direction. Up to reaching the yield point, the stresses and strains are coupled by the generalized Hooke's law, such that the relationships between yield stress and yield strain are coupled by this law

as well. The important consequence of this is that it enables prediction of the load-dependent yield stress based on information about bone anisotropy, as represented by Hooke's law, and yield strain of the bone tissue itself, which is virtually constant (52). An interesting aspect of these relationships is that they might only be valid for trabecular bone, but not for porous structures in general (278).

2.3.3 Healthy Versus Osteoporotic Bone

In most of the studies mentioned here, the bone material used either represented samples from healthy bone or from a mixed population. This raised the question of whether the relationships developed would be valid for osteoporotic bone. In a recent study, Homminga et al. (106) applied the stochastic relationships determined by Kabel et al. (122) for healthy bone to predict the mechanical properties of bone samples from fracture patients. They found that the relations obtained by Kabel et al. could well predict the mechanical properties of the bone samples from fracture patients. Hence, it was concluded that morphology-based relations that predict the elastic properties are not different for trabecular bone from women with or without osteoporotic fractures.

The application of these relationships to patients requires the measurement of bone density (or volume fraction). This can be done using quantitative imaging techniques such as DEXA, or QCT. The determination of MIL or other morphometric parameters requires imaging methods such as high-resolution CT or MR (153,157).

2.4 Mechanical Imaging of Bone Strength

The title of this section is contradictory: Obviously it is not possible to "see" the strength of bones. Nevertheless, mechanical properties (stiffness and strength) of bones are fully determined by only two factors: the mechanical properties of the bone tissue itself and the structural organization of the trabeculae (which also comprises bone density). Hence, quantifying bone structures by imaging already provides most of the information required to assess bone strength or stiffness. As clarified in the previous section, variations in tissue mechanical properties are only modest and the structural organization of the bone can be accounted for by micro-FEA. Hence, by assuming reasonable values for bone tissue mechanical properties, it is possible to calculate mechanical properties of the whole bone by using micro-FEA models that are solely based on high-resolution images of the bone: mechanical imaging!

In this section we show how this approach can lead to an improved understanding of the role of bone architecture, improved predictions of bone strength, and new insights in the function of trabecular bone.

2.4.1 The Role of Trabecular Structure for Its Apparent Stiffness and Strength

The strong dependence of trabecular bone mechanical properties on bone mass already indicates that trabecular structure plays a prominent role in the mechanical behavior of trabecular bone. Nevertheless, none of the relationships found so far could provide an accurate and generally valid prediction of mechanical properties based on mass. The question arises as to whether this is due to the material properties of the bone

tissue itself that are not accounted for by these relationships, to errors in the determination of the mechanical properties of the bone, to the fact that bone mass and its structural parameters do not sufficiently describe the structure, or to other, yet unknown factors.

A definite answer to this question was obtained with the use of micro-FEA methods. The anisotropic stiffness of bone specimens was first measured in experimental compression tests. It was then calculated from micro-FEA models of the same specimens, using isotropic material properties for the bone tissue itself, and found predictive for the experimental anisotropy. As the FEA anisotropy values did not depend on variations in bone tissue stiffness, it could only be an effect of architecture. So these studies demonstrated that excellent agreement between anisotropic stiffness calculated from micro-FEA and measured with accurate experimental methods can be obtained, as illustrated in Fig. 4-12 (118,150,281). This implies that, first, the elastic properties of trabecular bone depend on its structure and a single "effective" tissue Young's modulus (122); second, that variations in tissue moduli are small enough to be neglected; and third, that the anisotropy of cancellous bone is fully due to its architecture. In other words, anisotropy at the bone tissue level plays no role at the bone apparent level.

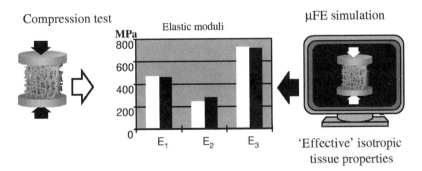

FIGURE 4-12. Mechanical imaging of bone strength: three perpendicular elastic moduli, measured from a cube of trabecular bone in compressive testing, in comparison with the moduli values determined by micro-FEA. From the moduli the strength can be estimated. (Adapted from van Rietbergen, et al. Determination of trabecular bone tissue elastic properties by comparison of experimental and finite element results. In: Sol H, Oomens CWJ, eds. *Material identification using mixed numerical experimental methods*. Dordrecht: Kluwer Academic Publishers, 1997:183–192.)

Based on micro-FEA results of a large number of specimens from different donors and different sites, several other new conclusions about the anisotropic elastic behavior of cancellous bone could be reached. First, in a study by Yang et al. (302) it was proven that cancellous bone can be described as orthotropic at the 95% confidence level. The important implication of this is that the elastic behavior of cancellous bone can be described by the nine common engineering elastic constants (three Young's moduli, three shear moduli, and three Poisson's ratios). Second, it was shown that fabric and orthotropic principal directions of trabecular bone are closely related (209). Although the coincidence of fabric and orthotropic principal axes, as well as the orthotropic elastic behavior itself, were generally assumed to be valid for a long time, it was not possible earlier to prove these assumptions.

Micro-FEAs were also used to elucidate the role of trabecular bone structure for its strength (133,201,202). In these studies, a specific strain-dependent yield criterion was specified for the bone tissue. Micro-FEA models of bone specimens were then loaded by a stepwise-increasing external force and the local loading conditions calculated at each step. As soon as the local strains exceeded the yield strain, a reduction of bone stiffness resulted, according to the prescribed yield criterion. At the apparent level, the yielding of bone tissue resulted in loss of stiffness, and the apparent stress-strain curve started to deviate from linear. Recent studies showed that this micro-FEA approach can accurately predict the compressive and tensile strengths, and failure strains, of bovine specimens. For this purpose, asymmetric tissue yield strains, with a higher yield strain for compression than for tension—typical of cortical bone—must be implemented (201).

A unique feature of the micro-FEA technique is that a specimen can be tested to failure multiple times, something that is clearly impossible with laboratory experiments. This enabled the development of a multiaxial failure criterion, which then can be tested against a small set of laboratory experiments. In a recent study,

Niebur et al. (200) investigated the biaxial failure behavior of bovine tibial bone and found that the biaxial yield properties were best described by independent curves for on-axis and transverse loading. Presently, these techniques are used for the development of a complete multi-axial failure criterion for human trabecular bone. Results obtained thus far indicated that trabecular bone has almost uncoupled failure behavior along its three main axes, leading to a failure envelope that is nearly cuboid in shape (6,7). Such uncoupling of yield behavior is indicative of bone adaptive isolation of the effects of damage from non-habitual loading, such as a fall. Such behavior will allow healing, while preserving nearly intact material properties along habitual loading directions.

2.4.2 Micro-FEA for Improved Strength Diagnoses

The application of micro-FEA techniques to analyze bone *in vivo* is complicated by the limited resolution of images that can be obtained from people. Presently, only peripheral quantitative ; computer tomography (pQCT) and MRI techniques can produce high-resolution images of bone *in vivo*, albeit with a resolution that is less than generally required for micro-FEA models. In a number of validation studies, it was found that micro-FEA with models based on pQCT and MR images can provide accurate results when care is taken that elements in the resulting micro-FEA model are well connected to each other and that the load-carrying bone mass is preserved (105,221,268).

Using a pQCT scanner, Ulrich et al. (266) were able to generate a micro-FEA model of the distal radius of a young healthy volunteer. After solving this model for external loading conditions representing a fall, they found that regions for which high bone tissue loading was calculated corresponded well with the regions in which typical collus-type fractures occur. In a follow-up study, Pistoia et al. (222) used the same pQCT scanner and the same FEA approach to analyze the distal radii of 20 post-mortem arms (Fig. 4-13). After imaging, these arms were

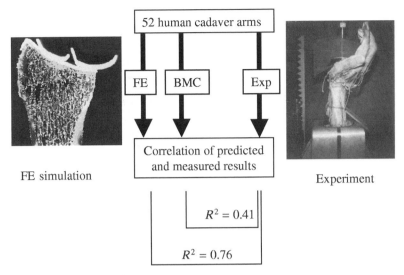

FIGURE 4-13. Mechanical imaging of bone strength: The strength of the radius bone was measured experimentally and then correlated with its apparent density and with the elastic properties obtained with a micro-FEA model. Micro-FEA gives a more dependable prediction for bone strength than bone density (Adapted from Pistoia et al. Estimation of distal radius failure load with micro-finite element analysis models based on three-dimensional peripheral quantitative computed tomography images. *Bone* 2002;30:842–848.)

compressed in a testing machine and the loads at which the first signs of fracture occurred were measured. They found a fairly good correlation between the fracture load measured in experiments for each of the 54 cadaver arms and a predicted fracture load, based on micro-FEA calculated tissue loading ($R^2 = 0.75$). The fact that this correlation was higher than the correlation between fracture load and bone density ($R^2 = 0.48$) indicates that micro-FEA can improve on estimates of bone fracture risk.

Recently, micro-FEA based on *in vivo* MR images was introduced in longitudinal clinical trial studies to investigate the efficacy of drugs for the treatment of osteoporosis (282). In this study a total of 56 patients was subdivided in a group that received a new drug for the treatment of osteoporosis (idoxifene) and an untreated group. High-resolution MR images were made at baseline and after 1 year. Micro-FEA models were made to estimate elastic properties of cubic volumes of interest from radius and calcaneus. The results of these analyses indicated changes in elastic properties of bone *in vivo* between baseline

and 1 year, which could not be detected from changes in volume fraction. It is presently investigated if the results of such analyses are sensitive and accurate enough to enhance the evaluation of treatment efficacy.

2.4.3 Stresses and Strains at the Bone Tissue Level

Another application in this field is mechanical imaging of stresses and strains at the level of the bone tissue. There are several reasons why stresses and strains at this level are so interesting. First, these are the stresses that are sensed by the bone cells. Hence, stresses and strains at these levels directly govern load adaptive bone modeling and remodeling processes. Second, because bone fractures are initiated at the level of the bone tissue, knowledge about stresses and strains at this level could enhance predictions of bone fractures. Third, based on "Wolff's law" it is generally assumed that, in the healthy situation, bone tissue is loaded rather uniformly. Knowledge about the magnitude and distribution of

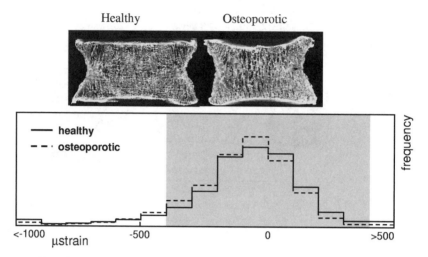

FIGURE 4-14. 'Mechanical' imaging of bone strength: Three-dimensional micro-FEA models were constructed from 2 post-mortem lumbar vertebral bodies, one with normal bone density and one with osteoporotic bone density. The (vertical) loads for the micro-FEA evaluations were scaled to the body weights of the persons concerned. The results show that the predicted strain distributions in the trabeculi hardly differ. This suggests that the trabecular densities were simply adapted to mechanical usage. Note that in the osteoporotic vertebra the horizontal trabeculi in particular have thinned, so that this person's bone could easily fail due to 'error' loads. This example nicely illustrates that (disuse) osteoporosis is not a disease, but rather the result of a normal load-adaptive process. (Adapted from Homminga et al. The osteoporotic vertebral structure is well adapted to the loads of daily life, but not to infrequent "error" loads. *Bone* 2004;34:510–516. ref. 108.)

tissue-level stresses and strains could help to decide whether a bone is healthy or osteoporotic.

To quantify healthy and osteoporotic load distributions, van Rietbergen et al. (280) calculated bone tissue-level stresses in the femoral head of a healthy and an osteoporotic post-mortem femur. It was found that the average strain in the healthy femur was 304 μstrain and in the osteoporotic femur 520 μstrain. Calculated safety factors of 8.6 for the healthy and 4.9 for the osteoporotic femur also demonstrated that the former was much stronger. It is interesting that the average stresses and strains calculated for the healthy human femur were very similar to those calculated earlier for a canine femur (283), suggesting that stresses and strains in trabeculae might be similar among species.

Homminga et al. (108) used a similar approach to determine stresses and strains in the bone tissue of both a healthy vertebral body and an osteoporotic vertebral body (Fig. 4-14). In this study, however, very similar tissue-level stresses and strains were found for both cases. This was due to the fact that, although it had much less bone tissue, the osteoporotic bone managed to organize all its material in the predominant loading orientation. A consequence of this behavior is that the osteoporotic bone would be prone to failure for loads applied in nonhabitual directions.

Recently, a new mechanical imaging concept was developed, enabling the calculation of strains in bone tissue without assuming its material properties (287). For this purpose high-resolution imaging is used to create three-dimensional reconstructions of bone samples in both the unloaded and loaded states. By correlating these three-dimensional reconstructions, it is possible to determine deformations throughout the bone tissue. Presently, this method can only produce accurate results if the deformations are rather large ($>1\%$), implying strains in the post-yield region.

3 BONE MECHANOBIOLOGY— MODELING, REMODELING, AND ADAPTATION

Skeletal gestation, growth, development and maintenance are intricately choreographed processes involving many cell and tissue types. During growth in the embryo, the long bones initially form as mesenchymal condensations, which chondrify to become cartilaginous anlagen. As development progresses, the cartilage cells—*chondrocytes*—hypertrophy and their extracellular matrices mineralize, forming the primary ossification center. The chondrocytes die by apoptosis and the mineralized cartilage is modeled to bone by the coordinated activity of bone-forming cells—*osteoblasts*—and bone-resorbing cells—*osteoclasts*. Most osteoblasts continue to produce extracellular matrix and become trapped within the matrix as *osteocytes*. Other osteoblasts close off the bone surface as *lining cells*. The cycle of chondrocyte hypertrophy, extracellular mineralization, chondrocyte apoptosis, and bone formation proceeds spatially from the middiaphysis toward the epiphyses. In some bones, as the primary center progresses axially, secondary centers form that mineralize through the same endochondral process. The growth plate is where the two growth fronts meet. Longitudinal growth at the growth plate occurs through chondrocyte division and hypertrophy, and continues until skeletal maturity. Concurrently, radial diaphyseal growth occurs through direct apposition of bone by osteoblasts on the periosteal surface and resorption by osteoclasts on the endosteal surface. In parallel with the formation of the mineralized skeleton, layers of cartilage at the joint surfaces develop into articular cartilage and fibrous anlagen develop into tendons and ligaments. Joints form at the interzones between the cartilage anlagen. The premise of mechanobiology is that these biological processes are regulated by sig-nals to cells generated by mechanical loading, a concept dating back to Roux (235). The relevant questions include how external and muscle loads are transferred to the tissues, how the cells sense these loads, and how the signals are translated into the cascade of biochemical reactions to produce cell expression or differentiation.

The process of cartilage differentiation and bone development continues in the mature organism during bone regeneration in fracture healing (Chapter 13) and during skeletal adaptation to implants (Chapter 14). These processes again involve tissue differentiation from granulation through fibrous connective tissue and cartilage to bone. The differentiation pathway from granulation tissue to cartilage is a gradual process that can be influenced over time. Mineralization, however, is a "catastrophic[2] event," occurring almost instantly and irreversibly (255, 256). This event transforms the mechanical and morphological status of the tissue dramatically and completely; not a single chondrocyte survives.

After ossification, bone differentiation continues within the tissue. Osteoclasts and osteoblasts now build the characteristic microstructures of cortical or cancellous bone tissue. This process of structural modulation and growth is called *modeling* (73). Mechanics also modulates the bone modeling process, as evident from the trabecular patterns that line up with external forces, suggesting an optimized structure of minimal weight and maximal strength (296,297). After the tissue has matured, osteoclast resorption and subsequent osteoblast formation continually maintain bone, in a process called *remodeling* (73). One purpose of this process is the removal of microcracks and microdamage (286), hence the term "maintenance." Osteoclasts are believed to be attracted by microcracks, through the apoptosis of osteocytes (203). At maturity, bone modeling continues

---

[2] A "catastrophic event" implies a sudden, violent change in the conditions of a system, in a time frame that is almost infinitely small compared with a typical time constant for that system.

due to variations in physical activity; exercise enhances bone mass, while inactivity reduces it. In the elderly, osteoporosis can develop, the etiology of which is also thought to be affected by mechanobiology. Finally, the development of osteoarthrosis in the elderly may be related to mechanical loading as well.

To understand how a mechanical stimulus produces a biological signal for cells to differentiate or adapt a tissue, we need to understand the relevant stimuli, the signal transduction pathways and the response processes (62). As in many sciences, the integration of experimental and analytical models is critical to gaining an understanding of the skeletal response to mechanical factors. Experiments provide insights and measures, which can then be interpreted within the context of analytical frameworks. Analytical simulations permit investigation of possible explanations that require *in vivo* validation and will suggest further experimental investigations. These investigations are greatly impacted by recent technological advances in imaging, computational mechanics, genetics, and molecular biology. The integration of these techniques can provide many important insights into skeletal development and diseases (276).

3.1 Bone Gestation

During embryonic development of long bones, cartilaginous tissue develops into bone tissue (Fig. 4-15). This endochondral ossification process passes the subsequent stages of chondrocyte proliferation, chondrocyte hypertrophy—which is primarily achieved by accumulation of water (20,216)—and mineralization of the cartilage matrix. The mineralization process starts in the primary ossification center, in the middle of the rudiment, extends toward the periphery and subsequently toward the distal ends of the bone. Matrix vesicles play an important role in the initiation of mineral deposition (141), but the actual mineralization process is a physical one, occurring in the extracellular matrix by deposition of a calcium phosphate. Mineralization proceeds very fast. In embryonic metatarsals of the mouse, for example, about one-fourth of the metatarsal is mineralized within 1 day (25,87,252, 279).

Development of bone

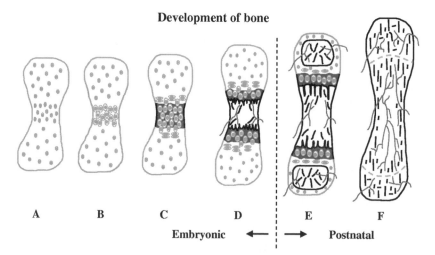

A   B   C   D   E   F

Embryonic ←⋮→ Postnatal

FIGURE 4-15. Schematic illustration of the development of long bones from embryonic to mature (figures not to scale). **(A)** Cartilaginous rudiment; **(B)** chondrocytes in the center swell; **(C)** cartilage mineralization occurs around hypertrophic chondrocytes, proliferating, flattened cells develop; **(D)** blood vessels penetrate the tissue, mineralized cartilage is resorbed, bone formation takes place, and longitudinal growth commences; **(E)** secondary ossification centers develop and growth plates remain in between; **(F)** the bone is mature, the growth plates are closed. (Adapted from Tanck et al. Increase in bone volume fraction precedes architectural adaptation in growing bone. *Bone* 2001;28:650–654.)

It was shown that cultures of metatarsals under microgravity conditions, i.e., during space flight, reduced mineralization compared with controls (279). It was also observed that the mineralization process in the metatarsals starts at 16 days of gestational age, just when the first muscle contractions in the feet occur (24,223). How are the external loads transferred to the cell level, and to which mechanical stimuli do they react? Several studies showed that mechanical stimulation influences chondrocyte metabolism (82,84,162,241,300). Evidence was found for the presence of stretch-activated membrane ion channels in articular chondrocytes, so that deformations may affect cell activity (300). Guilak et al. showed that cell deformation changes the Ca^{2+} concentration in the cytoplasm (84). Static compression of articular cartilage generally leads to dose-dependent reductions in cell activity, but the response to dynamic loading is not consistent (82). Dynamic *strains* applied to articular chondrocytes embedded in agarose increased chondrocyte proliferation (162). It was also shown that chondrocytes *in vitro* can alter their activities by changes in *osmotic pressure* (269,270), *fluid flow* (139,140), *hydrostatic pressure* (156,213,214,269,270), *electrical potential gradients* (69,139), and pH (81). All these signals are not necessarily independent. From these *in vitro* experiments it is clear that chondrocytes can react to many biophysical stimuli in their environment. It should be noted that *in vivo* cells are not isolated but embedded in a matrix, which affects cell activity. *In vivo*, loads are transferred to the cells through the matrix they are embedded in. The mechanical matrix properties determine in what form, relative to magnitudes and dynamic characteristics, they arrive at the cell. The effects of these attenuative mechanisms are not known. And then the question is still what property of the load, applied to the cell, stimulates the relevant cell activities: magnitude, velocity (frequency), energy, or only the resulting deformation.

Based on FEA results, Carter et al. (37,40) and Wong and Carter (298,299) proposed that cyclic shear stresses accelerate the endochondral ossification process, while dynamic hydrostatic pressure inhibits the process (see also Chapter 13 for alternative theories). For the combination of shear stress (S) and hydrostatic stress (D) they defined an "osteogenic index" as $I = S + kD$, in which k is an empirical constant. Using this rule, the start of secondary ossification centers could be predicted (40), indicating that the hypothesis could be true. In their FEA model, linear-elastic material properties were assumed for the cartilaginous tissue. As cartilage consists of a solid phase, mainly collagen and proteoglycans, and a fluid phase of interstitial water, biphasic or poroelastic FEA models (187), including both solid and fluid components, would produce more realistic information. The advantage of such models is also that, in addition to stresses and strains, variables like pressure gradients and interstitial fluid flow can be studied. The choice of using biphasic or linear-elastic FEA models for a particular analysis depends, of course, on the question or hypothesis for the study.

Example 3. Mechanical signals for enchondral ossification. Tanck et al. used poroelastic FEA models to study the effects of mechanical forces on cartilage mineralization effects found experimentally (254). From *in vitro* organ culture experiments, there were indications that cartilage mineralization is stimulated by mechanical loads. Loaded metatarsals had mineralized diaphyseal parts two to three times longer than those of the unloaded controls (143). Tanck et al. studied which factor was the most likely one to have stimulated the mineralization process in these *in vitro* experiments. *Distortional strains* occurred in the region where mineralization proceeded. Hence, distortional strain could have enhanced the mineralization process. Its value was, however, very sensitive to the intrinsic compressibility modulus of the solid matrix; for realistic values probably too small (about 2 μstrain) to have stimulated the mineralization. *Hydrostatic pressure* seemed the only candidate variable left to have enhanced the mineralization process.

In another study embryonic mouse metatarsal rudiments were cultured as whole organs, and the geometry of the primary ossification center was compared with rudiments that had developed in utero (252). The mineralization geometry in the presence of muscular forces differed from that *in vitro*, in the absence of muscular forces. Using FEA, the local distributions of distortional strain and fluid pressure at the mineralization front were calculated in the metatarsal as a result of muscle contraction in the embryonic hind limbs *in vivo*, but could not explain the difference in mineralization shape. The most likely candidate to explain the difference was the *distortional strain*, resulting from muscle contraction. These examples illustrate how studies designed to discover what variable determines tissue differentiation can provide different answers, depending on experimental design.

Shortly after the cartilage matrix is mineralized in the gestational bone phase the chondrocyte cells die by apoptosis (19). Blood vessels penetrate the tissue (Fig.15D), the mineralized cartilage is resorbed by osteoclasts, and bone tissue is formed by osteoblasts on remnants of mineralized cartilage. At the distal ends of the bone, the secondary ossification centers develop, in which the same cascade of processes takes place. These centers create the trabecular bone of the epiphyses. Between the primary and secondary ossification centers, cartilaginous growth plates remain, in which the endochondral ossification process continues. In this way, the lengths of bones increase. During growth to maturity, cell proliferation, matrix production, and cell swelling determine the longitudinal growth rate (114). At maturity, chondrocyte proliferation stops and the growth plates are closed. All cartilage is then replaced by bone tissue, except at the joint surfaces, where a layer of articular cartilage remains present.

In conclusion, the role of mechanics in cartilage mineralization is not fully explained yet, although combinations of animal experiments and FEAs produced promising results. If the role of mechanics in cartilage mineralization could be elucidated, the knowledge can be applied to fracture healing and implant incorporation as well because similar processes are involved (see also Chapters 13 and 14).

3.2 Bone Modeling and Remodeling—Adaptation and Maintenance

After new bone is formed from the growth plate toward the marrow cavity (Fig. 4-15E) the bone tissue on the remnants grows and subsequently fuses into a trabecular structure, initially consisting of woven bone. In that stage bone resorption hardly occurs, but later woven bone is replaced by lamellar trabecular bone, in which both resorption and formation take place. Frost (73) defined growth and development of the cortical and trabecular structures—and later morphological adaptation—as "modeling." The later stage of dynamic morphological equilibrium of the trabecular architecture (metabolic homeostasis), was defined as "remodeling." In contemporary biomechanics the term "remodeling" is often used to mean "adaptation." However, remodeling is definitely related to renewal—*maintenance*—of the bone matrix. Modeling, in Frost's theories, means morphological *adaptation*, as it occurs in growth or reactions to reduced and increased external loads.

The metabolic capacities of bone modeling and remodeling have several advantages, like the competence to repair itself, but also the ability to adapt to environmental changes. If the mechanical load increases by, for instance, increased physical activity, then bone mass increases (5). If, however, bed rest or immobilization decrease load, this leads to decreased bone mass (160). Not only bone mass, but also bone architecture adapts to external loads. In the adult stage, the trabeculae are aligned to the principal stress directions, as Wolff described it (296,297). In this way, trabecular bone is believed to be adapted to the typical–dynamic–external loads of daily living in both density and architecture.

3.2.1 Bone Maintenance—Remodeling

Bone remodeling (or maintenance) is the process of ongoing replacement of old bone by new. Its role is to maintain bone mechanical competence, as it prevents microdamage accumulating to structural failure. The remodeling process is expressed by bone-resorbing osteoclasts and bone-forming osteoblasts. It begins at a quiescent bone surface with the appearance of osteoclasts. These are large multinucleated cells that form by fusion of mononuclear precursors of haematopoietic origin (271). They attach to the bone tissue matrix and form a ruffled border at the bone/osteoclast interface that is completely surrounded by a "sealing" zone, creating an isolated microenvironment. The osteoclasts acidify the microenvironment and dissolve the organic and inorganic compounds of the bone (272). Briefly after the resorptive process stops, osteoblasts appear at the same surface site, derived from mesenchymal stem cells found in the bone marrow, periosteum, and soft tissues. These deposit osteoid and mineralize it to actually form new bone. Some of the osteoblasts are encapsulated in the osteoid matrix and differentiate to osteocytes. Others continue to synthesize bone until they eventually transform to quiescent lining cells that completely cover the newly formed bone surface. These lining cells are highly interconnected with the osteocytes in the bone matrix through a network of canaliculi (164).

It appears that osteoclasts and osteoblasts closely collaborate in the remodeling process, in what is called "basic multicellular units," or BMUs. This indicates that a coupling mecha-

nism must exist between formation and resorption (71). The organization of the BMUs in cortical and trabecular bone differs, but only in geometric parameters, not in a biological sense. In cortical bone a BMU forms a cylindrical canal about 2,000 μm long, on average, and 150–200 μm wide (Fig. 4-16). It gradually burrows through the bone at a speed of 20–40 μm/day. In its tip on the order of ten osteoclasts dig a circular tunnel (*cutting cone*). They are followed by several thousands of osteoblasts that fill the tunnel (*closing cone*) to produce a (secondary) osteon of renewed bone (211). Thus, between 2% and 5% of cortical bone is remodeled each year.

The remodeling process in trabecular bone is a surface event. Due to its large surface-to-volume ratio, trabecular bone is more actively remodeled than cortical bone, with remodeling rates up to ten times higher (161). Again osteoclasts appear, travel along the trabecular surface, but dig a trench rather than a tunnel, with depths of 40–60 μm. As in cortical bone, they are followed by osteoblasts forming bone (Fig. 4-17). Active remodeling sites cover areas of varying sizes from some 50×20 up to $1,000 \times 1,000 \, \mu m$ (183). The trabecular BMU can be regarded as half a cortical BMU. The resulting structure formed is called a trabecular osteon or hemiosteon (64,72).

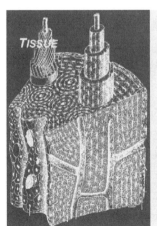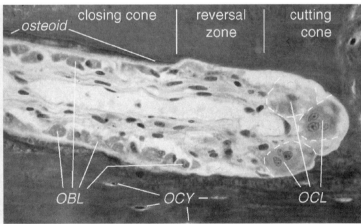

FIGURE 4-16. *Left*: Drawing of a cortical bone segment, indicating the circular, haversian osteons, produced as an effect of cortical remodeling. *Right*: Actual longitudinal section through a cortical remodeling canal. (From Schenk R, Willenegger H. On the histology of primary bone healing. *Langenbecks Arch Klin Chir Ver Deutsch Z Chir* 1964;308:440–452, with permission.)

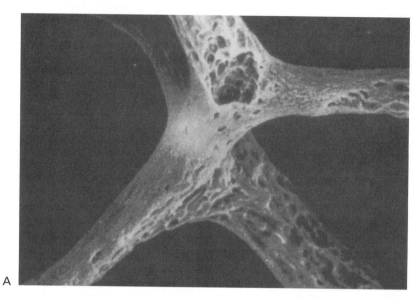

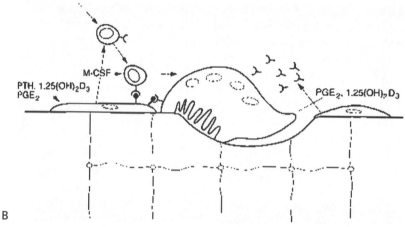

FIGURE 4-17. A: The photograph shows several trabecular resorption cavities. **B:** The artist impression shows trabecular surface resorption by an osteoclast, forming a resorption cavity. Lining cells are indicated on either side and osteocytes within the matrix. Biochemical signaling pathways are shown, as discussed in the text. (Courtesy of Dr. Chambers, UK.)

In recent years much information was obtained about the cell-signaling pathways through which osteoclasts are attracted from the marrow and activated in bone resorption (22,41,43). It is now established that cells of the osteoblast lineage, which express RANKL, are involved in maturation and activation of osteoclasts. Osteoclast precursors expressing RANK, a receptor for RANKL, recognize RANKL through direct cell-to-cell interaction and then differentiate to osteoclasts (127,264). Despite this information, it

is not known what triggers the onset of the remodeling processes. It is generally assumed that microcracks and damage, due to sustained mechanical usage, play an important role (26,182). It may be that osteoclast recruitment signals are initialized by lining cells when their communication with the osteocytic network is interrupted by mechanical damage or lack of mechanical "pumping" (22). Alternatively, it was hypothesized that osteoclast recruitment signals are generated by osteocytes or lining cells in case of microdamage in the bone matrix, or damage to the osteocytes themselves (203,246,285). A correlation was indeed found between microdamage, osteocyte apoptosis, and subsequent bone resorption sites (286). Once the remodeling process has been initiated, osteoclasts resorb bone in the dominant mechanical loading direction. This was concluded from the observation that osteons are aligned to that direction (219). The pathways along which external forces are translated to local osteoclast activity are unknown, however.

Another unresolved issue is what couples bone formation to resorption. It was suggested that this coupling mechanism has a biochemical origin. During the resorption phase, growth factors like TGF-β are released. These factors are potent stimulators of osteoblast bone formation and thus may couple formation to resorption (16,196). However, it was also suggested that coupling finds its origin in mechanical factors (233). Local stress concentrations, surrounding resorption lacunae, may initiate signals from the osteocytic network to stimulate bone formation. That osteocyte processes are in contact with bone-forming osteoblasts supports this hypothesis, but also the observation that lack of mechanical loading uncouples formation from resorption, makes the hypothesis plausible (183).

3.2.2 Bone Adaptation—modeling

It has long been known that bones adapt to the functional mechanical requirements to which they are exposed. Reduced mobility and lack of gravity cause osteoporosis-loss of bone mass. Excessive training increases bone mass, bones affected by trauma outgrow their maldeformities, and teeth subjected to abnormal external forces migrate through the jaw bone. This principle of functional adaptation in bones became known as Wolff's law (297), illustrated in Fig. 4-18. Many orthopaedic surgical procedures are based on its workings, as they have as their main objective "...to restore musculoskeletal function by creating the mechanical and biological environment in the musculoskeletal tissues which allows them to heal, adapt and maintain

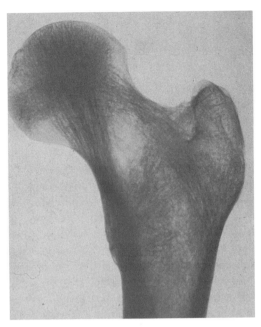

FIGURE 4-18. Radiograph of the hip, showing the typical density distributions of trabecular patterns and cortical shells. This, by itself, intuitively associates bone morphology with mechanical optimality, as Wolff (296) understood it.

themselves"; Wolff's law is a significant factor for reaching that goal.

At maturity, trabecular bone mass and architecture are adapted to the typical external loads of daily living. Little quantitative data are available on the development of architecture and mechanical adaptation in juvenile trabecular bone. Using radiographs and digital imaging, Korstjens et al. (148) analyzed the two-dimensional trabecular patterns of the distal radius in children, ages 4 to 14 years. Their study showed that the refined trabecular patterns of young children had coarsened in the older ones. Nafei et al. (197,198) analyzed trabecular bone in epiphyseal proximal tibiae of immature and mature sheep. Using mechanical tests and serial sectioning, they found that architectural and mechanical properties changed significantly with skeletal maturity. A study in rats showed that the highest bone formation rates were present directly after birth (249). From there on, the formation rates decreased continuously with increasing age in both epiphysis and metaphysis, whereby formation rates were higher than resorption rates during the first 150 days of age. The development of micro-computed tomography (micro-CT) made it possible to analyze the three-dimensional architecture of trabecular bone accurately (67).

Example 4. Using micro-CT, the development of trabecular structure during growth in pigs was investigated (253). Pigs between 6 and 230 weeks of age, and between 12 and 212 kg of body weight, were used. During growth, body weight, hence load, increased gradually, which implies that density and architecture would change as well. As an increase in trabecular density due to increased loading would only have to involve bone formation, but the adaptation of trabecular architecture must involve both formation and resorption, we hypothesized that there is a time lag between these processes during the development. To test this hypothesis, three-dimensional morphological and mechanical parameters of trabecular bone samples from the vertebra and proximal tibia were studied using micro-CT and micro-FEA (253).

The results of the micro-CT showed clear differences in trabecular structure with age (Fig. 4-19). For the youngest bones, the structure was refined, whereas in older bones it had developed into a much coarser trabecular structure. The three-dimensional morphological parameters showed that the bone volume fraction (BV/TV) increased rapidly in the initial growth phase, whereas the morphological anisotropy started increasing somewhat later during the development (Fig. 4-20).

In addition, the maximal value of BV/TV was reached earlier in time than the maximal value of anisotropy. The development of stiffness, resulting from the micro-FEA calculations, could be explained by the combined development of volume fraction and anisotropy (Fig. 4-20). As stiffness and strength are highly correlated (132), trabecular bone also becomes stronger during growth. Interestingly, BV/TV and total body weight did not exactly follow the same trend: although total body weight reached a maximum at 104 weeks of age (Table C.1), BV/TV reached its maximum at 56 weeks of age (Fig. 4-20). Adaptation of the trabecular architecture to the weight increase between 6 and 56 weeks of age could be explained by the increase in BV/TV. Between 56 and 104 weeks of age, adaptation of the trabecular architecture to the weight increase could be explained by the increase in anisotropy, i.e., that the trabeculae aligned to the primary loading direction. By increasing the anisotropy and decreasing, or stabilizing, the trabecular density, the trabecular structure becomes more efficient to resist load in the primary loading direction. We concluded that the hypothesis was supported by the time lag between the increase in trabecular density and the adaptation of the trabecular architecture (253).

This is an example of the versatility of micro-CT in bone research. It also elucidates the role

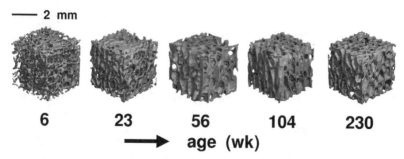

FIGURE 4-19. Micro-CT images of 2 × 2 × 2 mm trabecular bone cubes, taken from the tibial epiphyses of pigs at ages 6 weeks through 230 weeks. Initially, many thin trabeculae, unorganized in directionality, preside. In the course of time they reduce in number, become thicker and orient themselves in the (vertical) predominant loading direction. (Adapted from Tanck et al. Increase in bone volume fraction precedes architectural adaptation in growing bone. *Bone* 2001; 28:650–654.)

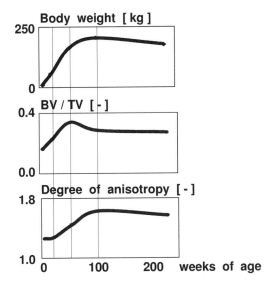

FIGURE 4-20. Results of measurements performed on series of micro-CT images of tibial, epiphyseal bone cubes from growing pigs (see Fig. 4-19.) There is an obvious increase of body weight between 6 and 230 weeks of age. Trabecular density (BV/TV) increases sharply in early youth, reaches a peak around 50 weeks, and then stabilizes at a somewhat lower value. Degree of anisotropy peaks at around 100 weeks. It is thought that the overshot in density reflects the addition of bone mass occurring much faster than reorientation of trabecular structure, which illustrates the role of mechanical loading in morphological adaptation. (Adapted from Tanck et al. Increase in bone volume fraction precedes architectural adaptation in growing bone. *Bone* 2001; 28:650–654.)

mechanical loading has, or can have, in the maturation of the skeleton. In the next section its role in adaptation of the mature skeleton is discussed. Although, in our minds, maturity is for the skeleton not really a new phase, but rather a continuation of the force-adaptive processes already evident in early childhood.

3.3 Experimental and Computational Studies of Mechanical Bone Adaptation

3.3.1 Animal Models and Theories for Mechanical Bone Adaptation

In order to be adapted to external loads, in mass and structure, bone requires a load sensorial capacity in the form of "mechanosensors." This function could be located in the bone matrix itself, or in the bone cells. Potential strain-mechanosensory mechanisms in the bone matrix are piezoelectricity and streaming potentials (146,220), but presently the mechanosensory function is thought to reside in bone cells. The permanent cells in bone are osteocytes and lining cells. Osteoblasts and osteoclasts are attracted to the bone from the marrow, and responsible for bone formation and resorption, respectively. In other words, they are able to change bone mass and bone architecture, but cannot be the sensors that initiate these processes. They are both attracted to and active at the bone surface. Some of the osteoblasts become osteocytes when encapsulated by the bone matrix they produce. Others cover the new bone matrix as lining cells. Osteocytes are matured osteoblasts, surrounded by calcified bone. The osteocytes in the bone matrix are regularly distributed throughout the bone. They are connected to each other and to the lining cells at the bone surface by their canalicular processes. Through this canalicular network, nutrients can be transported from the lining cells to the osteocytes and vice versa. In addition, biochemical products can be transported between the osteocytes, and from osteocytes to lining cells. With these properties, osteocytes would be excellent candidates to serve as the mechanosensors of bone (23,143). Many experiments were performed and several theories developed to test this hypothesis. Mechanical strain is an important regulator of bone homeostasis, but the mechanism whereby bone tissue detects the strain, and how this results in anabolic or catabolic responses, is only partially understood (21).

Skerry et al. (246) found an increased enzyme activity of osteocytes following bone loading *in vivo*. This increase was proportional to the strain magnitude in the bone tissue. Weinbaum et al. (293) proposed that *in vivo* strains in the calcified matrix could be sensed by the osteocytes through small fluid shear stresses. Bone fluid flows through the bone pores, which are filled with a proteoglycan matrix (54,293). The combination of bone fluid and matrix is thought to function as a gel, which acts on the membranes of the osteocytic processes. The intracellular actin cytoskeleton could also amplify the deformation of osteocytes by fluid drag forces (304). Klein-Nulend et al. (142) studied the effect of pulsating fluid flow and intermittent hydrostatic pressure on isolated osteocytes, osteoblasts, and periosteal fibroblasts. Pulsating fluid flow increased the prostaglandin E_2 production of the osteocytes, whereas osteoblasts and fibroblasts did not react to the applied flow. The effects of hydrostatic pressure were less pronounced; osteocytes as well as osteoblasts reacted to hydrostatic pressure, although the production of prostaglandin was less, relative to the reaction of osteocytes to fluid flow. It was concluded that osteocytes were the most mechano-sensitive cells in bone, reacting most profoundly to pulsating fluid flow (142). Jacobs et al. (120) tested the effects of oscillating and pulsating fluid flows on bone cells with 0.5, 1.0, and 2.0 Hz frequencies. They showed that oscillating and pulsating flow were both stimulatory to bone cells and that dynamic flows became less stimulatory with increasing frequency. Oscillating flow was less stimulatory than pulsing flow, suggesting that different cellular mechanisms could be involved in these flow modalities (120). The effects of load-induced fluid flow were observed and quantified after four-point bending tests on rat tibiae *in vivo* by Knothe-Tate et al. (145). Mechanical loading enhanced the transport of small and large molecular mass tracers, but the small molecules showed the fastest transport through the tissue. These results indicated that mechanical loading is able to modulate the distribution and concentration of bone-fluid tracers within the tissue. In summary, strain-induced fluid flow is a prominent candidate for the primary stimulus for osteocyte mechanosensation.

Bone adaptation was studied using a wide variety of experimental models. Approaches used to increase loading include exercise, osteotomy, and devices to apply controlled loading (14,47). Decreased loading was achieved by casting, neurectomy, hind-limb suspension, or space flight (180,265,288). Several common concepts emerged from the past century of *in vivo* experimentation. Bone adaptation occurs in response to cyclic not static loading. The outcome mainly changes cortical bone quantity, not quality. Cancellous adaptation is less well characterized but has a similar response, present as changes in the tissue apparent density. In general, demonstrating a definitive increase in bone mass or strength is more difficult than demonstrating a loss. Increased bone mass and strength are also harder to achieve with physiological than with non-physiological loading conditions. Finally, the adaptive response is generally greater in growing than in mature animals, but growth may have confounded the results of the experiments.

Precise quantitative predictions of the skeletal response to mechanical stimuli are often desirable, but currently impossible to generate. Much of our inability to predict adaptation arises from experimental logistics: Until recently, most skeletal functional adaptation experiments could not identify the driving feature of the mechanical stimulus, or the contributing elements of the response pathways (62). For example, when the loading environment is altered by exercise and a skeletal effect is observed, does the response result from the increased applied forces, the increased numbers of loading cycles, the increased loading rates, another exercise-induced parameter, or a combination of these and other factors? Can one design an exercise study to distinguish these features of the stimulus? Increasing bone mass and strength with *in vivo* physiological loading, such as exercise, is notoriously difficult. Exercise studies produced contradictory results: Running chickens at one speed was shown to increase cortical area and moments of inertia (15), while running for a longer duration at a similar intensity suppressed bone growth and reduced strength over a similar experimental period (174). Differences from one skeletal site to the next, within the same animal, were also found in these studies (163). Whether these differences were caused by differences in the local mechanical environment or by fundamentally different adaptive responses is unknown. Answering these questions experimentally is difficult, because the *in vivo* loads cannot be measured directly. In adult animals, physiological exercise generally produced bone hypertrophy or no response. The absence of a response may indicate that the exercise protocol did not sufficiently elevate the loads above habitual levels.

These unknowns all point toward the need for a better understanding of the applied mechanical loads.

To improve the effectiveness of studies for identifying the mechanical stimulus underlying bone adaptation, noninvasive experimental models were developed recently, which control the stimulus applied to cortical diaphyses (83,186,259,261). Most commonly used are the ulnar compression model of Lanyon and coworkers (Fig. 4-21) and the tibial four-point bending approach developed by Turner and colleagues. The ulnar compression model likely creates more physiological stresses and strains within the bone and has load application points that are farther from the point of interest than the tibial four-point bending model. Both models were initially developed for the rat and were modified for the mouse (2,70). Neither model requires surgery, as previous controlled loading models often did (47,100,236). In both systems, dynamic loads are applied and load magnitude, rate, number of cycles, and duration are well controlled. These noninvasive models, combined with increased computing power, higher resolution imaging, and new molecular and genetic techniques enable systematic evaluation of loading parameters to understand the nature of the

osteogenic stimuli and pathways. For the cortical diaphysis, stimuli characteristics that induce bone modeling are becoming evident: The applied strain rates and magnitudes need to be high (185,186); the strain rate contributes to the morphology of the bone formed (263); distinct, temporally separated loading episodes are required, not just increased numbers of loading cycles (232); and gender and genetic background influence the nature of the response (2,217).

Similar questions need to be examined in cancellous bone, a site of more clinical relevance than the cortical diaphyses. Applying controlled loading to cancellous bone is more difficult than to the cortical diaphyses. Trabecular bone adaptation models include direct stimulation of the site of interest as well as in encapsulating bone chambers (42,79,85,103,133,155). Nearly all models require surgical intervention at the trabecular site; the rat-tail vertebra model is an exception because only the adjoining vertebral bodies are operated on. Systematic application of dynamic loading needs to be performed to address the same questions as posed above for cortical bone. For example, the rodent ulna model can presumably be extended to also examine cancellous bone, and perhaps also the response of the cartilage in the growth plate to mechanical loading.

Compared with questions about the nature of the stimulus, even less is known regarding the transduction of osteogenic signals to stimulate bone formation or resorption. This pathway is hard to delineate, particularly when using *in vivo* models. However, recent molecular advances allow examination of whether individual genes and molecules contribute to the adaptation pathways. The mouse provides a unique opportunity to examine genetic factors through manipulation of murine embryonic stem cells and because significant portions of the genome were characterized (48). Transgenic technology led to the creation of both knockout and transgenic animals, either missing or overexpressing genes, and previously recorded natural mutations can now be identified. One can now directly determine whether a given protein is important to skeletal adaptation by removing it. Transgenic

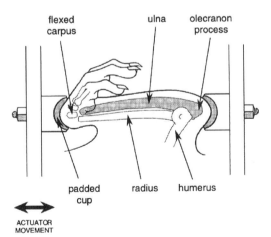

FIGURE 4-21. Artist interpretation of the ulnar compression model, used by several laboratories to investigate strain-related bone mass adaptation. (From Mosley JR, Lanyon LE. Strain rate as a controlling influence on adaptive modeling in response to dynamic loading of the ulna in growing male rats. *Bone*1998;23:313–318.)

technology allows the role of potential regulatory factors (65), cell surface receptors (306), and matrix constituents (138) to be examined.

Increasingly, mouse genetic studies are demonstrating extreme redundancy within the genome under normal conditions; simply characterizing the normal phenotype may be unrevealing or insufficient. However, manipulating the system by changing the applied loads can require cellular/tissue adaptation above and beyond normal development and can demonstrate significant phenotypic effects. Examples include the osteopontin-knockout mouse and the bone morphogenetic protein-5–deficient *short ear* mouse. The former has no obvious phenotype, but does not lose bone when subjected to hindlimb suspension (116). The phenotype of the latter is an overall reduced body size, and these mice respond to increased loads more slowly than heterozygous controls (179,274). Unfortunately, developing transgenic or knockout mice and examining all potential regulatory factors will consume many research careers. However, further strengths of these genetic models will become evident when we start to examine genetic control of skeletal responses by not only expression but also linkage analyses (8,144, 303).

In summary, many questions remain regarding the role of mechanics in the formation and adaptation of skeletal tissues. For functional adaptation, we need global descriptions of adaptive responses at different skeletal sites and ages, for example. To do so requires understanding the nature of an osteogenic mechanical stimulus and characterizing the molecular pathway this stimulus activates. More generally, in skeletal tissue formation these same questions apply focused on the mechanical stimuli that induce cell and tissue differentiation. Answering these questions will require carefully controlled experiments with well-characterized mechanical environments.

When designing and interpreting experiments, consideration must be given to contributing factors, including the type of model (*in vitro* or *in vivo*), species, type of loading (physiological or invasive), the nature of loading (tension/compression, cyclic/static, controlled/

natural, etc.), and level of analysis (cell, organ, or tissue level).

3.3.2 Computational Models and Theories for Mechanical Bone Adaptation

One could say that Wolff's law (296,297) was already based on the comparison between trabecular morphology and the results of a computational analysis, i.e., graphic statics (109). Modern developments in biomechanics started with the "theory of adaptive elasticity" for cortical bone (53), which was later used for an FEA simulation model by Hart et al. (93). These studies examined the adaptation of cortical form to external forces. Alternative theories were proposed and used by Huiskes et al. (111), Mattheck (175), Prendergast & Taylor (225), van der Meulen et al. (275), and Martin (173). Adaptation of (trabecular) bone density was simulated by several groups, using different isotropic (9,10,36,111,291,292) or anisotropic theories (94,119,169). Hart (92) wrote an excellent historical overview of these theories and computational models.

These trabecular computational models were phenomenological in nature and simulated the outcome of coordinated osteoclast and osteoblast activities as either a net increase or decrease in apparent density. Hence, the simulations implied an optimization of bone density distributions, with a local mechanical-loading variable— e.g., strain, stress, strain-energy density—as input. This does imply the use of recursive mathematical formulas, as each change in density would automatically change the distributions of local stress and strain—hence, optimization. Such computer simulation studies can have their uses for predicting bone density—hence, strength—adaptations around orthopaedic implants, in preclinical testing (137), discussed in Chapter 14. They can also be used to estimate net trabecular bone loss due to reduced mechanical loading in disuse. However, they are useless for basic research in bone physiology because they lack realistic descriptions of bone cell biology. A more mechanistic approach is necessary to represent the true physiology of the adaptation process, which occurs only on trabecular surfaces and is executed by osteoclasts and osteoblasts. Only if they are included in the workings of a simulation theory can biological mechanisms be considered.

Later, theories and computational models were developed for trabecular bone that came closer to the biological reality. Adachi et al. (1) proposed a phenomenological adaptation model for the trabecular structure using nonuniformity of the local surface stress distribution as the regulatory feedback signal, but does include parameters that tie the process to bone physiological parameters. A theory to simulate local trabecular adaptation based on surface metabolism only, that also includes a biological osteocyte-mechanosensory and signaling function, was developed by Mullender and Huiskes (189). A later theory that also includes separate descriptions of osteoclast resorption and osteoblast formation, enabling simulation of mechanobiologically modulated growth, adaptation, and maintenance (remodeling) was published recently (110,239). These developments are discussed in more detail below.

3.3.3 Bone Density Controlled by Mechanical Factors

In the work of Fyhrie and Carter (74) bone tissue was considered as a continuum, characterized by apparent density distributions. It was assumed to be a self-optimizing material with the objective to adapt its apparent density ρ to an "effective stress" σ_{eff}. Based on strength or strain optimization criteria, they derived

$$\rho = A\sigma_{eff}^{\alpha}, \tag{12}$$

where A and α are constants, and the effective stress is determined from either a failure or an elastic energy criterion. In later publications (31,74) they assumed $\alpha = 0.5$ and for the effective stress they postulated

$$\sigma_{eff}^2 = 2EU, \tag{13}$$

where E is the apparent elastic modulus and U the apparent strain-energy density (SED). By assuming a modulus-density relation of $E = c\rho^3$ (35), with c a constant, the optimization

function transforms to

$$\rho = c'U, \tag{14}$$

where c' is a constant. Applying this optimization criterion allowed predictions of density distributions in the proximal femur assumed optimal (31,74). To test the theory they visually compared the resulting density patterns with those in radiograms of a real femur, and observed similarities.

Originally, bone density was described as adapting toward reference states of deformation caused by single loads. To incorporate variable loading, a stimulus S was defined that took account of individual loading configurations by averaging their individual contributions (36), as

$$S = \frac{1}{n}\frac{1}{\rho}\sum_{i=1}^{n} U_i, \tag{15}$$

where U_i is the SED value for loading case i, n the total number of loading cases, and ρ the apparent density. In order to estimate the actual SED values in the trabeculae the remodeling signal was approximated by U/ρ as the strain energy per unit of bone mass (36).

3.3.4 Pattern Formation

In 1992, Weinans et al. (291) applied this theory to a two-dimensional finite element model of a proximal femur. Bone was represented as a continuum, capable of adapting its apparent density due to mechanical stimulation. The stimulus value S was measured per element, and the apparent density ρ was adapted per element according to

$$d\rho/dt = B(S - k), \tag{16}$$

with B and k constants and S the stimulus value in the element. This theory produced density distributions that showed good resemblance with those in a real proximal femur. However, this became only visible if these distributions were locally averaged from discontinuous density patterns in trabecular bone (Fig. 4-22). In fact, the underlying patchwork of either full or empty elements is inadmissible relative to the mathematical basis of FEA. However,

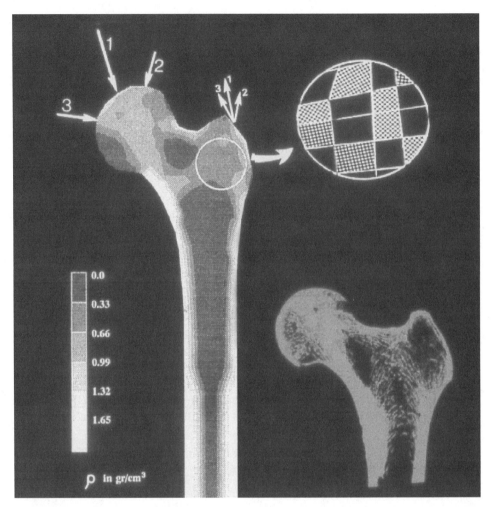

FIGURE 4-22. Applied to a two-dimensional femur FEA model, starting from a uniform density distribution, the simulation model of Weinans et al. (282) produced density distributions similar to those in a real femur. However, the density results were computationally smoothed from a patchwork of full (maximal density) and empty (zero density) elements. This phenomenon, that makes the results of the FEA-computation invalid, is called 'checkerboarding.' An adaptation algorithm that regulates density for each element separately, which makes the elements mutually 'compete,' causes this. This formulation, besides computationally unstable, is also unrealistic. In reality, strain sensation is likely to be an osteocyte function, away from the osteoclast and osteoblast locations. This was implemented in a new theory (189,192).

Weinans et al. (292) also showed that it is in the nature of the differential equations used to mathematically describe the adaptive remodeling process that the simulation produces discontinuous end-configurations, a phenomenon called "checkerboarding." Using an analytical two-unit model they showed that the differential equations have an unstable uniform solution and that the slightest non-uniformity causes stress shielding by the stiffer elements.

Hence, in the ongoing process the stiffer elements will even become stiffer, while the others lose density, until they are virtually empty, so that a "checkerboard" results (Fig. 4-22). This phenomenon is the result of capturing both sensation of the local mechanical stimulus and actual adaptation of bone mass in that same location, in one equation, which make the elements—which are artifacts for biology—work for themselves.

3.3.5 Osteocyte Mechanosensation

Besides being mathematically unstable, the previous theory was also biologically naïve because osteoblasts and osteoclasts, the bone production and removal cells, do not reside within the bone, but only appear at the trabecular surface as an effect of mechanical signals, which must be sensed within the bone matrix. Hence, sensation of mechanical stimuli and adaptation of material properties should be separated in the theory, as was shown by Mullender et al. (188–193). Osteocytes within the tissue matrix were assumed to be mechanosensitive and capable of translating signals to the bone surface to attract so-called basic multicellular units (BMUs) (i.e., osteoclasts and osteoblasts, the actor cells of bone biology), which control the net apposition or removal of bone tissue. The signal sent to the surface by an osteocyte was assumed to decay exponentially with increasing distance d (mm), according to

$$f(x, x') = e^{-d(x,x')/D}, \qquad (17)$$

where x is the location in which the signal strength is determined, x' is the location of the osteocyte concerned, and D (mm) determines the decay in signal strength. The relative density m (-) at location x was regulated by the BMUs. Relative to the total amount of stimulus P in that location they adapt bone density according to

$$dm(x, t)/dt = \tau P(x, t), \qquad (18)$$

where τ (MPa^{-1}·s^{-1}) is a rate constant. All osteocytes N located within the region surrounding x contribute to the stimulus P, so that its value in x is determined by

$$p(x, t) = \sum_{i=1}^{N} f(x, x_i)(S(x_i, t) - k), \qquad (19)$$

where x_i is the location of osteocyte i, $S_{(x_i, t)}$ is the mechanical signal this osteocyte senses, and k is a reference value.

Although hypothetical, the mechanosensory role of osteocytes is not controversial. Osteocytes are shown to be sensitive to mechanical loading. They derive from osteoblasts that are encapsulated in the tissue matrix they produce. They are interconnected by a network of canaliculi that seems perfectly equipped for signal transmission (22).

A two-dimensional computational model was developed to test this theory, applied at a microscopic level to a square plate of 2×2 mm^2, divided in 80×80 elements. The separation of sensation and density adaptation into two different functions prevented the so-called checkerboarding phenomenon. The theory produced configurations with characteristics that resemble actual trabecular bone structures, with average density correlating to the loading magnitude and trabecular orientation directly related to the external loading direction. The influence parameter D in Eq. 17 had a prominent role; variations affected the resulting morphology. The smaller the influence distance D, the more refined the resulting architectures, with thinner trabeculae. The model was able to realign its trabeculae to alternative loads and so explained both modeling and adaptation. After the structure was optimized, adapted to the external loads, the activity of the BMUs stopped.

3.3.6 Separation of Osteoclast and Osteoblast Activity

In actual bone, however, the activities of osteoclasts and osteoblasts continue throughout life. In the growth stage, or during adaptation, these cells shape the bone structure (modeling), while in homeostatic conditions (or adulthood) they maintain the bone structure by tissue renewal through constant osteoclast resorption and subsequent refilling of the cavities by osteoblasts (remodeling). In metabolic diseases (e.g., osteoporosis) it is the activities of these cells that are deregulated. How are the separate actions of these cells controlled? How is coupling between activity of these cells established, and how does this relate to bone maintenance? In order to answer such questions a more refined theory was required, in which the separate activities of osteoclasts and osteoblasts were incorporated (110,239). Again it was assumed that osteocytes act as sensors of strain and generate signals to the bone surface, through the canaliculi, that stimulates osteoblast bone formation, like in the earlier theory from Mullender et al. (188–193).

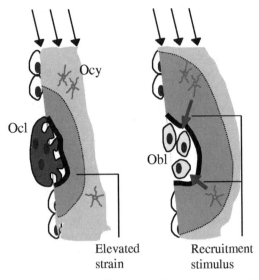

FIGURE 4-23. Paradigms to explain mechanical effects on bone remodeling (107). Lining cells cover the trabecular surface, and inside the mineralized tissue are the osteocytes (Ocy). Osteoclasts (Ocl) are recruited, it is assumed, through a lack of osteocyte signaling due to disruption of canaliculi caused by microcracks in the bone matrix. After an osteoclast (Ocl) is recruited to resorb bone, a cavity is made. This causes a local elevation of strain, through "notching" effects, which is felt by the osteocytes (Ocy) around the resorption cavity and makes them send bone signals to the environment to attract osteoblasts (Obl). This, it is assumed, is the "coupling factor" that starts the biochemical cascade of events, coupling osteoclast (Ocl) resorption to osteoblast (Obl) formation, choreographed by osteocyte (Ocy) signaling. During the bone formation process some of the osteoblasts are entrapped in the bone matrix, where they differentiate to new osteocytes. After repair, the remaining osteoblasts become lining cells, covering the new bone surface.

Resorption, however, was described as a separate osteoclast function, triggered by microcracks or damage in the bone matrix and a subsequent lack of osteocyte signaling. The coupling factor between osteoclasts and osteoblasts in remodeling was specified based on the fact that an osteoclast resorption cavity produces a "notch" (177,199,224), as illustrated in Fig. 4-23. The new theory is summarized in the regulation scheme depicted in Fig. 4-24, and the mathematical equations are specified below.

Tissue adaptation on a specific location x at time t was supposed to be the result of osteoclast bone resorption and osteoblast bone formation,

hence

$$dm_{tot}(x, t)/dt = dm_{cl}(x, t)/dt + dm_{bl}(x, t)/dt. \quad (20)$$

What exactly initiates resorption is not known. In the theory it was assumed that osteoclasts are attracted toward the bone surface by microdamage, and that microdamage occurs spatially random—i.e., it can happen anywhere at any time—so that bone resorption is determined according to

$$dm_{cl}(x, t)/dt = -r_{cl}, \quad (21)$$

where r_{cl} [mm³/day] represents a stochastic function. Osteoblast activity is controlled by an osteocyte bone formation signal P (mol·mm⁻²·day⁻¹). If the stimulus exceeds a certain threshold value k_{tr} (mol·mm⁻²·day⁻¹) there is assumed to be tissue formation at the trabecular surface according to

$$dm_{bl}(x, t)/dt = \tau(P(x, t) - k_{tr}), \quad (22)$$

where τ (mm⁵·mol⁻¹) is a proportionality factor that determines the formation rate. The formation stimulus P in location x is determined by all osteocytes N located within the influence region, the signal R (J·mm⁻³·s⁻¹) sensed by each osteocyte i, with mechanosensitivity μ_i (mol·mm·J⁻¹·s·day⁻¹) and location x_i, according to

$$P(x, t) = \sum_{i=1}^{N} f(x, x_i)\mu_i R(x_i, t), \quad (23)$$

where $f(x, x_i)$ determines the decay in signal strength according to Eq. 17. Until now computational models of bone adaptation used static loads to evaluate the mechanical signals. It is, however, known that bone only reacts to dynamic loads. In the new theory the stimulus sensed by osteocytes is assumed to be a typical SED rate $R(x, t)$ in a recent loading history. Cyclic loading conditions, characterized by frequency and magnitude, were imposed and it was assumed that osteocytes react to the maximal SED rate during the loading cycle. It was shown that the maximal SED rate is related to the SED value for some substitute static load and

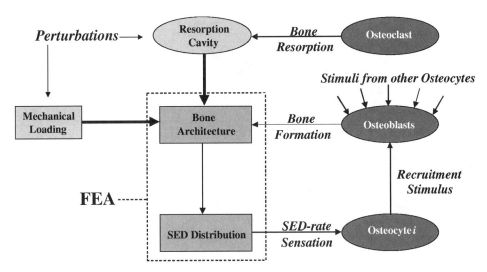

FIGURE 4-24. A scheme of the proposed regulatory process (110). Osteoclasts are assumed to resorb bone in a spatially random manner. The cavities they produce alter the local strain-energy density (SED) rate distributions, transferred by the external mechanical loads. These effects can be calculated with finite element analysis (FEA). The SED rate elevations are sensed by osteocytes, it is assumed, which dissipate a biochemical stimulus for osteoblast bone formation. Apart from the mechanical effects of the resorption cavities, also elevation in external-loading intensity can perturbate the system in producing additional bone. If load is decreased, due to disuse, osteoblast formation will not be stimulated, and bone mass will reduce through continuous resorption, until a new balance between mass and trabecular strain is reached.

that it could be calculated by static FEA (109, 239).

The relationships were incorporated in a two-dimensional computer simulation model. Starting from different initial configurations the structures remodeled toward similar homeostatic configurations, in which the process of resorption and formation continued, but no more architectural changes occurred (Fig. 4-25). Trabeculae were aligned to the loading direction. The regulatory mechanism was able to adapt the structure to alternative loading conditions. Increasing the magnitude led to apposition of bone tissue while decreasing it led to bone loss. After rotating the direction of the external load, the trabeculae realigned their orientations accordingly (Fig. 4-25). From the simulation model it was concluded that the theory was able to explain both modeling (formation and adaptation) as well as remodeling (maintenance) of trabecular-like architectures as governed by external forces. Several additional conclusions could be drawn from the theory. Osteoblasts and osteoclasts are often assumed to collaborate in so-called BMUs. In our theory, the "coupling factor" between

these cells is established only implicitly through mechanics. The resorption cavities produced by osteoclasts cause local stress and strain concentrations. Consequently, osteocytes within the tissue matrix sense elevated mechanical signals and locally recruit osteoblasts to form bone tissue until the mechanical signal has decreased to normal levels, i.e., until the cavity is refilled (Fig. 4-23). The important biochemical pathways are only implicitly involved in the theory (264), as triggered through mechanical feedback, which obviously can be a coupling factor for the relevant biochemical processes to take place. Another conclusion came from the observation that both modeling (growth and adaptation) and remodeling (maintenance) can be explained by one unifying theory. Indeed both processes are based on the same cellular mechanisms, and it could be concluded that both modeling and remodeling are similar in nature and just different stages of the metabolic cascade.

Applied in a two-dimensional computer simulation model the theory could explain morphological adaptations observed in trabecular bone as related to load-induced cell activities,

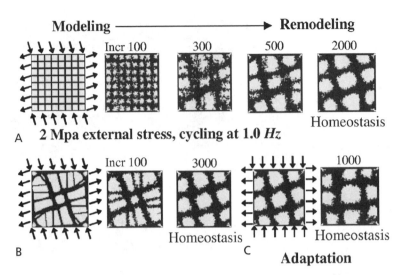

FIGURE 4-25. Development of bone architecture in the simulation model, started from two different initial configurations, **(A)** and **(B)**, shown in a few iterations. Eventually, homeostasis is obtained, where only remodeling occurs, during which the architecture at large does not change anymore, although resorption cavities are still made and filled. When the external load is rotated to vertical/horizontal, the trabecular orientation gradually adapts accordingly **(C)**. (Adapted from Huiskes et al. Effects of mechanical forces on maintenance and adaptation of form in trabecular bone. *Nature* 2000;405:704–706.)

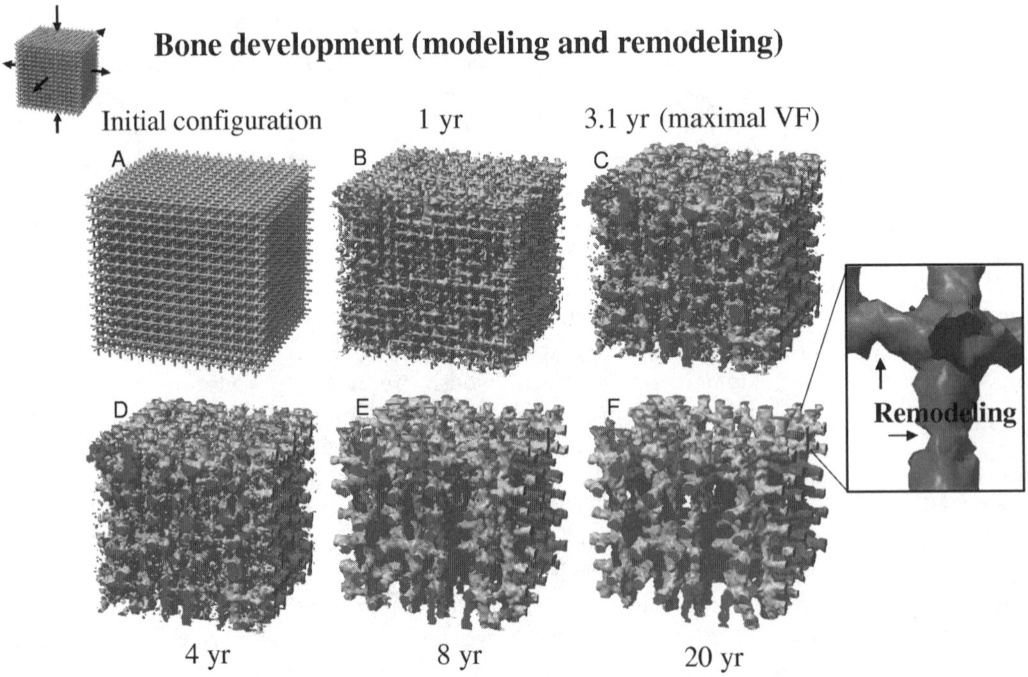

Bone development (modeling and remodeling)

Initial configuration   1 yr   3.1 yr (maximal VF)

A   B   C

Remodeling

D   E   F

4 yr   8 yr   20 yr

FIGURE 4-26. Starting from a porous initial configuration representing bone in the postmineralized fetal stage **(A)** the structure developed to a mature structure **(E)** in approximately 8 years (modeling). From this point the structure was maintained **(F)** in remodeling, while no more large architectural changes occurred. (Adapted from Ruimerman et al. A theoretical framework for strain-related trabecular bone maintenance and adaptation. *J Biomech* 2004;35:(*in press*)).

however, only in a conceptual sense. To actually validate the theory in a quantitative sense, and to apply it for valid predictions that are useful and falsifiable, its application in a three-dimensional geometry is required. Computer capacity is a limiting factor for this requirement, and it is currently not possible to simulate bone modeling and remodeling with this computational theory in complete bones at the trabecular level. In order to test whether our theory can produce trabecular-like structures in three dimensions, with morphological characteristics in a quantitative realistic range, for actual trabecular bone, we developed a three-dimensional computer simulation model that can be applied to a small domain of bone tissue. The results show that the theory mimics the real morphological expressions of bone cell metabolism in a robust way, in growth, adaptation, and remodeling, when applied to a small cube (4.5 × 4.5 × 4.5 mm³) of bone tissue with external loads imposed (238). When started from an initial porous configuration, the theory produced structures with trabecular alignment in the loading directions (Fig. 4-26). Volume fraction, trabecular thickness, remodeling rate and remodeling space values were all in realistic ranges, while the development of volume fraction in early modeling mimicked what was found in studies of growing pig bones (Fig. 4-27; com-

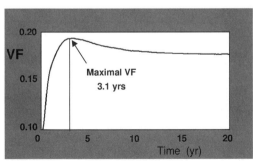

FIGURE 4-27. Development of volume fraction during the simulation of modeling (growth) and remodeling (Fig. 4-26). These results show the same overshot as found in the study of bone development in pigs, shown in Fig. 4-20. (Adapted from ref. 238.)

pare Fig. 4-20). The theory describes growth and adaptation of complex three-dimensional structures similar to actual trabecular bone and can also generate osteoporosis as effects of both disuse and post-menopausal osteoporosis (238) as illustrated in Fig. 4-28.

3.3.7 Application to Cortical Remodeling—The "Cutting Cone"

Because osteocytes, osteoblasts, and osteoclasts are the same cells in cortical and in trabecular bone, presumably reacting in the same way to similar stimuli, it stands to reason that the above theory should be applicable to the haversian "cutting cone" in cortical remodeling as well. It is assumed that cortical remodeling is initiated by osteoclast resorption in the same way as described for trabecular bone, through the presence of microcracks or damage. The question is then: Why does it proceed in the cutting cone in such an orderly fashion, straight along the direction of predominant cortical loading? Smit and Burger (247) showed in an FEA that near the tip of the cutting cone, where the osteoclasts resorb bone, the bone strain is low, while around the closing cone, where the osteoblasts form new bone, the strain is high. In comparison to the trabecular bone remodeling theory described above, this can be translated into lack of osteocyte signals at the resorption site, and high signals at the formation site, hence, compatibility with the trabecular theory. In fact, we were able to unify the theory for both cortical and trabecular remodeling in this way (240) as illustrated in Fig. 4-29.

3.3.8 Discussion

Initially, theories for bone adaptation related bone density changes directly to mechanical, strain-derived variables as effects of external forces. The computational simulation models based on these theories proved useful tools for prosthetic design. They were empirical models on a macroscopic level and the underlying biological processes involved were not taken into account. In the past decade the focus shifted from biomechanics to mechanobiology, as it is likely

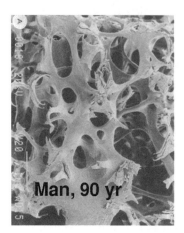
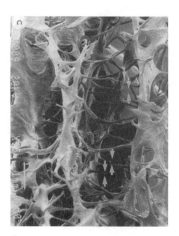

Man, 90 yr

Reduced "error loads"

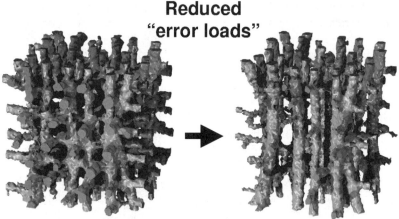

FIGURE 4-28. A simulation of disuse osteoporosis. In the mature morphology of Fig. 4-26 the horizontal forces (error loads) on the bone cube were reduced by 75%. As a result the horizontal trabeculae thinned or resorbed altogether, during the FEA simulation. The bone pictures show a comparison between similar cases in reality. (Adapted from ref. 238.)

that actual intervention in metabolic processes, to cure bone diseases, requires understanding of the relationship between mechanics and cell biology. Knowledge of bone biology has expanded enormously over the past 15 years. This, combined with increased computer capacities and efficient FEA algorithms enabled the application of realistic theories, that include realistic aspects of bone biology. The theory relates cellular activity in bone modeling and remodeling to external forces, and explains adaptive behavior of trabecular bone at a microscopic level. Although the most important relationships are captured in the theories, it should still be considered as a computational framework. The relationships are captured in simple mathematical equations, but actually encompass complex biological processes, the biochemical components of which are largely unknown. Nevertheless, the computational models based on the theory will enable us to investigate the morphological consequences of alternative loading conditions, metabolic disorders, and their pharmaceutical interventions. They are useful tools for the development and investigation of hypotheses and for efficient designs of experiments. Potentially, they are useful for prosthetic design, as the adaptation of bone tissue to alternative mechanical

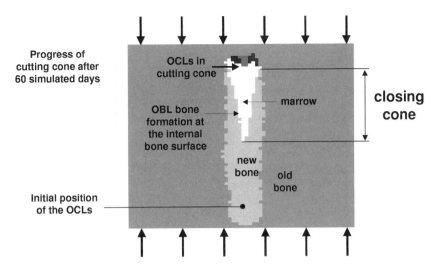

FIGURE 4-29. Result of a two-dimensional FEA simulation of cortical remodeling ('cutting cone,' compare Fig. 4-16). These results were based on the same theoretical framework as used for trabecular modeling and remodeling, whereby a unified theory was obtained (from [Ruimerman et al. Mechanically induced osteocyte signals explain osteoclast resorption direction and coupling of formation to resorption in cortical bone. *Proceedings of the EORS.* 2004;29, ref. 240).

environments can be preclinically tested. They can also be used in the development of treatment methods for osteoporosis, either based on physical exercise or in combination with pharmaceutics. In the near future, the three-dimensional computational model can be used to investigate questions like: Can the morphological changes seen in disuse osteoporosis be explained by reduced physical activity alone? Can antiresorptive drug administration prevent loss of bone tissue and preserve trabecular connectivity, and at what stage should such a treatment start? Another area where the computational framework can be applied is in postmenopausal osteoporosis. Can the theory mimic the phenomena observed in postmenopausal osteoporotic bone (loss of bone density and trabecular connectivity at a higher remodeling rate), and what is the role of mechanical coupling between osteoclasts and osteoblasts for this condition? Can osteoporosis be an effect of reduced osteocyte mechanosensitivity? Can the morphology of osteopetrotic bone be predicted as an effect of dysfunctioning osteoclasts? Can the loss of trabeculae in older ages be prevented? Could high-frequency vibrations replace the effects of physical activity? These are impor-

tant questions in bone biology and pharmacology for which computational frameworks could be useful.

REFERENCES

1. Adachi T, Tsubota K, Tomita Y, et al. Trabecular surface remodeling simulation for cancellous bone using microstructural voxel finite element models. *J Biomech Eng* 2001;123:403–409.
2. Akhter MP, Cullen DM, Pedersen EA, et al. Bone response to in vivo mechanical loading in two breeds of mice. *Calcif Tissue Int* 1998;63:442–449.
3. Ashman RB, Rho JY. Elastic modulus of trabecular bone material. *J Biomech* 1988;21:177–181.
4. Ashman RB, Rho JY, Turner CH. Anatomical variation of orthotropic elastic moduli of the proximal human tibia. *J Biomech* 1989;22:895–900.
5. Bailey AJ, Sims TJ, Ebbesen EN, et al. Age-related changes in the biochemical properties of human cancellous bone collagen: relationship to bone strength. *Calcif Tissue Int* 1999;65:203–210.
6. Bayraktar HH, Gupta A, Kwon RY, et al. Multiaxial failure behavior of human femoral trabecular bone. *Proceedings of the ORS* 2003;28.
7. Bayraktar HH, Morgan EF, Niebur GL, et al. Comparison of the elastic and yield properties of

human femoral trabecular and cortical bone tissue. *J Biomech* 2004;37:27–35.

8. Beamer WG, Shultz KL, Donahue LR, et al. Quantitative trait loci for femoral and lumbar vertebral bone mineral density in C57BL/6J and C3H/HeJ inbred strains of mice. *J Bone Miner Res* 2001;16:1195–1206.

9. Beaupre GS, Orr TE, Carter DR. An approach for time-dependent bone modeling and remodeling—theoretical development. *J Orthop Res* 1990;8:651–661.

10. Beaupre GS, Orr TE, Carter DR. An approach for time-dependent bone modeling and remodeling-application: a preliminary remodeling simulation. *J Orthop Res* 1990;8:662–670.

11. Beck JD, Canfield BL, Haddock SM, et al. Three-dimensional imaging of trabecular bone using the computer numerically controlled milling technique. *Bone* 1997;21:281–287.

12. Bergmann G, Graichen F, Rohlmann A, et al. Frictional heating of total hip implants. Part 2: finite element study. *J Biomech* 2001;34:429–435.

13. Bergot C, Laval-Jeantet AM, Hutchinson K, et al. A comparison of spinal quantitative computed tomography with dual energy X-ray absorptiometry in European women with vertebral and nonvertebral fractures. *Calcif Tissue Int* 2001;68:74–82.

14. Biewener AA, Bertram JE. Skeletal strain patterns in relation to exercise training during growth. *J Exp Biol* 1993;185:51–69.

15. Biewener AA, Swartz SM, Bertram JE. Bone modeling during growth: dynamic strain equilibrium in the chick tibiotarsus. *Calcif Tissue Int* 1986;39:390–395.

16. Bonewald LF, Mundy GR. Role of transforming growth factor-beta in bone remodeling. *Clin Orthop* 1990;261:276.

17. Boutry N, Cortet B, Dubois P, et al. Trabecular bone structure of the calcaneus: preliminary in vivo MR imaging assessment in men with osteoporosis. *Radiology* 2003;227:708–717.

18. Bouxsein ML, Courtney AC, Hayes WC. Ultrasound and densitometry of the calcaneus correlate with the failure loads of cadaveric femurs. *Calcif Tissue Int* 1995;56:99–103.

19. Bronckers AL, Goei W, Luo G, et al. DNA fragmentation during bone formation in neonatal rodents assessed by transferase-mediated end labeling. *J Bone Miner Res* 1996;11:1281–1291.

20. Buckwalter JA, Mower D, Ungar R, et al. Morphometric analysis of chondrocyte hypertrophy. *J Bone Joint Surg Am* 1986;68:243–255.

21. Burger EH, Klein-Nulend J. Microgravity and bone cell mechanosensitivity. *Bone* 1998;22:127S–130S.

22. Burger EH, Klein-Nulend J. Mechanotransduction in bone—role of the lacuno-canalicular network. *FASEB J* 1999;13[Suppl]:S101–S112.

23. Burger EH, Klein-Nulend J, van der Plas A, Nijwcide PJ. Function of osteocytes in bone—their role in mechanotransduction. *J Nutr* 1995;125:2020S–2023S.

24. Burger EH, Klein-Nulend J, Veldhuijzen JP. Modulation of osteogenesis in fetal bone rudiments by mechanical stress in vitro. *J Biomech* 1991;24[Suppl 1]:101–109.

25. Burger EH, Klein-Nulend J, Veldhuijzen JP. Mechanical stress and osteogenesis in vitro. *J Bone Miner Res* 1992;7[Suppl 2]:S397–S401.

26. Burr DB, Forwood MR, Fyhrie DP, et al. Bone microdamage and skeletal fragility in osteoporotic and stress fractures. *J Bone Miner Res* 1997;12:6–15.

27. Burstein AH, Currey JD, Frankel VH, et al. The ultimate properties of bone tissue: the effects of yielding. *J Biomech* 1972;5:35–44.

28. Burstein AH, Reilly DT, Martens M. Aging of bone tissue: mechanical properties. *J Bone Joint Surg Am* 1976;58:82–86.

29. Burstein AH, Zika JM, Heiple KG, et al. Contribution of collagen and mineral to the elastic-plastic properties of bone. *J Bone Joint Surg Am* 1975;57:956–961.

30. Caler WE, Carter DR. Bone creep-fatigue damage accumulation. *J Biomech* 1989;22:625–635.

31. Carter DR. Mechanical loading history and skeletal biology. *J Biomech* 1987;20:1095–1109.

32. Carter DR, Caler WE, Spengler DM, et al. Fatigue behavior of adult cortical bone: the influence of mean strain and strain range. *Acta Orthop Scand* 1981;52:481–490.

33. Carter DR, Hayes WC. Bone compressive strength: the influence of density and strain rate. *Science* 1976;194:1174–1176.

34. Carter DR, Hayes WC. Compact bone fatigue damage—I. Residual strength and stiffness. *J Biomech* 1977;10:325–337.

35. Carter DR, Hayes WC. The compressive behavior of bone as a two-phase porous structure. *J Bone Joint Surg Am* 1977;59:954–962.

36. Carter DR, Orr TE, Fyhrie DP. Relationships between loading history and femoral cancellous bone architecture. *J Biomech* 1989;22:231–244.

37. Carter DR, Orr TE, Fyhrie DP, et al. Influences of mechanical stress on prenatal and postnatal skeletal development. *Clin Orthop* 1987;237–250.

38. Carter DR, Schwab GH, Spengler DM. Tensile fracture of cancellous bone. *Acta Orthop Scand* 1980;51:733–741.

39. Carter DR, Spengler DM. Mechanical properties and composition of cortical bone. *Clin Orthop* 1978;192–217.

40. Carter DR, Wong M. The role of mechanical loading histories in the development of diarthrodial joints. *J Orthop Res* 1988;6:804–816.

41. Chambers TJ. The direct and indirect effects of estrogen on bone formation. *Adv Organ Biol* 1998;5B:627–638.

42. Chambers TJ, Evans M, Gardner TN, et al. Induction of bone formation in rat tail vertebrae by mechanical loading. *Bone Miner* 1993;20:167–178.

43. Chambers TJ, Fuller K. Bone cells predispose bone surfaces to resorption by exposure of mineral to osteoclastic contact. *J Cell Sci* 1985;76:155–165.

44. Choi K, Goldstein SA. A comparison of the fatigue behavior of human trabecular and cortical bone tissue. *J Biomech* 1992;25:1371–1381.

45. Choi K, Kuhn JL, Ciarelli MJ, et al. The elastic moduli of human subchondral, trabecular, and cortical bone tissue and the size-dependency of cortical bone modulus. *J Biomech* 1990;23:1103–1113.

46. Chrischilles EA, Butler CD, Davis CS, et al. A model of lifetime osteoporosis impact. *Arch Intern Med* 1991;151:2026–2032.

47. Churches AE, Howlett CR. Functional adaptation of bone in response to sinusoidally varying controlled compressive loading of the ovine metacarpus. *Clin Orthop* 1982;168:265–280.

48. Clark S, Rowe DW. Transgenic animals. In: Bilizikian JP, Rais LG, Rodan GA, eds. *Principles of bone biology.* New York: Academic Press, 1996:1161–1172.

49. Cooper C, Atkinson EJ, Jacobsen SJ, et al. Population-based study of survival after osteoporotic fractures. *Am J Epidemiol* 1993;137:1001–1005.

50. Cooper C, Campion G, Melton LJ III. Hip fractures in the elderly: a world-wide projection. *Osteoporos Int* 1992;2:285–289.

51. Cowin SC. The relationship between the elasticity tensor and the fabric tensor. *Mech Mat* 1985;4:137–147.

52. Cowin SC, He QC. Tensile and compressive yield criteria for cancellous bone. *J Biomech* 2004;35 (*in press*).

53. Cowin SC, Hegedus DH. Bone remodeling I: theory of adaptive elasticity. *J Elast* 1976;6:313–326.

54. Cowin SC, Weinbaum S, Zeng Y. A case for bone canaliculi as the anatomical site of strain generated potentials. *J Biomech* 1995;28:1281–1297.

55. Currey JD. *The mechanical adaptation of bones.* Princeton, NJ: Princeton University Press, 1984.

56. Currey JD. The effect of porosity and mineral content on the Young's modulus of elasticity of compact bone. *J Biomech* 1988;21:131–139.

57. Currey JD. The effects of drying and re-wetting on some mechanical properties of cortical bone. *J Biomech* 1988;21:439–441.

58. Dalen N, Hellstrom LG, Jacobson B. Bone mineral content and mechanical strength of the femoral neck. *Acta Orthop Scand* 1976;47:503–508.

59. Dalstra M, Huiskes R, Odgaard A, et al. Mechanical and textural properties of pelvic trabecular bone. *J Biomech* 1993;26(4/5), 523–535.

60. Dambacher MA, Ruegsegger P. Bone density measurements and their indications. *Orthopade* 1994;23:38–44.

61. Duboeuf F, Jergas M, Schott AM, et al. A comparison of bone densitometry measurements of the central skeleton in post-menopausal women with and without vertebral fracture. *Br J Radiol* 1995;68:747–753.

62. Duncan RL, Turner CH. Mechanotransduction and the functional response of bone to mechanical strain. *Calcif Tissue Int* 1995;57:344–358.

63. Engelke K, Hahn M, Takada M, et al. Structural analysis of high resolution in vitro MR images compared to stained grindings. *Calcif Tissue Int* 2001;68:163–171.

64. Eriksen E, Kassem M. *Sandoz J Med Sci* 1992;Triangle:45–57.

65. Erlebacher A, Derynck R. Increased expression of TGF-beta 2 in osteoblasts results in an osteoporosis-like phenotype. *J Cell Biol* 1996;132:195–210.

66. Fazzalari NL, Forwood MR, Manthey BA, et al. Three-dimensional confocal images of microdamage in cancellous bone. *Bone* 1998;23:373–378.

67. Feldkamp LA, Goldstein SA, Parfitt AM, et al. The direct examination of three-dimensional bone architecture in vitro by computed tomography. *J Bone Miner Res* 1989;4:3–11.

68. Fondrk M, Bahniuk E, Davy DT, et al. Some viscoplastic characteristics of bovine and human cortical bone. *J Biomech* 1988;21:623–630.

69. Frank EH, Grodzinsky AJ. Cartilage electromechanics—I. Electrokinetic transduction and the effects of electrolyte pH and ionic strength. *J Biomech* 1987;20:615–627.

70. Fritton JC, Myers ER, van der Meulen MC, et al. Validation of a loading apparatus: characterization of murine tibial surface strains in vivo. *Transactions of the ORS* 2001;26.

71. Frost HM. Dynamics of bone remodeling. In: Frost HM, ed. *Bone biodynamics.* Boston: Little, Brown and Company, 1964:315–333.

72. Frost HM. *Intermediary organization of the skeleton.* Boca Raton: CRC Press, 1986.

73. Frost HM. Bone "mass" and the "mechanostat": a proposal. *Anat Rec* 1987;219:1–9.

74. Fyhrie DP, Carter DR. A unifying principle relating stress to trabecular bone morphology. *J Orthop Res* 1986;4:304–317.

75. Genant HK, Cooper C, Poor G, et al. (1999). Interim report and recommendations of the World Health Organization Task-Force for Osteoporosis. *Osteoporos Int* 1999;10:259–264.

76. Gibson LJ. The mechanical behaviour of cancellous bone. *J Biomech* 1985;18:317–328.

77. Gibson LJ. Cancellous bone. In: *Cellular solids.* New York: Pergamon Press, 1988:316–331.

78. Goldstein SA. The mechanical properties of trabecular bone: dependence on anatomic location and function. *J Biomech* 1987;20:1055–1061.

79. Goldstein SA, Matthews LS, Kuhn JL, et al. Trabecular bone remodeling: an experimental model. *J Biomech* 1991;24[Suppl 1]:135–150.

80. Goulet RW, Goldstein SA, Ciarelli MJ, et al. The relationship between the structural and orthogonal compressive properties of trabecular bone. *J Biomech* 1994;27:375–389.

81. Gray ML, Pizzanelli AM, Grodzinsky AJ, et al. Mechanical and physiochemical determinants of the chondrocyte biosynthetic response. *J Orthop Res* 1988;6:777–792.

82. Gray ML, Pizzanelli AM, Lee RC, et al. Kinetics of the chondrocyte biosynthetic response to compressive load and release. *Biochim Biophys Acta* 1989;991:415–425.

83. Gross T, Srinivasan S, Bailey M, et al. Non-invasive activation of bone formation in the murine tibia. *Transactions of the ORS* 2000;25.

84. Guilak F, Donahue H, Zell R, et al. Deformation-induced calcium signaling in articular chondrocytes. In: Mow et al., eds. *Cell mechanics and cellular engineering.* New York: Springer-Verlag, 1994:380–397.

85. Guldberg RE, Caldwell NJ, Guo XE, et al. Mechanical stimulation of tissue repair in the hydraulic bone chamber. *J Bone Miner Res* 1997;12:1295–1302.

86. Guo XE. Mechanical properties of cortical bone and cancellous bone tissue. In: Cowin SC, ed. *Bone mechanics handbook.* Boca Raton: CRC Press, 2001:10-1–10-23.

87. Haaijman A, D'Souza RN, Bronckers AL, et al. OP-1 (BMP-7) affects mRNA expression of type I, II, X collagen, and matrix Gla protein in ossifying long bones in vitro. *J Bone Miner Res* 1997;12:1815–1823.

88. Hansson TH, Keller TS, Panjabi MM. A study of the compressive properties of lumbar vertebral trabeculae: effects of tissue characteristics. *Spine* 1987;12:56–62.

89. Hara T, Tanck E, Homminga J, et al. The influence of microcomputed tomography threshold variations on the assessment of structural and mechanical trabecular bone properties. *Bone* 2002;31:107–109.

90. Harrigan TP, Jasty M, Mann RW, et al. Limitations of the continuum assumption in cancellous bone. *J Biomech* 1988;21:269–275.

91. Harrigan TP, Mann RW. Characterization of microstructural anisotropy in orthotropic materials using a second rank tensor. *J Mat Sci: Mater Med* 1984;19:761–767.

92. Hart RT. Bone remodeling and remodeling: theories and computation. In: Cowin SC, ed. *Bone mechanics handboo.k* Boca Raton: CRC Press, 2001:31-1–31-42.

93. Hart RT, Davy DT, Heiple KG. A computational method for stress analysis of adaptive elastic materials with a view toward applications in strain-induced bone remodeling. *J Biomech Eng* 1984;106:342–350.

94. Hart RT, Fritton SP. Introduction to finite element based simulation of functional adaptation of cancellous bone. *Forma* 1997;12:277–299.

95. Hayes WC. Biomechanics of cortical and trabecular bone: implications for assessment of fracture risk. In: Mow VC Hayes WC, eds. *Basic orthopaedic biomechanics.* New York: Raven Press, 1991:93–142.

96. Hayes WC, Carter DR. Biomechanics of bone. In: *Skeletal research: an experimental approach.* New York: Academic Press, 1979:263–300.

97. Hayes WC, Gerhart TN. Biomechanics of bone: applications for assessment of bone strength. In: Peck WA, ed. *Bone and mineral research.* Amsterdam: Elsevier Science, 1985:259–294.

98. Hayes WC, Myers ER, Morris JN, et al. Impact near the hip dominates fracture risk in elderly nursing home residents who fall. *Calcif Tissue Int* 1993;52:192–198.

99. Hayes WC, Piazza SJ, Zysset PK. Biomechanics of fracture risk prediction of the hip and spine by quantitative computed tomography. *Radiol Clin North Am* 1991;29:1–18.

100. Hert J, Liskova M, Landrgot B. Influence of the long-term, continuous bending on the bone. An experimental study on the tibia of the rabbit. *Folia Morphol (Praha)* 1969;17:389–399.

101. Hildebrand T, Ruegsegger P. Quantification of bone microarchitecture with the structure model index. *Comput Methods Biomech Biomed Engin* 1997;1:15–23.

102. Hodgskinson R, Currey JD. Young's modulus, density and material properties in cancellous bone over a large density range. *J Mat Sci: Mater Med* 1992;3:377–381.

103. Hollister SJ, Guldberg RE, Kuelske CL, et al. Relative effects of wound healing and mechanical stimulus on early bone response to porous-coated implants. *J Orthop Res* 1996;14:654–662.

104. Hollister SJ, Kikuchi N. Direct analysis of trabecular bone stiffness and tissue level mechanics using an element-by-element homogenization method. *Transactions of the ORS* 1992;17:559.

105. Homminga J, Huiskes R, van Rietbergen B, et al. Introduction and evaluation of a gray-value voxel conversion technique. *J Biomech* 2001;34:513–517.

106. Homminga J, McCreadie BR, Ciarelli TE, et al. Cancellous bone mechanical properties from normals and patients with hip fractures differ on the structure level, not on the bone hard tissue level. *Bone* 2002;30:759–764.

107. Homminga J, McCreadie BR, Weinans H, et al. The dependence of the elastic properties of osteoporotic cancellous bone on volume fraction and fabric. *J Biomech* 2003;36:1461–1467.

108. Homminga J, van Rietbergen B, Lochmuller EM, et al. The osteoporotic vertebral structure is well adapted to the loads of daily life, but not to infrequent "error" loads. *Bone* 2004;34:510–516.

109. Huiskes R. If bone is the answer, then what is the question? *J Anat* 2000;197(Pt 2):145–156.

110. Huiskes R, Ruimerman R, van Lenthe GH, et al. Effects of mechanical forces on maintenance and adaptation of form in trabecular bone. *Nature* 2000;405:704–706.

111. Huiskes R, Weinans H, Grootenboer HJ, et al. Adaptive bone-remodeling theory applied to prosthetic-design analysis *J Biomech* 1987;20:1135–1150.

112. Huiskes R. On the modelling of long bones in structural analyses. *J Biomech* 1982;15:65–69.

113. Huiskes R. Some fundamental aspects of human joint replacement. *Acta Orthop Scand Suppl* 1980;185:1–209.

114. Hunziker EB, Schenk RK. Physiological mechanisms adopted by chondrocytes in regulating longitudinal bone growth in rats. *J Physiol* 1989;414:55–71.

115. Hvid I. Mechanical strength of trabecular bone at the knee. *Dan Med Bull* 1988;35:345–365.

116. Ishijima M, Rittling SR, Yamashita T, et al. Enhancement of osteoclastic bone resorption and suppression of osteoblastic bone formation in response to reduced mechanical stress do not occur in the absence of osteopontin. *J Exp Med* 2001;193:399–404.

117. Iwamoto J, Takeda T. Stress fractures in athletes: review of 196 cases. *J Orthop Sci* 2003;8:273–278.

118. Jacobs CR, Davis BR, Rieger CJ. NACOB presentation to ASB Young Scientist Award: postdoctoral. The impact of boundary conditions and mesh size on the accuracy of cancellous bone tissue modulus determination using large-scale finite-element modeling. North American Congress on Biomechanics. *J Biomech* 1999;32:1159–1164.

119. Jacobs CR, Simo JC, Beaupre GS, et al. Adaptive bone remodeling incorporating simultaneous density and anisotropy considerations. *J Biomech* 1997;30:603–613.

120. Jacobs CR, Yellowley CE, Davis BR, et al. Differential effect of steady versus oscillating flow on bone cells. *J Biomech* 1998;31:969–976.

121. Kabel J, van Rietbergen B, Dalstra M, et al. The role of an effective isotropic tissue modulus in the elastic properties of cancellous bone. *J Biomech* 1999;32:673–680.

122. Kabel J, van Rietbergen B, Odgaard A, et al. Constitutive relationships of fabric, density, and elastic properties in cancellous bone architecture. *Bone* 1999;25:481–486.

123. Kanatani KI. Distribution of directional data and fabric tensors. *Int J Eng Sci* 1984;22:149–164.

124. Kanatani KI. Stereological determination of structural anisotropy. *Int J Eng Sci* 1984;22:531–546.

125. Kanatani KI. Procedures for stereological estimation of structural anisotropy. *Int J Eng Sci* 1985;23:587–598.

126. Kaplan SJ, Hayes WC, Stone JL, et al. Tensile strength of bovine trabecular bone. *J Biomech* 1985;18:723–727.

127. Katagiri T, Takahashi N. Regulatory mechanisms of osteoblast and osteoclast differentiation. *Oral Dis* 2002;8:147–159.

128. Keaveny TM. Strength of trabecular bone. In: Cowin SC, ed. *Bone mechanics handbook.* Boca Raton: CRC Press, 2001:16-1–16-42.

129. Keaveny TM, Borchers RE, Gibson LJ, et al. Theoretical analysis of the experimental artifact in trabecular bone compressive modulus. *J Biomech* 1993;26:599–607.

130. Keaveny TM, Guo XE, Wachtel EF, et al. Trabecular bone exhibits fully linear elastic behavior and yields at low strains. *J Biomech* 1994;27:1127–1136.

131. Keaveny TM, Hayes WC. Mechanical properties of cortical and trabecular bone. In: *Bone, volume VII: bone growth-B.* Boca Raton: CRC Press, 1992:285–344.

132. Keaveny TM, Hayes WC. A 20-year perspective on the mechanical properties of trabecular bone. *J Biomech Eng* 1993;115:534–542.

133. Keaveny TM, Morgan EF, Niebur GL, et al. Biomechanics of trabecular bone. *Annu Rev Biomed Eng* 2001;3:307–333.

134. Keaveny TM, Pinilla TP, Crawford RP, et al. Systematic and random errors in compression testing of trabecular bone. *J Orthop Res* 1997;15:101–110.

135. Keaveny TM, Wachtel EF, Ford CM, et al. Differences between the tensile and compressive strengths of bovine tibial trabecular bone depend on modulus. *J Biomech* 1994;27:1137–1146.

136. Keenan MJ, Hegsted M, Jones KL, et al. Comparison of bone density measurement techniques: DXA and Archimedes' principle. *J Bone Miner Res* 1997;12:1903–1907.

137. Kerner J, Huiskes R, Lenthe GH, et al. Correlation between pre-operative periprosthetic bone density and post-operative bone loss in THA can be explained by strain-adaptive remodelling. *J Biomech* 1999;32(7):695–703.

138. Khillan JS, Olsen AS, Kontusaari S, et al. Transgenic mice that express a mini-gene version of the human gene for type I procollagen (COL1A1) develop a phenotype resembling a lethal form of osteogenesis imperfecta. *J Biol Chem* 1991;266:23373–23379.

139. Kim YJ, Bonassar LJ, Grodzinsky AJ. The role of cartilage streaming potential, fluid flow and pressure in the stimulation of chondrocyte biosynthesis during dynamic compression. *J Biomech* 1995;28:1055–1066.

140. Kim YJ, Sah RL, Grodzinsky AJ, et al. Mechanical regulation of cartilage biosynthetic behavior: physical stimuli. *Arch Biochem Biophys* 1994;311:1–12.

141. Kirsch T, Nah HD, Shapiro IM, et al. Regulated production of mineralization-competent matrix vesicles in hypertrophic chondrocytes. *J Cell Biol* 1997;137:1149–1160.

142. Klein-Nulend J, van der, PA, Semeins CM, et al. Sensitivity of osteocytes to biomechanical stress in vitro. *FASEB J* 1995;9:441–445.

143. Klein-Nulend J, Veldhuijzen JP, Burger EH. Increased calcification of growth plate cartilage as a result of compressive force in vitro. *Arthritis Rheum* 1986;29:1002–1009.

144. Klein OF, Carlos AS, Vartanian KA, et al. Confirmation and fine mapping of chromosomal regions influencing peak bone mass in mice. *J Bone Miner Res* 2001;16:1953–1961.

145. Knothe Tate ML, Steck R, Forwood MR, et al. In vivo demonstration of load-induced fluid flow in the rat tibia and its potential implications for processes associated with functional adaptation. *J Exp Biol* 2000;203(Pt 18):2737–2745.

146. Konikoff JJ. Origin of the osseous bioelectric potentials: a review. *Ann Clin Lab Sci* 1975;5:330–337.

147. Kopperdahl DL, Keaveny TM. Yield strain behavior of trabecular bone. *J Biomech* 1998;31:601–608.

148. Korstjens CM, Geraets WG, van Ginkel FC. Longitudinal analysis of radiographic trabecular pattern by image processing. *Bone* 1995;17:527–532.

149. Kuhn JL, Goldstein SA, Feldkamp LA. Evaluation of a microcomputed tomography system to study trabecular bone structure. *J Orthop Res* 1990;8:833–842.

150. Ladd AJ, Kinney JH, Haupt DL, et al. Finite-element modeling of trabecular bone: comparison with mechanical testing and determination of tissue modulus. *J Orthop Res* 1998;16:622–628.

151. Laib A, Hauselmann HJ, Ruegsegger P. In vivo high resolution 3D-QCT of the human forearm. *Technol Health Care* 1998;6:329–337.

152. Laib A, Hildebrand T, Hauselmann HJ, et al. Ridge number density: a new parameter for in vivo bone structure analysis. *Bone* 1997;21:541–546.

153. Laib A, Ruegsegger P. Calibration of trabecular bone structure measurements of in vivo three-dimensional peripheral quantitative computed tomography with 28-microm-resolution microcomputed tomography. *Bone* 1999;24:35–39.

154. Laib A, Ruegsegger P. Comparison of structure extraction methods for in vivo trabecular bone measurements. *Comput Med Imaging Graph* 1999;23:69–74.

155. Lamerigts NM, Buma P, Huiskes R, et al. Incorporation of morsellized bone graft under controlled loading conditions. A new animal model in the goat. *Biomaterials* 2000;21:741–747.

156. Lammi MJ, Inkinen R, Parkkinen JJ, et al. Expression of reduced amounts of structurally altered aggrecan in articular cartilage chondrocytes exposed to high hydrostatic pressure. *Biochem J* 1994;304 (Pt 3):723–730.

157. Lang T, Augat P, Majumdar S, et al. Noninvasive assessment of bone density and structure using computed tomography and magnetic resonance. *Bone* 1998;22:149S–153S.

158. Langton CM, Njeh CF. Quantitative ultrasound. In: Langton CM, Njeh CF, eds. *The physical measurement of bone*. Bristol: IOP, 2004:412–474.

159. Lappe JM, Stegman MR, Recker RR. The impact of lifestyle factors on stress fractures in female Army recruits. *Osteoporos Int* 2001;12:35–42.

160. LeBlanc A, Schneider V, Spector E, et al. Calcium absorption, endogenous excretion, and endocrine changes during and after long-term bed rest. *Bone* 1995;16:301S–304S.

161. Lee DA, Einhorn T. In: Marcus, Feldman, and Kelsey, eds. *Osteoporosis* 2001:3–20.

162. Lee DA, Bader DL. Compressive strains at physiological frequencies influence the metabolism of chondrocytes seeded in agarose. *J Orthop Res* 1997;15:181–188.

163. Li KC, Zernicke RF, Barnard RJ, et al. Differential response of rat limb bones to strenuous exercise. *J Appl Physiol* 1991;70:554–560.

164. Lian J, Stein G. In: Marcus, Feldman, and Kelsey, eds. *Osteoporosis.* 2001:21–71.

165. Linde F. Elastic and viscoelastic properties of trabecular bone by a compression testing approach. *Dan Med Bull* 1994;41:119–138.

166. Link TM, Majumdar S, Grampp S, et al. Imaging of trabecular bone structure in osteoporosis. *Eur Radiol* 1999;9:1781–1788.

167. Lochmuller EM, Lill CA, Kuhn V, et al. Radius bone strength in bending, compression, and falling and its correlation with clinical densitometry at multiple sites. *J Bone Miner Res* 2002;17:1629–1638.

168. Lotz JC, Gerhart TN, Hayes WC. Mechanical properties of trabecular bone from the proximal

femur: a quantitative CT study. *J Comput Assist Tomogr* 1990;14:107–114.

169. Luo ZP, An KN. A theoretical model to predict distribution of the fabric tensor and apparent density in cancellous bone. *J Math Biol* 1998;36:557–568.

170. Magaziner J, Simonsick EM, Kashner TM. Survival experience of aged hip fracture patients. *Am J Public Health* 1989;79:274–278.

171. Majumdar S. A review of magnetic resonance (MR) imaging of trabecular bone microarchitecture: contribution to the prediction of biomechanical properties and fracture prevalence. *Technol Health Care* 1998;6:321–327.

172. Majumdar S, Genant HK. High resolution magnetic resonance imaging of trabecular structure. *Eur Radiol* 1997;7:51–55.

173. Martin RB. Toward a unifying theory of bone remodeling. *Bone* 2000;26:1–6.

174. Matsuda JJ, Zernicke RF, Vailas AC, et al. Structural and mechanical adaptation of immature bone to strenuous exercise. *J Appl Physiol* 1986;60:2028–2034.

175. Mattheck C. *Design in nature*. Berlin: Springer-Verlag, 1998.

176. McBroom RJ, Hayes WC, Edwards WT, et al. Prediction of vertebral body compressive fracture using quantitative computed tomography. *J Bone Joint Surg Am* 1985;67:1206–1214.

177. McNamara LM, van der Linden JC, Weinans H, et al. High stresses occur in bone trabeculae under low loads! A study using micro-serial sectioning techniques and finite element analysis. Wroclaw, Poland: *Proceedings of the 13th Conference of the ESB*, 2002.

178. Melvin JW. Fracture mechanics of bone. *J Biomech Eng* 1993;115:549–554.

179. Mikic B, van der Meulen MC, Kingsley DM, et al. Mechanical and geometric changes in the growing femora of BMP-5 deficient mice. *Bone* 1996;18:601–607.

180. Morey-Holton ER, Whalen RT, Arnaud SB, et al. The skeleton and its adaptation to gravity. In: *Handbook of physiology: environmental physiology, part III: the gravitational environment, section 1: microgravity*. Oxford: Oxford University Press, 1996:691–719.

181. Morgan EF, Bayraktar HH, Keaveny TM. Trabecular bone modulus-density relationships depend on anatomic site. *J Biomech* 2003;36:897–904.

182. Mori S, Harruff R, Ambrosius W, et al. Trabecular bone volume and microdamage accumulation in the femoral heads of women with and without femoral neck fractures. *Bone* 1997;21:521–526.

183. Mosekilde L. Consequences of the remodelling process for vertebral trabecular bone structure: a scanning electron microscopy study (uncoupling

of unloaded structures). *Bone Miner* 1990;10:13–35.

184. Mosekilde L, Bentzen SM, Ortoft G, et al. The predictive value of quantitative computed tomography for vertebral body compressive strength and ash density. *Bone* 1989;10:465–470.

185. Mosley JR, Lanyon LE. Strain rate as a controlling influence on adaptive modeling in response to dynamic loading of the ulna in growing male rats. *Bone* 1998;23:313–318.

186. Mosley JR, March BM, Lynch J, et al. Strain magnitude related changes in whole bone architecture in growing rats. *Bone* 1997;20:191–198.

187. Mow VC, Kuei SC, Lai WM, et al. Biphasic creep and stress relaxation of articular cartilage in compression? Theory and experiments. *J Biomech Eng* 1980;102:73–84.

188. Mullender M, van Rietbergen B, Ruegsegger P, et al. Effect of mechanical set point of bone cells on mechanical control of trabecular bone architecture. *Bone* 1998;22:125–131.

189. Mullender MG, Huiskes R. Proposal for the regulatory mechanism of Wolff's law. *J Orthop Res* 1995;13:503–512.

190. Mullender MG, Huiskes R. Osteocytes and bone lining cells: which are the best candidates for mechano-sensors in cancellous bone? *Bone* 1997;20:527–532.

191. Mullender MG, Huiskes R, Versleyen H, et al. Osteocyte density and histomorphometric parameters in cancellous bone of the proximal femur in five mammalian species. *J Orthop Res* 1996;14:972–979.

192. Mullender MG, Huiskes R, Weinans H. A physiological approach to the simulation of bone remodeling as a self-organizational control process. *J Biomech* 1994;27:1389–1394.

193. Mullender MG, van der Meer DD, Huiskes R, et al. Osteocyte density changes in aging and osteoporosis. *Bone* 1996;18:109–113.

194. Muller R, Hahn M, Vogel M, et al. Morphometric analysis of noninvasively assessed bone biopsies: comparison of high-resolution computed tomography and histologic sections. *Bone* 1996;18:215–220.

195. Muller R, Hildebrand T, Hauselmann HJ, et al. In vivo reproducibility of three-dimensional structural properties of noninvasive bone biopsies using 3D-pQCT. *J Bone Miner Res* 1996;11:1745–1750.

196. Mundy GR. The effects of TGF-beta on bone. *Ciba Found Symp* 1991;157:137–143.

197. Nafei A, Danielsen CC, Linde F, et al. Properties of growing trabecular ovine bone. Part I: mechanical and physical properties. *J Bone Joint Surg Br* 2000;82:910–920.

198. Nafei A, Kabel J, Odgaard A. Properties of growing trabecular ovine bone. Part II: architectural

and mechanical properties. *J Bone Joint Surg Br* 2000;82:921–927.

199. Nicolella D, Lankford J. Strain concentration effects of osteocyte lacunae. *Proceedings of the ORS* 2002.

200. Niebur GL, Feldstein MJ, Keaveny TM. Biaxial failure behavior of bovine tibial trabecular bone. *J Biomech Eng* 2002;124:699–705.

201. Niebur GL, Feldstein MJ, Yuen JC, et al. High-resolution finite element models with tissue strength asymmetry accurately predict failure of trabecular bone. *J Biomech* 2000;33:1575–1583.

202. Niebur GL, Yuen JC, Hsia AC, et al. Convergence behavior of high-resolution finite element models of trabecular bone. *J Biomech Eng* 1999;121:629–635.

203. Noble BS, Stevens H, Loveridge N, et al. Identification of apoptotic changes in osteocytes in normal and pathological human bone. *Bone* 1997;20:273–282.

204. Norman TL, Vashishth D, Burr DB. Fracture toughness of human bone under tension. *J Biomech* 1995;28:309–320.

205. Odgaard A. Three-dimensional methods for quantification of cancellous bone architecture. *Bone* 1997;20:315–328.

206. Odgaard A. Quantification of cancellous bone architecture. In: Cowin SC, ed. *Bone mechanics handbook.* Boca Raton: CRC Press, 2001:14-1–14-19.

207. Odgaard A, Andersen K, Melsen F, et al. A direct method for fast three-dimensional serial reconstruction. *J Microsc* 1990;159(Pt 3):335–342.

208. Odgaard A, Andersen K, Ullerup R, et al. Three-dimensional reconstruction of entire vertebral bodies. *Bone* 1994;15:335–342.

209. Odgaard A, Kabel J, van Rietbergen B, et al. Fabric and elastic principal directions of cancellous bone are closely related. *J Biomech* 1997;30:487–495.

210. Odgaard A, Linde F. The underestimation of Young's modulus in compressive testing of cancellous bone specimens. *J Biomech* 1991;24:691–698.

211. Parfitt AM. Osteonal and hemi-osteonal remodeling: the spatial and temporal framework for signal traffic in adult human bone. *J Cell Biochem* 1994;55:273–286.

212. Parfitt AM, Mathews CH, Villanueva AR, et al. Relationships between surface, volume, and thickness of iliac trabecular bone in aging and in osteoporosis. Implications for the microanatomic and cellular mechanisms of bone loss. *J Clin Invest* 1983;72:1396–1409.

213. Parkkinen JJ, Lammi MJ, Inkinen R, et al. Influence of short-term hydrostatic pressure on organization of stress fibers in cultured chondrocytes. *J Orthop Res* 1995;13:495–502.

214. Parkkinen J, Lammi M, Tammi M, et al. Proteoglycan synthesis and cytoskeleton in hydrostat-

ically loaded chondrocytes. In: Mow et al., eds. *Cell mechanics and cellular engineering.* New York: Springer-Verlag, 1994:420–444.

215. Pattin CA, Caler WE, Carter DR. Cyclic mechanical property degradation during fatigue loading of cortical bone. *J Biomech* 1996;29:69–79.

216. Pauwels F. *Biomechanics of fracture healing.* Berlin: Springer-Verlag, 1980:106–120.

217. Pedersen EA, Akhter MP, Cullen DM, et al. Bone response to in vivo mechanical loading in C3H/HeJ mice. *Calcif Tissue Int* 1999;65:41–46.

218. Pester S, Smith PC. Stress fractures in the lower extremities of soldiers in basic training. *Orthop Rev* 1992;21:297–303.

219. Petrtyl M, Hert J, Fiala P. Spatial organization of the haversian bone in man. *J Biomech* 1996;29:161–169.

220. Pienkowski D, Pollack SR. The origin of stress-generated potentials in fluid-saturated bone. *J Orthop Res* 1983;1:30–41.

221. Pistoia W, van Rietbergen B, Laib A, et al. High-resolution three-dimensional-pQCT images can be an adequate basis for in-vivo microFE analysis of bone. *J Biomech Eng* 2001;123:176–183.

222. Pistoia W, van Rietbergen B, Lochmuller EM, et al. Estimation of distal radius failure load with micro-finite element analysis models based on three-dimensional peripheral quantitative computed tomography images. *Bone* 2002;30:842–848.

223. Platzer AC. The ultrastructure of normal myogenesis in the limb of the mouse. *Anat Rec* 1978;190:639–657.

224. Prendergast PJ, Huiskes R. Microdamage and osteocyte-lacuna strain in bone: a microstructural finite element analysis. *J Biomech Eng* 1996;118:240–246.

225. Prendergast PJ, Taylor D. Prediction of bone adaptation using damage accumulation. *J Biomech* 1994;27:1067–1076.

226. Reilly DT, Burstein AH. Review article. The mechanical properties of cortical bone. *J Bone Joint Surg Am* 1974;56:1001–1022.

227. Reilly DT, Burstein AH. The elastic and ultimate properties of compact bone tissue. *J Biomech* 1975;8:393–405.

228. Reilly DT, Burstein AH, Frankel VH. The elastic modulus for bone. *J Biomech* 1974;7:271–275.

229. Rho JY, Ashman RB, Turner CH. Young's modulus of trabecular and cortical bone material: ultrasonic and microtensile measurements. *J Biomech* 1993;26:111–119.

230. Rice JC, Cowin SC, Bowman JA. On the dependence of the elasticity and strength of cancellous bone on apparent density. *J Biomech* 1988;21:155–168.

231. Riggs BL, Melton LJ, III. Evidence for two distinct syndromes of involutional osteoporosis. *Am J Med* 1983;75:899–901.

232. Robling AG, Burr DB, Turner CH. Partitioning a daily mechanical stimulus into discrete loading bouts improves the osteogenic response to loading. *J Bone Miner Res* 2000;15:1596–1602.

233. Rodan GA. Mechanical loading, estrogen deficiency, and the coupling of bone formation to bone resorption. *J Bone Miner Res* 1991;6:527–530.

234. Rohl L, Larsen E, Linde F, et al. Tensile and compressive properties of cancellous bone. *J Biomech* 1991;24:1143–1149.

235. Roux W. *Der Kampf der Teile im Organismus.* Leipzig: Engelman, 1881.

236. Rubin CT, Lanyon LE. Regulation of bone formation by applied dynamic loads. *J Bone Joint Surg Am* 1984;66:397–402.

237. Ruegsegger P, Koller B, Muller R. A microtomographic system for the nondestructive evaluation of bone architecture. *Calcif Tissue Int* 1996;58:24–29.

238. Ruimerman R, Hilbers P, van Rietbergen B, et al. A theoretical framework for strain-related trabecular bone maintenance and adaptation. *J Biomech* 2004;35 (*in press*).

239. Ruimerman R, Huiskes R, van Lenthe G, et al. A computer-simulation model relating bone-cell metabolism to mechanical adaptation of trabecular architecture. *Comput Methods Biomech Biomed Eng* 2001;4:433–448.

240. Ruimerman R, van Oers R, Tanck E, et al. Mechanically induced osteocyte signals explain osteoclast resorption direction and coupling of formation to resorption in cortical bone. *Proceedings of the EORS* 2004;29.

241. Sah RL, Kim YJ, Doong JY. Biosynthetic response of cartilage explants to dynamic compression. *J Orthop Res* 1989;7:619–636.

242. Schaffler MB, Burr DB. Stiffness of compact bone: effects of porosity and density. *J Biomech* 1988;21:13–16.

243. Schaffler MB, Choi K, Milgrom C. Aging and matrix microdamage accumulation in human compact bone. *Bone* 1995;17:521–525.

244. Schaffler MB, Radin EL, Burr DB. Mechanical and morphological effects of strain rate on fatigue of compact bone. *Bone* 1989;10:207–214.

245. Schenk R, Willenegger H. On the histology of primary bone healing. *Langenbecks Arch Klin Chir Ver Dtsch Z Chir* 1964;308:440–452.

246. Skerry TM, Bitensky L, Chayen J, et al. Early strain-related changes in enzyme activity in osteocytes following bone loading in vivo. *J Bone Miner Res* 1989;4:783–788.

247. Smit TH, Burger EH. Is BMU-coupling a strain-regulated phenomenon? A finite element analysis. *J Bone Miner Res* 2000;15:301–307.

248. Snyder BD, Hayes WC. Multiaxial structure-property relations in trabecular bone. In: *Biomechanics of diarthrodial joints.* New York: Springer-Verlag, 1990:31–59.

249. Sontag W. Age-dependent morphometric alterations in the distal femora of male and female rats. *Bone* 1992;13:297–310.

250. Stanczyk M, van Rietbergen B. Thermal analysis of bone cement polymerisation at the cement-bone interface. *J Biomech* 2004;(*in press*).

251. Stone JL, Beaupre GS, Hayes WC. Multiaxial strength characteristics of trabecular bone. *J Biomech* 1983;16:743–752.

252. Tanck E, Blankevoort L, Haaijman A, et al. Influence of muscular activity on local mineralization patterns in metatarsals of the embryonic mouse. *J Orthop Res* 2000;18:613–619.

253. Tanck E, Homminga J, van Lenthe GH, et al. Increase in bone volume fraction precedes architectural adaptation in growing bone. *Bone* 2001;28:650–654.

254. Tanck E, van Driel WD, Hagen JW, et al. Why does intermittent hydrostatic pressure enhance the mineralization process in fetal cartilage? *J Biomech* 1999;32:153–161.

255. Tanck E, van Dijk ME, Errington RJ, et al. Proposal for the effect of chondrocyte volume on the mineralization rate. *J Musculoskel Res* 2001;5:37–44.

256. Tanck E, van Donkelaar CC, Jepsen KJ, et al. The mechanical consequences of mineralization in embryonic bone. *Bone* 2004;35:186–190.

257. Taylor D, Prendergast PJ. A model for fatigue crack propagation and remodelling in compact bone. *Proc Inst Mech Eng [H]* 1997;211:369–375.

258. Thompson DW. *On growth and form.* Cambridge: Cambridge University Press, 1961.

259. Torrance AG, Mosley JR, Suswillo RF, et al. Noninvasive loading of the rat ulna in vivo induces a strain-related modeling response uncomplicated by trauma or periosteal pressure. *Calcif Tissue Int* 1994;54:241–247.

260. Turner CH. Yield behavior of bovine cancellous bone. *J Biomech Eng* 1989;111:256–260.

261. Turner CH, Akhter MP, Raab DM, et al. A noninvasive, in vivo model for studying strain adaptive bone modeling. *Bone* 1991;12:73–79.

262. Turner CH, Cowin SC, Rho JY, et al. The fabric dependence of the orthotropic elastic constants of cancellous bone. *J Biomech* 1990;23:549–561.

263. Turner CH, Forwood MR, Rho JY, et al. Mechanical loading thresholds for lamellar and woven bone formation. *J Bone Miner Res* 1994;9:87–97.

264. Udagawa N, Takahashi N, Jimi E, et al. Osteoblasts/stromal cells stimulate osteoclast activation through expression of osteoclast differentiation factor/RANKL but not macrophage

colony-stimulating factor: receptor activator of NF-kappa B ligand. *Bone* 1999;25:517–523.

265. Uhthoff HK, Jaworski ZF. Bone loss in response to long-term immobilisation. *J Bone Joint Surg Br* 1978;60-B:420–429.

266. Ulrich D, van Rietbergen B, Laib A, et al. Load transfer analysis of the distal radius from in-vivo high- resolution CT-imaging. *J Biomech* 1999;32:821–828.

267. Ulrich D, van Rietbergen B, Laib A, et al. The ability of three-dimensional structural indices to reflect mechanical aspects of trabecular bone. *Bone* 1999;25:55–60.

268. Ulrich D, van Rietbergen B, Weinans H, et al. Finite element analysis of trabecular bone structure: a comparison of image-based meshing techniques. *J Biomech* 1998;31:1187–1192.

269. Urban JP. The chondrocyte: a cell under pressure. *Br J Rheumatol* 1994;33:901–908.

270. Urban J. The effects of hydrostatic and osmotic pressures on chondrocyte metabolism. In: Mow et al., eds. *Cell mechanics and cellular engineering.* New York: Springer-Verlag, 1994:398–419.

271. Vaananen HK, Horton M. The osteoclast clear zone is a specialized cell-extracellular matrix adhesion structure. *J Cell Sci* 1995;108(Pt 8):2729–2732.

272. Vaananen HK, Zhao H, Mulari M, et al. The cell biology of osteoclast function. *J Cell Sci* 2000; 113(Pt 3):377–381.

273. van den Bergh JPW, van Lenthe GH, Hermus ARMM, et al. Speed of sound reflects Young's modulus as assessed by microstructural finite element analysis. *Bone* 2000;26(5):519–524.

274. van der Meulen MC. Differential bone adaptation to mechanical loading: role of bone morphogenetic protein-5. In: *Proceedings of the Bioengineering Conference.* New York: ASME, 1999:689–690.

275. van der Meulen MC, Beaupre GS, Carter DR. Mechanobiologic influences in long bone crosssectional growth. *Bone* 1993;14:635–642.

276. van der Meulen MC, Huiskes R. Why mechanobiology? A survey article. *J Biomech* 2002;35:401–414.

277. van Lenthe GH, van den Bergh JP, Hermus AR, et al. The prospects of estimating trabecular bone tissue properties from the combination of ultrasound, dual-energy X-ray absorptiometry, microcomputed tomography, and microfinite element analysis. *J Bone Miner Res* 2001;16:550–555.

278. van Lenthe GH, Huiskes R. How morphology predicts mechanical properties of trabecular structures depends on intra-specimen trabecular thickness variation. *J Biomech* 2002;35:1191–1197.

279. Van Loon JJ, Bervoets DJ, Burger EH, et al. Decreased mineralization and increased calcium release in isolated fetal mouse long bones under near

weightlessness. *J Bone Miner Res* 1995;10:550–557.

280. van Rietbergen B, Huiskes R, Eckstein F, et al. Trabecular bone tissue strains in the healthy and osteoporotic human femur. *J Bone Miner Res* 2003;18:1781–1788.

281. van Rietbergen B, Kabel J, Odgaard A, et al. Determination of trabecular bone tissue elastic properties by comparison of experimental and finite element results. In: Sol H, Oomens CWJ, eds. *Material identification using mixed numerical experimental methods.* Dordrecht: Kluwer Academic Publishers, 1997:183–192.

282. van Rietbergen B, Majumdar S, Newitt D, et al. High-resolution MRI and micro-FE for the evaluation of changes in bone mechanical properties during longitudinal clinical trials: application to calcaneal bone in postmenopausal women after one year of idoxifene treatment. *Clin Biomech (Bristol, Avon)* 2002;17:81–88.

283. van Rietbergen B, Muller R, Ulrich D, et al. Tissue stresses and strain in trabeculae of a canine proximal femur can be quantified from computer reconstructions. *J Biomech* 1999;32:165–173.

284. van Rietbergen B, Weinans H, Huiskes R, et al. A new method to determine trabecular bone elastic properties and loading using micromechanical finite-element models. *J Biomech* 1995;28:69–81.

285. Vashishth D, Verborgt O, Divine G, et al. Decline in osteocyte lacunar density in human cortical bone is associated with accumulation of microcracks with age. *Bone* 2000;26:375–380.

286. Verborgt O, Gibson GJ, Schaffler MB. Loss of osteocyte integrity in association with microdamage and bone remodeling after fatigue in vivo. *J Bone Miner Res* 2000;15:60–67.

287. Verhulp E, van Rietbergen B, Huiskes R. A three-dimensional digital image correlation technique for strain measurements in microstructures. *J Biomech* 2004;37(9):1313–1320.

288. Vico L, Hinsenkamp M, Jones D, et al. Osteobiology, strain, and microgravity. Part II: studies at the tissue level. *Calcif Tissue Int* 2001;68:1–10.

289. Wehrli FW, Hwang SN, Song HK, et al. Visualization and analysis of trabecular bone architecture in the limited spatial resolution regime of in vivo micro-MRI. *Adv Exp Med Biol* 2001;496:153–164.

290. Weibel ER. *Stereological methods: vol. 2: theoretical foundations.* New York: Academic Press, 1980.

291. Weinans H, Huiskes R, Grootenboer HJ. Effects of material properties of femoral hip components on bone remodeling. *J Orthop Res* 1992;10:845–853.

292. Weinans H, Huiskes R, Grootenboer HJ. The behavior of adaptive bone-remodeling simulation models. *J Biomech* 1992;25:1425–1441.

293. Weinbaum S, Cowin SC, Zeng Y. A model for the excitation of osteocytes by mechanical loading-induced bone fluid shear stresses. *J Biomech* 1994;27:339–360.

294. Wenzel TE, Schaffler MB, Fyhrie DP. In vivo trabecular microcracks in human vertebral bone. *Bone* 1996;19:89–95.

295. Whitehouse WJ. The quantitative morphology of anisotropic trabecular bone. *J Microsc* 1974; 101(Pt 2):153–168.

296. Wolff J. *Das gesetz der Transformation de Knochen.* Berlin: Hirschwald, 1892.

297. Wolff J. *The law of bone remodeling.* Berlin: Springer-Verlag, 1986.

298. Wong M, Carter DR. A theoretical model of endochondral ossification and bone architectural construction in long bone ontogeny. *Anat Embryol (Berl)* 1990;181:523–532.

299. Wong M, Carter DR. Theoretical stress analysis of organ culture osteogenesis. *Bone* 1990;11:127–131.

300. Wright M, Jobanputra P, Bavington C, et al. Effects of intermittent pressure-induced strain on the electrophysiology of cultured human chondrocytes: evidence for the presence of stretch-activated membrane ion channels. *Clin Sci (Lond)* 1996;90:61–71.

301. Wright TM, Hayes WC. Tensile testing of bone over a wide range of strain rates: effects of strain rate, microstructure and density. *Med Biol Eng* 1976;14:671–680.

302. Yang G, Kabel J, van Rietbergen B, et al. The anisotropic Hooke's law for cancellous bone and wood. *J Elast* 1998;53:125–146.

303. Yershov Y, Baldini TH, Villagomez S, et al. Bone strength and related traits in HcB/Dem recombinant congenic mice. *J Bone Miner Res* 2001;16:992–1003.

304. You L, Cowin SC, Schaffler MB, et al. A model for strain amplification in the actin cytoskeleton of osteocytes due to fluid drag on pericellular matrix. *J Biomech* 2001;34:1375–1386.

305. Yu W, Gluer CC, Grampp S, et al. Spinal bone mineral assessment in postmenopausal women: a comparison between dual X-ray absorptiometry and quantitative computed tomography. *Osteoporos Int* 1995;5:433–439.

306. Zimmerman D, Jin F, Leboy P, et al. Impaired bone formation in transgenic mice resulting from altered integrin function in osteoblasts. *Dev Biol* 2000;220:2–15.

307. Zioupos P. Accumulation of in-vivo fatigue microdamage and its relation to biomechanical properties in ageing human cortical bone. *J Microsc* 2001;201:270–278.

308. Zioupos P, Casinos A. Cumulative damage and the response of human bone in two-step loading fatigue. *J Biomech* 1998;31:825–833.

309. Zioupos P, Wang XT, Currey JD. The accumulation of fatigue microdamage in human cortical bone of two different ages in vitro. *Clin Biomech (Bristol Avon)* 1996;11:365–375.

5

STRUCTURE AND FUNCTION OF ARTICULAR CARTILAGE AND MENISCUS

VAN C. MOW
WEI YONG GU
FAYE HUI CHEN

Cartilage is a soft connective tissue that is composed of a single cell type, chondrocyte, and a highly specialized extracellular matrix (ECM). Three major types of cartilaginous tissues are present in the body: hyaline cartilage, elastic cartilage, and fibrocartilage. These tissues are distinguished by their respective ECMS. The biochemical composition and molecular structure of the matrix give rise to distinct biomechanical properties of different types of cartilage required by their functions.

Hyaline cartilage is the most common type of cartilage. As the name implies, hyaline cartilage is glassy smooth, glistening, and bluish-white in appearance, although older tissues tend to lose this appearance. The most common hyaline cartilage, and the most studied, is articular cartilage (295,350). This tissue covers the articulating surfaces of long bones and sesamoid bones within synovial joints, e.g., the surfaces of the tibia, the femur, and the patella of the knee joint. Another example of hyaline cartilage is the growth plate, which develops into bones by the process of endochondral ossification during skeletal development (81,507,534). Hyaline cartilage is also found in the larynx, the trachea, the nasal septum, and the sternal end of the rib (costal cartilage) (171,172,534). Elastic cartilage is generally yellowish and opaque in appearance (534) and can be found in the epiglottis, the external ear, the external auditory canal, the eustachian tube, and the larynx. Elastic cartilage is distinguished by the presence of elastic fibers, which make this cartilage more flexible than hyaline cartilage. Fibrocartilage contains thick layers of larger collagen fibers in the ECM that contribute to its relatively rough and fibrous appearance. Two major fibrocartilage tissues are the annulus fibrosus of the intervertebral disc, which provides the flexible junctions between the vertebral bodies in the spine (2,36,461,470,509, 510,534; see Chapter 12 for more details on the spine) and the meniscus of the knee (see following section on the meniscus of the knee, and references 3,4,15,123,131,234,317,344, 388,400,432,469,551). Other fibrocartilage can be found in the symphysis pubis, the sternoclavicular and temporomandibular joints, and some places where tendons insert into bones.

Articular cartilage and meniscus are vital to the maintenance of normal joint motion, and both are significantly involved in degenerative disease of the knee such as osteoarthritis (OA). Articular cartilages in freely movable joints, such as hip and knee, can withstand very large loads (5,6,155,198,199; also see Chapter 2 by Prendergast et al., and Chapter 3 by Andriacchi et al.) while providing a smooth, lubricating bearing material with minimal wear (see Chapter 10 on joint lubrication by Ateshian and Mow). The major motivation for the study of articular cartilage and meniscus has been the development of an understanding of the OA disease processes that can afflict most of the load-bearing joints (10,46,116,209,256,273,295,404,465, 475). More recently, tissue engineering as it pertains to cartilage repair has become another motivating factor for innovative studies of cartilage biology (348,527; also see the section later in this chapter for more details on chondrocyte function, Chapter 6 by Guilak and Hung on physical regulation of cartilage metabolism, and Chapter 8 by Vunjak-Novakovic and Goldstein on biomechanical principles of cartilage and bone tissue engineering).

The breakdown of cartilage leading to OA can result from a multitude of mechanical, biochemical, and humoral factors, and can occur in an acute and traumatic form, or in a chronic fashion, occurring over many years. These changes ultimately result in alterations of the biomechanical properties of the tissue and a reduction in its ability to function in the highly stressed environment of the joint (5,6,57,116,209,273,295, 347,350,465,490,517). Therefore, it is important to understand (a) the mechanical properties of normal cartilage and meniscus, (b) the manner in which biochemical and microstructural factors contribute to the material properties of cartilage, and (c) the manner in which changes in tissue composition affect the mechanical properties of cartilage. Furthermore, in order to understand how knees, hips, and other diarthrodial joints carry and support load, and provide lubrication and protection against friction and wear, one must know, in a quantitative manner, the exact shape of each of these joints (see Chapter 9 by Ateshian and Eckstein for a description of a quantitative determination of joint anatomy and Chapter 10 by Ateshian and Mow for details of diarthrodial joint tribology). In this chapter, we describe the biochemical composition and ultrastructural organization of the two important tissues of the knee (articular cartilage and meniscus) and relate these to their mechanical properties in order to provide an understanding of the structure-function relationships of these tissues.

1 STRUCTURE OF A DIARTHRODIAL JOINT

All diarthrodial joints have common structural features. First, all diarthrodial joints are enclosed in a strong fibrous capsule (Fig. 5-1) (350). Second, the inner surfaces of the joint capsules are lined with the highly vascularized synovium,

which secretes the synovial fluid and provides the nutrients required by the various tissues within the joint (485). It has long been thought that the synovial fluid also serves as the lubricant for diarthrodial joints (419), particularly in more recent times, with its viscoelastic properties better understood (see Chapter 10 by Ateshian and Mow for more details on joint lubrication). Recently, joint lubrication has reemerged as an important issue with such injected viscoelastic supplements as Synvise® as a clinical treatment modality for some early stages of OA (27). Third, each articulating bone end within the joint is lined with a thin layer of hydrated soft tissue, i.e., the articular cartilage. These linings, i.e., the synovium and the two articular cartilage layers, form the joint cavity, which contains the synovial fluid (385,422). Thus, the synovial fluid, articular cartilage, and supporting bone in the mature animal form a "closed" biomechanical system that

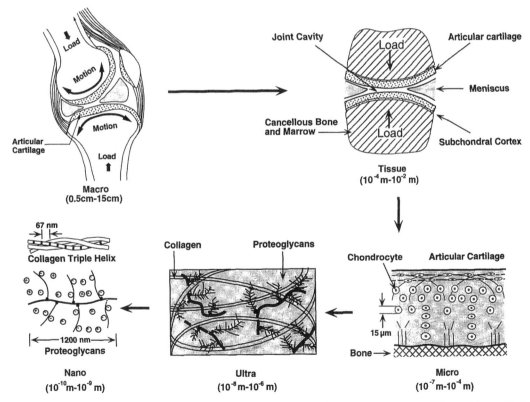

FIGURE 5-1. Some of the important structural features of a typical diarthrodial joint at different hierarchical scale: macro (0.5 to 15 cm), tissue (10^{-4} to 10^{-2} m), micro (10^{-7} to 10^{-4} m), ultra (10^{-8} to 10^{-6} m), and nano (10^{-10} to 10^{-9} m) (350).

provides the smooth, nearly frictionless bearing system of the body. Although diarthrodial joints are subjected to an enormous range of loading conditions (see Chapter 2 by Prendergast et al. for muscle loading, and Chapter 3 by Andriacchi et al. for dynamics of locomotion and joint loading), particularly with slow cyclical conditions and high loads (5,6,155,385), the load-bearing articulating cartilage surfaces have the potential to remain unimpaired and functional, with extraordinarily low coefficients of friction and wear rates (see Chapter 10) for the lifetime of an individual.

Two geometric features of diarthrodial joints are most important for their biomechancial function: (a) the anatomic forms of the articulating surfaces and (b) the thickness contours of the cartilage layers (16,17,22,83,106–108,259, 272,329,387,479,480; also see Chapter 9 by Ateshian and Eckstein on quantitative anatomy and imaging). The overall anatomic form largely dictates the types of motion (rolling, sliding, or a combination of both) that a joint may have, and the thickness contours of the articular cartilage layers (along with their material properties and loadings) dictate the types of stresses and their magnitudes existing *within* the tissue. Note that stresses within the tissue cannot be measured by any experimental technique, but rather, even if the deformation field is measured, e.g., by optical microscopic techniques (448), the stresses and material properties within the tissue must be *calculated* (73,449,529) by using an appropriate constitutive (stress–strain) law (20,264,338, 340) as described in this chapter.

The hip, for example, is a close-fitting ball-and-socket joint that is nearly spherical, and because the acetabulum (socket) is normally a deep cup, this is a very stable joint. However, at times, congenital childhood abnormalities of acetabulum shape (shallow cup) lead to severe hip diseases. Also, deviations from sphericity of the articular and subchondral bone surfaces on the acetabulum and femoral head (ball) have been noted, and hypothesized as being an important factor in the etiology of OA (60,434). In severe arthritis, both sides of the hip become grossly distorted by the formation of bony spurs (osteophytes), which, in their advanced stages,

severely restrict the motion of the hip (46,209). The glenohumeral joint of the shoulder is also a close-fitting, spherical, ball-and-socket joint, though here the glenoid surface on the scapula is a very shallow spherical sector covering only one-third of the spherical humeral head (479). This is necessary because of all the joints in the body, the shoulder must provide the largest range of motion required by the activities of daily living. Because of this, however, the shoulder is very susceptible to instability and dislocation, i.e., shifting of contact region within the joint to the periphery (480), which could often lead to the development of severe cartilage wear, and eventually OA. For both the hip and the shoulder, under normal conditions, the articulation is characterized by a sliding motion of one articular surface over the other (155,233,480). These close-fitting sliding articulations also provide the necessary geometric forms for the formation of fluid-film lubrication in these joints (for more details on joint lubrication, see Chapter 10 by Ateshian and Mow on lubrication and wear of diarthrodial joints).

Other joint surfaces have more complex geometric forms. For example, the knee is actually composed of three joints: the patello-femoral joint and the two femoro-tibial joints (lateral and medial). The anatomic arrangement of the knee, characterized by a lever arm, can produce the large moments required for knee function (e.g., the extension moments required to rise from deep knee bends). To produce these moments, very large forces must be generated by the surrounding muscles, thus creating very large joint reaction forces (see Chapter 2 by Prendergast et al. and Chapter 3 by Andriacchi for more information on joint reaction forces). These large joint reaction forces significantly deform and stress the articular cartilage and the subjacent bony structures.

Factors affecting the magnitude and type of stresses and strains in articular cartilage are its form, thickness contour, loading, and material properties (16–20,82,83,350,529). Recently, there has been much interest in developing MRI methods to quantitatively assess articular cartilage thickness contours *in vivo*, in normal subjects and in patients with OA (22,83,106–108,

272,329,387; also see Chapter 9 by Ateshian and Eckstein on quantitative anatomy and imaging). Over the past few years, the accuracies of these MRI methods for determining the articular surface contours, using commercially available MRI, have increased to 200 to 300 μm *in vivo* (see Chapter 9). These methods, along with further refinements of MRI technology, offer opportunities for researchers to develop realistic joint models to calculate precisely the stresses and strains in the cartilaginous layers *in vivo*. Recently, accurate *in vitro* methods (less than 100 μm) for assessing joint anatomy and cartilage thickness maps have also been developed using stereophotogrammetry (16,17,40,213,479, 480; also see Chapter 9). The results of these studies are very accurate (less than 90 μm for knees and less than 25 μm for wrist joints); and still represent the state of the art in quantitative imaging. An important finding from these studies is that the articular cartilage layer thicknesses are, in general, not uniform and that the surfaces have high curvatures with regular patterns of ridges and grooves running across their surfaces (259). Obviously, these features will have pronounced effects on the stresses and strains developed in the cartilage layer during joint loading and the lubrication mechanisms that exist between the two articulating surfaces (see Chapter 10).

2 COMPOSITION AND STRUCTURE OF ARTICULAR CARTILAGE AND MENISCUS

Articular cartilage and meniscus, in their young, normal, and healthy state, are glistening, smooth, intact, and substantial tissues. In older individuals and in preclinical disease states, the tissues lose this appearance and often look dull, roughened, and fibrillated (320). Meniscus degenerates in the form of tears and fraying (93,349). Articular cartilage fibrillates, forms deep fissures, and, in advanced OA, is entirely lost at weight-bearing sites over the joint surface; the remaining bone becomes eburnated, dense, and extremely hard (e.g., 46,209,295,475). The origins of these readily evident macroscopic manifestations of pathologies (often simplistically referred to as "wear and tear") have not yet been fully explained in mechanical, molecular, and cellular terms. However, to provide a basis for understanding this disease process, it is necessary first to understand the structure–material property–function relationships existing for articular cartilage and meniscus. This necessarily means knowing the stress–strain behaviors of these materials. Thus, in the following sections, the biochemical composition and microorganization of articular cartilage and meniscus are described, and these will be related to the mechanical properties of the tissue.

Articular cartilage and meniscus should be regarded as multiphasic materials with two major phases: a fluid phase composed of water and electrolytes and a solid phase composed of collagen, trapped proteoglycans, other proteins, and the chondrocytes (264,278,302,303,338,340, 350,356,484,485) (see Table 5-1). For an understanding of cartilage swelling, the dissolved electrolytes (Na^+, Ca^{2+}, Cl^-, etc.) within the interstitial fluid must be considered as a separate third phase, and the solid phase must be charged (159–161,264,266,351,353,365). Indeed, each phase of the tissue contributes significantly to its known mechanical and physicochemical properties. Table 5-2 provides a summary of the biochemical components of cartilage and meniscus. Of the organic components, the collagens (120,325,367–369,515) provide the quantitatively major organic component, followed by

TABLE 5-1. COMPOSITION OF ARTICULAR CARTILAGE AND MENISCUS

Tissue	Water	Collagen (Wet Wt.)	Proteoglycan (Wet Wt.)
Articular cartilage	68–85%	10–20% (type II)	5–10%
Meniscus	60–70%	15–25% (type I)	1–2%

TABLE 5-2. A SUMMARY OF THE COMPONENTS OF ARTICULAR CARTILAGE AND/OR MENISCUS

Component	Wet Weight
Quantitatively major	
Water	60–85%
Collagen, type II	15–22%
Aggrecan	4–7%
Quantitatively minor (<5%)	
Link protein	
Hyaluronan	
Collagen type I	
Collagen type V	
Collagen type VI	
Collagen type IX	
Collagen type XI	
Decorin	
Biglycan	
Fibromodulin	
Perlican	
Thrombospondin	
COMP/TSPS	

aggrecans and proteoglycan aggregates (55,56, 140,174–179,181–183,185,190–192,291,356, 357,392,396,407,513). Quantitatively minor components include hyaluronan, link protein, the smaller proteoglycans versican, biglycan, decorin, fibromodulin, perlican, fibronectin, thrombospondins including thrombospondin5/ cartilage oligomeric matrix protein (COMP), and cartilage matrix protein (90,104,130,158, 176,189,192,218,270,520). Although these are not major components in terms of the absolute mass of the solid phase, some of them may approach the molar concentrations of collagen and aggrecan and serve important biological regulating functions. It should be noted that much of the noncollagenous component of articular cartilage and meniscus is yet to be accounted for, and it is likely that only when these, as yet undescribed, molecules are characterized, and their biological and mechanical functions defined, will a comprehensive understanding of the structure–function relations for articular cartilage and meniscus be developed.

2.1 Interstitial Water

By far, water is the most abundant component of articular cartilage (42,110,111,278,300, 302,307,315,340,498,499,518). It is believed that in normal cartilage a portion of this water (approximately 30%) resides within the intrafibrillar space of collagen, and for normal tissue this proportion appears not to vary with age (231,232,305,306,496,526). The diameter of collagen fibers, and thus the amount of water within the intrafibrillar compartment, is modulated by the swelling pressure generated by the fixed charge density (FCD) of the surrounding proteoglycans (232,305,526). In the native tissue, it appears that most of this intrafibrillar water is not available for transport under mechanical loading and is believed to be excluded from the proteoglycans (304,498). This exclusion effectively raises the density of the fixed charges within the tissue, thus raising the interstitial osmotic pressure (by the Donnan osmotic pressure law) or equivalently by charge–charge repulsion (62; for more details, see discussions in Section 7, "Swelling of Articular Cartilage"). In contrast, there is a significant increase of water content in degenerating articular cartilages (12,42,48,141,294,301,303,340,350,365,518, 519). It is not known, however, whether the same proportion of water exists in the intrafibrillar space within these degenerating cartilages. Scanning electron microscopic examinations of some canine articular cartilages subsequent to high-impact loading have shown the collagen fibers in the traumatized tissue to be highly swollen (101,119,490,500), but no information exists about whether the water in these swollen fibers is free to flow and be available for proteoglycan solvation. If either or both occur, then there will be an increased permeability (which is biomechanically highly detrimental) and a decrease of FCD (which decreases the swelling pressure and its concomitant load support). It is known, phenomenologically, that changes in the total water content have strong influences in the mechanical, swelling, and fluid-transport properties exhibited by the tissue (7,8,12,19–21,141,159, 168,302,304,308,350,351,462). From the recently developed triphasic theory, mathematical relationships have now been derived for the dependence of hydraulic permeability, electric conductivity, swelling pressure, streaming potential, and other physicochemical and electromechanical phenomena on the water content in articular cartilage (159–161,264,351). Details of these functional relationships are described below.

The amount of water present depends largely on several factors: (a) the concentration of the proteoglycans, i.e., FCD, and the resultant swelling pressure exerted by the negative charge groups on the proteoglycans and the ions dissolved in the interstitial fluid—the Donnan osmotic pressure (264,302,351); (b) the organization of the collagen network; and (c) the strength and stiffness of this network, which surrounds the proteoglycan molecules and resists the swelling pressure (8,112,156,264,302,308, 351,360,362,365,464). The predominant ions within the interstitial fluid are sodium, chloride, potassium, and calcium (278,473). In cartilage from osteoarthritic joints, disruption of the collagen network can cause the water content of the tissue to increase by more than 10% (8,12, 42,141,294,301,308,316,365). This increase greatly affects the mechanical properties of the tissue (8,10,13,46,116,141,168,195,197,225–227,273,340,350,462,465).

Most of the fluid and ions within the tissue are freely exchangeable by diffusion with the bathing solution surrounding the tissue (160,161,278, 294,300,302,496,498,499). The interstitial fluid may also be extruded from the tissue by applying a pressure gradient across the tissue (141,160, 161,296,297,315) or by simply compressing the tissue (12,23,82,110,111,117,195,202–204, 278,315,345,350,351,473). As the interstitial fluid flows through the pores of the collagen-proteoglycan solid matrix, significant frictional drag forces are exerted on the walls of the pores of the solid matrix, thus causing compaction (20,202–204,264,338,350). This nonlinear flow-induced compression effect (often referred to as the strain-dependent permeability) is very important in the physiology of articular cartilage because it means that it becomes more difficult to squeeze fluid from such tissues with prolonged compression. For both cartilage and meniscus, the frictional drag force not only dominates their compressive viscoelastic behaviors, e.g., creep and stress relaxation, but also provides the mechanism for energy dissipation (264,315,

338,340,342,343,400). A major focus of this chapter is the description of this flow-dependent, i.e., biphasic, viscoelastic phenomenon, and the swelling behavior of the tissue.

2.2 Collagens

In articular cartilage and meniscus, the primary function of the collagen appears to be to provide the tensile stiffness and strength for the tissues. However, because there is an array of different collagens present, mostly in quantitatively minor amounts, it is likely that other, as yet undefined biomechanical and biological functions exist. The importance of the collagens for cartilage to tissue function is easily demonstrated by the evidence of collagen mutations contributing to heritable disorders, including precocious OA (9,47,71,359,363,373,398,399,523,524,531).

2.2.1 Collagen Types

Collagens are a family of the most abundant proteins in human. Their critical roles in maintaining the structural integrity of various tissues are demonstrated by the wide spectrum of diseases caused by collagen mutations (see 363 and 373 for review). At least 20 different collagen types have been identified so far (398,399,489,515), with at least 38 genetically different polypeptide chains (363,373,398,399,489,515). Collagens comprise three polypeptide α chains forming a characteristic tight right-handed collagen triple helix. The nomenclature for the collagen superfamily consists of a Roman numeral that indicates the genetic type with the α-chain composition. The three α chains in each collagen can be identical, or different. For example, type II collagen, the primary collagen of articular cartilage, contains three $\alpha 1(II)$ polypeptide chains $[\alpha 1(II)]_3$; type I collagen, the major collagen of meniscus, ligaments, and tendons, is composed of two $\alpha 1(I)$ and one $\alpha 2(I)$ polypeptide chains $[\alpha 1(I)]_2 \alpha 2(I)$ (120, 367); and type IX collagen contains three distinct α chains $\alpha 1(IX)\alpha 2(IX)\alpha 3(IX)$ (Table 5-3) (514). Type X is a low-molecular-weight collagen with three identical $\alpha 1(X)$ chains.

The collagen α chains all contain segments of the basic structural repeat motif of Gly-X-Y

TABLE 5-3. A SUMMARY OF THE FIBRILLAR ORGANIZATION OF THE GENETICALLY DISTINCT COLLAGENS IN CARTILAGE AND MENISCUS

Collagen Type	Chain Organization
Type I	$[\alpha 1(\text{I})]_2 \, \alpha 2(\text{I})$
Type II	$[\alpha 1(\text{II})]_3$
Type V	$[\alpha 1(\text{V})]_2 \, \alpha 2(\text{V})$
Type VI	$\alpha 1(\text{VI}) \, \alpha 2(\text{VI}) \, \alpha 3(\text{VI})$
Type IX	$\alpha 1(\text{IX}) \, \alpha 2(\text{IX}) \, \alpha 3(\text{IX})$
Type X	$[\alpha 1(\text{X})]_3$
Type XI	$\alpha 1(\text{XI}) \, \alpha 2(\text{XI}) \, \alpha 3(\text{XI})$

that form a left-handed helix. However, there is considerable variability in the structure of the collagens that presumably provides for extensive differences in function (Table 5-3). The family of collagen is usually divided into several subclasses based on their structures and biological functions. Most collagens in articular cartilage and meniscus belong to the class of fibril-forming collagens, which include types I, II, III, V, and XI. Type X collagen belongs to the second major class of collagen, the network-forming collagens. This class also includes types IV and VIII. Other cartilage collagens such as type IX belong to a group called FACIT (*F*ibril-*A*ssociated *C*ollagens with *I*nterrupted *T*riple helices) collagens, which also include type XII, XIV, XVI, and XIX. Other classes are beaded filament-forming collagens (type VI), collagens of anchoring fibrils (type VII), collagens with a transmembrane domain (types XIII and XVII), and collagen types XV and XVIII.

Articular cartilage contains primarily type II collagen, with smaller amounts of other types of collagens, including types VI, IX, XI, XII, and XIV. Other than articular cartilage, type II collagen is also present in nasal septum and the sternal cartilage as well as in the intervertebral disc. By comparison, 90% of the collagen found in fibrocartilaginous meniscus is type I, with small amounts of types II, III, V, and VI (120, 123). Type I collagen is the most abundant collagen in humans and is distributed widely throughout the body. It is found in copious amount in skin, bone, tendon, and ligament, as well as in fibrocartilage of the meniscus and intervertebral disc. Type X is one of the most specialized

collagens and is synthesized primarily by hypertrophic chondrocytes in the growth plate (325, 367–369,423). Types IX, XII, and XIV are unusual in the collagen family in that they also contain glycosaminoglycan (GAG) chains attached to the α chains.

2.2.2 Collagen Structure

The primary functions of collagen fibrils in cartilage are twofold. First, its structure provides tensile stiffness and strength to the tissue. Second, the collagen network also functions to restrain the swelling pressure of the embedded proteoglycans, which provides compression stiffness. Collagen structure is well suited for carrying out these functions.

Collagen is a rod-shaped molecule with a high degree of structural organization (Fig. 5-2). It is defined by the presence of a right-handed triple helical collagenous domain formed by three polypeptide α chains. Each α chain is composed of repeating $(\text{Gly-X-Y})_n$ triplets that form a natural left-handed helix, where X is often proline and Y is often hydroxyproline, an unusual amino acid rare in other proteins but plentiful in collagen. The number of repeats varies among collagen types. Whereas there is often a continuous helical (Gly-X-Y) structure over the approximately 1,000-amino-acid length in the fibril-forming collagen α chains, the repeats are commonly interrupted by other noncollagenous domains in the nonfibrillar collagens. The presence of glycine at every third residue and the presence of proline and hydroxylproline as well as hydroxylysine are responsible for the tightly packed, rigid triple helical structure that confers collagen's characteristic tensile strength (7,8, 238–242,257,399,427). The ring structures of proline and hydroxyproline keep the α chain in an extended configuration. The structure of the center of the helix is so spatially restricted that only glycine, the smallest amino acid, can be accommodated. Each of the α chains also contains a short sequence of about 25 amino acid residues at each end (telopeptides) that do not have a triple helix structure. Telopeptides play an important yet poorly defined role in assembly of the proteins into fibrils. This highly organized

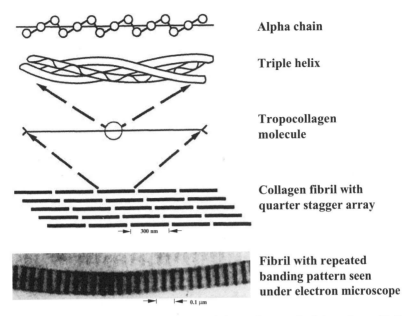

Alpha chain

Triple helix

Tropocollagen molecule

Collagen fibril with quarter stagger array

Fibril with repeated banding pattern seen under electron microscope

FIGURE 5-2. Schematic representation and photomicrograph of the collagen fibril structure.

collagen structure appears to have been specifically designed to resist tension (8,144,211,238–242,420,427,451,521,522,537–539).

The triple helical collagenous domains in fibrillar collagens can further polymerize extracellularly in a staggered lateral association to form collagen fibrils. These fibrils show a periodicity of 680 Å that can be visualized by transmission electron microscopy (72). This is called the D-period and is created by packing of the collagen molecules side by side with adjacent molecules staggered along the axis by 680 Å or 1.0 D. The fibrils can be further stabilized by covalent intermolecular cross-links. The cross-links further confer physical and mechanical properties of tensile strength fundamental to the structural and functional role of collagen fibrils in connective tissues (241,450,451). The diameter of a fibril ranges from 100 to 2,000 Å, depending on the types of collagens as well as tissue origin. In articular cartilage, small-diameter fibrils of 10 to 25 nm composed of type II tropocollagen molecules are formed in the pericellular region, and larger-diameter fibrils of up to 3,000 Å diameter are found in the territorial and interterritorial matrix (49–52,78,79). However, these are still much smaller than the collagen fibers

present in menisci or ligaments and tendons, where large-diameter fibers are formed by the type I collagen (59,132,400,537,538,546).

The collagen fibrils in tissues are often heterogenous, containing more than one type of collagen. For example, type I collagen fibrils often contain small amounts of types III, V, and XII collagens, with type V in the core and III and XII on the surface of the fibril (30,53,228, 373,399). In cartilage collagen fibrils, type II collagen is the main component, while type XI collagen can also be found in the core with type IX collagen decorating the surface of the fibril (41,89,322,373). Collagen XI is located largely within the fibrils and cross-linked to type II covalently. It is found in greater quantities in smaller fibrils. Its role in collagen fibrilogenesis has been proposed to act as the nuclei for type II fibril formation. Type IX collagen (Fig. 5-3) contributes only 1% of the total collagen in mature articular cartilage, although it is present at a much higher concentration in fetal tissues. It is covalently cross-linked to the type II collagen on the surface of the fibrils in an antiparallel fashion (125,514,543). These covalent links are similar to the intramolecular and intermolecular covalent cross-link of type II collagen,

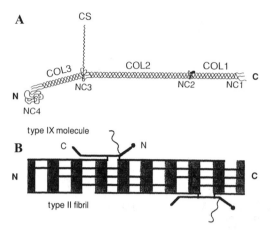

FIGURE 5-3. The structure of type IX collagen and its association with type II collagen. **(A)** Type IX collagen consists of three triple helical domains (COL1, COL2, COL3) with four nonhelical domains (NC1–NC4), and the molecule is stabilized by interchain disulfide bridges. The single chondroitin sulfate chain is attached at the NC3 domain. **(B)** The majority of type IX collagen molecules exist in the extracellular matrix covalently bound to the surface of the type II collagen fibrils in an antiparallel manner.

the trifunctional hydroxypyridinium cross-link (122,124,126,364,545). Type IX also projects into the matrix from the surface of type II fibrils and may interact with the other type IX covalently. This interaction may help to form and stabilize the collagen fibril meshwork. Type IX collagen therefore appears to have an important role in stabilizing the three-dimensional organization of the collagen network (125,514,543) and thus contributes to the ability of collagen to resist the swelling pressure of the proteoglycans and the tensile stresses developed within the tissue when it is loaded in situ (240,308,350,450,451). The importance of type IX collagen in collagen fibril formation is indicated by the fact that defects in this collagen results in chondrodysplasia. Furthermore, it has been shown that a reduction in function of type IX collagen has the potential to contribute to degeneration of articular cartilage (47,127,359).

2.2.3 Collagen Synthesis

Collagen biosynthesis, secretion, and aggregation into fibrils are complex processes. Extensive splicing occurs in chondrocyte cell nucleus where tissue-specific and developmentally regulated alternative splicing of the transcripts takes place for collagens, including collagen types II and IX (371,435,443). For fibril-forming collagens, collagen α chains are synthesized and translocated to the endoplasmic reticulum as prepro–α chains. After cleavage of the signal peptides, the procollagen chains undergo extensive and complex posttranslational modification, before chain assembly and folding of the triple helix take place. These include the hydroxylation of proline and lysine into hydroxyproline and hydroxylysine, and glycosylation. Chain assembly occurs from the noncollagenous COOH terminus and proceeds toward the NH_2 terminus, when one α chain combines with two other in the lumen of the endoplasmic reticulum to form the triple-helical molecule. Inter- and intrachain disulfide bridges also form in this process. Once the triple helix is formed, the procollagen enters into the secretory pathway.

After secretion into the extracellular space, the propeptides at both the COOH and NH_2 termini are cleaved. The cleaved amino and carboxyl propeptides may have a role in feedback regulation of procollagen synthesis. Collagen molecules then come together and self-aggregate into fibrils. The fibrils are strengthened by covalent cross-links within and between collagen molecules by lysyl oxidase (472).

The processing and assembly of other nonfibril-forming collagens follow similar steps, with a few variations. For example, types VI, IX, and XI collagens retain their amino and carboxyl noncollagenous domains after secretion. Some collagens also have additional processing steps such as adding the chondroitin sulfate chain, probably intracellularly in the Golgi apparatus (399).

2.3 Proteoglycans

Proteoglycans (PGs) are large complex molecules each formed by a core protein and one or more covalently attached GAG chains (135,177,179, 251,356,357,413,433,453). PGs are found in virtually all connective tissues to various extents. In the case of cartilage, a major component of the matrix is the large aggregating PG, aggrecan, which endows cartilage with the mechanical properties to withstand compressive stresses due to joint loading. Like collagen, PGs are vital for cartilage matrix assembly and cartilage structure. Disturbance to PG metabolism in cartilage also underlies many diseases. For example, degradation and loss of aggrecan results in a loss of functional integrity of cartilage, which leads to destructive joint diseases. The vital role of PG in cartilage matrix is readily displayed in the phenotypes of the cmd mouse and nanomelia chick that result from mutations in aggrecan core protein gene (11,275,532). In humans, mutations in aggrecan gene have not yet been reported.

PGs are a very diverse class of molecules. To date, more than 30 genes have been identified to encode the core proteins. There are many types of GAGs as well (Fig. 5-4), with further differences in their fine structure; see, for example, reference 179. Furthermore, the number of combinations between various core proteins and GAGs is huge, and GAG distribution on the core protein also varies to a great extent. Variation can also derive from the fact that while each protein core can carry a variety of GAGs, different cores may also bear the same type of GAG. There-fore, there is enormous diversity in proteoglycan structure.

2.3.1 Proteoglycans of Articular Cartilage and Meniscus

One of the major components of cartilage matrix is the large aggregating PG, aggrecan. Aggrecan has been studied extensively because of its role in skeletal growth, joint function, and the development of arthritis (56,177,181–183,185, 192,356,357,392). Aggrecan constitutes as much as 80% to 90% of proteoglycans in articular cartilage, and its presence is considered the hallmark of chondrogenesis. Aggrecan, along with versican, belongs to the large aggregating proteoglycan family, because of its ability to form large aggregates. Aggrecan in cartilage is found as large aggregates of numerous aggrecan monomers noncovalently attached to hyaluronan, which is further stabilized by the binding of a link protein. These large aggregates are responsible for the ability of cartilage to resist compressive loading. Other PGs existing in articular cartilage include the small PGs biglycan, decorin, fibromodulin, and lumican, which belong to a group of small leucine-rich proteoglycans

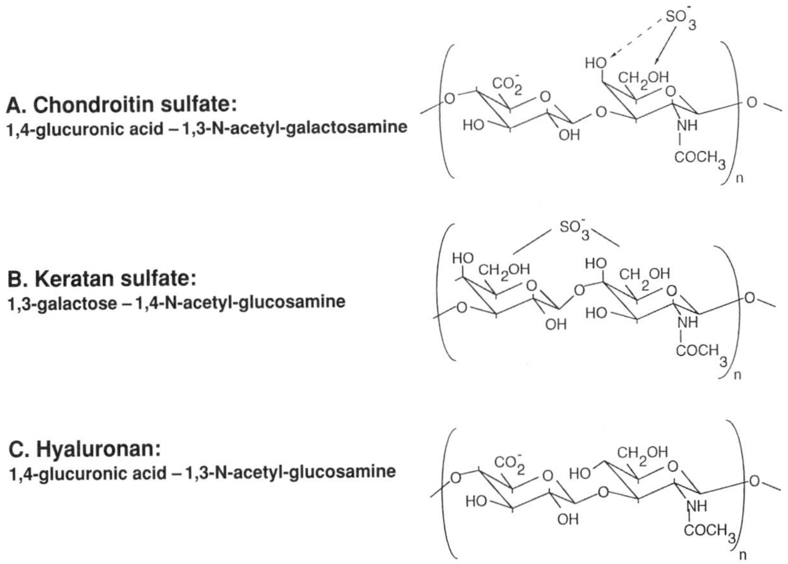

A. Chondroitin sulfate:
1,4-glucuronic acid – 1,3-N-acetyl-galactosamine

B. Keratan sulfate:
1,3-galactose – 1,4-N-acetyl-glucosamine

C. Hyaluronan:
1,4-glucuronic acid – 1,3-N-acetyl-glucosamine

FIGURE 5-4. The disaccharide units of the three primary glycosaminoglycan chains in cartilage (295).

(SLRPs) and related glycoproteins, as well as perlecan, a heparan sulfate PG (453,486). In meniscus, aggrecan, versican, decorin, biglycan, and fibromodulin are also present. They are expressed with patterns reflecting the age and health stage of the meniscus (194,314,457). Futhermore, type IX collagen is also considered a PG because of the presence of attached GAG side chain (251,433).

Hyaluronan, also known as hyaluronic acid (HA), is different from the other GAGs in that it is not sulfated (see later discussion). It is often considered as a PG, although it does not have a core protein. It consists solely of repeating disaccharide units of *N*-acetylglucosamine linked to glucuronic acid, and it can reach molecular masses of 10^2 to 10^4 kDa. The function of hyaluronan is to interact with aggrecan and link protein to form macromolecular aggregates that are immobilized within the collagen network (174–176,357) (see later discussion). HA further functions to link ECM to the chondrocytes through the interaction with chondrocyte

cell surface hyaluronan receptor CD44 (252). This forms a direct linkage between the cells and their surrounding matrix (see later discussion).

Aggrecan is comprised of a core protein and chondroitin sulfate and keratan sulfate GAG chains. The core protein of aggrecan constitutes only 10% of its molecular mass; the rest is made up of GAG chains. Two types of GAGs, keratan sulfate and chondroitin sulfate (Fig. 5-4), attach to the core protein primarily in the keratan sulfate and chondroitin sulfate attachment domain, respectively (Fig. 5-5). As many as 50 keratan sulfate and 100 chondroitin sulfate chains can be attached to a single core protein (98,99,177, 179,183,192,513). The fine structure of chondroitin sulfate chains in cartilage changes with age and depth of cartilage. The chain length decreases with age, with increased ratio of chondroitin 6-sulfate to chondroitin 4-sulfate and heterogeneity (31,32,430).

The core protein of aggrecan has been cloned from several species with similar molecular organization. It has a molecular mass of 210 to

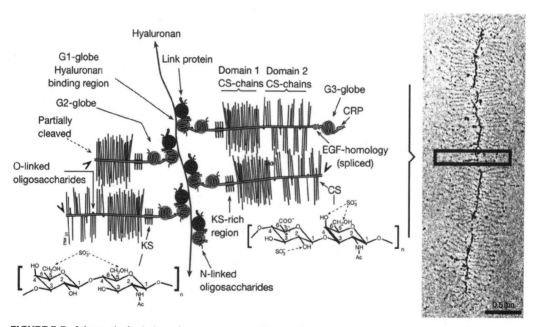

FIGURE 5-5. Schematic depiction of an aggrecan and its location on a proteoglycan aggregate. An aggrecan is composed of glycosaminoglycan chains (keratan sulfate and chondroitin sulfate) bound covalently to a core protein molecule. The proteoglycan aggregate that is composed of aggrecans that are noncovalently attached to hyaluronan with stabilizing link proteins. An electron micrograph of the macromolecule after rotary shadowing is shown at right – scale bar = 0.5 µm. (Adapted from Dick Heinegard D, Bayliss M, Lorenzo P. Pathogenesis of structural changes in the osteoarthritic joint. In: Brandt KD, Doherty M, Lohmander LS, eds. *Osteoarthritis*. Oxford: Oxford University Press, 2003;73–184.) (46)

250 kDa and contains three globular domains, G1 at the NH_2 terminus, followed by G2, and G3 at the COOH terminus; an interglobular domain between G1 and G2 domains; and a keratan sulfate and a chondroitin sulfate GAG attachment domain between G2 and G3 domains (Fig. 5-5). The function of the G1 domain serves to mediate the interaction with HA and link protein. The function of the other globular domains is currently unclear. The interaction of G1 domain with HA is further stabilized by a link protein, which itself is highly homologous to the G1 domain. The link protein binds to both HA and the G1 domain, forming aggrecan–HA–link protein complexes. The noncovalent interactions among these three molecules are extremely strong and cannot be dissociated under physiological conditions, unless chaotropic denaturants or proteases are present (174–176, 182,183,386,406,408). Many aggrecan molecules can attach to a single HA molecule to form aggregate. Some 300 aggrecan monomers have been found to form an aggregate in fetal cartilage. The aggregate size varies among different types of cartilage and depends on the length of HA and the number of aggrecans attached to it (55). The aggregate size also decreases with age and disease stage. As aggregates, the aggrecan molecules can form macromolecular complexes of 300 to 400×10^6 Da and make major contributions to the mechanical and physicochemical properties of cartilage (159,161,215,264,297–300,302,350–353). The extremely large stable complexes of this ternary PG aggregates keep the aggrecan in ECM and are critical for maintaining cartilage matrix architecture. Furthermore, the interaction of HA with its cell surface receptor CD44 also contributes to the retention of aggrecan in the ECM (250,253). For example, inhibition of CD44 leads to the loss of cartilage matrix (77). An additional function of this interaction is to provide a direct linkage between the chondrocytes and their surrounding matrix, and it may provide an important mechanism by which the chondrocyte can detect changes in the ECM and respond accordingly. It also provides a means for HA turnover through receptor-mediated endocytosis (210).

The primary amino acid sequence of the core proteins of biglycan (130,426,442) and decorin (90,520) show sequence homology of 55%. Their GAG chains are chondroitin sulfate and dermatan sulfate. Whereas there are two GAG chains attached to biglycan, there is one GAG chain attached to decorin, although the types of GAG in each PG vary. In adult cartilage, there are almost as many biglycan and decorin molecules as there are of aggrecan, although they probably contribute less than 10% to the total weight of PGs (426,431). The spatial and temporal expression patterns of biglycan and decorin seem to be divergent. For example, epiphyseal cartilage stains strongly for decorin and weakly for biglycan, whereas developing articular cartilage expresses biglycan in the pericellular matrix but not decorin. In adult articular cartilage, decorin is found in the interterritorial matrix while biglycan is found in the pericellular matrix. Decorin is also the dominant PG in meniscus (432). The small proteoglycans are important for collagen fibril formation. Decorin is associated with collagen fibrils. It has also been suggested that the dermatan sulfate chain on decorin has the ability to self-associate, providing a means by which adjacent collagen fibers can interact (456). In decorin-deficient mice, collagen fibril assembly is irregular and tensile strength of the skin and tendon are reduced (91). However, it should be noted that the major cartilage collagen, Col II, has not been reported to be affected by decorin deficiency. The distribution and role of biglycan is less well studied. Biglycan knockout mice show decreased postnatal skeletal growth, suggesting that biglycan may function as a positive regulator of bone formation (544).

2.3.2 *Glycosaminoglycan Side Chains*

The GAG chains of the proteoglycan impart many of the physical properties to the molecule (Fig. 5-4). The GAGs are among the most anionic molecules because of the presence of large numbers of negatively charged sulfate and carboxyl groups. The high negative charge attracts counterions and gives rise to Donnan osmotic pressure that favors tissue hydration. GAGs also have a natural tendency to repel each other, which is restrained by the collagen fibril network.

GAGs are linear unbranched polysaccharides consisting mainly of repeating disaccharide of alternating uronic acid and acetylated amino sugar such as hexamine (Fig. 5-4). Depending on the main repeating disaccharides, GAGs are classified into various families including heparan sulfate, chondroitin sulfate, dermatan sulfate, keratan sulfate, and hyaluronan. Within each of these families there is much detailed variation of precise sequences of sugars.

Chondroitin sulfate is composed of repeating disaccharide units of glucuronic acid and N-acetyl-galactosamine with a sulfate group per disaccharide and may reach a molecular mass of 20 kDa. Keratan sulfate consists of repeating disaccharide units of galactose and N-acetyl-glucosamine, again averaging approximately one sulfate group per disaccharide. The sulfate and carboxyl groups on the chondroitin sulfate and keratan sulfate chains become charged in solution and in situ. The total FCD in cartilage ranges from 0.05 to 0.3 mEq/g wet weight of tissue (297,298,302). Briefly, these charges provide the swelling properties of the tissue in the following way (a more detailed explanation is given later in this chapter). First, the fixed negative charges are placed close together in the dense solid matrix thereby creating charge–charge repulsion forces. At the same time, to maintain electroneutrality, counterions, e.g., Na^+, will be present, and these will cause a swelling pressure known as the Donnan osmotic pressure (100,230,264,297,302,351). These two phenomena define the swelling pressure (264), which has been measured and calculated to be approximately 0.25 MPa. The swelling pressure contributes equilibrium compressive stiffness of the ECM of cartilage, which usually ranges from 0.5 to 1.0 MPa, depending on the type of tissue (23,24,338,343,345,350,351). The FCD also largely determines the transport of electrolytes and electrokinetic properties of cartilage (112,113,136–138,159–164). Finally, the bulk properties of the proteoglycans will contribute to the flow-dependent viscoelastic properties that occur when cartilage or meniscus is loaded (346, 460,549).

The size, structural rigidity or flexibility, and complex molecular conformation of normal proteoglycan aggregates make important contributions to the mechanical behavior of articular cartilage. In dilute aqueous solution of pure proteoglycans, it has been shown that these molecules will occupy a large solvation domain, five to ten times larger than that available within the interfibrillar space of native cartilage (183, 357,384,424,425). Their sheer size, folded into their compacted state in situ, acts to retard their movement by diffusion and by hydrodynamic convective transport through the fine interfibrillar space by steric exclusion and by frictional drag (86,159,180,262,300,302,341,350,396). All these proteoglycan characteristics undoubtedly will promote proteoglycan–proteoglycan networking and collagen–proteoglycan interactions in situ (178,214,331,354,357,454,548, 549,552,553), which are important in stabilizing the collagen–proteoglycan solid matrix (5,6, 49,50,155), thus enabling it to function in the highly loaded environment of diarthrodial joints.

2.3.3 Biosynthesis of Proteoglycans

In cartilage, the single cell type (chondrocyte) is responsible for the synthesis, modification, assembly, and organization of the proteoglycan molecules. The synthesis of aggrecan is well studied and serves as an example for all of the proteoglycans synthesized in other cartilaginous tissues (Fig. 5-6). The protein core is synthesized by the normal secretory pathway in the endoplasmic reticulum, where N-linked oligosaccharides are added and GAG chains are initiated. The core protein is then passed to the Golgi apparatus where further elongation and complex posttranslational modification of the GAG chains take place. Specific serine residues are linked to long GAG chains that are synthesized in situ. These chains are then sulfated by sulfotransferase enzymes. After sulfation, the aggrecan molecule is secreted by the cells. The polysaccharide chains are assembled by the sequential action of a series of glycosyltransferases following a nontemplate mechanism that is not under direct genetic control. Because the protein core of aggrecan can have more than ten times its weight of carbohydrate attached to it (Fig. 5-5), there can be considerable modulation of structure during the posttranslational stages of processing (177). The

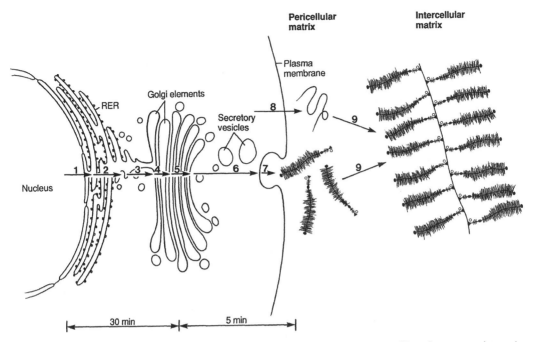

FIGURE 5-6. A schematic representation of a series of metabolic events controlling the proteoglycans in cartilage. The chondrocytes synthesize and secrete proteoglycan, link protein, and hyaluronan, which become incorporated into the matrix as functional aggregates. Enzymes released by the cells break down these aggregates into fragments, which are released from the matrix into the synovial fluid. The fragments are then taken up by the lymphatics and moved to the circulating blood (295).

number, size, and type of GAG chains that are added can be significantly modulated at the post-translational step.

Once secreted, the formation of aggrecan aggregates depends on the synthesis of two other molecules, link protein and hyaluronan (Fig. 5-5). Link protein plays a major role in contributing to the material properties exhibited by the proteoglycan networks in solution (346,549), and therefore, the control of the synthesis of link protein and proteoglycan is vital. Although the aggrecan and link protein are separate gene products, they are often synthesized together and at similar rates (409). However, it has been shown that the chondrocyte has the ability to control the biosynthesis of these two molecules independently (409).

The third component of the proteoglycan aggregate is HA. The enzymes responsible for HA synthesis, hyaluronan synthase (HAS), are localized on plasma membranes, and synthesis of HA occurs there and does not go through the endoplasmic reticulum–Golgi pathway used by pro-

teoglycan and link protein (397). Three HASs have been identified in the mammalian system, two of which are found in chondrocytes. How the HAS system regulates the synthesis of HA is not very clear; however, inhibition of HAS in chondrocytes can lead to impaired matrix assembly and retention of cartilage matrix (370). The synthesized HA is then exported into the pericellular environment directly. The association of aggrecan with HA and link protein occurs after secretion, in the ECM, probably including sites distant from the pericellular matrix. Portions of HA without attached aggrecan are free to bind to hyaluronan receptors CD44 on the surface of the chondrocytes, thus forming a defined and specific linkage between the cell and its ECM (250,253). Through this linkage, the cells can potentially receive signals from the cartilage ECM and respond correspondingly, although a precise mechanism by which this is mediated is still not defined. In synovial fluid, synoviocytes can also synthesize HA and secrete it into the joint, where it can act as a lubricant.

Expression of many PGs is also regulated in a tissue- and developmental-stage-specific manner. For example, meniscus expresses low levels of aggrecan, and ligaments and tendons usually also have low levels except in areas that are regularly subjected to compression (118). Although tissues have usually been shown to express aggrecan at low levels (414), high levels of expression can occur in some cartilaginous tissues, such as the intervertebral disc. Aggrecan expression is concomitant with the establishment of chondrocyte phenotype and is generally used as a biomarker of chondrocyte differentiation. However, further study is still needed to elucidate the tissue-specific or developmental-stage-specific regulation of aggrecan gene expression.

2.4 Collagen–proteoglycan Interactions

In articular cartilage and meniscus, collagen fibrils and proteoglycan networks show interaction not only within themselves, but also between the two components when they form the ECM network. Specific interactions between the collagen network and the proteoglycan aggregates are not well characterized; however, the interaction is considered to be primarily frictional in nature (240,350,451). The swelling pressure exerted by FCD (264,302,308) serves to inflate the collagen network and thus helps to maintain the ECM organization. This inflated state also allows the collagen network to sustain tensile loads and thus provides shear stiffness to the ECM (550).

In vitro, proteoglycans are able to interact with each other to form networks under physiological concentrations (178,341,346,549,552). Adding type II collagen and/or link protein seems to increase the interaction sites and strength, suggesting that these two proteins can also interact with the proteoglycan network and contribute directly to the mechanical properties of cartilage (549,553). The proteoglycan networks and the proteoglycan–collagen composite matrix formed *in vitro* are capable of storing elastic energy, but their shear stiffness of ~ 10 Pa is less than 10^{-5} times that of normal articular cartilage. Therefore, other factors, such

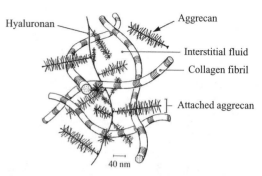

FIGURE 5-7. A schematic diagram indicating the collagen–proteoglycan matrix in cartilage (354).

as collagen cross-linking and interactions with type IX collagen, must have strong influences on the shear properties of cartilage and meniscus (482,550,551). The other aspect of interaction of PG and collagen lies in the fact that some SLRPs, including decorin and fibromodulin, can interact with and regulate collagen fibrillogenesis (see earlier discussion). Through these interactions, fibril assembly and diameter can be influenced. Also, it is known that aggrecan molecules can accelerate fibril formation, whereas aggrecan aggregates have little influence on fibril formation (232,454,455). Thus, it is possible that different proteoglycans in the matrix affect fibril formation differently, giving rise to the possibility of biologically controlled ECM architecture throughout the tissue (Fig. 5-7).

2.5 Cartilage Ultrastructure

From the material standpoint, the ECM of cartilage is a fiber-reinforced composite solid consisting of a dense stable network of collagen fibers embedded in a very high concentration of proteoglycan gel, which itself is also a viscoelastic network. The composition and structure of articular cartilage are inhomogeneous within the tissue and vary with depth. Along with the differences in collagen fiber and proteoglycan network, water content also changes. Chondrocyte shape and size also vary with the depth. This gives the tissue a layered appearance under electron microscopy (Fig. 5-8). In the superficial zone, which represents 10% to 20% of the total thickness of articular cartilage, there is the

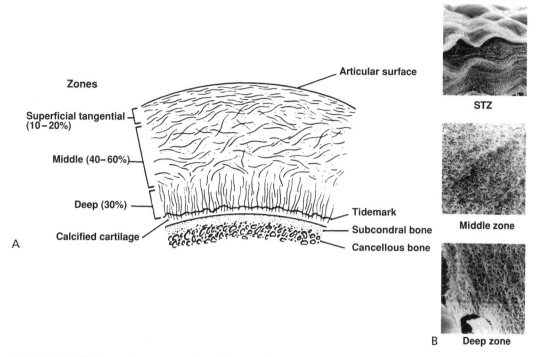

FIGURE 5-8. (A) Layered structure of cartilage collagen network showing three distinct regions, and **(B)** corresponding SEM collagen fibrillar arrangement. (SEMs are courtesy of Dr. T Takei; reference 354.)

highest content of water (75% to 80%) and the highest content of collagen (85% dry weight) (279,302,355,498,499). Aggrecan level is the lowest compared with the other zones (7,8,302, 303). Fine collagen fibrils are densely organized in parallel to the articular surface (78,79,267, 336,533). This is a region where tissue is exposed to the highest tensile and compressive stresses. Tensile strength has been shown to be the highest in this zone, too (8,238,241,427,537). The dense collagen fibrils lying in parallel to the joint surface in this zone may also help to resist shear forces generated during joint use (550). The next zone, which comprises 40% to 60% of the total thickness, is the middle zone. Collagen content decreases from the superficial zone to the middle zone and remains relatively constant in the deeper zones, whereas aggrecan content increases to its maximum in the middle zone (140,279, 302,303,407,484). Water content generally decreases with depth. The collagen fibrils in the middle zone have a larger diameter that is less tightly packed with random orientation (15,35,

49–52,78,79,267,336,533). In the deep zone (about 30% of the total thickness), the fibers appear to be woven together to form large fiber bundles organized perpendicular to the surface (51,78,79,417). These bundles cross the "tidemark" to insert into the calcified cartilage and subchondral bone, thus securely anchoring the uncalcified tissue onto the bone ends (58,79, 267,417). The inhomogeneous distribution of collagen and PG produces pronounced variations in the tensile stiffness and swelling behaviors of various zones of the cartilage, and causes swelling and curling when the tissue is removed from the bone (458,464).

2.6 Meniscus Ultrastructure

The fibrous structure of the meniscus also has a layered appearance, but it differs from that of articular cartilage. The menisci are semilunar in shape and are situated between the femoral condyles and tibial plateau of the knee (Fig. 5-9). The articulating surface of the meniscus is

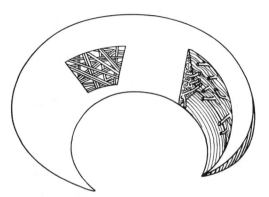

FIGURE 5-9. Collagen ultrastructure of the meniscus, showing the surface and deep zone fiber orientations. The surface zone fibers are arranged in a random fashion, whereas the deep zone fibers are large and arranged predominantly in a circumferential manner. Radial fibers are also shown (132).

composed of fine fibrils in a random meshlike woven matrix (15,59,546), although split lines are also present. Approximately 100 μm from the surface layers into the interior are large rope-like collagen fiber bundles that are principally arranged circumferentially around the semilunar meniscus. Smaller radial fibers appear to reinforce the structure of the meniscus by tying the large circumferential fiber bundles together (59, 234,400,469). This fibrillar organization predominates throughout the peripheral two-thirds of the tissue, whereas the inner region appears to contain more randomly arranged smaller collagen fibers and proteoglycans, resembling hyaline cartilage (147,364,546).

2.7 Inhomogeneous and Anisotropic Material Properties

The layered morphology of the collagen network (inhomogeneity) and the preferred orientation of collagen fibers (anisotropy) of both articular and meniscal cartilages provide a convenient means of examining how the collagen content and organization influence their strengths and stiffnesses. Anisotropic properties have been assessed by simply cutting test specimens oriented in a specific direction relative to the split-line pattern, whereas tissue inhomogeneity has been measured by testing tissue from different layers

and different regions of these tissues (Fig. 5-8). Anisotropic and inhomogeneous compressive, tensile, and shear properties of articular cartilage and the meniscus have been demonstrated (69, 73,74,132,241,274,350,400,427,448,449,451, 469,529,530,537,539,551). Details of various tensile tests and results are provided hereafter.

3 HOMEOSTASIS OF ARTICULAR CARTILAGE

Articular cartilage and meniscus, like all connective tissues, are metabolically active. The metabolic activities involve both anabolic and catabolic events. The anabolic activity refers to the synthesis, assembly, and organization of the matrix, and the catabolic process refers to the degradation and subsequent loss of the matrix (Fig. 5-6). The chondrocytes are responsible for the orchestration of these events. A balance between the two processes will result in the homeostasis and maintenance of the ECM and its biological function throughout life. However, this balance can be disturbed during disease processes, resulting in remodeling and degradation of the ECM as observed in articular cartilage during osteoarthritis. Chondrocytes are metabolically active and respond to changes in their environment, which include soluble mediators (e.g., cytokines, growth factors, hormones, proteases, pharmaceutical agents) and mechanical environment (e.g., stresses, strains, flow velocities, osmotic and hydraulic pressures, electric currents and potentials, and other physicochemical events) (33,67,154,167,378, 381,412,438; also see this chapter for more details on cell–matrix interactions). Although the following descriptions primarily refer to articular cartilage, it is hypothesized that similar processes are ongoing in meniscus, with the major difference involving the molecules synthesized.

The degradation of matrix is an integral and ongoing process during growth and development and matrix turnover in mature cartilage. It is normally under tight control of growth factors, cytokines and proteases that can regulate the synthesis of matrix proteins and various proteases and inhibitors. Normal healthy tissues have a balanced process of synthesis and degradation. Under pathological conditions, this balance is disturbed and matrix degradation prevails.

When degradation of healthy cartilage is induced, aggrecan is lost rapidly followed by type II collagen (37,68,94). Degradation products of aggrecan and collagen can be detected in synovial fluid. Generally, collagen fibrils have very long half-lives, with a small portion having more rapid turnover (292,293,418). PGs have a more rapid turnover rate than cartilage collagen, with a range of half-life from 8 days to 600 days (293, 299). The normal turnover of matrix components is consistent with the presence of matrix metalloproteases (MMPs), a class of degradative enzymes, in the cartilage.

3.1 Chondrocytes and Cell Surface Receptors

Chondrocytes are the single cell type in adult articular cartilage. They are highly specialized, terminally differentiated cells. In healthy cartilage, chondrocytes are normally surrounded by a layer of pericellular matrix that is 2 μm thick. This pericellular matrix is rich in type VI collagen and contains few well-defined collagen fibers. The chondrocyte and its pericellular matrix seem to act as a structural and functional unit, and therefore, are also called a chondron (394,395). In menisci, the cells are termed fibrochondrocytes (318,485). In skeletally mature cartilage and meniscus tissues, the ECM contributes the vast majority of the tissue volume (at least 90%). The cells occupy only a small proportion of the total volume (1% to 10%); however, the cells are responsible for the synthesis, assembly, and organization of the ECM, and for the maintenance of homeostasis in these tissues.

Chondrocytes have different size, shape, orientation, and biosynthetic activity in different zones of articular cartilage (25). In the superficial zone close to the articular surface, the cells are flattened and parallel to the surface. Chondrocytes in this layer synthesize a matrix that is high in collagen and low in proteoglycans.

Cells in this layer also turn over proteoglycans more rapidly. The middle zone contains cells that are rounded with seemingly higher synthetic activities. They synthesize and organize a matrix with a higher concentration of proteoglycans and larger collagen fibrils. In the deep zone, the chondrocytes are often lined up in columns perpendicular to the articular cartilage surface. The cell density decreases into the middle and the deep zone, and also decreases with age (328).

Chondrocyte interacts with its ECM through cell surface receptors such as integrins, annexin V, and CD44. Through these interactions, chondrocytes can sense the changes in the ECM, such as the deformation caused by mechanical loading, or the composition changes caused by the degradation and depletion of the matrix molecules. Chondrocytes are metabolically active and can adapt to these changes to a limited extent. This can be seen in the early stages of joint degeneration where cell proliferation and increased matrix synthesis are observed. However, in general, the metabolic activity of chondrocytes is relatively low and their ability to remodel is limited. Therefore lesions to the cartilage can often remain in the tissue without repair, which leads to impaired functions.

CD44, the receptor for HA, is important for the interaction of chondrocytes with ECM and for the retention of proteoglycan aggregates in the matrix. Its inhibition has been shown to lead to a loss of aggrecan, which is thought to be caused by increased aggrecan degradation by aggrecanase (77). HA can inhibit chondrocyte proteoglycan synthesis, probably also through interaction with CD44 (28, 478). Annexin V, also called anchorin CII, is a chondrocyte cell surface receptor for type II collagen (503). It binds to the telopeptide region and the C-propeptide of type II collagen. It can also interact with type X collagen (246,390). Annexin V is thought to function as a mechanotransduction receptor on the chondrocyte cell surface.

Another group of cell surface receptors, integrins, are a family of heterodimeric receptors for adhesive proteins that mediate a wide range of functions. They are heterodimeric because each integrin molecule consists of one α

and one β subunit. Integrin structure, function, and associated intracellular signaling events have been extensively reviewed (148,216). Their expression in chondrocyte has also been reviewed (282,441,540). Through the extracellular domain, integrins recognize a number of cartilage ECM proteins including collagen, fibronectin, thrombospondin, vitronectin, and laminin. The intracellular domain of integrin interacts with intracellular signaling molecules as well as cytoskeleton. Integrins are capable of transmitting molecular signals in both directions across the cell membrane, signaling events which are termed "inside-out" and "outside-in." Integrins can transmit signals from extracellular matrix to the cells to affect cellular function and gene expression (i.e., outside-in signaling). On the other hand, integrin expression pattern and ligand affinity can be modified by the cells to affect the interaction of cells with ECM (i.e., inside-out signaling) (148, 216). Therefore, integrins serve as a bridge that links the ECM to intracellular cytoskeleton as well as the intracellular signaling machinery.

Chondrocytes express a panel of integrins, including those containing β_1 subunits paired with $\alpha_1, \alpha_2, \alpha_3, \alpha_4, \alpha_5, \alpha_6,$ and α_{10} subunits, as well as integrins $\alpha_V\beta_5$ and $\alpha_V\beta_3$ (64,281,282, 441,540). Chondrocytes can bind the ECM molecules through integrins. For example, $\alpha_1\beta_1$ and $\alpha_{10}\beta_1$ have been reported to mediate the attachment of chondrocytes to type II collagen. Integrins $\alpha_1\beta_1$ can also mediate the cellular interaction with type VI collagen. Integrin $\alpha_5\beta_1$ is a major receptor on chondrocyte that recognizes fibronectin. The expression patterns of integrins vary with developmental stage and the layer of cartilage where the cells reside, and can be regulated by various growth factors and cytokines that regulate cartilage function, such as insulin-like growth factor-I (IGF-I) and transforming growth factor-β (TGF-β) (282). The interaction of chondrocyte with ECM through integrin has been implicated in mediating important functions of cartilage. Interfering with integrin function using functional blocking integrin antibodies can inhibit cartilage growth and differentiation (196,467). Integrins have also been suggested to function as a mechanotransducer

for cartilage, which may enable the cells to respond to external loading and mechanical stimuli (205,326,542).

3.2 Growth Factors and Cytokines Important for Cartilage

Chondrocytes are exposed to a complex array of growth factors, cytokines, and hormones that can have different effects on cell proliferation, differentiation, and matrix synthesis and degradation. These factors control chondrocyte metabolism and affect cartilage homeostasis in either an autocrine or a paracrine manner with either anabolic or catabolic effects on the chondrocytes. Some factors can have both effects and are considered having a regulatory function on chondrocytes. The cytokines with predominantly anabolic activities include IGF-I, members of the TGF-β/bone morphogenetic protein (BMP) family, and fibroblast growth factor (FGF). The cytokines that have catabolic activities include interleukin-1 (IL-1), tumor necrosis factor α (TNF-α), IL-17, IL-18, and leukemia inhibitory factor (LIF). Cytokines such as IL-6 can have dual effect on chondrocytes. Cartilage destruction is frequently linked with aberrant growth factor and cytokine expression and activity.

IGF-I is one of the most potent anabolic growth factors for cartilage (501). It belongs to a family of insulin-like growth factors consisting of IGF-I, IGF-II, and insulin. Both IGF-I and its receptor are expressed by chondrocytes (366). Through binding to its cell surface receptor, IGF-I triggers receptor tyrosine phosphorylation and a complex intracellular signaling pathway involving the insulin receptor substrate 1 (IRS-1) (for review, see reference 80). This ultimately leads to chondrocyte differentiation and proliferation (80,290). IGF-I potently stimulates the synthesis of collagen and proteoglycans (166,286,319,374,506) and inhibits cartilage catabolism (286,506). The extent of IGF-I effect on cells depends on the balance of the expression level of IGF, IGF-binding protein, and IGF-I receptor. IGF-I levels are found to increase along with increased levels of IGF-binding protein in the cartilage and synovial fluid of

OA patients (312,323,452). Interestingly, despite an increase in free IGF-I level and normal or increased receptor and IGF-binding protein levels, chondrocytes from experimental arthritis animals or OA patients show reduced responsiveness to the stimulation of exogenous IGF-I (75,102,128,446,488).

The TGF-β/BMP proteins are the other family of growth factors that act on chondrocytes to stimulate their anabolic activities. This family of growth factors bind to cell surface and stimulate intracellular signaling pathways that involve Smad proteins (for review, see references 311 and 421). TGF-β and its receptors are ubiquitously expressed on most cells; therefore, the bioactivity of TGF-β depends on its activation from the latent form. TGF-β is produced by articular cartilage (220,466). TGF-β maintains cartilage homeostasis by stimulating chondrocyte mitogenesis and increasing matrix synthesis as well as decreasing proteoglycan degradation (87,332, 416). It can stimulate chondrocyte differentiation and cartilage formation during development (76,92,258). TGF-β has also been shown to protect cartilage against IL-1-induced degradation process (see later discussion), possibly by down-regulating IL-1 receptor (87,103). However, TGF-β has also been shown to stimulate MMP-13 expression, which can in turn act on cartilage to initiate matrix degradation (see later discussion of MMPs) (330). The BMPs are important for development, and they seem to be more potent and specific on cartilage in stimulating proteoglycan and collagen matrix synthesis (134,200,287,439,541). BMPs also have chondroprotective activity to counteract matrix degradation induced by IL-1 or other matrix degradation products (212,254,287).

IL-1 is the best-characterized destructive cytokine for cartilage. It is the key regulator of matrix degradation in arthritis. It is synthesized by chondrocytes as well as mononuclear cells lining the synovium. IL-1 has a pronounced effect on cartilage matrix, including suppression of proteoglycan and type II, IX, and XI collagen synthesis and acceleration of proteoglycan degradation (152,153,333,408,504,505). Degradation of the collagen network seems to happen only after proteoglycan degradation is advanced.

IL-1 further cause the depletion of cartilage matrix through induction of the destructive proteases (97,229,389,393). In addition, IL-1 also increases production of inflammatory mediator including iNOS and COX-2, which can modulate chondrocyte activity. The net effects of IL-1 action on cartilage are reduced synthesis, increased degradation, and rapid matrix depletion. In animal models, IL-1 can induce cartilage damage when injected intraarticularly. There are also increased levels of IL-1 and its receptor in OA cartilage (309,321,471). The central role of IL-1 in cartilage destruction has been suggested by the experiment in which inhibition of IL-1 by antagonists prevented cartilage and bone destruction in animal models of arthritis (222).

The effect of TNF-α (tumor necrosis factor) is similar to and synergistic with that of IL-1 in inducing cartilage destruction. TNF-α inhibits type II collagen synthesis and plays a role in cartilage destruction, although less potently than IL-1 (63,440). TNF-α is also up-regulated in OA. Inhibition of TNF-α has been found to improve symptoms but does not prevent joint destruction (222).

3.3 Degradative Enzymes

MMPs, which are active at neutral pH, are suggested to be the key enzymes responsible for cartilage matrix protein degradation. However, other proteases may also play a role in joint destruction. For example, plasmin, cathepsin B, and kallikrein can cleave the proforms of MMPs into their active forms, which can lead to cartilage destruction.

MMPs are a class of endoproteinases whose activities depend on the presence of Zn^{2+}. MMPs comprise a family of about 20 proteases that degrade a wide range of ECM proteins that are important for regulating cellular functions, including collagen, proteoglycan, fibronectin, fibrinogen, and thrombospondin. MMPs, with the exception of MT1-MMP and MMP-11, are secreted as proenzymes by a variety of cells and are activated when the profragments are cleaved by a number of proteases such as plasmin, urokinase plasminogen activator, and membrane-type MMPs (34,38,149,525). MMPs are inhibited by tissue inhibitors of metalloproteinases (TIMPs). MMP activities therefore depend on their activation stage as well as the ratio of MMP versus TIMP and the other natural inhibitor that is present in serum, α2-macroglobulin. According to their substrate specificities, MMPs can be grouped into collagenases, gelatinases, stromelysins, and membrane-type MMPs. Collagenases, including MMPs 1, 8, and 13, can cleave helical collagens at a single site three-fourths of the way from the NH_2 terminus. These enzymes are considered to be critical in cartilage breakdown (84,324,415,468). MMP-13 may play an important role in degrading cartilage because it is the most efficient at cleaving type II collagen (249,327). This cleavage exposes neoepitopes that become more accessible after proteolysis and denaturing of the triple helix and can be recognized by a monoclonal antibody, COL2-3/4m (201). The cleaved and denatured collagen chains are then more susceptible to secondary cleavages by other MMPs such as gelatinases and stromelysin. Catabolic cytokines including IL-1 and TNF-α stimulate MMP synthesis and matrix degradation. In OA, increased expression and activity of various MMPs are also observed.

The core protein of aggrecan can be cleaved during joint catabolic process. The primary cleavage sites in human, Asn^{341}–Phe^{342} and Glu^{373}–Ala^{374}, are located in the IGD between the G1 and G2 domains of aggrecan core protein (133,445). Cleavage here separates the part of the proteoglycan involved in aggregation (the G1 domain) from the GAG-containing regions. This new nonaggregating GAG-containing fragment, although large, is able to pass through the matrix relatively rapidly and is lost to the synovial fluid (283,284,410–412). This appears to be an efficient mechanism of catabolism of aggrecan. The cleavage at these two sites also generates neoepitopes that can be recognized by specific antibodies, which have been employed to effectively detect the metabolism of aggrecan. The cleavage at the Asn^{341}–Phe^{342} bond has been attributed to the action of MMPs and can be reproduced *in vitro*. The cleavage of Glu^{373}–Ala^{374} has been shown to result from the aggrecanase activity. Aggrecanases have been cloned and have been shown to belong to a protein family called ADAMTS (A Disintegrin And Metalloproteinases with Thrombospondin motifs) (1,66,495). It has been suggested that during cartilage degradation, aggrecanase activity is responsible for primary cleavage of aggrecan. Cleavage at the MMP site occurs only as a late event in cartilage degradation (66,269,280, 516).

3.4 Effect of Mechanical Loading

Cartilage has been known to respond to mechanical stimuli and remodel. The pressure exerted on cartilage varies between 0 and 20 MPa during movement (5,6,155,199,385). The effects of applied forces are likely to modify cellular behavior by affecting metabolism, growth factor and cytokine secretion, and gene expression.

Chondrocytes can be considered cells under pressure (511). Chondrocytes are sensitive to mechanical forces. They require normal mechanical loading to maintain their normal balance of ECM. This is obvious in *in vivo* immobilization experiments. In animal models, when limbs are immobilized, the weight-bearing limbs often see increased cartilage matrix synthesis and content (223,247), while the immobilized limb incurs decreased matrix synthesis and content, which often leads to cartilage thinning (223, 247,376). The effect of loading also depends on loading magnitude as well as frequency. Static compression of the tissue to physiological strain magnitudes leads to the breakdown of cartilage proteoglycan (167,277,405). Moderate exercise increases cartilage matrix synthesis and content and has a protective effect on the joint (248, 375,377,487). This is supported by *in vitro* experiments showing that loading with moderate frequency and magnitude increases matrix synthesis and biomechanical properties (255,313, 437,511,536). However, a higher magnitude or frequency can cause the chondrocytes to break down their matrix. Matrix degradation can also be induced by changing the mechanical environment of the cells. For example, transection of the anterior cruciate ligament of the knee in dogs results in an increase in proteoglycan and collagen synthesis and an increase in matrix breakdown (65,121,412,444).

The mechanism leading from mechanical load stimulation to signal transduction and change in gene expression has yet to be elucidated clearly. The stimulus may be changes in cell shape and volume (169,170), or fluid flow (26,244,245), hydrostatic and osmotic pressure, shear, and electrical potential that are brought about by loading (352). Integrins that bridge the ECM to the intracellular cytoskeleton and stretch-activated ion channels (326,436,542) have been implicated in mediating the signaling events that lead to changes in cell metabolism and gene expression.

3.5 Articular Cartilage Pathology

Most of the collagen of cartilage matrix is type II, with minor collagens types IX and XI. Genetic mutations in all these forms of collagen have been identified in humans as causing defects in the cartilage. Mutation in type II results in cartilage degeneration and chondrodysplasia (71, 523). Mutation in type IX collagen leads to multiple epiphyseal dysplasia (47,359). Mutation in type X caused autosomal dominant Schmid metaphyseal chondrodysplasia (531). Mutation in type XI has been linked to an autosomal dominant Stickler's syndrome (524). These mutations affect the quality as well as the quantity of cartilage matrix, which renders the matrix inferior in its material properties and unable to withstand normal loading brought about by normal activities.

Joint pain and loss of mobility caused by the degeneration of articular cartilage are among the most common causes of disability in middle-age and older people. These pose a huge economic burden on society. Articular cartilage degeneration caused by joint injury or developmental or genetic or inflammatory disorders is most frequently associated with either primary or secondary OA. The understanding of the process of degeneration, and OA, in order to develop treatment modality depends on the understanding of the structure and biochemical and biomechanical properties of articular cartilage. OA, also referred to as arthrosis, is linked to age, genetics, gender, and occupation and can be caused by a multitude of factors, including disruption of joint integrity and cellular and molecular processes, mechanical force, and trauma (88). The process involves cartilage degradation and repair processes with a net outcome of degradation.

The earliest histological changes in OA include fibrillation of the superficial zone of the articular cartilage, along with decreased staining of proteoglycan, which extends into the middle zone. On a molecular level, the macromolecular matrix network is altered and disrupted. Decrease in PGs leads to the mechanical weakening of cartilage. As more PGs are depleted from the cartilage, cartilage loses its normal load-supporting mechanism (see later discussion) and becomes susceptible to mechanical microdamage that further disrupts the matrix integrity. One consequence of the loss of aggrecan from the tissue is loss of the FCD that is required to maintain the osmotic environment around chrocytes, and thus the ability to retain water is impaired. These are followed by the change and degradation of the collagen network. The net outcome of these changes is an increase in permeability, an increased water content, and a decrease in the stiffness of the tissues. The process may perpetuate itself, which in turn makes the cartilage more sensitive to the mechanical insult and impairs the ability of the cells to accomplish repair. The details of these biomechanical processes are described later.

4 BASIC CONCEPTS OF MATERIAL BEHAVIOR

4.1 Material Versus Structural Properties

When an object is subjected to an external load, it will move and deform. If all the external forces acting on the object sum up to zero, it will deform, but its center of mass will not move. The load and deformation responses of any material or structure depend on many factors, including the magnitude and direction of the applied load, the materials that constitute the body, and the size and shape of the body. Structural properties reflect the mechanical behavior of the body as a whole, including both material and geometric contributions to the load–deformation response (e.g., a bridge, an airplane wing, a femur or tibia, or a knee or hip is a structure). The mechanical properties describe the intrinsic characteristics of the material itself and depend on its composition, molecular structure, and ultrastructure (e.g., steel, aluminum, bone tissue, and cartilage tissue are different materials with different intrinsic material properties). Consequently, studies on the intrinsic mechanical properties of cartilage and meniscus have focused on the relationships between these properties and biochemical components and molecular organization (7,12, 132,240,264,340,400). These intrinsic material properties reflect the compositional and micro- and ultrastructural characteristics of the tissue (see Fig. 5-1) during its normal development and during aging and disease such as OA.

4.2 Stresses, Strains, and Constitutive Equations

Two types of physical quantities are necessary to determine the deformational response of a material body: stress and strain. Stress acting on or within an object is defined as force per unit area. Six components are required to completely define the state of stress at any point. There are three normal stress components, each of which could be tensile (positive) or compressive (negative), and three shear stress components. For the beginner, it is important to emphasize that stresses within an object can never be measured; i.e., there is no "stress gauge." Stress must be calculated. Strain is the local deformation at any point inside or on the surface of the object. There are also six components of strain: three lineal strains (change in length per original length) and three shear strains (change of angle between two mutually perpendicular line elements emanating from a material point). Strain on the surface of an object *can* be measured. There are strain gauges, and there are many techniques, mechanical, electronic, and optical, that are readily available for use in measuring strains on the surface of an object. For more details, the reader is referred to

standard engineering mechanics textbooks (142, 265,491).[1]

In general, when an object is under load, theoretical models and mathematical (or numerical) analyses are required to determine the states of stress (six components) and strain (six components) within the object. These analyses are based on Cauchy's equations (ca. 1830), which are derived from Newton's second and third laws of motion (ca. 1700), and on an *assumed* stress–strain relationship for the material. For each material (steel, wood, glass, PMMA, cartilage, meniscus, tendon, ligament, etc.), its stress–strain relationship must be individually experimentally measured in the laboratory. *There is no exception to this rule.* The mathematical expression used to describe the experimentally determined stress–strain response is known as the constitutive equation or constitutive law. Each constitutive equation or law is an idealization, or mathematical abstraction, of a measured stress–strain response of a real material. However, one cannot arbitrarily use any mathematical expression for the stress–strain law. Each stress–strain law must satisfy a set of fundamental and rigorous restrictions such as the laws of thermodynamics and observer independence (502).

The isotropic, linearly elastic constitutive law has most often been assumed to describe such material as steel, titanium, and bone. This mathematical relationship assumes that, for these materials, their stress and strain responses are related in a linear manner and that the stress–strain responses are not directionally dependent (i.e., the material is isotropic). For bone, however, the assumption of isotropy is not a good one in most cases. Nevertheless, because this constitutive law is the simplest 3D stress–strain law possible, known as the generalized Hooke's law (ca. 1680), it is the most frequently used law first employed by many to describe many materials. Two independent material coefficients are necessary to describe such isotropic materials: Young's modulus

---

[1] For birefringent photoelastic materials, polarized light is refracted as it passes through the strained material. In such cases, the strain field inside the object becomes visible via the pattern of color light. There have been photoelasticity studies of stress and strain fields in bone.

TABLE 5-4. CONVERSION OF CONSTANTS FOR ISOTROPIC LINEARLY ELASTIC MATERIAL

Basic Pairs	λ	μ	B	E	ν	H_A
λ, μ	λ	μ	$\lambda + (2/3)\mu$	$\mu(3\lambda + 2\mu)/(\lambda + \mu)$	$\lambda/2(\lambda + \mu)$	$\lambda + 2\mu$
E, ν	$\nu E /(1 + \nu)(1 - 2)$	$E/2(1 + \nu)$	$E/3(1 - 2\nu)$	E	ν	$\frac{E(1-\nu)}{(1+\nu)(1-2\nu)}$
μ, ν	$2\mu\nu/(1 - 2\nu)$	μ	$2\mu(1 + \nu)/3(1 - 2\nu)$	$2\mu(1 + \nu)$	ν	$\frac{2\nu(1-\nu)}{(1-2\nu)}$

Note: λ, Lame constant; μ, shear modulus; B, bulk modulus; E, Young's modulus; ν, Posisson's ratio: H_A, aggregate modulus.

(E) (ca. 1810) and shear modulus (μ). In engineering textbooks, the shear modulus is often referred to as the modulus of rigidity. For isotropic materials, these material coefficients are related to other coefficients such as the Poisson's ratio (ν) (ca. 1835), bulk modulus (k), aggregate modulus (H_A), and Lame's coefficients (λ, μ) (ca. 1850) (142,265,491). Depending on the convenience of the problem, these alternative material coefficients are often preferred. In other words, for isotropic, linearly elastic materials, there are only two independent material coefficients. Table 5-4 provides the relationships for these various commonly used isotropic elastic coefficients.

To begin analyzing the deformational behavior of any material, one must first assume a constitutive law for the material of interest and then use it to mathematically analyze its response in a laboratory experiment. If the mathematical predictions can accurately describe the experimentally measured strain or deformation or load response, then the coefficients of the constitutive law for the material can be determined. This is usually done by a curve-fitting procedure using a numerical algorithm, such as least square optimization, between the experimental data and the theoretical predictions. Such curve-fitting procedures, however, do not provide a unique solution. Therefore, it is always prudent to verify the validity of the calculated material coefficients with another *independent* experiment by using the material coefficients calculated from the first experiment to predict the results of a second experiment. For example, if the material coefficients are obtained from a creep experiment, then the response of an independent stress-relaxation experiment should be predicted

using these coefficients. This validation procedure is very important, especially in biomechanics, where the material stress–strain responses are often nonlinear and anisotropic. If an incorrect constitutive law has been assumed at the outset, this validation procedure will fail, and the analysis would render incorrect interpretations of the data. This situation is well recognized, and indeed, Y.C. Fung (1968) has gently advised that: "If no agreement is obtained, new analyses based on a different starting point would become necessary" (143).

4.3 History of Constitutive Modeling for Articular Cartilage

Various constitutive models have been used to describe cartilage. Some of the earliest models assumed the tissue to be isotropic and linearly elastic (29,150,187,195,206,236,474). This model can describe the mechanical behavior of soft hydrated tissues such as articular cartilage under static or equilibrium conditions, but it lacks the ability to describe the time-dependent creep and stress-relaxation behaviors exhibited by the tissue. Later, various viscoelastic models composed of springs and dashpots were proposed for cartilage to account for its creep and stress-relaxation behaviors (85,186,188,382,383,482,538). Although these viscoelasticity models are able to describe those behaviors successfully, they cannot describe the known effects of interstitial fluid flow. Early descriptions by Benninghoff (35) and studies by McCutchen (315), Sokoloff (473), Linn and Sokoloff (278), Edwards (110,111), and Maroudas (297,300) have demonstrated that when the tissue is compressed, it will lose water, and when soaked in fluid, it will absorb water. Further, the time rate of change of tissue hydration was shown to follow a pattern similar to that of compressive creep, suggesting that the compressive mechanical response of articular cartilage may be related to the fluid movement in the tissue (110,186,278,300,335). Thus, various poroelastic and biphasic models have been developed and used to account for interstitial fluid flow and its influence on the creep and stress-relaxation behaviors of cartilage (69,110, 164,211,288,315,338,340,342).

To date, the most successful theories for cartilage compressive behaviors are the biphasic theories developed by Mow and coworkers (20, 204,338,340,342,481). These mixture theories model soft hydrated tissues as composite materials consisting of two intrinsically incompressible and immiscible phases (a solid phase and a fluid phase) (44,45,204,338). The porous solid phase is elastic and permeable to fluid flow. It may be isotropic or anisotropic, linear or nonlinear. In this theory, the frictional drag associated with the interstitial fluid flow through the porous solid matrix is responsible for the compressive viscoelastic behavior of the tissue. The intrinsic viscoelastic nature of the solid matrix becomes important when interstitial fluid drag effects are not significant (285,456). A biphasic poroviscoelastic theory has also been developed to describe the compressive behavior of cartilage by incorporating the intrinsic viscoelasticity of the solid matrix and the biphasic nature of the tissue (95,96,288). This theory has been shown to be successful in describing tissues with high permeabilities (460,461). To account for the observed Donnan osmotic pressure effects (100,302,494, 509,510), the ion-induced swelling (or contracting) effects (112,113,360,362), ion transport through the tissue (159–162,230), and other streaming and diffusion potentials and electrokinetic effects (136–138), Lai and coworkers developed the triphasic theory in 1991 (264). This theory was further developed by Gu et al. to account for multiple species of ions in tissue (161). Note that a similar theory to the triphasic theory was also developed by Huyghe and Janssen in 1997 (215); this theory was given the name of quadriphasic theory. The biphasic and tripha-

sic constitutive equations are discussed in greater detail in later sections of this chapter.

Throughout the maze of equations and complexities, it is important to remember that each constitutive equation is only a model adopted to describe the most salient and idealized mechanical behavior of the material. It represents a simplification of the real stress–strain behavior of the specific material and has significant restrictions and limitations for its general applicability.

4.4 Elastic Solids, Viscous Fluids, and Viscoelastic Materials

A material is linear if the stress and strain are related in a linear manner and is elastic if the material always returns to its original shape when the applied stress is removed. The latter concept implies that all the energy stored in the material as a result of deformation is entirely recoverable, and the material response is insensitive to the time rate of the applied stress or strain. In other words, there is no internal energy dissipation within an elastic material. The mechanical behavior of an elastic material such as a metal spring can be entirely determined by a graph showing a linear load–deformation, $F = kX$, or stress–strain relationship, $\sigma = E\varepsilon$ (Fig. 5-10A). The slope of the linear region of the F-X graph is the structural stiffness k(N/m), and that of the σ–ε graph is the Young's modulus of elasticity E (N/m^2). For a straight prismatic elastic bar of cross-sectional area A and length L, the relationship between structural stiffness k and Young's modulus E is given by

$$k = EA/L. \tag{1}$$

We see that the structural stiffness k depends directly on A and inversely on L and hence is not an intrinsic property of the structure. The range of the Young's modulus for stainless steel is 106 to 114 GPa, for titanium-193 to 207 GPa, for poly(methyl methacrylate) (PMMA) 2.4 to 3.5 GPa, and for bone 0.1 to 15 GPa; note that 1.0 GPa = 10^3 MPa = 10^9 Pa (pascal). The shear moduli for steel and titanium are 73 GPa and 41 GPa, respectively. As will be seen later, the Young's modulus of the solid matrix of

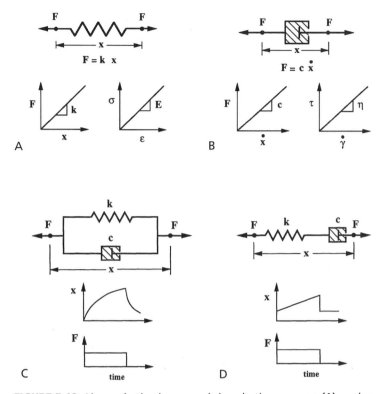

FIGURE 5-10. Linear elastic, viscous, and viscoelastic responses: **(A)** an elastic spring, **(B)** a viscous dashpot, **(C)** a Kelvin–Voigt body, and **(D)** a Maxwell body. Under constant load or stretch, the elastic solid responses are independent of time. Under constant stretching, the viscous dashpot response is independent of time. Viscoelastic materials show time-dependent responses (lower figures in **C** and **D**).

cartilage in compression ranges from 0.3 to 1.0 MPa, and that of the meniscus ranges from 0.1 to 0.6 MPa (12,23,24,115,141,338,340,400, 462).

A dashpot is a piston moving through a viscous fluid contained in a closed cylinder (Fig. 5-10B). The registered force F is linearly related to the piston's rate of displacement $\dot{x}$ (speed); i.e., $F = c\dot{x}$. Here, the constant of proportionality c (N-sec/m) is called the viscous (or frictional) damping coefficient of the dashpot. For a linear, purely viscous material the shear stress (τ) and shear rate ($\dot{\gamma}$) are linearly related; i.e., $\tau = \eta\dot{\gamma}$. This is known as a Newtonian fluid (see Chapter 8 on synovial fluid for discussions on more complex fluid flow behaviors). The slope of this linear graph is the viscosity coefficient η (N-sec/m^2) of the fluid. The viscosity coefficient η describes an intrinsic property of

the viscous fluid. A viscous fluid does not exhibit any tendency to recover its original shape when the applied stress is removed. This means no energy is stored in the material, and all the energy required to cause the flow is dissipated as heat by internal friction. Common viscous fluids are water, air, and low-molecular-weight oils. The viscosity coefficients of air and water at 20°C are 1.8×10^{-4} poise and 1.0×10^{-2} poise, respectively.[2]

Simple elastic or viscous responses are time-independent when subject to constant stress, constant strain, or constant strain rate. Most biological materials, however, exhibit time-dependent creep (i.e., deformation will increase with

---

[2] Poise is used as a measure of viscosity; 1.0 poise = 0.1 Pa-sec = 0.1 N-sec/m^2.

a constant applied stress) and stress relaxation (i.e., stress will decrease at constant applied strain) until an equilibrium is reached. Liquids that exhibit a shear stress response that decreases with time at a constant shear rate are known as thixotropic liquids.[3] Consequently, it is often necessary to use viscoelastic models to describe a material whose response to a constant applied load or constant deformation is time dependent.

A viscoelastic material, as the name suggests, combines the properties of both elastic and viscous substances. Using the elastic and viscous models described above, a viscoelastic material may be conceptualized as elastic springs and dashpots linked together. The Kelvin–Voigt body is defined by a spring and a dashpot connected in parallel (Fig. 5-10C), and a Maxwell body is one where a spring and dashpot are connected in series (Fig. 5-10D). The equation governing the force–displacement relation for a Kelvin–Voigt body is

$$F = kx + c\dot{x}, x = 0 \quad \text{at } t = 0 \qquad (2)$$

and for a Maxwell body, it is given by

$$(F/c) + (\dot{F}/k) = \dot{x}, x = F/k \quad \text{at } t = 0. \qquad (3)$$

When these equations are written in terms of stress and strain, they represent the intrinsic stress–strain response of the viscoelastic material.

The initial conditions are also given in Eqs. 2 and 3. When a load is applied to the Kelvin–Voigt body, its initial response is governed by that of the dashpot, i.e., $x(0)$ is zero, and when a load is applied to the Maxwell body, its initial response is the sudden deformation of the spring, i.e., $x(0) = F/k$. The creep is defined as the deformation produced by a sudden application of a constant force F at $t = 0$. Equations 4 and 5 give the creep response of the Kelvin–Voigt and Maxwell bodies, respectively:

$$x(t) = [F/k]\left[1 - e^{-(k/c)t}\right], t > 0 \qquad (4)$$

$$x(t) = F[(1/k) + (t/c)], t > 0. \qquad (5)$$

The creep and recovery curves of these two idealized viscoelastic bodies are also depicted in Figs. 5-10C and 5-10D. The reader is referred to standard engineering references on viscoelasticity for models in which more springs and dashpots are connected in series and parallel (39,40, 129,142). Whether or not any real material behaves in accord with the patterns predicted by these idealized viscoelastic laws can be ascertained by matching these predictions with the experimental data (502). If the patterns of these load–deformation responses are similar to those for a specific material, then the elastic and viscous material coefficients of the assumed constitutive law can be calculated for the material.

For single-phase materials such as polymeric plastics, the mechanisms responsible for their viscoelastic behaviors may include intermolecular friction, stretching and uncoiling of molecules, and random vibration (from thermal excitation) of the long-chain polymers comprising the material (39,129,142). However, by virtue of composition, molecular structure, and water and electrolyte contents, the viscoelastic behavior of cartilage and meniscus has another dimension. For example, in compression, their viscoelastic behaviors are dominated by the frictional drag of interstitial fluid flow through the porous–permeable collagen–proteoglycan solid matrix, thus causing viscous dissipation (202–204,315,338,340,460,462,473,481). Because viscous dissipation associated with interstitial fluid flow dominates the creep and stress-relaxation behaviors, the degree of hydration of these tissues and tissue permeability are important parameters governing their deformational behaviors. In fact, the earliest compositional change in articular cartilage that occurs during OA is an increase in hydration (42,141,294, 301), which has been shown to affect the intrinsic properties of articular cartilage (12,197,460, 462).

4.5 Biphasic Materials and Permeation Experiments

Permeation studies have demonstrated that water is capable of flowing through the porous–permeable solid matrix of cartilage and meniscus

---

[3] Thixotropic liquids are polymeric solutions that have a molecular network that breaks down during shearing. A common example is tomato catsup; it flows more easily after being shaken.

under an imposed pressure gradient (110,111, 262,296,297,300,315,358,400). In this experiment, a specimen is subjected to an applied pressure gradient ΔP across the thickness h of the specimen. The rate of volume discharge Q across an area A is related to the hydraulic permeability coefficient k by Darcy's law:

$$Q = kA \Delta P/h. \qquad (6)$$

The permeation speed V is related to Q by the expression $V = Q/A\phi^f$, where the parameter ϕ^f is the porosity of the tissue defined as the ratio of the interstitial fluid volume (V^f) to the total tissue volume (V^T). Results from this permeation experiment showed that for normal cartilage and meniscus, k ranges from 10^{-15} to 10^{-16} m^4/N-sec. The diffusive drag coefficient K is inversely related to the permeability coefficient k and is given by (262)

$$K = \left(\phi^f\right)^2/k. \qquad (7)$$

Because the porosity ϕ^f for cartilage and meniscus is approximately 0.75, the K ranges from 10^{14} to 10^{15} N-sec/m^4. The very large drag coefficient indicates that interstitial fluid flow will cause large drag forces to be generated in these tissues.

Water is also capable of flowing through the porous–permeable solid matrix as the tissue is compressed (12,23,110,278,315,338,340, 345,350,462). In this case, the compressive stress causes the solid matrix to be compacted, thus raising the pressure in the interstitium and forcing the fluid out of the tissue. The rate of efflux is controlled by the drag force generated during flow. In general, the manner with which an applied load is shared between the fluid phase (fluid pressure) and the solid phase (stress in the solid matrix) is determined, among other things, by the volumetric ratios of the tissue, i.e., the porosity ϕ^f and solidity $\phi^S(= V^S/V^T)$, the loading rates and the type of loading (tension, compression and shear), and load partition at the surface (13,202,203,207,208,263,338–340,380,476,477). The load-carrying capacity of each phase is determined by balancing the viscous drag forces against the elastic forces at each point within the tissue. For example, flow

of fluid through a very permeable solid matrix would cause little frictional drag or fluid pressurization. A compressive stress acting on very permeable materials would be predominantly supported by the stress developed within the solid matrix, such as a highly porous rigid steel filter. Conversely, flow of fluid through a solid matrix with very low permeability would cause high frictional drag forces, thus requiring high hydrodynamic pressures or large compressive loads to maintain the flow. In this case, fluid pressure can provide a significant component of total load support, thus minimizing the stress acting on the solid matrix. Such is the case for cartilage and meniscus (13,202,203,207,208,263,338–340,380,476,477).

The biphasic theory was developed by Mow and coworkers (204,338,340,342,351) to describe the flow and deformational behaviors of cartilage and meniscus under a variety of conditions. The theory may be conceptually understood by the following simplified constitutive assumptions:

1. The solid matrix may be linearly elastic or hyperelastic, and isotropic or anisotropic.
2. The solid matrix and interstitial fluid are intrinsically incompressible; that is, compression of the tissue as a whole is possible only if there is fluid exudation.
3. Viscous dissipation is a result mainly of interstitial fluid flow *relative* to the porous–permeable solid matrix.
4. Frictional drag is directly proportional to the relative velocity; the proportionality factor is known as the diffusive drag coefficient (K), and this may be strain dependent.

This general biphasic theory takes its simplest form under the condition of infinitesimal strain, where the stress–strain law of the solid matrix may be described by the generalized Hooke's law, and where the diffusive drag coefficient is a constant. These constitutive *assumptions* embody what is generally known as the linear biphasic theory for cartilage and meniscus (204,338, 340,351,400,539). Under strict laboratory testing conditions, the isotropic form of the linear biphasic theory has been shown to provide a very accurate description of the compressive creep and stress-relaxation behaviors of these tissues (12,23,24,36,202,338,340,400,462,476,477, 539).

It should be emphasized that these simple constitutive assumptions are not generally valid to describe the nonhomogeneous and anisotropic nature of articular cartilage and meniscus. There are many obvious areas for improving the sophistication of these assumptions. For example, a material symmetry could be introduced into the constitutive equations in order to describe the transversely isotropic or orthotropic or tension–compression nonlinear material properties of articular cartilage and meniscus (69, 82,239,274,350,400,401,427,530,537). Note that the material properties of cartilage are also inhomogeneous (73,74,448,449,529); see the review paper by Mow and Guo (353). However, to solve such problems is mathematically very challenging, and to perform the experiments to extract the material coefficients is nearly impossible. Further, if the material is subject to heavy loads, large deformations, and rapid loading rates, nonlinear finite deformational effects occur, and more advanced theories may be required (20,202,204,261,342). Because these types of biological tissues are soft and generally have high water contents, care must always be ex-

ercised to choose the correct form of the biphasic theory for the specific loading and deformational conditions (54,342,350). In this chapter, we discuss only the linear biphasic theory for articular cartilage and meniscus for the purpose of material property determinations.

4.6 Tension, Compression, and Shear

Uniaxial stress and uniaxial strain tests are often used to determine the mechanical response of a material. In these experiments, the loads or deformations are applied in only one direction. In general, an experiment with an applied uniaxial stress will yield multiaxial strains, and conversely, an experiment with uniaxial strain will generate multiaxial stresses in the tissue. These types of experiments greatly simplify the theoretical analyses required to describe the data.

In a uniaxial tension or compression test, a cylindrical specimen of known cross-sectional area (A) is placed in a testing machine and subjected to a tensile load (P) along one axis (Fig. 5-11A). The uniaxial stress σ acting in the specimen is P/A. With time, the specimen elongates along the direction of the applied tension. The stretch, $\lambda(t) = L(t)/L_o$, of the specimen

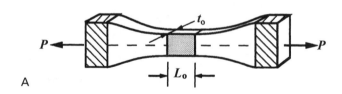

A

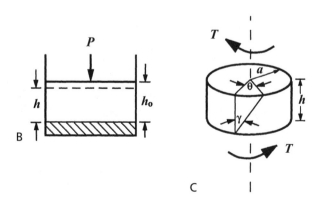

B

C

FIGURE 5-11. (A) Tensile testing of a specimen with gauge length L_o, thickness t_o, and cross-sectional area A. **(B)** Confined compression test of a specimen of thickness h_o. **(C)** Shear test of a circular specimen of radius a; γ is the shear strain.

is measured as the tensile test proceeds. Here, $L(t)$ is the deformed gauge length of the specimen at time t, and L_o is the original undeformed gauge length. The tensile strain ε is calculated by the relation $\varepsilon = (L - L_o)/L_o$.[4] For linearly elastic materials, the Young's modulus E is given by the expression

$$E = \sigma/\varepsilon = (P/A)/[(L - L_o)/L_o]. \quad (8)$$

For nearly all materials, tension would cause a lateral contraction, whereas compression would cause a lateral expansion. To be consistent with the laws of thermodynamics, tension must always produce an increase in volume. The Poisson's ratio ν is used as a measure of the lateral strain (ε_d) relative to the axial strain and is defined as

$$\nu = -\varepsilon_d/\varepsilon = -[(d - d_o)/d_o]/[(L - L_o)/L_o]. \quad (9)$$

Here, d is the deformed lateral dimension, and d_o is the original lateral dimension. For isotropic materials, the Poisson's ratio ranges from 0 to 0.5. A Poisson's ratio of 0.5 means the material is incompressible, and a Poisson's ratio of zero means the material is maximally compressible. The values of ν for some common isotropic materials are stainless steel, 0.30; titanium, 0.34; adult articular cartilage, 0.10 to 0.40; cork, 0; and rubber, 0.5. For anisotropic materials, there are no such restrictions on the Poisson's ratio.

Another type of uniaxial experiment is the confined compression experiment (Fig. 5-11B). In this experiment, the deformation is maintained in one direction. This is done by restricting the material from expanding in the lateral direction by placing the test sample in a confining chamber. The confining wall serves to exert a normal compressive force onto the lateral surface of the cylinder in order to maintain one-dimensional motion. Thus, the uniaxial confined compression experiment is actually a *multiaxial* stress experiment; the stress acting on the lateral surface has the effect of increasing the compressive modulus. This modulus is

known as the compressive aggregate modulus. For isotropic materials (338), the Young's modulus (E), Poisson's ratio (ν), and aggregate modulus (H_A) are related by the expression $H_A = E(1 - \nu)/(1 + \nu)(1 - 2\nu)$.

The third common experiment utilizes torsion to determine the shear properties of a material. Torsion of a circular cylinder of a homogeneous material yields a state of pure shear in the material, which experiences no volume change (Fig. 5-11C). The shear strain γ is related to the total angle of twist θ, the thickness h, and the radius of the disc a by $\gamma = \theta a/h$. The shear stress τ at a circumferential position is determined from the resulting torque T as $\tau = Ta/I_p$ where I_p is the polar area moment of inertia given by $\pi a^4/2$. These quantities can be used to calculate the shear modulus of an isotropic, linearly elastic material as

$$\mu = \tau/\gamma = Th/I_p\theta. \quad (10)$$

See Table 5-4 for the relationships among the elastic constants (E, ν, H_A, μ, λ) in terms of any of the basic pairs. With these general concepts, it is now possible to develop an understanding of the material properties of articular cartilage and meniscus. These topics occupy the remainder of this chapter.

5 MATERIAL PROPERTIES OF THE EXTRACELLULAR MATRIX OF CARTILAGINOUS TISSUES

The material coefficients most commonly used to describe the intrinsic or "flow-independent" properties of the porous–permeable solid matrix of cartilage and meniscus are Young's modulus, the compressive aggregate modulus, the shear modulus, and Poisson's ratio. The experiments used to determine these coefficients are (a) creep or stress-relaxation equilibrium measurements in confined compression or indentation; (b) slow, constant-strain-rate or equilibrium tensile tests; and (c) shear tests with infinitesimal shear strains. The specific choice of test depends on the size, shape, and amount of tissue available for study and the objectives of the study.

---

[4] For large deformation, the "strain" ε along the direction of applied stress is given by $(\lambda^2 - 1)/2$. See references 142 and 265 for more details.

TABLE 5-5A. EQUILIBRIUM TENSILE MODULUS (MPa) OF NORMAL HUMAN, BOVINE, AND CANINE ARTICULAR CARTILAGE: INHOMOGENEOUS VARIATIONS THROUGH THE DEPTH OF THE CARTILAGE LAYER[a]

	Bovine		Canine		Human	
	Glenoid	Humerus	Femoral Groove	Femoral Condyle	Femoral Groove	Femoral Condyle
Surface	5.9 (2.4)	13.4 (4.6)	27.4 (8.4)	23.3 (8.5)	13.9 (2.4)	7.8 (1.7)
Middle	0.9 (0.5)	2.7 (1.6)			3.4 (1.4)	4.0 (1.1)
Deep	0.2 (0.2)	1.7 (0.8)			1.0 (0.5)	

[a]All sample harvested in a direction parallel to the local split-line direction. Data are expressed as mean (SD). From Akizuki et al. (7) and Setton et al. (464), with permission. Data on bovine articular cartilage from Ebara et al. (105), with permission.

5.1 Tensile Properties of the Solid Matrix

5.1.1 Equilibrium Tensile Measurements

The tensile modulus of the solid matrix of cartilage and meniscus has been determined using the equilibrium data from the tensile stress-relaxation experiment (7,8,69,151,168,274, 362,462,492,535). For normal cartilage, the equilibrium stress–strain relationship is linear for strains up to 15%, from which the equilibrium tensile modulus is determined. Various studies showed that the tensile modulus of articular cartilage may vary from less than 1 MPa to over 30 MPa. This variation arises from a number of factors: (a) type of tissue (e.g., human, bovine, canine); (b) age of the animal; (c) type of joint in the body; (d) sample location in the joint (i.e., weight-bearing characteristics); (e) depth

of sample from the articular surface; (f) relative orientation with respect to the local split-line direction; (g) biochemical composition and molecular structure; and (h) state of degeneration (7,8, 105,168,239,240,242,427,462,537). For example, Table 5-5A shows the variation of this equilibrium tensile modulus for normal articular cartilage from bovine, canine, and human knee and shoulder joints (7,8,105,462), and Table 5-5B fibrillated and osteoarthritic human knee cartilage (7,8). Further, studies on canine knee joint cartilage from the surface zone, in which OA was experimentally induced by sectioning the anterior cruciate ligament, show dramatic decreases of the tensile modulus (Table 5-6) (168,361, 462).

Some general conclusions may be drawn: (a) The tensile modulus of cartilage from the surface zone is larger than that of the middle and deep zones in the skeletally mature animal. (b) The

TABLE 5-5B. EQUILIBRIUM TENSILE MODULUS (MPa) OF NORMAL, FIBRILLATED, AND OSTEOARTHRITIC HUMAN ARTICULAR CARTILAGE: INHOMOGENEOUS VARIATIONS THROUGH THE DEPTH OF THE CARTILAGE LAYER[a]

	Normal	Fibrillated	Osteoarthritic
Surface	7.79	7.15	1.36
	(1.37)	(1.89)	(0.09)
Subsurface	4.85	7.47	0.85
	(1.37)	(0.65)	(0.81)
Middle	4.00	4.90	2.11
	(1.05)	(1.03)	(0.30)

[a]All samples were harvested from the femoral condyle in an orientation parallel to the local split-line direction. Data are expressed mean (SD), from Akizuki et al. (7), with permission.

TABLE 5-6. EQUILIBRIUM TENSILE MODULUS (MPa) of surface-zone canine articular cartilage in an animal model of osteoarthritis[a]

	Greyhound Femoral Groove	Greyhound Femoral Condyle	Beagle Femoral Condyle
Control	27.4 (8.4)	23.3 (8.5)	15.5 (4.5)
6 weeks	23.3 (8.7)	13.2 (4.4)	
12 weeks	12.5 (2.9)	6.7 (2.5)	
16 weeks			8.6 (5.0)

[a]All cartilage is harvested from the surface and subsurface zones parallel to the split-line direction. Data are expressed as mean (SD). From Guilak et al. (167) and Setton et al. (464), with permission.

tensile modulus of specimens aligned parallel to the local split-line direction is larger than that of specimens aligned perpendicular to the split-line direction, and this is true regardless of the state of tissue degeneration. (c) The tensile modulus of normal cartilage is larger than that of fibrillated and OA cartilage. The presence of fibrillation and OA, whether occurring naturally in humans (Table 5-5B) or induced experimentally in animals (Table 5-6), greatly reduces the tensile modulus near the articular surface. Finally, (d) the tensile modulus is not affected by the proteoglycan content (238, 451). The first general conclusion is consistent with the idea that the surface zone of cartilage is rich in collagen. The second is consistent with the observation that there is a subtle preferred alignment of collagen fibers at the articular surface, though often

not observable by scanning electron microscopy (14,49–52,79,336,533). The third conclusion is consistent with the preponderant microscopic data on the morphology of tissue disruption occurring during OA. Finally, the last conclusion indicates that the bonding between collagen and proteoglycan in the solid matrix is not covalent.

These studies showed that there is a highly significant correlation between the tensile modulus and the ratio of collagen to proteoglycan in normal human articular cartilage ($r = 0.714$, $p < 0.001$) (Fig. 5-12). Clearly, specimens from the surface are stiffer than those from the midzone, and surface-zone specimens from high-weight-bearing areas (HWAs) are less stiff than those from the low-weight-bearing areas (LWAs). This is at least in part a result of the

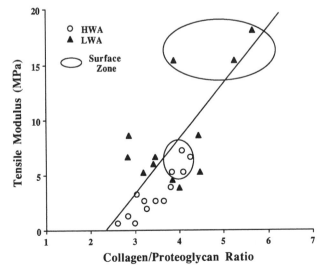

FIGURE 5-12. Relationship between intrinsic tensile modulus and collagen/proteoglycan ratio for normal human knee joint cartilage ($r = 0.714$, $p < 0.001$) (7).

lower collagen/proteoglycan ratio in the HWA than in the LWA. This physiological phenomenon seems to be true for other soft hydrated tissues, such as tendons (118,522). When tendons are under compressive load, they remodel by producing higher concentrations of aggrecan, proteoglycan aggregates, byglycan, and decorin.

5.1.2 Constant-strain-rate Tensile Measurements

When a strip of cartilage is stretched under a constant strain rate, the tensile stress–strain behavior is nonlinear. A typical nonlinear stress–strain (σ–ε) curve for cartilage, meniscus, and other soft tissues is depicted in Fig. 5-13. This figure also shows the cause of the nonlinear behavior; that is, the initial toe region of the σ–ε curve results from the straightening of the coiled collagen structure, and the linear region of the σ–ε curve represents the stretching of the straightened parallel array of collagen fibers (144,239, 241,420,427,521,522,537). It is thought that the linear region reflects the stiffness of the collagen fibers as they are pulled in uniaxial tension (see also Chapter 6 on tendons and ligaments), and the slope of this curve gives a tensile modulus (E) of the specimen. Beyond the linear region, the collagen fibrils will fracture, and the tensile failure stress is the measure of the strength of the collagen fibrils.

A number of investigators have shown that the nonlinear stress–strain data can be described by a two-parameter (A,B) exponential stress–strain relationship (144,243,334,420,427,538):

$$\sigma = A[\exp(B\varepsilon) - 1]. \qquad (11)$$

It can be shown from this representation that the derivative or tangent modulus is directly related to the stress:

$$d\sigma/d\varepsilon = B\varepsilon + C. \qquad (12)$$

This means that the increase in the stiffness of the specimen is directly related to the applied stress σ. The concept of fiber recruitment has long been proposed as an explanation for this stiffening effect (521). As illustrated in Fig. 5-13, as tension proceeds and more of the coiled or slack fibers are straightened and stretched, the number of fibers actively resisting the applied tensile load will increase, resulting in an increased tensile stiffness. The concept of fiber recruitment as the specimens are stretched is commonly used in tensile studies of tendons and ligaments (see Chapter 7 for more details on tendons and ligaments).

In Eq. 12, the tangent modulus ($d\sigma/d\varepsilon$) is proportional to the factor B, and C is the product AB and represents the tangent modulus as $\sigma \to 0$. Table 5-7 provides the coefficients A, B, and C and the tensile Young's modulus E determined from the linear portion of the tensile σ–ε curve for bovine cartilage. As expected, these

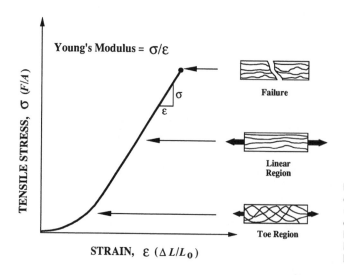

FIGURE 5-13. Typical stress–strain curve for articular cartilage in a uniaxial and uniform strain rate experiment. The toe region is marked by an increasing slope, whereas the linear region appears to be a straight line with a slope of σ/ε (354).

TABLE 5-7. PARAMETERS *A*, *B*, AND *C* (= *AB*) AND YOUNG'S MODULUS, *E*, OF BOVINE ARTICULAR CARTILAGE: DEPENDENCE ON DEPTH AND SPLIT-LINE ORIENTATION

	Slice	*A*(MPa)	*B*	*C*	*E* (MPa)
Group ‖	1	2.1	5.0	10.6	43.2
	2	1.0	3.2	3.3	13.0
	3	0.6	1.6	0.9	2.6
Group⊥	1	0.9	3.6	3.2	15.6
	2	0.5	2.2	1.0	4.7
	3	0.3	1.3	0.3	1.1

Note: ‖ and ⊥ represent parallel and perpendicular specimens, respectively, and 1, 2, and 3 represent the first three layers of tissue. Data from Roth et al. (428).

coefficients vary with the depth from the articular surface and the split-line direction. Specimens taken from the articular surface and parallel to the split-line direction have the greatest tensile modulus.

The uniaxial constant strain-rate experiments have also been used to determine the tensile stress–strain relationship for human and bovine meniscal tissues (59,131,132,344,400). As with cartilage, these tensile properties vary with respect to location (anterior, central, and posterior) and specimen orientation relative to the predominant collagen fiber direction (circumferential and radial). The regional variation in tensile modulus (*E*), as shown in Table 5-8, indicates that specimens from the posterior half of the medial meniscus are significantly less stiff and less strong in tension than specimens from all other regions. The rate of change (*B*) of the tangent modulus ($d\sigma / d\varepsilon$) is uniform throughout the meniscus, indicating the relative uniformity of collagen and proteoglycan content present in normal human meniscus. In contrast, the tangent modulus at very low stresses, *C*, varies in a manner similar to that seen for tangent modulus beyond the toe region.

Ultrastructural studies using polarized light (131) showed that in lateral meniscus, large type I collagen fiber bundles are highly oriented and are arranged parallel to the periphery of this semilunar-shaped tissue. However, in the posterior half of the medial meniscus, collagen fiber bundles have significantly reduced circumferential organization, that is, they are not highly aligned in the circumferential direction. This observation appears to explain the lower measured tensile modulus of the medial posterior specimens. This site has a high frequency of clinically observed tears, which may result from the inferior tensile properties of the meniscus in this region.

Although the collagen fibers of the meniscus are arranged predominantly in the circumferential direction, there is evidence of large radially oriented fibers within human and bovine menisci (Fig. 5-8). It has long been conjectured that these radial fibers act to "tie" the large circumferentially oriented collagen fibers together, thus providing the tissue with greater strength in the radial direction (59). This hypothesis was examined by Skaggs and coworkers (469), who harvested tensile specimens of meniscal tissue

TABLE 5-8. PARAMETERS *A*, *B*, AND *C* (= *AB*) AND TENSILE MODULUS, *E*, OF HUMAN MENISCUS: DEPENDENCE ON LOCATION[a]

Location	*A*	*B*	*C*	*E* (MPa)
MA	1.6	28.4	42.4	159.6
MC	0.9	27.3	23.7	93.2
MP	1.4	20.1	25.2	110.2
LA	1.4	28.8	30.2	159.1
LC	2.1	31.9	55.7	228.8
LP	3.2	27.5	67.5	294.1

[a]MA, medial anterior; MC, medial central; MP, medial posterior; LA, lateral anterior; LC, lateral central; LP, lateral posterior. Data from Fithian et al. (131).

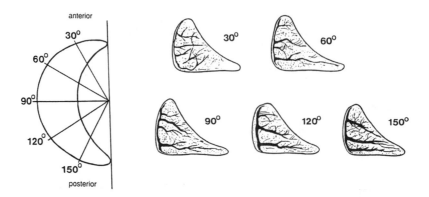

FIGURE 5-14. Schematic representations of the regional variation in the architecture of the radial tie fibers. The anterior region contains no radial tie fibers, and the posterior region often contained large multiple radial tie fibers (469).

oriented in the radial direction. From their histologic observations, it was noted that the size and density of the radial tie fibers in bovine meniscus gradually increased from the anterior region to the posterior region of the meniscus (Fig. 5-14). This gradual increase also manifested in the tensile modulus and ultimate tensile stress of radial specimens, those specimens containing full radial fibers being the stiffest (Fig. 5-15A, B).

The tensile σ–ε relationship for articular cartilage and the resulting tensile modulus are also dependent on the rate of strain. It has been

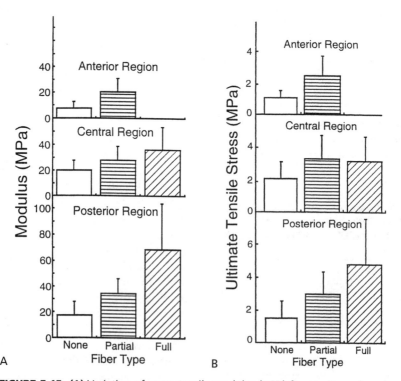

FIGURE 5-15. (A) Variation of mean tensile modulus ($\pm$SD) for specimens by region and by presence of the radial tie fibers. **(B)** Variation of mean tensile ultimate stress ($\pm$SD) for specimens by region and by presence of the radial tie fibers.

shown that substantial quantities of fluid are expressed from cartilage specimens during the stretching process (427). This fluid movement must necessarily cause fluid pressurization in the interstitium and frictional drag to be exerted onto the solid matrix. These effects increase as the rate of strain increases. Thus, the specimens would appear to stiffen with increasing strain rate. Conversely, as the strain rate becomes very low, the tensile modulus would decrease and would approach the equilibrium tensile modulus measured from stress relaxation. This hypothesis was examined and verified experimentally (7,8,276).

5.2 Compressive Properties of the Solid Matrix

The equilibrium compressive properties of the solid matrix have been most extensively studied in confined compression and indentation tests (12,20,29,73,74,112,113,115,150,186,195, 197,211,224,236,237,261,285,289,338,345, 449,529). In the confined compression experiment, a small cylindrical cartilage-bone plug is placed in a cylindrical confining chamber, schematically shown in Fig. 5-16. Ideally, the lateral expansion of cartilage is prevented. A constant compressive load is applied to the specimen through a rigid porous filter; the liquid in the pores of this filter is maintained at an ambient level. Creep deformation occurs as the fluid is forced to flow from the tissue. The aggregate modulus is determined at creep equilibrium. Just as in tension, for small strains (<20%),

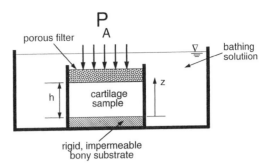

FIGURE 5-16. Confined compression test. Load (P_A) is applied to the cartilage surface with a rigid-porous filter, allowing free escape of the interstitial fluid (h is cartilage thickness, z is displacement coordinate). Lateral extension of the specimen is prevented by the confining test chamber.

human and bovine cartilage tissues demonstrate a linear stress–strain relationship (20,23, 24,115,202,203,261,338,342). The average aggregate modulus for the lateral condyle and femoral groove cartilages of normal human, canine, cynomolgus monkey, and rabbit knees, and bovine meniscus is given in Table 5-9 (23,400). These data indicate significant species and site variations of the aggregate modulus. To illustrate the site variations on a specific joint, Fig. 5-17 provides a map of the aggregate modulus and cartilage thickness on a normal 21-year-old male human tibial plateau.

Besides variations related to tissue location and species, other factors such as tissue composition, ultrastructure, and pathology also have strong influences on tissue properties. The equilibrium aggregate modulus for human articular cartilage correlates in an inverse manner with

TABLE 5-9. EQUILIBRIUM AGGREGATE MODULUS (MPa) OF LATERAL CONDYLE AND PATELLAR GROOVE CARTILAGE AND MENISCUS

	Human[a]	Bovine[b]	Canine[c]	Monkey[d]	Rabbit[e]
Lateral condyle	0.70	0.89	0.60	0.78	0.54
Patellar groove	0.53	0.47	0.55	0.52	0.51
Meniscus	NA[f]	0.41	NA	NA	NA

[a] Young normal.
[b] 18 months to 2 years old.
[c] Mature beagles and greyhounds.
[d] Mature cynomologus monkeys.
[e] Mature New Zealand White rabbits.
[f] Not available. Data shown were obtained from indentation creep tests.

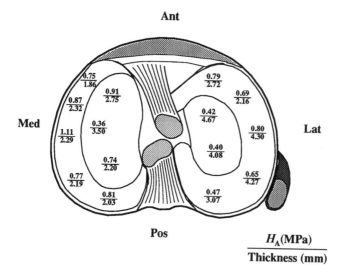

FIGURE 5-17. Variation of equilibrium compressive modulus and thickness of cartilage with joint location on the tibial plateau. (Courtesy of Dr. Shaw Akizuki; normal, human, 21-year-old specimen.)

water content ($r = -0.74$) (Fig. 5-18) and in a direct manner with proteoglycan content per wet weight ($r = 0.69$) (Fig. 5-19) (347,428). No correlation exists between the compressive stiffness and collagen content. Thus, these correlations suggest that proteoglycans are responsible for providing compressive stiffness of the tissue. Recent investigations have revealed that the highly loaded regions of articular cartilage generally have a greater proteoglycan content (7,226). These results are consistent with the fact that highly loaded regions of articular cartilages are stiffer in compression than the less-loaded regions, as mentioned previously (Fig. 5-17) (5,67). Degenerative changes of the ECM during OA often include loss of proteoglycan and thus have a profound influence on cartilage material properties and joint function

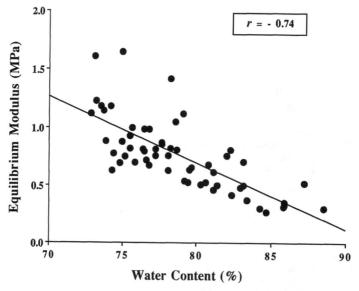

FIGURE 5-18. Variation of the confined compression equilibrium modulus with water content for articular cartilage from the lateral facet of human patellae (12).

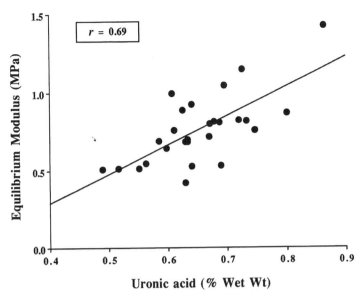

FIGURE 5-19. Variation of the confined compression equilibrium modulus of human patellar articular cartilage specimens with uronic acid content (347).

(140,235,236). Indeed, removal of proteoglycans from articular cartilage samples *in vitro* has been shown to result in a tenfold decrease of tissue compressive modulus (239,483).

5.3 Shear Properties of the Solid Matrix

The intrinsic viscoelastic properties of the solid matrix of cartilage can be determined in a pure shear experiment and under small strain conditions. When these two conditions exist, no volumetric change or hydrodynamic pressures are produced in the tissue; thus, no interstitial fluid flow can occur (188,429,463,482,547,550). The intrinsic or flow-independent viscoelastic behavior of the cartilage matrix has been measured under these two conditions, and both stress-relaxation and dynamic oscillatory shear behaviors have been characterized.

In the pure shear experiment, a circular specimen is subjected to a torsional shear deformation. The mechanical response of a cartilage specimen to a sudden change of angular displacement is an instantaneous increase in shear stress followed by a rapid decay until an equilibrium is reached. This stress-relaxation behavior is the manifestation of the intrinsic viscoelastic behavior of the solid matrix exhibited in shear. Figure 5-20 shows a typical mean of a normalized shear stress-relaxation function $G(t)$ calculated from ten levels of step shear strain (0.002 to 9.02 rads) for normal human patellar cartilage specimens (547–550). Using the quasilinear viscoelastic theory (144), this normalized stress-relaxation function yields the spectrum parameters: $C = 0.13$, $\tau_1 = 0.0004$ sec, and $\tau_2 = 36.2$ sec. Clearly, the quasilinear viscoelastic theory provides an excellent description of the intrinsic stress-relaxation behavior of normal human patellar cartilage. Equilibrium stress–strain relationships from this shear stress-relaxation test are linear for shear strains up to 0.03 rad. The average equilibrium shear modulus for human patellar cartilage is 0.23 MPa (547,550), although patellar cartilage is known to be particularly soft when compared with other cartilages in the knee. For canine femoral condylar cartilage at 6 or 12 weeks following anterior cruciate ligament transection, the equilibrium shear modulus was found to decrease from 0.22 MPa to 0.07 MPa and 0.06 MPa, respectively (463).

The dynamic viscoelastic shear behaviors of the solid matrix of cartilage and meniscus have

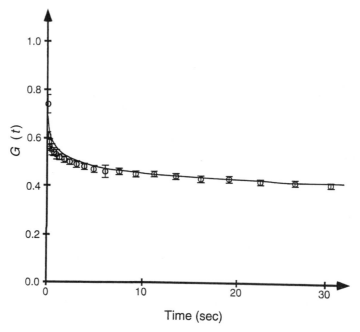

FIGURE 5-20. Analysis of articular cartilage reduced shear stress-relaxation function using the quasilinear viscoelastic (QLV) theory proposed by Fung (144). The three material parameters of the QLV theory for this specimen are $C = 0.13$, $\tau_1 = 0.0004$ sec, and $\tau_2 = 36.2$ sec (547).

also been determined using the pure shear experiment. In this test, the specimen is subjected to a steady sinusoidal torsional strain of small amplitude over a range of frequencies (429,463, 547,550). A sinusoidal angular displacement $\theta = \theta_0 e^{i\omega t}$ is applied to the specimen, and the torque response $T = T_o \exp(i\omega t + \delta)$ is registered. Here, ω is the circular frequency in radians per second (frequency $f = \omega/2\pi$ in hertz; the period $p = 2\pi/\omega = 1/f$ in seconds), and δ is the phase-shift angle between the sinusoidal displacement input and torque output. To calculate the dynamic shear modulus (G^*), the following formula is used:

$$G^* = G' + iG'' = \frac{T_o h}{I_p \theta_o}(\cos \delta + i \sin \delta) \quad (13)$$

where $i = \sqrt{-1}$. The storage modulus G' is proportional to elastically stored strain energy, and the loss modulus G'' is proportional to dissipated strain energy in the material over one cycle of periodic oscillation. Often, it is convenient to calculate the magnitude of dynamic shear modu-

lus $|G^*|$ and phase-shift angle δ. They are related to G' and G'' by

$$|G^*| = \sqrt{G'^2 + G''^2} = \frac{T_o h}{I_p \theta_o}, \delta = \tan^{-1}\left(\frac{G''}{G'}\right) \quad (14)$$

The magnitude of the shear modulus $|G^*|$ reflects the overall stiffness of the tissue in shear. The phase-shift angle characterizes the energy dissipation relative to energy storage within the tissue. For more details, the reader is referred to standard engineering texts on continuum mechanics or viscoelasticity (39,129,142,265).

The values of $|G^*|$ vary from 0.2 MPa to 2.5 MPa for bovine articular cartilage (550) under infinitesimal strain (<0.001 rad). We note that a material is purely elastic when $\delta = 0°$ and purely viscous when $\delta = 90°$, whereas δ lies somewhere between 0° and 90° for a general viscoelastic material. The solid matrix of both normal human and bovine articular cartilage exhibits a slightly viscoelastic behavior (188,429,463,547,550). The phase-shift angle

Pure Shear

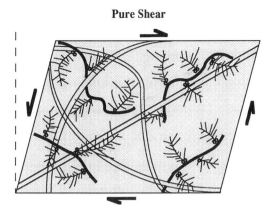

FIGURE 5-21. A schematic representation of cartilage in pure shear. The tension of collagen provides shear stiffness (340).

δ lies between 9° and 20° over a frequency range of 0.01 to 20 Hz.

The collagen network plays an active mechanical role in contributing to the shear stiffness and energy storage in cartilage. Conceptually, the role played by collagen when the specimen is in shear may be visualized as shown in Fig. 5-21. The tension in the diagonally oriented collagen acts to increase the shear stiffness of the solid matrix. This effect is confirmed by the result shown in Fig. 5-22, where $|G^*|$ is directly and significantly related to the collagen content of articular cartilage (550).

In the recent canine OA studies of Setton and coworkers (463), the $|G^*|$ of the tissue at the femoral condyle decreased from 0.8 MPa at 10 rad/sec for controls to 0.25 MPa at 6 and 12 weeks following anterior cruciate ligament transection, and tan δ increased from 0.22 for controls to 0.31 at 12 weeks postoperative. These findings are consistent with the major drop in tensile modulus and loss of collagen cross-linking of the superficial tangential zone in this canine OA model (168) and a general disorganization of the collagen–proteoglycan solid matrix.

For the most part, collagen stores energy like an elastic material. Based on the work of Woo and coworkers (538,539) on canine medial collateral ligaments (composed mainly of collagen), the energy dissipation of these tissues in tension is very slight, with a phase-shift angle δ of about 3.6°. The energy dissipation of pure proteoglycan solutions at high concentrations (10 to 50 mg/mL) has also been determined. These phase-shift angles range from 50° to 75° (178, 341,346,549). Thus, from these results, we may

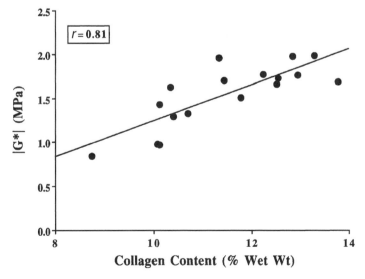

FIGURE 5-22. A direct correlation between the collagen content (by wet weight) and magnitude of dynamic modulus $|G^*|$ for bovine articular cartilage. The compressive clamping strain is 20%, and frequency $f = 1.0$ Hz.

conclude that the ability of collagen to resist tension provides the strength of solid matrix in shear, and energy dissipation in collagen fibrils is minimal when it is stretched. Furthermore, the interaction of proteoglycans with collagen fibrils functions to maintain collagen fibrils in proper spatial orientations, thus providing cartilage with its strength and stiffness in shear (451,550). Note that the magnitude of the dynamic shear modulus is significantly greater than the equilibrium shear modulus. This situation is similar to any viscoelastic material where stiffness increases with increasing rates of deformation.

The viscoelasticity of meniscus in response to shear is qualitatively similar to that exhibited by articular cartilage, although the magnitudes of the material coefficients of these tissues are significantly different. First, meniscus shear properties exhibited an orthotropic symmetry, that is, the three planes of symmetry defined by its fibrous architecture dominate the shear properties of the meniscus. The equilibrium shear moduli are 36.8 kPa, 29.8 kPa, and 21.4 kPa in the circumferential, axial, and radial directions, respectively. The circumferential, perpendicular, and radial specimens relative to the collagen fiber orientation for these shear tests are defined in Fig. 5-23. It is to be noted that these shear values are ten times less than those observed for articular cartilage. For these tests, the $|G^*|$ and δ for circumferential, axial, and radial specimens reflect orthotropic symmetry as well (Fig. 5-24).

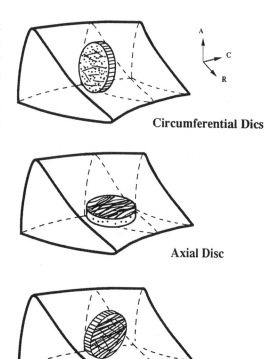

Circumferential Dics

Axial Disc

Radial Disc

FIGURE 5-23. Orientation of meniscal test specimens for anisotropic shear studies (551).

As with tension, the dynamic shear modulus is stiffer than the equilibrium shear modulus.

In summary, the collagen-proteoglycan solid matrix of articular cartilage and meniscus are

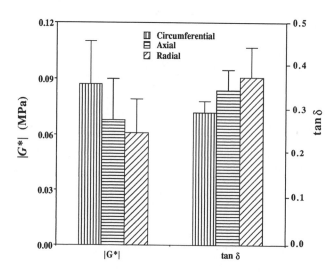

FIGURE 5-24. The magnitude of dynamic shear modulus $|G^*|$ and tan δ for circumferentially, axially, and radially oriented meniscal specimens at 1 rad/sec.

viscoelastic. However, the contribution of these intrinsic viscoelasticity behaviors appears to be minor when one examines the mechanical response of these tissues in compression (288,460). Thus, in compression, the predominant loading mode, the creep and stress-relaxation responses of normal cartilage and meniscus are dominated by the frictional drag of interstitial fluid flow. For pathologic tissues, where the permeability is increased (reduced frictional drag force), the intrinsic viscoelasticity of the solid matrix becomes important (460). These observations have been recently theoretically and experimentally validated (211).

6 BIPHASIC VISCOELASTIC PROPERTIES OF ARTICULAR CARTILAGE IN COMPRESSION

In this section, the transient compressive creep and stress-relaxation behaviors of cartilage and meniscus are discussed. We have shown that the dominant physical mechanism affecting these time-dependent responses is the frictional drag caused by interstitial fluid flow through the porous-permeable solid matrix. These are the *flow-dependent* properties of the tissue, and they

are best described and understood using the biphasic theory.

6.1 Strain-dependent Permeability

As described previously, the permeability coefficient of the soft-hydrated tissue can be determined from the permeation experiment using Darcy's law (Eq. 6). The values of permeability for cartilage and meniscus obtained are very low (10^{-15} to 10^{-16} m^4/N-sec), and by Eq. 7, the diffusive drag coefficients were very high (10^{15} to 10^{16} N-sec/m^4). Thus, very large drag forces are exerted by interstitial fluid as it flows through the porous–permeable solid matrix. These large drag forces can cause significant compaction of the porous–permeable solid matrix (202,204,262,296); this phenomenon is known as flow-induced compaction of the solid matrix. Indeed, for articular cartilage, the permeability is highly dependent on the compressive strain and applied pressures. As can be seen in Fig. 5-25, the permeation measurements show the dramatic effects of compressive strain ε_c and pressure gradient ΔP on the permeability coefficient k of the tissue (204,262,296, 338).

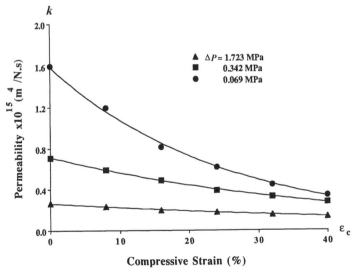

FIGURE 5-25. Variation of the apparent permeability *k* with compressive clamping strain (ε_c) and pressure gradient ΔP. This is known as the strain-dependent permeability effect (262,338).

These experimental observations indicate that a reduction in the dimensions of the cartilage would lead to a reduction of fluid content and thus in the porosity and permeability of the solid matrix. This nonlinear strain-dependent permeability effect plays an important physiological role in regulating the transient compressive responses of cartilage and in dissipating energy. It serves to prevent rapid and excessive fluid exudation from the tissue by compression (20, 202,204,262,338,342).

6.2 The Mechanism of Biphasic Creep and Stress Relaxation

6.2.1 Confined Compression Experiment and Analysis

The observed creep and stress-relaxation behaviors of articular cartilage and meniscus result from the balance of stresses between that carried by the drag force of interstitial fluid flow and that supported by the solid matrix. An estimate of the drag force can be made using data on cartilage permeability and the diffusive drag coefficient relationship (Eq. 7). Consider the case of a cartilage specimen with permeability coefficient of 1.5×10^{-15} m^4/N-sec and porosity of 0.75, then the diffusive drag coefficient is 0.375 $\times 10^{15}$ N-sec/m^4. For a fluid filtration velocity of 15 μm/sec, according to Eq. 6, this drag force would require a pressure differential of 7.5 MPa to move a 1-mm column of fluid through the tissue at that speed (262). Thus, even for this very low flow speed, very large drag forces and hydraulic pressures are exerted on the solid matrix. Further, we note that for normal cartilage with a compressive modulus less than 1.0 MPa (Table 5-9), a compressive stress of approximately 0.25 MPa is required to compress the tissue by 25% (a normal occurrence *in vivo*). In this example, the ratio of the stress from fluid drag to the stress required to compress the tissue is about 30:1. Thus, the drag force of interstitial fluid flow and the associated fluid pressure appear to be the major mechanisms for load support in the joint. This is the most important fact in understanding how cartilage and meniscus support load in the joint. This observation of fluid load

support has been recently theoretically predicted and experimentally validated (476,477).

The compressive creep behaviors of articular cartilage, intervertebral disc and meniscus have been studied extensively in the confined compression test (23,115,202,203,224,260,263, 338,340,342,345,400,539). In the creep experiment, the surface of a small cylindrical plug of the tissue specimen is loaded against a free-draining, rigid, porous–permeable filter (Fig. 5-16). The pressure in the pore fluid of the filter is kept at ambient; thus, a free-draining condition is maintained that allows fluid exudation from the tissue to occur in an unimpeded manner. A load is suddenly applied to, and constantly maintained on, the specimen. Exudation of the interstitial fluid begins immediately. As fluid leaves the tissue, compressive creep deformation occurs. A typical creep curve, on a semi-log scale for intervertebral disc is shown in Fig. 5-26. The rate of creep is controlled by the rate of fluid exudation and thus by tissue permeability. In the confined compression experiment, ideally, the fluid movement and solid matrix deformation occur only in the axial direction. From the linear biphasic formulation for cartilage (338), the principle of conservation of mass yields an explicit relationship between

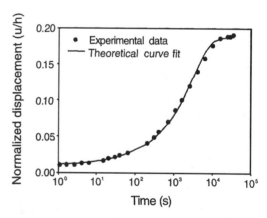

FIGURE 5-26. Curve-fitted and experimental results of the biphasic viscoelastic creep in confined compression for a plug of intervertebral disc. The solid line represents the creep response calculated by the linear biphasic model, Eq. 18. The results of the curve fit yielded a confined compression modulus of 0.52 MPa and an average hydraulic permeability of 0.17×10^{-15} m^4/N sec (36).

fluid exudation velocity $v^f(0,t)$ and surface creep velocity $v^s(0,t)$. This is given by

$$\phi^s v^s(0,t) = -\phi^f v^f(0,t), \qquad (15)$$

where $z = 0$ defines the position of the surface. The negative sign means compression of the solid matrix that would yield fluid exudation. From this expression, it is clear that creep will reach equilibrium when fluid exudation ceases. Thus, at creep equilibrium (i.e., no interstitial fluid flow), the load applied via the rigid–porous filter will be entirely borne by the solid matrix. This result also shows that the kinetics of creep may be used as a convenient way to determine tissue permeability.

According to the biphasic constitutive law, the total stress σ^T acting on the tissue is given by:

$$\sigma^T = \sigma^S + \sigma^f, \qquad (16)$$

where σ^S is the stress acting on the elastic collagen–proteoglycan solid matrix, and σ^f is the stress acting on the interstitial fluid. The stress differential on σ^T is balanced by the frictional drag force acting on the solid and fluid phases, which are given respectively by

$$f^s = -f^f = K(v^s - v^f) + p\nabla\phi^f. \quad (17)$$

These fundamental concepts provide the basis for understanding the creep and stress-relaxation behaviors of any hydrated soft tissues. For creep, the analytic solution for the surface displacement $u(0,t)$ in the axial direction is obtained:

$$\frac{u(0,t)}{h} =$$
$$\frac{F_o}{H_A}\left\{1 - 2\sum_{n=0}^{\infty}\frac{\exp\left(-\left(n+\tfrac{1}{2}\right)^2\pi^2 H_A kt/h^2\right)}{\left(n+\tfrac{1}{2}\right)^2\pi^2}\right\} \quad (18)$$

where h is the thickness of the specimen, F_o is the applied compressive stress, and H_A is the aggregate modulus. Equation 18 predicts that at time $t = 0$, the surface displacement $u(0,0) = 0$; that is, there is no instantaneous displacement of cartilage at the surface under confined compression conditions (Fig. 5-26). Physically, this is because fluid flux (volume/time/area) through the interstitium can not occur instantaneously because of the frictional drag. This situation is analogous to

the viscous dashpot (Fig. 5-10B), which cannot respond instantaneously. Equation 18 also shows that the kinetics of creep from $t = 0^+$ (shortly after loading) to $t \to \infty$ is governed by the time constant T defined by

$$T = \frac{h^2}{H_A k} = \frac{h^2 K}{(\phi^f)^2 H_A} \qquad (19)$$

This constant is known as the characteristic time for a biphasic material. It is proportional to the ratio of the frictional drag coefficient K to the compressive aggregate modulus H_A. Theoretically, it has been shown that this time constant T is the most important parameter governing the kinetics of creep and stress relaxation in compression (203). With material coefficients for normal and osteoarthritic cartilages, their characteristic times ($\approx 1,500$ sec versus 500 sec) differ considerably, as does the manner of their load support (Problem 14). This means that normal cartilage would take more than three times longer to reach creep equilibrium than does degenerative cartilage; that is, the fluid pressurization effect is more important in load carriage for normal tissue than for OA tissue. This observation has been recently validated experimentally (476,477). This characteristic time also shows that a tissue that is twice as thick will take four times as long to reach creep equilibrium. An increase of permeability would decrease creep time, and a decrease of compressive modulus would increase creep time.

The solution given by Eq. 18 provides the explicit expression to determine the properties of the test specimens under the uniaxial confined compression creep condition. Note that as time approaches infinity, the specimen would reach a compressive equilibrium strain given by $u/h = F_o/H_A$. Therefore, the compressive aggregate modulus H_A can be determined from the equilibrium displacement, the thickness of the tissue, and the applied compressive stress.[5] The permeability coefficient of the specimen may be determined from the kinetics of the

---

[5] From the expresssion $u/h = F_o/H_A$, it can be seen that for the linear biphasic theory to be valid, F_o must be $<< H_A$.

TABLE 5-10A. PERMEABILITY COEFFICIENT (10^{-15} m⁴/N sec) OF LATERAL CONDYLE AND PATELLAR GROOVE CARTILAGE

	Human[a]	Bovine[b]	Canine[c]	Monkey[d]	Rabbit[e]
Lateral condyle	1.18	0.43	0.77	4.19	1.81
Patellar groove	2.17	1.42	0.93	4.74	3.84

[a]Young normal.
[b]18 months to 2 years old.
[c]Mature beagles and greyhounds.
[d]Mature cynomologus monkeys.
[e]Mature New Zealand White rabbits.
Data shown were obtained from indentation creep tests.

confined compression creep data. This is done by analyzing the experimental data with Eq. 18 and by using a least-squares numerical curve-fitting procedure (12,36,141,338,350,400). As shown in Fig. 5-26, the experimental creep data are compared with the predictions of Eq. 18. To check the accuracy of this curve-fitting procedure, the calculated value of k may be compared with the values of k determined from the uniaxial permeation experiment. Indeed, the average permeability coefficient k determined from the confined compression experiment is consistent with those obtained from the direct permeation experiment (262,296,345). The permeability coefficients determined from this creep test for various tissues are presented in Table 5-10A. The corresponding thickness of the articular cartilage is presented in Table 5-10B. The average value of permeability of normal bovine meniscus is 0.81×10^{-15} m⁴/N-sec (400). The variations with time of the aggregate modulus, shear modulus, Poisson's ratio, permeability, and thickness of greyhound tibial plateau cartilage following anterior cruciate ligament (ACL) transection (control, 6 weeks, 12 weeks) are shown

in Table 5-10C (462). Clearly, injuries of this type have significant detrimental effects on knee joint cartilage.

The compressive stress-relaxation test has the same experimental setup as the uniaxial confined compression creep test. In this test, a displacement function $u(0,t)$ is imposed at the specimen surface via the rigid porous-permeable platen. During the ramp phase ($0 < t < t_o$), the tissue is compressed at a constant rate, $u(0,t) = Rt$, where R is the rate of compression. Fluid exudation occurs across the surface (see Fig. 5-27, points A and B). Because of the large frictional drag associated with fluid flow through the solid matrix, large loads are needed to compress the tissue. Figure 5-27 (bottom right) depicts the stress rising during the ramp phase. During the relaxation phase ($t > t_o$), the compressive strain is held constant. Thus, by Eq. 15, no fluid exudation occurs (Fig. 5-27C, D, E). The compressive stress at the surface decays with time as solid compaction at the surface is relieved. This results in a transfer of stress away from the compacted regions. This phenomenon also indicates that it is difficult to maintain high stresses

TABLE 5-10B. AVERAGE CARTILAGE THICKNESS (mm) OF LATERAL CONDYLE AND PATELLAR GROOVE

	Human[a]	Bovine[b]	Canine[c]	Monkey[d]	Rabbit[e]
Lateral condyle	2.31	0.94	0.58	0.57	0.25
Patellar groove	3.57	1.38	0.52	0.41	0.20

[a]Young normal.
[b]18 months to 2 years old.
[c]Mature beagles and greyhounds.
[d]Mature cynomologus monkeys.
[e]Mature New Zealand White rabbits.
Data shown were obtained from indentation creep tests.

TABLE 5-10C. PROPERTIES OF GREYHOUND TIBIAL PLATEAU AT TWO TIME PERIODS FOLLOWING ACL TRANSECTION[a]

Mean (SD)	Control	6 Weeks Post-ACLT	12 Weeks Post-ACLT
$\kappa(\times 10^{-15}$ m^4/N sec)	2.4 (1.3)	2.6 (0.4)	4.1 (1.0)[b]
H (MPa)	0.56 (0.19)	0.31 (0.10)[b]	0.42 (0.10)[b]
μ_s (MPa)	0.25 (0.08)	0.14 (0.03)[b]	0.19 (0.05)[b]
ν_s	0.07 (0.10)	0.08 (0.07)	0.09 (0.06)
Thickness (mm)	0.85 (0.17)	0.85 (0.11)	0.94 (0.24)

[a]Data from Setton et al. (464).
[b]Result of biphasic indentation testing of cartilage sites on the tibial plateau covered by the meniscus significantly different from control ($p < 0.05$).

in the solid matrix of normal cartilage. It has been shown that the rate of stress relaxation in such a material occurs four times faster than the rate of creep (202,203). At equilibrium, the compressive aggregate modulus computed from the stress-relaxation experiment reflects the intrinsic material stiffness and is therefore equal to that determined from the compressive creep experiment.

It is important to emphasize that during the creep and stress-relaxation processes, a severely nonhomogeneous compressive strain field is developed in the solid matrix, and because of the porous–permeable loading platen, the surface region will experience the most severe compaction. This nonhomogeneous strain field has three important physiological consequences: (a) the permeability at the surface is significantly reduced as a result of the strain-dependent permeability effect; (b) the frictional drag force caused by fluid exudation is exerted most severely at the surface; and (c) the nominal strain in an experiment (e.g., grip-to-grip strain measurement) does *not* provide an accurate assessment of the actual nonhomogeneous compressive strains experienced by the tissue. However, as the compacted region

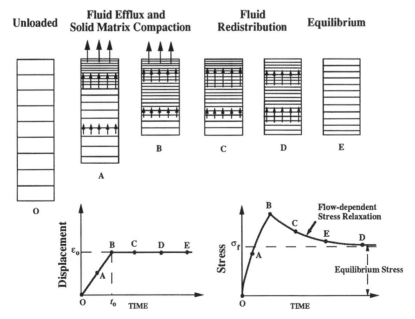

FIGURE 5-27. Schematic representation of fluid exudation and redistribution within cartilage during a rate-controlled compression stress-relaxation experiment *(lower left)*. The horizontal bars in the upper figures indicate the distribution of strain in the tissue. The lower graph *(right)* shows the stress response during the compression phase (O, A, B) and the relaxation phase (B, C, D, E).

gradually diffuses into the deeper zones of the tissue, the creep and stress-relaxation processes eventually cease; at equilibrium, for a homogeneous material, there will be a homogeneous state of compressive strain in the material. Thus, in measuring the intrinsic material properties of soft hydrated tissues, grip-to-grip motion may only be used at equilibrium for homogeneous materials.

6.2.2 Indentation Creep Experiment

The indentation experiment is the most frequently used method worldwide for studying the biomechanical properties of articular cartilage (10, 23, 24, 29, 85, 117, 141, 150, 195, 197, 206, 226, 236, 237, 285, 345, 382, 383, 473, 474). A schematic diagram of an articular cartilage indentation experiment, where the tissue is compressed by a circular rigid, smooth, porous, free-draining indenter of radius *a*, is shown in Fig. 5-28. This experiment is attractive because it does not require special specimen preparation techniques such as microtoming precise strips required for the tensile tests or preparing precise cartilage–bone plugs for the confined compression tests. Further, the indentation test has the added advantage that the material properties of cartilage are determined in situ on the bone, a condition more closely resembling the physi-

ological situation. It also provides a method to determine the variation of cartilage properties over the joint surface (10,23,24,29,85,117,141, 150,195,197,206,226,236,237,285,345,382,383, 473,474) and does not affect the ultrastructure or composition of the tissue. It is this relative simplicity that has led many investigators to adopt the indentation test as the method of choice for determining cartilage material properties.

The mathematics of modeling the indentation experiment of cartilage-on-bone configuration is very complex because of the multidimensional deformations in the layer of tissue as well as the biphasic nature of the tissue (289,345). Because of the mathematical difficulties involved with modeling the indentation test, early investigators resorted to the use of a linearly elastic constitutive law to analyze and interpret the experimental viscoelastic creep data without accounting for the interstitial fluid flow in the tissue (187,195,226,227,236,237,473,474). Because elastic analyses cannot predict time-dependent behavior, these models necessarily cannot describe the creep and stress-relaxation behaviors exhibited by cartilage. Hence, researchers introduced the use of elastic modulus determined at a specific time, for example, Kempson's 2-sec creep modulus (236,237). Clearly the choice of any arbitrary time means that the data are subjective, and therefore, not a true measure of the material property. Such arbitrariness has led to significant controversies in the cartilage biomechanics literature. For a detailed discussion of the history of the indentation experiment, the reader is referred to reviews by Mow and coworkers (345) and Mak and coworkers (289) on this subject.

As discussed earlier, in the specific case of uniaxial confined compression, two material coefficients (H_A and k) can be determined using the linear biphasic theory. In general, however, the biphasic theory contains three material coefficients (H_A, v, k); these three coefficients are equivalent to any other set, such as (E, v, k) or (E, μ, k) (see Table 5-4). In the application of the early model such as the mathematical solutions of elastic theory for indentation (187), a priori assumptions for Poisson's ratio must be made.

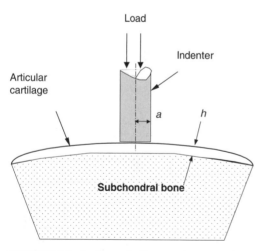

FIGURE 5-28. A schematic diagram showing a layer of articular cartilage of thickness *h* being indented by a circular, rigid, porous-permeable, free-draining indenter of radius *a*.

Various investigators have chosen the Poisson's ratio to be between 0.4 and 0.5 (197,236,474). Such an arbitrary choice (see Table 5-4) means that all calculated values of material parameters from the study would also be arbitrary, and therefore, invalid. However, the indentation creep test, analyzed using the linear biphasic theory, provides the determination of all three material coefficients simultaneously (23,24,141,345) without any arbitrary choice of the Poisson's ratio. The mathematics of modeling the indentation experiment is very complex and is beyond the scope of this chapter. The reader is referred to published references (187,285,289,345) for a complete mathematical description of the problem.

The nature of the mathematical solution showing the dependence of biphasic indentation creep on the aggregate modulus, Poisson's ratio, and permeability is shown in Fig. 5-29A. From this result, we now know that: (a) the equilibrium displacement value, $u(\infty)$, defines a relationship for the intrinsic compressive modulus (H_A) and the Poisson's ratio (ν); (b) the shape of the creep curve is also defined by the Poisson's ratio; and (c) the rate of the creep curve (i.e., the kinetics of creep) is defined by the shift factor $S = \log_{10}(H_A k t / a^2)$, where a is the radius of the indenter tip. This shift factor provides the third necessary relationship to determine the permeability (k) of the tissue from the creep data. These three relationships have been used to determine the three intrinsic properties of articular cartilage (H_A, ν, k) (289,345). This problem has been solved numerically from the exact mathematical formulation. To determine these three coefficients at the indentation site, the numerical solutions are curve-fitted using a least-squares procedure. Typical curve-fitting results are shown in Fig. 5-29B on a semilog$_{10}(t)$ scale. Tables 5-9 and 5-10A,C provide the aggregate modulus and permeability determined by this method. Table 5-11 provides the Poisson's ratio for the same population of animals.

The available data on Poisson's ratio reflects some important characteristics of cartilage: (a) it varies with species and location; (b) it almost always falls outside of the 0.4 to 0.5 range, the commonly *assumed range*; and (c) a priori es-

timates of Poisson's ratio in the range 0.4 to 0.5 may lead to significant errors in calculating the aggregate modulus. For example, errors as large as 200% can occur if one assumes $\nu = 0.4$ in the calculation for H_A and the actual Poisson's ratio is zero (345). For an isotropic porous–permeable solid matrix, Poisson's ratio is a measure of the compressibility of its pores: $\nu = 0$ means the pores are maximally compressible, and $\nu = 0.5$ means the pores are incompressible. For isotropic biphasic materials, a measure of the volume efflux of fluid through the tissue when it is compressed is Poisson's ratio. For a biphasic material with $\nu = 0.5$, no fluid flow can occur, and thus no creep and stress-relaxation behaviors are possible. The species and anatomic site variation of Poisson's ratio over the joint surface may in fact reflect the fluid efflux requirement at a specific location on the joint surface, say for purposes of joint lubrication (see Chapter 10 for more details on lubrication).

7 SWELLING OF ARTICULAR CARTILAGE

7.1 Mechanism of Swelling: Change of Hydration and Dimensions

In cartilage, proteoglycan aggregates are immobilized and restrained in the collagen meshwork. They contain a large number of negatively charged groups (SO_3^- and COO^-) along their GAG chains. For normal and degenerate femoral head cartilage, the FCD ranges from 0.04 to 0.18 mEq/g wet tissue at physiological pH (297,298,302). Each negative charge requires a counterion to be nearby to maintain electroneutrality. Thus, the total ion concentration inside the tissue is greater than the ion concentration in the external bathing solution. This imbalance of ions gives rise to a pressure in the interstitial fluid that is higher than the ambient pressure in the external bath. This is known as the Donnan osmotic pressure (100). This osmotic pressure is one of the causes of cartilage swelling and maintenance of hydration.

In the ECM, it is estimated that the proteoglycans are restrained to one fifth of their

TABLE 5-11. AVERAGE POISSON'S RATIO (ν) OF LATERAL CONDYLE AND PATELLAR GROOVE CARTILAGE

	Human[a]	Bovine[b]	Canine[c]	Monkey[d]	Rabbit[e]
Lateral condyle	0.10	0.40	0.30	0.24	0.34
Patellar groove	0.00	0.25	0.09	0.20	0.21

[a]Young normal.
[b]18 months to 2 years old.
[c]Mature beagles and greyhounds.
[d]Mature cynomologus monkeys.
[e]Mature New Zealand White rabbits.

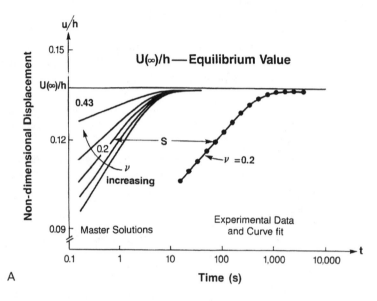

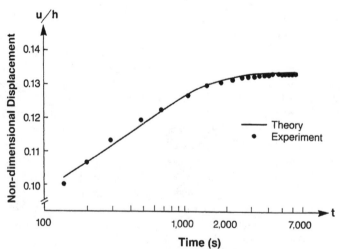

FIGURE 5-29. (A) Representation of the time-shift method in which a master solution is shifted by an amount S along the logarithmic time axis. Diagram illustrates how the shape of the displacement curve is controlled by the Poisson's ratio ν. **(B)** A typical nonlinear regression curve fit using the bicubic spline interpolation for biphasic creep indentation solution in logarithmic time scale.

volume in free solution (182,357). Thus, the charge groups fixed along the GAG chains of the solid matrix are very close to each other, causing large charge–charge repulsive forces to be exerted against each other. The electrostatic interactions between fixed charges and mobile ions are primarily responsible for tissue swelling. The electrostatic forces are modulated by the counterions and coions swarming around the proteoglycan molecules in solution. With increasing ion concentration within the tissue, the equivalent Debye length between the ion cloud and the fixed charges is decreased. This results in charge shielding, which decreases the net charge–charge repulsive force (62,145). Decrease of the size of the PG molecule in solution with charge shielding has been measured (384). Changes in the di-

mensions and shape of the tissue specimen and isometric stress caused by NaCl concentration changes in the external bathing solution have also been measured (8,112,113,156,350,360, 362,458,459,462,464,493).

Maroudas and coworkers were the first to provide significant amounts of data on changing tissue hydration and interstitial ion concentration (c) with changing external bathing solution c^* (297,298,300). In those studies the cartilage swelling is measured by weight. Later, Mow and coworkers (362,459,464) measured the tendency for cartilage to swell dimensionally or curl when c^* is changed. The results of these dimensional swelling studies show that swelling of articular cartilage is nonhomogeneous (Fig. 5-30A) and anisotropic (Fig. 5-30B),

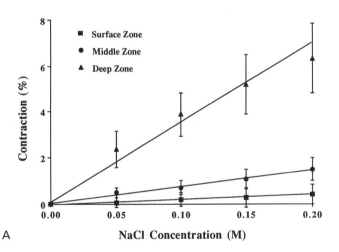

A

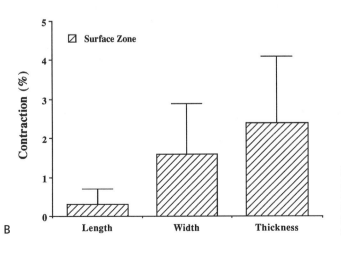

B

FIGURE 5-30. Free swelling of articular cartilage strips: **(A)** along the length axis as a function of depth (surface, middle, and deep zones); **(B)** in the directions of length, width, and thickness of the specimen (362).

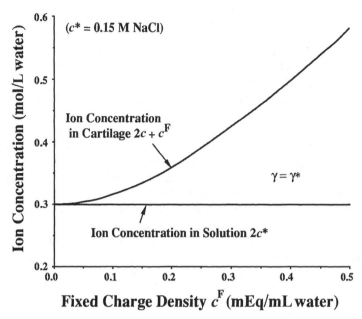

FIGURE 5-31. Ion concentration in the interstitium versus fixed charged density.

which would produce curling when the tissue is excised from the bone. The length and width directions correspond to directions parallel and perpendicular to the local split-line directions. The magnitude of contraction is largest along the thickness direction and in the deep zone of the tissue. Further, as can be seen in Fig. 5-30A, the ion-induced contractions of cartilage under free swelling conditions vary linearly with c^*. This result is described by the relationship $\varepsilon_s = -\alpha_c c^*$, where α_c is known as the coefficient of chemical contraction, and ε_s is the ioninduced contraction (360,362). For articular cartilage, the value α_c ranges from 0.05 M^{-1} to 0.3 M^{-1}.

7.2 Donnan Equilibrium, Ion Distribution, and Osmotic Pressure

If the tissue is bathed in deionized water (i.e., very low electrolyte solution), the total internal counterion concentration c^+ would be approximately equal to the total FCD. If the tissue is bathed in an external NaCl solution of concentration c^*, the total concentrations of c^- and c^+

within the interstitium would be determined by the ideal Donnan equilibrium ion distribution law:

$$c^- c^+ = (c^*)^2. \qquad (20a)$$

This equation was derived by Donnan in 1924 (100) and governs the ion concentration in an ideal polyelectrolyte solution. This law has been used extensively for articular cartilage (297,300, 302).[6] In Eq. 20a, c^- and c^+ are concentrations of Cl^- and Na^+ ions, respectively. These ion concentrations are related to the FCD (c^F) by the electroneutrality condition (230,264):

$$c^+ = c^- + c^F \qquad (20b)$$

The total internal ion concentration ($c^+ + c^-$) in cartilage as a function of the FCD c^F at an external concentration $c^* = 0.15$ M NaCl is shown in Fig. 5-31. If, however, the tissue is bathed in a very high-concentration NaCl solution, that

---

[6] Cartilage, by virtue of its solid matrix, is not an ideal polyelectrolyte solution. However, predictions of total ion concentrations using Eqs. 20a and 20b seem to be accurate.

is, if $c^* >> c^F$, the difference between the total number of ions within the tissue $(c^+ + c^-)$ $(= 2c^- + c^F)$ and the total number of ions outside $(2c^*)$ is given by (264):

$$(2c^- + c^F) - 2c^* = (c^F)^2/(4c^*). \quad (21)$$

Thus, this difference approaches zero as the external concentration $c^* \to \infty$. From the classical relationship for osmotic pressure, the Donnan osmotic pressure (π) that results from the excess of ion particles inside the tissue (see Fig. 5-31) is given by:

$$\pi = RT[\Phi(2c^- + c^F) - 2\Phi^*c^*] + P_\infty, \quad (22)$$

where R is the universal gas constant, T is the absolute temperature, Φ and Φ^* are osmotic coefficients, and P_∞ is the osmotic pressure attributable to the concentration of proteoglycan particles in the tissue (109,494). Usually, because of the size of proteoglycan molecules, P_∞ is negligibly small. We emphasize that this expression is for polyelectrolyte solutions, where there is no solid matrix. However, it has nevertheless been used extensively to describe the swelling pressures of cartilage and the intervertebral disc (297, 300,302,509).

7.3 Triphasic Swelling Theory

A triphasic theory (comprising a miscible ion phase along with the two immiscible fluid and solid phases of the biphasic theory) has been developed to account for the ion-induced swelling effects and the biphasic deformational effects (264). This theory describes (a) all biphasic viscoelastic effects; (b) the Donnan equilibrium ion distributions (c^F, c); (c) the dimensional swelling effect (ε_s); (d) the Donnan osmotic pressures (π); (e) kinetics of swelling (i.e., transient effects); and (f) all electrokinetic effects (e.g., diffusion and streaming potentials (266)).

Typical experimental or theoretical swelling studies of cartilage are performed under confined compression (260,338,340,351), unconfined compression (13,300,302,438,528), or the free (unloaded and unconstrained) condi-

tion (360,459). For the confined-compression swelling experiment, the tissue specimen is held at a fixed compressive strain by a rigid, free-draining loading platen. Under these conditions, the triphasic theory predicts that the total equilibrium axial stress σ^T at the loading platen will be equal to:

$$\sigma^T = \sigma^S + \pi \quad (23)$$

Here, σ^S is the stress in the elastic solid matrix caused by the imposed uniaxial compression (i.e., from the biphasic theory), and π is the Donnan osmotic swelling pressure (i.e., Eq. 22). This swelling pressure has a significant effect on tissue stiffness and other equilibrium material properties (264,285,351,528). The stress-relaxation behavior of cartilage has also been influenced by the swelling pressure effect (351,528).

8 EFFECTS OF WATER CONTENT AND FIXED CHARGE DENSITY ON TRANSPORT PROPERTIES

8.1 Hydraulic Permeability

Hydraulic permeability of cartilage is one of the most important properties of soft-hydrated tissues, especially in the load-carrying capacity that is physiologically required of articular cartilage (see Chapter 10, and references 20,211, 350,476,477). Many studies have been conducted to determine this property (e.g., 12,70, 110,111,159–165,203,204,262–264,296,297, 299,302,338,340,345). In these experiments, generally the permeability is determined under zero-current conditions (i.e., open-circuit conditions). Because of the coupling of mechanical and electrical effects, the measured hydraulic permeability of charged tissues such as articular cartilage also depends on the electrical current flow (157,161,215,230). That is, the tissue with electrical current flow (closed-circuit case) is more permeable than the tissue without electrical current flow (open-circuit case). Open-circuit permeability (a more general case) depends on the FCD (70,114,161,297). For example, Maroudas (in 1968 and 1975) showed experimentally that measured open-circuit hydraulic permeability of human cartilage decreases with increasing its FCD (297,300). The relationship between closed-circuit permeability and open-circuit permeability is given as follows (159,163):

$$\frac{\kappa_o}{\kappa} = 1 - \frac{RT(c^F)^2}{\phi^f(c^+ D^+ + c^- D^-)}\left(\frac{\kappa_o}{\eta}\right) \quad (24)$$

where κ is the closed-circuit Darcy permeability and κ_o is the open-circuit Darcy permeability. The Darcy permeability is related to the hydraulic permeability (k) in the biphasic theory and the viscosity coefficient of fluid (η) by $\kappa = k \cdot \eta$. In Eq. 24, D^+ and D^- are the intrinsic diffusion coefficients of the Na^+ and Cl^- ions in the interstitial fluid of the tissue, respectively. Figure 5-32 shows the effect of FCD on the ratio of open-circuit permeability to closed-circuit permeability (κ_o/κ) as a function of open-circuit permeability (κ_o). The curves in Fig. 5-32 indicate there is an upper limit for κ_o for charged hydrated tissues ($c^F \neq 0$) (163). That is, more highly permeable tissues must have a lower value of FCD because the ratio (κ_o/κ) cannot be negative.

Note that closed-circuit permeability κ is a function of tissue composition and structure, independent of tissue FCD. Thus, the closed-circuit permeability is an intrinsic material property, while the open-circuit permeability depends on the FCD as described by Eq. 24. Recently, a new model for intrinsic permeability of fibrous porous media was proposed (163, 164):

$$\kappa = a \left(\frac{\phi^f}{\phi^s}\right)^n, \quad (25)$$

where a and n are material parameters whose values depend on the structure and composition of the porous medium. This form of polynomial dependence of permeability on the volume fraction of solid and fluid within the biphasic medium is similar to that proposed in the theoretical study of Holmes and Mow (204).

Equation 25 states that a tissue would be impermeable if its porosity ϕ^f approaches zero. Because tissue porosity is related to the tissue deformation, Eq. 25 can also be used to predict the well-known nonlinear strain-dependent

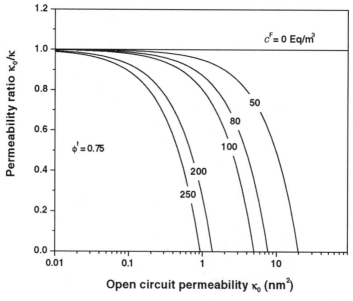

FIGURE 5-32. The ratio of biphasic open-circuit permeability (κ_o) to triphasic closed-circuit permeability (κ) is dependent on the tissue fixed charge density (c^F) and open-circuit permeability. The effect of c^F on the ratio of κ_o/κ decreases with decreasing κ_o.

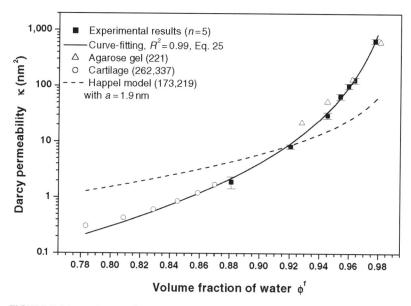

FIGURE 5-33. Variation of intrinsic Darcy permeability (κ) with water volume fraction (ϕ^f). The solid symbols are the mean $\pm$ SD $n = 5$ specimens at each agarose gel concentration (164). The best fit line is given by $\kappa = 0.00339(\phi^f/\phi^s)^{3.236}$ (nm²), $R^2 = 0.9995$. Happel's model (173), Johnson and Deen's data for agarose gel (221), and how Mow and Lai's data (337) for bovine articular cartilage ($\phi_o^f = 0.87$ and $\eta = 0.001$N-sec/m²) are also plotted for comparison. There is an excellent agreement between our model prediction and the experimental data for bovine articular cartilage (262,337).

permeability behavior of the tissue under deformation (20,159,202–204,238,239,263,296).

Equation 24 together with Eq. 25 provides the mathematical relationships for the measured (open-circuit) permeability to tissue porosity and FCD. Recent analysis of FCD-dependent permeability data reported by Maroudas in 1968 and 1975 showed that the measured open-circuit permeability is more sensitive to changes in tissue porosity (water content) than in FCD (163). Thus, it is not a surprise that Eq. 25 (with $a = 0.00339$ nm² and $n = 3.236$) can accurately predict variations in permeability for agarose gels (221) and bovine articular cartilage (262,337–340) as a function of water volume fraction in a wide range (approximately four orders of magnitude variation in permeability) (164); see Fig. 5-33. In Fig. 5-33, a microstructure model, that is, a Happel model (173,219) with fiber radius $a = 1.9$ nm for agarose gels (221) is also plotted for comparison.

8.2 Electrical Conductivity

Electrical conductivity is one of the material properties of charged, hydrated, soft tissues. Its value governs the electrokinetic phenomena observed in cartilage and other charged hydrated soft tissues (such as streaming potential; see

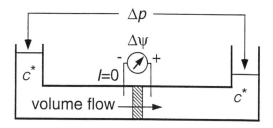

FIGURE 5-34. A one-dimensional permeation experiment on a permeable, charged, hydrated tissue specimen under an open-circuit condition to determine the streaming potential $\Delta\psi$. Here Δp is the pressure differential, I is the current ($= 0$), and c^* is the concentration of neutral salt (e.g., NaCl) in the permeating fluid (159).

Fig. 5-34). Under a zero fluid flow condition, the measured tissue electrical conductivity (χ) of a tissue in NaCl solution is related to intrinsic ion diffusivities (D^+, D^-), ion concentrations (c^+ and c^-), FCD (c^F), volume fraction of water, and temperature by (139,193,297):

$$\chi = F_c^2 \phi^f (c^+ D^+ + c^- D^-)/RT, \qquad (26)$$

where F_c is the Faraday constant, c^+ is the cation ion concentration, and c^- is the anion concentration. For negatively charged tissues, the ion concentrations in the tissues are related to the absolute value of c^F through the electroneutrality condition, i.e., Eq. 20b.

The ion concentrations within the cartilaginous tissues or any charged gel can be calculated using the ideal Donnan equation (20a) together with Eq. 20b (268,300,302), given as follows:

$$c^+ = \frac{c^F + \sqrt{(c^F)^2 + 4c^{*2}}}{2},$$

$$c^- = \frac{-c^F + \sqrt{(c^F)^2 + 4c^{*2}}}{2}, \qquad (27)$$

where c^* is the concentration of bathing (NaCl) solution.

Electrical conductivity of cartilage is not sensitive to FCD (184). Rather, it is sensitive to tissue porosity ϕ^f as observed in many other hydrated soft tissues (162,447). For charged hydrated soft tissues with high water content ($\phi^f > 0.7$), the correlation of electrical conductivity to water content is almost linear (162,447). Thus, one may use the conductivity method to determine tissue hydration *in vivo* or *in vitro*. The variation of electrical conductivity with porosity is mainly due to the dependence of ion diffusivity on tissue porosity (139,165).

8.3 Solute Diffusivity

The diffusion coefficients of solutes in cartilaginous tissues are generally smaller than those in aqueous solutions (43,61,146,271,300,402, 497,508). For small solutes, the value of diffusion coefficient in cartilage and intervertebral disc is about 35% to 60% of the value in aqueous solution (61,302,512). For human articu-

lar cartilage, Maroudas reported that the relative diffusivity of Cl^- is in the range of 0.35 to 0.45 and the relative diffusivity for Na^+ is at most 10% lower than that for Cl^- (302). The relative diffusivity of Na^+ in bovine articular cartilage is found to be around 0.6 (61). Studies show that solute diffusivity in cartilaginous tissues depends on tissue compression (43,61,271,372, 402,403). The measured ion diffusivity seems not sensitive to FCD (61,268,300).

In spite of the fact that numerous studies have been conducted to investigate solute diffusion in gels and soft tissues, to date there is no theoretical model capable of satisfactorily describing the diffusion behavior of solutes in gels or biological soft tissues (310). Recently, Gu and coworkers proposed an empirical model for the intrinsic diffusivity (D) of spherical solutes in porous fibrous media, given by:

$$\frac{D}{D_0} = \exp\left[-\alpha \left(\frac{r_s}{\sqrt{\kappa}}\right)^\beta\right], \qquad (28)$$

where D_0 is the diffusivity of the solute in an aqueous solution, r_s is the solute Stokes radius, κ is the Darcy permeability of the medium, and α and β are two positive material parameters that depend on the structure of the porous medium. Equation 28 indicates that relative diffusivity (D/D_0) decreases as solute size increases. In this model, the structural information of media is embedded in the Darcy permeability (κ). Because Darcy permeability depends on tissue porosity (Eq. 25), it follows that solute diffusivity is a function of tissue porosity as well, i.e., strain dependent (165,204,262,338, 340).

This model, Eq. 28, can satisfactorily predict the diffusivity data of spherical macromolecules in agarose gels reported in the literature (165,221,391). This model has also been successfully used to investigate ion diffusivity in porcine annulus fibrosus using the electrical conductivity method (165). These fundamental relationships can be profitably applied for the theoretical studies of molecular transport through normal or pathological articular cartilage for pharmacological studies.

9 SUMMARY

Articular cartilage, intervertebral discs, and meniscus are three of the specialized load-bearing soft tissues of the body that possess fixed charges and are hydrated. Each tissue is endowed with a specific biochemical composition, molecular conformation, and ultrastructure that govern its deformational behaviors. The biomechanical properties of these three tissues have been extensively studied, and they are different because of their specific biochemical composition and their molecular and ultrastructural arrangements. (Although this chapter has extensively covered the structure–function relationships for articular cartilage and meniscus, the reader may wish to refer to the existing references on the intervertebral disc, since intervertebral discs possesses similar general deformational characteristics. For example, see Iatridis et al. (217), Setton et al. (461), and Gu and Yao (163). Almost always, these compositional and molecular features are altered during diseases or when the tissues are injured. These tissues exhibit biphasic mechanical properties, with the frictional drag force of interstitial fluid flow being the dominant factor controlling their compressive viscoelastic creep and stress-relaxation behaviors. The aggregate modulus and permeability of normal cartilage are on the order of 1.0 MPa and 1 to 10 × 10^{-15} m^4/N-sec, and for degenerate cartilage, they are 0.35 MPa and 10^{-14} m^4/N-sec, respectively. There are significant variations in these material properties with anatomical sites as well as with species. For the meniscus, the aggregate modulus and permeability are 0.4 MPa and 0.5 to 1.0 × 10^{-15} m^4/N-sec, respectively. These differences have strong implications for the manner in which loads are supported by cartilage and meniscus in the joint. The permeability is strain dependent; that is, it decreases with compressive strain. This effect serves to restrict excessive fluid exudation when prolonged compression occurs.

All three tissues have anisotropic and non-homogeneous properties. The intrinsic tensile properties of the collagen–proteoglycan solid matrix of both tissues are nonlinear, and their shear properties are viscoelastic. The magnitude of the complex shear modulus of normal carti-

lage is of the order of 0.5 MPa, whereas for the meniscus this is less than 0.15 MPa. Viscoelastic dissipation in shear is slight; the phase shift angle is approximately 15° for both tissues. These viscoelastic shear properties appear to be of little significance unless the permeability of the solid matrix becomes large, i.e., when the frictional drag effects are minimized. The Poisson's ratio of the solid matrix of articular cartilage may range anywhere from 0 to 0.4.

Pressure is a colligative property of atoms and molecules colliding against a surface. Donnan osmotic pressure is due to the difference of the total number of particles of ions (i.e., concentration) in the interstitium and the total number of particles of ions (i.e., concentration) in the external bathing solution. The Donnan equilibrium ion distribution in the interstitium depends on the FCD of the negative charge groups on the proteoglycans and on the external ion concentration of bathing solution. Strictly speaking, these two concepts are valid only for charged polymeric *liquids,* although they have been widely adopted for cartilage, a solid. In cartilage, the swelling pressure has significant effect on equilibrium compressive stiffness of cartilage. Recent results show that Donnan osmotic pressure may account for up to 50% of the equilibrium compressive modulus, and minimally during transient load support (see Chapter 10).

Also, recent studies on the effect of tissue porosity and FCD on transport properties in charged hydrated soft tissues and gels have provided additional insights into transport of fluid and solute within cartilage. This knowledge is important for understanding nutrition during tissue growth and remodeling, and, for example, the transport of pharmacological agents. Articular cartilage, intervertebral disc, and meniscus are three examples of charged, hydrated soft tissues exhibiting multiphasic properties that depend on the nature of the tissues' biochemical composition, molecular structure, and fibrous architecture. Other important connective tissues such as ligaments and tendons offer new opportunities for future investigation for advances in the understanding of mechanism of trauma and degenerative diseases. Some examples of recent results from the biomechanics literature on these complex and intriguing tissues have been introduced in this book as well.

ACKNOWLEDGMENTS

The materials and data presented in this chapter are based on studies sponsored by grants from the National Science Foundation, the National Institutes of Health, and the Orthopaedic Research and Education Foundation. The authors thank Ms. Diana E. Arnold and Ms. Suma Tumuluri for their excellent work on the final preparation of this manuscript and the editors of Lippincott Williams & Wilkins for their patience and support during the long process of the preparation of this book.

PROBLEMS

1. a. Read reference (357) and write a three-page summary of this paper.
   b. Sketch and describe the molecular architecture of a proteoglycan aggrecan and aggregate.
2. a. Read reference (325) and write a three-page summary of this paper.
   b. Sketch and describe the molecular architecture of a collagen fibril.
3. a. Read reference (79) and write a three-page summary of this paper.
   b. Sketch the collagen ultrastructure of adult articular cartilage.
4. Derive Eqs. 2 and 3 governing the force–displacement relationship of the Kelvin–Voigt and Maxwell bodies. Explain why the Kelvin–Voigt body behaves as a solid and why the Maxwell body behaves as a fluid.
5. Given Eqs. 2 and 3 for Kelvin–Voigt and Maxwell bodies, derive the solutions for their stress-relaxation behaviors for $t > 0$ if the applied initial displacement is $x(0) = 1$.
6. Given Eqs. 2 and 3 for Kelvin–Voigt and Maxwell bodies, derive the solutions for their creep behaviors for $t > 0$, if the applied initial load is $F(0) = 1$.
7. A standard three-element linear viscoelastic body is one for which a spring is connected in series with the Kelvin–Voigt body.
   a. Sketch a spring–dashpot arrangement for the standard body.
   b. Derive the force–displacement relationship for this material.
   c. Show that this arrangement is equivalent to a spring connected in parallel with a Maxwell body.
   d. Does the standard three-element body behave as a solid or a fluid? Explain why.
8. The fluid transport Q (volume discharge per unit time, m^3/sec) is given by Darcy's linear relationship $Q = kA\Delta P/h$, where ΔP is the applied pressure differential, A is the area of perfusion, and h is the thickness of the tissue.
   a. For a cartilage tissue with the thickness $h = 1.75$ mm and the perfusion area $A = 6.25$ mm^2, and the permeability $k = 4.6 \times 10^{-15}$ m^4/N-sec, calculate the volume flux across the tissue if $\Delta P = 0.5$ MPa and 1.0 MPa. (Ans. 8.2×10^{-12} m^3/sec; 16.4×10^{-12} m^3/sec)
   b. For a meniscus tissue with $h = 10$ mm, $A = 15$ mm^2, and the permeability $k = 0.8 \times 10^{-15}$ m^4/N-sec calculate the volume flux across the tissue. (Ans. 0.6×10^{-12} m^3/sec; 1.2×10^{-12} m^3/sec)
   c. How long will it take for a fluid particle to travel across the cartilage and the meniscus at $\Delta P = 1.0$ MPa, assuming $\phi^f = 0.75$? (Ans. 500 sec; 9.4×10^4 sec)
9. If normal cartilage and meniscus have water contents of 80% and 74%, respectively, calculate the diffusive drag coefficient for these two tissues. Water content, defined as the ratio of water weight to total weight, is equivalent to porosity. (Ans. 0.14×10^{15} N-sec/m^4, 0.69×10^{15} N-sec/m^4)
10. The Poiseuille's law for volume discharge per unit time (Q) of a fluid with viscosity η through a cylindrical circular tube of radius a and length l is given by $Q = \pi a^4(\Delta p)/8\eta l$. If cartilage and meniscus are modeled by uniform collections of identical cylindrical circular tubes, given the permeabilities of cartilage and meniscus, calculate the

average pore size for these tissues. Use the viscosity of water for this calculation. (Hint: The ratio *l/h* is known as the tortuosity. It is the actual path traveled by a fluid particle as it flows through the tissue of thickness *h*. Assume this value to be no more than 2.) (Ans. 68 to 86 Å; 29 to 42 Å)

11. Rubber is an incompressible material. Its Young's modulus is 1.5 MPa, and its Poisson's ratio is 0.5. Using Table 5-4, determine the aggregate modulus of rubber. Explain your result.

12. Using Table 5-4, calculate the aggregate modulus for steel and cork. Give a physical explanation of your result for cork. (Ans. 1.35*E*, *E*)

13. From the data given in Table 5-7 for bovine articular cartilage, calculate the tangent modulus for slices 1 and 3, || specimens at 5%, 10%, and 15% tensile strains. Compare this result with the Young's modulus *E*. Explain similarities and differences. (Ans. Slice 1 : 13.6, 17.4, 22.3 MPa; Slice 3 : 0.98, 1.07, 1.16 MPa)

14. Assume normal human tibial plateau cartilage has an equilibrium aggregate modulus of 0.79 MPa. If the average in situ compression of cartilage in the medial compartment of the tibial plateau cartilage is 15%, using Eq. 8, calculate the size of the total contact area required to support a joint load of 375 N (75 lb) in this knee. Is this a reasonable answer? Explain.

15. If, as in Problem 14, the individual had the medial meniscus removed during surgery, causing the contact area to be reduced by a factor of 3, calculate the average compressive strain acting in the collagen–proteoglycan solid matrix of cartilage. Is this a reasonable answer? Explain.

16. Use the equation in Problem 10 for calculating the average pore size and the permeability results in Fig. 5-25, and assume a tortuosity of 2.

  a. Find the change in pore size in cartilage at 8% compressive strain between $\Delta P = 0.069$ MPa and 1.723 MPa. (Ans. 69 Å and 28 Å)

  b. Find the change in pore size in cartilage

at $\Delta p = 0.069$ MPa between clamping strains $\varepsilon_s = 0\%$ and 31%. (Ans. 80 Å and 45 Å)

17. The permeability, porosity, and compressive modulus of cartilage are changed during OA. If, for a diseased tissue, the permeability is increased by a factor of 10 to 1.5×10^{-14} m^4/N-sec, the porosity increased to 85%, and the compressive aggregate modulus decreased to 0.35 MPa:

  a. Calculate the pressure differential required to cause 1 mm of fluid to flow through this diseased tissue at 15 μm/sec. (Ans. 0.85 MPa) How does this compare with a normal tissue when $\phi^f = 0.75$ and $k = 1.5 \times 10^{-15}$ m^4/N-sec?

  b. Calculate the stress required to produce 25% compression of this diseased tissue. (Ans. 0.0875 MPa)

  c. What is the ratio of stress from fluid drag to stress required to deform the solid matrix? How does this compare with normal cartilage? (Ans. 10:1)

18. The surface of cartilage in a joint is covered by synovial fluid, and during joint motion a pressure of $P = 4$ MPa is generated in this fluid. From theoretical considerations, it can be shown that the pressure at the articular surface is partitioned according to the porosity ϕ^f, i.e., the pressure acting on the interstitial fluid at the articular surface is $\phi^f P$, and the pressure acting on the solid matrix at the articular surface is $(1 - \phi^f)P$.

  a. For normal cartilage, the porosity ϕ^f is 75%, the permeability is 1.5×10^{-15} m^4/N-sec, and the aggregate modulus is 1.0 MPa. How much pressure is acting on the interstitial fluid at the articular surface? What is the filtration speed of the interstitial fluid across a layer of cartilage of thickness $h = 1.5$ mm (assuming the downstream pressure is zero)? At equilibrium, how much compressive strain exists in the solid matrix? Comment on this result. (Ans. 3 MPa; 5.3 μm/sec; 1.)

  b. For abnormal cartilage, the porosity ϕ^f is 85%, the permeability is 1.5×10^{-14}

m^4/N-sec, and the aggregate modulus is 0.35 MPa. Repeat the questions of part a. All other variables remain the same. Compare the results of parts a and b. (Ans. 3.4 MPa; 0.47 μm/sec; 1.7)

19. Show that $T = h^2/H_A k$ has the dimension of time.

20. Calculate the characteristic time T for human, bovine, and rabbit lateral condyle and patellar groove cartilage. From Eq. 18, explain which tissue will creep the fastest and which will creep the slowest.

21. Describe some circumstances under which the composition and structure of articular cartilage might change. How would the biphasic properties (H_A, v, k,ϕ^f) of the tissue be changed with these changes in composition and tissue structure? How would these changes affect the creep behavior of the tissue?

22. If the FCD of cartilage $c^F = 0.2$ mEq/mL (i.e., 0.2 mol/L), and the external NaCl concentration is 0.15 mol/L, using Eq. 20, calculate the total concentration of NaCl within the tissue. Hint: First determine c from data given and that sodium and chlorine are both monovalent ions. (Ans. $c = 0.216$ mol/L)

23. For a cartilage specimen with $c^F = 0.2$ mEq/mL, bathed in an external electrolyte solution of $c^* = 0.3$ mol/L, calculate the Donnan osmotic pressure π at room temperature ($T = 24°C$). In this calculation, assume the osmotic coefficients $\Phi = \Phi^* = 0.8$, $P_\infty = 0$, R (universal gas constant) = 8.314 Nm/mol-K, and K = 273°C. (Ans. $\pi = 0.063$MPa) Describe justification for the assumption $P_\infty = 0$.

24. If the inequality $c^F >> c^*$ holds true, derive the expression for open-circuit permeability κ_o using Eq. 24.

25. Using Eqs. 26 and 27, calculate the conductivity χ of cartilage equilibrated with a normal saline ($c^* = 150$ mole/m^3) at body temperature. The parameters are $\phi^f = 0.8$, $c^F = 0.2$ mEq/mL, $D^+ = 0.5 \times 10^{-9}$ m^2/sec, $D^- = 0.9 \times 10^{-9}$ m^2/sec, $R = 8.314$ Nm/mole-K, and the Fara-

day constant $F_c = 9.648 \times 10^4$ amp-sec/mole.

26. Using Eqs. 25 and 28, calculate the relative diffusivity (D/D$_o$) of sodium ion (radius $r_s = 0.2$ nm) in cartilage with water content $\phi^f = 0.8$. Assuming $\alpha = 1.2$ and $\beta = 0.3$ in Eq. 28.

REFERENCES

1. Abbaszade I, Liu RQ, Yang F, et al. Cloning and characterization of ADAMTS11, an aggrecanase from the ADAMTS family. *J Biol Chem* 1999;274:23443–23450.
2. Acaroglu ER, Iatridis JC, Setton LA, et al. Degeneration and aging affect the tensile behavior of human lumbar anulus fibrosus. *Spine* 1995;20:2690–2701.
3. Adams ME, Muir H. The glycosaminoglycans of canine menisci. *Biochem J* 1981;197:385–389.
4. Adams ME, Ho YA. Localization of glycosaminoglycans in human and canine menisci and their attachments. *Connect Tissue Res* 1987;16:269–279.
5. Ahmed AM, Burke DL. In-vitro measurement of static pressure distribution in synovial joints—part I: tibial surface of the knee. *J Biomech Eng* 1983;105:216–225.
6. Ahmed AM, Burke DL, Yu A. In-vitro measurement of static pressure distribution in synovial joints—part II: retropatellar surface. *J Biomech Eng* 1983;105:226–236.
7. Akizuki S, Mow VC, Muller F, et al. Tensile properties of human knee joint cartilage: I influence of ionic conditions, weight bearing, and fibrillation on the tensile modulus. *J Orthop Res* 1986;4:379–392.
8. Akizuki S, Mow VC, Muller F, et al. Tensile properties of human knee joint cartilage: II correlations between weight bearing and tissue pathology and the kinetics of swelling. *J Orthop Res* 1987;5:173–186.
9. Ala-Kokko L, Baldwin CT, Moskowitz RW, et al. Single base mutation in the type II procollagen gene (COL2A1) as a cause of primary osteoarthritis associated with a mild chondrodysplasia. *Proc Natl Acad Sci U S A* 1990;87:6565–6568.
10. Altman RD, Tenenbaum J, Latta L, et al. Biomechanical and biochemical properties of dog cartilage in experimentally induced osteoarthritis. *Ann Rheum Dis* 1984;43:83–90.
11. Argraves WS, McKeown-Longo PJ, Goetinck PF. Absence of proteoglycan core protein in

the cartilage mutant nanomelia. *FEBS Lett* 1981;131:265–268.

12. Armstrong CG, Mow VC. Variations in the intrinsic mechanical properties of human articular cartilage with age, degeneration, and water content. *J Bone Joint Surg* 1982;64:88–94.

13. Armstrong CG, Lai WM, Mow VC. An analysis of the unconfined compression of articular cartilage. *J Biomech Eng* 1984;106:165–173.

14. Aspden RM, Hukins DW. Collagen organization in articular cartilage, determined by X-ray diffraction, and its relationship to tissue function. *Proc R Soc Lond* 1981;212:299–304.

15. Aspden RM, Yarker YE, Hukins DW. Collagen orientations in the meniscus of the knee joint. *J Anat* 1985;140:371–380.

16. Ateshian GA, Soslowsky LJ, Mow VC. Quantitation of articular surface topography and cartilage thickness in knee joints using stereophotogrammetry. *J Biomech* 1991;24:761–776.

17. Ateshian GA, Rosenwasser MP, Mow VC. Curvature characteristics and congruence of the thumb carpometacarpal joint: differences between female and male joints. *J Biomech* 1992;25:591–607.

18. Ateshian GA, Lai WM, Zhu WB, et al. An asymptotic solution for the contact of two biphasic cartilage layers. *J Biomech* 1994;27:1347–1360.

19. Ateshian GA, Wang H. A theoretical solution for the frictionless rolling contact of cylindrical biphasic articular cartilage layers. *J Biomech* 1995;28:1341–1355.

20. Ateshian GA, Warden WH, Kim JJ, et al. Finite deformation biphasic material properties of bovine articular cartilage from confined compression experiments. *J Biomech* 1997;30:1157–1164.

21. Ateshian GA, Wang H, Lai WM. The role of interstitial fluid pressurization and surface porosities on the boundary friction of articular cartilage. *J Tribol* 1998;120:241–248.

22. Ateshian GA, Cohen ZA, Kwak SD, et al. Determination of in-situ contact in diarthrodial joints by MRI. *Adv Bioeng Trans ASME* 1995;BED31:225–226.

23. Athanasiou KA, Rosenwasser MP, Buckwalter JA, et al. Interspecies comparisons of in situ intrinsic mechanical properties of distal femoral cartilage. *J Orthop Res* 1991;9:330–340.

24. Athanasiou KA, Agarwal A, Muffoletto A, et al. Biomechanical properties of hip cartilage in experimental animal models. *Clin Orthop* 1995;254–266.

25. Aydelotte MB, Schumacher BL, Kuettner KE. Heterogeneity of articular chondrocytes. In: Kuettner KE, ed. *Articular cartilage and osteoarthritis.* New York: Raven Press, 1992:237–249.

26. Bachrach NM, Valhmu WB, Stazzone E, et al. Changes in proteoglycan synthesis of chondrocytes in articular cartilage are associated with the time-dependent changes in their mechanical environment. *J Biomech* 1995;28:1561–1569.

27. Balazs EA, Denlinger JL. Viscosupplementation: a new concept in the treatment of osteoarthritis. *J Rheumatol Suppl* 1993;39:3–9.

28. Bansal MK, Ward H, Mason RM. Proteoglycan synthesis in suspension cultures of Swarm rat chondrosarcoma chondrocytes and inhibition by exogenous hyaluronate. *Arch Biochem Biophys* 1986;246:602–610.

29. Bar E. Elasticitatsprufungen der Gelenknorpel. *Arch Entwicklungsmech Organ* 1926;108:739–760.

30. Bateman JF, Lamande ER, Ramshaw JAM. Collagen superfamily. In: Comper WD, ed. *Extracellular matrix.* Amsterdam: Harwood, 1996:22–67.

31. Bayliss MT, Davidson C, Woodhouse SM, et al. Chondroitin sulphation in human joint tissues varies with age, zone and topography. *Acta Orthop Scand Suppl* 1995;266:22–25.

32. Bayliss MT, Osborne D, Woodhouse S, et al. Sulfation of chondroitin sulfate in human articular cartilage. The effect of age, topographical position, and zone of cartilage on tissue composition. *J Biol Chem* 1999;274:15892–15900.

33. Behrens F, Kraft EL, Oegema TR Jr. Biochemical changes in articular cartilage after joint immobilization by casting or external fixation. *J Orthop Res* 1989;7:335–343.

34. Benaud C, Dickson RB, Thompson EW. Roles of the matrix metalloproteinases in mammary gland development and cancer. *Breast Cancer Res Treat* 1998;50:97–116.

35. Benninghoff, A. Form und Bau der Gelenkknorpel in ihren Beziehungen zu Funktion. II. Der Aufbau des Gelenkknorpel in seinen Beziehungen zu Funktion. *Z Zellforsch* 1925;2:783–862.

36. Best BA, Guilak F, Setton LA, et al. Compressive mechanical properties of the human anulus fibrosus and their relationship to biochemical composition. *Spine* 1994;19:212–221.

37. Billinghurst RC, Wu W, Ionescu M, et al. Comparison of the degradation of type II collagen and proteoglycan in nasal and articular cartilages induced by interleukin-1 and the selective inhibition of type II collagen cleavage by collagenase. *Arthritis Rheum* 2000;43:664–672.

38. Birkedal-Hansen H. Proteolytic remodeling of extracellular matrix. *Curr Opin Cell Biol* 1995;7:728–735.

39. Bland DR. *The theory of linear viscoelasticity.* Oxford: Pergamon Press, 1960.

40. Blankevoort L, Kuiper JH, Huiskes R, et al. Articular contact in a three-dimensional model of the knee. *J Biomech* 1991;24:1019–1031.

41. Blaschke UK, Eikenberry EF, Hulmes DJ, et al. Collagen XI nucleates self-assembly and limits lateral growth of cartilage fibrils. *J Biol Chem* 2000;275:10370–10378.

42. Bollet, AJ, Nance, JL. Biochemical findings in normal and osteoarthritic articular cartilage. II. Chondroitin sulfate concetration and chain length, water and ash content. *J Clin Invest* 1966;45:1170–1177.

43. Bonassar LJ, Grodzinsky AJ, Srinivasan A, et al. Mechanical and physicochemical regulation of the action of insulin-like growth factor-I on articular cartilage. *Arch Biochem Biophys* 2000;379:57–63.

44. Bowen RM. Continuum theory of mixtures. *Nat Technol Inf Ser* 1971;BRL45:1–170.

45. Bowen RM. Incompressible porous media models by use of the theories of mixtures. *Int J Eng Sci* 1980;18:1129–1148.

46. Brandt KD, Doherty M, Lohmander LS. *Osteoarthritis*. Oxford: Oxford University Press, 2003.

47. Briggs MD, Choi H, Warman ML, et al. Genetic mapping of a locus for multiple epiphyseal dysplasia (EDM2) to a region of chromosome 1 containing a type IX collagen gene. *Am J Hum Genet* 1994;55:678–684.

48. Brocklehurst R, Bayliss MT, Maroudas A, et al. The composition of normal and osteoarthritic articular cartilage from human knee joints. With special reference to unicompartmental replacement and osteotomy of the knee. *J Bone Joint Surg* 1984;66:95–106.

49. Broom ND. Structural consequences of traumatizing articular cartilage. *Ann Rheum Dis* 1986;45:225–234.

50. Broom ND, Marra DL. Ultrastructural evidence for fibril-to-fibril associations in articular cartilage and their functional implication. *J Anat* 1986;146:185–200.

51. Broom ND. The collagen framework of articular cartilage: its profound influence on normal and abnormal load-bearing function. In: Nimni ME, ed. *Collagen: chemistry, biology and biotechnology*. Boca Raton, FL: CRC Press, 1988:243–265.

52. Broom ND, Silyn-Roberts H. Collagen–collagen versus collagen–proteoglycan interactions in the determination of cartilage strength. *Arthritis Rheum* 1990;33:1512–1517.

53. Brown JC, Timpl R. The collagen superfamily. *Int Arch Allergy Immunol* 1995;107:484–490.

54. Brown TD, Singerman RJ. Experimental determination of the linear biphasic constitutive coefficients of human fetal proximal femoral chondroepiphysis. *J Biomech* 1986;19:597–605.

55. Buckwalter JA, Rosenberg LC. Electron microscopic studies of cartilage proteoglycans. Direct evidence for the variable length of the chondroitin sulfate-rich region of proteoglycan subunit core protein. *J Biol Chem* 1982;257:9830–9839.

56. Buckwalter JA, Kuettner KE, Thonar EJ. Age-related changes in articular cartilage proteoglycans: electron microscopic studies. *J Orthop Res* 1985;3:251–257.

57. Buckwalter JA, Mow VC, Ratcliffe A. Restoration of injured or degenerated articular cartilage. *J Am Acad Orthop Surg* 1994;2:192–201.

58. Bullough P, Goodfellow J. The significance of the fine structure of articular cartilage. *J Bone Joint Surg Br* 1968;50:852–857.

59. Bullough PG, Munuera L, Murphy J, et al. The strength of the menisci of the knee as it relates to their fine structure. *J Bone Joint Surg* 1970;52:564–567.

60. Bullough PG. The geometry of diarthrodial joints, its physiologic maintenance, and the possible significance of age-related changes in geometry-to-load distribution and the development of osteoarthritis. *Clin Orthop Rel Res* 1981;156:61–66.

61. Burstein D, Gray ML, Hartman AL, et al. Diffusion of small solutes in cartilage as measured by nuclear magnetic resonance (NMR) spectroscopy and imaging. *J Orthop Res* 1993;11:465–478.

62. Buschmann MD, Grodzinsky AJ. A molecular model of proteoglycan-associated electrostatic forces in cartilage mechanics. *J Biomech Eng* 1995;117:179–192.

63. Campbell IK, Piccoli DS, Roberts MJ, et al. Effects of tumor necrosis factor alpha and beta on resorption of human articular cartilage and production of plasminogen activator by human articular chondrocytes. *Arthritis Rheum* 1990;33:542–552.

64. Camper L, Hellman U, Lundgren-Akerlund E. Isolation, cloning, and sequence analysis of the integrin subunit alpha10, a beta1-associated collagen binding integrin expressed on chondrocytes. *J Biol Chem* 1998;273:20383–20389.

65. Carney SL, Billingham ME, Muir H, et al. Demonstration of increased proteoglycan turnover in cartilage explants from dogs with experimental osteoarthritis. *J Orthop Res* 1984;2:201–206.

66. Caterson B, Flannery CR, Hughes CE, et al. Mechanisms involved in cartilage proteoglycan catabolism. *Matrix Biol* 2000;19:333–344.

67. Caterson B, Lowther DA. Change in the metabolism of the proteoglycans from sheep articular cartilage in response to mechanical stress. *Biochim Biophys Acta* 1978;540:412–422.

68. Cawston TE, Ellis AJ, Humm G, et al. Interleukin-1 and oncostatin M in combination promote the release of collagen fragments from bovine nasal cartilage in culture. *Biochem Biophys Res Commun* 1995;215:377–385.

69. Chahine NO, Wang CC, Hung CT, et al. Anisotropic strain-dependent material properties of bovine articular cartilage in the transitional range from tension to compression. *J Biomech* 2004;37:1251–1261.

70. Chammas P, Federspiel WJ, Eisenberg SR. A microcontinuum model of electrokinetic coupling in the extracellular matrix: perturbation formulation and solution. *J Colloid Interface Sci* 1994;168:526–538.

71. Chan D, Cole WG, Chow CW, et al. A COL2A1 mutation in achondrogenesis type II results in the replacement of type II collagen by type I and III collagens in cartilage. *J Biol Chem* 1995;270:1747–1753.

72. Chapman JA, Hulmes DJ. Electron microscopy of the collagen fibril. In: Ruggeri A, Motta PM, eds. *Ultrastructure of the connective tissue matrix.* Boston: Martinus Nijhoff, 1984:1–33.

73. Chen AC, Bae WC, Schnagl RM, et al. Depth- and strain-dependent mechanical and electromechanical properties of full-thickness bovine articular cartilage in confined compression. *J Biomech* 2001;34:1–12.

74. Chen SS, Falcovitz YH, Schneiderman R, et al. Depth-dependent compressive properties of normal aged human femoral head articular cartilage: relationship to fixed charge density. *Osteoarthritis Cartilage* 2001;9:561–569.

75. Chevalier X, Tyler JA. Production of binding proteins and role of the insulin-like growth factor I binding protein 3 in human articular cartilage explants. *Br J Rheumatol* 1996;35:515–522.

76. Chimal-Monroy J, Diaz de Leon L. Differential effects of transforming growth factors beta 1, beta 2, beta 3 and beta 5 on chondrogenesis in mouse limb bud mesenchymal cells. *Int J Dev Biol* 1997;41:91–102.

77. Chow G, Nietfeld JJ, Knudson CB, et al. Antisense inhibition of chondrocyte CD44 expression leading to cartilage chondrolysis. *Arthritis Rheum* 1998;41:1411–1419.

78. Clark JM. The organization of collagen in cryofractured rabbit articular cartilage: a scanning electron microscopic study. *J Orthop Res* 1985;3:17–29.

79. Clarke IC. Articular cartilage: a review and scanning electron microscope study. 1. The interterritorial fibrillar architecture. *J Bone Joint Surg Br* 1971;53:732–750.

80. Clemmons DR. Insulin-like growth factors—their binding proteins and growth regulation. In: Canalis E, ed. *Skeletal growth factors.* Philadelphia: Lippincott Williams & Wilkins, 2000:79–99.

81. Cohen B, Chorney GS, Phillips DP, et al. Compressive stress-relaxation behavior of bovine growth plate may be described by the nonlinear biphasic theory. *J Orthop Res* 1994;12:804–813.

82. Cohen B, Lai WM, Mow VC. A transversely isotropic biphasic model for unconfined compression of growth plate and chondroepiphysis. *J Biomech Eng* 1998;120:491–496.

83. Cohen ZA, McCarthy DM, Kwak SD, et al. Knee cartilage topography, thickness, and contact areas from MRI: in-vitro calibration and in-vivo measurements. *Osteoarthritis Cartilage* 1999;7:95–109.

84. Cole AA, Chubinskaya S, Schumacher, B, et al. Chondrocyte matrix metalloproteinase-8. Human articular chondrocytes express neutrophil collagenase. *J Biol Chem* 1996;271:11023–11026.

85. Coletti JM Jr, Akeson WH, Woo SL. A comparison of the physical behavior of normal articular cartilage and the arthroplasty surface. *J Bone Joint Surg* 1972;54:147–160.

86. Comper WD, Williams RP, Zamparo O. Water transport in extracellular matrices. *Connect Tissue Res* 1990;25:89–102.

87. Crabb ID, O'Keefe RJ, Puzas JE, et al. Synergistic effect of transforming growth factor beta and fibroblast growth factor on DNA synthesis in chick growth plate chondrocytes. *J Bone Miner Res* 1990;5:1105–1112.

88. Creamer P, Hochberg MC. Osteoarthritis. *Lancet* 1997;350:503–508.

89. Cremer MA, Rosloniec EF, Kang AH. The cartilage collagens: a review of their structure, organization, and role in the pathogenesis of experimental arthritis in animals and in human rheumatic disease. *J Mol Med* 1998;76:275–288.

90. Danielson KG, Fazzio A, Cohen I, et al. The human decorin gene: intron—exon organization, discovery of two alternatively spliced exons in the 5' untranslated region, and mapping of the gene to chromosome 12q23. *Genomics* 1993;15:146–160.

91. Danielson KG, Baribault H, Holmes DF, et al. Targeted disruption of decorin leads to abnormal collagen fibril morphology and skin fragility. *J Cell Biol* 1997;136:729–743.

92. Denker AE, Nicoll SB, Tuan RS. Formation of cartilage-like spheroids by micromass cultures of murine C3H10T1/2 cells upon treatment with transforming growth factor-beta 1. *Differentiation* 1995;59:25–34.

93. Dicarlo EF. Pathology of the meniscus. In: Mow VC, Arnoczky SP, Jackson DL, eds. *Knee meniscus: basic and clinical foundation.* New York: Raven Press, 1992:117–130.

94. Dingle JT, Horsfield P, Fell HB, et al. Breakdown of proteoglycan and collagen induced in pig articular cartilage in organ culture. *Ann Rheum Dis* 1975;34:303–311.

95. DiSilvestro MR, Suh JK. Biphasic poroviscoelastic characteristics of proteoglycan-depleted articular cartilage: simulation of degeneration. *Ann Biomed Eng* 2002;30:792–800.

96. DiSilvestro MR, Zhu Q, Suh JK. Biphasic poroviscoelastic simulation of the unconfined compression of articular cartilage: II—effect of variable strain rates. *J Biomech Eng* 2001;123:198–200.

97. Dodge GR, Poole AR. Immunohistochemical detection and immunochemical analysis of type II collagen degradation in human normal, rheumatoid, and osteoarthritic articular cartilages and in explants of bovine articular cartilage cultured with interleukin 1. *J Clin Invest* 1989;83:647–661.

98. Doege KJ, Sasaki M, Kimura T, et al. Complete coding sequence and deduced primary structure of the human cartilage large aggregating proteoglycan, aggrecan. Human-specific repeats, and additional alternatively spliced forms. *J Biol Chem* 1991;266:894–902.

99. Doege KJ, Garrison K, Coulter SN, et al. The structure of the rat aggrecan gene and preliminary characterization of its promoter. *J Biol Chem* 1994;269:29232–29240.

100. Donnan FG. The theory of membrane equilibria. *Chem Rev* 1924;1:73–90.

101. Donohue JM, Buss D, Oegema TR Jr, et al. The effects of indirect blunt trauma on adult canine articular cartilage. *J Bone Joint Surg* 1983;65:948–957.

102. Dore S, Pelletier JP, DiBattista JA, et al. Human osteoarthritic chondrocytes possess an increased number of insulin-like growth factor 1 binding sites but are unresponsive to its stimulation. Possible role of IGF-1-binding proteins. *Arthritis Rheum* 1994;37:253–263.

103. Dubois CM, Ruscetti FW, Palaszynski EW, et al. Transforming growth factor beta is a potent inhibitor of interleukin 1 (IL-1) receptor expression: proposed mechanism of inhibition of IL-1 action. *J Exp Med* 1990;172:737–744.

104. Dudhia J, Bayliss MT, Hardingham TE. Human link protein gene: structure and transcription pattern in chondrocytes. *Biochem J* 1994;303 (Part 1):329–333.

105. Ebara S, Kelkar R, Bigliani LU, et al. Bovine glenoid cartilage is less stiff than humeral head cartilage in tension. *Trans Orthop Res Soc* 1994;19:146.

106. Eckstein F, Muller-Gerbl M, Putz R. Distribution of subchondral bone density and cartilage thickness in the human patella. *J Anat* 1992;180(pt 3):425–433.

107. Eckstein F, Sittek H, Milz S, et al. The morphology of articular cartilage assessed by magnetic resonance imaging (MRI). Reproducibility and anatomical correlation. *Surg Radiol Anat* 1994;16:429–438.

108. Eckstein F, Sittek H, Gavazzeni A, et al. Magnetic resonance chondro-crassometry (MR CCM); a method for accurate determination of articular cartilage thickness? *Magn Reson Med* 1996;35:89–96.

109. Edmond E, Ogston AG. An approach to the study of phase separation in ternary aqueous systems. *Biochem J* 1968;109:569–576.

110. Edwards J. Physical characteristics of articular cartilage. *Proc Inst Mech Eng* 181-1967;3J:16–24.

111. Edwards J, Smith AU. The uptake of fluid by living cartilage after compression. *J Physiol* 1966;183:5P–6P.

112. Eisenberg SR, Grodzinsky AJ. Swelling of articular cartilage and other connective tissues: electromechanochemical forces. *J Orthop Res* 1985;3:148–159.

113. Eisenberg SR, Grodzinsky AJ. The kinetics of chemically induced nonequilibrium swelling of articular cartilage and corneal stroma. *J Biomech Eng* 1987;109:79–89.

114. Eisenberg SR, Grodzinsky AJ. Electrokinetic micromodel of extracellular-matrix and other polyelectrolyte networks. *Physicochem Hydrodynam* 1988;10:517–539.

115. Eisenfeld J, Mow VC, Lipshitz H. Mathematical analysis of stress relaxation in articular cartilage during compression. *J Math Biosci* 1978;39:97–112.

116. Elliott DM, Guilak F, Vail TP, et al. Tensile properties of articular cartilage are altered by meniscectomy in a canine model of osteoarthritis. *J Orthop Res* 1999;17:503–508.

117. Elmore SM, Sokoloff L, Norris G, et al. Nature of "imperfect" elasticity of articular cartilage. *J Appl Physiol* 1962;18:393–396.

118. Evanko SP, Vogel KG. Proteoglycan synthesis in fetal tendon is differentially regulated by cyclic compression in vitro. *Arch Biochem Biophys* 1993;307:153–164.

119. Ewers BJ, Dvoracek-Driksna D, Orth MW, et al. The extent of matrix damage and chondrocyte death in mechanically traumatized articular cartilage explants depend on rate of loading. *J Orthop Res* 2001;19:779–784.

120. Eyre DR. Collagen: molecular diversity in the body's protein scaffold. *Science* 1980;207:1315–1322.

121. Eyre DR, McDevitt CA, Billingham ME, et al. Biosynthesis of collagen and other matrix proteins by articular cartilage in experimental osteoarthrosis. *Biochem J* 1980;188:823–837.

122. Eyre DR, Oguchi H. The hydroxypyridinium crosslinks of skeletal collagens: their measurement, properties and a proposed pathway of formation. *Biochem Biophys Res Commun* 1980;92:403–410.

123. Eyre DR, Wu JJ. Collagen of fibrocartilage: a distinctive molecular phenotype in bovine meniscus. *FEBS Lett* 1983;158:265–270.

124. Eyre DR, Koob TJ, Van Ness KP. Quantitation of hydroxypyridinium crosslinks in collagen by high-performance liquid chromatography. *Anal Biochem* 1984;137:380–388.

125. Eyre DR, Apon S, Wu JJ, et al. Collagen type IX: evidence for covalent linkages to type II collagen in cartilage. *FEBS Lett* 1987;220:337–341.

126. Eyre DR, Dickson IR, Van Ness K. Collagen crosslinking in human bone and articular cartilage. Age-related changes in the content of mature hydroxypyridinium residues. *Biochem J* 1988;252:495–500.

127. Fassler R, Schnegelsberg PN, Dausman J, et al. Mice lacking alpha 1 (IX) collagen develop non-inflammatory degenerative joint disease. *Proc Natl Acad Sci U S A* 1994;91:5070–5074.

128. Fernihough JK, Billingham ME, Cwyfan-Hughes S, et al. Local disruption of the insulin-like growth factor system in the arthritic joint. *Arthritis Rheum* 1996;39:1556–1565.

129. Ferry JD. *Viscoelastic properties of polymers.* New York: John Wiley & Sons, 1970.

130. Fisher LW, Heegaard AM, Vetter U, et al. Human biglycan gene. Putative promoter, intron—exon junctions, and chromosomal localization. *J Biol Chem* 1991;266:14371–14377.

131. Fithian DC, Zhu WB, Ratcliffe A, et al. Exponential law representation of tensile properties of human meniscus. *Proc Inst Mech Eng* 1989;c384/058:85–90.

132. Fithian DC, Kelly MA, Mow VC. Material properties and structure–function relationships in the menisci. *Clin Orthop* 1990;19–31.

133. Flannery CR, Lark MW, Sandy JD. Identification of a stromelysin cleavage site within the interglobular domain of human aggrecan. Evidence for proteolysis at this site in vivo in human articular cartilage. *J Biol Chem* 1992;267:1008–1014.

134. Flechtenmacher J, Huch K, Thonar EJ, et al. Recombinant human osteogenic protein 1 is a potent stimulator of the synthesis of cartilage proteoglycans and collagens by human articular chondrocytes. *Arthritis Rheum* 1996;39:1896–1904.

135. Fosang AJ, Hardingham TE. Matrix proteoglycans. In: Comper WD, ed. *Extracellular matrix.* Amsterdam: Harwood Academic, 1996.

136. Frank EH, Grodzinsky AJ. Cartilage electromechanics—II. A continuum model of cartilage electrokinetics and correlation with experiments. *J Biomech* 1987;20:629–639.

137. Frank EH, Grodzinsky AJ. Cartilage electromechanics—I. Electrokinetic transduction and the effects of electrolyte pH and ionic strength. *J Biomech* 1987;20:615–627.

138. Frank EH, Grodzinsky AJ, Koob TJ, et al. Streaming potentials: a sensitive index of enzymatic degradation in articular cartilage. *J Orthop Res* 1987;5:497–508.

139. Frank EH, Grodzinsky AJ, Phillips SL, et al. Physiochemical and bioelectrical determinants of cartilage material properties. In: Mow VC, Wood DO, Woo SL, eds. *Biomechanics of diarthrodial joints* New York: Springer-Verlag, 1990:261–282.

140. Franzen A, Inerot S, Hejderup SO, et al. Variations in the composition of bovine hip articular cartilage with distance from the articular surface. *Biochem J* 1981;195:535–543.

141. Froimson MI, Ratcliffe A, Gardner TR, et al. Differences in patellofemoral joint cartilage material properties and their significance to the etiology of cartilage surface fibrillation. *Osteoarthritis Cartilage* 1997;5:377–386.

142. Fung YC. *Foundations of solid mechanics.* Upper Saddle River, NJ: Prentice-Hall, 1965.

143. Fung YC. Biomechanics: its scope, history, and some problems of contiuum mechanics in physiology. *Appl Mech Rev* 1968;21:1–20.

144. Fung YC. *Mechanical properties of living tissues.* New York: Springer-Verlag, 1981.

145. Gabler R. *Electrical interactions in molecular biophysics: an introduction.* New York: Academic Press, 1978.

146. Garcia AM, Frank EH, Grimshaw PE, et al. Contributions of fluid convection and electrical migration to transport in cartilage: relevance to loading. *Arch Biochem Biophys* 1996;333:317–325.

147. Ghosh P, Taylor TK, Pettit GD, et al. Effect of postoperative immobilisation on the regrowth of the knee joint semilunar cartilage: an experimental study. *J Orthop Res* 1983;1:153–164.

148. Giancotti FG, Ruoslahti E. Integrin signaling. *Science* 1999;285:1028–1032.

149. Gilles C, Polette M, Seiki M, et al. Implication of collagen type I—induced membrane-type 1-matrix metalloproteinase expression and matrix metalloproteinase-2 activation in the metastatic progression of breast carcinoma. *Lab Invest* 1997;76:651–660.

150. Gocke E. Elastizitasstudien an jungen und alten Gelenkknorpel. *Verh Dtsch Orthop Ges* 1927;22:130–147.

151. Goertzen DJ, Budney DR, Cinats JG. Methodology and apparatus to determine material properties of the knee joint meniscus. *Med Eng Phys* 1997;19:412–419.

152. Goldring MB, Birkhead J, Sandell LJ, et al. Interleukin 1 suppresses expression of cartilage-specific types II and IX collagens and increases types I and III collagens in human chondrocytes. *J Clin Invest* 1988;82:2026–2037.

153. Goldring MB. The role of cytokines as inflammatory mediators in osteoarthritis: lessons from animal models. *Connect Tissue Res* 1999;40:1–11.

154. Gray ML, Pizzanelli AM, Grodzinsky AJ, et al. Mechanical and physiochemical determinants of the chondrocyte biosynthetic response. *J Orthop Res* 1988;6:777–792.

155. Greenwald AS, O'Connor JJ. The transmission of load through the human hip joint. *J Biomech* 1971;4:507–528.

156. Grodzinsky AJ, Roth V, Myers E, et al. The significance of electromechanical and osmotic forces in the nonequilibrium swelling behavior of articular cartilage in tension. *J Biomech Eng* 1981;103:221–231.

157. Grodzinsky AJ. Electromechanical and physicochemical properties of connective tissue. *Crit Rev Biomed Eng* 1983;9:133–199.

158. Grover J, Roughley PJ. Versican gene expression in human articular cartilage and comparison of mRNA splicing variation with aggrecan. *Biochem J* 1993;291(pt 2):361–367.

159. Gu WY, Lai WM, Mow VC. Transport of fluid and ions through a porous–permeable charged–hydrated tissue, and streaming potential data on normal bovine articular cartilage. *J Biomech* 1993;26:709–723.

160. Gu WY, Lai WM, Mow VC. A triphasic analysis of negative osmotic flows through charged hydrated soft tissues. *J Biomech* 1997;30:71–78.

161. Gu WY, Lai WM, Mow VC. A mixture theory for charged–hydrated soft tissues containing multi-electrolytes: Passive transport and swelling behaviors. *J Biomech Eng* 1998;120:169–180.

162. Gu WY, Justiz MA, Yao H. Electrical conductivity of lumbar anulus fibrosis: effects of porosity and fixed charge density. *Spine* 2002;27:2390–2395.

163. Gu WY, Yao H. Effects of hydration and fixed charge density on fluid transport in charged hydrated soft tissues. *Ann Biomed Eng* 2003;31:1162–1170.

164. Gu WY, Yao H, Huang CY, et al. New insight into deformation-dependent hydraulic permeability of gels and cartilage, and dynamic behavior of agarose gels in confined compression. *J Biomech* 2003;36:593–598.

165. Gu WY, Yao H, Vega AL, et al. Diffusivity of ions in agarose gels and intervertebral disc: effect of porosity. *Ann Biomed Eng (in press)*.

166. Guenther HL, Guenther HE, Froesch ER, et al. Effect of insulin-like growth factor on collagen and glycosaminoglycan synthesis by rabbit articular chondrocytes in culture. *Experientia* 1982;38:979–981.

167. Guilak F, Meyer BC, Ratcliffe A, et al. The effects of matrix compression on proteoglycan metabolism in articular cartilage explants. *Osteoarthritis Cartilage* 1994;2:91–101.

168. Guilak F, Ratcliffe A, Lane N, et al. Mechanical and biochemical changes in the superficial zone of articular cartilage in canine experimental osteoarthritis. *J Orthop Res* 1994;12:474–484.

169. Guilak F, Ratcliffe A, Mow VC. Chondrocyte deformation and local tissue strain in articular cartilage: a confocal microscopy study. *J Orthop Res* 1995;13:410–421.

170. Guilak F, Jones WR, Ting-Beall HP, et al. The deformation behavior and mechanical properties of chondrocytes in articular cartilage. *Osteoarthritis Cartilage* 1999;7:59–70.

171. Hall BK. *Cartilage: structure function and biochemistry*. New York: Academic Press, 1983.

172. Hall BK. *Cartilage: development, differentiation and growth*. New York: Academic Press, 1983.

173. Happel J. Viscous flow relative to arrays of cylinders. *AIChE J* 1959;5:174–177.

174. Hardingham TE, Muir H. The specific interaction of hyaluronic acid with cartilage proteoglycans. *Biochim Biophys Acta* 1972;279:401–405.

175. Hardingham TE, Muir H. Hyaluronic acid in cartilage and proteoglycan aggregation. *Biochem J* 1974;139:565–581.

176. Hardingham TE. The role of link-protein in the structure of cartilage proteoglycan aggregates. *Biochem J* 1979;177:237–247.

177. Hardingham TE. Proteoglycans: their structure, interactions and molecular organization in cartilage. *Biochem Soc Trans* 1981;9:489–497.

178. Hardingham TE, Muir H, Kwan MK, et al. Viscoelastic properties of proteoglycan solutions with varying proportions present as aggregates. *J Orthop Res* 1987;5:36–46.

179. Hardingham TE, Fosang AJ. 1992; Proteoglycans: many forms and many functions. *FASEB J* 6:861–870.

180. Harper GS, Comper WD, Preston BN. Dissapative structures in proteoglycan solutions. *J Biol Chem* 1984;259:10582–10589.

181. Hascall VC, Sajdera SW. Proteinpolysaccharide complex from bovine nasal cartilage. The function of glycoprotein in the formation of aggregates. *J Biol Chem* 1969;244:2384–2396.

182. Hascall VC. Interactions of cartilage proteoglycans with hyaluronic acid. *J Supramol Struct* 1977;7:101–120.

183. Hascall VC, Hascall GK. Proteoglycans. In: Hay ED, ed. *Cell biology of extracellular matrix*. New York: Plenum, 1981:39–63.

184. Hasegawa I, Kuriki S, Matsuno S, et al. Dependence of electrical conductivity on fixed charge density in articular cartilage. *Clin Orthop* 1983;283–288.

185. Hassell JR, Kimura JH, Hascall VC. Proteoglycan core protein families. *Annu Rev Biochem* 1986;55:539–567.

186. Hayes WC, Mockros LF. Viscoelastic properties of human articular cartilage. *J Appl Physiol* 1971;31:562–568.

187. Hayes WC, Keer LM, Herrmann G, et al. A mathematical analysis for indentation tests of articular cartilage. *J Biomech* 1972;5:541–551.

188. Hayes WC, Bodine AJ. Flow-independent viscoelastic properties of articular cartilage matrix. *J Biomech* 1978;11:407–419.

189. Hedbom E, Antonsson P, Hjerpe A, et al. Cartilage matrix proteins. An acidic oligomeric protein (COMP) detected only in cartilage. *J Biol Chem* 1992;267:6132–6136.

190. Heinegard D, Axelsson I. Distribution of keratan sulfate in cartilage proteoglycans. *J Biol Chem* 1977;252:1971–1979.

191. Heinegard D, Paulsson M, Inerot S, et al. A novel low-molecular weight chondroitin sulphate

proteoglycan isolated from cartilage. *Biochem J* 1981;197:355–366.

192. Heinegard D, Oldberg A. Structure and biology of cartilage and bone matrix noncollagenous macromolecules. *FASEB J* 1989;3:2042–2051.

193. Helfferich F. *Ion exchange.* New York: McGraw-Hill, 1962.

194. Hellio Le Graverand MP, Reno C, Hart DA. Gene expression in menisci from the knees of skeletally immature and mature female rabbits. *J Orthop Res* 1999;17:738–744.

195. Hirsch C. The pathogenesis of chondromalacia of the patella. *Acta Chir Scand* 1944;83:1–106.

196. Hirsch MS, Lunsford LE, Trinkaus-Randall V, et al. Chondrocyte survival and differentiation in situ are integrin mediated. *Dev Dyn* 1997;210:249–263.

197. Hoch DH, Grodzinsky AJ, Koob TJ, et al. Early changes in material properties of rabbit articular cartilage after meniscectomy. *J Orthop Res* 1983;1:4–12.

198. Hodge WA, Carlson KL, Fijan RS, et al. Contact pressures from an instrumented hip endoprosthesis. *J Bone Joint Surg Am* 1989;71:1378–1386.

199. Hodge WA, Fijan RS, Carlson KL, et al. Contact pressures in the human hip joint measured in vivo. *Proc Natl Acad Sci U S A* 1986;83:2879–2883.

200. Hogan BL. Bone morphogenetic proteins: multifunctional regulators of vertebrate development. *Genes Dev* 1996;10:1580–1594.

201. Hollander AP, Heathfield TF, Webber C, et al. Increased damage to type II collagen in osteoarthritic articular-cartilage detected by a new immunoassay. *J Clin Invest* 1994;93:1722–1732.

202. Holmes MH, Lai WM, Mow VC. Singular perturbation analysis of the nonlinear, flow-dependent compressive stress relaxation behavior of articular cartilage. *J Biomech Eng* 1985;107:206–218.

203. Holmes MH, Lai WM, Mow VC. Compression effects on cartilage permeability. In: Hargins AR, ed. *Tissue nutrition and viability.* New York: Springer-Verlag, 1985:73–100.

204. Holmes MH, Mow VC. The nonlinear characteristics of soft gels and hydrated connective tissues in ultrafiltration. *J Biomech* 1990;23:1145–1156.

205. Holmvall K, Camper L, Johansson S, et al. Chondrocyte and chondrosarcoma cell integrins with affinity for collagen type II and their response to mechanical stress. *Exp Cell Res* 1995;221:496–503.

206. Hori RY, Mockros LF. Indentation tests of human articular cartilage. *J Biomech* 1976;9:259–268.

207. Hou JS, Holmes MH, Lai WM, et al. Boundary conditions at the cartilage–synovial fluid interface for joint lubrication and theoretical verifications. *J Biomech Eng* 1989;111:78–87.

208. Hou JS, Mow VC, Lai WM, et al. An analysis of the squeeze-film lubrication mechanism for articular cartilage. *J Biomech* 1992;25:247–259.

209. Howell DS, Treadwell BV, Trippel SB. Etiopathogenesis of osteoarthritis. In: Moskowitz RW, Howell DS, Goldberg VM, et al., eds., *Osteoarthritis Diagnosis, and medical/surgical management.* Philadelphia: WB Saunders, 1992.

210. Hua Q, Knudson CB, Knudson W. Internalization of hyaluronan by chondrocytes occurs via receptor-mediated endocytosis. *J Cell Sci* 1993;106:365–375.

211. Huang CY, Soltz MA, Kopacz M, et al. Experimental verification of the roles of intrinsic matrix viscoelasticity and tension–compression nonlinearity in the biphasic response of cartilage. *J Biomech Eng* 2003;125:84–93.

212. Huch K, Wilbrink B, Flechtenmacher J, et al. Effects of recombinant human osteogenic protein 1 on the production of proteoglycan, prostaglandin E2, and interleukin-1 receptor antagonist by human articular chondrocytes cultured in the presence of interleukin-1beta. *Arthritis Rheum* 1997;40:2157–2161.

213. Huiskes R, Kremers J, de Lange A, et al. Analytical stereophotogrammetric determination of three-dimensional knee-joint geometry. *J Biomech* 1985;18:559–570.

214. Hunziker EB, Schenk RK. Structural organization of proteoglycans in cartilage. In: Wight TW, Mecham RP, eds. *Biology of proteoglycans.* New York: Academic Press, 1987:155–183.

215. Huyghe JM, Janssen JD. Quadriphasic mechanics of swelling incompressible porous media. *Int J Eng Sci* 1997;35:793–802.

216. Hynes RO. Integrins: bidirectional, allosteric signaling machines. *Cell* 2002;110:673–687.

217. Iatridis JC, Setton LA, Foster RJ, et al. Degeneration affects the anisotropic and nonlinear behaviors of the human anulus fibrosus in compression. *J Biomech* 1998;31:535–544.

218. Iozzo RV, Cohen IR, Grassel S, et al. The biology of perlecan: the multifaceted heparan sulphate proteoglycan of basement membranes and pericellular matrices. *Biochem J* 1994;302(pt 3):625–639.

219. Jackson GW, James DF. The permeability of fibrous porous media. *Can J Chem Eng* 1986;64:364–374.

220. Jakowlew SB, Dillard PJ, Winokur TS, et al. Expression of transforming growth factor-beta s 1–4 in chicken embryo chondrocytes and myocytes. *Dev Biol* 1991;143:135–148.

221. Johnson EM, Deen WM. Hydraulic permeability of agarose gels. *AIChE J* 1996;42:1220–1224.

222. Joosten LA, Helsen MM, Saxne T, et al. IL-1 alpha beta blockade prevents cartilage and bone destruction in murine type II collagen-induced arthritis, whereas TNF-alpha blockade only ameliorates joint inflammation. *J Immunol* 1999;163:5049–5055.

223. Jortikka MO, Inkinen RI, Tammi MI, et al. Immobilisation causes longlasting matrix changes both in

the immobilised and contralateral joint cartilage. *Ann Rheum Dis* 1997;56:255–261.

224. Joshi MD, Suh JK, Marui T, et al. Interspecies variation of compressive biomechanical properties of the meniscus. *J Biomed Mater Res* 1995;29:823–828.

225. Jurvelin J, Kiviranta I, Tammi M, et al. Softening of canine articular cartilage after immobilization of the knee joint. *Clin Orthop* 1986;246–252.

226. Jurvelin J, Kiviranta I, Arokoski J, et al. Indentation study of the biochemical properties of articular cartilage in the canine knee. *Eng Med* 1987;16:15–22.

227. Jurvelin J, Arokoski J, Hunziker EB, et al. Topographical variation of the elastic properties of articular cartilage in the canine knee. *J Biomech* 2000;33:669–675.

228. Kadler K. Extracellular matrix 1: fibril-forming collagens. *Protein Profile* 1995;2:491–619.

229. Kandel RA, Dinarello CA, Biswas C. The stimulation of collagenase production in rabbit articular chondrocytes by interleukin-1 is increased by collagens. *Biochem Int* 1987;15:1021–1031.

230. Katchalsky A, Curran PF. *Non-equilibrium thermodynamics in biophysics.* Cambridge, MA: Harvard University Press, 1975.

231. Katz EP, Li ST. The intermolecular space of reconstituted collagen fibrils. *J Mol Biol* 1973;73:351–369.

232. Katz EP, Wachtel EJ, Maroudas A. Extrafibrillar proteoglycans osmotically regulate the molecular packing of collagen in cartilage. *Biochim Biophys Acta* 1986;882:136–139.

233. Kelkar R, Flatow EL, Bigliani LU, et al. The effect of articular congruence and humeral head rotation on glenohumeral kinematics. *Adv Bioeng Trans ASME* 1994;BED28:19–20.

234. Kelly MA, Fithian DC, Chern KY, et al. Structure and function of the meniscus: basic and clinical implications. In: Mow VC, Ratcliffe A, Woo SLY, eds. *Biomechanics of diarthrodial joints.* New York: Springer-Verlag, 1990:191–211.

235. Kempson GE, Muir H, Swanson SA, et al. Correlations between stiffness and the chemical constituents of cartilage on the human femoral head. *Biochim Biophys Acta* 1970;215:70–77.

236. Kempson GE, Freeman MA, Swanson SA. The determination of a creep modulus for articular cartilage from indentation tests of the human femoral head. *J Biomech* 1971;4:239–250.

237. Kempson GE, Spivey CJ, Swanson SA, et al. Patterns of cartilage stiffness on normal and degenerate human femoral heads. *J Biomech* 1971;4:597–609.

238. Kempson GE, Muir H, Pollard C, et al. The tensile properties of the cartilage of human femoral condyles related to the content of collagen and glycosaminoglycans. *Biochim Biophys Acta* 1973;297:456–472.

239. Kempson GE. Mechanical properties of articular cartilage and their relationship to matrix degeneration and age. *Ann Rheum Dis* 1975;34:111–113.

240. Kempson GE, Tuke MA, Dingle JT, et al. The effects of proteolytic enzymes on the mechanical properties of adult human articular cartilage. *Biochim Biophys Acta* 1976;428:741–760.

241. Kempson GE. Mechanical properties of articular cartilage. In: Freeman MAR, ed. *Adult articular cartilage.* Kent, UK: Pitman Medical, 1979:333–414.

242. Kempson GE. Age-related changes in the tensile properties of human articular cartilage: a comparative study between the femoral head of the hip joint and the talus of the ankle joint. *Biochim Biophys Acta* 1991;1075:223–230.

243. Kenedi RM, Gibson T, Daly CH. Bioengineering studies of the human skin, the effects of unidirectional tension. In: Jackson SF, Harkness SM, Tristrain GR, eds. *Structure and function of connective and skeletal tissues.* St. Andrews, Scotland: Scientific Committee, 1964:388–395.

244. Kim YJ, Sah RL, Grodzinsky AJ, et al. Mechanical regulation of cartilage biosynthetic behavior: physical stimuli. *Arch Biochem Biophys* 1994;311:1–12.

245. Kim YJ, Bonassar LJ, Grodzinsky AJ. The role of cartilage streaming potential, fluid flow and pressure in the stimulation of chondrocyte biosynthesis during dynamic compression. *J Biomech* 1995;28:1055–1066.

246. Kirsch T, Pfaffle M. Selective binding of anchorin CII (annexin V) to type II and X collagen and to chondrocalcin (C-propeptide of type II collagen). Implications for anchoring function between matrix vesicles and matrix proteins. *FEBS Lett* 1992;310:143–147.

247. Kiviranta I, Jurvelin J, Tammi M, et al. Weight bearing controls glycosaminoglycan concentration and articular cartilage thickness in the knee joints of young beagle dogs. *Arthritis Rheum* 1987;30:801–809.

248. Kiviranta I, Tammi M, Jurvelin J, et al. Moderate running exercise augments glycosaminoglycans and thickness of articular cartilage in the knee joint of young beagle dogs. *J Orthop Res* 1988;6:188–195.

249. Knauper V, Lopez-Otin C, Smith B, et al. Biochemical characterization of human collagenase-3. *J Biol Chem* 1996;271:1544–1550.

250. Knudson CB, Nofal GA, Pamintuan L, et al. The chondrocyte pericellular matrix: a model for hyaluronan-mediated cell–matrix interactions. *Biochem Soc Trans* 1999;27:142–147.

251. Knudson CB, Knudson W. Cartilage proteoglycans. *Cell Dev Biol* 2001;12:69–78.

252. Knudson W, Knudson CB. Assembly of a chondrocyte-like pericellular matrix on non-chondrogenic cells. Role of the cell surface hyaluronan receptors in the assembly of a pericellular matrix. *J Cell Sci* 1991;99(pt 2):227–235.

253. Knudson W, Aguiar DJ, Hua Q, et al. CD44-anchored hyaluronan-rich pericellular matrices: an ultrastructural and biochemical analysis. *Exp Cell Res* 1996;228:216–228.

254. Koepp HE, Sampath KT, Kuettner KE, et al. Osteogenic protein-1 (OP-1) blocks cartilage damage caused by fibronectin fragments and promotes repair by enhancing proteoglycan synthesis. *Inflamm Res* 1999;48:199–204.

255. Korver TH, van de Stadt RJ, Kiljan E, et al. Effects of loading on the synthesis of proteoglycans in different layers of anatomically intact articular cartilage in vitro. *J Rheumatol* 1992;19:905–912.

256. Kuettner KE, Schleyerbach R, Peyron JG, et al., eds. *Articular cartilage and osteoarthritis*. New York: Raven Press, 1992.

257. Kuhn K. The classical collagens: types I, II, and III. In: Mayne R, Burgeson RE, eds. *Structure and function of collagen types*. Orlando: Academic Press, 1987:1–42.

258. Kulyk WM, Rodgers BJ, Greer K, et al. Promotion of embryonic chick limb cartilage differentiation by transforming growth factor-beta. *Dev Biol* 1989;135:424–430.

259. Kwak SD, Colman WW, Ateshian GA, et al. Anatomy of the human patellofemoral joint articular cartilage: Surface curvature analysis. *J Orthop Res* 1997;15:468–472.

260. Kwan MK, Wayne JS, Woo SL, et al. Histological and biomechanical assessment of articular cartilage from stored osteochondral shell allografts. *J Orthop Res* 1989;7:637–644.

261. Kwan MK, Lai WM, Mow VC. A finite deformation theory for cartilage and other soft hydrated connective tissues—I. Equilibrium results. *J Biomech* 1990;23:145–155.

262. Lai WM, Mow VC. Drug-induced compression of articular cartilage during a permeation experiment. *Biorheology* 1980;17:111–123.

263. Lai WM, Mow VC, Roth V. Effects of nonlinear strain-dependent permeability and rate of compression on the stress behavior of articular cartilage. *J Biomech Eng* 1981;103:61–66.

264. Lai WM, Hou JS, Mow VC. A triphasic theory for the swelling and deformation behaviors of articular cartilage. *J Biomech Eng* 1991;113:245–258.

265. Lai WM, Rubin D, Krempel E. *Introduction to continuum mechanics*. London: Pergamon, 1993.

266. Lai WM, Mow VC, Sun DN, et al. On the electric potentials inside a charged soft hydrated biological tissue: streaming potential versus diffusion potential. *J Biomech Eng* 2000;122:336–346.

267. Lane JM, Weiss C. Review of articular cartilage collagen research. *Arthritis Rheum* 1975;18:553–562.

268. Lanir Y, Seybold J, Schneiderman R, et al. Partition and diffusion of sodium and chloride ions in soft charged foam: the effect of external salt concentration and mechanical deformation. *Tissue Eng* 1998;4:365–378.

269. Lark MW, Gordy JT, Weidner JR, et al. Cell-mediated catabolism of aggrecan. Evidence that cleavage at the "aggrecanase" site (Glu373-Ala374) is a primary event in proteolysis of the interglobular domain. *J Biol Chem* 1995;270:2550–2556.

270. Lawler J, Chen H. Cartilage oligomeric matrix protein. In: *Encyclopedia of molecular medicine*. New York: John Wiley & Sons, 2002:481–484.

271. Leddy HA, Guilak F. Site-specific molecular diffusion in articular cartilage measured using fluorescence recovery after photobleaching. *Ann Biomed Eng* 2003;31:753–760.

272. Lehner KB, Rechl HP, Gmeinwieser JK, et al. Structure, function, and degeneration of bovine hyaline cartilage: assessment with MR imaging in vitro. *Radiology* 1989;170:495–499.

273. LeRoux MA, Arokoski J, Vail TP, et al. Simultaneous changes in the mechanical properties, quantitative collagen organization, and proteoglycan concentration of articular cartilage following canine meniscectomy. *J Orthop Res* 2000;18:383–392.

274. LeRoux MA, Setton LA. Experimental and biphasic FEM determinations of the material properties and hydraulic permeability of the meniscus in tension. *J Biomech Eng* 2002;124:315–321.

275. Li H, Schwartz NB, Vertel BM. cDNA cloning of chick cartilage chondroitin sulfate (aggrecan) core protein and identification of a stop codon in the aggrecan gene associated with the chondrodystrophy, nanomelia. *J Biol Chem* 1993;268:23504–23511.

276. Li JT, Armstrong CG, Mow VC. The effect of strain rate on mechanical properties of articular cartilage in tension. *Proc Biomech Symp Trans ASME* 1983;AMD56:117–120.

277. Li KW, Williamson AK, Wang AS, et al. Growth responses of cartilage to static and dynamic compression. *Clin Orthop* 2001;S34–48.

278. Linn FC, Sokoloff L. Movement and composition of interstitial fluid of cartilage. *Arthritis Rheum* 1965;8:481–494.

279. Lipshitz H, Etheredge R III, Glimcher MJ. Changes in the hexosamine content and swelling ratio of articular cartilage as functions of depth from the surface. *J Bone Joint Surg* 1976;58:1149–1153.

280. Little CB, Flannery CR, Hughes CE, et al. Aggrecanase versus matrix metalloproteinases in the catabolism of the interglobular domain of aggrecan in vitro. *Biochem J* 1999;344(pt 1):61–68.

281. Loeser RF, Carlson CS, McGee MP. Expression of beta 1 integrins by cultured articular

chondrocytes and in osteoarthritic cartilage. *Exp Cell Res* 1995;217:248–257.

282. Loeser RF. Chondrocyte integrin expression and function. *Biorheology* 2000;37:109–116.

283. Lohmander LS, Dahlberg L, Ryd L, et al. Increased levels of proteoglycan fragments in knee joint fluid after injury. *Arthritis Rheum* 1989;32:1434–1442.

284. Lohmander LS, Roos H, Dahlberg L, et al. Temporal patterns of stromelysin-1, tissue inhibitor, and proteoglycan fragments in human knee joint fluid after injury to the cruciate ligament or meniscus. *J Orthop Res* 1994;12:21–28.

285. Lu XL, Sun DD, Guo XE, et al. Indentation determined mechanoelectrochemical properties and fixed charge density of articular cartilage. *Ann Biomed Eng* 2004;32:370–379.

286. Luyten FP, Hascall VC, Nissley SP, et al. Insulin-like growth factors maintain steady-state metabolism of proteoglycans in bovine articular cartilage explants. *Arch Biochem Biophys* 1988;267:416–425.

287. Majumdar MK, Wang E, Morris EA. BMP-2 and BMP-9 promote chondrogenic differentiation of human multipotential mesenchymal cells and overcomes the inhibitory effect of IL-1. *J Cell Physiol* 2001;189:275–284.

288. Mak AF. The apparent viscoelastic behavior of articular cartilage—the contributions from the intrinsic matrix viscoelasticity and interstitial fluid flows. *J Biomech Eng* 1986;108:123–130.

289. Mak AF, Lai WM, Mow VC. Biphasic indentation of articular cartilage—I. Theoretical analysis. *J Biomech* 1987;20:703–714.

290. Makower AM, Wroblewski J, Pawlowski A. Effects of IGF-I, rGH, FGF, EGF and NCS on DNA-synthesis, cell proliferation and morphology of chondrocytes isolated from rat rib growth cartilage. *Cell Biol Int Rep* 1989;13:259–270.

291. Manicourt DH, Pita JC, Pezon CF, et al. Characterization of the proteoglycans recovered under nondissociative conditions from normal articular cartilage of rabbits and dogs. *J Biol Chem* 1986;261:5426–5433.

292. Mankin HJ. The structure, chemistry and metabolism of articular cartilage. *Bull Rheum Dis* 1967;17:447.

293. Mankin HJ, Lippiello L. The turnover of adult rabbit articular cartilage. *J Bone Joint Surg Am* 1969;51:1591–1600.

294. Mankin HJ, Thrasher AZ. Water content and binding in normal and osteoarthritic human cartilage. *J Bone Joint Surg* 1975;57:76–80.

295. Mankin HJ, Mow VC, Buckwalter JA, et al. Articular cartilage structure, composition and function. In: Buckwalter JA, Einhorn TA, Simon SR, eds. *Orthopaedic basic science: biology and biomechanics of the musculoskeletal system.* Rosemont,

IL: American Academy of Orthopaedic Surgeons, 2000:443–470.

296. Mansour JM, Mow VC. The permeability of articular cartilage under compressive strain and at high pressures. *J Bone Joint Surg* 1976;58:509–516.

297. Maroudas A. Physicochemical properties of cartilage in the light of ion exchange theory. *Biophys J* 1968;8:575–595.

298. Maroudas A, Muir H, Wingham J. The correlation of fixed negative charge with glycosaminoglycan content of human articular cartilage. *Biochim Biophys Acta* 1969;177:492–500.

299. Maroudas A. Transport through articular cartilage and some physiological implications. In: Ali SY, Elves MW, Leaback DH, eds. *Normal and osteoarthrotic articular cartilage.* London: Institute of Orthopaedics, 1974:33.

300. Maroudas A. Biophysical chemistry of cartilaginous tissues with special reference to solute and fluid transport. *Biorheology* 1975;12:233–248.

301. Maroudas A, Venn M. Chemical composition and swelling of normal and osteoarthrotic femoral head cartilage. II Swelling. *Ann Rheum Dis* 1977;36:399–406.

302. Maroudas A. Physicochemical properties of articular cartilage. In: Freeman MAR, ed. *Adult articular cartilage.* Kent, UK: Pitman Medical Publishing, 1979:215–290.

303. Maroudas A, Bayliss MT, Venn MF. Further studies on the composition of human femoral head cartilage. *Ann Rheum Dis* 1980;39:514–523.

304. Maroudas A, Bannon, C. Measurement of swelling pressure in cartilage and comparison with the osmotic pressure of constituent proteoglycans. *Biorheology* 1981;18:619–632.

305. Maroudas A, Schneiderman R. "Free" and "exchangeable" or "trapped" and "non-exchangeable" water in cartilage. *J Orthop Res* 1987;5:133–138.

306. Maroudas A, Wachtel E, Grushko G, et al. The effect of osmotic and mechanical pressures on water partitioning in articular cartilage. *Biochim Biophys Acta* 1991;1073:285–294.

307. Maroudas A, Grushko G. Measurement of swelling pressure of cartilage. In: Maroudas KKA, ed. *Methods in cartilage research.* San Diego: Academic Press, 1990:298–302.

308. Maroudas AI. Balance between swelling pressure and collagen tension in normal and degenerate cartilage. *Nature* 1976;260:808–809.

309. Martel-Pelletier J, McCollum R, DiBattista J, et al. The interleukin-1 receptor in normal and osteoarthritic human articular chondrocytes. Identification as the type I receptor and analysis of binding kinetics and biologic function. *Arthritis Rheum* 1992;35:530–540.

310. Masaro L, Zhu XX. Physical models of diffusion for polymer solutions, gels and solids. *Prog Polymer Sci* 1999;24:731–775.

311. Massague J, Blain SW, Lo RS. TGT-beta signaling in growth control, cancer, and heritable disorders. *Cell* 2000;103:295–309.

312. Matsumoto T, Gargosky SE, Iwasaki K, et al. Identification and characterization of insulin-like growth factors (IGFs), IGF-binding proteins (IGFBPs), and IGFBP proteases in human synovial fluid. *J Clin Endocrinol Metab* 1996;81:150–155.

313. Mauck RL, Soltz MA, Wang CC, et al. Functional tissue engineering of articular cartilage through dynamic loading of chondrocyte-seeded agarose gels. *J Biomech Eng* 2000;122:252–260.

314. McAlinden A, Dudhia J, Bolton MC, et al. Age-related changes in the synthesis and mRNA expression of decorin and aggrecan in human meniscus and articular cartilage. *Osteoarthritis Cartilage* 2001;9:33–41.

315. McCutchen CW. The frictional properties of animal joints. *Wear* 1962;5:1–17.

316. McDevitt CA, Muir H. Biochemical changes in the cartilage of the knee in experimental and natural osteoarthritis in the dog. *J Bone Joint Surg Br* 1976;58:94–101.

317. McDevitt CA, Webber RJ. The ultrastructure and biochemistry of meniscal cartilage. *Clin Orthop* 1990;8–18.

318. McDevitt CA, Miller A, Spindler KP. The cells and and cell matrix interaction of the meniscus. In: Mow VC, Arnoczky SP, Jackson DW, eds. *Knee meniscus: basic and clinical foundations.* New York: Raven Press, 1992:29–36.

319. McQuillan DJ, Handley CJ, Campbell MA, et al. Stimulation of proteoglycan biosynthesis by serum and insulin-like growth factor-I in cultured bovine articular cartilage. *Biochem J* 1986;240:423–430.

320. Meachim G. Surface morphology and topography of patello-femoral cartilage fibrillation in Liverpool necropsies. *J Anat* 1973;116:103–120.

321. Melchiorri C, Meliconi R, Frizziero L, et al. Enhanced and coordinated in vivo expression of inflammatory cytokines and nitric oxide synthase by chondrocytes from patients with osteoarthritis. *Arthritis Rheum* 1998;41:2165–2174.

322. Mendler M, Eich-Bender SG, Vaughan L, et al. Cartilage contains mixed fibrils of collagen types II, IX, and XI. *J Cell Biol* 1989;108:191–197.

323. Middleton JF, Tyler JA. Upregulation of insulin-like growth factor I gene expression in the lesions of osteoarthritic human articular cartilage. *Ann Rheum Dis* 1992;51:440–447.

324. Miller EJ, Harris ED Jr, Chung E, et al. Cleavage of type II and III collagens with mammalian collagenase: site of cleavage and primary structure at the NH2-terminal portion of the smaller fragment released from both collagens. *Biochemistry* 1976;15:787–792.

325. Miller EJ. Collagen types: structure, distribution and functions. In: Nimni ME, ed. *Collagen: bio-chemistry.* Boca Raton, FL: CRC Press, 1988:139–156.

326. Millward-Sadler SJ, Salter DM. Integrin-dependent signal cascades in chrondocyte mechanotransduction. *Ann Biomed Eng* 2004;32:435–446.

327. Mitchell PG, Magna HA, Reeves LM, et al. Cloning, expression, and type II collagenolytic activity of matrix metalloproteinase-13 from human osteoarthritic cartilage. *J Clin Invest* 1996;97:761–768.

328. Mitrovic D, Quintero M, Stankovic A, et al. Cell density of adult human femoral condylar articular cartilage. Joints with normal and fibrillated surfaces. *Lab Invest* 1983;49:309–316.

329. Modl JM, Sether LA, Haughton VM, et al. Articular cartilage: correlation of histologic zones with signal intensity at MR imaging. *Radiology* 1991;181:853–855.

330. Moldovan F, Pelletier JP, Hambor J, et al. Collagenase-3 (matrix metalloprotease 13) is preferentially localized in the deep layer of human arthritic cartilage in situ: in vitro mimicking effect by transforming growth factor beta. *Arthritis Rheum* 1997;40:1653–1661.

331. Montes GS, Jungeria LCU. Histochemical localization of collagen and proteglycans in tissues. In: Nimni ME, ed. *Collagen: biochemistry and biomechanic.* Boca Raton, FL: CRC Press, 1988:41–72.

332. Morales TI, Roberts AB. Transforming growth factor beta regulates the metabolism of proteoglycans in bovine cartilage organ cultures. *J Biol Chem* 1988;263:12828–12831.

333. Morales TI, Hascall VC. Effects of interleukin-1 and lipopolysaccharides on protein and carbohydrate metabolism in bovine articular cartilage organ cultures. *Connect Tissue Res* 1989;19:255–275.

334. Morgan FR. The mechanical properties of collagen fibers: stress–strain curves. *J Soc Leather Trades Chem* 1960;44:171–182.

335. Mow VC. The role of lubrication in biomechanical joints. *J Lubr Tech Trans* 1969;91:320–329.

336. Mow VC, Lai WM. Some surface characteristics of articular cartilage. IA scanning electron microscopy study and a theoretical model for the dynamic interaction of synovial fluid and articular cartilage. *J Biomech* 1974;7:449–456.

337. Mow VC, Lai WM. Selected unresolved problems in synovial joint biomechanics. In: Van Buskirk W, ed. *Proceedings of Biomechanics Symposium.* New York: ASME, 1979:19–52.

338. Mow VC, Kuei SC, Lai WM, et al. Biphasic creep and stress relaxation of articular cartilage in compression: theory and experiments. *J Biomech Eng* 1980;102:73–84.

339. Mow VC, Lai WM. Recent developments in synovial joint biomechanics. *SIAM Rev* 1980;22:275–317.

340. Mow VC, Holmes MH, Lai WM. Fluid transport and mechanical properties of articular cartilage: a review. *J Biomech* 1984;17:377–394.

341. Mow VC, Mak AF, Lai WM, et al. Viscoelastic properties of proteoglycan subunits and aggregates in varying solution concentrations. *J Biomech* 1984;17:325–338.

342. Mow VC, Kwan MK, Lai WM, et al. A finite deformation theory for nonlinearly permeable soft hydrated biological tissues. In: Schmid-Schonbein G, Woo SL-Y, Zweifach B, eds. *Frontiers in biomechanics*. New York: Springer-Verlag, 1986:153–179.

343. Mow VC, Holmes MH, Lai WM. Influence of load bearing on the fluid transport and mechanical properties of articular cartilage. In: Helminen HK, Kiviranta I, Saamanen AM, et al., eds. *Joint loading: biology and health of articular structure*. Kuopio, Finland: Butterworth, 1987:264–286.

344. Mow VC, Proctor CS, Schmidt MB, et al. Tensile and compressive properties of normal meniscus. In: Fung YC, Hayashi K, Seguchi Y, eds. *Progress and new directions of biomechanics*. Tokyo: Mita Press, 1988:107–122.

345. Mow VC, Gibbs MC, Lai WM, et al. Biphasic indentation of articular cartilage—II. A numerical algorithm and an experimental study. *J Biomech* 1989;22:853–861.

346. Mow VC, Zhu W, Lai WM, et al. The influence of link protein stabilization on the viscometric properties of proteoglycan aggregate solutions. *Biochim Biophys Acta* 1989;992:201–208.

347. Mow VC, Setton LA, Howell DS, et al. Structure–function relationships of articular cartilage and the effects of joint instability and trauma on cartilage function. In: Brandt KD, ed. *Cartilage changes in osteoarthritis*. Indianapolis: Ciba-Geigy Corp., 1990:22–42.

348. Mow VC, Ratcliffe A, Rosenwasser MP, et al. Experimental studies on repair of large osteochondral defects at a high weight bearing area of the knee joint: a tissue engineering study. *J Biomech Eng* 1991;113:198–207.

349. Mow VC, Ratcliffe A, Chern KY, et al. Structure and function relationships of the menisci of the knee. In: Mow VC, Arnoczky SP, Jackson DW, eds. *Knee meniscus: basic and clinical foundations*. New York: Raven Press, 1992:37–57.

350. Mow VC, Ratcliffe A, Poole AR. Cartilage and diarthrodial joints as paradigms for hierarchical materials and structures. *Biomaterials* 1992;13:67–97.

351. Mow VC, Ateshian GA, Lai WM, et al. Effects of fixed charges on the stress-relaxation behavior of hydrated soft tissues in a confined compression problem. *Int J Solids Struct* 1998;35:4945–4962.

352. Mow VC, Wang CC, Hung CT. The extracellular matrix, interstitial fluid and ions as a mechanical signal transducer in articular cartilage. *Osteoarthritis Cartilage* 1999;7:41–58.

353. Mow VC, Guo XE. Mechano-electrochemical properties of articular cartilage: their inhomogeneities and anisotropies. *Annu Rev Biomed Eng* 2002;4:175–209.

354. Mow VC, Proctor CS, Kelly MA. Biomechanics of articular cartilage. In: Nordin M, Frankel VH, eds. *Basic biomechanics of the locomotor system*. Philadelphia: Lea and Febiger, 1989:31–58.

355. Muir H, Bullough P, Maroudas A. The distribution of collagen in human articular cartilage with some of its physiological implications. *J Bone Joint Surg* 1970;52:554–563.

356. Muir H. Biochemistry. In: Freeman MA, ed. *Adult articular cartilage*. Kent, UK: Pittman Medical, 1979:145–214.

357. Muir H. Proteoglycans as organizers of the intercellular matrix. *Biochem Soc Trans* 1983;11:613–622.

358. Mulholland R, Millington PF, Manners J. Some aspects of the mechanical behavior of articular cartilage. *Ann Rheum Dis* 1975;34:104–107.

359. Muragaki, Y, Mariman, EC, van Beersum, SE, et al. A mutation in the gene encoding the alpha 2 chain of the fibril-associated collagen IX, COL9A2, causes multiple epiphyseal dysplasia (EDM2). *NatGenet* 1996;12:103–105.

360. Myers E, Armstrong CG, Mow VC. Swelling pressure and collagen tension. In: Hukins DWL, ed. *Connective tissue matrix*. London: Macmillan, 1984:161–186.

361. Myers E, Hardingham T, Billingham ME, et al. Changes in the tensile and compressive properties of cartilage in a canine model of osteoarthritis. *Trans Orthop Res Soc* 1986;11:231.

362. Myers ER, Lai WM, Mow VC. A continuum theory and an experiment for the ion-induced swelling behavior of articular cartilage. *J Biomech Eng* 1984;106:151–158.

363. Myllyharju J, Kivirikko KI. Collagens and collagen-related diseases. *Ann Med* 2001;33:7–21.

364. Nakano T, Thompson JR, Aherne FX. Distribution of glycosaminoglycans and the nonreducible collagen crosslink, pyridinoline in porcine menisci. *Can J Vet Res* 1986;50:532–536.

365. Narmoneva DA, Wang JY, Setton LA. A noncontacting method for material property determination for articular cartilage from osmotic loading. *Biophys J* 2001;81:3066–3076.

366. Nilsson A, Isgaard J, Lindahl A, et al. Regulation by growth-hormone of number of chondrocytes containing IGF-I in rat growth plate. *Science* 1986;233:571–574.

367. Nimni ME, ed. *Collagen: biochemistry*. Vol. 1. Boca Raton, FL: CRC Press, 1988.

368. Nimni ME, ed. *Collagen: biochemistry and biomechanics*. Vol. 2. Boca Raton, FL: CRC Press, 1988.

369. Nimni ME, ed. *Collagen: biotechnology*. Vol. 3. Boca Raton, FL: CRC Press, 1988.

370. Nishida, Y, Knudson CB, Nietfeld JJ, et al. Antisense inhibition of hyaluronan synthase-2 in human articular chondrocytes inhibits proteoglycan retention and matrix assembly. *J Biol Chem* 1999;274:21893–21899.

371. Nishimura I, Muragaki Y, Olsen BR. Tissue-specific forms of type IX collagen–proteoglycan arise from the use of two widely separated promoters. *J Biol Chem* 1989;264:20033–20041.

372. O'Hara BP, Urban JP, Maroudas A. Influence of cyclic loading on the nutrition of articular cartilage. *Ann Rheum Dis* 1990;49:536–539.

373. Olsen BR. New insights into the function of collagens from genetic analysis. *Curr Opin Cell Biol* 1995;7:720–727.

374. Osborn KD, Trippel SB, Mankin HJ. Growth-factor stimulation of adult articular-cartilage. *J Orthop Res* 1989;7:35–42.

375. Otterness IG, Eskra JD, Bliven ML, et al. Exercise protects against articular cartilage degeneration in the hamster. *Arthritis Rheum* 1998;41:2068–2076.

376. Palmoski M, Perricone E, Brandt KD. Development and reversal of a proteoglycan aggregation defect in normal canine knee cartilage after immobilization. *Arthritis Rheum* 1979;22:508–517.

377. Palmoski MJ, Colyer RA, Brandt KD. Joint motion in the absence of normal loading does not maintain normal articular cartilage. *Arthritis Rheum* 1980;23:325–334.

378. Palmoski MJ, Brandt KD. Running inhibits the reversal of atrophic changes in canine knee cartilage after removal of a leg cast. *Arthritis Rheum* 1981;24:1329–1337.

379. Palotie A, Vaisanen P, Ott J, et al. Predisposition to familial osteoarthrosis linked to type II collagen gene. *Lancet* 1989;1:924–927.

380. Park S, Krishnan R, Nicoll SB, et al. Cartilage interstitial fluid load support in unconfined compression. *J Biomech* 2003;36:1785–1796.

381. Parkkinen JJ, Ikonen J, Lammi MJ, et al. Effects of cyclic hydrostatic pressure on proteoglycan synthesis in cultured chondrocytes and articular cartilage explants. *Arch Biochem Biophys* 1993;300:458–465.

382. Parsons JR, Black J. The viscoelastic shear behavior of normal rabbit articular cartilage. *J Biomech* 1977;10:21–29.

383. Parsons JR, Black J. Mechanical behavior of articular cartilage: quantitative changes with alteration of ionic environment. *J Biomech* 1979;12:765–773.

384. Pasternack SG, Veis A, Breen M. Solvent-dependent changes in proteoglycan subunit conformation in aqueous guanidine hydrochloride solutions. *J Biol Chem* 1974;249:2206–2211.

385. Paul JP. Joint kinetics. In: Sokoloff L, ed. *The joints and synovial fluid.* New York: Academic Press, 1980:139–176.

386. Perkins SJ, Miller A, Hardingham TE, et al. Physical properties of the hyaluronate binding region of proteoglycan from pig laryngeal cartilage. Densitometric and small-angle neutron scattering studies of carbohydrates and carbohydrate–protein macromolecules. *J Mol Biol* 1981;150:69–95.

387. Peterfy CG, van Dijke CF, Janzen DL, et al. Quantification of articular cartilage in the knee with pulsed saturation transfer subtraction and fat-suppressed MR imaging: optimization and validation. *Radiology* 1994;192:485–491.

388. Peters TJ, Smillie IS. Studies on the chemical composition of the menisci of the knee joint with special reference to the horizontal cleavage lesion. *Clin Orthop Rel Res* 1972;86:245–252.

389. Pettipher ER, Higgs GA, Henderson B. Interleukin 1 induces leukocyte infiltration and cartilage proteoglycan degradation in the synovial joint. *Proc Natl Acad Sci U S A* 1986;83:8749–8753.

390. Pilar Fernandez M, Selmin O, Martin GR, et al. The structure of anchorin CII, a collagen binding protein isolated from chondrocyte membrane. *J Biol Chem* 1988;263:5921–5925.

391. Pluen A, Netti PA, Jain RK, et al. Diffusion of macromolecules in agarose gels: comparison of linear and globular configurations. *Biophys J* 1999;77:542–552.

392. Poole AR. Proteoglycans in health and disease: structures and functions. *Biochem J* 1986;236:1–14.

393. Poole AR, Alini M, Hollander AP. Cellular biology of cartilage degradation. In: Henderson B, Pettifer R, Edwards J, eds. *Mechanisms and models in rheumatoid arthritis.* London: Academic Press, 1995:163–204.

394. Poole CA, Flint MH, Beaumont BW. Chondrons in cartilage: ultrastructural analysis of the pericellular microenvironment in adult human articular cartilages. *J Orthop Res* 1987;5:509–522.

395. Poole CA. Articular cartilage chondrons: form, function and failure. *J Anat* 1997;191:1–13.

396. Pottenger LA, Lyon NB, Hecht JD, et al. Influence of cartilage particle size and proteoglycan aggregation on immobilization of proteoglycans. *J Biol Chem* 1982;257:11479–11485.

397. Prehm P. Synthesis of hyaluronate in differentiated teratocarcinoma cells. Mechanism of chain growth. *Biochem J* 1983;211:191–198.

398. Prockop DJ. What holds us together? Why do some of us fall apart? What can we do about it? *Matrix Biol* 1998;16:519–528.

399. Prockop DJ, Kivirikko KI. Collagens: molecular biology, diseases, and potentials for therapy. *Annu Rev Biochem* 1995;64:403–434.

400. Proctor CS, Schmidt MB, Whipple RR, et al. Material properties of the normal medial bovine meniscus. *J Orthop Res* 1989;7:771–782.

401. Puso MA, Weiss JA, Maker BN, et al. A transversely isotropic hyperelastic shell finite element. *Adv Bioeng Trans ASME* 1995;BED29:103–104.

402. Quinn TM, Kocian P, Meister JJ. Static compression is associated with decreased diffusivity of dextrans in cartilage explants. *Arch Biochem Biophys* 2000;384:327–334.

403. Quinn TM, Morel V, Meister JJ. Static compression of articular cartilage can reduce solute diffusivity and partitioning: implications for the chondrocyte biological response. *J Biomech* 2001;34:1463–1469.

404. Radin EL, Rose RM. Role of subchondral bone in the initiation and progression of cartilage damage. *Clin Orthop* 1986;34–40.

405. Ragan PM, Badger AM, Cook M, et al. Downregulation of chondrocyte aggrecan and type-II collagen gene expression correlates with increases in static compression magnitude and duration. *J Orthop Res* 1999;17:836–842.

406. Ratcliffe A, Hardingham T. Cartilage proteoglycan binding region and link protein. Radioimmunoassays and the detection of masked determinants in aggregates. *Biochem J* 1983;213:371–378.

407. Ratcliffe A, Fryer PR, Hardingham TE. The distribution of aggregating proteoglycans in articular cartilage: comparison of quantitative immunoelectron microscopy with radioimmunoassay and biochemical analysis. *J Histochem Cytochem* 1984;32:193–201.

408. Ratcliffe A, Tyler JA, Hardingham TE. Articular cartilage cultured with interleukin 1. Increased release of link protein, hyaluronate-binding region and other proteoglycan fragments. *Biochem J* 1986;238:571–580.

409. Ratcliffe A, Hughes C, Fryer PR, et al. Immunochemical studies on the synthesis and secretion of link protein and aggregating proteoglycan by chondrocytes. *Collagen Rel Res* 1987;7:409–421.

410. Ratcliffe A, Doherty M, Maini RN, et al. Increased concentrations of proteoglycan components in the synovial fluids of patients with acute but not chronic joint disease. *Ann Rheum Dis* 1988;47:826–832.

411. Ratcliffe A, Billingham ME, Saed-Nejad F, et al. Increased release of matrix components from articular cartilage in experimental canine osteoarthritis. *J Orthop Res* 1992;10:350–358.

412. Ratcliffe A, Beauvais PJ, Saed-Nejad F. Differential levels of synovial fluid aggrecan aggregate components in experimental osteoarthritis and joint disuse. *J Orthop Res* 1994;12:464–473.

413. Ratcliffe A, Mow VC. The structure and function of articular cartilage. In: Comper WD, ed. *Structure and function of connective tissues*. Amsterdam: Harwood Academic Press, 1996:234–302.

414. Re P, Valhmu WB, Vostrejs M, et al. Quantitative polymerase chain reaction assay for aggrecan and link protein gene expression in cartilage. *Anal Biochem* 1995;225:356–360.

415. Reboul P, Pelletier JP, Tardif G, et al. The new collagenase, collagenase-3, is expressed and synthesized by human chondrocytes but not by synoviocytes. A role in osteoarthritis. *J Clin Invest* 1996;97:2011–2019.

416. Redini F, Galera P, Mauviel A, et al. Transforming growth factor beta stimulates collagen and glycosaminoglycan biosynthesis in cultured rabbit articular chondrocytes. *FEBS Lett* 1988;234:172–176.

417. Redler I, Mow VC, Zimny ML, et al. The ultrastructure and biomechanical significance of the tidemark of articular cartilage. *Clin Orthop* 1975;357–362.

418. Repo RU, Mitchell N. Collagen synthesis in mature articular cartilage of the rabbit. *J Bone Joint Surg Br* 1971;53:541–548.

419. Reynolds O. On the theory of lubrication and its application to Mr. Beauchamp Tower's experiment, including an experimental determination of the viscosity of olive oil. *Proc Phil Trans R Soc* 1886;177:157–234.

420. Ridge MD, Wright V. The description of skin stiffness. *Biorheology* 1964;2:67–74.

421. Roberts AB. Transforming growth factor beta. In: Canalis E, ed. *Skeletal growth factors*. Philadelphia: Lippincott Williams & Wilkins, 2000:221–232.

422. Ropes MW, Bauer W. *Synovial fluid changes in joint diseases*. Cambridge, MA: Harvard University Press, 1953.

423. Rosati R, Horan GS, Pinero GJ, et al. Normal long bone growth and development in type X collagen-null mice. *Nat Genet* 1994;8:129–135.

424. Rosenberg L. Structure of cartilage proteoglycans. In: Burleigh PMC, Poole AR, eds. *Dynamics of connective tissue macromolecules*. Amsterdam: North-Holland, 1974:105–128.

425. Rosenberg L, Hellmann W, Kleinschmidt AK. Electron microscopic studies of proteoglycan aggregates from bovine articular cartilage. *J Biol Chem* 1975;250:1877–1883.

426. Rosenberg LC, Choi HU, Tang LH, et al. Isolation of dermatan sulfate proteoglycans from mature bovine articular cartilages. *J Biol Chem* 1985;260:6304–6413.

427. Roth V, Mow VC. The intrinsic tensile behavior of the matrix of bovine articular cartilage and its variation with age. *J Bone Joint Surg* 1980;62:1102–1117.

428. Roth V, Mow VC, Lai WM, et al. Correlation of intrinsic compressive properties of bovine articular cartilage with its uronic acid and water content. *Trans Orthop Res Soc* 1981;6:21.

429. Roth V, Schoonbeck JM, Mow VC. Low frequency dynamic behavior of articular cartilage under torsional shear. *Trans Orthop Res Soc* 1982;7:150.

430. Roughley PJ, White RJ. Age-related changes in the structure of the proteoglycan subunits from human articular cartilage. *J Biol Chem* 1980;255:217–224.

431. Roughley PJ, White RJ. Dermatan sulphate proteoglycans of human articular cartilage. The properties of dermatan sulphate proteoglycans I and II. *Biochem J* 1989;262:823–827.

432. Roughley PJ, White RJ. The dermatan sulfate proteoglycans of the adult human meniscus. *J Orthop Res* 1992;10:631–637.

433. Roughley PJ, Lee ER. Cartilage proteoglycans: structure and potential functions. *Microsc Res Tech* 1994;28:385–397.

434. Rushfeldt PD, Mann RW, Harris WH. Improved techniques for measuring in vitro the geometry and pressure distribution in the human acetabulum—I. Ultrasonic measurement of acetabular surfaces, sphericity and cartilage thickness. *J Biomech* 1981;14:253–260.

435. Ryan MC, Sandell LJ. Differential expression of a cysteine-rich domain in the amino-terminal propeptide of type II (cartilage) procollagen by alternative splicing of mRNA. *J Biol Chem* 1990;265:10334–10339.

436. Sachs F. Mechanical transduction by membrane ion channels: a mini review. *Mol Cell Biochem* 1991;104:57–60.

437. Sah RL, Kim YJ, Doong JY, et al. Biosynthetic response of cartilage explants to dynamic compression. *J Orthop Res* 1989;7:619–636.

438. Sah RL, Doong JY, Grodzinsky AJ, et al. Effects of compression on the loss of newly synthesized proteoglycans and proteins from cartilage explants. *Arch Biochem Biophys* 1991;286:20–29.

439. Sailor LZ, Hewick RM, Morris EA Recombinant human bone morphogenetic protein-2 maintains the articular chondrocyte phenotype in long-term culture. *J Orthop Res* 1996;14:937–945.

440. Saklatvala J. Tumour necrosis factor alpha stimulates resorption and inhibits synthesis of proteoglycan in cartilage. *Nature* 1986;322:547–549.

441. Salter DM, Hughes DE, Simpson R, et al. Integrin expression by human articular chondrocytes. *Br J Rheumatol* 1992;31:231–234.

442. Sampaio Lde O, Bayliss MT, Hardingham TE, et al. Dermatan sulphate proteoglycan from human articular cartilage. Variation in its content with age and its structural comparison with a small chondroitin sulphate proteoglycan from pig laryngeal cartilage. *Biochem J* 1988;254:757–764.

443. Sandell LJ, Morris N, Robbins JR, et al. Alternatively spliced type II procollagen mRNAs define distinct populations of cells during vertebral development: differential expression of the aminopropeptide. *J Cell Biol* 1991;114:1307–1319.

444. Sandy JD, Adams ME, Billingham ME, et al. In vivo and in vitro stimulation of chondro- cyte biosynthetic activity in early experimental osteoarthritis. *Arthritis Rheum* 1984;27:388–397.

445. Sandy JD, Flannery CR, Neame PJ, et al. The structure of aggrecan fragments in human synovial fluid. Evidence for the involvement in osteoarthritis of a novel proteinase which cleaves the Glu 373–Ala 374 bond of the interglobular domain. *J Clin Invest* 1992;89:1512–1516.

446. Schalkwijk J, Joosten LA, van den Berg WB, et al. Chondrocyte nonresponsiveness to insulin-like growth factor-1 in experimental arthritis. *Arthritis Rheum* 1989;32:894–900.

447. Schepps JL, Foster KR. The UHF and microwave dielectric properties of normal and tumour tissues: variation in dielectric properties with tissue water content. *Phys Med Biol* 1980;25:1149–1159.

448. Schinagl RM, Ting MK, Price JH, et al. Video microscopy to quantitate the inhomogeneous equilibrium strain within articular cartilage during confined compression. *Ann Biomed Eng* 1996;24:500–512.

449. Schinagl RM, Gurskis D, Chen AC, et al. Depth-dependent confined compression modulus of full-thickness bovine articular cartilage. *J Orthop Res* 1997;15:499–506.

450. Schmidt MB, Schoonbeck JM, Mow VC, et al. The relationship between collagen cross-linking and the tensile properties of articular cartilage. *Trans Orthop Res Soc* 1987;12:134.

451. Schmidt MB, Mow VC, Chun LE, et al. Effects of proteoglycan extraction on the tensile behavior of articular cartilage. *J Orthop Res* 1990;8:353–363.

452. Schneiderman R, Rosenberg N, Hiss J, et al. Concentration and size distribution of insulin-like growth factor-I in human normal and osteoarthritic synovial fluid and cartilage. *Arch Biochem Biophys* 1995;324:173–188.

453. Schwartz NB, Pirok EW III, Mensch JR Jr, et al. Domain organization, genomic structure, evolution, and regulation of expression of the aggrecan gene family. *Prog Nucleic Acid Res Mol Biol* 1999;62:177–225.

454. Scott JE. Proteoglycan–fibrillar collagen interactions. *Biochem J* 1988;252:313–323.

455. Scott JE. Proteoglycan:collagen interactions and subfibrillar structure in collagen fibrils. Implications in the development and ageing of connective tissues. *J Anat* 1990;169:23–35.

456. Scott JE. Proteodermatan and proteokeratan sulfate (decorin, lumican/fibromodulin) proteins are horseshoe shaped. Implications for their interactions with collagen. *Biochemistry* 1996;35:8795–8799.

457. Scott PG, Nakano T, Dodd CM. Isolation and characterization of small proteoglycans from different zones of the porcine knee meniscus. *Biochim Biophys Acta* 1997;1336:254–262.

458. Setton LA, Gu WY, Lai WM, et al. Pre-stress in articular cartilage due to internal swelling pressures. *Adv Bioeng Trans ASME* 1992;BED19:485–492.

459. Setton LA, Lai WM, Mow VC. Swelling-induced residual stress and the mechanism of curling in articular cartilage in vitro. *Adv Bioeng Trans ASME* 1993;BED26:59–62.

460. Setton LA, Zhu W, Mow VC. The biphasic poroviscoelastic behavior of articular cartilage: role of the surface zone in governing the compressive behavior. *J Biomech* 1993;26:581–592.

461. Setton LA, Zhu W, Weidenbaum M, et al. Compressive properties of the cartilaginous endplate of the baboon lumbar spine. *J Orthop Res* 1993;11:228–239.

462. Setton LA, Mow VC, Muller FJ, et al. Mechanical properties of canine articular cartilage are significantly altered following transection of the anterior cruciate ligament. *J Orthop Res* 1994;12:451–463.

463. Setton LA, Mow VC, Howell DS. Mechanical behavior of articular cartilage in shear is altered by transection of the anterior cruciate ligament. *J Orthop Res* 1995;13:473–482.

464. Setton LA, Tohyama H, Mow VC. Swelling and curling behaviors of articular cartilage. *J Biomech Eng* 1998;120:355–361.

465. Setton LA, Elliott DM, Mow VC. Altered mechanics of cartilage with osteoarthritis: human OA and animal model of joint degeneration. *Osteoarthritis Cartilage* 1999;7:2–14.

466. Seyedin SM, Thompson AY, Bentz H, et al. Cartilage-inducing factor-A. Apparent identity to transforming growth factor-beta. *J Biol Chem* 1986;261:5693–5695.

467. Shakibaei M. Inhibition of chondrogenesis by integrin antibody in vitro. *Exp Cell Res* 1998;240:95–106.

468. Shlopov BV, Lie WR, Mainardi CL, et al. Osteoarthritic lesions: involvement of three different collagenases. *Arthritis Rheum* 1997;40:2065–2074.

469. Skaggs DL, Warden WH, Mow VC. Radial tie fibers influence the tensile properties of the bovine medial meniscus. *J Orthop Res* 1994;12:176–185.

470. Skaggs DL, Weidenbaum M, Iatridis JC, et al. Regional variation in tensile properties and biochemical composition of the human lumbar anulus fibrosus. *Spine* 1994;19:1310–1319.

471. Smith MD, Triantafillou S, Parker A, et al. Synovial membrane inflammation and cytokine production in patients with early osteoarthritis. *J Rheumatol* 1997;24:365–371.

472. Smith-Mungo LI, Kagan HM. Lysyl oxidase: properties, regulation and multiple functions in biology. *Matrix Biol* 1998;16:387–398.

473. Sokoloff L. Elasticity of articular cartilage: effect of ions and viscous solutions. *Science* 1963;141:1055–1057.

474. Sokoloff L. Elasticity of aging cartilage. *Fed Proc* 1966;25:1089–1095.

475. Sokoloff L. *The biology of degenerative joint disease.* Chicago: University of Chicago Press, 1969.

476. Soltz MA, Ateshian GA. Experimental verification and theoretical prediction of cartilage interstitial fluid pressurization at an impermeable contact interface in confined compression. *J Biomech* 1998;31:927–934.

477. Soltz MA, Ateshian GA. Interstitial fluid pressurization during confined compression cyclical loading of articular cartilage. *Ann Biomed Eng* 2000;28:150–159.

478. Solursh M, Vaerewyck SA, Reiter RS. Depression by hyaluronic acid of glycosaminoglycan synthesis by cultured chick embryo chondrocytes. *Dev Biol* 1974;41:233–244.

479. Soslowsky LJ, Flatow EL, Bigliani LU, et al. Articular geometry of the glenohumeral joint. *Clin Orthop* 1992;181–190.

480. Soslowsky LJ, Flatow EL, Bigliani LU, et al. Quantitation of in situ contact areas at the glenohumeral joint: a biomechanical study. *J Orthop Res* 1992;10:524–534.

481. Spilker RL, Suh JK, Mow VC. A finite element analysis of the indentation stress-relaxation response of linear biphasic articular cartilage. *J Biomech Eng* 1992;114:191–201.

482. Spirt AA, Mak AF, Wassell RP. Nonlinear viscoelastic properties of articular cartilage in shear. *J Orthop Res* 1989;7:43–49.

483. Stahurski TM, Armstrong CG, Mow VC. Variation of the intrinsic aggregate modulus and permeability of articular cartilage with trypsin digestion. *Proc Biomech Symp Trans ASME* 1981;AMD43:137–140.

484. Stockwell RA, Scott JE. Distribution of acid glycosaminoglycans in human articular cartilage. *Nature* 1967;215:1376–1378.

485. Stockwell RA. *Biology of cartilage cells.* Cambridge, UK: Cambridge University Press, 1979.

486. SundarRaj N, Fite D, Ledbetter S, et al. Perlecan is a component of cartilage matrix and promotes chondrocyte attachment. *J Cell Sci* 1995;108:2663–2672.

487. Tammi M, Kiviranta I, Peltonen L, et al. Effects of joint loading on articular cartilage collagen metabolism: assay of procollagen prolyl 4-hydroxylase and galactosylhydroxylysyl glucosyltransferase. *Connect Tissue Res* 1988;17:199–206.

488. Tardif G, Reboul P, Pelletier JP, et al. Normal expression of type 1 insulin–like growth factor receptor by human osteoarthritic chondrocytes with increased expression and synthesis of insulin-like growth factor binding proteins. *Arthritis Rheum* 1996;39:968–978.

489. Thomas JT, Ayad S, Grant ME. Cartilage collagens: strategies for the study of their organisation

and expression in the extracellular matrix. *Ann Rheum Dis* 1994;53:488–496.

490. Thompson RC Jr, Oegema TR Jr, Lewis JL, et al. Osteoarthrotic changes after acute transarticular load. An animal model. *J Bone Joint Surg* 1991;73:990–1001.

491. Timoshenko S, Goodier JN. *Theory of elasticity.* New York: McGraw-Hill, 1970.

492. Tissakht M, Ahmed AM. Tensile stress–strain characteristics of the human meniscal material. *J Biomech* 1995;28:411–422.

493. Tohyama H, Gu WY, Setton LA, et al. Ion-induced swelling behavior of articular cartilage in tension. *Trans Orthop Res Soc* 1995;20:702.

494. Tombs MP, Peacocke AR. *The osmotic pressure of biological macromolecules.* Oxford: Clarendon Press, 1974.

495. Tortorella MD, Burn TC, Pratta MA, et al. Purification and cloning of aggrecanase-1: a member of the ADAMTS family of proteins. *Science* 1999;284:1664–1666.

496. Torzilli PA. Influence of cartilage conformation on its equilibrium water partition. *J Orthop Res* 1985;3:473–483.

497. Torzilli PA, Adams TC, Mis RJ. Transient solute diffusion in articular cartilage. *J Biomech* 1987;20:203–214.

498. Torzilli PA. Water content and equilibrium water partition in immature cartilage. *J Orthop Res* 1988;6:766–769.

499. Torzilli PA, Askari E, Jenkins JT. Water content and solute diffusion properties in articular cartilage. In: Mow VC, Ratcliffe A, Woo SL-Y, eds. *Biomechanics of diarthrodial joints.* New York: Springer Verlag, 1990:363–390.

500. Torzilli PA, Grigiene R, Borrelli JJ, et al. Effect of impact load on articular cartilage: cell metabolism and viability and matrix water content. *J Biomech Eng* 1999;121:433–441.

501. Trippel SB. Insulin-like growth factor 1 can decrease degradation and promote synthesis of proteoglycan in cartilage exposed to cytokines. *J Rheumatol Suppl* 1995;43:129–132.

502. Truesdell C, Noll W. The nonlinear field theories of mechanics. In: Flügge S, eds. *Handbuch der Physik,* Vol. 3. Berlin: Springer Verlag, 1965.

503. Turnay J, Pfannmuller E, Lizarbe MA, et al. Collagen binding activity of recombinant and N-terminally modified annexin V (anchorin CII). *J Cell Biochem* 1995;58:208–220.

504. Tyler JA. Articular cartilage cultured with catabolin (pig interleukin 1) synthesizes a decreased number of normal proteoglycan molecules. *Biochem J* 1985;227:869–878.

505. Tyler JA, Benton HP. Synthesis of type II collagen is decreased in cartilage cultured with interleukin 1 while the rate of intracellular degradation remains unchanged. *Collagen Rel Res* 1988;8:393–405.

506. Tyler JA. Insulin-like growth factor 1 can decrease degradation and promote synthesis of proteoglycan in cartilage exposed to cytokines. *Biochem J* 1989;260:543–548.

507. Uhthoff HK, Wiley JJ. *Behavior of the growth plate.* New York: Raven Press, 1988.

508. Urban JP, Holm S, Maroudas A. Diffusion of small solutes into the intervertebral disc: as in vivo study. *Biorheology* 1978;15:203–221.

509. Urban JP, Maroudas A. Swelling of the intervertebral disc in vivo. *Connect Tissue Res* 1981;9:1–10.

510. Urban JP, McMullin JF. Swelling pressure of the inervertebral disc: influence of proteoglycan and collagen contents. *Biorheology* 1985;22:145–157.

511. Urban JP. The chondrocyte: a cell under pressure. *Br J Rheumatol* 1994;33:901–908.

512. Urban JPG. Fluid and solute transport in the intervertebral disc. PhD thesis, London University, 1977.

513. Valhmu WB, Palmer,GD, Rivers PA, et al. Structure of the human aggrecan gene: exon–intron organization and association with the protein domains. *Biochem J* 1995;309(pt 2):535–542.

514. van der Rest M, Mayne R. Type IX collagen proteoglycan from cartilage is covalently cross-linked to type II collagen. *J Biol Chem* 1988;263:1615–1618.

515. van der Rest M, Garrone R. Collagen family of proteins. *FASEB J* 1991;5:2814–2823.

516. van Meurs JB, van Lent PL, Holthuysen AE, et al. Kinetics of aggrecanase- and metalloproteinase-induced neoepitopes in various stages of cartilage destruction in murine arthritis. *Arthritis Rheum* 1999;42:1128–1139.

517. Vener MJ, Thompson RC Jr, Lewis JL, et al. Subchondral damage after acute transarticular loading: an in vitro model of joint injury. *J Orthop Res* 1992;10:759–765.

518. Venn M, Maroudas A. Chemical composition and swelling of normal and osteoarthrotic femoral head cartilage. I Chemical composition. *Ann Rheum Dis* 1977;36:121–129.

519. Venn MF. Variation of chemical composition with age in human femoral head cartilage. *Ann Rheum Dis* 1978;37:168–174.

520. Vetter U, Vogel W, Just W, et al. Human decorin gene: intron–exon junctions and chromosomal localization. *Genomics* 1993;15:161–168.

521. Viidik A. An ideological model for uncalcified parallel fibered collagenous tissues. *J Biomech* 1968;1:3–11.

522. Viidik A. Mechanical properties of parallel fibered collagenous tissues. In: Viidik A, Vuusst J, eds. *Biology of collagen.* New York: Academic Press, 1980:237–255.

523. Vikkula M, Metsaranta M, Ala-Kokko L. Type II collagen mutations in rare and common cartilage diseases. *Ann Med* 1994;26:107–114.

524. Vikkula M, Mariman EC, Lui VC, et al. Autosomal dominant and recessive osteochondrodysplasias associated with the COL11A2 locus. *Cell* 1995;80:431–437.

525. Vu TH, Werb Z. Matrix metalloproteinases: effectors of development and normal physiology. *Genes Dev* 2000;14:2123–2133.

526. Wachtel E, Maroudas A, Schneiderman R. Age-related changes in collagen packing of human articular cartilage. *Biochim Biophys Acta* 1995;1243:239–243.

527. Wakitani S, Goto T, Pineda SJ, et al. Mesenchymal cell-based repair of large, full-thickness defects of articular cartilage. *J Bone Joint Surg* 1994;76:579–592.

528. Wan LQ, Miller C, Guo XE, et al. Fixed electrical charges and mobile ions affect the measurable mechano-electrochemical properties of charged-hydrated biological tissues: the articular cartilage paradigm. *Mech Chem Biosys* 2004;1:81–99.

529. Wang CB, Hung CT, Mow VC. An analysis of the effects of depth-dependent aggregate modulus on articular cartilage stress-relaxation behavior in compression. *J Biomech* 2001;34:75–84.

530. Wang CC, Chahine NO, Hung CT, et al. Optical determination of anisotropic material properties of bovine articular cartilage in compression. *J Biomech* 2003;36:339–353.

531. Warman ML, Abbott M, Apte SS, et al. A type X collagen mutation causes Schmid metaphyseal chondrodysplasia. *Nat Genet* 1993;5:79–82.

532. Watanabe H, Kimata K, Line S, et al. Mouse cartilage matrix deficiency (cmd) caused by a 7 bp deletion in the aggrecan gene. *Nat Genet* 1994;7:154–157.

533. Weiss C, Rosenberg L, Helfet AJ. An ultrastructural study of normal young adult human articular cartilage. *J Bone Joint Surg* 1968;50:663–674.

534. Williams PL. *Gray's anatomy.* New York: Churchill Livingston, 1995.

535. Williamson AK, Chen AC, Masuda K, et al. Tensile mechanical properties of bovine articular cartilage: variations with growth and relationships to collagen network components. *J Orthop Res* 2003;21:872–880.

536. Wong M, Siegrist M, Cao X. Cyclic compression of articular cartilage explants is associated with progressive consolidation and altered expression pattern of extracellular matrix proteins. *Matrix Biol* 1999;18:391–399.

537. Woo SL, Akeson WH, Jemmott GF. Measurements of nonhomogeneous, directional mechanical properties of articular cartilage in tension. *J Biomech* 1976;9:785–791.

538. Woo SL, Simon BR, Kuei SC, et al. Quasi-linear viscoelastic properties of normal articular cartilage. *J Biomech Eng* 1980;102:85–90.

539. Woo SL, Mow VC, Lai WM. Biomechanical properties of articular cartilage. In: Skalak R, Chien S, eds. *Handbook of bioengineering.* New York: McGraw-Hill, 1987:4.1–4.44.

540. Woods VL Jr, Schreck PJ, Gesink DS, et al. Integrin expression by human articular chondrocytes. *Arthritis Rheum* 1994;37:537–544.

541. Wozney JM, Rosen V. Bone morphogenetic protein and bone morphogenetic protein gene family in bone formation and repair. *Clin Orthop* 1998;26–37.

542. Wright MO, Nishida K, Bavington C, et al. Hyperpolarisation of cultured human chondrocytes following cyclical pressure-induced strain: evidence of a role for alpha 5 beta 1 integrin as a chondrocyte mechanoreceptor. *J Orthop Res* 1997;15:742–747.

543. Wu JJ, Woods PE, Eyre DR. Identification of cross-linking sites in bovine cartilage type IX collagen reveals an antiparallel type II–type IX molecular relationship and type IX to type IX bonding. *J Biol Chem* 1992;267:23007–23014.

544. Xu T, Bianco P, Fisher LW, et al. Targeted disruption of the biglycan gene leads to an osteoporosis-like phenotype in mice. *Nat Genet* 1998;20:78–82.

545. Yamauchi M, Mechanic G. Cross-linking of collagen. In: Nimni ME, ed. *Collagen: biochemistry.* Boca Raton, FL: CRC Press, 1988:157–172.

546. Yasui K. Three-dimensional architecture of human normal mensci. *J Jpn Orthop Assoc* 1978;52:391–399.

547. Zhu W, Lai WM, Mow VC. Intrinsic quasilinear viscoelastic behavior of the extracellular matrix of cartilage. *Trans Orthop Res Soc* 1986;11:407.

548. Zhu W, Mow VC, Lai WM, et al. Influence of composition, size and structure of cartilage proteoglycans on the strength of molecular network formed in solution. *Trans Orthop Res Soc* 1988;13:67.

549. Zhu W, Lai WM, Mow VC. The density and strength of proteoglycan–proteoglycan interaction sites in concentrated solutions. *J Biomech* 1991;24:1007–1018.

550. Zhu W, Mow VC, Koob TJ, et al. Viscoelastic shear properties of articular cartilage and the effects of glycosidase treatments. *J Orthop Res* 1993;11:771–781.

551. Zhu W, Chern KY, Mow VC. Anisotropic viscoelastic shear properties of bovine meniscus. *Clin Orthop* 1994;34–45.

552. Zhu W, Mow VC, Rosenberg LC, et al. Determinations of kinetic changes of aggrecan–hyaluronan interactions in solution from its rheological properties. *J Biomech* 1994;27:571–579.

553. Zhu W, Iatridis JC, Hlibczuk V, et al. Determination of collagen–proteoglycan interactions in vitro. *J Biomech* 1996;29:773–783.

PHYSICAL REGULATION OF CARTILAGE METABOLISM

FARSHID GUILAK
CLARK T. HUNG

1 INTRODUCTION

Under normal physiological conditions, articular cartilage provides a nearly frictionless surface for the transmission and distribution of joint loads, exhibiting little or no wear over decades of use (219,221) (also see Chapter 10 for more details on friction, lubrication, and wear of articular cartilage). These unique properties of cartilage are determined by the structure and composition of the fluid-filled extracellular matrix (ECM). The fluid component consists primarily of water with dissolved solutes and mobile ions (184). The solid material of the ECM is composed largely of collagen (mainly type II) and polyanionic glycosaminoglycans that are covalently attached to a core protein to form aggrecan, which in turn is stabilized as proteoglycan aggregates (120,195,223) (also see Chapter 5 on articular cartilage and meniscus for more details). The remainder of the solid matrix includes smaller amounts of other collagens, proteoglycans, proteins, and glycoproteins.

The composition and structure of articular cartilage is maintained through a balance of the anabolic and catabolic activities of the chondrocyte cell population, which comprises a small fraction of the tissue volume (300,301). Chondrocyte activity is controlled not only by biochemical factors (e.g., growth factors, cytokines, and hormones), but also by physical factors such as joint loading. Chondrocytes are able to perceive and respond to signals generated by the normal load-bearing activities of daily living, such as walking and running (125). The physical mechanisms involved in this transduction process potentially involve mechanical, chemical, and electrical signals. Joint loading produces deformation of the cartilage layer, and associated changes in the mechanical environment of the cell within the ECM, such as spatially varying tensile, compressive, and shear stresses and strains (219). In addition, the presence of a large fluid phase containing mobile ions, as well as a high density of negatively charged proteoglycans in the solid matrix (i.e., fixed charge density (FCD)), gives rise to coupled electrical and chemical phenomena during joint loading (79,99,168). The ability of the chondrocytes to regulate their metabolic activity in response to the mechanical, electrical, or chemical signals of their physical environment provides a means by which articular cartilage can alter its structure and composition to the physical demands of the body. In this sense, the mechanical environment of the chondrocytes plays a major role in the health and function of the diarthrodial joint (125,238–241,323).

A number of different approaches have been used to decipher the role of physical stimuli in regulating cartilage and chondrocyte activity, ranging from *in vivo* studies to experiments at the cell and molecular level (125,303,323). Each level of study provides specific advantages and disadvantages. *In vivo* animal studies based on emulating the physiological relevant loading conditions provide a means to study long-term (i.e., weeks to years) tissue changes associated with growth, remodeling, or aging (215,252). These studies are limited, however, by the difficulties in determining the precise loading history within the joint and on the articular cartilage. Further, such studies may be complicated by the effect of systemic factors or local soluble mediators (e.g., hormones, cytokines, enzymes), which are difficult to control *in vivo*. These confounding effects make it difficult to relate specific mechanical stimuli directly to the biological response within the joint.

At the next level, *in vitro* studies on the regulation of chondrocyte metabolism provide a system where both the applied loading and biochemical environment of the chondrocyte can be better controlled over time periods generally ranging from hours up to several months. These studies have used a variety of model systems (323), including cartilage explants and isolated chondrocytes grown in three-dimensional (3D) matrices. In explant cultures, the chondrocytes maintain their differentiated phenotype, and interactions between the cells and the ECM that are naturally present in articular cartilage are also maintained (17,297,304). These and other studies have provided information on the relationships between matrix loading and chondrocyte anabolic and catabolic activities. However, the presence of the dense ECM generates physical signals associated with applied stress or strain, which vary markedly in space and time (113, 219,221,222). Chondrocytes that are cultured in a 3D matrix such as agarose, also tend to retain their phenotype in terms of aggrecan and collagen synthesis (17,56,131,304), and allow for a means to assess the role of the ECM in transducing physical stimuli and inducing metabolic responses. However, the loading of an explant or artificial matrix in a controlled and isolated manner *in vitro* (e.g., uniaxial compression) will not completely reproduce the *in vivo* environment of the chondrocytes. It is difficult, therefore, to extrapolate information to physiologically relevant situations characteristic of daily living in an intact joint. Furthermore, many of the biophysical phenomena that the chondrocytes are exposed to, and to which they respond, cannot be uncoupled in most *in situ* configurations (29, 222).

Studies at the cellular level are the most useful for examining involvement of single pathways of signal transduction (303), or for isolating the effects of a single biophysical stimulus (e.g., osmotic or hydrostatic pressure, pH, deformation). Studies of isolated chondrocytes in monolayer culture allow for direct stimulation of cells as well as rapid isolation of cells for analysis. However, in such cultures, chondrocytes tend to dedifferentiate and lose the chondrocyte phenotype (17,131). As with explant studies, single-cell systems are further removed from the *in vivo* situation and they present significant difficulties in extrapolating results to a physiologically relevant condition.

It is important to take into account the advantages and limitations associated with experimental models at each level and to evaluate the implications of the results from each of these different systems. Taken together, these culture systems have allowed a variety of studies of the mechanisms by which physical forces may regulate chondrocyte metabolism at the molecular, cellular, tissue, and organ levels.

In this chapter, we present a review of the effects of various physical factors on articular cartilage chondrocytes in three model systems: *in vivo* human and animal studies, *in vitro* 3D culture systems, and *in vitro* two-dimensional (2D) cell culture systems. The primary mechanism for altering the physical environment of cartilage *in vivo* is through joint. Therefore, studies of chondrocyte response to physical stimulus seek to examine the role of mechanical strains, stresses, pressures, fluid flows, electric fields (currents and potentials), and altered solute transport properties, individually or in combination, as all these aspects necessarily relate to the natural loading condition in the joint. Together, these studies present us with a broad range of understanding of chondrocyte behavior, and its interactions with its native environment. This information, in turn, provides the basis for ongoing and future studies of cell-based repair and remodeling mechanisms for maintaining the healthy and normal function of articular cartilage. Moreover, knowledge gained from such basic science studies of cartilage mechanical signal transduction provides the underlying framework for efforts aimed at the functional tissue engineering of articular cartilage (36,114).

2 *IN VIVO* STUDIES OF CARTILAGE RESPONSE TO LOAD

In the 19th century, it was generally believed that articular cartilage was inert and without structure (51,327). However, by the turn of the century, many investigators had hypothesized that articular cartilage not only had form and structure, but also that changes in the normal physical environment of the joint could alter the composition and morphology of the tissue (for more details see Chapter 5) [125,297]). By the mid-20th century, it was suggested that specific relationships existed between the structural characteristics and functional history of articular cartilage, and with increased knowledge of the composition and structure of cartilage, investigators began to hypothesize how these properties may be affected by alterations in the mechanical environment *in vivo*. Further, it was suggested that physiological loading was necessary for the proper maintenance of the joint, and that deviations from normal loading patterns could be a source of significant joint degeneration (27,72,125,158,277,297,308).

A number of more recent *in vivo* investigations have been undertaken to examine the effects of altering the normal pattern of joint loading using models of disuse and immobilization, overuse, impact loading, and joint "instability" (215,252). These studies have provided strong evidence that "abnormal" joint loading can significantly affect the composition, structure, metabolic activity, and mechanical properties of articular cartilage and other joint tissues.

For example, disuse of the joint, achieved through immobilization, casting, or muscle transection, may result in changes in cartilage composition and mechanical behavior that are characteristic of degeneration. Important changes observed in the cartilage include a loss of proteoglycans and changes in proteoglycan molecular conformation, a decrease in cartilage thickness, and material property changes including a decreased compressive stiffness and increased tensile stiffness (16,27,40,151–153,224,238–240, 268,269,287,288,306,329). In addition, there is direct evidence of decreased proteoglycan and collagen biosynthesis and elevated levels of metalloproteinases suggesting an altered metabolic balance following periods of unloading and disuse in both human and experimental animal tissue (40,100,238,306,307,329). Many of these changes are localized to specific sites and depths in the cartilage layer, and some of these changes have been shown to be partly reversible with remobilization of the joint (152,161,238).

In contrast to studies of joint disuse, moderate exercise seems to have few deleterious effects on the cartilage, and has been shown to increase proteoglycan content, reduce the extractability of proteoglycans, and increase the cartilage thickness (150,151,159,171). More strenuous exercise has been shown to cause site-specific changes in proteoglycan content and cartilage stiffness, although it is not clear that these changes affect cartilage function (153,160).

Experimental models of altered joint loading have been developed for studies of cartilage degeneration in response to observations for natural degeneration in the human joint following traumatic loading, joint instability, or isolated injury. These studies have provided a means for tracking the time sequence of events in cartilage that occurs with degeneration, and also an important tool for isolating aging changes from the degenerative process of osteoarthritis (OA). In one experimental model of joint degeneration, an impact load delivered to the joint (i.e., a rapid increase of force across the joint) has been shown to cause both immediate and progressive damage to the articular cartilage (6,57,233,259,260,309,328). These studies have utilized single or repetitive impact loading to emulate different loading conditions in the human related to injury or repetitive daily activity, respectively. In studies of the canine or porcine patellofemoral joint following isolated impact, cartilage changes included altered cellular activity and histological appearance, and increased hydration and proteoglycan content within 2 weeks after loading (6,57). Subfracture impact loads also cause a significant decrease in the tensile stiffness of the surface zone cartilage, but no detectable changes in either the compressive modulus or hydraulic permeability of the full-thickness cartilage (6). Impact loading to the articular surface can be expected to produce a combination of tensile, compressive and shear stresses and strains, as well as very high hydrostatic pressure (6). The mechanical environment during and following impact or injurious compression can be expected to vary significantly with depth in the cartilage layer (43, 47,57,143,144,255). These studies suggest that changes in the mechanical environment due to impact loads delivered to the cartilage layer may serve as a cellular signal that alters cell viability and biosynthetic activities in a manner that will modify tissue composition and mechanical behavior.

Damage to the pericapsular and intracapsular soft tissues, such as ligaments and menisci, has often been observed to produce degenerative changes in the knee joint under both clinical and experimental conditions. Alterations in the mechanisms of force attenuation in the joint, such as occurs with meniscal or ligamentous injuries, will alter the magnitude and distribution of forces applied to the cartilage layers *in vivo*. It has been well documented that the clinical phenomena of "joint laxity" and "joint instability" leads to alterations in contact areas and stresses (165,183), and therefore, surgical destabilization of the joint has been used as an animal model to study the effects of altered joint loading on cartilage degeneration (3,27,38,59, 77,93,110,127,172,206,207,214,235,249,285, 287,288,290,302).

Transection of the anterior cruciate ligament has been the most widely used model for studying degenerative changes in articular cartilage that occur following "destabilization" of the joint (3,27,38,59,93,110,206,207,214, 235,249,285,287,302). This model has been studied by Brandt and co-workers over an extended time course of 54 months, and has been found to produce degenerative changes in the joint very similar to those of human OA (27). In general, morphologic and histologic changes include fibrillation of the articular surface, loss of proteoglycan content and collagen fibril organization, regional changes (increased or decreased) of cellularity, meniscal changes, and joint capsule thickening. Compositional and metabolic changes include an increase in water content, increased rates of proteoglycan and collagen synthesis, decreased concentration of collagen cross links, decreased content of hyaluronan, and alterations in the number and size of proteoglycan aggregates (38,59,71,110, 194,206,224,264,279). These compositional and structural changes are accompanied by distinct changes in the biomechanical properties of the articular cartilage, including a decrease in the tensile, compressive, and shear moduli, increased evidence of swelling behavior, and

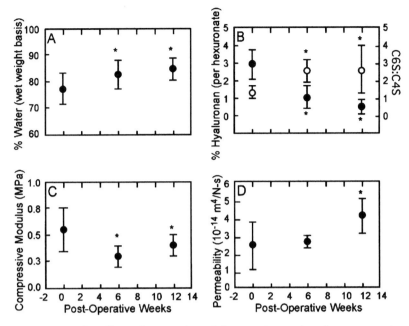

FIGURE 6-1. The effect of transection of the anterior cruciate ligament on the composition and properties of canine articular cartilage. Data are shown for changes in **(A)** water content, **(B)** hyaluronate (closed circles) and GAG composition (ratio of chondroitin 6 to chondroitin 4 sulfates; open circles), **(C)** compressive modulus, and **(D)** hydraulic permeability of canine cartilage following transection of the anterior cruciate ligament. Data are presented as mean ± SD, * = significantly different from control by a Student Neuman-Keul's test. All data were measured in full-thickness cartilage from covered regions of the tibial plateau of the operated knee. Increased hydration and changes in proteoglycan content and structure are known to contribute to the observed changes in the compressive behavior of articular cartilage. (Adapted with permission from Muller FJ, Setton LA, Manicourt DH, et al. Centrifugal and biochemical comparison of proteoglycan aggregates from articular cartilage in experimental joint disuse and joint instability. *J Orthop Res* 1994;12: 498–508 and, Setton LA, Mow VC, Muller FJ, et al. Mechanical properties of canine articular cartilage are significantly altered following transection of the anterior cruciate ligament. *J Orthop Res* 1994;12:451–463).

increased hydraulic permeability of the tissue (3,88,110,285,287) (Fig. 6-1).

Surgical resection of the meniscus has also proved to be a valuable experimental system for studying altered joint loading, and cartilage degeneration, in a number of animal models (7,77,127,142,214,290). Degenerative changes following meniscectomy are observed in the articular cartilage, including signs of cartilage fibrillation (i.e., a roughening of the cartilage surface as collagen fiber bundles become frayed), increased hydration and decreased proteoglycan content of the ECM, and elevated collagen and proteoglycan synthesis rates (19,77,127,191,290). In addition, changes in the mechanical behavior of the cartilage layer have been observed, including alterations in the magnitude of streaming potentials and changes in both the compressive and tensile properties (66,127,172,181). As with the experimental models of impact loading or ligament transection, it is unclear what specific role is played by the chondrocytes in eliciting these changes in the composition and mechanical behavior of the ECM. The changes in biosynthetic rates provide indirect evidence that altered physical and/or biological factors following meniscectomy-induced chondrocyte activity.

Recent studies suggest that changes in the mechanical loading history of the cartilage caused by loss of joint congruity due to a "step-off" defect may also lead to progressive joint degeneration. Twenty weeks after the creation of 3-mm-wide sagittal defect displaced 5 mm from the joint surface, rabbit knee joints exhibited progressive osteoarthritic changes such as osteophytes, cartilage fibrillation, hypocellularity, and severe loss of safranin-O staining (179). A similar defect, displaced 2 mm from the joint surface, showed cartilaginous and bony repair and resulted in closure of the surgical defect with restoration of femoral congruity and did not lead to progressive degeneration (180).

In all of these experimental *in vivo* models, it has been observed that the articular cartilage chondrocytes exhibit altered biologic activity following changes in the joint loading history. These *in vivo* studies emphasize the relationship between joint loading and the function of articular cartilage, and suggest that the chondrocyte population plays an active role in maintaining this relationship. It is important to note that a critical level, and manner of joint loading, is required to provide physical signals to the chondrocyte, which will, in turn, maintain the composition, material properties, and mechanical function of the cartilage ECM. Although these studies demonstrate important characteristics of chondrocyte function *in vivo,* they also point to the many unknowns in the chondrocyte-matrix relationship. Related studies are needed to determine the detailed nature of the metabolic response of the chondrocyte to physical signals, as well as the precise relationships between isolated factors of mechanical loading and specific physical signaling mechanisms.

3 AGGRECAN METABOLISM AND GENE EXPRESSION IN CARTILAGE EXPLANTS AND CHONDROCYTE CULTURES

With the knowledge that the loading history of the joint has an important influence on health of articular cartilage, considerable research effort has been directed toward understanding the processes by which physical signals are converted to a biochemical signal by the chondrocyte population (i.e., the mechanical signal transduction process). Clarification of the specific signaling mechanisms in cartilage would not only provide a better understanding of the processes that regulate normal and pathological cartilage physiology, but would also be expected to yield new insights on the pathogenesis of joint disease.

Studies of cartilage in an *in vitro* system allow for control of sample geometry, physical environment, and biochemical environment, so that changes in metabolic activity can be correlated with physical phenomena that can be either measured directly or predicted by theoretical models (113,221,333,344). Because load-induced physical phenomena in cartilage consist of time-averaged and time-varying components, studies are naturally divided into those that examine the metabolic responses during one or a combination of the following conditions: (a) prolonged static loading; (b) the onset or release of a load, and (c) cyclic or intermittent ("dynamic") loading. The use of alternative mechanical, electrical, and physicochemical test protocols, such as imposed displacements or hydrostatic or osmotic pressures, or application of electrical fields or current densities, have been used to assess the regulatory effects of specific static or cyclic physical signals on chondrocyte metabolism.

Experimental studies of the physical regulation of cartilage matrix metabolism have focused primarily on the large aggregating proteoglycan, aggrecan (120,223). The regulation of aggrecan metabolism is of particular interest because of the contribution of aggrecan to the critical load-bearing functions of articular cartilage, including compressive and shear behaviors, hydraulic permeability, and hydration of the ECM (154,200,219,222,258,351). The maintenance of aggrecan in the ECM is a dynamic process and dependent on the coordinated synthesis, assembly, and degradation of this macromolecule. This is in contrast to the relatively slow turnover of the collagen macromolecule *in vivo* (195,201,203). In the following sections, the regulation of aggrecan biosynthesis by physical factors is reviewed as one measure of chondrocyte activity in *in vitro* culture systems.

The effects of physical factors on aggrecan metabolism have been studied extensively by examining the incorporation and release of radiolabeled sulfate using pulse-chase techniques (201). In such studies, ^{35}S-sulfate is included in the culture medium prior to, during, or following application of the physical stimulus. Because sulfate is a relatively small anion, it diffuses quickly through the matrix where it rapidly equilibrates with intracellular sulfate pools and is incorporated primarily into the glycosaminoglycans of newly synthesized aggrecan (121,200). Although aggrecan turnover does occur, the quantity of sulfate reutilized from degraded glycosaminoglycan is small compared with the utilization of sulfate from the extracellular medium. Therefore, the kinetics of ^{35}S-sulfate incorporation into macromolecules, and the subsequent release of ^{35}S, is highly indicative of aggrecan

metabolism. To examine the effects of various physical factors on aggrecan metabolism, radio-label incorporation studies have been performed in each of the *in vitro* culture systems discussed above—explant cultures, chondrocytes in 3D matrices, and isolated cell culture systems. Complementary studies of aggrecan gene expression and transcriptional regulation have also been performed in these culture systems using polymerase chain reaction (PCR) and reporter gene assays.

3.1 Static Compression

In studies of cartilage explants, static compression has been shown to produce a dose-dependent inhibition of proteoglycan synthesis (30,96,97,109,148,155,273,283,316,341) (Figs. 6-2 and 6-3). In studies where tissue

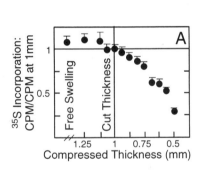
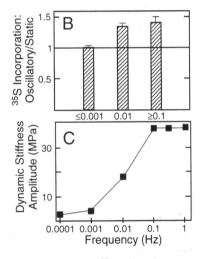

FIGURE 6-2. Effect of static and oscillatory compression on ^{35}S-sulfate incorporation (as a measure of aggrecan synthesis rates) into discs of articular cartilage. **A:** Discs were radiolabeled during 12 hours of static compression. Incorporation is expressed relative to discs held at 1 mm (the original cartilage thickness). Static compression showed a dose-dependent decrease in the rate of ^{35}S-sulfate incorporation. Data are expressed as mean ± SEM (*n* = 9–12). **B:** Discs were radiolabeled during the last 8 hours of 23 hours of oscillatory compression protocols. Experimental discs were statically compressed to a thickness of 1 mm with a superimposed oscillatory strain of 1% to 2% at frequencies of 0.0001–1.0 Hz; controls were statically compressed at 1 mm. A significant increase in the rate of ^{35}S-sulfate incorporation was observed at frequencies of 0.01 Hz and higher. Incorporation data are expressed as oscillatory/static (*n* = 12–72). **C:** Dynamic stiffness amplitude was measured during oscillatory compression experiments. (Adapted with permission from Sah RL, Grodzinsky AJ, Plaas AHK, et al. Effects of static and dynamic compression on matrix metabolism in cartilage explants. In: Kuettner KE, Schleyerbach R, Peyron JG, et al., eds. *Articular cartilage and osteoarthritis.* New York: Raven Press, 1992:373–392).

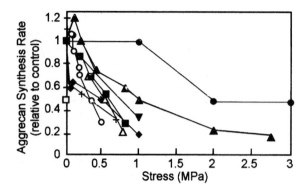

	Stimulus	Duration	Tissue	Ref.
●	mech. comp.	6 hrs	calf AC	148
□	mech. comp.	2 hrs	dog AC	241
■	osmotic press.	4 hrs	human AC	283
△	mech. comp.	4 hrs	human AC	283
▲	mech. comp.	12 hrs	calf EP	96
○	mech. comp.	12 hrs	calf AC	273
▼	mech. comp.	28 hrs	calf AC	173
+	mech. comp.	24 hrs	dog AC	30
◆	mech. comp.	24 hrs	calf AC	109

FIGURE 6-3. Summary of the effects of different magnitudes of static physical stimuli (mechanical and osmotic) on aggrecan synthesis rates as measured by the rate of ^{35}S-sulfate incorporation. Data are expressed relative to control studies. Nearly all studies show a trend of decreasing aggrecan synthesis rates with increasing stress. AC, articular cartilage; EP, epiphyseal plate cartilage. (Adapted with permission from Gray ML, Pizzanelli AM, Lee RC, et al. Kinetics of the chondrocyte biosynthetic response to compressive load and release. *Biochim Biophys Acta* 1989;991:415–425).

compression is maintained for at least several hours and as long as several days, the magnitude of the biosynthetic inhibition is relatively stable. Furthermore, the inhibition of aggrecan synthesis within different zones of immature articular cartilage appears to be similarly affected by various levels of applied stress (109). Static compression of cylindrical cartilage explants will generate stresses and strains in the solid matrix of articular cartilage, and a decrease in cartilage hydration, or an increase in the solid volume fraction of the ECM (184,216). These changes are associated with an increase in the density of matrix-associated negative charges, or fixed charge density, which produce an altered osmotic and ionic environment within the ECM and surrounding the cell (96,168,200,318). Although transient changes in hydrostatic pressure may occur shortly after loading (5,8,11,113, 218,298), the pressure will equilibrate with the external environment for long times after loading, so that the long-term effects of osmotic pressure changes are presumed to dominate over hydrostatic pressure changes. Because a similar inhibition has been observed by mechanical

compression of cartilage explants or by incubation of cartilage explants in medium containing osmotically active solutes such as polyethylene glycol (283,317,318), the inhibition of biosynthesis by static compression is predominantly associated with tissue consolidation and the associated osmotic effects.[1] Nutrient and waste product transport limitations due to compression, i.e., decrease of permeability and diffusivity (102,167,216–219,222), may be a cause for these inhibition effects.

The contributory role of the cartilage ECM in chondrocyte signaling has been elucidated by studies of cartilage chondrocytes in 3D hydrogel matrices such as agarose, alginate, and type I collagen (31,136,262). In addition, because the depth-dependent variation of biochemical and material properties (112,281,282) gives rise to a complex environment around chondrocytes in situ that makes it difficult to study

---

[1] It should be noted, however, that mechanical loading in general does not produce the same internal fluid pressure as osmotic loading (171). It is therefore difficult to make direct comparisons between the results of these two types of biosynthesis studies.

chondrocyte response with specificity, thus cell encapsulation in these matrices permits study of chondrocyte mechanical signal transduction in a homogeneous physiologic environment prior to matrix elaboration (163,174,221). In these studies, static compression resulted in an inhibition of biosynthesis similar to that observed in cartilage explants, but only after prolonged culture in which a proteoglycan-rich ECM had formed (31,262). At earlier times of culture, static compression did not alter biosynthesis, providing further support for the notion that the biosynthesis changes that occur with static compression are due to the associated longer-term osmotic effects or development of cell-matrix interactions (e.g., integrin attachment [187,188]).

In studies of cartilage under compression, the regulatory roles of a number of physical factors have been examined, such as matrix stresses or strains, altered electrostatic effects, and decreased hydration or increased solid volume fraction (i.e., associated with a decrease in apparent porosity). One factor that has been discounted as a major regulatory factor in short-term, *in vitro* experiments is the hindered transport of nutrients or regulatory molecules to the chondrocytes during compression (102,167,216–219,222). Evidence for this stems from the findings that the dose-dependent inhibition of aggrecan biosynthesis is not sensitive to sample dimensions, and therefore, the available pathway for diffusion and fluid convection transport of regulatory molecules. This finding applies to compression of cartilage test samples of various dimensions, ranging from thin slices of cartilage (200–400 μm), and large cartilage explants ($\sim$5 mm diameter), to full thickness cartilage from the human femoral head (97,148, 155,283). Recent studies suggest, however, a possible role for transport limitations of relatively large molecular weight solutes through the ECM in mediating the biological response of chondrocytes to cartilage compression (256). Furthermore, matrix consolidation that decreases diffusion and convection through the matrix (102,167,216–219,222), may be the cause of a decrease of release of proteoglycans from articular cartilage during prolonged cyclic loading that involves a "static" offset (311).

Studies have also indicated that articular cartilage chondrocytes can respond to short-term compressive loads by transiently up-regulating expression of the aggrecan gene (11,261,321). Interestingly, Valhmu and co-workers reported that long-term compression did not significantly alter aggrecan mRNA levels, suggesting that previously observed inhibitory effects of prolonged static compression on proteoglycan synthesis in articular cartilage may be, for the most part, mediated through mechanisms other than suppression of aggrecan mRNA levels (321). Ragan and co-workers reported that aggrecan and type II collagen mRNA expression increased during the initial 0.5 hours of static compression; however, 4 to 24 hours after compression was applied, total mRNA levels had significantly decreased. The synthesis of aggrecan and collagen protein decreased more rapidly than did mRNA levels after the application of a step compression (261). The nature of loading (i.e., the boundary conditions) as well as any compositional or material property inhomogeneity of the tissue properties define the spatial and time-varying stimuli that arise in cartilage explant and chondrocyte-seeded matrices following mechanical loading (106,107,219,221,222,333,335). Using quantitative autoradiography techniques (32), the biosynthetic activity of chondrocytes has been shown to be correlated with the local strain environment in statically loaded explants (254,340).

3.2 Compression and Release

The biosynthetic responses of cartilage to an applied compression are different after application and removal of the static load (i.e., during the loading and unloading stage). The time course of the inhibitory effect of compression occurs within several hours of mechanical equilibration (97,273). However, the release of an applied static compression has more variable effects on subsequent proteoglycan synthesis (30,97,109,148,155,241,273). The release of a relatively low level of compressive load may result in the return of suppressed proteoglycan synthetic rates to uncompressed control levels (96,109,173). However, the release of a somewhat higher level of compressive load can lead to a stimulation of proteoglycan biosynthesis to levels higher than that of unloaded control samples (30,109,273). Finally, the application and then release of extremely high levels of compression (~50% or 1 MPa) may require a prolonged duration for proteoglycan synthesis rates to return to unloaded control levels or, alternatively, may result in cell death (30,109). A variable effect of release from static compression has also been reported for chondrocyte-seeded type I collagen matrices (136). Interestingly, step hypertonic loading of cultured chondrocytes induced suppression of aggrecan promoter activity, which was followed by increased activity upon reintroduction of isotonic conditions (237).

3.3 Osmotic Pressure

Proteoglycan synthesis rates have been shown to be maximal when the osmolality of the extracellular media matches the in situ osmolality of cartilage (350–450 mOsmol), suggesting that the normal interstitial environment is optimal for maintaining chondrocyte activity (317,318). These findings are consistent with earlier studies that have shown that the composition of the matrix (e.g., proteoglycan concentration) exerts a strong influence on chondrocyte biosynthetic activity (117,119,278).

In studies of static compression, the regulatory roles of physicochemical factors, such as pH, FCD, and osmotic pressure, appear to predominate over the transient mechanical or electrokinetic factors such as hydrostatic pressure, interstitial fluid-flow, or streaming potential. The role of the extracellular ionic environment has been examined by comparing the biosynthetic response of explants subjected to compression with the response to alterations in the extracellular ion composition or osmotic pressure in the absence of mechanical loading (96,283, 316,317). Cartilage explants that were placed under osmotic pressure using various concentrations of polyethylene glycol showed similar decreases in aggrecan synthesis rates to those placed under static compression (283). Although the two loading conditions do not produce identi-

cal pressures and deformations (169), both osmotic and mechanical stress also resulted in a similar decrease in tissue water content, suggesting that factors related to hydration were responsible for the observed effects. As in the application of mechanical stress, osmotic loading gives rise to non-uniform strains in cartilage that are dependent on the distribution of FCD and material properties within the tissue (227,289,333, 334).

In other studies, biosynthesis has been found to be inhibited by increasing the hydrogen ion concentration (decreasing the pH) and reducing the concentration of bicarbonate (96,338), suggesting a pH-mediated inhibition of biosynthesis. More recent data indicate differing dynamics of pH-induced and mechanically induced changes in biosynthesis, suggesting that pH is not the persisting mechanism in this process (25,26). It is possible that local changes in FCD are sufficient to cause these changes in pH, despite the relatively high intracellular buffering capacity of chondrocytes (337). Biosynthesis may also be inhibited by deviations in the extracellular osmotic pressure from the normal value of the cartilage matrix. The osmotic pressure in cartilage has been altered by incubation of explants in dilute or concentrated media (316) or by the addition of sodium chloride (315). Direct osmotic compression of the chondrocytes within cartilage by the addition of sucrose to the bathing media has been shown to modulate chondrocyte biosynthesis as well (317).

3.4 Hydrostatic Pressure

The role of hydrostatic pressure as a physical factor in modulating cartilage biosynthesis can be isolated for study, because physiological levels of hydrostatic pressure can be applied without inducing confounding physical factors such as fluid flow, electrokinetic effects, or cell deformation. High pressures, up to those estimated to occur *in vivo*, have been shown to modulate proteoglycan biosynthesis depending on the amplitude, frequency, and duration of pressurization. Continuous pressures of <3 MPa do not generally affect aggrecan biosynthesis (116,157), although other studies show variable effects in this pressure range (185). During the application of higher pressures for 2 hours (116), aggrecan biosynthesis depended on the amplitude of pressure. In these studies, pressures of 5–10 MPa were found to stimulate synthesis relative to non-pressure control samples, although higher pressures of 30–50 MPa were found to inhibit biosynthesis. The application of a single pulse of pressure of 10–20 MPa for only 20 seconds stimulated aggrecan biosynthesis in the subsequent two hours, but did not markedly alter synthesis at lower pressures or 50 MPa of pressure. The frequency of applied load appears important because pressure of 5 MPa applied at 0.5 Hz has been found to stimulate biosynthesis, while lower frequencies of pressurization (0.017–0.25 Hz) did not affect biosynthesis (242).

High-density primary cultures of bovine chondrocytes exposed to hydrostatic pressure applied intermittently at 1 Hz or constantly for 4 hours at 10 MPa (294) increased aggrecan mRNA, and constant pressure decreased type II collagen mRNA when bathed in serum-free medium. In the presence of 1% fetal bovine serum, intermittent pressure increased aggrecan and type II collagen mRNA, whereas constant pressure had no effect on either mRNA. In studies using the same hydrostatic pressure regimen applied for 4 hours/day for 4 days (295), type II collagen mRNA exhibited a biphasic pattern, approximately 5-fold at 4 and 8 hours that subsequently decreased by 24 hours. In contrast, aggrecan mRNA signals increased progressively 3-fold throughout the loading period. Application of intermittent loading increased type II collagen 9-fold and aggrecan 20-fold, when compared with unloaded cultures.

In early studies of embryonic epiphyseal chick cartilage, intermittent pressures of 0.01–0.02 MPa applied for an extended period were shown to stimulate chondrocyte growth and proteoglycan biosynthesis (162,324). In these studies, hydrostatic pressurization was achieved through a pressurized gas phase, which also resulted in preferential stimulation of cartilage explants from osteoarthritic tissue but not normal articular cartilage (166). However, because these hydrostatic pressures were applied via a gas phase, it may be that changes in the concentration of dissolved

gas, rather than pressure itself, were the stimulatory signal.

3.5 Cyclic and Intermittent Compression

Cyclic and intermittent compression of cartilage explants and chondrocyte-seeded 3D agarose matrices can produce a range of effects depending on the characteristics of the loading conditions, such as the loading amplitude and frequency (30,31,155,164,173,236,241,242,273, 325) (Fig. 6-4). In contrast to static compression, physical factors that may regulate the biosynthetic response to cyclic compression are related to time-varying behaviors, including fluid flow, electric fields, matrix stresses and strains, hydrostatic pressure, and cellular deformations (31,155,168,216–219,221,222,273).

Theoretical analyses of cylindrical cartilage explants in the unconfined compression configuration (5,156) have been performed for the condition of a time-varying compressive load applied to the explant through two impermeable platens, as is frequently the case in *in vitro* culture systems. For these precise loading conditions, the magnitude of the physical phenomena is predicted to vary with position within the disk and also with the frequency of applied compression (5,106,113,156). At very low frequencies, the ECM may be axially compressed in a radially uniform manner with minimal fluid pressurization. With increasing compression frequency, the magnitude of the fluid velocity and streaming potential increases at the disc periphery (near the tissue-bath solution interface) while the hydrostatic pressure increases near the center of the disc. In addition, at the higher frequencies, cyclic changes in cell shape and volume may vary with radial position. In some cases, it may be difficult to distinguish between the effects of signals associated with cyclic compression, with time-averaged signals associated with a time-averaged compression, particularly in studies where frequency and amplitude of the load is varied without controlling the time-averaged load (173,241). Nevertheless, a number of studies using a variety of cyclic compression conditions have suggested a potential

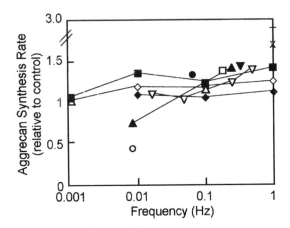

	Stimulus	Duration	Stress or Strain	Tissue	Ref.
X	tension	8 hrs	10%	chick embr. chond.	178
○	mech. comp.	2 hrs	1-11 kPa	dog AC	241
●	mech comp.	2 hrs	5.5 kPa	human AC	241
□	mech. comp.	24 hrs	5.5%	chick EP cells	54
▣	mech. comp.	23 hrs	1-5%	calf AC	273
▲	mech. comp.	28 hrs	1.0 MPa	calf AC	173
▼	mech. comp.	7 days	0.2 MPa	calf AC	164
▽	mech. comp.	1.5 hrs	0.5 MPa	cow AC	242
△	mech. comp.	23 hrs	4-7%	calf AC	155
◆	mech. comp.	10 hrs*	3%	calf chond.	31
◇	mech. comp.	10 hrs**	3%	calf chond.	31

FIGURE 6-4. Summary of the effects of different frequencies of cyclic (dynamic) mechanical stimuli on aggrecan synthesis rates as measured by the rate of ^{35}S-sulfate incorporation. Nearly all studies show a trend of increasing synthesis rates with increasing loading frequency. AC, articular cartilage; EP, epiphyseal plate cartilage; * tests were performed 2 days following seeding of chondrocytes in agarose gel; ** tests were performed 41 days following seeding of chondrocytes in agarose gel. (Adapted with permission from Gray ML, Pizzanelli AM, Lee RC, et al. Kinetics of the chondrocyte biosynthetic response to compressive load and release. *Biochim Biophys Acta* 1989;991:415–425).

regulatory role for dynamic physical stimuli of cyclic compression protocols in the unconfined compression configuration have been used to study specific physical factors, such as fluid flow, streaming potentials, and cell deformation, and their role in modulating aggrecan biosynthesis. In protocols with low-magnitude amplitudes of applied compression, matrix deformation is relatively small so that biosynthetic stimulation is not likely to occur through mechanisms related to changes in solid volume fraction, such as os-motic effects associated with increased FCD. In the radially unconfined compression configuration of cylindrical test samples, compression frequencies of 0.01–1 Hz and amplitudes of 1–5% stimulated aggrecan biosynthesis above control levels, while lower compression frequencies or amplitudes appear not to elicit a biosynthetic response (31,155,271,274) (Fig. 6-2). Because the biosynthetic stimulation is highest in the circumferential areas of the cyclically compressed samples and the peak stress in the experiments was <1 MPa, physical factors such as fluid flow, streaming, and diffusion-driven electrical potentials, and cell deformation, rather than hydrostatic pressure, appear to be responsible for the stimulation of biosynthesis [113,170,219,222]. Buschmann and co-workers have used quantitative autoradiography techniques to demonstrate a correlation of chondrocyte aggrecan biosynthesis with these circumferential regions, associated with high interstitial fluid flow, in cartilage explants subjected to dynamic compressive loading in unconfined compression [32,33]. Dynamic compression has also been shown to stimulate proteoglycan synthesis most rapidly in the pericellular matrix that exhibited the greatest sensitivity to mechanical compression (156,254,275). In a different test configuration, the central region of cartilage discs were loaded with a non-porous plane-ended indenter, and a variety of compressive stress amplitudes and frequencies were examined (242). This geometry and test condition do not correspond to that described mathematically by the unconfined compression solution (5,156), although similar types of physical signals may be expected to occur. Aggrecan synthesis was stimulated beneath and nearby the loaded site as compared with regions away from the loaded site. In another configuration, osteochondral bovine sesamoid samples were cultured and subjected to load against a nylon surface, resulting in contact of a portion of the articular cartilage surface (164). Here, cyclic compression at 0.33 Hz stimulated aggrecan synthesis, especially in the superficial layers of the articular cartilage. In yet another configuration, cartilage disks were compressed between a porous platen and the non-porous base of a culture dish (173). Here, cyclic loads of 1 MPa at a frequency of 0.25 Hz stimulated aggrecan synthesis, whereas a frequency of 0.008 Hz slightly inhibited aggrecan synthesis, emphasizing the sensitivity of the cellular environment to frequency of loading. The generation of physical signals in these experimental geometries, however, has not been well characterized so that it is difficult to assess the role of potential physical regulators of cartilage metabolism. For example, under the same magnitude of applied stress, different loading frequencies will result in a different magnitude of tissue strain within the tissue sample, thus emphasizing the fact that cyclic loading experiments that are "load controlled" must be interpreted separately from those which are "deformation controlled".

3.6 Impact Loading

A number of *in vivo* studies have shown that a single or repeated impact loading of the joint can damage the articular cartilage, initiating a process that may ultimately lead to progressive joint degeneration characteristic of OA (6,10,230, 259,260). Complementary to the *in vivo* models of cartilage degeneration (OA or disuse) described earlier, morphological analyses of *in vitro* cartilage injury models have revealed characteristics similar to those of early-stage OA. A number of *in vitro* studies have investigated supraphysiologic loading of cartilage using a single impact load (6,143,144,209,257, 312) or repeated impact loading (45,73,190, 259,260).

Chen and co-workers (1999,2001) demonstrated that stress rate and loading duration are important determinants of cartilage damage (44,45). Impact is more destructive than smoothly arising compression to the same peak stress ($\geq$2.5 MPa), stress rate ($\geq$30 MPa/sec), and loading duration ($\geq$120 sec or 36 cycles for 5 MPa) (44). With increasing impact stress, decreased proteoglycan biosynthesis and increased water content have been reported with a critical threshold level (15–20 MPa for moderate applied loading rates) above which cell death and apparent rupture of the collagen fiber network were observed at the time of impact (6,312). Water loss in these studies increased linearly with strain amplitude, reaching swelling (i.e., imbibition equilibrium at 1 hour). Jeffrey and co-workers have previously reported significant water loss (up to 60%) from cartilage loaded in unconfined compression (143). More recently, Quinn and co-workers (2001) found that single subimpact loads (constant strain rate of $0.7 \, sec^{-1}$ to a peak stress between 3.5 and 14 MPa) resulted in tissue fissures and cell deactivation that was most pronounced near the cartilage superficial zone. In contrast, these authors found that low strain rate loading (3×10^{-5} sec^{-1}) resulted in cell deactivation throughout the tissue depth in the absence of visible matrix damage (257). In a subsequent study, the same investigators subjected explants to a level of 50% injurious strain (6 one-hour loading/recovery cycles over 12 hours, 0.07 mm/sec compression velocity) and found two populations of cells; one viable, larger, and metabolically active, and the other apparently dead (255). The surviving cells exhibited increased cell volume and mediated an acceleration of proteoglycan degradation. Mechanical testing of explants (loaded in unconfined compression) showed that the collagen fibrillar network was more affected than the proteoglycan component of the matrix.

The cumulative effects of repetitive loading can also lead to an injurious cartilage and chondrocyte response. Lucchinetti and co-workers (190) reported matrix damage only in the uppermost layer of the superficial zone in response to static or cyclic (0.5 Hz) continuous loading for 24 hours with a maximum stress of 1 MPa. Static loads promoted early cell death (e.g., at 3 hours) compared with cyclic loads (at 6 hours), with no apparent apoptosis but some necrosis (190). In another study, Farquhar and co-workers reported swelling and fibronectin accumulation in cartilage explants after cyclical impact loading (50 MPa once every 5 seconds for 30 minutes, loading rate 100 MPa/sec) (73). Cell death and matrix damage has been reported by Chen and co-workers for cyclic continuously loaded (confined compression, cyclic stress of 1 or 5 MPa at 0.5 Hz for 0.2–48 hours) cartilage to be time and depth dependent (45). Surprisingly, the region of cell death did not go beyond the superficial zone for even the highest compressive strains of 40% at 60 MPa; cell depth occurring first in the uppermost region of the superficial tangential zone (STZ) and appeared to be progressing toward the middle zone (45,209). The finding of dramatic changes to the superficial zone, a hallmark of early-stage OA, is reminiscent of that observed in an experimental canine model of OA

(110,285) and in human osteoarthritic tissue (88,130). The collapse of the superficial zone has been attributed to its lower compressive modulus (112,281) and the trapping of interstitial fluid, which act as a protective mechanism for the underlying middle and deep zones, bolstering their interstitial load support. This explanation is consistent with a multiphasic theoretical framework (5,9,168,216,217,219) as well as experimental measurements of interstitial fluid pressurization in cartilage explants (298). Shifting of the load support mechanism from interstitial fluid pressurization to that of one supported by the solid matrix (where the cells are attached) will increase the magnitude of matrix deformation and subject chondrocytes to supraphysiologic levels of deformation (217,219). Cyclic impact loading of the 2 mm core of 4 mm discs were performed for 20–120 minutes at an impact stress of 5 MPa and at a maximum loading rate of 60 MPa/sec at a frequency of 0.3 Hz. Cell death was initially confined to regions of direct impact and extended to the outer core with extended culture time. When outer rings were physically isolated from central cores after impact, cell death in the outer ring was similar to control levels. These results suggest the role of soluble factors and intercellular signaling as a mechanism for propagating cell death into the interior of the tissue after impact (182).

3.7 Tensile Stretch

The response of chondrocytes to applied tensile loading has been studied using chondrocyte-seeded collagen sponges (345,346). Mechanical stimulation of 5% elongation for 15 min/hr at 1 Hz increased proliferation and cartilage matrix protein (CMP/matrilin-1) mRNA levels in immature chondrocytes. The response of chondrocytes to tensile stretch has also been examined using 2D cell culture systems (54,90,132, 178,313). In one model of cyclic tensile stretch, the collagen matrix generated by epiphyseal chondrocytes in high-density culture was stretched at strains of 5.5% at 0.2 Hz, and significant increases were observed in aggrecan synthesis rates following 24 hours of applied strains (54). In other studies, tensile strains of

10% applied to a supportive elastin membrane at 1 Hz resulted in a two- to three-fold increase in the rates of aggrecan synthesis in chick sternal chondrocytes (178). Further, agitation of the substrate had similar effects on cellular activity as stretching of the substrate, implying that fluid motion may have contributed to the observed effects (178,331). More recent studies have also observed a significant increase in aggrecan synthesis by chondrocytes isolated from rat ribs as induced by tensile deformation of an underlying substrate, although the magnitude of applied strain was not reported (313). Substratum stretch using the Flexercell Strain System (13) has been shown to up-regulate metalloproteinase activity (89,132). Specifically, excessive and continuous cyclic mechanical stress induces the production of IL-1 and MMP-9, which may result in cartilage degradation (89). RNA levels of MMP-1, MMP-3, MMP-9, IL-1beta, TNF-alpha, and TIMP-1 were elevated in the cultured chondrocytes, while the mRNA level of MMP-2 and TIMP-2 was unchanged (89). It is important to note, however, that even if the strain in the substrate is precisely characterized in studies such as these, the relationship between substrate strain and cellular strain may be complex (14).

3.8 Shear Loading

To better understand the role of deformation-induced fluid flow in explant loading studies, Frank and co-workers have studied the effect of simple shear loading of cartilage explants (83). The simple shear loading configuration has minimal associated fluid flow compared with axial loading configurations (5,216,218). Tissue shear loading at 1% to 3% strain amplitudes (with a 0% to 10% compressive offset strain) at frequencies of 0.01–1.0 Hz was observed to increase protein and proteoglycan synthesis uniformly across the central core region and the outer annular region of the explants (in contrast to dynamic compressive loading described above). These findings suggest that chondrocytes can respond to shear stress-initiated pathways, in the absence of macroscopic (bulk) tissue-level fluid flow that mediate ECM production (146).

3.9 Electric Fields

The role of electric fields on chondrocyte activity has also been studied in culture conditions (1,138,178,192), and has led investigators to hypothesize that mechanically induced electric fields may serve as a mechanism for the regulation of aggrecan biosynthesis. Studies of chick sternal chondrocytes in culture showed that extremely low-level electric currents induced qualitatively similar changes in aggrecan synthesis rates as those induced by cyclic stretching of the substrate, suggesting that similar mechanisms were involved in transducing tension or externally applied electric fields (178). To determine if electric fields modulate cartilage metabolism, it is important to distinguish thermal effects due to the method of electric field application from the effects of the electric fields themselves because the induction of currents using pulsed electromagnetic fields may be associated with heating (138). In calf cartilage explants, current densities up to 1 mA/cm^2 at frequencies of 1–10 Hz did not affect aggrecan biosynthesis (272), while higher amplitude current densities of 10–30 mA/cm^2 at a frequency of 10–1,000 Hz stimulated aggrecan biosynthesis (192). These effects were not due to heating because the medium temperature was not detectably altered and there was no evidence for the production of characteristic heat-shock proteins. Pulsed electromagnetic fields, as used to stimulate fracture healing, also appear to stimulate aggrecan biosynthesis in cartilage explants (1). Due to the nature of the electromagnetic stimulus, such protocols would be predicted to induce electric currents of a variety of amplitudes and frequencies within cartilage. Recent experimental and theoretical studies have shown that compression of cartilage samples can induce both fluid flow-driven (streaming) and deformation-driven (diffusion) electrical potentials across the samples whose magnitudes are of the order of several mA (42,170).

3.10 Metabolism of Other ECM and Soluble Products

The results of numerous *in vitro* culture studies have demonstrated extensive evidence that changes in the physical environment can modulate the metabolic response of the chondrocyte, whether the cell is within the native tissue or an artificial 3D construct. The application of static changes in the physical environment seems to decrease synthesis rates in a dose-dependent manner (Fig. 6-3), while cyclic and dynamic stimuli seem to increase synthesis rates at higher frequencies (Fig. 6-4). Although this chapter has focused on aggrecan biosynthesis as a marker of chondrocyte metabolism, there are data available on the biosynthesis of a number of metabolic products, including collagen, noncollagenous proteins, and metalloproteinases. It should be emphasized that biosynthetic regulation of these other matrix molecules by physical factors may not be similar to that of aggrecan, as presented in this section. Studies of aggrecan metabolism provide a model system for understanding the involvement of the variety of physical signals associated with static and cyclic compression; a full understanding awaits a more thorough investigation of the long-term influences on aggrecan metabolism as well as the physical influences on other matrix macromolecules. Cartilage oligomeric matrix protein (COMP), a pentameric extracellular protein, is primarily localized to the musculoskeletal system where it is an abundant component of the chondrocyte and tendon ECM, with expression also found in ligament and synovium (124,225). Altered levels of COMP and its degradation products in serum and synovial fluid have been proposed to be used as markers for cartilage destruction in OA and rheumatoid arthritis (339). COMP levels and fibronectin have been shown to increase in articular cartilage explants subjected to cyclic loading (0.1 Hz and higher, 45 hours) in unconfined compression whereas static compression decreased fibronectin synthesis over free-swelling controls (341). In other studies, cyclic matrix deformation of growth plate chondrocytes cultured in 3D type I collagen sponge matrices stimulated proliferation and synthesis of cartilage matrix protein (CMP/matrilin-1), a mature chondrocyte marker, and type X collagen (345).

Nitric oxide (NO), NO synthase (NOS), and leukotrienes regulate a variety of processes in joint tissues and are frequently elevated in arthritis. NO production has been shown to be influenced by dynamic compressive loading in chondrocyte-seeded agarose and agarose hydrogel cultures (74–76,175). In porcine cartilage explant studies, static compression significantly increased NO production at 0.1 MPa stress for 24 hours. Intermittent compression at 0.5 Hz for 6 hours followed by 18 hours of recovery also increased NO production and NOS activity at 1.0 MPa stress. Intermittent compression at 0.5 Hz for 24 hours at a magnitude of 0.1 or 0.5 MPa caused an increase in NO production and NOS activity. Addition of 1400W (a specific NOS2 inhibitor) reduced NO production by 51% with no loss of cell viability (75). In explant studies where mechanical compression was applied for 1 hour followed by 23 hours, dynamic compression significantly increased LTB(4) and LOX protein production in the presence of 1400W. Increased LOX protein but not LTB(4) occurred in response to compression alone. These findings provide a direct link between mechanical stress and inflammation in cartilage and may have implications in the pathogenesis and treatment of arthritis (74). Related dynamic loading studies (0.3,1, or 3 Hz) of chondrocyte-seeded agarose suggest that NO appears to be a constituent of mechanical signal transduction pathways that influence proliferation of bovine chondrocytes (175). Fluid-induced shear of cultured osteoarthritic chondroctyes up-regulated the NO synthase gene and NO release, which contributed to an observed decrease in collagen type II and aggrecan mRNA levels (177). NO may be important in cartilage repair, playing a role in chondrocyte migration and cytoskeletal assembly in culture conditions (87), as well as in cellular communication as an extracellular messenger. Chondron pellet cultures (176) have been loaded (~35% deformation at 15 kPa loading) and observed to transiently increase release of adenosine trisphosphate (ATP), which may act as an extracellular signaling molecule between chondrocytes (65,95).

Metalloproteinase (MMP) expression and activation has been shown to be modulated in cartilage explants by compressive loading (20).

Mechanically loaded bovine cartilage explants (0.5 MPa, 1 Hz, 3 hours) showed increased MMP-2 and MMP-9 expression and activation, whereas expression of tissue inhibitors of MMPs (TIMPs) was unaffected. This imbalance of proteinases and their inhibitors may upset tissue homeostasis (20). MMP expression has also been observed in cultured chondrocytes subjected to fluid-induced shear (145).

4   MECHANICALLY INDUCED SIGNALS AT THE CELL AND MOLECULAR LEVEL

From these *in vivo* and *in vitro* studies, it is evident that mechanical loading has a strong influence on the metabolic activity of the chondrocytes. However, the precise events, and their sequence, and the mechanisms involved in regulating the synthesis and breakdown of matrix components are still unclear (222). One difficulty in isolating the effects of specific biophysical phenomena on chondrocyte activity is the intrinsic coupling of these phenomena in the physiological situation. Furthermore, the physicochemical, electrical, and fluid flow environments of the chondrocytes will be dependent on the specifics of the loading configuration to which the cartilage is exposed (Fig. 6-5). In the following sections, we present a review of several biophysical factors, which are evoked by mechanical loading of articular cartilage and the potential roles that they may play in signaling mechanisms to the chondrocyte.

4.1 Physicochemical Effects

The physicochemical environment within articular cartilage is determined by parameters such as matrix hydration, FCD, interstitial ion concentrations, and activity coefficients for specific ions within the cartilage ECM, etc. (101–103, 168,170,196–201,219,222). The negatively charged groups on the glycosaminoglycans in cartilage influence the concentrations of electrolytes (Na^+, Cl^-, Ca^{++}, etc.) are governed by Donnan equilibrium ion concentration law (170,196,200). This physicochemical state,

which can be described theoretically using Donnan or Boltzmann or mixture theory approaches, confers the tissue with an osmotic pressure that gives the tissue a propensity to swell and is responsible for electrokinetic effects including electroosmosis, streaming potentials, and streaming currents (79,99,101–103,168,170, 196–201,219,222). The swelling pressure in cartilage is therefore directly coupled to the state of stress and strain in the solid matrix, because the density of negative charges explicitly depends on the water volume fraction, and therefore, the dilatation of the cartilage solid matrix (168,170,218,332,335). As an example, when a cylindrical cartilage explant is deformed in compression by 20%, the negative FCD may increase from 15% to 20% (168), depending on other material parameters of the solid matrix such as the Poisson's ratio; conversely the FCD also strongly influence the Poisson's ratio (332).

In general, such changes in both the mechanical environment and electrical environment (i.e., FCD) would be expected to vary spatially throughout the explant during deformation. The associated changes in local ionic environment with compression will give rise to increases in overall and local osmotic swelling pressures and decreases in intratissue pH. These changes in the local physicochemical environment may modify the mechanical behaviors of the tissue because physicochemical factors have been strongly linked to material parameters such as hydraulic permeability and compressive modulus (3,4,99,102,103,168,170, 196,200,219,222,332). Chondrocyte biosynthetic activity is very sensitive to extracellular osmolarity, suggesting that coupling of the mechanical and physicochemical environments may be important as a process for transducing signals associated with applied loads.

4.2 Cell Deformation

One mechanism by which mammalian cells may perceive alterations in their physical environment is through cellular deformation (i.e., changes in shape and volume) (18,55,141, 270,318,336). Under physiological levels of matrix deformation, chondrocyte volume in situ

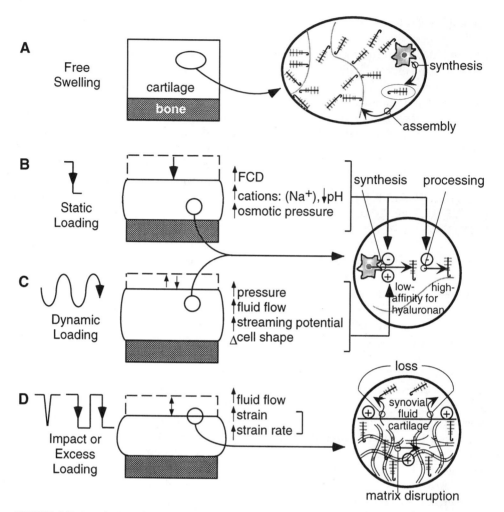

FIGURE 6-5. Regulation of matrix metabolism by physical phenomena in free-swelling and compressed cartilage. **A:** In free-swelling cartilage, local regions of low proteoglycan content (and low fixed-charge density (FCD)) attract a relatively low concentration of positive counterions (Na$^+$, H$^+$, Ca^{2+}), and may thereby stimulate aggrecan synthesis and deposition. **B:** During static compression, there is an increase in the FCD, the concentration of positive counterions, and the osmotic pressure in the tissue, which may inhibit aggrecan synthesis. **C:** Dynamic loading conditions such oscillatory or intermittent compression may affect chondrocyte metabolic activity through other biophysical mechanisms, such as hydrostatic pressure, fluid flow, streaming potentials, or oscillations in cell shape. **D:** During excessive compression or impact loading, high levels of strain or strain rate may cause tissue disruption, tissue swelling, increased diffusion, and potentially increased loss of matrix macromolecules due to fluid convection. (Adapted with permission from Sah RL, Grodzinsky AJ, Plaas AHK, et al. Effects of static and dynamic compression on matrix metabolism in cartilage explants. In: Kuettner KE, Schleyerbach R, Peyron JG, et al., eds. *Articular cartilage and osteoarthritis.* New York: Raven Press, 1992:373–392).

can be altered by as much as ~20% (26, 86,109,111,112) (Fig. 6-6A–C). Theoretical predictions and experimental measurements of cellular deformation in response to applied loading also indicate that the magnitude and distribution of cell deformations will vary with depth in the cartilage layer (11,107,112,284). The mechanism for chondrocyte volumetric decrease may be related to mechanical and osmotic effects associated with matrix compression (111,112), or may be an active cellular response to loading (86).

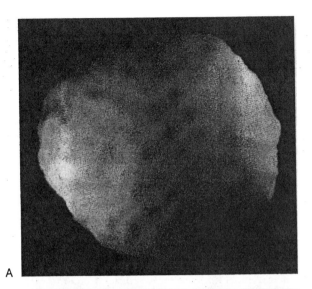

A

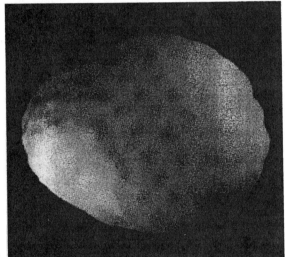

B

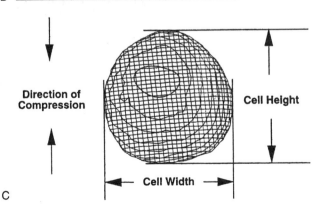

C

Direction of
Compression

Cell Height

Cell Width

FIGURE 6-6. Three-dimensional confocal microscopy images of viable chondrocytes in situ from the middle zone of articular cartilage of the canine patello femoral groove before **(A)** and after **(B)** compression of the ECM. Chondrocytes were imaged by introducing fluorescein dextran (MW 10,000 Da) to the extracellular media. This fluorescent indicator diffuses rapidly within the ECM, but is excluded from an intact cell membrane of viable chondrocytes. A series of 32 confocal images spaced at 0.5-μm intervals was recorded of a chondrocyte in the undeformed tissue. The tissue was then compressed in a direction perpendicular to the cartilage surface (vertical direction as shown in the figure) and the same chondrocyte was imaged again. A 15% surface-to-surface compression of the tissue resulted in significant decreases in cell height of 26%, 19%, and 20% and cell volume of 22%, 16%, and 17% in the surface, middle, and deep zones, respectively (112). Removal of compression resulted in a complete recovery of cell shape and volume. (From Guilak F. Compression-induced changes in the shape and volume of the chondrocyte nucleus. *J Biomech* 1995;28:1529–1542, with permission.)

Volume changes in other mammalian cells have been associated with mechanical transduction and signaling through the transport of ions and organic compounds (48,270, 280,326). In the chondrocyte, volume also seems to exert a strong influence on biosynthetic activity (318). Cell volume increases significantly by 30% to 40% when chondrocytes are removed from the ECM (318), and chondrocytes in situ (as well as the tissue itself—see Chapter 5 for more details) will shrink or swell in proportion to changes in the ionic composition of the ECM. Further, chondrocytes exhibit active volume recovery mechanisms in response to osmotic shock, i.e., a rapid change in the osmotic environment of the extracellular fluid (55,226,237). It may be difficult, however, to uncouple direct cellular deformation from ion-specific osmotic activity changes in these studies of volumetric changes induced by osmotic shock because physicochemical factors are known to be important in regulating chondrocyte activity (226). Such a decoupling may be possible in studies that investigate volume regulation of chondrocytes in 3D culture using confocal microscopy (112). The chondrocyte aggrecan gene expression response in monolayer or in agarose to an applied step hypotonic loading is similar (135), despite the fact that chondrocytes seeded in uncharged agarose exhibited nominal changes to cell size/shape (i.e., subjected to confined-swelling conditions due to the stiffer hydrogel matrix) (204), whereas isolated chondrocytes exhibited cell swelling (135). The role of cell-matrix interactions in this response has been studied using isolated chondrons encapsulated in agarose. Chondrocytes in their type VI collagen-rich pericellular environment associated with the chondron (250,251) can also change size in response to applied osmotic loading (126). The volume regulatory response of chondrocytes and chondrons in this agarose system were dependent on existence of the local microenvironment, with mechanically extracted chondrons changing their volume the least and exhibiting maximum volume regulation compared with enzymatically extracted chondrons and isolated chondrocytes (126).

The regulatory volume increases of chondrocytes in cartilage do not appear to be mediated by cell-matrix interactions (34,35). Chondro-

cytes from the middle zone of articular cartilage have been shown to behave as "perfect osmometers" (over the extracellular osmolarity range of ~250 to ~600 mOsmol) with the much stiffer ECM not restraining cell volume changes. With a relative isotonic value of 280 mOsmol, the three zones showed greatest swelling in the superficial zone, followed by the middle and deep zones, whereas cell shrinking at 180 mOsmol resulted in similar cell shrinking in all three zones. This heterogeneous swelling is similar to that exhibited by the three zones of the tissue (226). Moreover, no difference between the regulatory volume regulation response of chondrocytes from different zones (although differences in initial dimensions were found) nor differences between the response of chondrocytes in explants or monolayer was reported (34). These findings are particularly interesting in light of the development of non-uniform strain fields within articular cartilage, reflecting its inhomogeneous biochemical and material properties (112,282), in response to osmotic loading (227, 334).

Osmotic loading provides a means for modulating cell volume/shape in a time-varying way without the need for direct contact of an instrument with the tissue or cell. Intracellular signaling in response to cell volume changes may be occurring through changes in cell shape (likely from inhomogeneous cellular properties) and the accompanying deformation of the cell membrane and cytoplasm. The latter may be dependent on chondrocyte material properties, which appear to change with the extracellular osmotic environment (115,134). It is known that chondrocyte shape influences phenotypic expression (131,231) through what is apparently a secondary response to changes in cytoskeletal architecture (141,193,291). Further, stretching of an underlying substrate, which presumably cause changes in the shape of chondrocytes grown on the substrate, has been shown to modify chondrocyte metabolism, proliferation, and second messenger activity (89,132,178,313).

4.3 Hydrostatic Pressure

Due to the incompressible nature of the fluid-filled solid matrix at physiological pressures, hydrostatic fluid pressurization of cartilage will not cause appreciable deformation of the ECM or chondrocytes (12). Unlike the deforming loads of normal joint loading, (uniform) hydrostatic pressures will not induce interstitial fluid flow or osmotic changes because no dilatation of the ECM occurs (105). These points would suggest that somehow the chondrocyte itself is sensitive to the effects of static and intermittent hydrostatic pressures.

Hydrostatic pressure appears to modulate aggrecan biosynthesis through membrane-mediated pathways such as the transport of cations, amino acids, and macromolecules (318). Relatively low hydrostatic pressures (0.006 MPa) have been shown to inhibit the accumulation of cyclic adenosine $3',5'$ monophosphate (cAMP) in isolated chick epiphyseal chondrocytes in a manner that was mediated by the uptake of calcium ion (Ca^{2+}) (23), and it was hypothesized that these effects were regulated through pressure-induced changes in the structure of various membrane components. It has also been suggested that hydrostatic pressure may alter the action of the membrane Na^+/K^+ pump, thus altering intracellular K^+ concentrations (318). This hypothesis is supported by the finding that hydrostatic pressure has a direct effect on the transmembrane potential of chondrocytes (343). Continuous and low-frequency (<0.08 Hz) pressures of 120 mm Hg (0.016 MPa) caused membrane depolarization in chondrocytes, while higher frequency compression (0.33 Hz) significantly increased membrane resting potentials. Both Ca^{2+}-dependent K^+ channels and Na^+ channels were involved in these responses.

In addition to these membrane-related effects, there is evidence for involvement of the cytoskeleton in chondrocyte response to hydrostatic pressure (245,343), although separation of membrane and cytoskeletal effects is difficult due to the interactions between these components. Treatment with cytochalasin B, which disrupts actin microfilaments, abolished pressure-induced hyperpolarization of the chondrocyte membrane, suggesting that the actin cytoskeleton is involved in this phenomenon (343). Continuous pressures of up to 30 MPa alter the organization of stress fibers, microtubules, and

the Golgi apparatus in isolated chondrocytes. Treatment with nocodazole, which inhibits microtubule assembly, has been shown to block pressure-induced alterations of the Golgi apparatus (244). In monolayer cultures, nocodozole and taxol were observed to both prevent stimulation of proteoglycan synthesis in response to intermittent cyclic pressure (0.5 Hz, 5 MPa). Continuous high hydrostatic pressure caused inhibition of proteoglycan synthesis that was not dependent on microtubules (149). Considering that the ECM may influence cytoskeletal function (291), differences in chondrocyte shape and cytoskeletal structure may explain the differential response of isolated chondrocytes and explants to hydrostatic pressure (243,318).

4.4 Fluid Transport

One mechanism by which joint loading may regulate chondrocyte metabolism is through the induction of interstitial fluid flow. Cyclic and intermittent loading of articular cartilage produce spatial gradients in the hydrostatic fluid pressure within the cartilage matrix, resulting in convective transport and redistribution of the interstitial fluid phase. In explant models, physiologic frequencies of compression can generate interstitial fluid flow velocities, which are predicted to be in excess of 1 to 10 μm/sec (106,156,216–219,222,299). These velocities may be 1 to 2 orders of magnitude higher during joint contact and sliding (8) or in degenerative cartilage (286), although little is known regarding actual interstitial flow velocities *in vivo*.

Fluid flow within cartilage may modulate chondrocyte activity by accelerating the transport of solutes and macromolecules that regulate cartilage metabolism (22,91,102,196,200,218). Although the nutrition to the chondrocytes is achieved primarily through diffusion mechanisms, many essential macromolecules exhibit a very low diffusivity within cartilage compared with that in free solution (170,196,197,234). In addition, macromolecules that are greater than several kDa are largely excluded from partitioning into cartilage due to the small "effective pore size" of the ECM (199,200,218). This apparent pore size may be decreased even further in response to matrix deformations that increase the solid volume fraction (e.g., compression) (216–219). In addition, changes in FCD with matrix deformation may affect the diffusion properties, partition coefficients, or matrix permeabilities for select solutes (102,103,167,168, 196,200,216–219,222). Macromolecules that may be affected through such mechanisms and that are important to chondrocyte metabolism include a number of polypeptide growth factors, such as insulin-like growth factor I (22,202, 212).

There is little evidence that these factors play a role in transport of small solutes and nutrient molecules because they diffuse rapidly through the cartilage matrix and are unaffected by matrix loading (196–200,283,310,311). For these reasons, convective transport associated with time-varying or cyclic loading of articular cartilage appears to enhance the transport of larger molecules (e.g., growth factors, cytokines, or enzymes), as has been demonstrated experimentally (22,50,91,234).

In addition to enhanced nutrient supply, fluid flows may alter chondrocyte metabolism by directly exerting shear stresses on the chondrocyte membrane. This mechanism of cellular signal transduction has been studied extensively in other cells (53,78,228), with a growing number of reports showing direct evidence of shear stress effects on chondrocytes (293–296). For example, fluid-induced shear stress has been shown to affect chondrocyte metabolism (296). Shear stresses of 1.6 Pa applied to human chondrocytes in monolayer using a cone-on-plate viscometer caused cellular alignment with the direction of flow and induced a significant elevation of mRNA levels of tissue inhibitor of metalloproteinase (293). Fluid-induced shear also stimulated aggrecan synthesis two-fold and increased the length of newly synthesized chains. Downregulation of aggrecan gene expression has been observed in response to 1.6 Pa of applied steady shear flow for 2 hours using a parallel-plate flow chamber (133). It has also been found to regulate gene expression of matrix metalloproteinase-9 (MMP-9), a mediator of the progressive degradation of articular cartilage in OA (145). NO release in a manner dependent on the duration and the magnitude of the fluid-induced

shear has been reported as well (52). Although the aforementioned studies have applied nonphysiologic fluid flow rates, the well-defined conditions associated with the flow devices provide a tool for study of chondrocyte mechanical signal transduction. With this caveat, these findings imply that fluid flow, in and of itself, can modulate chondrocyte activity. An important question that remains is the process by which shear stresses interact at the cellular and intracellular levels to invoke these observed changes. Indeed, a variety of cell signaling pathways has been shown to mediate the fluid flow-induced response of chondrocytes (52,133,145,347,348).

4.5 Electromechanical Transduction

Another physical mechanism by which loading may regulate chondrocyte activity is through mechanical to electrical transduction phenomena that occur naturally within cartilage due to the presence of the negative FCD associated with its proteoglycan content. As a result, deformation of the cartilage solid matrix, a non-uniform distribution of FCD, is produced in response to applied loads giving rise to gradients in both fluid pressure and ionic composition (168,170, 222). Interstitial fluid and ion fluxes will result with associated electrokinetic phenomena such as electrical potentials and currents from such mechanisms as fluid convection (known as streaming) or diffusion (Nernst) (15,81,98,102, 168,170,189,196,200,305). These effects arise from the flow of migration of cations and anions relative to the fixed negative charge groups on the glycosaminoglycans in cartilage, which are restrained from flow by their large size and physical and chemical interactions with the solid matrix. Other examples of electrokinetic phenomena that occur in articular cartilage are mechanical stresses in response to an applied current density (i.e., current-generated stress) and electroosmosis (81,99). Various theoretical models have been developed to describe these phenomena in a variety of experimental geometries and to relate the measured potentials to the charged proteoglycan components of the tissue (63,80, 81,102,103,168,170,196,305). The streaming potential of cartilage tissue may be modulated by alteration in the proteoglycan content that result, for example, from enzymatic digestion, modulation of chondrocyte metabolism, or cartilage compression (21,42,82,102).

Although the magnitude and frequency of the electric fields *within* articular cartilage have not been directly measured, estimates of these field quantities have been made. Peak streaming potentials of ~15 mV have been predicted based on estimates of applied loading encountered during normal walking (see Chapter 1 by PJ Prendergast et al., and Chapter 3 by TP Andriacchi; also (128,129,200)). The spatial gradient in electrical potential, and the corresponding magnitude of local electric fields, are more difficult to estimate as they would depend on the distribution of the FCD, geometry of the cartilage layer and boundary conditions during joint loading *in vivo* (42,80,102,168,170,305,332). However, electric field strengths of up to 1,500 V/m and current densities of ~100 mA/cm^2 have been estimated to occur in cartilage during loading (79,122,170,196). Interestingly, cultured articular chondrocytes subjected to electric field strengths on this order have been observed to migrate to the negative pole or cathode (41). Based on more conservative estimates of fluid flow *in vivo*, current densities of 0.1–1 mA/cm^2 have also been predicted (272). Estimates of the magnitude and frequency of electric fields that occur naturally within articular cartilage provide a framework for examining the role of electric fields in modulating cartilage metabolism. As these phenomena are directly related to the magnitude of the interstitial fluid velocity (80,101–103,168,170,305), there is some indirect evidence supporting their involvement in elevating biosynthetic activity during cyclic loading (155,178). In addition to flow- and diffusion-mediated electrokinetic effects, several studies have provided evidence that low-level electric fields can directly influence chondrocyte activity (1,28,178,192,232,266). Possible mechanisms through which these fields interact with chondrocytes include gating of voltage-dependent ion channels, hyper- or hypopolarization of the membrane, or in some cases, thermal effects.

5 INTRACELLULAR SIGNALING PATHWAYS

To affect chondrocyte activity and gene expression, all potential physical signals described above must be transduced across the cell membrane to an intracellular biochemical signal. The chondrocyte plasma membrane is the host of numerous receptors, adhesion molecules, and ion channels, and thus serves as a critical component of cellular function (186,276,301,314). Hence, it is not surprising that the chondrocyte membrane is apparently involved in multiple physical signaling pathways, including osmotic and ionic changes, cell deformation, or hydrostatic pressure. In this section, we describe a variety of signaling pathways that have been studied in chondrocytes and could be potentially involved in the process of transducing physical signals (Fig. 6-7).

The plasma membrane in all cells seems to be critical to the transduction of cell deformation and volume change, possibly through mechanosensitive, or "stretch-activated" ion channels (213,270). These channels are defined as ion transport pathways whose gating characteristics are dependent on stretch of the plasma membrane (104). By activating or inactivating these channels, cellular deformation or volume change could directly regulate specific ion transport pathways, which could conceivably affect second messenger activity or membrane potential (18,48,270,280,336). Recent studies provide indirect evidence that chondrocytes possess stretch-activated ion channels (342). Furthermore, direct perturbation of the chondrocyte membrane has been shown to cause a rapid increase in the concentration of cytosolic calcium ion ($[Ca^{2+}]_i$) (108), an intracellular second messenger. Stretch-activated ion channel blockers such as gadolinium or amiloride significantly attenuated the peak increase of fluorescence in deformed cells, suggesting that this calcium signaling was regulated through stretch of the chondrocyte membrane. These findings provide support for the hypothesis that chondrocytes have the ability to transduce isolated deformations, in the absence of other matrix-related effects.

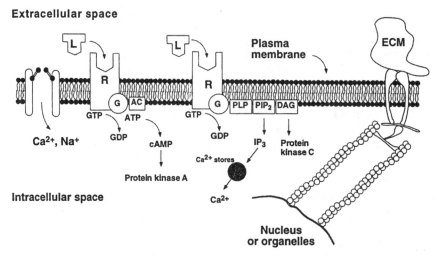

FIGURE 6-7. Potential signaling pathways by which physical factors may be transduced into an intracellular signal. Intracellular signaling may be occurring through one or more of the traditional second messenger systems such as the adenylate cyclase/cAMP system, the IP_3 system, or the Ca^{2+} system. The concentration of these intracellular messengers may be modulated by gating of membrane ion channels (e.g., voltage-activated or stretch-activated channels) or by a G-protein pathway that leads to increased levels of cytosolic cAMP or IP_3. Alternatively, transmembrane signaling may be occurring through a direct link between ECM molecules and intracellular organelles through membrane-spanning molecules (i.e., integrins). R, receptor; G, G protein; AC, adenylate cyclase; GDP or GTP, guanosine 5′-di- or triphosphate; ATP, adenosine triphosphate; cAMP, cyclic adenosine 3′, 5′ monophosphate; IP_3, inositol triphosphate; DAG, diacylglycerol; PIP_2, phophoinositolphosphate; PLP, phospholipase C.

Alternatively, chondrocytes may be responding to ECM deformation by sensing apparent changes in local tissue composition through plasma membrane binding proteins (receptors) for specific macromolecules such as hyaluronic acid (hyaluronan), aggrecan, collagen, or fibronectin (186,276,314,330). Changes in the local concentrations or conformations of these molecules through consolidation of the ECM could significantly affect the kinetics of ligand-receptor binding and ultimately influence cell activity through intracellular second messengers.

These membrane-related phenomena support the involvement of the traditional second messenger pathways and transmembrane enzymatic mechanisms such as the adenylate cyclase system, the inositol triphosphate system, and cytosolic calcium (Fig. 6-7) (303). The transport of even a relatively small number of ions may have a substantial biological effect through second messengers such as cAMP or Ca^{2+}. These messengers could affect levels of protein kinase A or phospholipase C, and subsequently, inositol

phosphate metabolism. This would result in the mobilization of Ca^{2+} from intracellular stores and the activation of protein kinase C, affecting phosphorylation of cytosolic proteins.

These pathways appear to be involved in the chondrocyte mechanical signal transduction cascade (303). Calcium is a nearly ubiquitous regulator of cell metabolism and is involved in the control of a large number of cellular functions (37,263). In chondrocytes, it has been suggested that an increase in $[Ca^{2+}]_i$ may initiate matrix vesicle biogenesis (139,267), alter type I and type II collagen ratios (56), and affect proteoglycan synthesis rates (49,61,62,229).

Cyclic AMP, which has been identified as an important mediator of proteoglycan synthesis and cartilage growth (58,210), also seems to play a direct role in the mechanical stimulation of matrix biosynthesis. Constant hydrostatic pressures that inhibit proteoglycan synthesis also inhibit cAMP accumulation through a calcium-mediated process (23,232). Conversely, mechanical factors, which increase cAMP levels, also seem to increase proteoglycan synthesis rates. For example, intermittent hydrostatic pressures in chondrocyte cell culture systems result in concurrent increases in both cAMP and proteoglycan synthesis rates (326), and continuous tension of chondrocytes causes a rapid increase of cAMP levels (313).

It is important to note that the ultimate second messenger response to mechanical stimuli may be a result of the interaction of multiple signal transduction pathways. For example, cAMP accumulation can be decreased by increased $[Ca^{2+}]_i$ (24), and IP_3 is an important mediator of cytosolic Ca^{2+} release from intracellular stores (208,253). Such signal "cross talk" may include interaction of the adenylate cyclase/cAMP and Ca^{2+} or IP_3 and Ca^{2+} pathways (140,322,350). Changes to intracellular calcium concentration, $[Ca^{2+}]_i$, have been observed in cultured articular chondrocytes subjected to fluid-induced shear stress and osmotic loading. Yellowley and co-workers have reported $[Ca^{2+}]_i$ response to fluid flow increases with peak flow rate and decreases with increasing frequency (0.05 to 4.4Pa with frequencies ranging from 0.5 to 5 Hz) with serum potentiating flow responsiveness (347). Steady flows (rather than oscillatory) have the greatest response, suggesting a role for agonist delivery or convective transport (2), and roles of extracellular calcium and gadolinium-sensitive channels were also observed. In a subsequent study, the authors report that (with steady shear of 3.7Pa) ryanodine and caffeine had no effect, whereas neomycin (an inhibitor of phospholipase C) and thapsigargin (inhibitor of calcium release from internal stores) significantly decreased calcium response, suggesting an IP_3 pathway (348). Pertussis toxin-sensitive G proteins were also found to be involved. G-protein activation and phospholipase C activation, along with NOS have also been observed to influence glycosaminoglycan metabolism in fluid-sheared (1.6Pa) chondrocytes (52).

Bovine articular chondrocytes exhibit swelling-activated membrane currents and increased intracellular calcium ($[Ca^{2+}]_i$) levels when subjected to hypotonic shock. Gadolinium and thapsigargin blocked the response, suggesting a role by stretch-activated channels

and intracellular Ca^{2+} stores (349). Guilak and co-workers reported significant increases and oscillations of $[Ca^{2+}]_i$ in mature pig knee chondrocytes to hypo- and hyper-osmotic stress (67–70). Similarly, Yellowley and Donahue (2000) reported that gadolinium blocked the peak $[Ca^{2+}]_i$ response to hyperosmotic shock but had no effect on hypo-osmotic shock (349). Chondrocytes strained in 3D agarose constructs (20% uniaxial unconfined compression at a rate of 5%/sec) also respond with transient increases of intracellular Ca^{2+} (265), which are inhibited significantly by gadolinium or EGTA (ethylene glycol bis(2-aminoethyl ether)-N,N,N′N′-tetraacetic acid). These inhibitor results suggest the potential role of stretch-activated channels as well as voltage-operated calcium channels.

Mitogen-activated protein kinases (MAPKs) play diverse roles in the transduction of environmental cues to the cell. The various MAPKs are activated by an assortment of physical and biological stimuli. These stimuli elicit a number of physical and biosynthetic responses from the cells. The MAPK family of protein kinases contains many subfamilies. Hung and co-workers showed that fluid-induced shear stress suppression of aggrecan gene expression in cultured bovine chondrocytes is mediated in part by calcium-independent extracellular signal-regulated kinase 1/2 (Erk-1 and Erk-2) regulation (133). Shear stimulation of chondrocytes stimulates Ras, Rac, and Cdc42, which subsequently activate c-Jun NH2-terminal kinase to induce a 12-0-tetradecanoylphorbol 13-acetate-responsive element-mediated expression of MMP-9 (145). ERK regulation is involved in strain-induced proliferation response of immature chondrocytes to mechanical stretch in collagen sponges (46). Recently, explants subjected to simple shear (83) have also been shown to elevate MAPK levels and transcriptional levels of type II collagen and aggrecan core protein (147).

In cartilage explants, the stimulatory effect of 0.1 MPa compressive stress on aggrecan mRNA levels was blocked by Rp-cAMP and U-73122, indicating the involvement of the classical signal transduction pathways (cAMP and IP_3) in the mechanical modulation of aggrecan gene expression. The responses of link protein mRNA to compression paralleled those of aggrecan (321). In support of these findings, compressive stress (0.1 MPa for 1 hour) induced increase of aggrecan mRNA was blocked by W-7, an inhibitor of calmodulin and KN-93, an inhibitor of CaM-dependent protein kinase II (CaMKII), as well as tetra-acetic acid (tetrakis acetoxymethyl ester) (BAPTA-AM) (322).

3D collagen sponges seeded with immature chondrocytes that were dynamically strained (5% elongation for 15 min/hour at 1 Hz for periods of 2, 4, 6, and 8 days) induced cell proliferation. Gadolinium blocked mechanical stimulation of chondrocyte proliferation but did not affect elevation of cartilage matrix protein (CMP/matrilin-1) mRNA levels. In contrast, nifedipine inhibited proliferation as well as CMP mRNA expression (345). This indicates that stretch-activated channels, channels transporting calcium, and sodium ions are involved in matrix-induced deformation chondrocyte proliferation. In the same loading system, Indian hedgehog (Ihh), a member of the vertebrate hedgehog morphogen family, was found to be a key signaling molecule that controls chondrocyte proliferation and differentiation. Cyclic mechanical strain induces the expression of Ihh by chondrocytes, which is blocked by gadolinium-sensitive stretch-activated channels, suggesting that the Ihh gene is mechanoresponsive (346).

Alternatively, mechanical and physical signaling may be occurring through a transmembrane pathway, which bypasses the traditional second messenger cascades. One hypothesis proposes that normal cellular activity and mechanical signal transduction are regulated by a physical connection from intracellular organelles to the ECM via the cytoskeleton and the proteins of the adhesion plaque (e.g., α-actinin, vinculin, talin) (18,141,246). The connection between the ECM and the cytoskeleton is believed to occur through the integrins, a family of membrane-spanning heterodimeric glycoproteins (137). Chondrocytes show strong expression of the $\beta 1$ and $\alpha 5$ integrin subunits, which mediate cellular attachment to extracellular collagen and fibronectin (186,276). The role of integrins in chondrocyte proliferation and biosynthesis has been studied in 2D using GRGDSP

or GRADSP oligopeptides (211) and 3D using RGD-alginate hydrogel constructs (92). The hydrophilic nature of agarose and alginate hydrogels discourages protein adsorption, preventing cell attachment via integrins during initial cell encapsulation (292). As chondrocytes elaborate a local matrix (e.g., pericellular matrix), cell-matrix interactions via integrins are established. Chondrocytes suspended in RGD-bonded alginate, for example, exhibited decreased biosynthetic activity and proteoglycan content, indicating that cell attachment may inhibit matrix biosynthesis by a negative feedback mechanism (92).

These molecular links provide a physical pathway through which changes in the extracellular mechanical environment could directly alter the shape or structure of the cell nucleus or other organelles (141,248). The direct influence of mechanical forces on nuclear function is not known, although hypothetically, mechanical signals from the ECM could modulate nuclear function (e.g., gene expression, mitosis) in a manner that bypasses or complements traditional second messenger systems. For example, direct deformation of the nucleus may be responsible for distortion of nuclear pores, and therefore, alter the transport of molecules responsible for cell cycling (118). This hypothesis is supported indirectly by the finding that the chondrocyte nucleus is deformed within the cartilage ECM (111) (Fig. 6-8). Clearly, chondrocyte mechanical signal transduction is complex and may involve interaction between traditional signaling cascades as well as mechanisms associated with direct extracellular-intracellular linkages. Mechanical stimulation of human articular chondrocytes in monolayer culture has been shown to stimulate levels of aggrecan mRNA and suppresses levels of MMP-3 mRNA that is dependent on integrins, stretch-activated ion channels, and interleukin-4. This chondroprotective response is absent in chondrocytes from osteoarthritic cartilage (211).

5.1 Reporter Constructs

Transcriptional regulation of physiologically relevant genes has been studied using luciferase reporter constructs and transient transfection

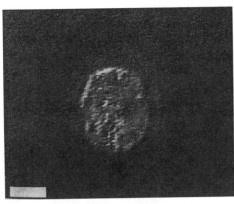 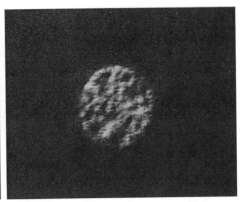

FIGURE 6-8. Digitally enhanced confocal microscopy section through the center of a chondrocyte nucleus in situ before (left) and after (right) 15% compression of the ECM. Chondrocyte nuclei were stained with acridine orange, and a 3D volume image of the cells and nuclei was recorded before and after application of compression. A 15% surface-to-surface tissue compression resulted in nuclear height and volume decreases of 9% and 10%, respectively, as well as significant changes in nuclear shape. Pre-treatment of the tissue with cytochalasin D to disrupt actin microfilament altered the relationship between matrix compression and nuclear height and shape changes, but not volume changes, suggesting that osmotic effects may play a role in the observed cell and nuclear volume changes.

techniques. Monolayer bovine articular chondrocytes transfected with a chimeric luciferase construct containing a 2.4-kb promoter fragment and 5'UTR (exon 1) of the human aggrecan gene, pAGC1(−2368)/5UTR has demonstrated that aggrecan promoter activity is down-regulated by fluid-induced shear stress (133). More recently, aggrecan gene transcription of cultured chondrocytes was observed to be suppressed in response to hypertonic loading and elevated by hypotonic loading. These changes to promoter activity mirrored changes in aggrecan message levels. As deletion of exon 1, using construct pAGC1(−2368/+25), eliminated the hypertonic loading response and had no effect on hypotonic loading, chondrocyte swelling, and shrinkage-induced regulation of aggrecan gene expression appear to be mediated by disparate mechanisms and/or cell signaling pathways (135). The 5'UTR of the human aggrecan gene contains several putative binding sites for the ubiquitous transcription factors, including PDGF, AP-1/CREB (cAMP response element-binding protein), NF-κB, STAT, and at least three shear stress response elements (SSRE) (319,320). Dynamic osmotic loading of monolayer cultures (300 mOsmol to 580 mOsmol at 0.0017 Hz) blocks hypertonic loading-induced aggrecan promoter suppression (237).

In similar studies on cultured rabbit chondrocytes, luciferase reporter assays suggest that the fluid-induced shear induction of MMP-9 is dependent on a region in the 5' promoter of the gene that contains a 12-0-tetradecanoylphorbol 13-acetate-responsive element (145). Transfection of MMP-9-luciferase construct together with the dominant negative mutant of c-Jun NH2-terminal kinase, but not with that of extracellular signal-regulated kinase or p38, attenuated the shear-induced MMP-9 promoter activity. In addition, transfection of constructs encoding dominant negative mutants of Ras, Rac, and Cdc42 attenuated the induction of c-Jun transcriptional activity by shear stress.

6 FUNCTIONAL TISSUE ENGINEERING OF ARTICULAR CARTILAGE

There is great interest in the development of cell-based therapies to address the limited healing capacity of articular cartilage. The majority of cartilage tissue engineering has been performed using rotating wall vessel (RWV) bioreactors. These RWV bioreactors provide a low shear environment and enhanced nutrient transport that is conducive for cartilage-like tissue growth

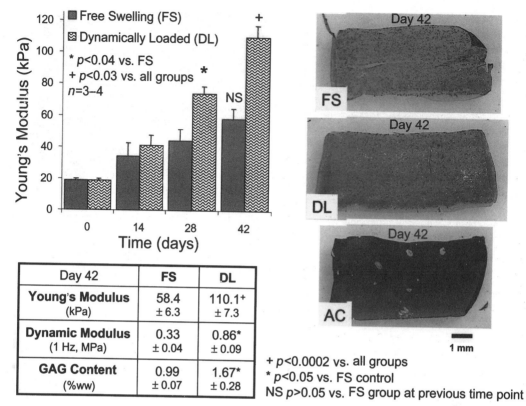

Day 42	FS	DL
Young's Modulus (kPa)	58.4 ± 6.3	110.1+ ± 7.3
Dynamic Modulus (1 Hz, MPa)	0.33 ± 0.04	0.86* ± 0.09
GAG Content (%ww)	0.99 ± 0.07	1.67* ± 0.28

+ p<0.0002 vs. all groups
* p<0.05 vs. FS control
NS p>0.05 vs. FS group at previous time point

FIGURE 6-9. Beneficial effects of applied physiologic deformational loading on the development of equilibrium Young's Modulus in chondrocyte-seeded agarose hydrogel constructs seeded at 10 million cells/ml (205). Dynamic loading (DL) was carried out in a custom deformational loading bioreactor in a volume of 5 ml DMEM with a loading regime of ~10% strain, at 1Hz, 1 hour on/1 hour off, 3 hours of loading/day, for 5 days/week (204). Free-swelling (FS) controls were maintained in the same amount of media adjacent to the loading device. After loading, discs were cultured in 30 ml of media for overnight culture. Every two weeks, 3-4 discs were removed for analysis over a six-week period. Mechanical testing was carried out using stress relaxation tests in unconfined compression with a ramp displacement of 10% strain, after which a sinusoidal displacement of 40 microns was applied at frequencies ranging from 1–0.005 Hz. The Young's modulus and dynamic modulus were calculated from specimen geometry and the resulting load/deformation profiles. Safranin-O staining demonstrates a corresponding increase of GAG-rich matrix elaboration that is consistent with measurements of GAG content.

(84,85,331) as well as a number of other tissue types (94). Perfusion bioreactors have also been used to stimulate construct growth (60,247). Recently, there have been expanding efforts to grow replacement tissues that can perform load-bearing function of native cartilage through application of physiologic levels of loading to cell-seeded constructs in custom bioreactors (36,114). The concept of functional tissue engineering (FTE) is rooted in our understanding of the importance of physical loading as a necessary component in maintaining cartilage homeostasis that has been gained from

decades of *in vivo* and *in vitro* basic science studies of cartilage mechanical signal transduction (110,112–116,221,222,238–249). The goal for FTE of articular cartilage is to grow a tissue that has the mechanical properties that permit the development of significant interstitial fluid pressurization within the tissue, responsible for its creep and stress-relaxation properties, as well as the lubrication properties of articular cartilage (see Chapter 10 by Ateshian and Mow [9,219,220,298]). Hydrostatic pressurization and deformational loading represent two significant components of the chondrocyte physical environment. Long-term application of intermittent hydrostatic pressurization using chondrocyte-seeded polyglycolic acid scaffolds (39,123) has enhanced elaboration of construct material and biochemical properties. Long-term deformational loading has also been shown to enhance matrix elaboration and material properties of chondrocyte-seeded agarose constructs (204,205) (Fig. 6-9). Such physical loading is also being used to spur differentiation of cell type (64).

7 SUMMARY AND CONCLUSIONS

It is evident that the process of mechanical signal transduction in cartilage involves a complex sequence of both mechanical and biochemical processes. Many other detailed studies must be performed before the disparate and scattered data can be eventually sorted out, and before we can fully understand the processes of mechanical signal transduction in cartilage. In summarizing the effects of physical factors on chondrocyte activity, consistent findings among different studies and model systems suggest the following broad conclusions:

- The mechanical environment of the chondrocytes plays an important role in the health and function of the diarthrodial joint *in vivo*. Significant deviations from the normal pattern of joint loading seem to result in deleterious and often irreversible changes in the articular cartilage and surrounding joint tissues.
- Under normal physiologic conditions, the chondrocyte population is exposed to changes in the mechanical, physicochemical, and electrical environment of the ECM, resulting in spatial and temporal variations in stress, strain, fluid flow, fluid pressure, osmotic pressure, FCD, pH, and electric field effects within the cartilage ECM. These physical phenomena have the potential to activate multiple cellular signaling pathways.
- In general, static compression of articular cartilage results in a suppression of biosynthesis. This effect is presumed to be related to

the changes in the physicochemical environment of the chondrocytes in response to matrix deformation, such as increase of FCD and its associated increase of osmotic pressure and intra-tissue pH, and/or changes in cell shape. Cyclic or intermittent (i.e., time-varying) compression of articular cartilage or chondrocytes *in vitro* significantly increases biosynthetic activity. Indirect evidence suggests that this stimulatory effect is related to factors involving interstitial fluid and ion flows in response to gradients in the mechanical stress-strain field and/or the development of a non-homogeneous distribution of the FCD. These factors include enhanced nutrient transport, flow-induced shear stresses and frictional drag forces, and electrokinetic signals such as electrical potentials due to fluid streaming and ion transport due to diffusion.

- Static and intermittent hydrostatic pressure can affect chondrocyte activity in a manner that is dependent on several factors such as the duration, magnitude, and frequency of loading.
- Externally applied electric fields can affect chondrocyte activity, supporting the notion that mechanically induced electric fields *in vivo* may play a role in the process of mechanical signal transduction.
- Cellular shape and volume change in response to ECM deformation or volumetric changes may affect biosynthesis. Deformations may be transduced to the cell through several different signaling mechanisms, including stretch-activated ion channels on the cell membrane or through a physical link between the ECM and the cytoskeleton. The plasma membrane is also likely to be involved in the transduction of hydrostatic pressure, osmotic and ionic changes, and ECM composition. Intracellular signaling in these cases seems to be occurring through transmembrane enzymatic and second messenger pathways (i.e., Ca^{2+}, IP_3, cAMP, MAPKs).
- Using a functional tissue engineering approach, the application of physiologic loadings to cell-seeded constructs can enhance the development of cartilage-like tissues *in vitro*.

8 ACKNOWLEDGMENTS

The authors would like to acknowledge the support of National Institutes of Health, the North Carolina Biotechnology Center, the Department of Veteran's Affairs, the National Science Foundation, and the Whitaker Foundation. We would like to thank Drs. Robert Sah and Lori Setton for important input into this chapter.

REFERENCES

1. Aaron RK, Ciombor DM. Enhancement of extracellular matrix synthesis in cartilage explant cultures by exposure to an electric field. *Trans Orthop Res Soc* 1993;18:630.

2. Allen FD, Hung CT, Pollack SR, et al. Mechanochemical coupling in the flow-induced activation of intracellular calcium signaling in primary cultured bone cells. *J Biomech* 2000;33:1585–1591.

3. Altman RD, Tenenbaum J, Latta L, et al. Biomechanical and biochemical properties of dog cartilage in experimentally induced osteoarthritis. *Ann Rheum Dis* 1984;43:83–90.

4. Armstrong CG, Mow VC. Variations in the intrinsic mechanical properties of human articular cartilage with age, degeneration, and water content. *J Bone Joint Surg Am* 1982;64:88–94.

5. Armstrong CG, Lai WM, Mow VC. An analysis of the unconfined compression of articular cartilage. *J Biomech Eng* 1984;106:165–173.

6. Armstrong CG, Mow VC, Wirth CR. Biomechanics of impact-induced microdamage to articular cartilage: a possible genesis for chondromalacia patella. In: Finerman G, ed. *AAOS symposium on sports medicine: the knee.* St. Louis: WB Saunders, 1985:70–84.

7. Arnoczky SP, Warren RF, Kaplan N. Meniscal remodeling following partial meniscectomy—an experimental study in the dog. *Arthroscopy* 1985;1:247–252.

8. Ateshian GA, Lai WM, Zhu WB, et al. An asymptotic solution for the contact of two biphasic cartilage layers. *J Biomech* 1994;27:1347–1360.

9. Ateshian GA. A theoretical formulation for boundary friction in articular cartilage. *J Biomech Eng* 1997;119:81–86.

10. Atkinson PJ, Haut RC. Subfracture insult to the human cadaver patellofemoral joint produces occult injury. *J Orthop Res* 1995;13:936–944.

11. Bachrach NM, Valhmu WB, Stazzone E, et al. Changes in proteoglycan synthesis of chondrocytes in articular cartilage are associated with the time-dependent changes in their mechanical environment. *J Biomech* 1995;28:1561–1570.

12. Bachrach NM, Mow VC, Guilak F. Incompressibility of the solid matrix of articular cartilage under high hydrostatic pressures. *J Biomech* 1998;31:445–451.

13. Banes AJ, Gilbert J, Taylor D, et al. A new vacuum-operated stress-providing instrument that applies static or variable duration cyclic tension or compression to cells *in vitro. J Cell Sci* 1985;75:35–42.

14. Barbee KA, Macarak EJ, Thibault LE. Strain measurements in cultured vascular smooth muscle cells subjected to mechanical deformation. *Ann Biomed Eng* 1994;22:14–22.

15. Bassett CA, Pawluk RJ. Electrical behavior of cartilage during loading. *Science* 1972;178:982–983.

16. Behrens F, Kraft EL, Oegema TR. Biochemical changes in articular cartilage after joint immobilization by casting and external fixation. *J Orthop Res* 1989;7:335–343.

17. Benya PD, Shaffer JD. Dedifferentiated chondrocytes reexpress the differentiated collagen phenotype when cultured in agarose gels. *Cell* 1982;30:215–224.

18. Ben-Ze'ev A. Animal cell shape changes and gene expression. *Bioessays* 1991;13:207–212.

19. Berjon JJ, Munera L, Calvo M. Degenerative lesions in articular cartilage after meniscectomy. *Traumatol* 1991;31:342–350.

20. Blain EJ, Gilbert SJ, Wardale RJ, et al. Up-regulation of matrix metalloproteinase expression and activation following cyclical compressive loading of articular cartilage *in vitro. Arch Biochem Biophys* 2001;396:49–55.

21. Bonassar LJ, Frank EH, Murray JC, et al. Changes in cartilage composition and physical properties due to stromelysin degradation. *Arthritis Rheum* 1995;38:173–183.

22. Bonassar LJ, Grodzinsky AJ, Srinivasan A, et al. Mechanical and physicochemical regulation of the action of insulin-like growth factor-I on articular cartilage. *Arch Biochem Biophys* 2000;379:57–63.

23. Bourret LA, Rodan GA. Inhibition of cAMP accumulation in epiphyseal cartilage cells exposed to physiological pressure. *Calcif Tissue Res* 1976;21:431–436.

24. Bourret LA, Rodan GA. The role of calcium in the inhibition of cAMP accumulation in epiphyseal cartilage cells exposed to physiological pressure. *J Cell Physiol* 1976;88:353–361.

25. Boustany NN, Gray ML, Black AC, et al. Time-dependent changes in the response of cartilage to static compression suggest interstitial pH is not the only signaling mechanism. *J Orthop Res* 1995;13:740–750.

26. Boustany NN, Gray ML, Black AC, et al. Correlation between synthetic activity and glycosaminoglycan concentration in epiphyseal cartilage raises

questions about the regulatory role of interstitial pH. *J Orthop Res* 1995;13:733–739.

27. Brandt KD, Myers SL, Burr D, et al. Osteoarthritic changes in canine articular cartilage, subchondral bone, and synovium fifty-four months after transection of the anterior cruciate ligament. *Arthritis Rheum* 1991;34:1560–1570.

28. Brighton CT, Unger AS, Stambough JL. In vitro growth of bovine articular cartilage chondrocytes in various capacitively coupled electrical fields. *J Orthop Res* 1984;2:15–22.

29. Brown TD. Techniques for mechanical stimulation of cells in vitro: a review. *J Biomech* 2000;33:3–14.

30. Burton-Wurster N, Vernier-Singer M, Farquhar T, et al. Effect of compressive loading and unloading on the synthesis of total protein, proteoglycan, and fibronectin by canine cartilage explants. *J Orthop Res* 1993;11:717–729.

31. Buschmann MD, Gluzband YA, Grodzinsky AJ, et al. Mechanical compression modulates matrix biosynthesis in chondrocyte/agarose culture. *J Cell Sci* 1995;108:1497–1508.

32. Buschmann MD, Maurer AM, Berger E, et al. A method of quantitative autoradiography for the spatial localization of proteoglycan synthesis rates in cartilage. *J Histochem Cytochem* 1996;44:423–431.

33. Buschmann MD, Kim YJ, Wong M, et al. Stimulation of aggrecan synthesis in cartilage explants by cyclic loading is localized to regions of high interstitial fluid flow. *Arch Biochem Biophys* 1999;366:1–7.

34. Bush PG, Hall AC. Regulatory volume decrease (RVD) by isolated and in situ bovine articular chondrocytes. *J Cell Physiol* 2001;187:304–314.

35. Bush PG, Hall AC. The osmotic sensitivity of isolated and in situ bovine articular chondrocytes. *J Orthop Res* 2001;19:768–778.

36. Butler DL, Goldstein SA, Guilak F. Functional tissue engineering: the role of biomechanics. *J Biomech Eng* 2000;122:570–575.

37. Carafoli E. Intracellular calcium homeostasis. *Annu Rev Biochem* 1987;56:395–433.

38. Carney SL, Billingham ME, Muir H, et al. Demonstration of increased proteoglycan turnover in cartilage explants from dogs with experimental osteoarthritis. *J Orthop Res* 1984;2:201–206.

39. Carver SE, Heath CA. Semi-continuous perfusion system for delivering intermittent physiological pressure to regenerating cartilage. *Tissue Eng* 1999;5:1–11.

40. Caterson B, Lowther DA. Changes in the metabolism of the proteoglycans from sheep articular cartilage in response to mechanical stress. *Biochim Biophys Acta* 1978;540:412–422.

41. Chao P-HG, Roy R, Mauck RL, et al. Chondrocyte translocation response to direct current electric fields. *J Biomech Eng Trans ASME* 2000;122:261–267.

42. Chen AC, Nguyen TT, Sah RL. Streaming potentials in normal and degraded articular cartilage. *Trans Orthop Res Soc* 1995;20:336.

43. Chen AC, Bae WC, Schinagl RM, et al. Depth- and strain-dependent mechanical and electromechanical properties of full-thickness bovine articular cartilage in confined compression. *J Biomech* 2001;34:1–12.

44. Chen CT, Burton-Wurster N, Lust G, et al. Compositional and metabolic changes in damaged cartilage are peak-stress, stress-rate, and loading-duration dependent. *J Orthop Res* 1999;17:870–879.

45. Chen C-T, Burton-Wurster N, Borden C, et al. Chondrocyte necrosis and apoptosis in impact damaged articular cartilage. *J Orthop Res* 2001;19:703–711.

46. Chen Q, Zhen X, Wu QQ, et al. Activation of extracellular signal-regulated kinase and P38 MAP kinase is required for mechanical stimulation of chondrocyte proliferation. *Trans Orthop Res* 1999;45:7.

47. Chen SS, Falcovitz YH, Schneiderman R, et al. Depth-dependent compressive properties of normal aged human femoral head articular cartilage: relationship to fixed charge density. *Osteoarthritis Cartilage* 2001;9:561–569.

48. Christensen O. Mediation of cell volume by $Ca2+$ influx through stretch-activated channels. *Nature* 1987;330:66–68.

49. Clark CC, Iannotti JP, Misra S, et al. Effects of thapsigargin, an intracellular calcium-mobilizing agent, on synthesis and secretion of cartilage collagen and proteoglycan. *J Orthop Res* 1994;12:601–611.

50. Cohen S, Snir E, Schneiderman R, et al. Solute transport in cartilage: effect of static compression. *Trans Orthop Res Soc* 1993;18:622.

51. Cruveilhier J. Observations sur les cartilages diarthrodiaux et les maladies des articulations diarthrodiales. *Arch Gen Med (Paris)* 1824;4:161–198.

52. Das P, Schurman DJ, Smith RL. Nitric oxide and G proteins mediate the response of bovine articular chondrocytes to fluid-induced shear. *J Orthop Res* 1997;15:87–93.

53. Davies PF, Tripathi SC. Mechanical stress mechanisms and the cell. An endothelial paradigm. *Circ Res* 1993;72:239–245.

54. De Witt MT, Handley CJ, Oakes BW, et al. In vitro response of chondrocytes to mechanical loading. The effect of short term mechanical tension. *Connect Tissue Res* 1984;12:97–109.

55. Deshayes CMP, Hall AC, Urban JPG. Effects of extracellular osmolality on porcine articular chondrocyte volume. *J Physiol* 1993;467:214P.

56. Deshmukh K, Kline WG, Sawyer BD. Role of calcium in the phenotypic expression of rabbit articular chondrocytes in culture. *FEBS Lett* 1976;67:48–51.

57. Donohue JM, Buss D, Oegema TR Jr, et al. The effects of indirect blunt trauma on adult canine articular cartilage. *J Bone Joint Surg Am* 1983;65:948–957.

58. Drezner MK, Neelon FA, Lebovitz HE. Stimulation of cartilage macromolecule synthesis by adenosine 3′,5′-monophosphate. *Biochim Biophys Acta* 1976;425:521–531.

59. Dunham J, Shackleton D, Nahir A, et al. Altered orientation of glycosaminoglycans and cellular changes in the tibial cartilage in the first two weeks of experimental osteoarthritis. *J Orthop Res* 1985;3:258–268.

60. Dunkelman NS, Zimber MP, LeBaron RG, et al. Cartilage production by rabbit articular chondrocytes on polyglycolic acid scaffolds in a closed bioreactor system. *Biotech Bioeng*, 1995;46:299–305.

61. Eilam Y, Beit-Or A, Nevo Z. Decrease in cytosolic free Ca2+ and enhanced proteoglycan synthesis induced by cartilage derived growth factors in cultured chondrocytes. *Biochim Biophys Res Commun* 1985;132:770–779.

62. Eilam Y, Beit-Or A, Nevo Z. Cytosolic free Ca++ as a signal for proteoglycan synthesis and cell proliferation in cultured chondrocytes. In: Horowitz S, Sela I, eds. *Current advances in skeletogenesis.* Jerusalem: Heiliger, 1987:127–139.

63. Eisenberg S, Grodzinsky A. Electrokinetic micromodel of extracellular matrix and other polyelectrolyte networks. *Physicochem Hydrodynam* 1988;10:517–530.

64. Elder SH, Kimura JH, Soslowsky LJ, et al. Effect of compressive loading on chondrocyte differentiation in agarose cultures of chick limb-bud cells. *J Orthop Res* 2000;18:78–86.

65. Elfervig MK, Graff RD, Lee GM, et al. ATP induces Ca2+ signaling in human chondrons cultured in three-dimensional agarose films. *Osteoarthritis Cartilage* 2001;9:518–526.

66. Elliott DM, Guilak F, Vail TP, et al. Tensile properties of articular cartilage are altered by meniscectomy in a canine model of osteoarthritis. *J Orthop Res* 1999;17:503–508.

67. Erickson GR, Caribardi A, Guilak F. Calcium dependent and independent volume regulation in articular chondrocytes. *Trans Orthop Res Soc* 2000;25:922.

68. Erickson GR, Guilak F. Osmotic stress initiates intracellular calcium waves in chondrocytes through calcium influx, the inositol phosphate, and a G-protein mediated pathway. *Trans Orthop Res Soc* 2000;25:923.

69. Erickson GR, Alexopoulos LG, Guilak F. Hyperosmotic stress induces volume change and calcium transients in chondrocytes by transmembrane, phospholipid, and G-protein pathways. *J Biomech* 2001;34:1527–1535.

70. Erickson GR, Guilak F. Dissociation and remodeling of the actin cytoskeleton of chondrocytes in response to hypo-osmotic stress. *Trans Orthop Res Soc* 2001;26:180.

71. Eyre DR, McDevitt CA, Billingham ME, et al. Biosynthesis of collagen and other matrix proteins by articular cartilage in experimental osteoarthrosis. *Biochem J* 1980;188:823–837.

72. Fairbank TJ. Knee joint changes after meniscectomy. *J Bone Joint Surg* 1948;30B:664–670.

73. Farquhar T, Xia Y, Mann K, et al. Swelling and fibronectin accumulation in articular cartilage explants after cyclical impact. *J Orthop Res* 1996;14:417–423.

74. Fermor B, Haribabu B, Brice Weinberg J, et al. Mechanical stress and nitric oxide influence leukotriene production in cartilage. *Biochem Biophys Res Commun* 2001;285:806–810.

75. Fermor B, Weinberg JB, Pisetsky DS, et al. The effects of static and intermittent compression on nitric oxide production in articular cartilage explants. *J Orthop Res* 2001;19:729–737.

76. Fermor B, Weinberg JB, Pisetsky DS, et al. Induction of cyclooxygenase-2 by mechanical stress through a nitric oxide-regulated pathway. *Osteoarthritis Cartilage* 2002;10:792–798.

77. Floman Y, Eyre DR, Glimcher MJ. Induction of osteoarthrosis in the rabbit knee joint: biochemical studies on the articular cartilage. *Clin Orthop* 1980;278–286.

78. Frangos JA, Eskin SG, McIntire LV, et al. Flow effects on prostacyclin production by cultured human endothelial cells. *Science* 1985;227:1477–1479.

79. Frank E, Grodzinsky A, Phillips S, et al. Physicochemical and bioelectrical determinants of cartilage material properties. In: Mow VC, Ratcliffe A, Woo SLY, eds. *Biomechanics of diarthrodial joints.* New York: Springer-Verlag, 1990:261–282.

80. Frank EH, Grodzinsky AJ. Cartilage electromechanics–II. A continuum model of cartilage electrokinetics and correlation with experiments. *J Biomech* 1987;20:629–639.

81. Frank EH, Grodzinsky AJ. Cartilage electromechanics–I. Electrokinetic transduction and the effects of electrolyte pH and ionic strength. *J Biomech* 1987;20:615–627.

82. Frank EH, Grodzinsky AJ, Koob TJ, et al. Streaming potentials: a sensitive index of enzymatic degradation in articular cartilage. *J Orthop Res* 1987;5:497–508.

83. Frank EH, Jin M, Loening AM, et al. A versatile shear and compression apparatus for mechanical stimulation of tissue culture explants. *J Biomech* 2000;33:1523–1527.

84. Freed LE, Vunjak-Novakovic G, Langer R. Cultivation of cell-polymer cartilage implants in bioreactors. *J Cell Biochem* 1993;51:257–264.
85. Freed LE, Martin I, Vunjak-Novakovic G. Frontiers in tissue engineering. In vitro modulation of chondrogenesis. *Clin Orthop* 1999;367:S46–58.
86. Freeman PM, Natarjan RN, Kimura JH, et al. Chondrocyte cells respond mechanically to compressive loads. *J Orthop Res* 1994;12:311–320.
87. Frenkel SR, Clancy RM, Ricci JL, et al. Effects of nitric oxide on chondrocyte migration, adhesion, and cytoskeletal assembly. *Arthritis Rheum* 1996;39(11):1905–1912.
88. Froimson MI, Ratcliffe A, Gardner TR, et al. Differences in patellofemoral joint cartilage material properties and their significance to the etiology of cartilage surface fibrillation. *Osteoarthritis Cartilage* 1997;5:377–386.
89. Fujisawa T, Hattori T, Takahashi K, et al. Cyclic mechanical stress induces extracellular matrix degradation in cultured chondrocytes via gene expression of matrix metalloproteinases and interleukin-1. *J Biochem* 1999;125:966–975.
90. Fukuda K, Asada S, Kumano F, et al. Cyclic tensile stretch on bovine articular chondrocytes inhibits protein kinase C activity. *J Lab Clin Med* 1997;130:209–215.
91. Garcia AM, Frank EH, Grimshaw PE, et al. Contributions of fluid convection and electrical migration to transport in cartilage: relevance to loading. *Arch Biochem Biophys* 1996;333:317–325.
92. Genes N, Rowley JA, Mooney DJ, et al. Culture of chondrocytes in RGD-bonded alginate: effects of mechanical and biosynthetic properties. ASME *Adv Bioeng* 1999;BED-42:1–2.
93. Gilbertson EMM. Development of periarticular osteophytes in experimentally induced osteoarthrosis in the dog. *Ann Rheum Dis* 1975;34: 12–25.
94. Goodwin TJ, Prewett TL, Wolf DA, et al. Reduced shear stress: a major component in the ability of mammalian tissues to form three-dimensional assemblies in simulated microgravity. *J Cell Biochem* 1993;51:301–311.
95. Graff RD, Lazarowski ER, Banes AJ, et al. ATP release by mechanically loaded porcine chondrons in pellet culture. *Arthritis Rheum* 2000;43:1571–1579.
96. Gray ML, Pizzanelli AM, Grodzinsky AJ, et al. Mechanical and physiochemical determinants of the chondrocyte biosynthetic response. *J Orthop Res* 1988;6:777–792.
97. Gray ML, Pizzanelli AM, Lee RC, et al. Kinetics of the chondrocyte biosynthetic response to compressive load and release. *Biochim Biophys Acta* 1989;991:415–425.
98. Grodzinsky AJ, Lipshitz H, Glimcher MJ. Electromechanical properties of articular cartilage during compression and stress relaxation. *Nature* 1978;275:448–450.
99. Grodzinsky AJ. Electromechanical and physicochemical properties of connective tissue. *Crit Rev Biomed Eng* 1983;9:133–199.
100. Grumbles RM, Howell DS, Howard GA, et al. Cartilage metalloproteases in disuse atrophy. *J Rheumatol* 1995;22:146–148.
101. Gu W, Lai WM, Mow VC. Theoretical basis for measurements of cartilage fixed-charge density using streaming current and electro-osmosis effects. *ASME Adv Bioeng* 1993;26:55–58.
102. Gu WY, Lai WM, Mow VC. Transport of fluid and ions through a porous-permeable charged-hydrated tissue, and streaming potential data on normal bovine articular cartilage. *J Biomech* 1993;26:709–723.
103. Gu WY, Lai WM, Mow VC. A mixture theory for charged hydrated soft tissues containing multielectrolytes: passive transport and swelling behaviors. *J Biomech Eng* 1998;120:169–180.
104. Guharay F, Sachs F. Stretch-activated single ion channel currents in tissue-cultured embryonic chick skeletal muscle. *J Physiol* 1984;352:685–701.
105. Guilak F, Hou JS, Ratcliffe A, et al. Articular cartilage under hydrostatic loading. *ASME Adv Bioeng* 1988;BED-8:183–186.
106. Guilak F. *Cell-matrix interactions and metabolic changes in articular cartilage under compression.* New York: Columbia University, Ph.D. Dissertation, 1992.
107. Guilak F, Mow VC. Determination of the mechanical response of the chondrocyte *in situ* using finite element modeling and confocal microscopy. *ASME Adv Bioeng* 1992;BED-20:21–23.
108. Guilak F, Donahue HJ, Zell R, et al. Deformation-induced calcium signaling in articular chondrocytes. In: Mow VC, Guilak F, Tran-Son-Tay R, et al., eds. *Cell mechanics and cellular engineering.* New York: Springer-Verlag, 1994:380–397.
109. Guilak F, Meyer BC, Ratcliffe A, et al. The effects of matrix compression on proteoglycan metabolism in articular cartilage explants. *Osteoarthritis Cartilage* 1994;2:91–101.
110. Guilak F, Ratcliffe A, Lane N, et al. Mechanical and biochemical changes in the superficial zone of articular cartilage in canine experimental osteoarthritis. *J Orthop Res* 1994;12:474–484.
111. Guilak F. Compression-induced changes in the shape and volume of the chondrocyte nucleus. *J Biomech* 1995;28:1529–1542.
112. Guilak F, Ratcliffe A, Mow VC. Chondrocyte deformation and local tissue strain in articular cartilage: a confocal microscopy study. *J Orthop Res* 1995;13:410–421.
113. Guilak F, Mow VC. The mechanical environment of the chondrocyte: a biphasic finite element model

of cell-matrix interactions in articular cartilage. *J Biomech* 2000;33:1663–1673.

114. Guilak F, Butler DL, Goldstein SA. Functional tissue engineering: the role of biomechanics in articular cartilage repair. *Clin Orthop* 2001;S295–305.

115. Guilak F, Erickson GR, Ting-Beall HP. The effects of osmotic stress on the viscoelastic and physical properties of articular chondrocytes. *Biophys J* 2002;82:720–727.

116. Hall AC, Urban JP, Gehl KA. The effects of hydrostatic pressure on matrix synthesis in articular cartilage. *J Orthop Res* 1991;9:1–10.

117. Handley CJ, Lowther DA. Extracellular metabolism by chondrocytes. III. Modulation of proteoglycan synthesis by extracellular levels of proteoglycan in cartilage cells in culture. *Biochim Biophys Acta* 1977;500:132–139.

118. Hansen LK, Ingber DE. Regulation of nucleocytoplasmic transport by mechanical forces transmitted through the cytoskeleton. In: Feldher C, ed. *Nuclear trafficking.* San Diego: Academic Press, 1992:71–86.

119. Hardingham TE, Fitton-Jackson S, Muir H. Replacement of proteoglycans in embryonic chicken cartilage in organ culture after treatment with testicular hyaluronidase. *J Biochem* 1972; 129:101–112.

120. Hardingham TE, Fosang AJ, Dudhia J. Aggrecan: the chondroitin sulfate/keratan sulfate proteoglycan from cartilage. In: Kuettner KE, Schleyerbach R, Peyron JG et al., eds. *Articular cartilage and osteoarthritis.* New York: Raven Press, 1992:5–20.

121. Hascall V, Handley C, McQuillan D, et al. The effect of serum on biosynthesis of proteoglycans by bovine articular cartilage in culture. *Arch Biochem Biophys* 1983;224:206–223.

122. Hasegawa I, Kuriki S, Matsuno S, et al. Dependence of electrical conductivity on fixed charge density in articular cartilage. *Clin Orthop* 1983;177:283–288.

123. Heath CA, Magari SR. Mini-review—mechanical factors affecting cartilage regeneration *in vitro.* *Biotechnol Bioeng* 1996;50:430–437.

124. Hecht JT, Deere M, Putnam E, et al. Characterization of cartilage oligomeric matrix protein (COMP) and cell death in redifferentiated pseudoachondroplasia chondrocytes. *Matrix Biol* 1998;17:625–633.

125. Helminen HJ, Jurvelin J, Kiviranta I, et al. Joint loading effects on articular cartilage: a historical review. In: Helminen HJ, Kiviranta I, Tammi M, et al., eds. *Joint loading: biology and health of articular structures.* Bristol: Wright and Sons, 1987:1–46.

126. Hing WA, Poole CA, Jensen CG, et al. An integrated environmental perfusion chamber and heat-

ing system for long-term, high resolution imaging of living cells. *J Microsc* 2000;199:90–95.

127. Hoch DH, Grodzinsky AJ, Koob TJ, et al. Early changes in material properties of rabbit articular cartilage after meniscectomy. *J Orthop Res* 1983;1:4–12.

128. Hodge W, Fijan R, Carlson K, et al. Contact pressures in the human hip joint measured *in vivo.* *Proc Natl Acad Sci U S A* 1986;83:2879–2883.

129. Hodge WA, Carlson KL, Fijan RS. et al. Contact pressures from an instrumented hip endoprosthesis. *J Bone Joint Surg* 1989;71A:1378–1386.

130. Hollander AP, Pidoux I, Reiner A, et al. Damage to type II collagen in aging and osteoarthritis starts at the articular surface, originates around chondrocytes, and extends into the cartilage with progressive degeneration. *J Clin Invest* 1995;96:2859–2869.

131. Holzer H, Abbot J, Lash J, et al. The loss of phenotypic traits by differentiated cells *in vitro.* I. Dedifferentiation of cartilage cells. *Proc Natl Acad Sci U S A* 1960;46:1533–1542.

132. Honda K, Ohno S, Tanimoto K, et al. The effects of high magnitude cyclic tensile load on cartilage matrix metabolism in cultured chondrocytes. *Eur J Cell Biol* 2000;79:601–609.

133. Hung CT, Henshaw DR, Wang C, et al. Mitogen-activated protein kinase signaling in bovine articular chondrocytes in response to fluid flow does not require calcium mobilization. *J Biomech* 2000;33:73–80.

134. Hung CT, Costa KD, Guo XE. Apparent and transient mechanical properties of chondrocytes during osmotic loading using triphasic theory and AFM indentation. *Adv Bioeng* 2001;BED-50:625–626.

135. Hung CT, Palmer GD, Leroux MA, et al. Disparate aggrecan gene expression in chondrocytes subjected to hypotonic and hypertonic loading. *Biorheology* 2003;40:61–72.

136. Hunter CJ, Imler SM, Malaviya P, et al. Mechanical compression alters gene expression and extracellular matrix synthesis by chondrocytes cultured in collagen I gels. *Biomaterials* 2002;23:1249–1259.

137. Hynes RO. Integrins, A family of cell surface receptors. *Cell* 1987;48:549–554.

138. Iannacone WM, Pienkowski D, Pollack SR, et al. Pulsing electromagnetic field stimulation of the *in vitro* growth plate. *J Orthop Res* 1988;6:239–247.

139. Iannotti JP, Naidu S, Noguchi Y, et al. Growth plate matrix vesicle biogenesis. The role of intracellular calcium. *Clin Orthop* 1994;306:222–229.

140. Iino M, Endo M. Calcium-dependent immediate feedback control of inositol 1,4,5-triphosphate-induced Ca2+ release. *Nature* 1992; 360:76–78.

141. Ingber D. Integrins as mechanochemical transducers. *Curr Opin Cell Biol* 1991;3:841–848.

142. Jackson DW, McDevitt CA, Simon TM, et al. Meniscal transplantation using fresh and cryopreserved allografts. An experimental study in goats. *Am J Sports Med* 1992;20:644–656.

143. Jeffrey JE, Gregory DW, Aspden RM. Matrix damage and chondrocyte viability following a single impact load on articular cartilage. *Arch Biochem Biophys* 1995;322:87–96.

144. Jeffrey JE, Thomson LA, Aspden RM. Matrix loss and synthesis following a single impact load on articular cartilage *in vitro*. *Biochim Biophys Acta* 1997;1334:223–232.

145. Jin G, Sah RL, Li YS, et al. Biomechanical regulation of matrix metalloproteinase-9 in cultured chondrocytes. *J Orthop Res* 2000;18:899–908.

146. Jin M, Frank EH, Quinn TM, et al. Tissue shear deformation stimulates proteoglycan and protein biosynthesis in bovine cartilage explants. *Arch Biochem Biophys* 2001;395:41–48.

147. Jin M, Fanning P, Emkey G, et al. Upregulation of ERK 1/2 phosphorylation and transcriptional level of type II collagen and aggrecan core protein in response to tissue shear deformation in cartilage explant. *48th Trans Orthop Res Soc* 2002;27:31.

148. Jones IL, Klamfeldt A, Sanstrom, T. The effect of continuous mechanical pressure upon the turnover of articular cartilage proteoglycans *in vitro*. *Clin Orthop* 1982;165:283–289.

149. Jortikka MO, Parkkinen JJ, Inkinen RI, et al. The role of microtubules in the regulation of proteoglycan synthesis in chondrocytes under hydrostatic pressure. *Arch Biochem Biophys* 2000;374:172–180.

150. Jurvelin J, Helminen HJ, Lauritsalo S, et al. Influences of joint immobilization and running exercise on articular cartilage surfaces of young rabbits. A semiquantitative stereomicroscopic and scanning electron microscopic study. *Acta Anat (Basel)* 1985;122:62–68.

151. Jurvelin J, Kiviranta I, Tammi M, et al. Effect of physical exercise on indentation stiffness of articular cartilage in the canine knee. *Int J Sports Med* 1986;7:106–110.

152. Jurvelin J, Kiviranta I, Saamanen AM, et al. Partial restoration of immobilization-induced softening of canine articular cartilage after remobilization of the knee (stifle) joint. *J Orthop Res* 1989;7:352–358.

153. Jurvelin J, Kiviranta I, Saamanen AM, et al. Indentation stiffness of young canine knee articular cartilage—influence of strenuous joint loading. *J Biomech* 1990;23:1239–1246.

154. Kempson GE, Muir H, Pollard C, et al. The tensile properties of the cartilage of human femoral condyles related to the content of collagen and glycosaminoglycans. *Biochim Biophys Acta* 1973;297:456–472.

155. Kim YJ, Sah RL, Grodzinsky AJ, et al. Mechanical regulation of cartilage biosynthetic behavior: physical stimuli. *Arch Biochem Biophys* 1994;311:1–12.

156. Kim YJ, Bonassar LJ, Grodzinsky AJ. The role of cartilage streaming potential, fluid flow and pressure in the stimulation of chondrocyte biosynthesis during dynamic compression. *J Biomech* 1995;28:1055–1066.

157. Kimura J, Schipplein O, Kuettner K, et al. Effects of hydrostatic loading on extracellular matrix formation. *Trans Orthop Res Soc* 1985;9:365.

158. King D. The healing of semilunar cartilages. *Clin Orthop* 1936;4–7.

159. Kiviranta I, Tammi M, Jurvelin J, et al. Moderate running exercise augments glycosaminoglycans and thickness of articular cartilage in the knee joint of young beagle dogs. *J Orthop Res* 1988;6:188–195.

160. Kiviranta I, Tammi M, Jurvelin J, et al. Articular cartilage thickness and glycosaminoglycan distribution in the canine knee joint after strenuous running exercise. *Clin Orthop* 1992;283:302–308.

161. Kiviranta I, Tammi M, Jurvelin J, et al. Articular cartilage thickness and glycosaminoglycan distribution in the young canine knee joint after remobilization of the immobilized limb. *J Orthop Res* 1994;12:161–167.

162. Klein-Nulend J, Veldhuijzen JP, van de Stadt RJ, et al. Influence of intermittent compressive force on proteoglycan content in calcifying growth plate cartilage *in vitro*. *J Biol Chem* 1987;262:15490–15495.

163. Knight MM, Lee DA, Bader DL. The influence of elaborated pericellular matrix on the deformation of isolated articular chondrocytes cultured in agarose. *Biochim Biophys Acta* 1998;1405:67–77.

164. Korver TH, van de Stadt RJ, Kiljan E, et al. Effects of loading on the synthesis of proteoglycans in different layers of anatomically intact articular cartilage *in vitro*. *J Rheumatol* 1992;19:905–912.

165. Kurosawa H, Fukubayashi T, Nakajuma H. Load-bearing mode of the knee joint: physical behavior of the knee joint with or without menisci. *Clin Orthop* 1980;149:283–290.

166. Lafeber F, Veldhuijzen JP, Vanroy JL, et al. Intermittent hydrostatic compressive force stimulates exclusively the proteoglycan synthesis of osteoarthritic human cartilage. *Br J Rheumatol* 1992;31:437–442.

167. Lai WM, Mow VC. Drag-induced compression of articular cartilage during a permeation experiment. *Biorheology* 1980;17:111–123.

168. Lai WM, Hou JS, Mow VC. A triphasic theory for the swelling and deformation behaviors of

articular cartilage. *J Biomech Eng* 1991;113:245–258.

169. Lai WM, Gu WY, Mow VC. On the conditional equivalence of chemical loading and mechanical loading on articular cartilage. *J Biomech* 1998;31:1181–1185.

170. Lai WM, Mow VC, Sun DN, et al. On the electric potentials inside a charged soft hydrated biological tissue: streaming potential vs. diffusion potential. *J Biomech Eng* 2000;122:336–346.

171. Lammi MJ, Hakkinen TP, Parkkinen JJ, et al. Adaptation of canine femoral head articular cartilage to long distance running exercise in young beagles. *Ann Rheum Dis* 1993;52:369–377.

172. Lane JM, Chisena E, Black J. Experimental knee instability: early mechanical property changes in articular cartilage in a rabbit model. *Clin Orthop* 1979;140:262–265.

173. Larsson T, Aspden RM, Heinegard D. Effects of mechanical load on cartilage matrix biosynthesis in vitro. *Matrix* 1991;11:388–394.

174. Lee DA, Bader DL. The development and characterization of an *in vitro* system to study strain-induced cell deformation in isolated chondrocytes. *In Vitro Cell Dev Biol* 1995;31:828–835.

175. Lee DA, Frean SP, Lees P, et al. Dynamic mechanical compression influences nitric oxide production by articular chondrocytes seeded in agarose. *Biochem Biophys Res Commun* 1998;251:580–585.

176. Lee GM, Poole CA, Kelley SS, et al. Isolated chondrons: a viable alternative for studies of chondrocyte metabolism in vitro. *Osteoarthritis Cartilage* 1997;5:261–274.

177. Lee MS, Trindade MC, Ikenoue T, et al. Effects of shear stress on nitric oxide and matrix protein gene expression in human osteoarthritic chondrocytes in vitro. *J Orthop Res* 2002;20:556–561.

178. Lee RC, Rich JB, Kelley KM, et al. A comparison of *in vitro* cellular responses to mechanical and electrical stimulation. *Am Surg* 1982;48:567–574.

179. Lefkoe TP, Trafton PG, Ehrlich MG, et al. An experimental model of femoral condylar defect leading to osteoarthrosis. *J Orthop Trauma* 1993;7:458–467.

180. Lefkoe TP, Walsh WR, Anastasatos J, et al. Remodeling of articular step-offs. Is osteoarthrosis dependent on defect size? *Clin Orthop* 1995;314:253–265.

181. LeRoux MA, Arokoski J, Vail TP, et al. Simultaneous changes in the mechanical properties, quantitative collagen organization, and proteoglycan concentration of articular cartilage following canine meniscectomy. *J Orthop Res* 2000;18:383–392.

182. Levin A, Burton-Wurster N, Chen C-T, et al. Intercellular signaling as a cause of cell death in cyclically impacted cartilage explants. *Osteoarthritis Cartilage* 2001;9:702–711.

183. Levy IM, Torzilli PA, Fisch ID. The contribution of the menisci to the stability of the knee. In: Mow VC, Jackson DW, Arnoczky SP, eds. *Knee meniscus: basic and clinical foundations.* New York: Raven Press, 1992:107–115.

184. Linn FC, Sokoloff L. Movement and composition of interstitial fluid of cartilage. *Arthritis Rheum* 1965;8:481–494.

185. Lippiello L, Kaye C, Neumata T, et al. *In vitro* metabolic response of articular cartilage segments to low levels of hydrostatic pressure. *Connect Tissue Res* 1985;13:99–107.

186. Loeser RF. Integrin-mediated attachment of articular chondrocytes to extracellular matrix proteins. *Arthritis Rheum* 1993;36:1103–1110.

187. Loeser RF. Modulation of integrin-mediated attachment of chondrocytes to extracellular matrix proteins by cations, retinoic acid, and transforming growth factor beta. *Exp Cell Res* 1994;211:17–23.

188. Loeser RF, Carlson CS, McGee MP. Expression of beta 1 integrins by cultured articular chondrocytes and in osteoarthritic cartilage. *Exp Cell Res* 1995;217:248–257.

189. Lotke P, Black J, Richardson S. Electromechanical properties in human articular cartilage. *J Bone Joint Surg Am* 1974;56A:1040–1046.

190. Lucchinetti E, Adams CS, Horton WE Jr., Torzilli PA. Cartilage viability after repetitive loading: a preliminary report. *Osteoarthritis Cartilage* 2002;10:71–81.

191. Lufti AM. Morphological changes in the articular cartilage after meniscectomy: an experimental study in the monkey. *J Bone Joint Surg* 1975;57B:525–528.

192. MacGinitie LA, Gluzband YA, Grodzinsky AJ. Electric field stimulation can increase protein synthesis in articular cartilage explants. *J Orthop Res* 1994;12:151–160.

193. Mallein-Gerin F, Garrone R, van der Rest M. Proteoglycan and collagen synthesis are correlated with actin organization in dedifferentiating chondrocytes. *Eur J Cell Biol* 1991;56:364–373.

194. Manicourt DH, Thonar EJ-M, Pita JC, et al. Changes in the sedimentation profile of proteoglycan aggregates in early experimental canine osteoarthritis. *Connect Tissue Res* 1989;23:33–50.

195. Mankin HJ, Brandt KD. Biochemistry and metabolism of articular cartilage in osteoarthritis. In: Moskowitz RW, Howell DS, Goldberg VM, et al., eds. *Osteoarthritis: diagnosis and medical/surgical management.* Philadelphia: WB Saunders, 1992:109–154.

196. Maroudas A. Physicochemical properties of cartilage in the light of ion exchange theory. *Biophys J* 1968;8:575–595.

197. Maroudas A. Distribution and diffusion of solutes in articular cartilage. *Biophys J* 1970;10:365–379.

198. Maroudas A. Physical chemistry and the structure of cartilage. *J Physiol* 1972;223:21P–22P.

199. Maroudas A. Mechanisms of fluid transport in cartilaginous tissues. In: Freeman M, ed. *Adult*

articular cartilage. Tunbridge Wells: Pitman Medical, 1973:47–72.

200. Maroudas A. Physicochemical properties of articular cartilage. In: Freeman M, ed. *Adult articular cartilage.* Tunbridge Wells: Pitman Medical, 1979:215–290.

201. Maroudas A. Determination of the rate of glycosaminoglycan synthesis *in vivo* using radioactive sulfate as tracer: comparison with *in vitro* results. In: Maroudas A, Kuettner KE, eds. *Methods in cartilage research.* New York: Academic Press, 1990:143–148.

202. Maroudas A, Popper O, Grushko G. Partition coefficients of IGF-I between cartilage and external medium in the presence and absence of FCS. *Trans Orthop Res Soc* 1991;16:398.

203. Maroudas A, Palla G, Gilav E. Racemization of aspartic acid in human articular cartilage. *Connect Tissue Res* 1992;28:161–169.

204. Mauck RL, Soltz MA, Wang CC, et al. Functional tissue engineering of articular cartilage through dynamic loading of chondrocyte-seeded agarose gels. *J Biomech Eng* 2000;122:252–260.

205. Mauck RL, Wang CC-B, Oswald ES, Ateshian GA, Hung CT. The role of cell seeding density and nutrient supply for articular cartilage tissue engineering with deformational loading. *Osteoarthritis Cartilage* 2003;11(12):879–890.

206. McDevitt C, Gilbertson E, Muir H. An experimental model of osteoarthritis: early morphological and biochemical changes. *J Bone Joint Surg* 1977;59B:24–35.

207. McDevitt CA, Muir H. Biochemical changes in the cartilage of the knee in experimental and natural osteoarthritis in the dog. *J Bone Joint Surg* 1976;58B:94–101.

208. Meyer T, Holowka D, Stryer L. Highly cooperative opening of calcium channels by inositol 1,4,5-trisphosphate. *Science* 1988;240:653–656.

209. Milentijevic D, Torzilli PA. Influence of strain magnitude on water loss and chondrocyte viability in impacted cartilage. *ASME Adv Bioeng* 2001;BED-50:781–782.

210. Miller RP, Husain M, Lohin S. Long acting cAMP analogues enhance sulfate incorporation into matrix proteoglycans and suppress cell division of fetal rat chondrocytes in monolayer culture. *J Cell Physiol* 1979;100:63–76.

211. Millward-Sadler SJ, Wright MO, Davies LW, et al. Mechanotransduction via integrins and interleukin-4 results in altered aggrecan and matrix metalloproteinase 3 gene expression in normal, but not osteoarthritic, human articular chondrocytes. *Arthritis Rheum* 2000;43(9):209–219.

212. Morales T, Hascall V. Factors involved in the regulation of proteoglycan metabolism in articular cartilage. *Arthritis Rheum* 1989;32:1197–1201.

213. Morris CE. Mechanosensitive ion channels. *J Membr Biol* 1990;113:93–107.

214. Moskowitz RW, Davis W, Sammarco J. Experimentally induced degenerative joint lesions following partial meniscectomy in the rabbit. *Arthritis Rheum* 1973;16:397–405.

215. Moskowitz RW. Experimental models of osteoarthritis. In: Moskowitz RW, Howell DS, Goldberg VM, et al., eds. *Osteoarthritis: diagnosis and medical/surgical management.* Philadelphia: WB Saunders, 1992:213–232.

216. Mow VC, Kuei SC, Lai WM, et al. Biphasic creep and stress relaxation of articular cartilage in compression: theory and experiments. *J Biomech Eng* 1980;102:73–84.

217. Mow VC, Lai WM. Recent developments in synovial joint biomechanics. *SIAM Rev* 1980;22:275–317.

218. Mow VC, Holmes MH, Lai WM. Fluid transport and mechanical properties of articular cartilage: a review. *J Biomech* 1984;17:377–394.

219. Mow VC, Ratcliffe A, Poole AR. Cartilage and diarthrodial joints as paradigms for hierarchical materials and structures. *Biomaterials* 1992;13:67–97.

220. Mow VC, Ateshian GA, Spilker RL. Biomechanics of diarthrodial joints: a review of twenty years of progress. *J Biomech Eng* 1993;115:460–467.

221. Mow VC, Bachrach N, Setton LA, et al. Stress, strain, pressure, and flow fields in articular cartilage. In: Mow VC, Guilak F, Tran-Son-Tay R, et al., eds. *Cell mechanics and cellular engineering.* New York: Springer-Verlag, 1994:345–379.

222. Mow VC, Wang CC, Hung CT. The extracellular matrix, interstitial fluid and ions as a mechanical signal transducer in articular cartilage. *Osteoarthritis Cartilage* 1999;7:41–58.

223. Muir H, Hardingham TE. Structure of proteoglycans. In: Whelan WJ, ed. *MTP international review of science: biochemistry of carbohydrates.* London: Butterworth, 1975:152–222.

224. Muller FJ, Setton LA, Manicourt DH, et al. Centrifugal and biochemical comparison of proteoglycan aggregates from articular cartilage in experimental joint disuse and joint instability. *J Orthop Res* 1994;12:498–508.

225. Murray RC, Smith RK, Henson FM, et al. The distribution of cartilage oligomeric matrix protein (COMP) in equine carpal articular cartilage and its variation with exercise and cartilage deterioration. *Vet J* 2001;162:121–128.

226. Myers ER, Lai WM, Mow VC. A continuum theory and an experiment for the ion-induced swelling behavior of articular cartilage. *J Biomech Eng* 1984;106:151–158.

227. Narmoneva DA, Wang JY, Setton LA. Nonuniform swelling-induced residual strains in articular cartilage. *J Biomech* 1999;32:401–408.

228. Nerem RM, Harrison DG, Taylor WR, et al. Hemodynamics and vascular endothelial biology. *J Cardiovasc Pharmacol* 1993;21:S6–10.

229. Nevo Z, Beit-Or A, Eilam Y. Slowing down aging of cultured embryonal chick chondrocytes by maintenance under lowered oxygen tension. *Mech Ageing Dev* 1988;45:157–165.

230. Newberry WN, Mackenzie CD, Haut RC. Blunt impact causes changes in bone and cartilage in a regularly exercised animal model. *J Orthop Res* 1998;16:348–354.

231. Newman P, Watt FM. Influence of cytochalasin D-induced changes in cell shape on proteoglycan synthesis by cultured articular chondrocytes. *Exp Cell Res* 1988;178:199–210.

232. Norton LA, Rodan GA, Bourret LA. Epiphyseal cartilage cAMP changes produced by electrical and mechanical perturbations. *Clin Orthop* 1977;59–68.

233. Oegema TR Jr, Lewis JL, Thompson RC Jr. Role of acute trauma in development of osteoarthritis. *Agents Actions* 1993;40:220–223.

234. O'Hara BP, Urban JP, Maroudas A. Influence of cyclic loading on the nutrition of articular cartilage. *Ann Rheum Dis* 1990;49:536–539.

235. Orford CR, Gardner DL, O'Connor P. Ultrastructural changes in dog femoral condylar cartilage following anterior cruciate ligament section. *J Anat* 1983;137:653–663.

236. Ostendorf RH, van de Stadt RJ, van Kampen, GP. Intermittent loading induces the expression of 3-B-3(-) epitope in cultured bovine articular cartilage. *J Rheumatol* 1994;21:287–292.

237. Palmer GD, Chao P-HG, Raia F, et al. Time dependent aggrecan gene expression of articular chondrocytes in response to hyperosmotic loading. *Osteoarthritis Cartilage* 2001;9:761–770.

238. Palmoski MJ, Perricone E, Brandt KD. Development and reversal of a proteoglycan aggregation defect in normal canine knee cartilage after immobilization. *Arthritis Rheum* 1979;22:508–517.

239. Palmoski MJ, Colyer RA, Brandt KD. Joint motion in the absence of normal loading does not maintain normal articular cartilage. *Arthritis Rheum* 1980;23:325–334.

240. Palmoski MJ, Brandt KD. Running inhibits the reversal of atrophic changes in canine knee cartilage after removal of a leg cast. *Arthritis Rheum* 1981;24:1329–1337.

241. Palmoski MJ, Brandt KD. Effects of static and cyclic compressive loading on articular cartilage plugs *in vitro*. *Arthritis Rheum* 1984;27:675–681.

242. Parkkinen JJ, Lammi MJ, Helminen HJ, et al. Local stimulation of proteoglycan synthesis in articular cartilage explants by dynamic compression *in vitro*. *J Orthop Res* 1992;10:610–620.

243. Parkkinen JJ, Ikonen J, Lammi MJ, et al. Effects of cyclic hydrostatic pressure on proteoglycan synthesis in cultured chondrocytes and articular cartilage explants. *Arch Biochem Biophys* 1993;300:458–465.

244. Parkkinen JJ, Lammi MJ, Pelttari A, et al. Altered Golgi apparatus in hydrostatically loaded articular cartilage chondrocytes. *Ann Rheum Dis* 1993;52:192–198.

245. Parkkinen JJ, Lammi MJ, Inkinen R, et al. Influence of short-term hydrostatic pressure on organization of stress fibers in cultured chondrocytes. *J Orthop Res* 1995;13:495–502.

246. Pavalko FM, Otey CA, Simon KO, et al. Alpha-actinin: a direct link between actin and integrins. *Biochem Soc Trans* 1991;19:1065–1069.

247. Pazzano D, Mercier KA, Moran JM, et al. Comparison of chondrogenesis in static and perfused bioreactor culture. *Biotechnol Prog* 2000;16:893–896.

248. Pienta KJ, Coffey DS. Nuclear-cytoskeletal interactions: evidence for physical connections between the nucleus and cell periphery and their alteration by transformation. *J Cell Biochem* 1992;49:357–365.

249. Pond MJ, Nuki G. Experimentally induced osteoarthritis in the dog. *Ann Rheum Dis* 1973;32:387–388.

250. Poole CA, Flint MH, Beaumont BW. Chondrons in cartilage: ultrastructural analysis of the pericellular microenvironment in adult human articular cartilages. *J Orthop Res* 1987;5:509–522.

251. Poole CA. Articular cartilage chondrons: form, function and failure. *J Anat* 1997;191:1–13.

252. Pritzker KPH. Animal models for osteoarthritis: processes, problems and prospects. *Ann Rheum Dis* 1994;53:406–420.

253. Putney J, Takemura H, Hughes A, et al. How do inositol phosphates regulate calcium signaling? *FASEB J* 1989;3:1899–1905.

254. Quinn TM, Grodzinsky AJ, Buschmann MD, et al. Mechanical compression alters proteoglycan deposition and matrix deformation around individual cells in cartilage explants. *J Cell Sci* 1998;111:573–583.

255. Quinn TM, Grodzinsky AJ, Hunziker EB, et al. Effects of injurious compression on matrix turnover around individual cells in calf articular cartilage explants. *J Orthop Res* 1998;16:490–499.

256. Quinn TM, Kocian P, Meister JJ. Static compression is associated with decreased diffusivity of dextrans in cartilage explants. *Arch Biochem Biophys* 2000;384:327–334.

257. Quinn TM, Allen RG, Schalet BJ, et al. Matrix and cell injury due to sub-impact loading of adult bovine articular cartilage explants: effects of strain rate and peak stress. *J Orthop Res* 2001;19:242–249.

258. Quinn TM, Dierick P, Grodzinsky AJ. Glycosaminoglycan network geometry may contribute to anisotropic hydraulic permeability in cartilage under compression. *J Biomech* 2001;34:1483–1490.

259. Radin EL, Paul IL. Response of joints to impact loading. I: *in vitro* wear. *Arthritis Rheum* 1971;14:356–362.

260. Radin EL, Parker GH, Pugh JW, et al. Response of joints to impact loading. III. Relationship between trabecular microfractures and cartilage degeneration. *J Biomech* 1973;6:51–57.

261. Ragan PM, Badger AM, Cook M, et al. Down-regulation of chondrocyte aggrecan and type-II collagen gene expression correlates with increases in static compression magnitude and duration. *J Orthop Res* 1999;17:836–842.

262. Ragan PM, Chin VI, Hung HH, et al. Chondrocyte extracellular matrix synthesis and turnover are influenced by static compression in a new alginate disk culture system. *Arch Biochem Biophys* 2000;383:256–264.

263. Rasmussen H. The calcium messenger system. *N Engl J Med* 1986;17:1094–1170.

264. Ratcliffe A, Billingham ME, Saed-Nejad F, et al. Increased release of matrix components from articular cartilage in experimental canine osteoarthritis. *J Orthop Res* 1992;10:350–358.

265. Roberts S, Knight M, Lee D, et al. Mechanical compression influences intracellular Ca(2+) signaling in chondrocytes seeded in agarose constructs. *J Appl Physiol* 2001;90:1385–1391.

266. Rodan GA, Bourret LA, Norton LA. DNA synthesis in cartilage cells is stimulated by oscillating electric fields. *Science* 1978;199:690–692.

267. Rosier RN. The role of intracellular calcium in matrix vesicle biogenesis. *Orthop Trans* 1984;8:238.

268. Saamanen AM, Tammi M, Kiviranta I, et al. Maturation of proteoglycan matrix in articular cartilage under increased and decreased joint loading. A study in young rabbits. *Connect Tissue Res* 1987;16:163–175.

269. Saamanen AM, Tammi M, Jurvelin J, et al. Proteoglycan alterations following immobilization and remobilization in the articular cartilage of young canine knee (stifle) joint. *J Orthop Res* 1990;8:863–873.

270. Sachs F. Mechanical transduction by membrane ion channels: a mini review. *Mol Cell Biochem* 1991;104:57–60.

271. Sah RL, Doong JH, Kim YJ, et al. Biosynthetic response of cartilage explants to mechanical and physicochemical stimuli. *Trans Orthop Res Soc* 1988;13:70.

272. Sah RL, Grodzinsky AJ. Biosynthetic response to mechanical and electrical forces: calf articular cartilage in organ culture. In: Norton LA Burston CJ, eds. *Biology of tooth movement.* Boca Raton: CRC Press, 1989:335–347.

273. Sah RL, Kim YJ, Doong JY, et al. Biosynthetic response of cartilage explants to dynamic compression. *J Orthop Res* 1989;7:619–636.

274. Sah, RL, Grodzinsky AJ, Plaas AH, et al. Effects of tissue compression on the hyaluronate-binding properties of newly synthesized proteoglycans in cartilage explants. *J Biochem* 1990;267:803–808.

275. Sah RL, Grodzinsky AJ, Plaas AHK, et al. Effects of static and dynamic compression on matrix metabolism in cartilage explants. In: Kuettner KE, Schleyerbach R, Peyron JG, et al., eds. *Articular cartilage and osteoarthritis.* New York: Raven Press, 1992:373–392.

276. Salter DM, Hughes DE, Simpson R, et al. Integrin expression by human articular chondrocytes. *Br J Pharmacol* 1992;31:231–234.

277. Salter RB, Field P. The effects of continuous compression on living articular cartilage. *J Bone Joint Surg* 1960;42A:31–76.

278. Sandy JD, Brown HLG, Lowther DA. Control of proteoglycan synthesis. Studies on the activation of synthesis observed during culture of articular cartilages. *Biochem J* 1980;188:119–130.

279. Sandy JD, Adams ME, Billingham ME, et al. *In vivo* and *in vitro* stimulation of chondrocyte biosynthetic activity in early experimental osteoarthritis. *Arthritis Rheum* 1984;27:388–397.

280. Sarkadi B, Parker JC. Activation of ion transport pathways by changes in cell volume. *Biochim Biophys Acta* 1991;1071:407–427.

281. Schinagl RM, Ting MK, Price JH, et al. Video microscopy to quantitate the inhomogeneous equilibrium strain within articular cartilage during confined compression. *Ann Biomed Eng* 1996;24:500–512.

282. Schinagl RM, Gurskis D, Chen AC, et al. Depth-dependent confined compression modulus of full-thickness bovine articular cartilage. *J Orthop Res* 1997;15:499–506.

283. Schneiderman R, Keret D, Maroudas A. Effects of mechanical and osmotic pressure on the rate of glycosaminoglycan synthesis in the human adult femoral head cartilage: an *in vitro* study. *J Orthop Res* 1986;4:393–408.

284. Setton LA, Lai WM, Mow VC. Swelling-induced residual stresses in articular cartilage: A potential role for chondrocyte morphology. In: Vossoughi J, ed. *Biomedical engineering: recent developments.* Washington DC: Proceedings of the 13th Southern Biomedical Engineering Conference, 1994:1207–1210.

285. Setton LA, Mow VC, Muller FJ, et al. Mechanical properties of canine articular cartilage are significantly altered following transection of the anterior cruciate ligament. *J Orthop Res* 1994;12:451–463.

286. Setton LA, Mow VC. Contributions of flow-dependent and flow-independent viscoelasticity to the behavior of articular cartilage in oscillatory compression. *ASME Adv Bioeng* 1995;BED-29:307–308.

287. Setton LA, Mow VC, Howell DS. Mechanical behavior of articular cartilage in shear is altered by transection of the anterior cruciate ligament. *J Orthop Res* 1995;13:473–482.

288. Setton LA, Mow VC, Muller FJ, et al. Altered material properties of articular cartilage after periods of joint disuse and joint disuse followed by remobilization. *Osteoarthritis Cartilage* 1997;5:1–16.

289. Setton LA, Tohyama H, Mow VC. Swelling and curling behaviors of articular cartilage. *J Biomech Eng* 1998;120:355–361.

290. Shapiro F, Glimcher MJ. Induction of osteoarthrosis in the rabbit knee joint. Histologic changes following meniscectomy and meniscal lesions. *Clin Orthop* 1980;147:287–295.

291. Sims JR, Karp S, Ingber DE. Altering the cellular mechanical force balance results in integrated changes in cell, cytoskeletal and nuclear shape. *J Cell Sci* 1992;103:1215–1222.

292. Smetana K. Cell biology of hydrogels. *Biomaterials* 1993;14:1046–1050.

293. Smith RL, Donlon BS, Gupta MK, et al. Effects of fluid-induced shear on articular chondrocyte morphology and metabolism *in vitro. J Orthop Res* 1995;13:824–831.

294. Smith RL, Rusk SF, Ellison BE, et al. *In vitro* stimulation of articular chondrocyte mRNA and extracellular matrix synthesis by hydrostatic pressure. *J Orthop Res* 1996;14:53–60.

295. Smith RL, Lin J, Trindade MC, et al. Time-dependent effects of intermittent hydrostatic pressure on articular chondrocyte type II collagen and aggrecan mRNA expression. *J Rehabil Res Dev* 2000;37:153–161.

296. Smith RL, Trindade MC, Ikenoue T, et al. Effects of shear stress on articular chondrocyte metabolism. *Biorheology* 2000;37:95–107.

297. Sokoloff L. Repair of articular cartilage, Chapter 6. In: *The biology of degenerative joint disease.* Chicago: University of Chicago Press, 1969:61–68.

298. Soltz MA, Ateshian GA. Experimental verification and theoretical prediction of cartilage interstitial fluid pressurization at an impermeable contact interface in confined compression. *J Biomech* 1998;31:927–934.

299. Spilker RL, Suh JK, Mow VC. Effects of friction on the unconfined compressive response of articular cartilage: a finite element analysis. *J Biomech Eng* 1990;112:138–146.

300. Stockwell RA, Meachim G. The chondrocytes. In: Freeman MAR, ed. *Adult articular cartilage.* London: Pitman Medical, 1973:51–99.

301. Stockwell RA. Chondrocyte proliferation, cartilage growth and repair, Chapter 7. In: *Biology of cartilage cells.* Cambridge, UK: Cambridge University Press, 1979:213–238.

302. Stockwell RA, Billingham MEJ, Muir H. Ultrastructural changes in articular cartilage after experimental section of the anterior cruciate ligament of the dog knee. *J Anat* 1983;136:425–439.

303. Stockwell RA. Structure and function of the chondrocyte under mechanical stress. In: Helminen HJ, Kiviranta I, Tammi M, et al., eds. *Joint loading: biology and health of articular structures.* Bristol: Wright and Sons, 1987:126–148.

304. Sun D, Aydelotte MB, Maldonado B, et al. Clonal analysis of the population of chondrocytes from the Swarm rat chondrosarcoma in agarose culture. *J Orthop Res* 1986;4:427–436.

305. Sun DD, Guo XE, Likhitpanichkul M, et al. The influence of the fixed negative charges on mechanical and electrical behaviors in articular cartilage under unconfined compression. *J Biomech Eng* 2004;126:6–16.

306. Tammi M, Saamanen AM, Jauhiainen A, et al. Proteoglycan alterations in rabbit knee articular cartilage following physical exercise and immobilization. *Connect Tissue Res* 1983;11:44–55.

307. Tammi M, Kiviranta I, Peltonen L, et al. Effects of joint loading on articular cartilage collagen metabolism: assay of procollagen prolyl 4-hydroxylase and galactosylhydroxylysyl glucosyltransferase. *Connect Tissue Res* 1988;17:199–206.

308. Thaxter TH, Mann RA, Anderson CE. Degeneration of the immobilized knee joint in rats. *J Bone Joint Surg* 1965;47A:567–585.

309. Thompson RC Jr, Oegema TR Jr, Lewis JL, et al. Osteoarthrotic changes after acute transarticular load. An animal model. *J Bone Joint Surg Am* 1991;73:990–1001.

310. Torzilli PA. Effects of temperature, concentration and articular surface removal on transient solute diffusion in articular cartilage. *Med Biol Eng Comput* 1993;31:S93–98.

311. Torzilli PA, Grigiene R. Continuous cyclic load reduces proteoglycan release from articular cartilage. *Osteoarthritis Cartilage* 1998;6:260–268.

312. Torzilli PA, Grigiene R, Borrelli J Jr, et al. Effect of impact load on articular cartilage: cell metabolism and viability, and matrix water content. *J Biomech Eng* 1999;121:433–441.

313. Uchida A, Yamashita K, Hashimoto K, et al. The effect of mechanical stress on cultured growth cartilage cells. *Connect Tissue Res* 1988;17:305–311.

314. Underhill CB. The interaction of hyaluronate with the cell surface, the hyaluronate receptor and the core protein. In: Evered D Whelan J, eds. *The biology of hyaluronan.* Chichester: John Wiley and Sons, 1989:138–149.

315. Urban J, Hall A. Adaptive responses of chondrocytes to changes in their physical environment. *Trans Orthop Res Soc* 1993;18:260.

316. Urban JP, Bayliss MT. Regulation of proteoglycan synthesis rate in cartilage *in vitro*: influence of

extracellular ionic composition. *Biochim Biophys Acta* 1989;992:59–65.

317. Urban JP, Hall AC, Gehl KA. Regulation of matrix synthesis rates by the ionic and osmotic environment of articular chondrocytes. *J Cell Physiol* 1993;154:262–270.

318. Urban JPG, Hall AC. The effects of hydrostatic and osmotic pressures on chondrocyte metabolism. In: Mow VC, Guilak F, Tran-Son-Tay R, et al., eds. *Cell mechanics and cellular engineering.* New York: Springer-Verlag, 1994:398–419.

319. Valhmu WB, Rivers PA, Ebara S, et al. Structure of the human aggrecan gene: extron-intron organization and association with the protein domains. *J Biochem* 1995;309:535–542.

320. Valhmu WB, Palmer GD, Dobson J, et al. Regulatory activities of the 5'- and 3'-untranslated regions and promoter of the human aggrecan gene. *J Biol Chem* 1998;273:6196–6202.

321. Valhmu WB, Stazzone EJ, Bachrach NM, et al. Load-controlled compression of articular cartilage induces a transient stimulation of aggrecan gene expression. *Arch Biochem Biophys* 1998;353:29–36.

322. Valhmu WB, Raia FJ. myo-Inositol 1,4,5-trisphosphate and Ca(2+)/calmodulin-dependent factors mediate transduction of compression-induced signals in bovine articular chondrocytes. *Biochem J* 2002;361:689–696.

323. van Campen GPJ, van de Stadt RJ. Cartilage and chondrocytes responses to mechanical loading *in vitro*. In: Helminen HJ, Kiviranta I, Tammi M, et al., eds. *Joint loading: biology and health of articular structures.* Bristol: Wright and Sons, 1987:112–125.

324. van Kampen GP, Veldhuijzen JP, Kuijer R, et al. Cartilage response to mechanical force in high-density chondrocyte cultures. *Arthritis Rheum* 1985;28:419–424.

325. van Kampen GP, Korver GH, van de Stadt RJ. Modulation of proteoglycan composition in cultured anatomically intact joint cartilage by cyclic loads of various magnitudes. *Int J Tissue React* 1994;16:171–179.

326. Veldhuijzen JP, Bourret LA, Rodan GA. *In vitro* studies of the effect of intermittent compressive forces on cartilage cell proliferation. *J Cell Physiol* 1979;98:299–306.

327. Velpeau AALM. *Manuel d'anatomie chirurgicale, générale et topographique.* Paris: Méquignon-Marvis, 1837.

328. Vener MJ, Thompson RC Jr, Lewis JL, et al. Subchondral damage after acute transarticular loading: an *in vitro* model of joint injury. *J Orthop Res* 1992;10:759–765.

329. Videman T, Michelsson JE, Rauhamaki R, et al. Changes in the 35S-sulphate uptake in different tissues in the knee and hip regions of rabbits during immobilization, remobilization and the de-velopment of osteoarthritis. *Acta Orthop Scand* 1976;47:290–298.

330. von der Mark K, Mollenhauer J, Mueller PK, et al. Anchorin CII, a collagen-binding glycoprotein from chondrocyte membranes. *Ann N Y Acad Sci* 1985;460:214–223.

331. Vunjak-Novakovic G, Martin I, Obradovic B, et al. Bioreactor cultivation conditions modulate the composition and mechanical properties of tissue-engineered cartilage. *J Orthop Res* 1999;17:130–138.

332. Wan LQ, Miller C, Guo XE, et al. Fixed electrical charges and mobile ions affect the measurable mechano-electrochemical properties of charged-hydrated biological tissues: the articular cartilage paradigm. *Mechanics Chem Biosystems* 2004;1:81–89.

333. Wang C, Hung CT, Mow VC. Analysis of the effects of depth-dependent aggregate modulus on articular cartilage stress-relaxation behavior in compression. *J Biomech* 2000;34:75–84.

334. Wang CC-B, Guo XE, Deng JJ, et al. A novel non-invasive technique for determining distribution of fixed charge density within articular cartilage. *Trans Orthop Res Soc* 2001;26:129.

335. Wang CC-B, Guo XE, Sun D, et al. The functional environment of chondrocytes within cartilage subjected to compressive loading: theoretical and experimental approach. *Biorheology* 2002;39:39–45.

336. Watson PA. Function follows form: generation of intracellular signals by cell deformation. *FASEB J* 1991;5:2013–2019.

337. Wilkins R, Hall A. Measurement of intracellular pH in isolated bovine articular chondrocytes. *Exp Physiol* 1992;77:521–524.

338. Wilkins RJ, Hall AC, Urban JPG. The correlation between changes in intracellular pH and changes in matrix synthesis rates in chondrocytes. *Trans Orthop Res Soc* 1992,17:182.

339. Wollheim FA, Eberhardt KB, Johnson U. HLA DRB1* typing and cartilage oligomeric matrix protein (COMP) as predictors of joint destruction in recent-onset rheumatoid arthritis. *Br J Rheumatol* 1997;36:847–849.

340. Wong M, Wuethrich P, Buschmann MD, et al. Chondrocyte biosynthesis correlates with local tissue strain in statically compressed adult articular cartilage. *J Orthop Res* 1997;15:189–196.

341. Wong M, Siegrist M, Cao X. Cyclic compression of articular cartilage explants is associated with progressive consolidation and altered expression pattern of extracellular matrix proteins. *Matrix Biol* 1999;18:391–399.

342. Wright M, Jobanputra P, Bavington C, et al. Evidence for stretch-activated ion channels in human chondrocytes. *Bone Miner* 1994;S1:S37.

343. Wright MO, Stockwell RA, Nuki G. Response of plasma membrane to applied hydrostatic pressure

in chondrocytes and fibroblasts. *Connect Tissue Res* 1992;28:49–70.

344. Wu JZ, Herzog W, Epstein M. Modelling of location- and time-dependent deformation of chondrocytes during cartilage loading. *J Biomech* 1999;32:563–572.

345. Wu Q-Q, Chen Q. Mechanoregulation of chondrocyte proliferation, maturation, and hypertrophy: ion-channel dependent transduction of matrix deformation signals. *Exp Cell Res* 2000; 256:383–391.

346. Wu Q-Q, Zhang Y, Chen Q. Indian hedgehog is an essential component of mechanotransduction complex to stimulate chondrocyte proliferation. *J Biol Chem* 2001;276:35290–35296.

347. Yellowley CE, Jacobs CR, Li Z, et al. Effects of fluid flow on intracellular calcium in bovine articular chondrocytes. *Am J Physiol* 1997;273:C30–36.

348. Yellowley CE, Jacobs CR, Donahue HJ. Mechanisms contributing to fluid-flow induced Ca2+ mobilization in articular chondrocytes. *J Cell Physiol* 1999;180:402–408.

349. Yellowley CE, Donahue HJ. Hypotonic swelling increases internal calcium concentration and activates membrane ion channel currents in bovine articular chondrocytes. *Trans Orthop Res Soc* 2000;25:328.

350. Yoshimasa T, Sibley DR, Bouvier M, et al. Cross-talk between cellular signalling pathways suggested by phorbol ester-induced adenylate cyclase phosphorylation. *Nature* 1987;327:67–70.

351. Zhu W, Lai WM, Mow VC. The density and strength of proteoglycan-proteoglycan interaction sites in concentrated solutions. *J Biomech* 1991;24:1007–1018.

STRUCTURE AND FUNCTION OF LIGAMENTS AND TENDONS

SAVIO L-Y. WOO
THAY Q. LEE
STEVEN D. ABRAMOWITCH
THOMAS W. GILBERT

1   INTRODUCTION

Tendons and ligaments are soft connective tissues composed of closely packed, parallel collagen fiber bundles that connect bone to muscle and bone to bone, respectively. These unique tissues serve essential roles in the musculoskeletal system by transferring tensile loads to guide motion and stabilize diarthrodial joints. Rupture of tendons, such as the flexor digitorum profundus tendons of the hand and the Achilles tendon of the ankle, as well as ligaments, such as the collateral and cruciate ligaments of the knee and the inferior glenohumeral ligament of the shoulder, upsets this balance between mobility and stability. These injuries often result in abnormal joint kinematics and damage to other tissues around the joint that may lead to morbidity, pain, and osteoarthritis.

With regards to tendon injuries, the number and incidence have increased over the last few decades, and it is estimated that they account for 30% to 50% of all injuries related to sports (101). Similarly the incidence of ligament injuries has also increased and is estimated to be 2 per 1,000 people per year for the knee alone in the general population. These injuries primarily involve the anterior cruciate ligament (ACL) and the medial collateral ligament (MCL), accounting for as much as 90% of all sports-related ligaments injuries (132). Recent studies have documented that females are at a much greater risk for ACL injury, i.e., 2 to 8 times more frequent than their male counterparts, when participating in similar sports activities (11,13,167,198). Some have described this phenomenon as an epidemic.

Within the knee, the potential for healing varies from ligament to ligament. Injuries to the MCL generally heal sufficiently well such that nonsurgical management has become the treatment of choice (57,89,96,100,157,187,220, 235). Although some of the structural properties of the femur–MCL–tibia complex (FMTC), obtained experimentally from a uniaxial tensile test, can be restored within 3 months, the mechanical properties of the healed MCL remain inferior to those for the normal MCL for years after injury (57,74,148,157,187,220, 225,247,257). These changes have been associated with an altered histomorphological appearance and biochemical composition (57,74,148, 187,220,235,247,257). Hence, there is a major effort to improve these suboptimal properties of the healing MCL and to apply the learned principles to aid the repair of other ligaments and tendons (47,78,93,136,137,191,238).

However, nonsurgical management of a ruptured ACL is successful for only a limited number of patients (25,37,96,122). Because of this, ACL reconstruction by replacement grafts has been regularly recommended by surgeons to regain knee function (52,81,102,154). In the United States alone, ACL surgical procedures using autografts are performed on 75,000 to 100,000 patients per year. However, it has been shown that even after undergoing these reconstruction procedures, knees have abnormal kinematics including increases in anterior translation, axial tibial rotation, and valgus rotation that could lead to progressive damage to other knee structures (43,190,244,256). Long-term follow-up studies at 7 to 10 years following ACL reconstruction have revealed that 10% to 25% of patients experience unsatisfactory results (3,14,97,98,177). Thus, a better understanding of ACL function, and further knowledge about how its biology and healing potential differ from the MCL, may help investigators develop new strategies to improve ligament (and also tendon) healing.

This chapter will provide readers with a review of the basic ligament and tendon biology and those sound biomechanical methods used to analyze their tensile properties, joint motions, and the in situ forces in these tissues (59,114,119,181,232,236). Specifically, how the biomechanical properties of these tissues are affected by various experimental and biological factors will be discussed (68,233,234,237,239, 245,249–251). With this background knowledge, the readers are prepared to learn about the contribution of ligaments and tendons to joint kinematics. Examples will include evaluations of the phalangeal joints of the hand, the glenohumeral joint of the shoulder, and the femoral-tibial joint of the knee where the ACL and a few of the key surgical parameters that affect the performance of ACL replacement grafts will be discussed (34,45,185,244,256). The focus will then turn to the healing of ligaments and tendons where the effects of mechanical and biological factors to improve the healing process are elucidated (23,57,68,78,148,197,220,257). Finally, the new developments in the fields of functional tissue engineering and mechanobiology utilizing the interplay of mechanical factors and biology to enhance the quality, rate, and completeness of healing are discussed. To conclude, future directions as well as new technologies and research avenues that have the potential to enhance new treatment strategies for ligament and tendon injuries are suggested (16,78,87,94,136,188,191,197,217).

2 HISTOLOGY AND BIOCHEMICAL COMPOSITION

Ultrastructurally, ligaments and tendons have a hierarchy of fibrillar arrangement organized into a structure composed of fibrils, fibers, subfascicular units, fasciculi, and the tissue itself. Both ligaments and tendons are surrounded by a loose areolar connective tissue, referred to as periligament and paratenon, respectively (35,103).

Tendon and ligament insertions to bone are functionally adapted to distribute and dissipate forces by transmitting them through the fibrocartilage to bone. The bony attachments of ligaments and tendons are complex and vary considerably. Generally speaking, there are two types of insertions: direct and indirect. The former is more common as the transition of fibers from ligament to bone occurs in four distinct phases: ligament, fibrocartilage, mineralized fibrocartilage, and bone (Fig. 7-1A) (41,53,237). The size of each zone varies with particular ligaments; however, the total length of the transition zone is usually much less than 1 mm. Indirect insertions are more complex morphologically as there

are distinct superficial and deep fibers. The superficial fibers are connected to the periosteum (Fig. 7-1B) (41,111,237), whereas the deeper fibers, sometimes called Sharpey fibers, are anchored directly on the bone. Indirect insertions usually occur when the ligaments attach to bone after crossing the epiphyseal plate.

Biochemically, ligaments and tendons consist of collagen, elastin, proteoglycans (PGs), glycolipids, water (65% to 70% of the total weight), and cells. Roughly 70% to 80% of the dry weight of normal tendon or ligament is composed of type I collagen, also found in skin and bone. This collagen is thought to remain relatively inert metabolically, with a half-life of 300 to 500 days (143). Certain components of the collagen molecule may turn over faster than others and may thus be of greater functional importance

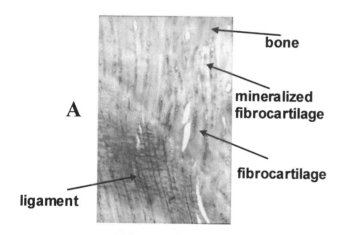

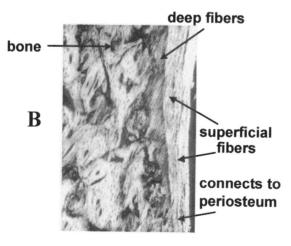

FIGURE 7-1. A: Photomicrograph demonstrating a direct insertion, i.e., the femoral insertion of rabbit MCL. The ligament passes acutely into bone through a well-defined zone of fibrocartilage. (Hematoxylin and eosin, ×50) **B:** Photomicrograph demonstrating an indirect insertion, i.e., the tibial insertion of rabbit MCL. The superficial fibrils of the ligament run parallel with the bone and insert in the periosteum. The deeper fibrils run obliquely and insert in the underlying bone (Hematoxylin and eosin, ×50). (Printed with permission from (237).)

in adaptations to environmental, traumatic, or pathologic processes (69). Collagen also has the ability to form covalent intramolecular (aldol) and intermolecular (Schiff base) cross-links, which are key to its tensile strength characteristics and resistance to chemical or enzymatic breakdown (17,130,204).

There are many other collagen types, including III, V, IX, X, XI, and XII, which exist only in minor amounts in ligaments and tendons. The significance of some of these minor collagen types has recently been elucidated. For example, type V collagen is believed to exist in association with type I collagen and serves as a regulator of collagen fibril diameter (22,117), whereas type III collagen is needed for wound healing (118). Our research has further identified that type XII collagen provides lubrication between collagen fibers (150). Last, collagen types IX, X, and XI have been identified to exist with type II collagen at the fibrocartilaginous zone of the ligament–bone and tendon–bone interface (61,149,183). It is hypothesized that these collagens exist in this zone to minimize the stress concentrations when loads are transmitted from soft tissue into bone (41,128,231).

The ground substance constituents of tendons or ligaments make up only a small percentage of the total dry tissue weight but are nevertheless quite significant because of their ability to imbibe water. The water and PGs provide lubrication and spacing that are crucial to the gliding function of fibers in the tissue matrix. Elastin, which is present in ligaments and tendons in a few percent by weight, allows the tissue to return to its prestretched length following physiological loading, but the detailed significance has yet to be elucidated. Collectively, these constituents serve to maintain fiber orientation and separation for optimal load distributions.

3 BIOMECHANICAL PROPERTIES

3.1 Structural Properties of Bone–ligament–bone Complexes

Because the main function of ligaments and tendons is to transmit tensile forces, experimental studies of the biomechanical properties of these tissues are generally performed in uniaxial tension. From this test, a load–elongation curve for the bone–ligament–bone complex (from which structural properties are determined) and a stress–strain curve of the tendon or ligament substance (from which the mechanical properties are determined) are obtained.

These tissues are complex, and there are many factors that have been shown to affect the outcome of tensile tests. Testing isolated ligament and tendon tissue is inherently difficult for several reasons. Slipping of the specimen from the clamp has been a common problem encountered by investigators. Although efforts have been made to limit this problem by using specially designed frozen, hydraulic, and pneumatic clamps with roughened gripping surfaces, slipping and the development of stress concentrations could result in premature failure of a test specimen. In addition, the substance of ligaments is often too short, making it impossible to accommodate clamps. As a result, tensile tests have been performed using the entire bone–ligament–bone complex with ligament insertion sites left anatomically intact. Bones are clamped such that the ligament can be aligned to the applied tensile load. A load–elongation curve that is typically nonlinear (concave upward) is obtained (Fig. 7-2A). Parameters obtained from this curve include stiffness, ultimate load, ultimate elongation, and energy absorbed at failure.

3.2 Mechanical Properties of the Ligament Substance

From the same uniaxial test, the mechanical properties (i.e., quality) of the ligament substance can also be obtained. This is done by normalizing the tensile load by the cross-sectional area (i.e, stress) and by normalizing the change in elongation in a defined region of the ligament midsubstance by the initial length (i.e., strain) (Fig. 7-2B). From the stress–strain curve, the tangent modulus, tensile strength, ultimate strain, and strain energy density of the ligament substance can be determined. The readers are encouraged to read chapter 24 of *The Orthopaedic Basic Science Book* published by the American

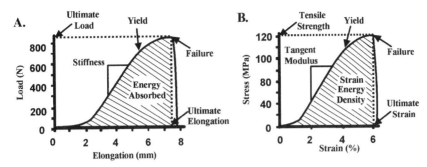

FIGURE 7-2. A: A typical load–elongation curve representing the structural properties of the bone–ligament–bone complex. **B:** A typical stress–strain curve representing the mechancial properties of a ligament or tendon substance.

Academy of Orthopaedic Surgeons (AAOS) for more detailed information (230).

3.3 Determination of Stress and Strain

As accurate measures of a specimen's cross-sectional area are required for stress calculations, the data on mechanical properties of ligaments and tendons could be compromised by an in-accurate method of measuring this parameter. The irregular, complex geometry of these tissues makes measurements difficult, and in some cases, the errors could be large.

Generally, techniques developed to measure the cross-sectional area of soft tissue can be separated into either contact or noncontact methods (49,72,88,151,228). Contact methods include the use of molding techniques, digital vernier calipers, and area micrometers (172,173). For these methods, errors may result from forcing the soft tissue into a rectangular shape by pressure or assuming a rectangular cross section (5,26,50,212,232).

To minimize distortion of tissue shape, other investigators have advocated the use of non-contact methods. These techniques include the shadow amplitude method (49), the profile method (72,151), and the use of a light source (88). In our laboratory, the laser micrometer system has been adopted as a method to measure both the cross-sectional area and the shape of soft tissues (114,232). This method has been shown to be highly accurate and reproducible with precision, and the reconstructed shapes

match histologic sections quite well. A new laser-reflectance system has also been developed to measure cross-sectional shape and area of soft tissue with concave surfaces (32).

Accurate experimental measurement of tissue elongation of ligaments and tendons also poses a number of hurdles including method of fixation, measurement of dimensions, and isolation of the properties of the tissue from its connecting structures. As in techniques for cross-sectional area measurement, tissue strains are determined by contact and noncontact methods. To avoid introducing possible errors during measurement, optical techniques to measure tissue strain, such as video tracking systems, which require no direct contact with the specimen, have been used. Two or more reference markers are drawn or fixed on the surface of the tendon or ligament by means of Verhoeff's stain (249), elastin stain (73,112), or reflective tape (187) to serve as gauge lengths. A camera is used to record marker motion, and the pixel coordinate output can be expressed as a function of the gauge length corresponding to percentage strain of the tissue (109,195,227,258).

To measure tissue elongation *in vivo*, contact techniques such as the use of a Differential Variable Reluctance Transducer (DVRT; MicroStrain, Inc., Burlington, VT) have been employed. This device tracks the position of a free-sliding transducer core by measuring the differential reluctance of coils, providing an analog output voltage that varies linearly with core position. Because of its small size and resistance to environmental factors, *in vivo* strain of the ACL during physiologic motions have been obtained using this technology (19,20).

3.4 Regional Strain Variation

The geometry, aspect ratio, and alignment of the MCL make it particularly suitable for an accurate determination of the stress–strain curve under uniaxial tensile loading. A recently developed finite element model of the MCL confirmed that this method of testing yields a homogenous stress and strain distribution in the central portion of the MCL, proximal and distal to the jointline (170). However, the strain along the MCL can vary with large strains occurring near the insertion sites (236).

3.5 Anisotropic Properties

Knowing ligaments and tendons are parallel fibered tissues, an appropriate representation of their mechanical behavior is transverse isotropy. Thus, a hyperelastic strain energy equation,

$$W(I_1, I_2, \lambda) = F_1(I_1, I_2) + F_2(\lambda) \\ + F_3(I_1, I_2, \lambda), \quad (1)$$

where I_1, I_2 are invariants of the right Cauchy stretch tensor and λ is the stretch along the collagen fiber direction, could be used (171). During a uniaxial tensile test, F_1 is represented by a two-coefficient Mooney-Rivlin material model that includes the behavior of the ground substance,

$$F_1 = \tfrac{1}{2}[C_1 (I_1 - 3) + C_2 (I_2 - 3)], \quad (2)$$

where C_1 and C_2 are constants. F_2 represents the strain energy of the collagen fibers and is described by separate exponential and linear functions of λ for the toe and linear regions of the stress versus stretch response, respectively. F_3 represents an interaction term accounting for shear coupling, and is assumed to be zero. Then, the Cauchy stress, $\mathbf{T}$, can be written as

$$\mathbf{T} = 2\{(W_1 + I_1 W_2)\mathbf{B} - W_2 \mathbf{B}^2\} \\ + \lambda W_\lambda a \otimes a + \rho \mathbf{1}, \quad (3)$$

where $\mathbf{B}$ is the left deformation tensor, and W_1, W_2, and W_λ are the partial derivatives of strain energy with respect to I_1, I_2, and λ, re-

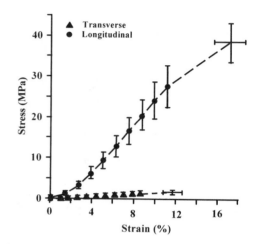

FIGURE 7-3. Stress–strain curves for human MCLs longitudinal and transverse to the collagen fiber direction (Printed with permission from (171)).

spectively. The unit vector field, a, represents the fiber direction in the deformed state, and ρ the hydrostatic pressure required to enforce incompressibility.

This form of hyperelastic strain energy equation has been demonstrated to fit both the longitudinal (tangent modulus of 332.2 ± 58.3 MPa and tensile strength of 38.6 ± 4.8 MPa) and transverse (tangent modulus of 11.0 ± 0.9 MPa and tensile strength of 11.0 ± 0.9 MPa) experimental data of the human MCL equally well, making it a good model for describing the three-dimensional behavior of the MCL (Fig. 7-3) (171).

3.6 Contribution of Experimental Factors

Functional support to the joint is provided by a tendon at the muscle–tendon–bone complex and by a ligament at the bone–ligament–bone unit. Clinically, failure in adult tissue–bone complexes is more common by substance tear rather than by avulsion, yet many investigators using cadavers and experimental animals have difficulty reproducing this failure mode and have frequently stated that the bony insertion is the weakest link (85,131,208,240,260). Upon closer examination, these discrepancies may result from (a) experimental factors, such as specimen orientation or strain rate; (b) handling, storage, or preparation of the tissue; and (c) biological factors, such as physiological changes associated with growth and development or the adaptation of ligaments and tendons to mobility.

3.6.1 Specimen Orientation

The structural properties of the bone–ligament–bone complex are significantly dependent on the loading axis. For human specimens, paired knees were tensile tested with the Femur-ACL-Tibia Complex (FATC) from one knee in the anatomic orientation and the contralateral FATC in the tibial orientation (239). In the anatomic orientation, the natural insertion angles of the ACL were maintained, which allowed for a smooth transition of load from bone to ligament as well as a more uniform load distribution within the ligament. For the tibial orientation, the insertion angles were not maintained, resulting in a nonuniform distribution of the tensile load within the ACL and more insertion site failures. The structural properties for the FATCs tested in the anatomic orientation were significantly different, showing a higher ultimate load, stiffness, and energy absorbed at failure from those tested in the tibial orientation. Similar results have also been observed for the FATC of the pig, dog, and rabbit (53,121,240).

3.6.2 Strain Rate

Considerable attention has been given to the effects of the extension rate on the failure mode of a bone–ligament–bone complex. Some investigators feel that the reason others have been unsuccessful in obtaining ligament substance failure is primarily due to the employment of slow strain rates (42,75,153). Others have shown that skeletal maturity can have a significant effect on the failure mode (250). These factors were investigated in studies that examined the effect of strain rate as a function of skeletal maturity on the mechanical properties of the MCL midsubstance as well as its effect on the mode of failure of the FMTC using a high-speed video recording system (160,161).

The FMTCs from two groups of New Zealand white rabbits—(a) open epiphysis ($3\frac{1}{2}$ months old) and (b) closed epiphysis ($8\frac{1}{2}$ months old)—were subjected to uniaxial tensile tests at extension rates of 0.008 to 113 mm/sec, corresponding to strain rates of the ligament substance of 0.01%/sec to over 200%/sec. For the open epiphysis group, the structural properties of the FMTC and the mechanical properties of the MCL substance in the prefailure range were found to be dependent on the extension rate, with increases in the range of 250% to 300% for most parameters (Figs. 7-4, 7-5). The closed epiphysis group followed similar trends, but the increases were less dramatic. For example, the tensile strength of the MCL in the closed-epiphysis group increased significantly with strain rate, but by only 60% from the lowest to the highest values. Regardless of the applied strain rate, all failures in animals with open

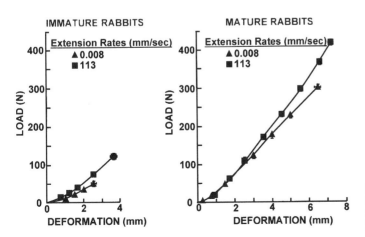

FIGURE 7-4. The structural properties of the FMTC in skeletally immature and mature rabbits as a function of extension rate (160).

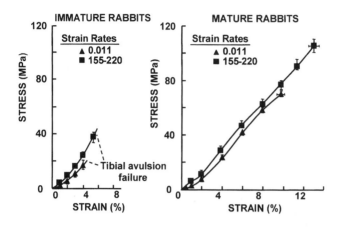

FIGURE 7-5. The mechanical properties of the MCL substance in skeletally immature and mature rabbits as a function of strain rate (160).

epiphyses occurred by tibial avulsion (therefore, no tensile strength of the MCL substance could be reported), whereas in animals with closed epiphyses, all failures occurred by ligamentous disruption either at midsubstance or near the tibial insertion site. Therefore, it can be concluded that the age of the animals is a much more important factor in determining failure mode than the strain rate.

Additional studies revealed similar results for failure mode and mechanical properties of the rabbit ACL and patellar tendon (PT) (44). However, the PT was found to have some sensitivity to strain rate, as its tangent modulus increased by 94% over four decades of strain rate. Overall, relative to the large range of strain rates studied, only comparatively small differences in both the mechanical properties of the ligament and tendon substances and the structural properties of the bone–ligament–bone complexes were found.

3.6.3 Temperature and Hydration

Environmental conditions, including temperature and hydration, are important considerations when testing ligaments and tendons. Testing specimens in air at room temperature will yield different results compared to immersing them in an aqueous bath of an isotonic solution where pH and temperature can be closely controlled. Using the adult canine FMTC, a linearly increasing stiffness was observed as the temperature declines (245). Further, there was less stress relaxation during cyclic loading. Tendons can also be affected by dehydration. For example, human PTs have a significantly higher tangent modulus and tensile strength when tested in a temperature-controlled saline bath than when tested in air with dripping saline (76).

3.6.4 Storage by Freezing

As biomechanical testing methodologies become more complex and time consuming, the necessity for storage of specimens by freezing becomes more frequent. Consequently, the effects of frozen storage on the mechanical properties of these tissues must be addressed. Several biomechanical studies comparing the properties of fresh soft tissues with those following storage have been conducted, but with conflicting results (127,194,209,221). A study was designed to evaluate possible changes in the mechanical properties of the rabbit MCL substance and of the structural properties of the FMTC following 3 months of frozen storage (249). The specimens were stored with muscle and other tissue left intact, rather than in the completely dissected state. Each specimen was double-wrapped in saline-soaked gauze, sealed in airtight plastic bags, and stored airtight at −20°C. The fresh contralateral limbs were dissected and tested immediately after sacrifice as controls.

There were no significant differences between fresh and frozen samples in most of the parameters measured (Table 7-1). The one exception was the area of hysteresis, where the frozen samples demonstrated significant decreases in area

TABLE 7-1. STRUCTURAL PROPERTIES OF THE FMTC (SKELETALLY MATURE RABBITS) COMPARING FRESH AND FROZEN BONE–LIGAMENT–BONE PREPARATIONS (REFER TO FIG. 7-2)

	Fresh (*n* = 5)	Stored 45 Days (*n* = 5)
Area of hysteresis		
First cycle (Nmm)	5.86 ± 1.60	2.20 ± 0.54[a]
Tenth cycle (Nmm)	1.36 ± 0.50	0.58 ± 0.30
Structural properties		
Ultimate load (N)	368 ± 15	316 ± 22
Ultimate elongation (mm)	6.6 ± 0.5	6.6 ± 0.5
Energy absorbed at failure (Nmm)	1,330.0 ± 200.0	1,170.0 ± 200.0

[a] $p < 0.05$.

during the first few cycles of loading and unloading when compared with fresh contralateral controls. These differences diminished and became insignificant with further cycling. It is thought that these changes may result from alterations in the ground substance (209) or from changes in fluid flow through the ligament in response to loading and unloading (199). However, it is necessary to reiterate that care must be taken in preparing the tissue sample prior to freezing in order to protect the sample from dehydration. Thawing was carried out at refrigerator temperatures (4°C) overnight, and specimens were prepared for testing soon after being removed from the refrigerator.

The experimental factors outlined in this section are of particular importance in explaining why findings may differ from study to study. It is important for specimens to be oriented anatomically such that loads are transferred from insertion, to midsubstance, to insertion mimicking the *in vivo* condition. Further, details regarding temperature, hydration, and storage must be provided in reports, as they can have profound effects on the outcome of soft tissue behavior.

3.7 Contribution of Biological Factors

Ligaments and tendons are subjected to morphological, biochemical, and biomechanical changes *in vivo* that are specific to their anatomical location, as well as the degree of skeletal maturation, age, and activity level of the animal. In addition,

the applied stress or tension can also influence the properties of ligaments. Based on these findings, a generalized statement similar to Wolff's law for bone (226) can be made about the adaptation of ligaments and tendons to stress and motion.

3.7.1 Anatomical Location

Because of the large range of motion and flexibility required of the glenohumeral joint, the mechanical behavior of ligaments that surround this joint is substantially different from that of ligaments that surround the knee. For example, the inferior glenohumeral ligament has a tangent modulus of 42 MPa as well as a tensile strength of 5 MPa, which are both approximately 10% of those for the MCL (21). Conversely, the interosseous ligament (IOL) of the forearm transmits load between the radius and ulna and has a relatively high tangent modulus of 528 ± 82 MPa (162). Similarly, the anterior longitudinal ligament of the spine has a tangent modulus that is comparable to that of the IOL (33,144,163). From these examples, it is clear that the properties of ligaments vary and these tissues are tailored to suit the functional demands and complex motions of each joint.

3.7.2 Maturation

Skeletal maturity has been shown to play a major role in the biomechanical properties of tendons, ligaments, and their insertions based on

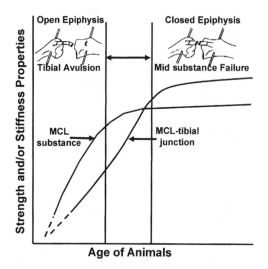

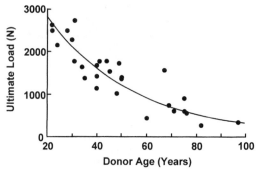

FIGURE 7-7. Ultimate load versus age for human FATC (Modified from Woo, SL-Y: *Am J Sports Med,* 1991;19:217–225 (239)).

FIGURE 7-6. A schematic diagram depicting the relationship between failure mode and age, hypothesizing the asynchronous rates of maturation between the bone–ligament–bone complex and the ligament substance (250).

animal models. Rat tail tendons were shown to have an age-dependent increase in collagen fibril size and tensile strength from puberty to adulthood (75,133,140), with little change observed until senescence (153). For the male New Zealand white rabbit, the structural properties of the FMTC under uniaxial tension changed dramatically from 1 to 7 months of age and remained relatively constant thereafter. The mechanical properties of the ligament substance demonstrated relatively early maturation in that by 4 to 5 months of age, the stress–strain curves in the functional range were similar to those of the adults. It was also noted through histological examination that the tibial insertion site of the MCL is affected by its proximity to the growth plate. The failure modes reflected that rapid remodeling activity in this region weakened the subperiosteal attachment for the younger animals (Fig. 7-6). All rabbits with open epiphyses failed by tibial avulsion, whereas in animals that had reached skeletal maturity (closed epiphyses), only 15% failed by tibial avulsion.

3.7.3 Aging

In addition to the changes in the biomechanical behavior of ligaments observed with skeletal maturation, changes associated with advancing age have also been documented. It has been hypothesized that factors including changes in the type and level of activity and/or the physical condition of the donor influence the properties of ligaments and tendons (179). The effects aging were studied in our laboratory using of human cadaveric knees obtained from young donors (22 to 41 years, mean age 35 years) and older donors (60 to 97 years, mean age 76 years) (239). The FATCs were tested to failure under uniaxial tension at a knee flexion angle of 30° with the ACL in the anatomic orientation. The mean stiffness and ultimate load of the younger specimens was 1.3 and 3.3 times higher than that of the older specimens, respectively (Fig. 7-7). Further, older specimens had a higher incidence of midsubstance failure than younger specimens (57% of the younger age group and 86% of the older age group).

On the other hand, there was little change in the load–elongation curve of the rabbit FMTC between skeletal maturity and the onset of senescence (248). In contrast to data from the human FATC, the structural properties of the rabbit FMTC and the tangent modulus of the MCL midsubstance did not decline with aging, illustrating that age-dependent changes are not uniform between ligaments.

In the shoulder, the biomechanical properties of the ligaments and joint capsule were also found to change with increasing age (21). Recent studies have shown that the mechanical properties of the shoulder joint capsule and its

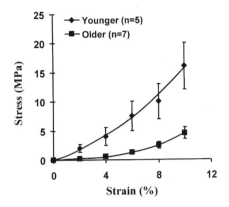

FIGURE 7-8. Graphs show the age-related mechanical properties the anterior band of the inferior glenohumeral ligament tested in tension. (Permission pending from (113)).

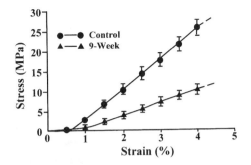

FIGURE 7-9. Mechanical properties of canine MCL from control and 9-week immobilization groups (Modified from Woo, SL-Y: *Am J Sports Med,* 1987;15:22–9 (242)).

ligaments became weaker (Fig. 7-8) (99,113). Failure modes shifted from either the glenoid–labrum region of the glenoid insertion site or the humeral insertion site for younger individuals to the midsubstance region close to the glenoid insertion site for older individuals.

3.7.4 Homeostatic Response

Connective tissues are known to respond to motion and stress. As many treatments of orthopaedic problems frequently involve a period of immobilization followed by rehabilitation, studies have investigated how these protocols affect the biomechanical properties of ligaments and tendons.

3.7.4.1 Effects of Immobilization

The effect of stress deprivation on synovial joints has been shown to be profound. Intraarticular changes include pannus formation, which leads to necrosis, erosion, and ulceration of articular cartilage (51,185). Increased joint stiffness is also well known clinically and has been demonstrated quantitatively in experimental animals (4,246). After 9 weeks of immobilization, the amount of torque required to initially extend the rabbit knee and the area of hysteresis were significantly increased (246). Yet, the ultimate loads and energy absorbed at failure of the FMTCs under uniaxial tension were only 31%

and 18%, respectively, of the contralateral non-immobilized controls (237). The tangent modulus of the MCL substance was significantly decreased, revealing a softening of the ligament substance after immobilization (Fig. 7-9). Failures occurred at the tibial insertion rather than the midsubstance.

For the ACL, there was also a significant decrease in the cross-sectional area following 9 weeks of immobilization (145). However, the changes in the tensile properties of the ACL were not as dramatic as with the MCL. Again, different ligaments may respond differently to immobilization, and therefore care must be taken when generalizing these results to other ligaments and tendons.

Remobilization of the knee joint following immobilization revealed that the mechanical properties of the MCL substance in the functional range rapidly returned to normal control values, while the structural properties of the experimental FMTCs remained inferior to those of controls (237). The mode of failure for the remobilized limb continued to occur by disruption at the bony insertion sites, suggesting incomplete recovery at these sites. The differences imply an asynchronous rate of recovery between the ligament and bony insertion.

3.7.4.2 Exercise

The positive effects of exercise on different ligaments and tendons have been investigated using dogs, rats, rabbits, and swine (8,28,88,205, 206,260), as well as anterior cruciate ligament preparations of monkeys (153,155). In a swine model, the effect of short- (3 months) and long-term (12 months) exercise on the biomechanical properties of digital tendons and the FMTC has been reported (233,251). After the animals were run on a track at speeds of 6 to 8 km/hr over an average distance of 40 km/wk, little or no effect was demonstrated with short-term exercise when compared with sedentary controls. However, long-term exercise resulted in positive changes including an increase in cross-sectional area as well as a 22% increase in tensile strength of the extensor tendons. Interestingly, for flexor tendons, the ultimate load of the exercised flexor–tendon complexes increased by 19% secondary to changes at the bony insertion sites. However, the mechanical properties of the tendon substance exhibited no statistical changes. For the FMTC, only the ultimate load at failure was significantly increased when normalized for the animal's body weight. Further, the concentrations of collagen and elastin in the MCL did not change with exercise.

3.7.4.3 Increased Tension

Altering the stress levels experienced by a ligament can elicit further changes in the biomechanical properties of its tissue (68). In a rabbit model, increased tension on the rabbit MCL by inserting a stainless steel pin beneath the MCL perpendicular to the long axis of the ligament was found to increase in situ strain of up to 4% with a corresponding 2- to 3.5-fold increase of the in situ stress (68). After 12 weeks, there was a positive increase of stress relative to strain compared to controls.

Based on these findings, it is possible to construct a hypothesis that schematically describes the homeostatic responses for soft tissues such as ligaments and tendons (Fig. 7-10). It is clear that highly nonlinear relationships exist between the level and duration of stress and motion and the dynamic biological activity that results in changes in tissue properties and tissue mass. With stress and motion deprivation (immobilization), a rapid reduction in tissue properties and mass would occur. In contrast, the positive changes following exercise and training are much more moderate.

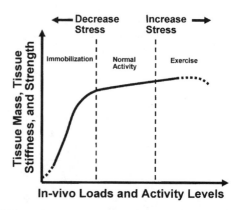

FIGURE 7-10. A schematic diagram describing the homeostatic responses of ligaments and tendons in response to different levels of stress and motion. (Printed with permission from (237).)

4   NONLINEAR VISCOELASTIC PROPERTIES

Ligaments and tendons display time- and history-dependent viscoelastic properties that reflect the complex interactions between proteins, ground substance, and water. The loading and unloading curves of these tissues do not follow the same path but instead form a hysteresis loop representing internal energy dissipation. Other important viscoelastic characteristics of ligaments and tendons include creep (i.e., an increase in deformation over time under a constant load) and stress relaxation (i.e., a decline in stress over time under a constant deformation). These viscoelastic behaviors for ligaments and tendons have important clinical significance. During walking or jogging, with the applied strains nearly constant, cyclic stress relaxation will soften the tissue substance with continuous decreases in peak stress per each cycle (Fig. 7-11) (54,101). This phenomenon may help to prevent fatigue failure of ligaments and tendons. Conversely, deformation will increase slightly during cycles between two constant loads, demonstrating creep behavior of ligaments and tendons (219). These changes have been noted clinically with an increased excursion in the exercised joints. After a short recovery period, there is a return to its apparent length, and thus, normal joint laxity.

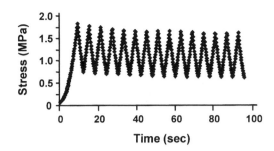

FIGURE 7-11. A typical cyclic stress–relaxation curve for ligaments and tendons demonstrating decreasing peak and valley stresses as a function of time.

4.1 Quasilinear Viscoelastic Theory

The quasilinear viscoelastic (QLV) theory developed by Dr. Y. C. Fung has been used successfully in the past to describe the time- and history-dependent viscoelastic properties for many soft tissues (30,36,63,64,92,106,164,193,203, 252,259), including ligaments and tendons (227,234). Recently, the QLV theory has been further refined to account for a constant strain rate in a stress relaxation experiment that results in a finite ramping phase instead of true step load that is physically impossible to achieve (108).

The QLV theory assumes that the stress relaxation function of the tissue can be expressed in the form

$$\sigma(t) = G(t)\sigma^e(\varepsilon) \qquad (4)$$

where $\sigma^e \varepsilon$ is the "elastic response," i.e., the maximum stress in response to an instantaneous step input of strain ε. $G(t)$ is the reduced relaxation function that represents the time-dependent stress response of the tissue normalized by the stress at the time of the step input of strain [i.e., $t = 0^+$, such that $G(t) = \sigma(t)/\sigma(0^+)$, and $G(0^+) = 1$].

If the strain history is considered as a series of infinitesimal step strains ($\Delta\sigma$), and the superposition principle is accepted as valid, then the overall stress relaxation function will be the sum of all individual relaxations. Thus, for a general strain history, the stress at time t, $\sigma(t)$, is given by the strain history and the convolution integral

over time of $G(t)$:

$$\sigma(t) = \int_{-\infty}^{t} G(t - \tau)\frac{\partial \sigma^e(\varepsilon)}{\partial \varepsilon}\frac{\partial \varepsilon}{\partial \tau}\partial\tau \qquad (5)$$

The lower limit of integration is taken as negative infinity to imply inclusion of all past strain history. In the experimental setting, we can assume that the history begins at $t = 0$. It is evident, then, that once $G(t)$, $\sigma^e(\varepsilon)$, and the strain history are known, the time- and history-dependent stress can be completely described by equation 5. For soft tissues, whose $\sigma - \varepsilon$ relationship and hysteresis are not overly sensitive to strain rates, Fung has proposed the following expression for $G(t)$:

$$G(t) = \frac{1 + C[E_1(t/\tau_2) - E_1(t/\tau_1)]}{1 + C\ln(\tau_2/\tau_1)} \qquad (6)$$

where $E_1(y) = \int_y^\infty \frac{e^{-z}}{z}dz$ is the exponential integral, and C, τ_1, and τ_2 are material coefficients. Because ligaments and tendons possess such properties, this formulation of $G(t)$ has been adopted for some musculoskeletal soft tissues (227).

An exponential approximation has been chosen to describe the elastic stress–strain relationship during a constant strain-rate test:

$$\sigma^e(\varepsilon) = A(e^{B\varepsilon} - 1) \qquad (7)$$

where A and B are material coefficients (227).

As noted previously, it is impossible to experimentally administer an instantaneous strain to the test material, and thus impossible to directly measure $\sigma^e(\varepsilon)$. To better approximate actual experimental conditions, it was necessary to develop a new procedure in which the instantaneous step load is replaced by a ramp load with a constant, finite strain rate γ to a strain level at time t_0. The corresponding stress rise during $0 < t < t_0$ can then be written by combining equations 6 and 7 as

$$\sigma(t) = \frac{AB\gamma}{1 + C\ln(\tau_2/\tau_1)}\int_0^t \{1 + C(E_1[(t - \tau)/\tau_2]$$

$$\times E_1[(t - \tau)/\tau_1])\}e^{B\gamma\tau}\partial\tau \qquad (8)$$

Similarly, the subsequent stress relaxation $\sigma(t)$, from t_0 to $t = \infty$, can be described as

$$\sigma(t) = \frac{AB\gamma}{1 + C\ln(\tau_2/\tau_1)}\int_0^{t_0}\{1 + C(E_1[(t - \tau)/\tau_2]$$
$$\times E_1[(t - \tau)/\tau_1])\}e^{B\gamma\tau}\partial\tau \tag{9}$$

These two equations are then normalized by dividing equations 8 and 9 by the peak stress $\sigma(t_0)$ to eliminate constant A.

$$\frac{\sigma(t)}{\sigma(t_0)} = \frac{\int_0^{\min(t,t_0)}\{1 + C(E_1[(t - \tau)/\tau_2]E_1[(t - \tau)/\tau_1])\}e^{B\gamma\tau}\partial\tau}{\int_0^0\{1 + C(E_1[(t_0 - \tau)/\tau_2]E_1[(t_0 - \tau)/\tau_1])\}e^{B\gamma\tau}\partial\tau} \tag{10}$$

However, the integrals of equation 10 are difficult for most nonlinear regression software packages to handle. Further, the upper limit of the integral in the denominator represents a removable singularity. By integrating both the numerator and denominator in equation 10 by parts and evaluating the denominator as the upper limit of the integral approaches t_0, a more expanded form can be obtained,

$$\frac{\sigma(t)}{\sigma(t_0)} = \frac{-1 + e^{\alpha Bt_0} - C\Gamma\left[\frac{t}{\tau_2}, \frac{t}{\tau_1}\right] + Ce^{\alpha Bt}\left(\Gamma\left[\alpha Bt + \frac{t}{\tau_2}, \alpha Bt + \frac{t}{\tau_1}\right] + \Gamma\left[\frac{(1+\alpha B\tau_1)(t-t_0)}{\tau_1}, \frac{(1+\alpha B\tau_2)(t-t_0)}{\tau_2}\right]\right) + Ce^{\alpha Bt_0}\Gamma\left[\frac{t-t_0}{\tau_2}, \frac{t-t_0}{\tau_1}\right]}{-1 - C\Gamma\left[\frac{t_0}{\tau_2}, \frac{t_0}{\tau_1}\right] + e^{\alpha Bt_0}\left(1 + C\left(\Gamma\left[\alpha Bt_0 + \frac{t_0}{\tau_2}, \alpha Bt_0 + \frac{t_0}{\tau_1}\right] + \ln\left[\frac{1+\alpha B\tau_2}{1+\alpha B\tau_1}\right]\right)\right)} \tag{11}$$

where $\Gamma[a,b]$ is the generalized incomplete gamma function $\int_a^b t^{-1}e^{-t}dt$. Equation 11 can be substituted for equation 10 to make nonlinear regression algorithms, such as those included in the software package Mathematica (Wolfram Research, Inc., Champaign, IL), run more efficiently.

With data from a stress–relaxation experiment, the material coefficients B, C, τ_1, and τ_2 can be determined by a nonlinear, least-square, curve-fitting procedure (108,115). Constant A can then be computed by using either equation 8 or 9. For a known strain history, these five constants, together with $G(t)$ and $\sigma^e(\varepsilon)$, can then be used to determine the stress at any time t, $\sigma(t)$, by using equation 5. The following example illustrates the method described (108,115).

The anteromedial bundles of porcine ACL were stretched to 5% strain at a strain rate of 2.5%/sec and allowed to stress relax up to 2 hours. By use of equation 10 and a nonlinear, least-square, curve-fitting procedure, the con-

stants B, C, τ_1, and τ_2 were found to be 0.63 $\pm$ 0.002, 0.146 $\pm$ 0.07, 0.097 $\pm$ 0.01 sec, and 0.808 $\pm$ 0.18 ($\times 10^5$ sec), respectively. Constant A was then determined to be 210 $\pm$ 36 MPa using equation 8. The time-dependent stress relaxation was then calculated from equation 6 as

$$G(t) = 0.858 - 0.049\ln t \tag{12}$$

The stress–strain relationship was then obtained using equation 7:

$$\sigma^e(\varepsilon) = 210(e^{0.063\varepsilon} - 1) \tag{13}$$

The theoretical prediction for the reduced relaxation function agrees well with the experimental findings, but these material constants must be verified by a second independent experiment. In this case, a more general cyclic strain history was used. The same anteromedial bundles of the ACL were cycled between 1% and 5% strains at a strain rate of 2.5%/sec for ten cycles. The peak stresses are plotted in Fig. 7-12 and the QLV theory compares well with the experimental data.

4.2 Single Integral Finite Strain Theory

Because there are numerous cases in which the deformation of the specimen is finite, a more general continuum model for nonlinear viscoelastic behavior of soft biological tissues is required (95). This model describes finite deformation of a nonlinearly viscoelastic material within the context of a three-dimensional model, called the single integral finite strain

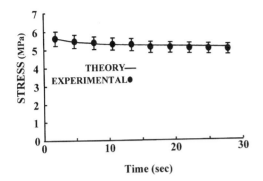

FIGURE 7-12. Theoretical versus experimental stress–relaxation values of the peak stress of the anteromedial bundle of a porcine ACL under a cyclic loading test (Modified from Lin, HC: *ASME Adv Bioeng,* 1987;BED 3:5–6.(115)).

(SIFS) viscoelastic model. It is fully nonlinear and reduces to an appropriate finite elasticity model for time zero. Moreover, if linearized, the SIFS model yields the equations for classical linear viscoelasticity.

A quite general integral series representation for nonlinear viscoelastic response was proposed by Pipkin and Rogers (166). It is proposed that the same constitutive equation can be applied to the modeling of ligaments and tendons. The development of the current model began with the assumption that the Cauchy stress **T** has the form (166)

$$\mathbf{T} = -p\mathbf{I} + \mathbf{F}(t)\{\mathbf{R}[\mathbf{C}(t), 0]$$
$$+ \int_0^t \frac{\partial}{\partial(t-s)}(\mathbf{R}[\mathbf{C}(s), t-s])ds\}\mathbf{F}^T(t)$$

$$(14)$$

where p is the indeterminate part of the stress arising from the constraint of incompressibility, **I** is the identity tensor, **F** is the deformation gradient tensor, and **C** is the Cauchy-Green strain tensor. The symbol **R** represents a strain-dependent tensorial relaxation function. The measures of deformation used here are properly frame indifferent (i.e., independent of the observer). All of the following results are consistent with this requirement, which is sometimes called the principle of objectivity or material frame indifference. The expression given by equation 14 incorporates the assumption that there has been no deformation prior to time $t = 0$. If deformation is

allowed for times $-\infty < t < 0$, then the lower limit of integration is changed, and equation 14 becomes

$$\mathbf{T} = -p\mathbf{I} + \mathbf{F}(t)x \int_\infty^t \frac{\partial}{\partial(t-s)}$$
$$\times (\mathbf{R}[\mathbf{C}(s), t-s])ds\}\mathbf{F}^T(t) \quad (15)$$

The term **R** [**C**(t),0] in equation 14 represents an instantaneous deformation occurring at $t = 0$. The strain-dependent tensorial relaxation function in the above equations has the form:

$$\mathbf{R} = \phi_0\mathbf{I} + \phi_1\mathbf{C} + \phi_2\mathbf{C}^2 \quad (16)$$

where ϕ_0, ϕ_1, and ϕ_2 are scalar functions of t and the tensorial invariants of **C**. If the equations are not linearized, QLV can be obtained by an appropriate selection of ϕ_0, ϕ_1, and ϕ_2. In fact, the formulation of QLV can be obtained as restrictions to one dimension for an infinite number of general models because the choices for ϕ_0, ϕ_1, and ϕ_2 that will yield QLV are not unique.

In general, the ϕ_i should be chosen so that the viscoelastic model will reduce to reasonable limits, such as an accepted model of finite elasticity. Here we are guided, as Fung was previously (62), by the similarities between the elasticity of rubber and of living tissues. The ϕ_i were chosen (223) such that

$$\mathbf{R}[\mathbf{C}(s), \xi] = G(\xi)\{[1 + \mu I(s)\mathbf{I} - \mu\mathbf{C}(s)\} \quad (17)$$

where

$$I(s) = \text{tr}\,\mathbf{C}(s) \quad (18)$$

and $G(\xi)$ is a relaxation function. The choice of relaxation function is based on the idea of fading memory; that is, events in the recent past have more influence on the current state of stress than those of the more distant past. Equation 15 can be rewritten by substituting the definitions in equations 17 and 18, as

$$\mathbf{T} = -p\mathbf{I} + \mathbf{C}_0\{[1 + \mu I(t)\mathbf{B}(t) - \mu\mathbf{B}^2(t)\}$$
$$- \mathbf{C}_0(1-\gamma)\int_0^t \dot{G}(t-s)\{[1 + \mu I(s)\mathbf{B}(t)$$
$$- \mu\mathbf{F}(t)\mathbf{C}(s)\mathbf{F}^T(s)\}ds \quad (19)$$

Here, $\mathbf{C}_0$ is the initial modulus, and $\gamma = C_\infty / C_0$, where C_∞ is the long-time modulus. The relaxation function, $\dot{G}(t-s)$, in the history integral ensures that more recent states of strain have greater weight in determining the stress than earlier states.

For uniaxial tension, equation 19 reduces to a single integral equation relating stress to stretch history:

$$\sigma(t) = C_0 \left(1 + \mu \frac{1}{\lambda(t)} \right) \left(\lambda^2(t) - \frac{1}{\lambda(t)} \right)$$

$$- C_0(1-\gamma) \left(\lambda^2(t) - \frac{1}{\lambda(t)} \right)$$

$$\times \int_0^t \dot{G}(t-s) \left(1 + \mu \frac{1}{\lambda(t)} \right) ds \tag{20}$$

where λ is the stretch ratio at time t. The shear modulus is assumed to be a function of the invariants of $\mathbf{B}$. For the present case, the following specific form can be used:

$$\mu = \mu_0 \left[\left(\lambda^2 - \frac{2}{\lambda} \right)^2 - 9 \right] \tag{21}$$

The function $G(t)$ was proposed based on empirical data in order to capture the physics of the stress–relaxation response exhibited by ligaments and tendons. The relaxation function was selected to be a decreasing function of time,

$$G(t) = \frac{\alpha}{t + \alpha} \tag{22}$$

Here α is a constant.

The model was applied to data from uniaxial extension of younger and older human PTs and canine MCLs (95,243). Model parameters were determined from curve-fitting stress–strain and stress–relaxation data and used to predict the time-dependent stress generated by cyclic extensions. Based on the parameters obtained from the stress–relaxation tests, there was very good agreement between model predictions and experimental results for an independent, cyclic stretching test to finite strain. SIFS theory can be used to model large deformations (greater than 5%) and structures in three dimensions. Thus, the robustness of this theory makes it useful for many future applications.

5 FUNCTION OF LIGAMENTS AND TENDONS IN SYNOVIAL JOINTS

The properties of ligaments and tendons are well suited to the physiological functions they perform. Multiple ligaments and tendons provide a mechanism for both locomotion and stability of joints. At low loads, ligaments and tendons have a relatively low modulus such that they can guide the joint to move normally, easily, and smoothly. Yet at high loads, the modulus of these tissues increases significantly such that stability can be maintained and damage to other tissues such as the articular cartilage and menisci avoided. By adding dynamic muscular control and neural feedback mechanisms, the static stabilizers are designed to place bones in their proper places and protect themselves from elongating beyond their limits. In the following sections, the hand, the glenohumeral joint, and the human knee joint will be used as primary examples to illustrate the key function of ligaments and tendons. However, the function of other important structures, such as the patellar and Achilles tendons and the spinal and wrist ligaments, are also available in the literature.

5.1 The Phalangeal Joints of the Hand

The normal gliding function of the flexor tendons can be described in terms of the relative moment arms of the flexor digitorum profundus and superficialis. The moment arms of these tendons are not equal at the proximal interphalangeal (PIP) and metacarpophalangeal (MCP) joints (9,10); thus, for a given degree of flexion, there will be nonequivalent excursions of the two flexors, and any movement of the joints will generate gliding motion between these tendons. When the distal interphalangeal (DIP) joint is flexed to 60°, there will be up to 4 mm of gliding motion in the distal palmar crease to the profundus tendon insertion (zone II region) (Fig. 7-13). If the PIP joint is flexed to 60°, as much as an additional 1.8 mm of relative gliding motion will occur. Larger motion of the DIP and PIP joints, such as in the "hook" and "fist" positions, will generate the

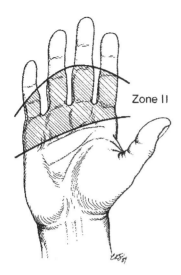

FIGURE 7-13. Diagram of human palm illustrating zone II region—distal palmar crease to the profundus tendon insertion.

greatest gliding motion between the two flexor tendons (218). The tendon excursion relative to the sheath in zone II has been considered a significant factor in the prevention of adhesion formation following injury.

The interrelationship of finger joint rotation and tendon excursion has been studied clinically, experimentally, and analytically. From the simple geometric relationship $\Delta\theta = r\Delta s$, the instantaneous moment arm of the tendon in the plane of motion (r) at a specific joint configuration can be obtained from the slope of a plot of tendon excursion (Δs) versus joint rotational displacement ($\Delta\theta$). The excursion–rotation relationship for both superficial and deep flexor tendons is relatively linear but becomes slightly nonlinear when the joint is close to full flexion. In other words, the moment arms of these two flexors increase as the joint flexion angle increases. Further, flexor tendon excursion is governed by the constraint of the pulley system (7). Therefore, any alteration in the flexor pulley system will result in a change in the normal relationship.

In our laboratory, the kinematics of the digital flexor tendons in the zone II region was examined in terms of tendon excursion, sheath displacement, and joint rotation in cadaveric human digits using radio-opaque markers placed in the flexor digitorum profundus and tendon sheath as well as the metacarpal and three phalangeal bones (84). Roentgenograms were taken in flexion and extension of the digit, with joint motion allowed initially at all joints, and then restricted to only the DIP, PIP, or MCP joint. The changes in the positions of the markers were determined, and the center of rotation, angle of rotation, tendon excursion, and sheath displacement were then calculated. Tendon excursion relative to sheath in zone II was maximized by motion of the PIP joint (1.7 mm/10° of joint flexion) relative to motion at DIP and MCP joints (Fig. 7-14) within zone II for which tendon excursion was determined. Little tendon excursion occurred distal to the joint in motion. This work suggests that flexion of joints distal to the repair site is more effective in achieving tendon excursion and therefore more effective in reducing scar formation after flexor tendon repair. Thus, the results of this research are essential to improving treatment options and rehabilitation protocols. In another study using canine digits, tendon excursions at the MCP, PIP, and DIP joints were found to be similar to the results obtained for human specimens, suggesting that the canine is a suitable model for studies of tendon kinematics and healing. As a result, a number of studies were done using this experimental animal model (23,66,70,84,152,233).

5.2 The Glenohumeral Joint of the Shoulder

Injuries about the shoulder girdle represent common occurrences in both the athletic and lay populations. The shoulder consists of four joints, the sternoclavicular, acromioclavicular, and glenohumeral joints and the scapulothoracic gliding plane, which function in a precise, synchronous manner to achieve a large range of motion. Indeed, the glenohumeral joint accounts for the greatest percentage of dislocations, and associated soft tissue damage of a tendinous or capsuloligamentous nature, of any major joint in the body (104). The glenohumeral joint lacks inherent bony stability and therefore relies heavily on the surrounding musculature

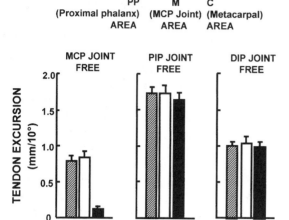

FIGURE 7-14. Tendon excursion relative to the sheath in zone II. The illustration depicts the three regions (PP, M, and C) within zone II for which tendon excursion was determined.

and capsuloligamentous structures for stabilization (126). The following research helped our understanding of glenohumeral instability, prevention, and treatment.

5.2.1 Shoulder Dislocation Model

The intricate and coordinated action of the shoulder muscles and the joint stability provided by the osteoarticular surfaces and the capsular ligaments are essential to normal joint function. In addition, the glenoid labrum, glenohumeral ligaments/capsule (Fig. 7-15), and normal intra-capsular pressure permit versatile motion while maintaining precise joint kinematics. The anterior band of the inferior glenohumeral ligament, located in the inferior, redundant part of the capsule, is a broad structure and is invariably present. It consists of closely packed collagen bundles that orient across the anterior glenohumeral joint and tighten with abduction and external rotation of the glenohumeral joint (67). It is the primary static restraint to anterior translation of the humeral head on the glenoid and is the primary site of pathology in joints with anterior instability (86,125,180,207). Tensile tests

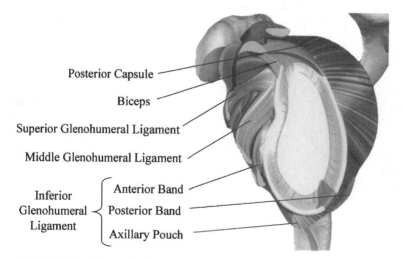

FIGURE 7-15. Schematic drawing shows the passive soft tissue restraints of the shoulder joint.

of glenoid–soft tissue–humerus (G-ST-H) complexes revealed that the rate of failure was higher at the glenoid insertion region, and that the permanent elongation of the tissue was greatest when injury occurred at this site (129).

Nevertheless, muscle forces are probably the most important stabilizer, especially in the midranges of shoulder motion when the capsule and glenohumeral ligaments are thought to be lax. Our laboratory simulated the forces in the rotator cuff muscles and the deltoid to study the glenohumeral joint forces and kinematics for shoulder abduction (45). Sectioning of the anterior joint capsule did not lead to dislocation of the glenohumeral joint while rotator cuff muscle action was simulated. Further, no dislocations were observed following division of the entire capsule, although a significant increase in posterior translation of the humerus with respect to the glenoid was demonstrated (12). These data suggest that dynamic stability can indeed

be maintained by rotator cuff muscle action and that the phenomenon of glenohumeral instability may include a combination of muscle imbalance and capsulolabral injury.

Until recently, there has been a lack of sufficient cadaveric models that are able to successfully dislocate the glenohumeral joint resulting in Bankart lesions similar to those seen *in vivo*. The necessity of shoulder muscle force simulation, including the pectoralis major, to create lesions similar to those seen *in vivo* with anterior shoulder dislocation was recently demonstrated (34). Fresh frozen human cadaveric shoulders were tested with the glenohumeral joint abducted 60° and the humerus externally rotated 90°. The humerus was then positioned 10° anterior to the plane of the scapula, in horizontal adduction. For shoulder dislocation, the humerus was horizontally abducted at a rate of 50 mm/sec until dislocation using a servomotor-controlled system (Fig. 7-16A,B). It was found

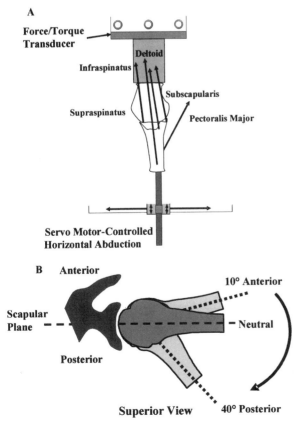

FIGURE 7-16. Using a servomotor-controlled system (**A**), the shoulder was dislocated by horizontally abducting the humerus at a rate of 50 mm/sec until dislocation occurred (**B**).

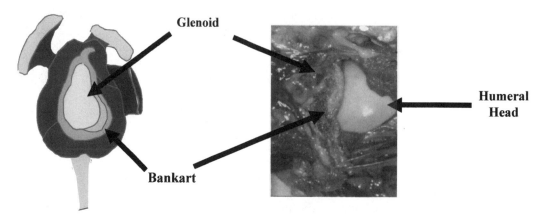

FIGURE 7-17. Schematic drawing and a photograph showing the Bankart lesion found in this study, which shows avulsion of the anteroinferior labrum from the bone of the glenoid rim as well as the soft tissues stripping off the glenoid neck (34).

that the glenohumeral joint was dislocated, either with a Bankart lesion, stretching of the capsuloligamentous structures, or capsuloligamentous avulsion from the humeral insertion site, providing pathology similar to that *in vivo*. The Bankart lesion showed avulsion of the anteroinferior labrum from the bone of the glenoid rim as well as the soft tissues stripping off the glenoid neck (Fig. 7-17). In addition, using a six-degree-of-freedom (6-DOF) load cell, the glenohumeral joint compression forces and the pectoralis major force were found for all three repeated dislocations (Fig. 7-18). The second dislocation resulted in only a 4.2%, 5.2%, 14.5%, and 4.7% decrease in compression, anterior, inferior, and pectoralis major forces with respect to the first dislocation, respectively. The third dislocation resulted in only a 13.8%, 23.1%, 31.4%, and 21.3% decrease in compression, anterior, inferior, and pectoralis major forces relative to the first dislocation, respectively. The fact that repeated anteroinferior shoulder dislo-

cations did not result in a significant decrease of glenohumeral joint forces suggests that more than one episode of traumatic anterior shoulder dislocation may be needed to have recurrent instability.

5.3 The Femoral–tibial Joint of the Knee

The ACL and the posterior cruciate ligament (PCL), which are located within the joint space surrounded by synovial fluid, restrain the anterior and posterior tibial displacement with respect to the femur, and more importantly, maintain the rotational stability of the knee. The other ligamentous structures including the MCL, lateral collateral ligament (LCL), posteromedial/lateral complexes, and joint capsule also serve collectively to stabilize the knee. In the following sections, we will focus on the MCL and ACL. A unique robotic/Universal Force-Moment Sensor (UFS) testing system has

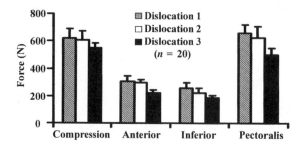

FIGURE 7-18. Graphs show the glenohumeral joint forces involved in repeated anterior inferior dislocations of the shoulder (34).

recently been developed such that the kinematics of the knee and in situ forces of ligaments can be measured. Thus, in our research center, experiments involving the ACL and ACL reconstructions can be compared.

5.3.1 Robotic/Universal Force-moment Sensor Testing System

In the past, in situ forces in the ACL were determined indirectly using a 6-DOF kinematic linkage, calculating ligament force by correlating the length–force relationship and the load–elongation curve obtained from tensile testing (82,83,202). Recently, we have developed a robotic/UFS testing system to directly determine the in situ forces in ligaments (59,181) (Fig. 7-19). The accuracy of this system is within 0.2 mm and 0.2° (positions) and 0.2 N and 0.01 Nm (forces and moments). The system can be operated in (a) position-control mode: moving the joint to a desired position in space and measuring the resulting forces (60); (b) force-control

mode: moving the joint to achieve a predetermined force-moment target using force feedback achieved by the UFS while recording the resulting knee kinematics (59,119,181); and (c) hybrid-control mode: combination of (a) and (b). With the use of this system, we are able to quantitatively evaluate joint kinematics in response to externally applied loads and the contributions of the specific ligaments that guide those complex motions (60).

During a test, the tibial portion of a knee specimen is rigidly connected to the UFS, which in turn is mounted to the end-effector of the robot. Meanwhile, the femur is fixed relative to the robot base. The 5-DOF path of passive flexion–extension of the intact knee is first determined from full extension to 90° of knee flexion (184). At each flexion angle, the positions that satisfy the condition of zero force and zero moment are recorded, and this motion is then repeated for 10 cycles to minimize viscoelastic effects. After this preconditioning is performed, the kinematics for the path of passive flexion–extension are

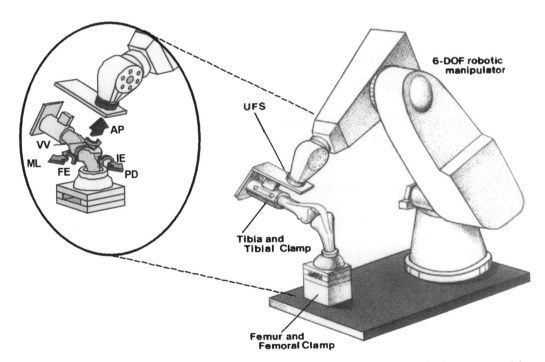

FIGURE 7-19. Schematic diagram of the robotic/UFS testing system showing a right knee mounted for testing. The arrows detail the anatomical axes of the knee joint (Printed with permission from Woo, SL-Y: *Knee Surgery*, Baltimore, MD: Williams & Wilkins, 1994: 155–173.)

recorded and serve as the reference (starting position) for subsequent tests where external loads are applied.

To determine the contribution of an individual ligament to joint kinematics, the in situ forces carried by that ligament in the intact joint can be measured during loading of the knee. After a known external load (F_1) is applied to the joint and the resulting motion is recorded, the ligament of interest is subsequently transected. The robot then reproduces the previously recorded path of joint motion, and a new set of force data (F_2) is obtained. Because the path of motion for both test conditions is identical, the principle of superposition can be applied and the in situ force of the ligament that was removed is the vectorial difference in recorded forces, i.e., ($F_1 - F_2$). We have validated and used this newly developed testing system to study the function of the cruciate ligaments (119).

5.3.2 Contribution of the ACL to Knee Kinematics

Because of the importance of understanding normal knee function as well as the changes that occur following ACL reconstruction, the forces in the ACL during physiologic knee function have received much attention. In the past, clinicians have tried to minimize the length changes (or loads) on the graft by seeking an isometric point for graft placement during ACL reconstruction. It was found that the changes in graft length were dependent on the femoral insertion site (27). Recently, isometry during clinical ACL reconstruction has been found to be less important as the native ACL exhibits nonisometric characteristics (186).

In our studies, we have shown that the force distribution between the anteromedial (AM) and posterolateral (PL) bundles of the ACL varied with knee flexion in response to an anterior tibial load (Fig. 7-20) (184). The AM bundle bears more load at high flexion angles of the knee, while the PL bundle has greater in situ force with the knee near extension. This work underscores the complexity of the ACL, the interrelationship of the two bundles, and the importance of the PL bundle in regards to ACL

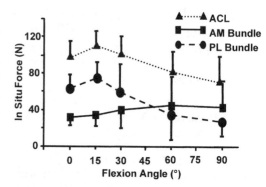

FIGURE 7-20. Magnitude of the in situ force in the intact anterior cruciate ligament (ACL), anteromedial bundle (AM), and posterolateral bundle (PL) under 110 N of applied anterior tibial load.

reconstruction. Furthermore, it suggests that the concept of "isometry" in ACL reconstruction being too simplistic.

Recent data further reveal the crucial role the ACL plays in knee stability in response to rotational loads. With an applied varus–valgus load to the knee at 15° and 30° of flexion, the ACL provided ATT stability. Also, the in situ force of the AM bundle of the ACL was larger than that of the PL bundle, but those for the PL bundle were still significant, i.e., greater than 30% of the total in situ force in the ACL (65). These findings substantiate an earlier study on canine knee joints which showed that the ACL was a primary restraint to valgus laxity (91). When the knee was allowed to move freely in 5 DOF (V—V and internal–external tibial rotation, proximal—distal, anteroposterior, and medial—lateral translations), there was a 123% increase in valgus rotation of the knee after the ACL was transected in contrast to only a 21% increase when the MCL was transected. The MCL was only found to be the "primary" restraint to valgus rotation when the knee joint is artificially restrained to 3 DOF, i.e., axial tibial rotation and anteroposterior translation (Fig. 7-21). As a result, after a MCL injury, the functional deficit in valgus rotation can be compensated for by the remaining structures, especially the ACL.

5.3.3 ACL Reconstruction

Most ACL reconstruction techniques have focused on reproducing the AM bundle. However,

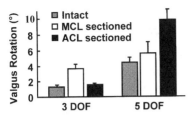

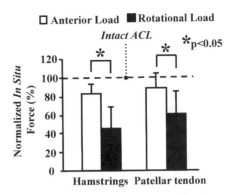

FIGURE 7-21. The increase in valgus rotation in response to 0.6 Nm of valgus torque after sectioning of either the MCL or ACL demonstrating the difference between 3-DOF and 5-DOF knee motion permitted by the test apparatus (Permission pending from (91).)

FIGURE 7-23. In situ force in the replacement grafts (normalized to the force in the intact ACL) in response to anterior tibial load and combined rotational load at 15° of knee flexion ($n = 12$). (Printed with permission from (244).)

because of the work demonstrating the importance of the PL bundle in the intact knee, it has been hypothesized that reconstruction of only the AM bundle may be insufficient to restore normal knee kinematics. In our research center, the robotic/UFS testing system was utilized to evaluate two popular ACL grafts (quadruple hamstring and bone-patellar tendon-bone) under two external loading conditions: (a) a 134 N anterior tibial load and (b) a combined rotational load of 10 Nm of valgus torque and 10 Nm of internal tibial torque. In response to the anterior tibial load, both grafts could restore the anterior tibial translations of the reconstructed knees close to those for the intact knee while in situ forces in the grafts also approached those for the intact knee (Figs. 7-22, 7-23). However, in response to the rotatory loads, the coupled an-

terior tibial translations measured only 10% to 15% less than those for the ACL-deficient knee (Fig. 7-22). This insufficiency was further supported by lower in situ forces in the grafts which ranged between 45% and 61% of those of the intact knee (Fig. 7-23) (244). It is thought that the grafts representing the AM bundle are too close to the central axis of the tibia and femur, making it inadequate for resisting rotational loads.

The above study suggests that an anatomical reconstruction, including reproduction of both the AM and PL bundles, may improve the results. This concept led to another study which compared the anatomical and single bundle reconstructions (256). The former was found to better reproduce the kinematics of the intact knee in response to the anterior tibial load as well as the combined rotatory load. Furthermore, the in situ forces in the anatomical reconstruction were significantly closer to those in the intact ACL as compared to those in the single bundle reconstruction in response to combined rotatory load (Fig. 7-24). This study clearly suggests the need to reproduce the normal anatomy of the ACL when considering the methods of ACL reconstruction.

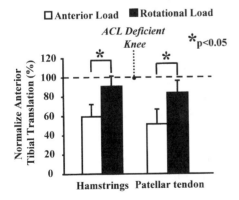

FIGURE 7-22. Anterior tibial translation (mean ± SD) in the reconstructed knee (normalized to the deficient knee) in response to anterior tibial load and combined rotational load at 30° of knee flexion ($n = 12$). (Printed with permission from (244).)

6 HEALING OF LIGAMENTS AND TENDONS

The management of torn ligaments and tendons is one of the most difficult and challenging

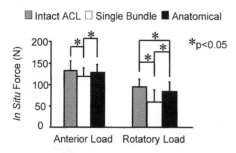

FIGURE 7-24. in situ forces of the intact ACL and ACL replacement grafts (Single Bundle and Anatomical) in response to anterior and combined rotatory loads at 30° of knee flexion. (Printed with permission from (256).)

clinical problems in orthopaedics. Although a great deal of work over the past 20 years has led to a better understanding of the problems related to ligament and tendon healing, many questions remain about enhancing the rate, quality, and completeness of healing. The reader is referred to *Injury and Repair of Musculoskeletal Soft Tissues* published by the American Academy of Orthopaedic Surgeons for specific reviews of research in this area (231). Two areas of particular clinical interest are (a) the efficacy of repair versus nonrepair, and (b) the effects of motion and activity levels following injury on function. The following are a few examples.

6.1   Flexor Tendons of the Hand

The digital flexor tendons of the hand are partially surrounded by synovial sheaths that provide lubrication and nutrition for the tendon. Mason and Allen (124) introduced the concept that after tendon injury and repair, the gliding surface between the flexor tendon and its fibrous sheath is compromised as a result of adhesion formation. Healing of flexor tendons involves the confounding need for protection from excessive motion so that the sutured tendon can heal, as well as for controlled mobilization so that adhesion formation can be limited while the healing mass can be sufficiently reduced to allow for adequate tendon motion. Hence, a dichotomy exists between the need for immobilization and mobilization, leading to the necessity of exploring fundamental questions regarding the process of

tendon healing and the response of the tendon to early controlled mobilization.

6.1.1   Effects of Controlled Passive Mobilization

The effects of mobilization on strength of repair, gliding function, and remodeling of the tendon were evaluated in a complete laceration of the canine flexor digitorum profundus (FDP) tendon model. After repair with a technique described by Kessler and Missim (105), the treatment methods included complete immobilization; delayed, passive mobilization; and early controlled mobilization (233). It was found that the early mobilization group had the best gliding function, returning to 97% to 100% of intact controls in 6 weeks (Fig. 7-25A). In addition, the tendons in the early mobilization group had a significantly higher stiffness and ultimate load at both 6 and 12 weeks (Fig. 7-25B). Microangiographic investigation demonstrated that the early mobilized group had vessels that were more normal in density and orientation. Furthermore, scanning electron microscopy showed that the early mobilized tendon and sheath repair sites had a smooth surface and were free of adhesions. This smooth, glistening surface remained unchanged and free of adhesions through 6 weeks. At the ultrastructural level, cells between the tendon ends were active in protein synthesis and collagen production between 3 and 6 weeks. DNA content at the repair site and in the digital sheath was significantly greater in the mobilized groups (66).

The higher frequency and shorter duration (12 cycles/min for 5 min/day) of controlled passive mobilization on tendon healing also significantly increased the tensile properties of the FDP tendon as compared to lower frequency and longer duration (1 cycle/min for 60 min/day). However, both maintained the same gliding function (201). These studies demonstrated that appropriate tensile forces and motion at the repair site provided by controlled passive mobilization could accelerate tendon repair. Of equal importance were the improvements in its gliding function. However, in order to successfully apply early controlled passive mobilization,

(A) Angular Rotation (ΔΘ)

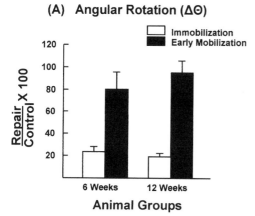

(B) Ultimate Load

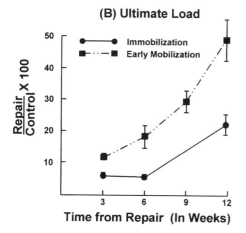

FIGURE 7-25. Comparison of normalized (experimental/control) **(A)** angular rotation and **(B)** ultimate load of repaired canine flexor tendon from immobilization), delayed mobilization, and early mobilization treatment groups (Modified from Woo, SL-Y: *Acta Orthop Scand,* 1981;52:615–22 (233)).

the repaired tendon must have adequate initial strength (189,211). Therefore, a number of suture techniques have been evaluated for gliding function and tensile properties at time zero and 3 and 6 weeks after laceration (152,224). It was found that a new low-profile, eight-strand repair method resulted in improved gliding function, joint rotation, and tendon excursion, as well as the best results for stiffness and strength (152). Moreover, this method significantly expands the safety zone for the application of increased *in vivo* load during the early stages of tendon healing (224).

6.1.2 Partial Lacerations—Repair versus Nonrepair

The appropriate management of partially lacerated FDP tendons has been debated. Although some authors have demonstrated a negative impact of repair, others have advocated repair of partial lacerations for the purpose of restoring gliding function (175). Using the canine model, the effect of tendon repair by the modified Kessler technique on 30% and 70% laceration of the FDP tendons was examined after 6 weeks of controlled passive motion. Although the structural properties of the bone–tendon complex were diminished postoperatively relative to control, the lacerated tendons still possessed good inherent stiffness and load-bearing capabilities. No significant differences were found in stiffness, ultimate load, or energy absorbed to failure between repaired and unrepaired groups at the 6-week postoperative interval regardless of the severity of the laceration (30% and 70%). The lack of ruptures confirmed the ability of the partial tendon laceration to tolerate postoperative mobilization whether or not the tendon was repaired (23).

6.2 Medial Collateral Ligament of the Knee

The medial collateral ligament (MCL) of the knee has been an excellent model for studying ligament healing because of its accessibility, its ability to heal spontaneously without surgical intervention, and the uniform cross-sectional area with a relatively large aspect ratio that is suitable to uniaxial tensile testing (187,220). As a result, extensive studies were done to elucidate the complex process of MCL healing. Generally, the healing process involves overlapping but distinct phases of acute inflammation, repair, and remodeling that lasts for 1 or more years postinjury. Interestingly, the mechanical properties of the healed tissue never recover to normal levels. As a review, the changes in the histological appearance, biochemical composition, and biomechanical properties of the healing MCL, as well as the effect of external factors involved in MCL healing, including repair versus nonrepair, mobilization versus immobilization, and multiple ligament injuries, are summarized below.

6.2.1 Histology

After a typical midsubstance tear of the MCL (characterized by the mop-end appearance of its torn ends), hemorrhage begins and a hematoma forms between the retracting ligament ends. Inflammatory and monocytic cells migrate into the injury site to convert the clot into granulation tissue and phagocytose necrotic tissue. Within about 2 weeks, the granulation tissue is replaced with a continuous network of immature, collagen fibers in the central region of the ligament, formed by randomly oriented fibroblasts. At this point, the torn ends of the ligament are no longer distinguishable, and angiogenesis begins, while fibroblasts continue to actively produce extracellular matrix.

Remodeling begins after several weeks and is marked by increased alignment of collagen fibers along the long axis of the ligament and continued collagen maturation. The longitudinal alignment of these fibers has been shown to correlate directly with an improvement in the structural properties of the bone–ligament complex.

Although the healing ligament remodels over time, long-term animal studies showed that the histological and morphological appearance of healed ligaments fails to return to its preinjury state. As demonstrated with transmission electron microscopy, the number of collagen fibrils increased in comparison to the uninjured ligament, but the diameters were uniformly small. This condition remained even after 2 years of healing (54,74). Additionally, the "crimp" patterns and collagen fiber alignment of the healing ligament remained abnormal for up to 1 year (54,56).

6.2.2 Biochemistry

The extracellular matrix of the healing ligament exhibits a number of important changes including elevated water content and glycosaminoglycan levels, and differences in elastin and other glycoproteins. There are also more types III and V collagen than in normal ligaments (57,148).

Recent work performed in our research center has also demonstrated in rabbits that the ratios of collagen types V/I and III/I in the healing MCL increased by 84% and 138%, respectively (148). After 52 weeks, the ratio of collagen type III/I had returned to normal levels, but collagen type V/I remained elevated. This elevation of minor collagen types, especially the persistent elevation of the type V/I ratio, serves to explain the uniform distribution of small collagen fibrils (74), as both collagen types III and V have been postulated to hinder cross-sectional growth of collagen fibrils (22,24,117,178,222). Furthermore, the number of mature collagen cross-links is only 45% of normal values after 1 year (55). A relationship has been demonstrated between inferior mechanical properties of the MCL and the smaller number of collagen cross-links, as well as the decrease in mass and diameter of the collagen fibers (55,229). It should also be noted that collagen types IX, X, and XIV have been identified at the bone–MCL interface (150), and further studies are needed to assess how the presence and amounts of these collagen types will affect the healing process.

6.2.3 Biomechanics

As a result of the changes in the histomorphological appearance and biochemical composition of the healing MCL, the biomechanical properties of the healing MCL are also altered. This has been demonstrated using a severe "mop-end" tear injury model developed by our laboratory in rabbits, which mimics injuries observed clinically (220). A "mop-end" tear of the MCL substance was created by placing a stainless steel rod beneath the MCL and pulling medially, rupturing the MCL in tension and causing a midsubstance tear and damage at the insertion sites. Immediately after injury (Time 0), the valgus rotation more than doubles as compared with sham-operated controls (Fig. 7-26), and is still approximately 20% greater than controls at 12 weeks of healing (220). The structural properties also differ from normal with the stiffness of the healing FMTC only approaching normal levels by 52 weeks after injury. This return to normal is largely due to an increase in the

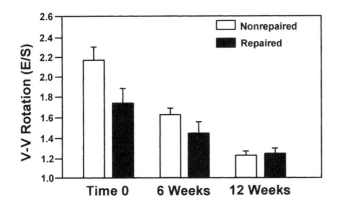

FIGURE 7-26. Normalized varus–valgus knee rotations from nonrepaired and repaired groups at 0, 6, and 12 weeks postoperatively. (Printed with permission from (220).)

cross-sectional area of the healing ligament to as much as $2\frac{1}{2}$ times its normal size (157). Thus, mechanical properties of the healing MCL midsubstance remain consistently inferior to those of the normal ligament and do not change with time (Table 7-2) (157,220). This means the healing process involves a larger quantity of lesser quality ligamentous tissue. Further, stiffness and strength of the insertion sites are below those for the ligament substance (Fig. 7-27). This is due to an asynchronous rate of healing between the ligament midsubstance and the insertion sites, which results from injury and lack of stress.

Studies have shown that the method of treatment can also have an impact on the process of ligament healing (38,39,156,205,241,242). Several animal studies have shown better results with nonoperative treatment and early mobilization than with surgical repair followed by immobilization (157,220,242). In the study

discussed above (220), which compared repair versus nonrepair, both with early mobilization, it was demonstrated that after 12 weeks of healing, there were no significant differences in varus–valgus rotation of the knee (Fig. 7-26), in situ force of the MCL, or tensile properties between repaired and nonrepaired MCL (Table 7-2) (220). As a result of the large body of research on the treatment of isolated MCL injuries, the paradigm of clinical management has shifted from surgical repair with immobilization to nonoperative management with early controlled range-of-motion exercises as soon as pain subsides (90,174).

6.2.4 New Animal Model

The sedentary nature of the rabbit model may not mimic healing as seen in the clinical situation. As a result, a goat model has been

TABLE 7-2. STRUCTURAL PROPERTIES OF THE FMTC FOR SHAM AND EXPERIMENTAL GROUPS AT 6 AND 12 WEEKS POSTOPERATIVELY (220)

	12 Weeks	
	Sham	Experimental
Nonrepaired		
Cross-sectional area (mm^2)	3.2 ± 0.1	5.5 ± 0.1[a]
Ultimate load (N)	294 ± 11	174 ± 24[a]
Stiffness (N/mm)	54.3 ± 4.4	39.9 ± 2.9[a]
Repaired		
Cross-sectional area (mm^2)	3.6 ± 0.2	7.0 ± 0.4[a]
Ultimate load (N)	313 ± 17	146 ± 16[a]
Stiffness (N/mm)	64.2 ± 5.2	42.7 ± 3.1[a]

[a] Significant difference from sham-operated control group.

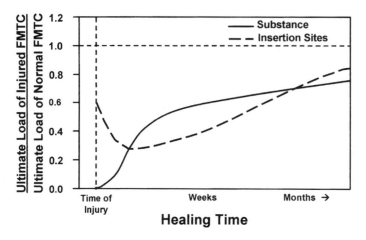

FIGURE 7-27. Changes in the stiffness and ultimate load characteristics of the medial collateral ligament and its insertions to bone as a function of time. (Printed with permission from (220).)

developed recently and used for study of MCL healing because of its large size, robust activity level, and the previously published success of ACL reconstructions using this animal (147). A comparison between tensile properties of the healing goat MCL and the healing rabbit MCL indicates that the stiffness and ultimate load of the healing goat FMTC are closer to control values at earlier time periods, probably due to the activity level of the former (225). However, the tangent modulus and morphology of the healing ligament for the goat and rabbit models demonstrate that the tissue is of similar quality. In addition, stress relaxation tests show that the percentage of static stress relaxation for the healing MCL was nearly double that for contralateral controls at 6 and 12 weeks of healing (1).

6.2.5 Combined Ligamentous Injuries

Clinical management of combined ligamentous injuries to the knee is obviously more difficult and remains controversial (58,79,90,96,). In the case of a combined ACL/MCL injury some have reported satisfactory results with nonoperative treatment while others advocate surgical reconstruction of the ACL with repair of the MCL to adequately restore knee stability. Still others choose to surgically reconstruct the ACL without addressing the MCL. Regardless, the prognosis for such injuries is generally worse than for the isolated MCL injury, and clinical and basic science studies continue to elucidate

the suitable treatments for this combined injury.

The effects of ACL deficiency on the healing of the injured MCL have been studied in our research center using canine, rabbit, and goat models (2,158,253,257). Laboratory studies have demonstrated that MCL repair combined with ACL reconstruction restored valgus laxity and improved the structural properties of the FMTC over those with ACL reconstruction alone in the short term (12 weeks). However, at longer term (52 weeks), the advantages of the MCL repair on the biomechanical properties of the FMTC disappeared (158,257). Therefore, it is apparent that only reconstruction of the ACL is necessary for successful healing of the MCL to take place after a combined injury due to the important role the ACL plays in maintaining valgus instability.

The difficulties of performing ACL reconstructions on smaller animals such as rabbits have led to the use of the goat model, and it is rapidly becoming the model of choice to study combined ligament injuries because ACL reconstructions have been shown to be successful both short- and long-term (146,147,159). Using the robotic/UFS testing system, a recent study performed in our research center has investigated the healing of a combined injury treated with ACL reconstruction using this model (2). It was demonstrated that the initially high in situ force in the ACL graft was transferred to the healing MCL during the early stages of healing (i.e., from

TABLE 7-3. STRUCTURAL PROPERTIES OF THE FMTC AND TANGENT MODULUS OF THE MCL FOR THE ISOLATED MCL (187) INJURY AND COMBINED ACL/MCL INJURY (2)

	Isolated MCL Injury	Combined ACL/MCL Injury
Stiffness (N/mm)	52.5 ± 19.4	40.1 ± 23.5
Ultimate load (N)	331 ± 130	206.2 ± 155.7
Tangent modulus (MPa)	205 ± 109	98 ± 64

time zero to 6 weeks). These excessively high loads likely contributed to the observed decrease in the structural properties of the FMTC and tangent modulus of the MCL substance when compared with the isolated MCL injury (Table 7-3) (2,187).

7 FUNCTIONAL TISSUE ENGINEERING OF LIGAMENTS AND TENDONS

As discussed in Section 6, it has been consistently found that healing results in a larger quantity of lesser quality tissue when compared with normal tissue in terms of histomorphological appearance, biochemical composition, and biomechanical behavior. Therefore, new treatment modalities are sought to improve the properties of healing ligaments and tendons to those of the intact condition. With the recent advances in the fields of molecular biology and biochemistry, new techniques, including application of growth factors, gene transfer, cell therapy, and the use of scaffolding or mechanical factors, are being developed for the treatment of ligament injuries.

7.1 Growth Factors

Growth factors are small polypeptides that bind to specific receptors on the surface of cells. They have been shown to activate pathways for complex intracellular signal transduction, resulting in changes in cell proliferation and migration, matrix synthesis, and the secretion of additional growth factors. The transforming growth factor-

β (TGF-β) has been shown to promote matrix synthesis, while platelet-derived growth factor-BB (PDGF-BB), basic fibroblast growth factor (b-FGF), and epidermal growth factor (EGF) are positive mitogens of fibroblasts of the ACL and MCL (47,78,123,134,135188,197,238). Although these growth factors have shown promising results *in vitro,* data from our research center have shown that their effect on the healing MCL is much different (31). This is likely due to infiltration of the healing tissue by inflammatory cells and other growth factors, as well as the milieu during the healing process. Furthermore, because the effectiveness of growth factors is short lived, repeated treatments are required. Therefore, work on the roles of growth factors, specifically the type, dosage, and time of administration, is in progress.

7.2 Gene Transfer and Gene Therapy

Gene transfer is the delivery of genetic material into cells for an increase or decrease in the production of specific proteins (e.g., growth factors) for longer-term expression. To promote efficient transfer of the sequence into the cell, viral vectors and liposomes have been used as delivery vehicles (139). Using the adenovirus as a vector, a marker gene (LacZ) was successfully introduced and expressed in the rabbit MCL and ACL (77). Further, growth factors, such as PDGF-BB and TGF-β, had also been successfully introduced and expressed in the patellar tendon (138,141). Gene transfer also resulted in the overexpression of the gene for focal adhesion kinase (pp125 FAK) in flexor tendons (120). However, with the concerns about the potential immune response to adenovirus, work is moving toward the use of others such as the adeno-associated virus (AAV) (254,255).

Antisense gene therapy using oligonucleotides (ODNs) is an alternative method to reduce undesirable proteins in the healing ligament or tendon. Because direct transfection of cells with naked ODNs is inefficient, liposomes are also being used as a vehicle to deliver therapeutic genes to healing ligaments. This methodology has been shown to be successful to reduce decorin in the healing MCL of a rabbit (138,139). As a result, its important role in fibrillogenesis was demonstrated (107,142), which led to an increase in the diameter of the collagen fibrils, and an 85% increase in the tensile strength of the healing MCL (137). Currently, antisense gene therapy using antisense ODNs is being used to reduce the expression of collagen types III and V in the healing MCL. Preliminary studies have shown that antisense ODNs are capable of reducing the gene expression and protein synthesis of collagen types III and V *in vitro* by approximately 40%, and that liposomal vectors can efficiently deliver antisense ODNs *in vivo* in a rat model (93,94,191,192).

7.3 Scaffolding

The use of both synthetic and biological materials as tissue scaffolding has been studied extensively for ligament and tendon repair. A successful scaffold should have characteristics that include adequate strength, as well as an appropriate modulus to effectively share the load with the healing host tissue. The scaffold should also provide a suitable environment for cell migration and production of new extracellular matrix in a controlled manner, as well as to deliver biological agents. Finally, the scaffold should degrade to allow the newly formed tissue to assume the mechanical function.

Although the major advantages of synthetic polymers include the ease of fabrication and reproducibility, their poor performance *in vivo* have discouraged their use for ligaments and tendons (18,71,176) in spite of their successful use when seeded with fibroblasts *in vitro*

(29,116). However, a variety of naturally derived collagen scaffolds derived from connective tissue have been considered for injury repair. Porcine small intestinal submucosa (SIS) has been studied extensively over the past 10 years, showing promise for musculoskeletal applications, and is now commercially available (15,16,40,46, 110,200). It consists of an organized type I collagen matrix with preferred alignment (16,182) and contains active growth factors (210), which both contribute to its ability to promote tissue healing. SIS has been used to replace a completely resected infraspinatus tendon in a dog model. After 3 months the histomorphological appearance was similar to the native infraspinatus tendon, while the load to failure was similar to the sham-operated controls, but with significantly smaller cross-sectional area (46). However, SIS was unsuccessful when used as an ACL replacement graft as the ultimate load dropped to approximately one third of that at the time of implantation (15).

In our research center, SIS was used for ligament healing following a gap injury (136). Using the rabbit MCL as a model, early data showed a more uniform appearance with a solid midsubstance when treated with SIS after 12 weeks. The stiffness of the FMTCs in the SIS treated group measured 56% higher than that in the nontreated group, while the ultimate load was nearly doubled. For mechanical properties, the tangent modulus and tensile strength of the healing MCL from the SIS treated group was nearly double that for the nontreated group, demonstrating a positive effect to improve the quality of the healing MCL. Current studies include the determination of whether this biological scaffold can be further enhanced by seeding it with fibroblasts and subjecting the construct to cyclic stretching prior to implantation.

7.4 Mechanical Factors

Mechanical forces are known to play a positive role in the etiology and healing of ligaments and tendons by a better organization of collagen fibers and alignment of fibroblasts (68). *In vitro* studies revealed that mechanical stretching of fibroblast-seeded collagen gels induces

FIGURE 7-28. Human patellar tendon fibroblasts grown on microgrooved silicone membrane become aligned and elongated in the direction of the microgrooves. (Adapted from Wang, JH-C: *Connect Tissue Res,* 2000;41:29–36 (214).)

alignment of the fibroblasts and collagen fibrils along the direction of stretching (48,87) and increases cell proliferation and expression of a variety of glycoproteins involved in tissue remodeling, including collagens and matrix metalloproteases (87,168,169).

A model to investigate the effect of mechanical factors on cell behavior based on tendon fibroblasts grown in microgrooved surfaces has been recently developed (214,215,217). Unlike the random distribution observed with fibroblasts cultured on smooth surfaces, cells become elongated and aligned in the microgrooves (Fig. 7-28). Collagen matrix formed by these cells was also highly aligned parallel to the microgrooves (216). Furthermore, when cyclically stretched uniaxially, the cells in the microgrooves remained aligned in the stretching direction and resembled those *in vivo.*

Because excessive repetitive loading can cause overuse injuries, most widely known as tendinopathy in tendons and ligaments, *in vitro* models of cyclic stretching have also been used to examine the effects of repetitive loading on cultured human tendon fibroblasts. Using these models, high levels of inflammatory mediators such as prostaglandin E_2 (PGE$_2$) were found (6).

Work from our research center has shown that when tendon fibroblasts are cyclically stretched in the microgrooved system described above, the production of PGE$_2$ increased in a stretching-magnitude dependent manner (213). Specifically, after 24 hours of stretching, no increase in PGE$_2$ was observed at 4% stretching; however, at 8% and 12% the PGE$_2$ levels increased 1.7- and 2.2-fold, respectively, compared with unstretched fibroblasts. Because PGE$_2$ is a known inflammatory mediator, the results of these studies suggest that tendinopathy may involve the release of PGE$_2$ following overstretching of tendon fibroblasts *in vivo.*

8 SUMMARY AND FUTURE DIRECTIONS

The biomechanical properties of ligaments and tendons are very difficult to measure accurately. With the utilization of new technologies such as the laser micrometer system and high-speed video recording systems, stress and strain of these tissues could be accurately determined. Even more important is that this improved technology will permit new areas to be explored in order to gain new insights into the biomechanical behavior of ligaments and tendons. This chapter has presented some of these findings, including the identification of the differences between the ligament substance and its insertion sites in relationship to skeletal maturation and aging. Further, it is important for bone–ligament–bone complexes to be oriented anatomically such that loads are transferred from insertion, to midsubstance, to insertion as they would be *in vivo*. Standardized and controlled testing procedures must be utilized, and proper documentation must be reported regarding temperature, hydration, and storage because they can have profound effects on soft tissue behavior.

The homeostasis of ligaments and tendons has been found to be dependent on the mechanical environment. Relatively short periods of immobilization on ligaments around the knee lead to substantial decreases in joint stiffness and significant weakening of the biomechanical properties of ligaments. Remobilization can restore the mechanical properties of ligaments fairly quickly; however, full recovery of the ligament–bone junction may require many months or years. Further, long periods of exercise can lead to positive effects on the properties of ligaments, but the gain is only gradual, in comparison to the rapid loss of properties observed with immobilization.

It has been demonstrated that in addition to acting as a restraint to ATT, the ACL also plays a crucial role in knee stability in response to combined rotatory loads, especially valgus and internal torques. With 5-DOF knee motion, the ACL has been shown to be more important than the MCL in providing valgus stability. Using a unique robotic/UFS testing system, the roles of the AM and PL bundles of the ACL have been elucidated. The importance of the PL bundle has been demonstrated, and thus, an anatomical reconstruction of both bundles could be shown to better restore the knee function than the traditional single-bundle reconstruction.

For the flexor tendons of the hand, relationships have been described among moment arms, excursions, and gliding functions. Further, it has been shown that flexor tendon excursion relative to the sheath in zone II was maximized by PIP joint motion, and this may provide a basis for a more complete understanding of tendon healing and treatment modalities.

Models of shoulder dislocation have shed light on the mechanism of dislocation and the importance of muscles, ligaments, and bony orientation in maintaining shoulder stability. However, it has also been demonstrated that under certain motions the force of the pectoralis major can actually contribute to anterior shoulder instability. Indeed, the development of new models to study ligament and tendon injury continues to generate much new information.

The development of the robotic/UFS testing system has enabled better understanding of the function of the knee ligaments and the results of different techniques for ACL reconstruction. The next step would involve the need to translate *in vivo* kinematics, e.g., motion from patients during activities of daily living and rehabilitation protocols, as inputs for cadaveric knee specimens on the robotic/UFS testing system such that more realistic in situ force in the ACL can be obtained. This approach should further improve our understanding of the function of the ACL, as well as mechanisms for its injury. It is hoped that this methodology can be further adapted for biomechanical studies of other synovial joints, such as the human shoulder, where motions are even more complex.

Complementary to the move from *in vitro* to *in vivo* studies is the development of computational models because they can offer more information than experiments. Several three-dimensional finite element models of the human ACL have been developed (80,165,196). Once a model is validated by experiments, it can be used to simulate more complex loading conditions such as those during activities of daily living, which may be beyond experimental capabilities. Further, the stress and strain distribution in the ligaments and tendons are calculated, which should provide further insight into the mechanisms of injury. It is hoped that this type of model can lead to a better understanding of knee ligament injuries and the development of strategies to optimize repair and reconstruction of ligaments and tendons.

In terms of treatment modalities after ligament injuries, it has been determined that conservative management with early mobilization offers the best results for healing of an isolated MCL rupture, and this has changed the paradigm of clinical management (157,187, 220). Immobilization has actually been shown to be detrimental to the healing process as well as to weaken the bone–ligament–bone complex. The MCL has been shown to heal spontaneously, even without reapproximation of the cut ends, and valgus stability is maintained by the remaining joint structures, especially the ACL. In addition, most of the structural properties of the FMTC approach normal levels within weeks after injury; however, the mechanical properties remain poor and do not improve over time. The prognosis is much worse for the more severe combined ACL/MCL injury (2,158,257). Clinically, the ACL rupture is reconstructed to provide stability to the knee, so that the MCL can be treated conservatively. Nevertheless, the outcome is that the biomechanical properties of the healing MCL are substantially lower after a combined injury when compared with the isolated MCL injury.

Functional tissue engineering approaches offer the opportunity to improve tissue quality during healing of ligaments and tendons. The potential of manipulating cellular and biochemical mediators to change the normal healing response clearly exists. A number of techniques have shown some promise, one of which is antisense gene therapy that blocks the production of specific proteins. Positive results have been demonstrated by decreasing decorin, which led to an increase in collagen fibril diameter and an increase in mechanical properties. Preliminary results are also encouraging for the inhibited production of collagen types III and V with antisense gene therapy with the help of delivery by liposomal vectors. Biomatrix scaffolds, such as porcine small intestinal submucosa, have demonstrated the ability to restore the histomorphological appearance and improve the biomechanical properties of healing ligaments and tendons. Further, several groups have also used cell seeding of scaffolds with the application of mechanical loading to develop ligament and tendon equivalents *in vitro*. It is likely that a combination of these approaches can be used to achieve even better results.

The biological and biomechanical story of ligaments and tendons is far from complete, and a wide variety of multidisciplinary studies are needed to build on the knowledge that

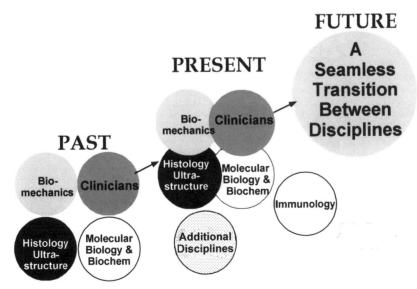

FIGURE 7-29. Timeline of the interactions between the multiple disciplines involved in the study of tendon and ligament biomechanics, with the future holding the potential for a seamless transition between disciplines.

we already have in order to improve the clinical outcome for patients. Further cooperation among biologists, biochemists, clinicians, and bioengineers will be needed to develop *in vitro, in vivo*, and computational models for the study of normal and injured ligaments and tendons. This will require respect for other disciplines and a willingness to learn the language of other fields. Through healthy collaborations and effective communication, we should be able to achieve our common goals much more rapidly (Fig. 7-29).

9 ACKNOWLEDGMENTS

The authors acknowledge the efforts of Peter Tang, MD, in the preparation of this book chapter, as well as funding from the National Institutes of Health (AR39683 and AR41820).

REFERENCES

1. Abramowitch SD, Clineff TD, Withrow JD, et al. The quasi-linear viscoelastic properties of the healing goat medial collateral ligament: an experimental and analytical approach. In: 23rd American Society for Biomechanics, Pittsburgh, PA. 1999:278–279.

2. Abramowitch SD, Yagi M, Tsuda E, et al. The healing medial collateral ligament following a combined anterior cruciate and medial collateral ligament injury—a biomechanical study in a goat model. *J Orthop Res* 2003;21(6):1124–1130.

3. Aglietti P, Buzzi R, Giron F, et al. Arthroscopic-assisted anterior cruciate ligament reconstruction with the central third patellar tendon. A 5–8-year follow-up. *Knee Surg Sports Traumatol Arthrosc* 1997;5:138–144.

4. Akeson WH, Amiel D, Woo SL-Y. Immobility effects on synovial joints the pathomechanics of joint contracture. *Biorheology* 1980;17:95–110.

5. Allard P, Thiry PS, Bourgault A, et al. Pressure dependence of "the area micrometer" method in evaluation of cruciate ligament cross-section. *J Biomed Eng* 1979;1:265–267.

6. Almekinders LC, Baynes AJ, Bracey LW. An in vitro investigation into the effects of repetitive motion and nonsteroidal antiinflammatory medication on human tendon fibroblasts. *Am J Sports Med* 1995;23:119–123.

7. An KN, Chao EY, Cooney WP III, et al. Normative model of human hand for biomechanical analysis. *J Biomech* 1979;12:775–788.

8. An KN, Cooney WP, Chao EY, et al. Determination of forces in extensor pollicis longus and flexor pollicis longus of the thumb. *J Appl Physiol* 1983;54:714–719.

9. An KN, Takahashi K, Harrigan TP, et al. Determination of muscle orientations and moment arms. *J Biomech Eng* 1984;106:280–282.

10. An KN, Ueba Y, Chao EY, et al. Tendon excursion and moment arm of index finger muscles. *J Biomech* 1983;16:419–425.

11. Anderson AF, Snyder RB, Lipscomb AB Jr. Anterior cruciate ligament reconstruction. A prospective randomized study of three surgical methods. *Am J Sports Med* 2001;29:272–279.

12. Apreleva M, Hasselman CT, Debski RE, et al. A dynamic analysis of glenohumeral motion after simulated capsulolabral injury. A cadaver model. *J Bone Joint Surg Am* 1998;80:474–480.

13. Arendt E, Dick R. Knee injury patterns among men and women in collegiate basketball and soccer. NCAA data and review of literature. *Am J Sports Med* 1995;23:694–701.

14. Bach BR Jr, Tradonsky S, Bojchuk J, et al. Arthroscopically assisted anterior cruciate ligament reconstruction using patellar tendon autograft. Five- to nine-year follow-up evaluation. *Am J Sports Med* 1998;26:20–29.

15. Badylak S, Arnoczky S, Plouhar P, et al. Naturally occurring extracellular matrix as a scaffold for musculoskeletal repair. *Clin Orthop Rel Res* 1999;367 Suppl:S333–343.

16. Badylak SF, Tullius R, Kokini K, et al. The use of xenogeneic small intestinal submucosa as a biomaterial for Achilles tendon repair in a dog model. *J Biomed Mater Res* 1995;29:977–985.

17. Bailey AJ. *Comprehensive biochemistry.* Amsterdam: Elsevier, 1968.

18. Bellincampi LD, Closkey RF, Prasad R, et al. Viability of fibroblast-seeded ligament analogs after autogenous implantation. *J Orthop Res* 1998;16:414–420.

19. Beynnon B, Howe JG, Pope MH, et al. The measurement of anterior cruciate ligament strain in vivo. *Int Orthop* 1992;16:1–12.

20. Beynnon BD, Fleming BC, Johnson RJ, et al. Anterior cruciate ligament strain behavior during rehabilitation exercises in vivo. *Am J Sports Med* 1995;23:24–34.

21. Bigliani LU, Pollock RG, Soslowsky LJ, et al. Tensile properties of the inferior glenohumeral ligament. *J Orthop Res* 1992;10:187–197.

22. Birk DE, Mayne R. Localization of collagen types I, III and V during tendon development. Changes in collagen types I and III are correlated with changes in fibril diameter. *Eur J Cell Biol* 1997;72:352–361.

23. Boardman ND III, Morifusa S, Saw SS, et al. Effects of tenorraphy on the gliding function and tensile properties of partially lacerated canine digital

flexor tendons. *J Hand Surg [Am]* 1999;24:302–309.

24. Bosch U, Decker B, Kasperczyk W, et al. The relationship of mechanical properties to morphology in patellar tendon autografts after posterior cruciate ligament replacement in sheep. *J Biomech* 1992;25:821–830.

25. Buss DD, Min R, Skyhar M, et al. Nonoperative treatment of acute anterior cruciate ligament injuries in a selected group of patients. *Am J Sports Med* 1995;23:160–165.

26. Butler DL, Kay MD, Stouffer DC. Comparison of material properties in fascicle-bone units from human patellar tendon and knee ligaments. *J Biomech* 1986;19:425–432.

27. Butler DL, Martin ET Kaiser AD, et al. The effects of flexion and tibial rotation on the 3-D orientation and lengths of human anterior cruciate ligament bundles. *Trans Orthop Res Soc* 1988;13:59.

28. Cabaud HE, Chatty A, Gildengorin V, et al. Exercise effects on the strength of the rat anterior cruciate ligament. *Am J Sports Med* 1980;8:79–86.

29. Cao Y, Vacanti JP, Ma X, et al. Generation of neotendon using synthetic polymers seeded with tenocytes. *Transplant Proc* 1994;26:3390–3392.

30. Carew EO, Talman EA, Boughner DR, et al. Quasi-linear viscoelastic theory applied to internal shearing of porcine aortic valve leaflets. *J Biomech Eng* 1999;121:386–392.

31. Celechovsky C, Niyibizi C, Watanabe N, et al. Analysis of collagens synthesized by cells harvested from MCL in the early stages of healing. *Trans Orthop Res Soc* 2001;26:703.

32. Chan SS, Livesay GA, Morrow DA, et al. The development of a low cost laser reflectance system to determine the cross sectional shape and area of soft tissues. *ASME Adv Bioeng* 1995;BED-31:123–124.

33. Chazal J, Tanguy A, Bourges M, et al. Biomechanical properties of spinal ligaments and a histological study of the supraspinal ligament in traction. *J Biomech* 1985;18:167–176.

34. Chow S, McMahon PJ, Yang BY, et al. A novel model of anterior glenohumeral dislocation. *Trans Orthop Res Soc* 2000;25:115.

35. Chowdhury P, Matyas JR, Frank CB. The "epiligament" of the rabbit medial collateral ligament: a quantitative morphological study. *Connect Tissue Res* 1991;27:33–50.

36. Chun KJ, Hubbard RP. Development of reduced relaxation function and stress relaxation with paired tendon. *ASME Adv Bioeng* 1986;BED2:162–163.

37. Ciccotti MG, Lombardo SJ, Nonweiler B, et al. Non-operative treatment of ruptures of the anterior cruciate ligament in middle-aged patients. Results after long-term follow-up. *J Bone Joint Surg Am* 1994;76:1315–1321.

38. Clayton ML, Miles JS, Abdulla M. Experimental investigations of ligamentous healing. *Clin Orthop Rel Res* 1968;61:146–153.

39. Clayton ML, Weir GJ. Experimental investigations of ligamentous healing. *Am J Surg* 1959;98:373–378.

40. Cook JL, Tomlinson JL, Kreeger JM, et al. Induction of meniscal regeneration in dogs using a novel biomaterial. *Am J Sports Med* 1999;27:658–665.

41. Cooper RR, Misol S. Tendon and ligament insertion. A light and electron microscopic study. *J Bone Joint Surg Am* 1970;52:1–20.

42. Crowninshield RD, Pope MH. The strength and failure characteristics of rat medial collateral ligaments. *J Trauma* 1976;16:99–105.

43. Daniel DM, Stone ML, Dobson BE, et al. Fate of the ACL-injured patient. A prospective outcome study. *Am J Sports Med* 1994;22:632–644.

44. Danto MI, Woo SL-Y. The mechanical properties of skeletally mature rabbit anterior cruciate ligament and patellar tendon over a range of strain rates. *J Orthop Res* 1993;11:58–67.

45. Debski RE, McMahon PJ, Thompson WO, et al. A new dynamic testing apparatus to study glenohumeral joint motion. *J Biomech* 1995;28:869–874.

46. Dejardin LM, Arnoczky SP, Ewers BJ, et al. Tissue-engineered rotator cuff tendon using porcine small intestine submucosa. Histologic and mechanical evaluation in dogs. *Am J Sports Med* 2001;29:175–184.

47. Duffy FJ Jr, Seiler JG, Gelberman RH, et al. Growth factors and canine flexor tendon healing: initial studies in uninjured and repair models. *J Hand Surg [Am]* 1995;20:645–649.

48. Eastwood M, Mudera VC, McGrouther DA, et al. Effect of precise mechanical loading on fibroblast populated collagen lattices: morphological changes. *Cell Motil Cytoskeleton* 1998;40:13–21.

49. Ellis DG. A shadow amplitude method for measuring cross sectional area of biological specimens. In: *21st Annual Conference on Engineering in Medicine and Biology,* Houston, TX. 1968:51–56.

50. Ellis DG. Cross sectional area measurements for tendon specimens—a comparison of several methods. *J Biomech* 1969;2:175–186.

51. Evans EB, Eggers GWN, Butler JK, et al. Experimental immobilization and remobilization of rat knee joints. *J Bone Joint Surg* 1960;42A:737–758.

52. Fetto JF, Marshall JL. The natural history and diagnosis of anterior cruciate ligament insufficiency. *Clin Orthop Rel Res* 1980;147:29–38.

53. Figgie HE III, Bahniuk EH, Heiple KG, et al. The effects of tibial-femoral angle on the failure mechanics of the canine anterior cruciate ligament. *J Biomech* 1986;19:89–91.

54. Frank C, McDonald D, Shrive N. Collagen fibril diameters in the rabbit medial collateral ligament scar: a longer term assessment. *Connect Tissue Res* 1997;36:261–269.

55. Frank C, McDonald D, Wilson J, et al. Rabbit medial collateral ligament scar weakness is associated with decreased collagen pyridinoline crosslink density. *J Orthop Res* 1995;13:157–165.

56. Frank C, Schachar N, Dittrich D. Natural history of healing in the repaired medial collateral ligament. *J Orthop Res* 1983;1:179–188.

57. Frank C, Woo SL-Y, Amiel D, et al. Medial collateral ligament healing. A multidisciplinary assessment in rabbits. *Am J Sports Med* 1983;11:379–389.

58. Frolke JP, Oskam, J, Vierhout PA. Primary reconstruction of the medial collateral ligament in combined injury of the medial collateral and anterior cruciate ligaments. Short-term results. *Knee Surg Sports Traumatol Arthrosc* 1998;6:103–106.

59. Fujie H, Livesay GA, Woo SL-Y, et al. The use of a universal force-moment sensor to determine in-situ forces in ligaments: a new methodology. *J Biomech Eng* 1995;117:1–7.

60. Fujie H, Mabuchi K, Woo SL-Y, et al. The use of robotics technology to study human joint kinematics: a new methodology. *J Biomech Eng* 1993;115:211–217.

61. Fukuta S, Oyama M, Kavalkovich K, et al. Identification of types II, IX and X collagens at the insertion site of the bovine achilles tendon. *Matrix Biol* 1998;17:65–73.

62. Fung YC. Stress strain history relations of soft tissues in simple elongation. In: Fung YC, Perrone N, Anliker M, eds. *Biomechanics: its foundations and objectives.* Englewood Cliffs, NJ: Prentice Hall, 1972:181–207.

63. Fung YC. Biorheology of soft tissues. *Biorheology* 1973;10:139–155.

64. Funk JR, Hall GW, Crandall JR, et al. Linear and quasi-linear viscoelastic characterization of ankle ligaments. *J Biomech Eng* 2000;122:15–22.

65. Gabriel MT, Wong EK, Yagi M, et al. Distribution of in situ forces in the anterior cruciate ligament in response to rotatory loads. *J Orthop Res* 2004;22(1):85–89.

66. Gelberman RH, Manske PR, Akeson WH, et al. Flexor tendon repair. *J Orthop Res* 1986;4:119–128.

67. Gohlke F, Essigkrug B, Schmitz, F. The patterns of the collagen fiber bundles of the capsule of the glenohumeral joint. *J Shoulder Elbow Surg* 1994;3:111–128.

68. Gomez MA, Woo SL-Y, Amiel D, et al. The effects of increased tension on healing medial collateral ligaments. *Am J Sports Med* 1991;19:347–354.

69. Grant ME, Prockop DJ. The biosynthesis of collagen. *N Engl J Med* 1972;286:194–199.

70. Grewal R, Saw SS, Bastidas JA, et al. Passive and active rehabilitation for partial lacerations of the canine flexor digitorum profundus tendon in zone II. *J Hand Surg [Am]* 1999;24:743–750.

71. Guidoin MF, Marois Y, Bejui J, et al. Analysis of retrieved polymer fiber based replacements for the ACL. *Biomaterials* 2000;21:2461–2474.

72. Gupta BN, Subramanian KN, Brinker WO, et al. Tensile strength of canine cranial cruciate ligaments. *Am J Vet Res* 1971;32:183–190.

73. Harner CD, Xerogeanes JW, Livesay GA, et al. The human posterior cruciate ligament complex: an interdisciplinary study. Ligament morphology and biomechanical evaluation. *Am J Sports Med* 1995;23:736–745.

74. Hart RA, Woo SL-Y, Newton PO. Ultrastructural morphometry of anterior cruciate and medial collateral ligaments: an experimental study in rabbits. *J Orthop Res* 1992;10:96–103.

75. Haut RC. Age-dependent influence of strain rate on the tensile failure of rat-tail tendon. *J Biomech Eng* 1983;105:296–299.

76. Haut RC, Powlison AC. The effects of test environment and cyclic stretching on the failure properties of human patellar tendons. *J Orthop Res* 1990;8:532–540.

77. Hildebrand KA, Deie M, Allen CR, et al. Early expression of marker genes in the rabbit medial collateral and anterior cruciate ligaments: the use of different viral vectors and the effects of injury. *J Orthop Res* 1999;17:37–42.

78. Hildebrand KA, Woo SL-Y, Smith DW, et al. The effects of platelet-derived growth factor-BB on healing of the rabbit medial collateral ligament. An in vivo study. *Am J Sports Med* 1998;26:549–554.

79. Hillard-Sembell D, Daniel DM, Stone ML, et al. Combined injuries of the anterior cruciate and medial collateral ligaments of the knee. Effect of treatment on stability and function of the joint. *J Bone Joint Surg Am* 1996;78:169–176.

80. Hirokawa S, Tsuruno R. Three-dimensional deformation and stress distribution in an analytical/computational model of the anterior cruciate ligament. *J Biomech* 2000;33:1069–1077.

81. Hirshman HP, Daniel DM, Miyasaka K. The fate of the unoperated knee ligament injuries. In: Daniel DM, Akeson WH, O'Connor JJ, eds. *Knee ligaments: structure, function, injury and repair.* New York: Raven Press, 1990:481–503.

82. Hollis JM, Marcin JP, Horibe S, et al. Load determination in ACL fiber bundles under knee loading. *Trans Orthop Res Soc* 1998;13:58.

83. Hollis JM, Takai S, Adams DJ, et al. The effects of knee motion and external loading on the length of the anterior cruciate ligament (ACL). A kinematic study. *J Biomech Eng* 1991;113:208–214.

84. Horibe S, Woo SL-Y, Spiegelman JJ, et al. Excursion of the flexor digitorum profundus tendon: a kinematic study of the human and canine digits. *J Orthop Res* 1990;8:167–174.

85. Horwitz MT. Injuries of the ligaments of the knee joint: an experimental study. *Arch Surg* 1939;38:946–954.

86. Hovelius L, Eriksson K, Fredin H, et al. Recurrences after initial dislocation of the shoulder. Results of a prospective study of treatment. *J Bone Joint Surg Am* 1983;65:343–349.

87. Huang D, Chang TR, Aggarwal A, et al. Mechanisms and dynamics of mechanical strengthening in ligament-equivalent fibroblast-populated collagen matrices. *Ann Biomed Eng* 1993;21:289–305.

88. Iaconis F, Steindler R, Marinozzi G. Measurements of cross-sectional area of collagen structures (knee ligaments) by means of an optical method. *J Biomech* 1987;20:1003–1010.

89. Indelicato PA. Non-operative treatment of complete tears of the medial collateral ligament of the knee. *J Bone Joint Surg Am* 1983;65:323–329.

90. Indelicato PA. Isolated medial collateral ligament injuries in the knee. *J Am Acad Orthop Surg* 1995;3:9–14.

91. Inoue M, McGurk-Burleson E, Hollis JM, et al. Treatment of the medial collateral ligament injury. I: the importance of anterior cruciate ligament on the varus-valgus knee laxity. *Am J Sports Med* 1987;15:15–21.

92. Jenkins RB, Little RW. A constitutive equation for parallel-fibered elastic tissue. *J Biomech* 1974;7:397–402.

93. Jia F, Shimomura T, Niyibizi C, et al. Regulating type III collagen gene expression using antisense gene therapy. *Trans Orthop Res Soc* 2002;27:588.

94. Jia F, Shimomura T, Westcott A, et al. Effects of antisense oligonucleotides with different target sites on type III collagen gene expression in HPTFs in vitro. In: Midwest Connective Tissue Workshop, Chicago, IL, 2001.

95. Johnson GA, Livesay GA, Woo SL-Y, et al. A single integral finite strain viscoelastic model of ligaments and tendons. *J Biomech Eng* 1996;118:221–226.

96. Jokl P, Kaplan N, Stovell P, et al. Non-operative treatment of severe injuries to the medial and anterior cruciate ligaments of the knee. *J Bone Joint Surg Am* 1984;66:741–744.

97. Jomha NM, Borton DC, Clingeleffer AJ, et al. Long-term osteoarthritic changes in anterior cruciate ligament reconstructed knees. *Clin Orthop Rel Res* 1999;358:188–193.

98. Jomha NM, Pinczewski LA, Clingeleffer A, et al. Arthroscopic reconstruction of the anterior cruciate ligament with patellar-tendon autograft and interference screw fixation. The results at seven years. *J Bone Joint Surg Br* 1999;81:775–779.

99. Kaltsas DS. Comparative study of the properties of the shoulder joint capsule with those of other joint capsules. *Clin Orthop Rel Res* 1983;173:20–26.

100. Kannus P. Long-term results of conservatively treated medial collateral ligament injuries of the knee joint. *Clin Orthop Rel Res* 1988;226:103–112.

101. Kannus P. Tendons—a source of major concern in competitive and recreational athletes. *Scand J Med Sci Sports* 1997;7:53–54.

102. Kannus P, Jarvinen M. Conservatively treated tears of the anterior cruciate ligament. Long-term results. *J Bone Joint Surg Am* 1987;69:1007–1012.

103. Kastelic J, Galeski A, Baer E. The multicomposite structure of tendon. *Connect Tissue Res* 1978;6:11–23.

104. Kazar B, Relovszky E. Prognosis of primary dislocation of the shoulder. *Acta Orthop Scand* 1969;40:216–224.

105. Kessler L, Missim, F. Primary repair without immobilization of flexor tendon division within the digital sheath. *Acta Orthop Scand* 1969;40:587–601.

106. Kim, SM, McCulloch TM, Rim, K. Comparison of viscoelastic properties of the pharyngeal tissue: human and canine. *Dysphagia* 1999;14:8–16.

107. Kuc IM, Scott PG. Increased diameters of collagen fibrils precipitated in vitro in the presence of decorin from various connective tissues. *Connect Tissue Res* 1997;36:287–296.

108. Kwan MK, Lin TH, Woo SL-Y. On the viscoelastic properties of the anteromedial bundle of the anterior cruciate ligament. *J Biomech* 1993;26:447–452.

109. Lam, TC, Frank CB, Shrive NG. Calibration characteristics of a video dimension analyser (VDA) system. *J Biomech* 1992;25:1227–1231.

110. Lantz GC, Badylak SF, Hiles MC, et al. Small intestinal submucosa as a vascular graft: a review. *J Invest Surg* 1993;6:297–310.

111. Laros GS, Tipton CM, Cooper RR. Influence of physical activity on ligament insertions in the knees of dogs. *J Bone Joint Surg Am* 1971;53:275–286.

112. Lee TQ, Dante M. Application of a continuous video digitizing system for tensile testing of bone soft tissue bone complex. *ASME Adv Bioeng* 1992;BED-22:87–90.

113. Lee TQ, Dettling J, Sandusky MD, et al. Age related biomechanical properties of the glenoid-anterior band of the inferior glenohumeral ligament-humerus complex. *Clin Biomech (Bristol, Avon)* 1999;14:471–476.

114. Lee TQ, Woo SL-Y. A new method for determining cross-sectional shape and area of soft tissues. *J Biomech Eng* 1988;110:110–114.

115. Lin HC, Kwan MK, Woo SL-Y. On the stress relaxation properties of anterior cruciate ligament (ACL). In: *ASME Adv Bioeng* 1987;BED 3:5–6.

116. Lin VS, Lee MC, O'Neal S, et al. Ligament tissue engineering using synthetic biodegradable fiber scaffolds. *Tissue Eng* 1999;5:443–452.

117. Linsenmayer TF, Gibney E, Igoe F, et al. Type V collagen: molecular structure and fibrillar

organization of the chicken a1(V) NH2-terminal domain, a putative regulator of corneal fibrillogenesis. *J Cell Biol* 1993;121:1181–1189.

118. Liu SH, Yang RS, al-Shaikh R, et al. Collagen in tendon, ligament, and bone healing. A current review. *Clin Orthop Rel Res* 1995;318:265–278.

119. Livesay GA, Rudy TW, Xerogeanes JW, et al. The use of robotic technology to examine the in situ force in the ACL. *Trans Orthop Res Soc* 1995;20:647.

120. Lou J, Kubota H, Hotokezaka S, et al. In vivo gene transfer and overexpression of focal adhesion kinase (pp125 FAK) mediated by recombinant adenovirus-induced tendon adhesion formation and epitenon cell change. *J Orthop Res* 1997;15:911–918.

121. Lyon RM, Woo SL-Y, Hollis JM, et al. A new device to measure the structural properties of the femur-anterior cruciate ligament-tibia complex. *J Biomech Eng* 1989;111:350–354.

122. Maffuli N. Rehabilitation of an anterior cruciate ligament [letter; comment]. *Clin Orthop Rel Res* 1997;343:253–255.

123. Marui T, Niyibizi C, Georgescu HI, et al. Effect of growth factors on matrix synthesis by ligament fibroblasts. *J Orthop Res* 1997;15:18–23.

124. Mason ML, Allen HS. The rate of healing of tendons. An experimental study of tensile strength. *Ann Surg* 1941;113:424–459.

125. Matsen FA, Thomas SC, Rockwood CA. Anterior glenohumeral instability. In: Matsen FA, ed. *The shoulder.* Philadelphia: WB Saunders, 1990:526–622.

126. Matsen FA, Fu, FH, Hawkins RJ. *The shoulder: a balance of mobility and stability.* Rosemont, IL: American Academy of Orthopaedic Surgeons, 1993.

127. Matthews LS, Ellis D. Viscoelastic properties of cat tendon: Effects of time after death and preservation by freezing. *J Biomech* 1968;1:65–71.

128. Matyas JR, Anton MG, Shrive NG, et al. Stress governs tissue phenotype at the femoral insertion of the rabbit MCL. *J Biomech* 1995;28:147–157.

129. McMahon PJ, Dettling JD, Sandusky MD, et al. Tensile properties of the glenoid-soft tissue-humerus complex: Analysis of deformation. *J Shoulder Elbow Surg* 2001;10:482–488.

130. Mechanic GL. An automated scintillation counting system with high efficiency for continuous analysis: cross-links of (^{3}H) NaBH$_4$-reduced collagen. *Anal Biochem* 1974;61:349–354.

131. Miltner LJ, Hu CH, Fang HC. Experimental joint sprain. Pathologic study. *Arch Surg* 1937;35:234–240.

132. Miyasaka KC, Daniel DM, Stone ML, et al. The incidence of knee ligament injuries in the general population. *Am J Knee Surg* 1991;4:3–8.

133. Morein G, Goldgefter L, Kobyliansky E, et al. Changes in the mechanical properties of rat tail tendon during postnatal ontogenesis. *Anat Embryol (Berl),* 1978;154:121–124.

134. Murphy PG, Loitz BJ, Frank CB, et al. Influence of exogenous growth factors on the expression of plasminogen activators by explants of normal and healing rabbit ligaments. *Biochem Cell Biol* 1993;71:522–529.

135. Murphy PG, Loitz, BJ, Frank CB, et al. Influence of exogenous growth factors on the synthesis and secretion of collagen types I and III by explants of normal and healing rabbit ligaments. *Biochem Cell Biol* 1994;72:403–409.

136. Musahl V, Abramowitch SD, Gilbert TW, et al. The use of porcine SIS to enhance the healing of the MCL: a functional tissue engineering study in rabbits. *J Orthop Res* 2004;22(1):214–220.

137. Nakamura N, Hart DA, Boorman RS, et al. Decorin antisense gene therapy improves functional healing of early rabbit ligament scar with enhanced collagen fibrillogenesis in vivo. *J Orthop Res* 2000;18:517–523.

138. Nakamura N, Shino K, Natsuume T, et al. Early biological effect of in vivo gene transfer of platelet-derived growth factor (PDGF)-BB into healing patellar ligament. *Gene Ther* 1998;5:1165–1170.

139. Nakamura N, Timmermann SA, Hart DA, et al. A comparison of in vivo gene delivery methods for antisense therapy in ligament healing. *Gene Ther* 1998;5:1455–1461.

140. Nathan H, Goldgefter L, Kobyliansky E, et al. Energy absorbing capacity of rat tail tendon at various ages. *J Anat* 1978;127:589–593.

141. Natsu-ume T, Nakamura N, Shino K, et al. Temporal and spatial expression of transforming growth factor-b in the healing patellar ligament of the rat. *J Orthop Res* 1997;15:837–843.

142. Neame PJ, Kay CJ, McQuillan DJ, et al. Independent modulation of collagen fibrillogenesis by decorin and lumican. *Cell Mol Life Sci* 2000;57:859–863.

143. Neuberger A, Slack HGB. The metabolism of collagen from liver, bones, skin and tendons in the normal rat. *Biochem J* 1953;53:47–52.

144. Neumann P, Keller TS, Ekstrom L, et al. Mechanical properties of the human lumbar anterior longitudinal ligament. *J Biomech* 1992;25:1185–1194.

145. Newton PO, Woo SL-Y, MacKenna DA, et al. Immobilization of the knee joint alters the mechanical and ultrastructural properties of the rabbit anterior cruciate ligament. *J Orthop Res* 1995;13:191–200.

146. Ng GY, Oakes BW, Deacon OW, et al. Biomechanics of patellar tendon autograft for reconstruction of the anterior cruciate ligament in the goat: three-year study. *J Orthop Res* 1995;3:602–608.

147. Ng GY, Oakes BW, Deacon OW, et al. Long-term study of the biochemistry and biomechanics of anterior cruciate ligament-patellar tendon autografts in goats. *J Orthop Res* 1996;14:851–856.

148. Niyibizi C, Kavalkovich K, Yamaji T, et al. Type V collagen is increased during rabbit medial collateral ligament healing. *Knee Surg Sports Traumatol Arthrosc* 2000;8:281–285.

149. Niyibizi C, Sagarrigo Visconti C, Gibson G, et al. Identification and immunolocalization of type X collagen at the ligament-bone interface. *Biochem Biophys Res Commun* 1996;222:584–589.

150. Niyibizi C, Visconti CS, Kavalkovich K, et al. Collagens in an adult bovine medial collateral ligament: immunofluorescence localization by confocal microscopy reveals that type XIV collagen predominates at the ligament-bone junction. *Matrix Biol* 1995;14:743–751.

151. Njus GO, Njus NM. A noncontact method for determining cross sectional area of soft tissues. *Trans Orthop Res Soc* 1968;11:126.

152. Noguchi M, Seiler JG III, Gelberman RH, et al. In vitro biomechanical analysis of suture methods for flexor tendon repair. *J Orthop Res* 1993;11:603–611.

153. Noyes FR, DeLucas JL, Torvik PJ. Biomechanics of anterior cruciate ligament failure: an analysis of strain-rate sensitivity and mechanisms of failure in primates. *J Bone Joint Surg Am* 1974;56:236–253.

154. Noyes FR, Mooar PA, Matthews DS, et al. The symptomatic anterior cruciate-deficient knee. Part I: the long-term functional disability in athletically active individuals. *J Bone Joint Surg Am* 1983;65:154–162.

155. Noyes FR, Torvik PJ, Hyde WB, et al. Biomechanics of ligament failure. II. An analysis of immobilization, exercise, and reconditioning effects in primates. *J Bone Joint Surg Am* 1974;56:1406–1418.

156. O'Donoghue DH, Frank CR, Jeter GL, et al. Repair and reconstruction of the anterior cruciate ligament in dogs: factors influencing long term results. *J Bone Joint Surg* 1971;43A:1167–1178.

157. Ohland KJ, Woo SL-Y, Weiss JA, et al. Healing of combined injuries of the rabbit medial collateral ligament and its insertions: a long term study on the effects of conservative vs. surgical treatment. *ASME Adv Bioeng* 1991;447–448.

158. Ohno K, Pomaybo AS, Schmidt CC, et al. Healing of the medial collateral ligament after a combined medial collateral and anterior cruciate ligament injury and reconstruction of the anterior cruciate ligament: comparison of repair and nonrepair of medial collateral ligament tears in rabbits. *J Orthop Res* 1995;13:442–449.

159. Papageorgiou CD, Ma CB, Abramowitch SD, et al. A multidisciplinary study of the healing of an intraarticular anterior cruciate ligament graft in a goat model. *Am J Sports Med* 2001;29:620–626.

160. Peterson RH, Gomez MA, Woo SL-Y. The effects of strain rate on the biomechanical properties of the medial collateral ligament: a study of immature and mature rabbits. *Trans Orthop Res Soc* 1987;12:127.

161. Peterson RH, Woo SL-Y. A new methodology to determine the mechanical properties of ligaments at high strain rates. *J Biomech Eng* 1986;108:365–367.

162. Pfaeffle HJ, Tomaino MM, Grewal R, et al. Tensile properties of the interosseous membrane of the human forearm. *J Orthop Res* 1996;14:842–845.

163. Pintar FA, Yoganandan N, Myers T, et al. Biomechanical properties of human lumbar spine ligaments. *J Biomech* 1992;25:1351–1356.

164. Pinto JG, Patitucci PJ. Visco-elasticity of passive cardiac muscle. *J Biomech Eng* 1980;102:57–61.

165. Pioletti DP, Rakotomanana LR, Benvenuti JF, et al. Viscoelastic constitutive law in large deformations: application to human knee ligaments and tendons. *J Biomech* 1998;31:753–757.

166. Pipkin AC, Rogers TC. A nonlinear integral representation for viscoelastic behavior. *J Mech Phys Solids* 1968;16:59–74.

167. Powell JW, Barber-Foss KD. Sex-related injury patterns among selected high school sports. *Am J Sports Med* 2000;28:385–391.

168. Prajapati RT, Chavally-Mis B, Herbage D, et al. Mechanical loading regulates protease production by fibroblasts in three-dimensional collagen substrates. *Wound Repair Regen* 2000;8:226–237.

169. Prajapati RT, Eastwood M, Brown RA. Duration and orientation of mechanical loads determine fibroblast cyto-mechanical activation: monitored by protease release. *Wound Repair Regen* 2000;8:238–246.

170. Puso MA, Weiss JA. Finite element implementation of anisotropic quasi-linear viscoelasticity using a discrete spectrum approximation. *J Biomech Eng* 1998;120:62–70.

171. Quapp KM, Weiss JA. Material characterization of human medial collateral ligament. *J Biomech Eng* 1998;120:757–763.

172. Race A, Amis AA. A molding method to find cross sections of soft tissue bundles with complex shapes. *Trans Orthop Res Soc* 1994;19:783.

173. Race A, Amis AA. The mechanical properties of the two bundles of the human posterior cruciate ligament. *J Biomech* 1994;27:13–24.

174. Reider B, Sathy MR, Talkington J, et al. Treatment of isolated medial collateral ligament injuries in athletes with early functional rehabilitation. A five-year follow-up study. *Am J Sports Med* 1994;22:470–477.

175. Reynolds B, Wray RC Jr, Weeks PM. Should an incompletely severed tendon be sutured? *Plast Reconstr Surg* 1976;57:36–38.

176. Richmond JC, Manseau CJ Patz R, et al. Anterior cruciate reconstruction using a Dacron ligament prosthesis. A long-term study. *Am J Sports Med* 1992;20:24–28.

177. Ritchie JR, Parker RD. Graft selection in anterior cruciate ligament revision surgery. *Clin Orthop Rel Res* 1996;325:65–77.

178. Romanic AM, Adachi E, Kadler KE, et al. Copolymerization of pNcollagen III and collagen I. pNcollagen III decreases the rate of incorporation of collagen I into fibrils, the amount of collagen I incorporated, and the diameter of the fibrils formed. *J Biol Chem* 1991;266:12703–12709.

179. Rowe CR. Acute and recurrent anterior dislocations of the shoulder. *Orthop Clin North Am* 1980;11:253–270.

180. Rowe CR, Zarins B, Ciullo JV. Recurrent anterior dislocation of the shoulder after surgical repair. Apparent causes of failure and treatment. *J Bone Joint Surg Am* 1984;66:159–68.

181. Rudy TW, Livesay GA, Woo SL-Y, et al. A combined robotic/universal force sensor approach to determine in situ forces of knee ligaments. *J Biomech* 1996;29:1357–1360.

182. Sacks MS, Gloeckner DC. Quantification of the fiber architecture and biaxial mechanical behavior of porcine intestinal submucosa. *J Biomed Mater Res* 1999;46:1–10.

183. Sagarriga Visconti C, Kavalkovich K, Wu, J, et al. Biochemical analysis of collagens at the ligament-bone interface reveals presence of cartilage-specific collagens. *Arch Biochem Biophys* 1996;328:135–142.

184. Sakane M, Fox, RJ, Woo SL-Y, et al. In situ forces in the anterior cruciate ligament and its bundles in response to anterior tibial loads. *J Orthop Res* 1997;15:285–293.

185. Salter RB, Field P. The effects of continuous compression on living articular cartilage: an experimental investigation. *J Bone Joint Surg* 1960;42A:31–49.

186. Sapega AA, Moyer RA, Schneck C, et al. Testing for isometry during reconstruction of the anterior cruciate ligament. Anatomical and biomechanical considerations. *J Bone Joint Surg Am* 1990;72:259–267.

187. Scheffler SU, Clineff TD, Papageorgiou CD, et al. Structure and function of the healing medial collateral ligament in a goat model. *Ann Biomed Eng* 2001;29:173–180.

188. Scherping SC Jr, Schmidt CC, Georgescu HI, et al. Effect of growth factors on the proliferation of ligament fibroblasts from skeletally mature rabbits. *Connect Tissue Res* 1997;36:1–8.

189. Seradge H. Elongation of the repair configuration following flexor tendon repair. *J Hand Surg [Am]* 1983;8:182–185.

190. Shelbourne KD, Klootwyk TE, Wilckens JH, et al. Ligament stability two to six years after anterior cruciate ligament reconstruction with autogenous patellar tendon graft and participation in accelerated rehabilitation program. *Am J Sports Med* 1995;23:575–579.

191. Shimomura T, Jia F, Niyibizi C, et al. Antisense oligonucleotides reduced type V collagen mRNA expression in human patellar tendon fibroblasts. In: Engineering Tissue Growth Conference, Pittsburgh, PA, 2002.

192. Shimomura T, Jia F, Niyibizi C, et al. Antisense oligonucleotides reduce synthesis of procollagen a1(V) chain in human patellar tendon fibroblasts: potential application in healing tendons and ligaments. *Connect Tissue Res* 2003;44(3–4):167–172.

193. Simon BR, Coats RS, Woo SL-Y. Relaxation and creep quasilinear viscoelastic models for normal articular cartilage. *J Biomech Eng* 1984;106:159–164.

194. Smith JW. The elastic properties of the anterior cruciate ligament of the rabbit. *J Anat* 1954;88:369–380.

195. Smutz, WP, Drexler M, Berglund LJ, et al. Accuracy of a video strain measurement system. *J Biomech* 1996;29:813–817.

196. Song Y, Debski RE, Musahl V, et al. A three-dimensional finite element model of the human anterior cruciate ligament: a computational analysis with experimental validation. *J Biomech* 2004;37(3):383–390.

197. Spindler KP, Dawson JM, Stahlman GC, et al. Collagen expression and biomechanical response to human recombinant transforming growth factor beta (rhTGF-b2) in the healing rabbit MCL. *J Orthop Res* 2002;20:318–324.

198. Stevenson H, Webster J, Johnson R, et al. Gender differences in knee injury epidemiology among competitive alpine ski racers. *Iowa Orthop J* 1998; 18:64–66.

199. Stouffer DC, Butler DL. Analysis of crimp unfolding, fluid expulsion and fiber failure in collagen fiber bundles. *ASME Adv Bioeng* 1984;46–47.

200. Suckow MA, Voytik-Harbin SL, Terril LA, et al. Enhanced bone regeneration using porcine small intestinal submucosa. *J Invest Surg* 1999;12:277–287.

201. Takai S, Woo SL-Y, Horibe S, et al. The effects of frequency and duration of controlled passive mobilization on tendon healing. *J Orthop Res* 1991;9:705–713.

202. Takai S, Woo SL-Y, Livesay GA, et al. Determination of the in situ loads on the human anterior cruciate ligament. *J Orthop Res* 1993;11:686–695.

203. Tanaka TT, Fung YC. Elastic and inelastic properties of the canine aorta and their variation along the aortic tree. *J Biomech* 1974;7:357–370.

204. Tanzer ML. Cross-linking of collagen. *Science* 1973;180:561–566.

205. Tipton CM, James SL, Mergner W, et al. Influence of exercise on strength of medial collateral knee ligaments of dogs. *Am J Physiol* 1970;218:894–902.

206. Tipton CM, Matthes RD, Maynard JA, et al. The influence of physical activity on ligaments and tendons. *Med Sci Sports* 1975;7:165–175.

207. Turkel SJ, Panio MW, Marshall JL, et al. Stabilizing mechanisms preventing anterior dislocation of the glenohumeral joint. *J Bone Joint Surg Am* 1981;63:1208–1217.

208. Viidik A, Lewin T. Changes in tensile strength characteristics and histology of rabbit ligaments induced by different modes of postmortal storage. *Acta Orthop Scand* 1966;37:141–155.

209. Viidik A, Sanquist L, Magi M. Influence of postmortem storage on tensile strength characteristics and histology of rabbit ligaments. *Acta Orthop Scand* [Suppl] 1965;79:1–38.

210. Voytik-Harbin SL, Brightman AO, Kraine MR, et al. Identification of extractable growth factors from small intestinal submucosa. *J Cell Biochem* 1997;67:478–491.

211. Wade PJ, Muir IF, Hutcheon LL. Primary flexor tendon repair: the mechanical limitations of the modified Kessler technique. *J Hand Surg [Br]* 1986;11:71–76.

212. Walker LB, Harris EH, Benedict JV. Stress strain relationship in human cadaveric plantaris tendon—a preliminary study. *Med Elect Biol Eng* 1964;2:31–38.

213. Wang JH-C, Jia F, Yang G, et al. Cyclic mechanical stretching of human tendon fibroblasts increases the production of prostaglandin E2 and levels of cyclooxygenase expression: a novel in vitro model study. *Connect Tissue Res* 2004;44(3–4):128–133.

214. Wang JH-C, Grood ES. The strain magnitude and contact guidance determine orientation response of fibroblasts to cyclic substrate strains. *Connect Tissue Res* 2000;41:29–36.

215. Wang JH-C, Grood ES, Florer J, et al. Alignment and proliferation of MC3T3-E1 osteoblasts in microgrooved silicone substrata subjected to cyclic stretching. *J Biomech* 2000;33:729–735.

216. Wang JH-C, Jia F, Gilbert TW, et al. Cell orientation determines the alignment of cell-produced collagenous matrix. *J Biomech* 2003;36(1):97–102.

217. Wang JH-C, Stone D, Jia F, et al. Biological responses of fibroblasts to cyclic stretching: a novel culture model study. *ASME Adv Bioeng* 2000;48:179–180.

218. Wehbe MA, Hunter JM. Flexor tendon gliding in the hand. Part II. Differential gliding. *J Hand Surg [Am]*, 1985;10:575–579.

219. Weisman G, Pope MH, Johnson RJ. The effect of cyclic loading on knee ligaments. *Trans Orthop Res Soc* 1979;4:24.

220. Weiss JA, Woo SL-Y, Ohland KJ, et al. Evaluation of a new injury model to study medial collateral ligament healing: primary repair versus nonoperative treatment. *J Orthop Res* 1991;9:516–528.

221. Wertheim, MG. Memoirs sur l'elasticité et la cohesion des principaux tissu du corps humain. *Ann Chim (Phys)* 1847;21:385–414.

222. White J, Werkmeister JA, Ramshaw JA, et al. Organization of fibrillar collagen in the human and bovine cornea: collagen types V and III. *Connect Tissue Res* 1997;36:165–174.

223. Wineman AS. Large axially symmetric stretching of a nonlinear viscoelastic membrane. *Int J Sols Structs* 1972;8:775–790.

224. Winters SC, Gelberman RH, Woo SL-Y, et al. The effects of multiple-strand suture methods on the strength and excursion of repaired intrasynovial flexor tendons: a biomechanical study in dogs. *J Hand Surg [Am]* 1998;23:97–104.

225. Withrow JD, Clineff TD, Abramowitch SD, et al. Biomechanical properties of healing goat medial collateral ligaments. In: *American Society for Biomechanics*, Pittsburgh, PA, 1999:202.

226. Wolff J. *Das Gesetz der Transformation der Kochen.* Berlin: Hirschwald, 1882.

227. Woo SL-Y Mechanical properties of tendons and ligaments. I. Quasi-static and nonlinear viscoelastic properties. *Biorheology* 1982;19:385–396.

228. Woo SL-Y, Akeson WH, Jemmott GF. Measurements of nonhomogeneous, directional mechanical properties of articular cartilage in tension. *J Biomech* 1976;9:785–791.

229. Woo SL-Y, An KN, Arnoczky SP, et al. Anatomy, biology, and biomechanics of tendon, ligament, and meniscus. In: Simon SR, ed. *Orthopaedic basic science.* Rosemont, IL: American Academy of Orthopaedic Surgeons, 1994:45–87.

230. Woo SL-Y, An KN, CD F, et al. Anatomy, biology, and biomechanics of tendon and ligament. In: Buckwalter JA, Einhorn TA, Simon SR, eds. *Orthopaedic basic science biology and biomechanics of the musculoskeletal system.* Rosemont, IL: American Academy of Orthopaedic Surgeons, 2000:581–616.

231. Woo SL-Y, Buckwalter JA, eds. *Injury and repair of musculoskeletal soft tissues.* Park Ridge, IL: American Academy of Orthopaedic Surgeons, 1988.

232. Woo SL-Y, Danto MI, Ohland KJ, et al. The use of a laser micrometer system to determine the cross-sectional shape and area of ligaments: a comparative study with two existing methods. *J Biomech Eng* 1990;112:426–431.

233. Woo SL-Y, Gelberman RH, Cobb NG, et al. The importance of controlled passive mobilization on flexor tendon healing. A biomechanical study. *Acta Orthop Scand* 1981;52:615–622.

234. Woo SL-Y, Gomez MA, Akeson WH. The time and history-dependent viscoelastic properties of the canine medical collateral ligament. *J Biomech Eng* 1981;103:293–298.

235. Woo SL-Y, Gomez MA, Inoue M, et al. New experimental procedures to evaluate the biomechanical properties of healing canine medial collateral ligaments. *J Orthop Res* 1987;5:425–432.

236. Woo SL-Y, Gomez MA, Seguchi Y, et al. Measurement of mechanical properties of ligament substance from a bone-ligament-bone preparation. *J Orthop Res* 1983;1:22–29.
237. Woo SL-Y, Gomez MA, Sites TJ, et al. The biomechanical and morphological changes in the medial collateral ligament of the rabbit after immobilization and remobilization. *J Bone Joint Surg Am* 1987;69:1200–1211.
238. Woo SL-Y, Hildebrand K, Watanabe N, et al. Tissue engineering of ligament and tendon healing. *Clin Orthop Rel Res* 1999;367(Suppl):S312–323.
239. Woo SL-Y, Hollis JM, Adams DJ, et al. Tensile properties of the human femur-anterior cruciate ligament-tibia complex. The effects of specimen age and orientation. *Am J Sports Med* 1991;19:217–225.
240. Woo SL-Y, Hollis JM, Roux RD, et al. Effects of knee flexion on the structural properties of the rabbit femur-anterior cruciate ligament-tibia complex (FATC). *J Biomech* 1987;20:557–563.
241. Woo SL-Y, Horibe S, Ohland KJ, et al. The response of ligaments to injury: healing of the collateral ligaments. In: Daniel DM, Akeson WH, O'Connor JJ, eds. *Knee ligaments: structure, function, injury, and repair.* New York: Raven Press, 1990;351–364.
242. Woo SL-Y, Inoue M, McGurk-Burleson E, et al. Treatment of the medial collateral ligament injury. II: structure and function of canine knees in response to differing treatment regimens. *Am J Sports Med* 1987;15:22–29.
243. Woo SL-Y, Johnson GA, Smith BA. Mathematical modeling of ligaments and tendons. *J Biomech Eng* 1993;115:468–473.
244. Woo SL-Y, Kanamori A, Zeminski J, et al. The effectiveness of anterior cruciate ligament reconstruction by hamstrings and patellar tendon: a cadaveric study comparing anterior tibial load versus rotational loads. *J Bone Joint Surg* 2002;84-A:907–914.
245. Woo SL-Y, Lee TQ, Gomez MA, et al. Temperature dependent behavior of the canine medial collateral ligament. *J Biomech Eng* 1987;109:68–71.
246. Woo SL-Y, Matthews JV, Akeson WH, et al. Connective tissue response to immobility. Correlative study of biomechanical and biochemical measurements of normal and immobilized rabbit knees. *Arthritis Rheum* 1975;18:257–264.
247. Woo SL-Y, Niyibizi C, Matyas J, et al. Medial collateral knee ligament healing. Combined medial collateral and anterior cruciate ligament injuries studied in rabbits. *Acta Orthop Scand* 1997;68:142–148.
248. Woo SL-Y, Ohland KJ, Weiss JA. Aging and sex-related changes in the biomechanical properties of the rabbit medial collateral ligament. *Mech Ageing Dev* 1990;56:129–142.
249. Woo SL-Y, Orlando CA, Camp JF, et al. Effects of postmortem storage by freezing on ligament tensile behavior. *J Biomech* 1986;19:399–404.
250. Woo SL-Y, Orlando CA, Gomez MA, et al. Tensile properties of the medial collateral ligament as a function of age. *J Orthop Res* 1986;4:133–141.
251. Woo SL-Y, Ritter MA, Amiel D, et al. The biomechanical and biochemical properties of swine tendons: long term effects of exercise on the digital extensors. *Connect Tissue Res* 1980;7:177–183.
252. Woo SL-Y, Simon BR, Kuei SC, et al. Quasi-linear viscoelastic properties of normal articular cartilage. *J Biomech Eng* 1980;102:85–90.
253. Woo SL-Y, Young EP, Ohland KJ, et al. The effects of transection of the anterior cruciate ligament on healing of the medial collateral ligament. A biomechanical study of the knee in dogs. *J Bone Joint Surg Am* 1990;72:382–392.
254. Xiao X, Li J, McCown TJ, et al. Gene transfer by adeno-associated virus vectors into the central nervous system. *Exp Neurol* 1997;144:113–124.
255. Xiao X, Li J, Tsao YP, et al. Full functional rescue of a complete muscle (TA) in dystrophic hamsters by adeno-associated virus vector-directed gene therapy. *J Virol* 2000;74:1436–1442.
256. Yagi M, Wong EK, Kanamori A, et al. The biomechanical analysis of anatomical ACL reconstruction. *Am J Sports Med* 2002;30(5):660–666.
257. Yamaji T, Levine RE, Woo SL-Y, et al. Medial collateral ligament healing one year after a concurrent medial collateral ligament and anterior cruciate ligament injury: an interdisciplinary study in rabbits. *J Orthop Res* 1996;14:223–227.
258. Yin FC, Tompkins WR, Peterson KL, et al. A video-dimension analyzer. *IEEE Trans Biomed Eng* 1972;19:376–381.
259. Zheng YP, Mak AF. Extraction of quasi-linear viscoelastic parameters for lower limb soft tissues from manual indentation experiment. *J Biomech Eng* 1999;121:330–339.
260. Zuckerman J, Stull GA. Effects of exercise on knee ligament separation force in rats. *J Appl Physiol* 1969;26:716–719.

8

BIOMECHANICAL PRINCIPLES OF CARTILAGE AND BONE TISSUE ENGINEERING

GORDANA VUNJAK-NOVAKOVIC
STEVEN A. GOLDSTEIN

Tissue engineering combines the principles of biology, engineering, and medicine to create biological substitutes or enhance the repair of lost or defective tissues. Cells, biomaterial scaffolds, and regulatory factors can be utilized in a variety of ways to generate functional tissue structures, either *in vitro* (using bioreactors) or *in vivo* (following surgical implantation). The primary functions of orthopaedic tissues are biomechanical in nature, and the main goal of all orthopaedic tissue engineering is the restoration of normal biomechanical functions. We discuss the biomechanical principles of cartilage and bone tissue engineering, in the context of clinical needs and the current state of the art of functional tissue engineering (FTE). We focus on representative studies that involved the utilization of physical and biological factors to enhance tissue development in vitro or in vivo, and the characterization of the engineered constructs and repair tissues toward the likelihood of their functional success following implementation. The paradigm of FTE (i.e., can an *in vitro* tissue engineered construct as a replacement within the highly loaded regions of the musculoskeletal system actually function *in vivo?*) is critically examined in order to identify standards of success, assess progress in the field, and outline some of the scientific, engineering, and clinical challenges and priorities. Three case studies are presented to illustrate the state of the art of FTE of cartilage and bone.

1 FUNCTIONAL TISSUE ENGINEERING OF CARTILAGE AND BONE

1.1 The Clinical Problem

Successful tissue engineering should begin with a precisely articulated definition of the specific attributes of the clinical problem, including the incidence, prevalence, and demographics of the conditions that demand therapeutic intervention. The existing treatment options and standards of clinical care should provide a baseline of comparison for any newly developed tissue engineering solution. The targeted properties of tissue-engineered constructs, or other alternatives, should provide an equal or better choice to that currently available in clinical practice. The identification of clinical issues is therefore the first step toward defining the required functional properties of tissue-engineered constructs.

The clinical demand for tissue-engineered cartilage and bone is extremely large and well distributed across the population in terms of gender and race, but clearly skewed toward older patients. For example, there are approximately 6 million bone fractures that occur annually in the United States (209). A subset of these fractures, estimated to be approximately 1 million, might be classified as fractures at risk of developing into delayed unions or nonunions if treated nonsurgically (86). Surgical intervention of bone fractures frequently involves the use of fixation devices and, in a large number of cases, the use of bone graft.

The incidence of osteoarthritis or degenerative joint disease is even more significant, as it affects approximately 20 million individuals in the United States (209). Most of these patients either developed degenerative joint disease from many years of wear and tear on their joints, or subsequent to trauma. Joint degeneration can range from localized bounded defects to the erosion of large surface areas of cartilage. In addition, the osteochondral resections due to neoplasms or severe trauma present substantial reconstructive challenges. The increasing incidence of these complex medical problems (due to an aging population) challenges our current technology and fuels the need for development of tissue engineering solutions.

1.2 Material Properties of Native Cartilage and Bone

Material properties of native cartilage and bone, described in Chapters 4 and 5 of this text, provide the basis for establishing the requirements and standards of success for cartilage and bone tissue engineering. The implications of material properties of native tissues for tissue engineering of cartilage and bone are summarized below.

Articular cartilage is *inhomogeneous* (properties vary with position within the tissue), *viscoelastic* (properties vary with time or the rate of loading), *nonlinear* (strain-dependent moduli (134,176), strain-dependent permeability (136), large differences between compressive and tensile moduli (238)), *inhomogeneous*, and *anisotropic* (properties vary with the site, depth, and direction (125,173,178)). There are four *zones* (superficial, middle, deep, calcified) within the tissue, demonstrating variations in matrix morphology and composition. Each zone consists of three distinct extracellular matrix (ECM) regions: pericellular, territorial, and interterritorial. The water and collagen contents decrease from the surface to the deep zone; the proteoglycan content is highest in the middle zone; collagen fibrils change orientation from parallel to the surface to perpendicular to the tidemark (see Chapter 5 for more details). Collagen content increases during tissue development and maturation, whereas the proteoglycan content remains largely unchanged (256). The onset of osteoarthritis involves degeneration of the tissue and various changes in its anatomical forms (see Chapter 9 for details), in the concentrations of the various biomacromolecules, and biomechanical and biophysical properties of tissue components (8–10,80,125,126,153,170–174, 176–179).

Bone tissue within the skeleton varies little with respect to its composition, in that the cells are embedded in a fibrous organic matrix composed primarily of collagen embedded in ground substance consisting of glycosaminoglycans (GAGs) and glycoproteins. This organic phase comprises approximately 50% of the volume of bone, while the other 50% of the volume is composed of mineral, primarily in the form of hydroxyapatite crystals and amorphous calcium phosphate (19) (also see Chapter 4 for more details). In contrast to the consistency in the matrix chemistry of bone, the organization of bone varies tremendously across various skeletal sites, and as a result, the biomechanical properties also vary greatly. In fact, the most striking feature of bone is the hierarchical organization of its architecture. Therefore, the structural properties of bone are best considered within this *hierarchical framework*. At a *macroscopic level*, bone can be divided into two compartments: a dense cortical compartment and a trabecular bone compartment resembling cellular foams. At a *microscopic level*, bone is organized into discrete assemblies: osteons in the cortical bone and trabecular packets. Within these structures the organization begins to appear the same: a parallel arrangement of lamellae. Each lamella is composed of cells (osteocytes) embedded within the mineralized collagen-type I dominated matrix.

The biomechanical behavior of cartilage is influenced by the balance between the swelling pressure of proteoglycan gel carrying fixed charge density and the restraining properties of the collagen network (137,153,154, 173,174,177,179). To fully describe cartilage, one would need to determine intrinsic biomechanical properties of the porous-permeable ECM, the frictional interactions between the interstitial fluid and the ECM, and the charge density and distribution within the tissue over a wide range of conditions associated with joint loading, anatomical location, developmental stage, and length scales (see Chapter 5 for more details). In adult cartilage, the equilibrium modulus increases with increasing wet weight fraction of proteoglycan (9,153,173–175,177,179)

and collagen (125,126,221) and decreasing wet weight fraction of water (80,153,173,174,176–179). The hydraulic permeability has been inversely correlated with the wet weight fraction of proteoglycans (153), directly correlated with water content (8,9,80,171,173) and the compressive strain (136); this is known as the nonlinear strain-dependent permeability effect (135,136). Compared with adult cartilage, immature cartilage and engineered constructs display relatively homogeneous and isotropic material properties, and microstructure contain lower fractions of collagen and lower compressive modulus (256). In developing cartilage, the increase in confined-compression modulus and decrease in hydraulic permeability were associated with an increase in collagen content and no detectable change in GAG content (256). The accumulation and functional assembly of collagen may thus be critical for cartilage tissue engineering (256). To date, however, no tensile data are available for tissue-engineered cartilage.

The biomechanical properties of bone are similarly related to the concentrations and inherent organization of its constituents. Although the mechanical function of whole bone depends on geometry and can be inferred by calculations of principle moments of inertia, the tissue-level properties depend on porosity, lamellar orientation, and mineral content. To fully describe bone, one would need to measure biomechanical properties of the tissue at multiple scales, (110). For example, whole bone biomechanical tests would provide information at the physiologic functional scale, whereas microscopic tests such as nanoindentation would provide an assessment of the local properties of the ECM of the bone. The formation or repair of bone follows two distinct cellular pathways: intramembranous bone formation, which occurs from mesenchymal condensation, and endochondral bone formation, which occurs through an intermediated cartilage state (223). Temporally, these two pathways create structures with very different functional properties and as such represent variations in targeted properties for tissue-engineered replacements. Intramembranous formation involves the direct expression of an ECM from fibroblastic and osteoblastic cells that is subsequently mineralized. The newly formed woven bone has lower modulus, lower strength, and less anisotropic structure as compared with mature bone, due to its disorganized matrix and compositional differences (89,91). Endochondral formation begins by producing a cartilage template that is eventually mineralized and replaced by bone. Physical forces as well as numerous biologic signaling molecules influence the character and geometry of the bone being formed or repaired, and as a result, its evolving mechanical properties.

1.3 Biomechanical Principles

The overall objective of orthopaedic tissue engineering is the restoration of normal tissue function. It is thought that lost or damaged tissue should be replaced by an engineered graft that can reestablish appropriate structure, composition, cell signaling and biomechanical function of the native tissue. In light of this paradigm, the clinical utility of tissue engineering will likely depend on our ability to replicate the *site-specific* properties of cartilage and bone across different *size scales*. In engineered constructs, the cells must conform to a specific *differentiated phenotype*, and the *composition and architectural organization* of the ECM must provide the necessary *biomechanical properties* inherent to the tissue being replaced, as well as contiguity and strength between the replacement constructs with the neighboring materials. Besides its dominant biomechanical role, an engineered tissue may also need to participate in physiological functions, such as metabolic remodeling in bone that supports mineral homeostasis. Ideally, an engineered graft should provide *regeneration*, rather than *repair*, and undergo orderly *remodeling* in response to environmental factors (Table 8-1).

For cartilage, these goals can be met through therapeutic manipulation of native cartilage to compensate for slow healing: by bringing in new cells capable of chondrogenesis and facilitating transport of nutrients (by convection and/or diffusion), metabolites, and regulatory signals (119). One approach involves filling the defect with cells alone (26,28) or with a cell seeded scaf-

fold (106,185). Another approach involves the implantation of functional tissue constructs engineered *in vitro* using cells, biomaterial scaffolds, and bioreactors (62,74,75,76,77,151,198, 199,229,230,233,236,247–250,256). For bone, it is often sufficient to approach tissue engineering *in vivo*, using scaffolds alone or in conjunction with various biofactors or cells.

To date, many tissue engineering constructs have successfully approached histological and biochemical similarity to a native tissue, but have failed to achieve normal mechanical properties. An evolving discipline called FTE is focused on the role of biomechanical factors in tissue regeneration, with an overall goal to develop a series of rational design principles to guide orthopaedic tissue engineering; this is particularly important in orthopaedics because most musculoskeletal tissues and structures must sustain very high loads for very long durations (10,97,128, 134,170,171); also see Chapters 2 to 5 for description of loadings on bone and cartilage, and Chapter 10 on the requirements of friction, lubrication, and wear. We believe that in order to sustain such magnitudes of loading, and over a lifetime of repetitive use with appropriate friction, lubrication, and wear properties, some principles of FTE must be established toward achieving viable surgical replacement for clinical use. In the body, there are numerous processes that can affect the clinical fate of the implanted engineered tissue constructs; they result in *repair, regeneration, and remodeling*—see Table 8-2 for definitions.

1.4 Standards of Success

To demonstrate the superiority of a certain technique, one would need to document the improved long-term clinical results as compared with either natural healing or currently accepted clinical treatment modalities. Diverse strategies for tissue engineering of cartilage have been evaluated using a variety of grading systems with variable success. Diagnostic and clinical criteria for cartilage lesions and rational goals for success of tissue regeneration therapies must be established; one set of criteria has been proposed by the International Cartilage Repair Society

TABLE 8-1. PRINCIPLES OF FUNCTIONAL TISSUE ENGINEERING

1. Define functional properties of native tissues
- Measure stresses and strains *in vivo*
  - Peak stresses/strains
  - Strain/stress histories
- Determine sub-failure and failure properties
  - Normal and pathological situations

2. Select and prioritize the pre-implantation requirements for engineered constructs
- Structure
  - Histomorphology
  - Biochemical composition
  - Molecular properties
- Presence of metabolically active differentiated cells capable of synthesizing and assembling functional tissue matrix
- Mechanical integrity
  - Handling
  - Implantation
- Mechanical behavior
  - Osmotic swelling
  - Static and dynamic properties in compression and tension
  - Shear
  - Electromechanical and physicochemical properties
  - Viscoelasticity and permeability
  - Subfailure and failure properties

3. Select and prioritize the therapeutic requirements for tissue regeneration
- Structural organization
  - Zonal distribution
  - Ultrastructure
  - Tissue micro-architecture
- Capacity to mature, remodel, regenerate (in response to *in vivo* environmental factors)
- Integration with surrounding native tissue (gold standard for cartilage repair)
- Mechanical behavior
  - Osmotic swelling
  - Static and dynamic properties in compression and tension
  - Shear
  - Electromechanical and physicochemical properties
  - Viscoelasticity and permeability
  - Subfailure and failure properties

4. Establish standards for the evaluation of engineered constructs and tissue repair
- How much is enough:
  - At the time of implantation?
  - At certain time points postoperatively?
- Which factors are critical for a successful regeneration in the long term?
- How can we assess these factors (methods and protocols)?

5. Physical regulatory factors of cell function
- *In vivo*
  - Study in developing and adult tissues
  - Use to enhance graft integration
- *In vitro*
  - Study under controlled conditions using bioreactors
  - Use to enhance formation of functional constructs

Adapted from Guilak F, Butler DL, Goldstein SA. Functional tissue engineering: the role of biomechanics in articular cartilage repair. *Clin Orthop* 2001;391[Suppl]:S295–S305, with permission.

TABLE 8-2. REPAIR, REGENERATION, AND REMODELING OF BONE AND CARTILAGE

- *Repair* is rapid replacement of the damaged, defective, or lost tissue with functional new tissue that resembles but does not replicate the structure, composition, and function of articular cartilage (30,196). Bone is unique in that its repair results in normal reconstitution of its constituents and properties. As such, bone repair is better characterized as regeneration.

- *Regeneration* is slow restoration of all components of the repair tissue to their original condition such that the new tissue is indistinguishable from normal articular cartilage or bone with respect to zonal organization, composition, and mechanical properties (30,64,196).

- *Remodeling* is the change in structure and composition of the constituent in response to the local and systemic environmental factors, that alters biomechanical tissue properties.

(117). Bone tissue engineering has had success in identifying targeted repair properties, which has led to therapeutic solutions. For example, clinical benefits have already been documented for the use of osteoconductive scaffolds made of naturally occurring or man-made carriers, with or without cells or growth factors. Current and future improvements in bone tissue engineering are focused on promoting rapid, predictable, and mechanically competent repair. Also, the clinical criteria for success have slowly evolved over the past several decades, and revolve around measures of geometry and density.

It is still an open question whether a true regeneration of cartilage or bone is necessary, or whether some form of repair would be acceptable (Table 8-1). If only a subset of the structural, material, and functional properties of the native tissue can be replicated, which ones are most important? For articular cartilage, the architecture of the repair tissue (e.g., zonal variation of composition and properties, columnar cells, tidemark at an appropriate depth), integration with adjacent cartilage and bone, and the ability to withstand physiological loading are perhaps more important landmarks of a successful repair than the reestablishment of exact biochemical properties. The current school of thought is that the restoration of native tissue structure is indispensable for a good long-term clinical prognosis, and that the transition from immature to mature cartilage is necessary for the tissue to assume its full physiological function. This is largely

based on the notion that, in response to loading, healthy native cartilage generates compressive, shear and tensile stresses, pressure gradients and interstitial fluid flow, streaming potentials and currents, and that the cartilaginous ECM mediates the presentation of physical signals to the cells (177,179). The specific mechanical properties of engineered cartilage that are essential for graft survival, development and remodeling, integration, and healthy function remain to be determined. For bone, a tissue-engineered construct must provide the appropriate chemical, physical, and biological signals to stimulate the natural and robust remodeling mechanisms that will result in eventual replacement of the construct with normal bone. When stimulated correctly, the remodeled or healed bone will have normal structural and mechanical properties. The specific mechanical properties of bone that need to be attained are dependent on the anatomic location being treated. For diaphyseal locations, the size and geometry of the cortical bone is critical. As described in Chapter 4, the area and polar moments of inertia provide the best assessment for diaphyseal bone function. The use of these geometrically dominated characteristics (i.e., structural characteristics) implies that the modulus of the bone tissue alone is insufficient to maintain integrity under physiological loading. The compressive moduli range from 12 to 20 GPa for cortical bone regions, and from 0.2 to 0.8 GPa for trabecular bone regions. The adaptation/remodeling in trabecular bone occurs rapidly, and results in a gradual and self-regulated adjustment to the required mechanical properties (6,85,110).

1.5 Testing Methods

The assessment of the biomechanical properties of native and engineered cartilage and bone requires attention to several experimental and theoretical issues.

1.5.1 Fresh or Frozen Tissue Samples

In tissues that have relatively high cell density (immature cartilage, engineered constructs at early stages of cultivation), freezing, storage, and thawing can result in cell lysis and breakdown of macromolecular matrix components. Two aspects of the freezing process can be manipulated to maintain cell viability in native and engineered cartilage: cooling rate (the initial freezing rate has to be slow enough to allow equilibration of water) and the use of cryoprotective agents are better controlled for isolated cells than for engineered tissues (119). For bone, freezing and thawing have small effect on its physical properties due to the low cellular density (6).

1.5.2 Biochemical Assays and Conversion Factors

Chondroitin sulfate is commonly used as a measure of GAGs in cartilage, and quantitative assays for hyaluronan and keratan sulfate are not routinely done. This assumption is acceptable for young cartilage and immature engineered constructs, but not necessarily for old or damaged cartilage, and mature engineered constructs (see Chapter 5 for more detailed descriptions of GAGs and proteoglycans in cartilage). Moreover, chondroitin sulfate correlates well with the fixed charge density in cartilage, which is the factor that endows the tissue with its swelling pressure (137,138,153,154,176,179). There have been a number of recent studies that have shown that Donnan osmotic swelling pressure and cell volume may be strong modulators of chondrocyte biosynthetic activities (98,107,177,256)(also see Chapter 6 for more details). These results argue for the necessity of pursuing basic science studies regarding the

above *assumption* of the influence of electrical charges attached to chondroitin sulfate on cell biosynthetic activities. Hydroxyproline is used as an indicator of total collagen, with hydroxyproline/collagen conversion factors ranging from 7.3 (107) to 10 (111,213).

1.5.3 Osmolality of the Testing Solution

Cartilage specimens can swell to variable degrees (young tissue tends to swell more than old; engineered tissue tends to swell more than native), depending on the osmolality of the bath, water content, and source of the tissue, and the properties of the bath solution (see Chapter 5 for more details) (95,98,137,138,153,154). Swelling can affect the measured material properties via related changes in the wet weight fractions of proteoglycan, water, and collagen, and the reference (free-swelling) dimensions to which the measured biomechanical data are normalized can also change (137,138). Previous studies have demonstrated that the osmotic environment of cartilage can significantly affect the tensile, compressive, and frictional properties of cartilage (137,138,153,173,179).

1.5.4 Duration and Conditions of Mechanical Testing

Prolonged testing can cause changes in cell metabolism and in some cases tissue composition (e.g., loss of proteoglycans from immature cartilaginous constructs (95,234)); also see Chapters 5 and 6. Experiments that last several hours and are performed in physiological buffer normally have no adverse effects (8,9).

The common intrinsic (flow- and geometry-independent) material properties of cartilage: Young's modulus, shear modulus, and the Poisson ratio (and a combination of these moduli—the aggregate modulus) can be assessed using a variety of established testing protocols (see Chapter 5 for details of cartilage testing). In general, the choice of the test depends on the material properties being assessed and, to some extent, on the size, shape, and amount of the tissue sample (173). For example, indentation may be an excellent choice for nondestructive testing of the tissue-engineered joint repair, whereas tensile properties of cartilage samples may be used to monitor age-related degradation of the tissue (125,126). With confined compression as a method of choice (170,171,174), the testing configuration necessarily requires an impermeable loading platen; the loads may be static or dynamic, stress, or displacement control. All these factors can affect the axial and radial distributions of strains, stresses, pressure, electric current, or potential within the tissue or construct. The added complexity of mechanical testing of engineered constructs is that the composition and functional assembly of the ECM are different from those in native cartilage, and that immature constructs, as with natural tissues, are spatially inhomogeneous. It is an open question what the appropriate controls are (e.g., with respect to the developmental stage and anatomical location) for evaluating engineered constructs.

The aggregate modulus H_A (a measure of the equilibrium resistance of the tissue to compressive forces in a radially confined testing configuration) and the hydraulic permeability k (a measure of the ease with which fluid flows through the tissue when driven by a pressure gradient) are two of the possible, and now routinely measured, biomechanical properties of cartilage (10,13,80,170,171). Static compression offset can affect both of these values. With an increase in strain, the wet weight fractions of proteoglycan and collagen increase, causing an increase in H_A and a decrease in k (i.e., the nonlinear strain-dependent permeability effect—Chapter 5). If different tissue samples are compared at a larger compressive strain, the differences in biomechanical properties tend to increase (10). It is possible that a certain factor may have a significant effect only at large strains. One notable example is the effect of the developmental stage of bovine cartilage on k, which was minimal at a static off-set of 0%–15% and became significant when measured at a static off-set of 30%–45% (256).

The assessments of the biomechanical properties of bone are dependent on a number of environmental factors, including, temperature, moisture content, ionic concentration, pH, and rate of loading or deformation. Biomechanical

testing protocols need to be designed as a function of the anatomic region or identity of bone (or cartilage) being replaced; cartilage from regions of high stress have higher proteoglycan content (therefore, lower collagen content) (3,9, 80,153,173). For bone, the testing protocols range from whole bone bending tests (diaphyseal locations) to uniaxial compression tests (metaphyseal bone), to bending and tensile or compression tests (metaphyseal bone), to bending and tensile or nanoindentation tests for in-depth evaluation of bone tissue (6).

An effective way to consider testing bone is within a hierarchical framework (110). The function of bone at the organ level provides an assessment of how the structure will withstand the functional demands of everyday usage. The whole bone testing can be done in either bending or torsion, and the choice of bending or torsional loading is dependent on the anatomic region and the typical usage of that region. Often, torsion is the most revealing test because it really represents a physiologically relevant loading mode and incorporates complex local stresses in tension, compression, and shear. For cortical bone, specimens can be machined and then tested in torsion, tension, (simple) shear, or bending. Note, aside from effects due to tissue microinhomogeneities and anisotropy, the torsion test yields a state of *pure* shear within the specimen whereas simple shear does not. Simple shear, by the law of conservation of angular momentum, must necessarily generate compression within the tested specimen. This becomes an important point of difference when testing cartilage in shear because compression will generate interstitial fluid flow and thus frictional dissipation within the tissue (for more details, see Chapter 5). For trabecular bone, the easiest and most common tests involve cubic specimens that are tested in axial compression.

1.5.5 Hierarchical Framework: Cartilage

In most cases, compression moduli for cartilage are determined from experimental data assuming tissue homogeneity. For full thickness cartilage, this would be an over-simplifying assumption, due to the gradients in tissue composition and mechanical properties over the depth of the tissue (3,125,126,146,153,178, 232)(see Chapter 5 for more details on articular cartilage inhomogeneities and anisotropies). For relatively thin samples, there is less change and the assumption may be acceptable. The surface of articular cartilage appears to be less stiff than the deep layers in compression (178,244), but in tension, the articular surface in mature animals is much stiffer than the deep layers (see Chapter 5 for more details). The results of mechanical testing are often biased by the procedure adopted for sample preparation, in particular immature engineered constructs seem to have spatially nonuniform compositions and mechanical properties. The standardization of the experimental protocols for sample cutting and mechanical testing would greatly enhance quantitative comparisons.

Any discontinuity in the structure or mechanical properties of cartilage or bone may alter stresses and strains quite significantly. For example, peak stresses measured at the interface with a prosthesis (18 MPa, (109)) were higher than peak stresses in intact joints (5–10 MPa, (29)). Integration at the graft-host interface represents a particularly complex situation for mechanical testing. The strains at the graft-host interface may be significantly higher than the nominal strains, as a result of different mechanical stiffnesses of the native and engineered tissue. Common experimental methods and theoretical models developed for native cartilage are difficult to apply to the integrative tissue repair, for several reasons. Tissue properties are inhomogeneous, in space and time, and it is not clear whether common material properties (e.g., equilibrium modulus) are indicative of the progression of integrative repair (2,172,178). It has been suggested that the adhesive strength of the interface, estimated from the adhesive failure of repair tissue, could be used to assess the quality of the integrative repair (2,189,211).

1.5.6 *Hierarchical Framework: Bone*

The most reliable measures of success of bone regeneration have been derived from biomechan-

ical testing of the repair tissue at several hierarchical scales (110). However, these assays are confined to use in preclinical models. Fortunately, noninvasive imaging techniques including computerized tomography (CT), magnetic resonance imaging (MRI), standard radiography, dual energy x-ray absorptiometry (DEXA), and potentially ultrasound have been excellent models for quantifying the structural and mechanical competence of regenerated bone tissue. For example, high-quality radiographs can be effectively interpreted to assess the degree of integration of a tissue-engineered bone construct with its surrounding native tissue. Furthermore, the density of the regenerated bone tissue as inferred from plain radiographs or quantitatively measured using CT or DEXA has been shown to correlate with the mechanical properties of bone (22,51,53,54,84,152). Bone tissue is capable of rapid remodeling in response to the changing metabolic and mechanical environment, and there is a need to monitor in situ the progression of bone regeneration toward a required mechanical integrity and load support capabilities.

1.6 Pre-clinical and Clinical Evaluation

The establishment of robust and reproducible pre-clinical and clinical outcome measures for tissue engineering applications is pivotal for assessing success or failure. For bone and cartilage, the incorporation of the construct into the native tissue and the evolution of biomechanical properties postimplantation are particularly important. Phase I or phase I/II clinical trials are performed to test the safety of a therapeutic intervention with a modest eye toward efficacy, while phase II and phase III studies have the primary goals of testing efficacy within a statistically robust experimental design; there is also a need to catalogue complications by a formal statistical comparison of the tissue-engineered construct properties to the prescribed targeted properties and desired clinical outcome.

For *clinical studies*, valid interpretation of the results requires controlled, prospective, randomized studies with defined inclusion and exclusion criteria, and standardized assessment methods.

In order to demonstrate the superiority of a specific approach to cartilage or bone regeneration, one would need to provide long-term results that are better than either the natural repair history or the current standard of care. Experience has taught us that many complications and failures occur after long periods of time (19,30,31,183). Because the life expectancy of a tissue engineered construct may likely exceed 20 to 30 years, short-term assessment strategies must be predictive of the long-term utility. It is widely assumed that therapeutic strategies that stimulate the regeneration of tissue that closely resembles native cartilage or bone with respect to overall morphology and hierarchical structure, biochemical composition, and biomechanical properties, will function well in situ, and have the highest probability of providing consistent and reliable symptom-free tissue repair in the long term. This fundamental hypothesis of FTE needs to be validated for both tissue-engineered bone and cartilage. One of the objectives of this chapter is to critically examine this perspective in light of the available data for prospective treatment modalities.

For *preclinical studies*, the most important aspect is the establishment of an experimental model that simulates clinical utility of the tissue-engineered construct, is compatible with human physiology, and allows the use of quantitative functional assays (e.g., biosynthesis rates of ECM components, mechanical properties, ultrastructure, and integration at the graft-host interfaces). In evaluating the repair tissue, comparisons should be made using controls that are age-, species-, and location-matched with the treated defects. Healthy native cartilage and bone have complex structural and ultrastructural organizational features that are generally not replicated within a repair tissue. Tissue homeostasis and the relative rates of synthesis and degradation of matrix components may be more important than the exact biochemical composition. For cartilage, integration between the repair tissue and subchondral bone is likely to be more important than the integration with adjacent cartilage (196). For bone, integration is a frequent and natural phenomenon that is essentially part of the normal process of fracture healing and repair. However, the relative importance of each

of these factors for normal physiological function and the specific cell-matrix interactions is not yet clear.

Animal models. For studies of tissue-engineered cartilage repair, the factors that are particularly important include the selection of animal species, defect site, and defect parameters (115). Partial defects are quite common in humans, and these defects rarely penetrate into the subchondral bone, even in cases of advanced osteoarthritis, and these defects rarely heal (30, 115). Human cartilage is 2 to 3 mm thick (medial femoral condyle), and may be as thick as 7 to 8 mm in the trochlea, in contrast to goat ($\sim$600 to 800 μm) or rabbit ($\sim$400 μm); see Chapter 9 for a quantitative description of joint topography and cartilage thickness variations over the knee joint surfaces. The cell density increases from human to goat to rabbit, with approximately the same cell size but fundamentally different structural organization of the tissue (115). In addition, the subchondral and medullary bone differ in density and structure, and load-bearing demand. The joint kinematics for various joints are also different, and there is no voluntary cooperation with immobilization and usage patterns (118). These multiple and complex differences make it nearly impossible to exactly mimic the human situation with an animal model of cartilage repair, and to scale down the dimensions of a human partial thickness lesion to a goat or a rabbit defect. If the same thickness of the defects is used, it corresponds to a partial thickness in a human and to a full thickness in an animal, a situation that is associated with major differences in environmental signals and cell recruiting for cartilaginous repair. Even if a partial thickness is studied in both models, the system geometry and transport distances are different. Additional factors that affect the repair are the lesion shape and volume, damage of the collagen mesh resulting from the creation of a lesion, and the age, activity, and biological response of the animal (118).

For bone tissue engineering, there have been a significant number of large and small animal models developed to test therapies for bone defects, non-unions, or fusions. Most investigators believe that a proposed therapy needs to be tested in both small and large animals, before pursuing clinical trials. There are a few principles to consider as a guide for preclinical studies of tissue-engineered bone repair. The *size, curvature of the surface*, and *location of the defect* or fracture created in the animal will dictate the type of healing that might take place (1). It is always possible to create a defect that is large enough that it will never heal, without intervention. These defects are called *critical size defects* and lead to fibrous non-unions. The animal model chosen should be evaluated with respect to its *ability to remodel bone*; the rate and degree of normal remodeling should be considered. The *loading environment* should be considered as an important part of the study design. For example, quadrupeds will subject their spines and their long bones to a different loading environment than humans. Similarly, animals in cages will have a lower demand then those that are allowed to run free on a farm.

The importance of the selection of animal species, age, defect design, and appropriate controls (age-, species-, and location-matched) cannot be overemphasized, and we still do not have universally accepted animal models for testing of engineered constructs. Although none of the existing animal models permits direct translation to human situation, many of them have yielded useful information and helped rationalize the design and interpretation of clinical studies.

2 REPRESENTATIVE STUDIES

An overview of representative studies of cartilage and bone tissue engineering that involved one or more of the following factors: utilization of physical forces to stimulate tissue development *in vitro*, utilization of scaffold chemistry or bioactive factors to stimulate tissue development *in vivo*, and functional evaluation of engineered constructs or the repair tissue (e.g., compressive, tensile or shear properties, integration with adjacent tissues) is given in Table 8-3.

2.1 Cartilage Engineered *In Vivo*

The only cell-based therapy for cartilage repair that has been Food and Drug Administration (FDA) approved for clinical use (Carticel™,

Genzyme, Cambridge, MA) involves harvesting and expansion of autologous articular chondrocytes from a minor load-bearing area, and reimplantation under a periosteal flap at the defect site (Fig. 8-1 (26)). The original study included 23 patients (14 to 48 years of age, full thickness cartilage defects 1.6 to 6.5 cm^2 in size). After 16 to 66 months after transplantation, 14 of the 16 patients with femoral condylar transplants and 2 of the 7 patients with patellar transplants had good-to-excellent clinical results. Biopsies showed hyaline cartilage in 11 of the 15 femoral transplants and 1 of the 7 patellar transplants. The clinical outcome of the 5-year follow-up has been good to excellent in 88% of cases of femoral implants and 29% of cases of patellar implants (26,212). More recently, the reported clinical outcome of the 2- to 10-year follow-up was good to excellent (84% to 90%) in patients with single condyle lesions, and less successful (average of 74%) for other types of lesions (28); the results of biopsies and indentation stiffness available for a limited number of patients correlated with the clinical outcome (205,206).

The original study report has been criticized for not being a prospectively controlled, randomized study, and for the lack of quantitative biochemical or mechanical data (169,183). Importantly, a 14-year follow-up of a similar patient group that underwent diagnostic arthroscopy in combination with one of several treatments (removal of loose bodies, shaving, Pride drilling) or no treatment had good-to-excellent knee function in 78% of patients (170). Further studies are thus needed to evaluate the function and durability of the new tissue, to determine if it prevents joint degeneration, to compare chondrocyte transplantation with alternative methods (including the use of periosteal transplants alone), and to test the utility of cell transplants in patients with osteoarthritis (30).

Long-term studies of this procedure in rabbits and dogs had limited success and showed degradation at the implant site (23,24,27,181). In adult rabbits, cultured autologous chondrocytes transplanted under a periosteal flap into partial or full thickness patellar defects formed cartilaginous repair tissue (27,90). In dogs, transplantation of cultured autologous chondrocytes

TABLE 8-3. REPRESENTATIVE EXAMPLES OF ORTHOPAEDIC TISSUE ENGINEERING

Cells and Tissues (Source, Preparation)	Scaffold (Material, Dimensions)	Regulatory Factors (Biochemical)	Regulatory Factors (Physical)	In Vitro Culture System (Duration)	In Vivo Host (Site, Defect Size)
A. Cartilage in vivo					
Articular chondrocytes (human, expanded 2–3 wk); periosteal flap	None	Autologous serum (15%) during cell expansion		Cell expansion (2–3 wk)	Human (14–48 yr) distal femur (n = 16), patella (n = 7) 1.6–6.5 cm^2, full thickness femoral condyle (n = 2)
Articular chondrocytes (rabbit, expanded 2 wk); periosteal flap	None or carbon fibers	10% FCS or NCS during cell expansion		Cell expansion (2 wk)	Rabbit (adult) patella, 3 mm dia, full thickness empty defects in young, adolescent and adult rabbits
Precursor cells from periosteum (rabbit, expanded 2–48 wk); periosteal grafts	None		CPM	Cell expansion (2–48 wk)	Rabbit (adult), several hundreds; free intra-articular CPM; free activity as control
Rib perichondrium and osteochondral plug	Bone plug covered with rib perichondrium 4 mm dia × 8 mm thick		CPM	None	Rabbit (adult), n = 100 medial femoral condyle 4 mm dia, full thickness CPM; free activity as control
Periosteal graft (rabbit)	Autologous bone or PMMA/HTR; 4 mm dia × 4 mm thick wrapped with periosteum	None	None	None	Rabbit (adult), n = 55 medial femoral condyle 4 mm dia × 4 mm thick empty defects as controls
Chondrocytes (1 mo old rabbit, primary or expanded 2 wk)	Collagen gel	10% FCS		Cell expansion (2 wk) or static culture in collagen (2 wk)	Rabbit (3–6 mo), n = 42+ 24 femoral condyle; patellar groove; 3 × 6 × 3 mm; 4 mm dia × 4 mm empty defects as controls
Precursor cells from bone marrow and periosteum (3–4 mo rabbit, expanded 2 wk)	Collagen gel	10% FCS during cell expansion		Cell expansion (2 wk)	Rabbit (3–4 mo), n = 68 distal femur; 3 × 6 × 3 mm cell-free collagen and empty defects as controls
Articular chondrocytes (adult dog, expanded 10–12 d) and periosteum	Type I or II collagen/GAG sponge (5 mm dia × 2 mm thick)	10% FCS during cell expansion and seeding		Cell expansion (10–12 d) scaffold seeding (12 h)	Dog (2–4 yr), n = 21 median and lateral femoral condyle 4 mm dia, full thickness; cell-seeded scaffolds under periosteal or type II collagen flap; unseeded scaffolds or periosteal flap alone; empty defects

Graft Type (Duration)	Assessment Methods	Result	Mechanical Properties; Integration; Geometry	References
Autograft, unilateral (16–66 mo)	Arthroscopy; clinical signs; H; IH indentation (qualitative)	Symptomatic relief (knee locking, pain, swelling) Femur repair better than patella. Zonal heterogeneity with hyaline-like cartilage in deep zone and fibrocartilage in the upper zone.	Knee: soft indentation and loose attachment at 3 mo; improved indentation stiffness, good attachment and visible borders at 12–46 mo Patella: intact articular surface in 1/7 cases at 19 mo	(26,27,169,212)
Autograft, bilateral (6 wk–1 yr)	H (semiquantitative) Mechanical properties (for empty defects)	Better repair in defects that received transplanted cells than in defects left empty. Poor integration with adjacent cartilage. No effect of carbon fibers.	At 12 wk in defects left empty, integration with adjacent cartilage and bone remodeling better for young animals; subnormal indentation stiffnesses (~one third of normal); no improvement over time.	(27,90,253)
Autograft, bilateral (2 wk–1 yr)	H (semiquantitative)	Regeneration of new hyaline cartilage integrated with the adjacent cartilage and subchondral bone. Endochondral ossification, in some cases extending into cartilage. CPM substantially enhanced cartilage regeneration.		(192,193,195)
Autograft, bilateral (6–52 wk)	H; mechanical properties (dynamic shear)	Hyaline cartilage repair; CPM group had better confluence and integration with adjacent cartilage, but contained cartilage layer devoid of PG; shear properties improved over time. CPM improved short-term but not long-term repair.	Dynamic shear moduli were initially higher for CPM group, increased over time and came into the range of values for articular cartilage at 52 wk; no long-term effect of CPM.	(133)
Autograft, bilateral (8 wk)	H; amounts of DNA, GAG and collagen; PG size; collagen typing; Mechanical properties (confined compression).	Cartilage and bone regeneration in 70% cases; lack of smooth articular surface and zonal distribution; inconsistent integration and mechanical properties.	Thickness, permeability and aggregate modulus of repair cartilage comparable to normal; incomplete integration with adjacent cartilage; fibrilated articular surface.	(173)
Autograft, bilateral (3 d to 48 wk)	H (semiquantitative); TEM thickness (needle penetration) compliance (microindentation)	Hyaline cartilage repair at 4–48 wk, but without zonal distribution, tidemark and bone remodeling; femoral groove morphology better than condyle. Normal compliance of repair cartilage after 12 wk.	Incomplete integration with adjacent cartilage. Irregular surface with major discontinuities. Compliance of repair cartilage in both groups comparable to normal cartilage after 12 wk.	(38,124,252)
Autograft, bilateral (2 to 24 wk)	H (semiquantitative) thickness (needle penetration) compliance (microindentation)	Hyaline cartilage (surface), new bone (deep); Repair with bone marrow and periosteum comparable, better than controls, but inferior to normal cartilage. Histological scores decreased with time	Incomplete integration with adjacent cartilage. Repair cartilage thinner than normal. At 24 wk, repair cartilage stiffer than controls but less stiff than adjacent cartilage.	(251)
Autograft, bilateral (15 wk; 6 months; 18 months)	H (semiquantitative)	Fibrocartilage repair prevailed in defects treated with cell-based grafts; some hyaline cartilage in untreated defects; incomplete integration. Suture damage; lack of regeneration in harvest sites. No bone remodeling.	Integration with subchondral plate fair (4–89%); integration with adjacent cartilage poor (16–32%). No difference between the groups.	(23,24,181)

(continued)

TABLE 8-3. (*continued*)

Cells and Tissues (Source, Preparation)	Scaffold (Material, Dimensions)	Regulatory Factors (Biochemical)	Regulatory Factors (Physical)	*In Vitro* Culture System (Duration)	*In Vivo* Host (Site, Defect Size)
Articular chondrocyte (adult bovine, expanded 3–4 wk)	Fibrin glue and PLGA (10 × 10 × 2 mm)	10% FCS during cell expansion		Cell expansion (3–4 wk)	Athymic (nude) mice, n = 33 subcutaneous pockets
Articular chondrocytes (2 wk old lambs)	Devitalized cartilage discs (5 mm dia × 1–1.5 mm thick) and chips; fibrin glue	10% FCS		Static culture of cells between two cartilage discs (3 wk),	Athymic (nude) mice, n = 74 subcutaneous pockets; cell-free cartilage discs, cells and cartilage chips in fibrin glue, cells in fibrin glue or fibrin alone
Perichondral chondrocyte (rabbit, expanded 3 wk)	(D,D,L,L) PLA 3.7 mm dia × 5 mm thick	10% FBS added to cell suspension		Cell adsorption onto scaffolds (2 hr)	Rabbit (9–12 mo) distal femur 3.7 mm dia, 5 mm deep
None (cell recruitment from subchondral plate)	Fibrous PGA 3 mm dia × 1–2 mm thick	10% HS during cell expansion			Rabbit (8 mo) distal femur, 3 mm dia, 1–2 mm deep right to subchondral plate empty defects as controls
None (cell recruitment from subchondral plate)	50/50 PLG sponge 7 mm dia × 7 mm thick	TGF•		None	Goat (adult), n = 46 medial femoral condyle 7 mm dia × 7 mm thick scaffold with or without absorbed TGF b empty defects
Articular chondrocyte (2–8 month old rabbits, expanded 10 d)	Fibrous PGA 10 mm dia × 2 mm thick	10% FCS during cell expansion		Static dish (2 or 4 wk)	Rabbit (8 mo) distal femur, 3 mm dia, full thickness PGA alone and empty defects as controls
Articular chondrocytes (expanded 8 d) and bone marrow (3 mo old rabbit)	Fibrous PGA 10 mm dia × 1 mm thick; Collagraft 7 × 5 × 4 mm	10% FBS during cell expansion and construct cultivation;	Convective mixing	Dynamic seeding onto PGA scaffolds (3 d); cultivation in orbitally mixed dishes (4–6 wk)	Rabbit (8 mo) femoropatellar grove: 7 × 5 × 5 mm; composites of engineered cartilage and Collagraft with or without bone marrow; PGA/Collagraft alone; empty defects

Graft Type (Duration)	Assessment Methods	Result	Mechanical Properties; Integration; Geometry	References
Allograft (6–12 wk)	H; mechanical properties (indentation)	Formation of cartilaginous matrix staining for PG and collagen; mechanical stiffness	At 12 wk, Young's modulus and failure load were approximately one third of normal.	(61)
Allograft (6–9 wk)	H; mechanical properties (adhesive strength of the interface for cell-disc constructs; equilibrium confined-compression modulus for all other constructs)	New cartilage formed only in grafts containing cells. New cartilaginous matrix provided a bond between two pieces of devitalized cartilage.	Adhesive and tensile properties of the cell-disc interface at 6 wks ~5–10% of normal. At 9 wks, equilibrium modulus of cell-based composites ~5–10% of normal.	(200,201)
Allograft (6 wk–12 mo)	H; amounts of GAG and collagen; IH (collagen types I, II); Mechanical properties (confined compression)	Cell alignment determined by scaffold geometry. Hyaline cartilage; collagen initially (6 wk) type I, later (52 wk) type II; GAG GAG subnormal; collagen content not reported. Biomechanics comparable to normal cartilage.	Confined-compression modulus and hydraulic permeability comparable to unoperated controls >12 wk. None of the specimens appeared normal at 1 yr; absence of subchondral bone restoration and surface fibrilation in some specimens; degradation of the repair tissue over time.	(115,196)
Autograft, bilateral (4 to 24 wk)	H (semiquantitative) Mechanical properties (indentation)	Fairly good repair in grafted defects at 24 wk; smooth articular surface, good integration. Surface fibrilation and degenerated matrix in controls.	Aggregate modulus and permeability of the repair tissue between controls and normal cartilage at 24 wk but the differences were NSD.	(94)
Unilateral (16 wk)	H (semiquantitative) Mechanical properties (indentation)	Incomplete repair in all groups at 16 wk, with defects partly and with fibrocartilage; poor integration; subnormal mechanical properties; TGF• improved tissue morphology (surface regularity, regularity, integration) and mechanical properties.	Discontinuities in the repair cartilage and bone. Surface integrity and bonding with adjacent tissues improved with TGF•. Mechanical properties (aggregate modulus, shear modulus, Poisson's ratio, permeability) subnormal but improved with TFG• treatment.	(11)
Allograft, bilateral (1 mo–2 yr)	H (semiquantitative) amounts of DNA, PG and total collagen;	Repair tissue a mixture of hyaline and fibrocartilage; cell-based grafts better than controls; immature constructs better than mature; Incomplete lateral integration and bone remodeling even after 2 yr.	Lack of integration for mature (4-wk) constructs; improved bone remodeling and lateral integration for immature (2-wk) constructs.	(70,94,233)
Allograft chondrocytes; autograft precursors; bilateral (6 wk–6 mo)	H (semiquantitative); morphometry; amounts of PG and total collagen; collagen typing; Mechanical properties (indentation)	Hyaline cartilage repair with characteristic architectural features and zonal distribution, tidemark and bone remodeling in grafts based on engineered cartilage. Good integration with bone, incomplete integration with adjacent cartilage; mechanical functionality.	Smooth and well developed cartilaginous surface, with tidemark and new subchondral bone; Mechanical properties developed over time. At 6 mo, Young's moduli were physiological in all groups except in defects left empty.	(230)

(continued)

TABLE 8-3. (*continued*)

Cells and Tissues (Source, Preparation)	Scaffold (Material, Dimensions)	Regulatory Factors (Biochemical)	Regulatory Factors (Physical)	*In Vitro* Culture System (Duration)	*In Vivo* Host (Site, Defect Size)
B. Cartilage *In Vitro*					
Articular chondrocyte (rabbit, 1–2 mo old)	None	15% FBS IL-1b		Static dish (4–10 wk)	
Articular chondrocyte (bovine, 3–2 wk old, expanded 4–6 d)	Agarose gel 16 mm dia × 1 mm thick	10% FBS	Mechanical compression (static and dynamic)	Static dish (7 wk); exposure to static or dynamic compression (once during culture); (static compression: 16 h, up to 50% strain) (dynamic compression: 10 h, static offset; 3% dynamic strain amplitude; 0.01–1 Hz)	
Articular chondrocyte (bovine, 18 mo old)	Agarose gel 5 mm dia × 5 mm thick	20% FBS	Mechanical compression (static or dynamic) (unconfined)	16 h of free swelling culture, followed by 48 h of static or dynamic unconfined compression strain: 15%; frequency: 0.3, 1, and 3 Hz	
Mesenchymal limb bud cells and chondrocytes (embryonic chick)	Agarose gel 11 mm dia × 2 mm thick; collagen sponge 20 mm × 20 mm × 2.5 mm	2% FBS	Mechanical compression (static or dynamic) (unconfined) dynamic stretch	Dishes with static compression (4.5 kPa for 2 h, once a day for 3 days) or dynamic compression (0.25–9 kPa; 0.03–0.33 Hz for 12 min–2 h, once a day for 3 days); both regimes were followed with 5 days of free-swelling culture. Dynamic stretch (5% elongation, 1 Hz, 15 min/h)	
Articular chondrocyte (bovine, 3–5 mo old)	Agarose gel 6.76 mm dia × 1.7 mm thick 4.76 mm × 1.6 mm thick	10% FBS	Mechanical compression (dynamic; unconfined; impermeable platens) free-swelling controls	Multiwell dishes (n = 16) (3 cycles per day; 1 h on 1 h off; 2% static offset; 5% strain amplitude; 1 Hz) (free swelling as control); 4 weeks of culture	
Articular chondrocyte	Agarose gel 4.76 mm × 1.6 mm thick	10% FBS plus 10 ng/mL TGF-β, or 300 ng/mL IGF-I	Mechanical compression (dynamic; unconfined; impermeable platens); free-swelling controls	60 mm dishes, 20–25 constructs per dish (3 cycles per day; 1 h on 1 h off; 2% static offset; 5% strain amplitude; 1 Hz) (free swelling as control); 5 weeks of culture	

Graft Type (Duration)	Assessment Methods	Result	Mechanical Properties; Integration; Geometry	References
	H; TEM; thickness; amounts of DNA, PG and collagen; synthesis rates; PG properties; collagen types; mechanical properties (in tension)	30–100 μm thick cartilaginous matrix containing subnormal amounts of PG and type II collagen; tensile properties; IL-1b reduced thickness and PG fraction and increased collagen fraction.	Tensile stiffness and modulus improved over time and with an increase in collagen fraction, and reached 1.3 Mpa after 8 wk of culture (physiological range: 0.9–27 MPa).	(68)
	H; SEM; GAG and DNA content Biosynthesis of PG and collagen (incorporation of ^{35}S and ^{3}H) Mechanical properties (confined compression)	Static compression decreased, dynamic compression increased biosynthesis, by amounts that increased with time in culture and strain amplitude. ECM structure and function developed over time;	Over 5–7 weeks of static (nonstimulated) culture, equilibrium modulus increased to 60–80 kPa; hydraulic permeability decreased to ~200% normal; streaming potential increased to ~20% of normal.	(34,35)
	Biosynthesis of DNA, glycosaminoglycan and protein	Compression at 0.3 or 3 Hz inhibited and at 1 Hz stimulated biosynthesis of GAG; stimulation of DNA synthesis; no stimulation of protein synthesis.		(141)
	Number of cartilage nodules; GAG synthesis; immunohistochemistry (typ[e II collagen); cell proliferation; expression of a variety of markers of chondrogenesis	Compressive loading doubled the number of cartilage nodules and enhanced sulfate incorporation (day 8). The effect depended on the frequency and duration of compressive loading (max for 0.33 Hz and 54 min). Dynamic stretch did not affect the rate but rather the extent of differentiation.		(66,67,260)
	GAG and collagen content Mechanical properties (confined and unconfined compression stress relaxation testing)	After 3–4 weeks, construct compositions and mechanical properties were better for dynamically stimulated constructs and for constructs seeded at a higher cell density (60 million cells per cm^3 as compared to 20 million cells per cm^3); effects of compression were higher at the lower cell density	After 4 weeks, constructs contained up to 2% wet weight GAG, <2% wet weight collagen and had an aggregate modulus of up to 75–100 kPa and a Young's modulus of up to 60 kPa	(163,164)
	GAG and collagen content Mechanical properties (confined compression stress relaxation testing) H; IH	Medium supplementation with either TGF-β or IGF-I improved the GAG and collagen contents and equilibrium moduli of both loaded and free-swelling constructs; a growth factor and mechanical loading had synergetic effects on construct properties	After 5 weeks, GAG fractions (% ww) were 0.5 (free-swelling), 1–1.2 (free-swelling + growth factor), 1 (loading), and 1.5 (loading + growth factor). Collagen contents (% ww) were 0.16, 0.6–1, 1 and 0.8–1, respectively. Equilibrium modulus (kPa) was 13, 20–24, 24, and 46–50, respectively.	(165)

(continued)

TABLE 8-3. (*continued*)

Cells and Tissues (Source, Preparation)	Scaffold (Material, Dimensions)	Regulatory Factors (Biochemical)	Regulatory Factors (Physical)	*In Vitro* Culture System (Duration)	*In Vivo* Host (Site, Defect Size)
Articular chondrocyte (bovine, 2–4 wk old)	fibrous PGA and PLGA; porous PLLA 10 mm × (5–10)mm × (2–3) mm fibrous PGA (10 mm dia × (1–5)mm thick)	10% FBS during cell expansion and construct cultivation	Convective mixing	Static and mixed dishes (2–12 wk); perfused bag (5 wk); perfused cartridges (4 wk); perfused chambers (2 wk)	
Articular chondrocyte (bovine, 2–4 wk old); cartilage explants (bovine, 2–4 wk old)	Fibrous PGA 5 mm dia × 2 mm thick	10% FBS during cultivation (constructs and explants)	Convective mixing; osmotic pressure	Mixed dishes (9 ± 1 wk)	
Articular chondrocyte (equine; young and adult)	Fibrous PGA 10 mm × 10 mm × 1 mm	10% FBS	Intermittent pressure; (3.4 or 6.9 MPa; 5 s on, 30 s off); flow	Compression chamber (5 wk); pre-culture in mixed flasks (0 or 1 wk)	
Articular chondrocyte (bovine, 2–4 wk old); human (30–65 yr old); rabbit	PLGA-coated fibrous PGA 12.7 mm dia × 1 mm thick; porous collagen (2 mm thick), PLGA or polydioxanon mesh embedded in agarose	10% FBS 2% FCS	Medium perfusion (interstitial velocity: 0.1–10 μm/s) medium perfusion (around constructs)	Perfused bioreactor (4 wk)	
Articular chondrocyte (bovine, 2–4 wk old)	Fibrous PGA 10 mm dia × 2 mm thick	10% FBS	mechanical compression (static and dynamic); (confined)	Free swelling culture in well plates (3 wk); static or dynamic confined compression between porous plates (24 h) (static offset: 0, 1, 300 or 50%; dynamic strain: 5%; frequency 0.001 or 0.1 Hz)	
Articular chondrocyte (bovine, 2–4 wk old)	Fibrous PGA 5 mm dia × 2 mm thick	10% FBS during construct cultivation		Rotating vessel (3 d–7 mo); seeding in mixed flasks (3 d)	

Graft Type (Duration)	Assessment Methods	Result	Mechanical Properties; Integration; Geometry	References
	H; IH (type II collagen) GAG, DNA, collagen, undegraded PGA incorporation of ^{35}S and ^{3}H Mechanical properties (confined compression; shear)	1–3.5 mm thick cartilaginous constructs. Scaffold and culture system affected biosynthesis. High initial cellularity, mixing and flow improved construct structures.	Over 12 wks of culture, aggregate modulus of cell-PGA constructs increased 40-fold to ~10% of normal; hydraulic permeability decreased four orders of magnitude to the range of values measured for native cartilage.	(72,73,92,148, 239)
	GAG, DNA and total collagen; collagen cross links; denaturation; Mechanical properties (confined compression; osmotic swelling)	Constructs and explants contained 50% and 65% of normal GAG, and 34% and 68% of normal collagen, respectively. Collagen fiber stiffness decreased from cartilage to constructs. Mechanical behavior in osmotic swelling and confined compression was consistent with the model of prestressed collagen network balanced by the swelling pressure of PGs.	In osmotic swelling, the strains increased from cartilage to explants and constructs; axial strain was twice as high as radial strain. The aggregate, lateral and shear moduli decreased from cartilage to explants and constructs; decreased with an increase in saline bath concentration; correlated with the compositions of tissue specimens.	(33)
	SEM; TEM; GAG and total collagen compressive stiffness (unconfined)	Cyclical loading promoted the production of GAG and collagen and increased compressive stiffness in constructs in a dose dependent manner. Constructs based on young cells better.	Compression moduli were 60–100 kPa for dynamically loaded constructs. Intermittent pressurization was more effective at 6.9 than at 3.4 MPa. Preculture in flasks enhanced the effects of intermittent pressure. Pressurized constructs had higher fractions of glycosaminoglycan and higher compressive moduli.	(42,104,105)
	H; IH (type II collagen) GAG, DNA and total collagen	Interstitial velocity of 1 μm/s increased the amounts of DNA, GAG and collagen after 4 weeks of culture 2-, 3- and 2.5-fold compared to static culture. Medium perfusion improved construct compositions.		(62,197,236)
	Incorporation/release of PG and protein; DNA content	Static compression inhibited biosynthesis; dynamic compression enhanced the synthesis of PG and protein by amounts that increased with static offset and compression frequency; no effect on the fraction of PG or collagen		(58)
	H; TEM; IH (collagen types II, IX) amounts of DNA, GAG, and collagen Incorporation of ^{35}S and ^{3}H. Mechanical properties (confined compression)	Development of 3–8 mm thick functional constructs. Biosynthesis rates intially high, decreased with time. Structure and function improved with time in culture. After 6 wk, ECM containing GAG (75% of normal) and type II collagen (40% of normal). After 7 months, normal PG content and compressive stiffness.	Over the period of 6 wks to 7 mo, the equilibrium modulus increased from ~0.2 MPa to 0.9 MPa; dynamic stiffness increased from ~3 to ~8 Mpa; permeability decreased from ~10 to ~5(10^{-15}m^4/Ns); streaming potential was ~0.08 mV/% at both time points.	(74,75,159)

(continued)

TABLE 8-3. (*continued*)

Cells and Tissues (Source, Preparation)	Scaffold (Material, Dimensions)	Regulatory Factors (Biochemical)	Regulatory Factors (Physical)	*In Vitro* Culture System (Duration)	*In Vivo* Host (Site, Defect Size)
Articular chondrocyte (bovine, 2–4 wk old)	Fibrous PGA 5 mm dia × 2 mm thick	10% FBS	Flow and mixing	Static and mixed flasks; rotating versel (6 wk)	
Articular chondrocyte (bovine, 2–4 wk old)	Fibrous PGA 5 mm dia × 2 mm thick	10% FBS oxygen; pH	Flow and mixing	Rotating vessel (5 wk) at oxygen tensions of 40 and 80 mm Hg, and various regimes of medium exchange	
Articular chondrocyte (bovine, 2–4 wk old)	Fibrous PGA 5 mm dia × 2 mm thick	10% FBS; IGF-I	Flow and mixing	Static and mixed dishes; static and mixed flasks; rotating vessel (4 wk)	
Articular chondrocyte (bovine, 2–4 wk old) transfected with human IGF-I, lacZ and nontransfected.	Fibrous PGA 5 mm dia × 2 mm thick	None	Flow and mixing	Rotating vessel (4 wk)	
Articular chondrocyte (bovine, 2–4 wk old)	Fibrous PGA 5 mm dia × 2 mm thick	10% FBS and either TGF-β + FGF-2 (days 3–10) or FGF-2 (days 1–28), or IGF-I (days 10–28)	Flow and mixing	Rotating vessel (4 wk)	
Articular chondrocyte	PGA (fibrous mesh; composite) Hyaff-11 (benzylated HA, porous sponge; fibrous mesh) 5 mm dia × 2 mm thick	10% FBS	Flow and mixing	Rotating vessel	

Graft Type (Duration)	Assessment Methods	Result	Mechanical Properties; Integration; Geometry	References
	SEM; H; amounts of DNA, GAG and total collagen; collagen typing (II, IX and X); collagen pyridinium crosslinks. Mechanical properties (confined compression)	Development of mechanically functional 5 mm thick cartilaginous matrix over 6 wks of culture. Mixed cultures better than static; laminar flow better than turbulent. Construct properties improved with time. GAG 80% of normal, acollagen 43% of normal. Structure of collagen normal; crosslinking subnormal. Construct properties odulated by flow and mixing. Mechanical parameters correlated with compositions.	Construct structure, electro/mechanical function depended on the conditions of *in vitro* cultivation. The equilibrium modulus, dynamic stiffness, hydraulic permeability and streaming potential correlated with the wet weight fractions of water, PG and total collagen. Best constructs had an equilibrium modulus of 175 kPa (articular surface: 270 kPa, apparent value: 470 kPa; deep zone: 710–949 kPa)	(159,213,248, 246)
	DNA, GAG and total collagen; biosynthesis and incorporation of GAG and protein; metabolic parameters. GAG distribution	Oxygen tension of 80 mm Hg and pH = 7 enhanced incorporation of GAG and collagen, and yieldfed markedly better construct structures. Mathematical model rationalized the effects of oxygen on chondrogenesis in engineered constructs.		(186,188)
	DNA, GAG and total collagen. Mechanical properties (confined compression)	Development of mechanically functional constructs. The mechanical environment and IGF-I interactively modulated tissue growth and mechanical properties. PG and collagen contents and equilibrium modulus up to 50% of normal.	IGF-I resulted in larger cartilaginous contructs. Equilibrium modulus ranged from 20 to 450 kPa and correlated with wet weight fraction of PG.	(87)
	DNA, GAG and total collagen; expression of IGF-I *in vitro* and *in vivo;* IH (chondrogenesis markers); mechanical properties (confined compression)	Transgene expression maintained *in vitro* and *in vivo;* At 4 weeks, IGF-I constructs contained 1.5–1.9-fold more DNA, 8–11.1-fold more GAG, and 2–2.4-fold more collagen than either control.	Overexpression of IGF-I resulted in 4-fold higher confined-compression equilibrium moduli (126 and 30–35 kPa for the IGF-I and control constructs, respectively).	(151)
	DNA, GAG and total collagen; H, IH and mRNA (collagens I and II); Mechanical properties (confined compression)	Sequential application of TGF-β/FGF-2 followed by IGF-I resulted in large cartilaginous constructs with high fractions of GAG and type II collagen and high compressive moduli; supplementation of FGF-2 suppressed chondrogenesis	After 4 weeks, GAG and collagen fractions were up to 3.5% ww each; Equilibrium moduli were up tp 400 kPa. i.e., comparable to those measured for native bovine cartilage.	(198)
	DNA, GAG and total collagen; H Mechanical properties (confined compression)	The hydrodynamic environment and the scaffold material and structure interactively modulated tissue growth and mechanical properties. Bioreactor hydrodynamics had the greatest effect on construct properties; scaffold structure was more important than scaffold composition.	After 4 weeks, the fractions of GAG and collagen were up to 4.4% ww and 3.6% ww, respectively. Equilbrium moduli were up to 540 kPa, i.e., comparable to those measured for native bovine cartilage.	(199)

(continued)

TABLE 8-3. (*continued*)

Cells and Tissues (Source, Preparation)	Scaffold (Material, Dimensions)	Regulatory Factors (Biochemical)	Regulatory Factors (Physical)	*In Vitro* Culture System (Duration)	*In Vivo* Host (Site, Defect Size)
Articular chondrocyte (bovine, 2–4 wk old); Cartilage explants (bovine, 2–4 wk old)	Constructs: fibrous PGA 5 mm dia × 2 mm thick Explants: 10/5 mm dia × 2 mm thick rings (intact or trypsin treated)	10% FBS during cultivation (constructs; composites); trypsin (to remove PG from explants)	Flow and mixing	Constructs: seeding in mixed flasks (3 d); cultivation in rotating vessels (5 d; 5 wk) Explants: intact or trypsin treated Construct/explant and explant/explant composites: rotating vessels (1–8 wk)	
Articular chondrocyte (bovine, 2–4 wk old; adult)	Explant pairs (9 mm × 5 mm × 0.5 mm each, with a 4 mm × 5 mm overlap)	None; 0.1% bovine serum albumin; 20% FBS	Static compression (0.06–0.4 Mpa, 24 h, at days 1 and 4)	Chondrocytes were seeded at the interface between two cartilage blocks and cultured for 3 wk, without or with static compression.	
C. Bone *in vivo*					
Human bone marrow stromal cells; 21–72 yr average age: 42 yr	None	None	Internal fixation device	No expansion or manipulation of cells prior to implantation	Human tibial non-union (no bone formation for three months with standard treatment)
None	PLA (50–100 mg strips; 100 mg capsules)	hBMP purified from human allograft bone (contains BMPs)	Fixation plates and nails	N/A	Human tibial non-unions approximately 2 × 1 × 1.5 cm 4 patients (29–35 yrs old), all with established non-unions for longer than 14 months.
None	Demineralized bone matrix 125 μg (rabbit)	rhop-1 in doses 3.13 to 400 μg	None	N/A	5 cm defect in ulna of adult (4–5 kg) rabbits; control implants were collagen scaffold alone (8 weeks)
None	OPLA (12 × 6 × 30 mm strips)	rhBMP-2	None	N/A	Canine spine fusion L4-L5 mature dogs; controls were polymer carrier alone or iliac crest autograft (positive control for 3 months; one group for 8 months)
None	Type I collagen and hydroxyapatite 7.5 mm diameter pellet	rhBMP-2	None	N/A	Pellets implanted into lower calf muscle pouch in 10 week old male rats. Evaluated at 3 weeks post-operatively
Human autogenous bone marrow	Composite of collagen type I and calcium phosphate	None	Internal or external fixator	no expansion or manipulation of cells prior to implantation/mixing	Long bone fractures in 303 human patients (352 fractures that required bone grafts randomized into autograft or implant groups.

Graft Type (Duration)	Assessment Methods	Result	Mechanical Properties; Integration; Geometry	References
	H (semiquantitative) amounts of DNA, PG and collagen. Mechanical properties (confined compression for constructs; adhesive strength at the interface of construct/explant composites)	Immature constructs integrated by progressive formation of cartilaginous tissue bond; mature constructs and native cartilage formed weaker bonds by secreting matrix components. Trypsin treatment enhanced integration.	The adhesive strengths of the integration interface were 80–160 kPa for mature (5 wk) constructs and explants and 250–380 kPa for immature constructs. Best integration for immature constructs and trypsin-treated cartilage.	(189)
	H; amounts of DNA and GAG; adhesive strength of the interface (uniaxial positive displacement applied at a constant rate to failure) Biosynthesis rates of GAG and protein.	Integration enhanced by the presence of viable cells and serum components. Most PG was lost into medium. Static compression inhibited proliferation. Adhesive strength correlated with collagen deposition.	Adhesive strength was up to 30 kPa after 3 weeks of culture.	(45,60,211)
Autograft	Radiographs	Good healing (90% of patients) based on radiographic and clinical examination	Radiographic evidence of incorporation in 9/10 cases based on mineralized callus bridging the fracture site	(123)
Allograft source of BMP	Radiographs	Good healing based on radiographic observation (bridging callus) and good patient function	Integration appeared good based on radiographic evidence of bone continuity across entire non-union site	(119)
Allograft source of matrix	Radiographs, histology, mechanical testing (torsion)	All healed radiographically except low dose (3.13 μg). Good torsional strength (47 to 155% of control). Normal histology, some increase in woven bone; larger callus and delay in complete remodeling	95% torsional strength of contralateral control at 8 weeks post implantation surgery	(56)
N/A	Computed tomography. Manual manipulation (to judge if stable by applied load) Radiographic mechanical testing Histology	Significant bone formation with OPLA/BMP. Greater mechanical integrity than autograft controls as evaluated by materials testing in non-destructive flexion-extension, bending and rotational loading	Exuberant bone formation and solid fusions induced	(226)
N/A	Radiographs; histology	Dose dependent (2, 10, 50 μg rhBMP-2). De novo bone formation	N/A	(132)
N/A	Radiographs; clinical assessment	95% Healing at 3 months based on radiographic evidence of callus healing by radiologist and surgeon	Excellent incorporation with 100% healing at 2 years	(43)

(continued)

TABLE 8-3. (*continued*)

Cells and Tissues (Source, Preparation)	Scaffold (Material, Dimensions)	Regulatory Factors (Biochemical)	Regulatory Factors (Physical)	In Vitro Culture System (Duration)	In Vivo Host (Site, Defect Size)
None	Poly[D1L1-(lactide-co-glycolide)]	rhBMP-2 and autogenous blood	Plate-screw fixation	N/A	2.5 cm mid diaphyseal femoral defect sheep (2 weeks–1 year); controls were polymer carrier and blood alone
W-20 murine stromal cell line	Demineralized rat bone matrix	BMP-2	Plate fixation in bone defects	W-20 cells infected for 4 hours with Ad-BMP-2 and cultured for an additional 12–14 hours	Intramuscular implant in SCID mice (2 wk) Nude rats bilateral femoral segmented defect (8 mm) (2 months) controls were carrier alone and carrier with cells transfected with LacZ
None	Viscose cellulose sponge	None	None	N/A	2.1 mm diameter defect Rat femoral diaphysis (1–6 weeks)
None	Type I collagen sponge (bovine collagen, lyophilized)	hPTH 1-34 DNA (plasmid)	Plate and screws in diaphyseal model	N/A	Canine 1–2.0 cm defects in mid tibial diaphysis (2–53 Weeks)
Bone marrow cells (rat, goat and human)	Porous calcium phosphate particles or calcium phosphate coated metallic plates	DEX and BMP-2 in culture	None	Cell expansion in monolayers. Second passage cells were seeded on particles or plates and cultured for 1 week.	Implanted in nude mice subcutaneously
None	Hydroxyapatite granules (300–600 um diameters) and combination with phospholipid-diacetyl-glycerol or sodium hyaluronan	None	None	N/A	4 mm diameter defects in bilateral tibias Rabbit (6 weeks)
None	None	Ad-BMP-2	Plate and wire fixation	N/A	1.3 cm segmental defect in femur Rabbit (7–12 weeks) Injected into defect (2 × 1010 particles of adenoviruses)
Calvaria osteoblasts (rat)	Hydrogels: PAG plus adipic acid (200 ul injected)	None	None	Rat calvarium cells were isolated and placed immediately in solution with the matrix and shaken for 20 min	Subcutaneous injection into SCID mice (9 weeks)

D. Bone *In Vitro*

Ros 17/2.8, osteoblast-like cells (rat)	Bioactive glass Synthetic hydroxyapatite	Fibronectin coating	None	Cells grown to confluence in flasks/dishes Attachment studies after 30 min. following cell seeding on biomaterials	N/A

Graft Type (Duration)	Assessment Methods	Result	Mechanical Properties; Integration; Geometry	References
N/A	Radiographs; histology	3/5 and 2/3 healed with BMP none healed in control based on radiographic assessment for bridging callus	N/A	(127)
Allograft matrix in rat studies	Radiographs; histology	Cell mediated gene therapy promotion of bone formation	Radiographic evidence of bone integration. Cortices appear thin	(144)
N/A	Histology	Bone formed by 3 weeks	Bone grew throughout sponge	(161)
N/A	Radiographs; histology	Successful *in-vivo* gene transfection from matrix containing plasmid DNA. Bone formed in defects	Radiographic and histologic evidence of bone integration in defect. Both endochondral and membranous bone formation.	(17)
N/A	Light and scanning electron microscopy	Bone spicules formed in all grafts. DEX and BMP treated cells induced bone earlier. Bone formed on both plates and around particles.	N/A	(59)
N/A	Histology X ray microfocus X-ray analysis	HA/PC composite handled well. Promoted (31%) bone fill; HA/phospholipid and HA/Hyaluronan formed 47–49% bone.	Good integration of bone. Carriers induce different robustness of response based on microradiographic and histologic evidence of bone formation in defect and healing across the defect	(145)
N/A	Radiographs; histology Biomechanical testing by 3 point bending to failure	All defects filled with bone by 7 weeks. Significant mechanical integrity by 12 weeks based on a significant increase in mechanical strength compared to controls.	Good integration. Large callus providing good mechanical integrity.	(12)
N/A	Histology	Bone formed in PAG/AAD matrix with osteoblasts Significant mineral formation	N/A	(142)
N/A	Adherence measures	Adherence mediated by RGD sequence Fibronectin density increase Increased adhesion Bioactive glasses more adherence	N/A	(83)

(continued)

TABLE 8-3. (*continued*)

Cells and Tissues (Source, Preparation)	Scaffold (Material, Dimensions)	Regulatory Factors (Biochemical)	Regulatory Factors (Physical)	*In Vitro* Culture System (Duration)	*In Vivo* Host (Site, Defect Size)
Bone marrow, stromal cells (rabbit)	Poly(caprolactone) PGLA HA	None	None	Cultured in flasks, confluence in 10–14 days Biomaterials incubated with cells for 2–8 weeks	N/A
Bone marrow cells (rat)	PGLA (5 mm × 7 mm × 7 mm)	None	None	Cells were expanded for 6 days seeded on scaffolds and cultured for 3–6 weeks.	N/A
Human osteoblasts	Bioglass 45S5 15 mm dia. By 3 mm. disks	None	None	Cells seeded on scaffolds (2–12 days) controls were bioinert plastic plates	N/A
MC3T3-E1 osteoblasts mouse	PLLA PLLA/HAP Composite foams (10 mm disks 1.5 mm thick)	None	Cultured in shaker with constructs in dishes	After 3 & 4 passages in monolayers cells were seeded on discs for 48 hours and cultured in orbital dishes (75 rpm). (6 weeks)	N/A
SaOs-2 cell line (human) (human)	PGLA (hollow spherical structures) Microcarriers (4 mm diameter × 2.5 mm long)	None	Rotating bioreactor	Cultured in rotating bioreactor at 25 rpm 2–7 days	N/A

AAD	adipic acid	PGA	polyglycolic acid
Ad	adenovirus	NCS	newborn calf serum
BMP	bone morphogenic protein	OPLA	open cell polylactic acid polymer
BMSC	bone marrow stromal cells	PAG	poly (aldehyde glucuronate)
CS	chondroitin sulfate	PLGA	polylactic-co-glycolic acid
DEX	dexamethasone	PLLA	poly (L) lactic acid
ECM	extracellular matrix	PTH	parathyroid hormone
GAG	glycosaminoglycan	r	recombinant
h	human	rhop-1	recombinant human osteogenic protein-1
H	histology	SEM	scanning electron microscopy
HA	hyaluronic acid	TEM	transmission electron microscopy
HAP	hydroxyapatite	*	review article
IH	immunohistochemistry	d	day
KS	keratan sulfate	wk	week
PG	proteoglycan	mo	month

Graft Type (Duration)	Assessment Methods	Result	Mechanical Properties; Integration; Geometry	References
N/A	Electron microscopy Histology	Polymer/ceramic composites supported bone cell growth as evidenced from observation of cells on surface that stained for collagen synthesis	N/A	(155)
N/A	Histology; Immunohistochemistry Fluorescent imaging osteocalcin, mineral (von Kossa), tetracycline labeling for bone formation	At optimal cell seeding density, bone formation throughout 3D structure 1×10^6 and 6×10^6 demonstrated complete formation while 0.5×10^6 did not	N/A	(112)
N/A	X ray analysis SEM Immunohistochemistry (collagen I, alkaline phosphatase, trap); TEM Biochemistry Flow Cytometry	Bioglass substantially supports proliferation and differentiation of osteoblastic cells	N/A	(261)
N/A	Histology DNA analysis Northern blot	PLLA/HAP induced increased bone cell number and bone tissue throughout 3D structure from histologic sampling	N/A	(148)
N/A	Immunohistochemistry Cell counting Scanning electron microscopy	Maintenance of osteoblast phenotype and increase in bone marker expression based on morphology and stain for mineralization	N/A	(20)

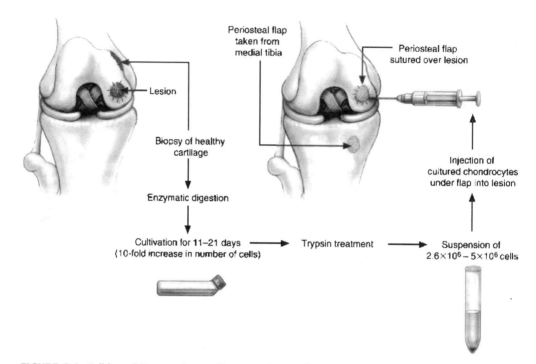

FIGURE 8-1. Cell-based therapy for cartilage repair. Autologous chondrocytes are obtained from an uninvolved area of the injured knee, isolated and cultured for 14 to 21 days, injected into the area of the defect and covered with a sutured periosteal flap taken from the proximal medial tibia (26). The therapy has had good clinical outcome (2- to 10-year follow up (28,206)). Further studies are needed to establish the scientific basis of chondrocyte transplants, collect quantitative data for the structural and mechanical properties of the new tissue, and test its utility in patients with osteoarthritis. Cell-based therapy for cartilage repair has been approved in 1996 by the FDA (Carticel®, Genzyme, Cambridge MA) and has been extensively used in the United States and Europe. (From Brittberg M, Lindahl A, Nilsson A, et al. Treatment of deep cartilage defects in the knee with autologous chondrocyte transplantation. *N Engl J Med* 1994;331:889–895, with permission.)

under periosteal flaps into femoral defects resulted in the initial formation of repair tissue (at 1.5 months) and remodeling (at 3 and 6 months), followed by degradation into fibrocartilage (at 12 and 18 months). Neither periosteum nor transplanted chondrocytes enhanced healing after 1 year, possibly due to the low cell retention and failure of immature repair tissue to withstand physiological loading (23,24,181). Implantation of allogeneic foal chondrocytes in fibrin glue into full-thickness cartilage defects in horses for 8 months resulted in the formation of cartilaginous tissue containing GAGS and type II collagen (106). Interestingly, mechanical properties of the repair tissue have not been assessed in any of these studies. An important related study of cartilage repair in untreated defects in rabbit knees (253) demonstrated that healing was morphologically better in skeletally immature than mature animals, but the mechanical quality of the regenerated tissue (assessed by indentation) remained subnormal in both groups. It has long been known that histomorphology is not necessarily indicative of biomechanical properties, and the biomechanical properties thus need to be used as the basis for evaluation of cartilage repair (8,9).

Periosteum alone transplanted into osteochondral defects in rabbit knees restored articular surface and subchondral bone (192,193). The repair depended on the orientation of the cambium layer of the tissue and the age of donor (immature animals healed better), and was enhanced by the postoperative continuous passive motion (CPM) (193). In patients with severe osteochondral defects, CPM resulted in symptomatic relief in only about 60% of cases (195), presumably due to the dynamic fluctuations of the fluid pressure (0.6 to 10 kPa in rabbit knees) (191). Repair of full thickness defects of condyles in mature rabbits using rib perichondrium, with or without CPM (133), resulted in repair tissues that were confluent with adjacent cartilage and had normal histological appearances and dynamic shear moduli. After 1 year *in vivo* postimplantation, CPM enhanced the initial tissue repair (at 6 weeks) but had no effects on long-term repair. In another study, repair tissue based on periosteum wrapped around a polymer scaffold was implanted in full thickness defects of condyles in mature rabbits, with or without CPM, and evaluated histologically, biochemically, and biomechanically (indentation) 8 weeks after surgery (173). The repair tissue had normal histological appearance and composition, but it was twice as thick as normal tissue, lacked the zonal organization characteristic of normal cartilage, had subnormal mechanical properties, and did not completely integrate with the adjacent tissues.

Caplan and co-workers pioneered the use of autologous mesenchymal stem cells in the repair of osteochondral defects (38). Progenitor cells were derived from bone marrow or periosteum, expanded in monolayers and delivered in collagen gels into full thickness defects (up to 3 mm × 6 mm × 3 mm) that were in some cases pretreated with proteolytic enzymes. Progenitor cells regenerated cartilaginous surface zone while tissue at the base of the defect hypertrophied, calcified, and was replaced by host-derived vasculature, marrow, and bone. In contrast, allografted chondrocytes in collagen gel or matrix rapidly formed plugs of hyaline cartilage that filled the entire defects but failed to develop subchondral bone or to integrate with the surrounding host tissue (124,252), and the compressive stiffness and permeability remained subnormal after 6 months *in vivo* (78). When allogeneic chondrocytes and bone marrow-derived osteoprogenitor cells were used in a hyaluronic acid gel to repair tibial defects in goats, autografts were better than allografts, but the repair tissue in both groups was different than adjacent articular cartilage (36). If the formation of subchondral

bone is delayed in allograft chondrocyte transplantation as suggested by these studies, this could have implications on the prescribed regime of postoperative weight-bearing function. Moreover, the mismatch between the thin layer of host cartilage and thick plug of the repair tissue and subnormal compliance of the regenerated tissue could contribute to implant failure (124). In addition, problems included progressive thinning and fibrillation of the articular surface, and poor integration with the host tissue (38). Despite the functional limitations, these studies established that regeneration of articular cartilage and subchondral bone can be achieved if some aspects of embryonic events are recapitulated by providing a sufficient number of reparative cells in a suitable delivery vehicle.

Scaffolds alone or in conjunction with growth factors promoted cell recruitment from the subchondral plate in goats and rabbits; and evaluated the repair tissue histologically and mechanically (by indentation). The use of fibrous polyglycolic acid (PGA) mesh improved tissue morphology but not the mechanical properties (94). Four-month repair in goats using a PLGA sponge resulted in fibrocartilage that was poorly integrated and had subnormal mechanical properties. The addition of TGF-β improved tissue repair, but the mechanical properties (aggregate and shear modulus, hydraulic permeability) remained sub-normal (11). A related study of osteochondral repair in condyles and patellar grooves of adult goats utilized two-phase scaffolds based on various PLGA polymers, in some cases with additional fibers and particles, alone or seeded with autologous chondrocytes (184). After 4 months, healing was better in the condyle (judged to be a high-weight bearing) than in the patella (intermittent and low-weight bearing).

Cell-polymer constructs obtained by seeding cultured bovine or lamb chondrocytes suspended in fibrin glue onto porous PLGA (61) or devitalized cartilage (200,201) were implanted subcutaneously in nude mice, and biomechanically tested. After 12 weeks *in vivo*, Young's moduli and failure load of the bovine constructs were approximately comparable to those measured for nasal cartilage. After 6 to 9 weeks, tensile and compressive properties of lamb constructs were

5% to 30% of normal, and the new tissue formed a bond that had 5% to 10% of the adhesive strength of normal tissue. A limitation of these studies is the animal model, which did not provide physiological loading conditions.

Perichondral cells seeded onto porous polylactic acid scaffolds and used for osteochondral repair in rabbits were evaluated histologically, biochemically, and biomechanically (48,49). After 1 year, the repair tissue had variable histological appearance and subnormal biochemical composition, but mechanical properties (i.e., confined-compression modulus and hydraulic permeability in confined compression) were comparable to those measured for the unoperated controls. Importantly, the repair tissue degraded over time and not a single specimen appeared normal after 1 year. In this case, mechanical testing appeared to be less sensitive than histological and biochemical assessments, reportedly due to the difficulties in mechanical testing of spatially inhomogeneous and geometrically irregular samples of the repair tissue.

Cartilaginous constructs obtained by culturing expanded allogeneic rabbit chondrocytes on PGA scaffolds for 3 to 4 weeks in static dishes (70) were implanted in rabbits for 6 months. As compared with the scaffold alone, cartilaginous constructs yielded repair tissue with better surface smoothness and cell columnarization (70). In a similar study, rabbit osteoprogenitor cells derived from skeletal muscle were cultured on PGA scaffolds for 2 to 3 weeks in static dishes to attach but not to differentiate. After 3 months, defects repaired with cell-PGA constructs consisted of a cartilaginous surface confluent with the host cartilage and normal-appearing subchondral bone, while implantation of PGA alone resulted in a patchy mixture of fibrous and hyaline cartilage (91). Allogeneic rabbit chondrocytes were cultured on PGA scaffolds in perfused cartilage implanted in rabbits (233). Repair of cartilage and bone based on immature (2-week) constructs was better than that based on mature (4-week) constructs. The lateral integration and bone remodeling remained incomplete even after 2 years. These results suggested that cell-polymer constructs can improve osteochondral repair, but the studies

were limited by inconsistent integration and the lack of biomechanical evaluation of the repair tissue.

Large osteochondral defects in adult rabbits ($7 \times 5 \times 5$ mm, femoropatellar groove) were repaired using *in vitro* engineered cartilage constructs (230). Articular chondrocytes were expanded, cultured for 4 to 6 weeks on PGA scaffolds, and sutured to an osteoconductive support; cell-free scaffolds and untreated defects served as controls. Repair tissue was evaluated histologically, biochemically, and biomechanically (by indentation). Over 6 months *in vivo*, defects implanted with engineered composites underwent orderly repair and yielded cartilage that had normal thickness, columnar cells, tidemark at an appropriate depth, and new subchondral bone. In contrast, controls repaired with fibrocartilage. The tissue-engineered cartilage had normal Young's moduli. Integration with subchondral bone was complete in most cases, whereas integration with cartilage was not consistently good. Functional cartilage engineered *in vitro* can thus provide a mechanically stable template that can yield osteochondral tissue with physiologically thick and stiff cartilage.

2.2 Cartilage Engineered *In Vitro*

Articular chondrocytes from immature rabbits cultured for up to 10 weeks in static dishes at high density without any scaffolding material formed 30–130 μm thick cartilaginous matrix (68). After 8 weeks of culture, the matrix contained subnormal fractions of GAGs and type II collagen, and had a "pseudolinear" elastic modulus in tension of 1.3 ± 0.2 MPa, as compared with the physiological range of 0.9–27 MPa.

Effects of long-term static and dynamic compression were studied using articular bovine calf chondrocytes embedded in agarose gel and cultured for up to 7 weeks (static strain amplitudes up to 50%, dynamic strain amplitudes of 6%, frequencies of 0.01–1 Hz) (34,35). The ECM was spatially discontinuous, contained wet weight fractions of DNA and GAG that were 25% of normal, and had confined-compression equilibrium moduli of up to 75 kPa. Constructs responded to mechanical forces in a manner similar to that of native cartilage: Static compression suppressed ECM synthesis by an amount that increased with increasing compression amplitude and culture time, whereas dynamic compression stimulated ECM synthesis by an amount that increased with ECM accumulation and culture time. In articular chondrocytes embedded in agarose and cultured for 2 days, dynamic compression (strain amplitudes of 15% and frequencies of 0.3–3 Hz) increased the rates of GAG and DNA synthesis, and decreased the rate of protein synthesis (141). Effects of intermittent dynamic compression (strain amplitudes of 10% and frequencies of 1 Hz in three consecutive cycles of 1 hour on/1 hour off once per day, 5 days per week) were studied in a similar system for 1 month (163). The equilibrium and Young's moduli (100 and 50 kPa, respectively) and biochemical compositions of dynamically stimulated constructs were all improved at 1 month of culture, as compared with free-swelling controls. An increase in cell seeding density from 10 to 60 million cells per cm^3 was associated with improved construct compositions and mechanical properties, an improvement that was counter-balanced with decreased beneficial effects of mechanical loading, such that the best constructs had equilibrium moduli in the range of 75–100 kPa (164).

Importantly, two growth factors known to mediate chondrogenesis, TGF-β and IGF-I, interacted with mechanical loading in a synergetic manner and improved the compositions and mechanical properties of cultured constructs to the extent greater than the sum of effects of either stimulus applied alone (165). Bovine chondrocytes were cultured in agarose gel for up to 5 weeks under the conditions of free swelling or with the application of mechanical loading. In either case, culture medium was supplemented either with 10% FBS, or with a combination of 10% FBS and either TGF-β or IGF-I. Overall, the equilibrium modulus of constructs increased from 13 kPa (free swelling conditions without supplemental growth factors) to 50 kPa (dynamic loading with the supplementation of growth factors). This study demonstrated that the beneficial effects of growth factors can be am-

plified by the application of dynamic mechanical loading.

Dynamic compression enhanced chondrogenesis of chick limb bud cells in a manner dependent on the frequency and duration of loading (66,67). Dynamic stretch affected the extent but not the rate of chondrogenesis of embryonic chick chondrocytes cultured on collagen sponges (260), whereas static compression increased both the rate and the extent of chondrogenesis in mouse limb-bud cells in collagen gel and promoted the expression of Sox9, a transcriptional activator of type II collagen (242). Intermittent hydrostatic pressure improved compositions and mechanical properties of young but not old chondrocytes cultured on PGA mesh and cultured in a perfused bioreactor for 5 weeks (40–42,104,105). Perfusion of culture medium alone, either through constructs or around constructs, also improved the tissue-engineered construct compositions; functional data were not reported (62,197,236).

Short-term (24 h) static or dynamic confined compression modulated the synthesis and retention of GAGs and protein in bovine calf chondrocytes cultured on PGA scaffolds for 3 weeks in static dishes (58). Static compression suppressed the matrix metabolism, whereas dynamic compression enhanced the synthesis and incorporation of both components by amounts that increased with an increase in static offset and dynamic compression frequency. Further studies are needed to explore if the stimulatory effect is only transitional, or can be sustained and utilized to augment the structure and function of engineered constructs.

The structural and functional properties of engineered constructs based on bovine calf chondrocytes and PGA scaffolds improved progressively and concomitantly over 12 weeks of cultivation in orbitally mixed dishes (147). The unconfined compression aggregate modulus increased 40-fold to 10% of normal, and the hydraulic permeability decreased four orders of magnitude to the range of values measured for native cartilage (147). In separate related studies, shear modulus of 8-week constructs positively correlated with GAG and collagen fractions but remained subnormal (239).

Mechanical behavior of engineered constructs based on bovine chondrocytes and PGA scaffolds, *in vitro* cultured cartilage explants and freshly explanted cartilage was recently characterized in radially confined axial compression and osmotic swelling (33). Constructs and explants cultured for 9 weeks in orbitally mixed dishes contained comparable amounts of proteoglycans (50% and 65% of normal, respectively), whereas the volumetric fractions of collagen in constructs were only one half of those in explants (34% and 68% of normal, respectively). In osmotic swelling, the axial and radial strains increased from cartilage to explants and constructs; for all tissues, the axial strain was twice as high as the radial strain, a finding consistent with tissue anisotropy. Consistently, the collagen fiber stiffness decreased from cartilage to explants and constructs. In confined compression, constructs, explants, and cartilage had similar stress-strain relationships, consistent with the model of prestressed collagen fibers balanced by swelling pressure of proteoglycans. The aggregate and shear moduli decreased from cartilage to explants and constructs, decreased with an increase in saline bath concentration, and correlated with wet weight fractions of proteoglycans and collagen.

The effects of bioreactor flow and mixing on construct structure and function were studied using static flasks (mass transport by molecular diffusion; no hydrodynamic shear), mixed flasks (convective mass transport; steady turbulent shear) and rotating vessels (convective mass transport; dynamic laminar shear) (248). Construct compositions and tested mechanical properties improved from static to mixed flasks, rotating vessels, and native cartilage. Constructs cultured in rotating vessels were uniformly cartilaginous, contained 75% as much GAG and 40% as much total collagen (hydroxyproline) per unit wet weight as normal cartilage, and had normal tissue morphology except for the lack of zonal organization and cell columnarization (75). The collagen network of 6-week constructs had normal fibril density and diameter, and the fractions of collagen types II, IX, and X, but the number of pyridinium cross-links per collagen molecule was only one third of normal (213).

The zero-strain compressive modulus of 6-week constructs was 175 kPa, as compared with 270 kPa measured for the articular surface (46), and 710 or 950 kPa measured for the deep zone of bovine articular cartilage (46,74). The dynamic stiffness, streaming potential, and hydraulic permeability were all different by a factor of 4 to 5 from the respective values measured for deep-zone bovine articular cartilage. Prolonged (7-month) cultivation yielded constructs with normal wet weight fractions of GAG and normal aggregate modulus and hydraulic permeability, but the fraction of collagen and dynamic stiffness remained subnormal (74). The relationships between constructs, compositions, and mechanical properties detected for chondrocyte-PGA constructs (248) appeared consistent with those reported for chondrocytes cultured in agarose gels (34), native calf cartilage (221), and in native adult human cartilage (9). These tissue engineering studies demonstrated that medium flow and mixing can be utilized to achieve spatially uniform initial cell distributions in thick constructs and to increase the rates of mass transport at construct surfaces, but also that the regime of flow (laminar and dynamic rather than turbulent and steady) is essential for the maintenance of differentiated cell function and cultivation of clinically sized, mechanically functional constructs.

Efficient gas exchange that maintained oxygen tension of $\sim$80 mm Hg and pH $\sim$7.0 markedly improved chondrogenesis in large (5 mm thick) constructs cultured in dynamic laminar flow as compared with oxygen tension of $\sim$40 mm Hg and pH $\sim$6.7 (186). The same effect was previously reported for cartilage formation by periosteum (chondrogenesis was maximal at oxygen tensions of 90–115 mm Hg) (194). In chondrocyte monolayers, oxygen tension of 40 mm Hg enhanced chondrogenesis more than oxygen tension of 160 mm Hg (101). A mathematical model of chondrogenesis in engineered constructs reconciled these apparent contradictions (188).

The interactive effects of the insulin-like growth factor-I IGF-I and mechanical environment (static and orbitally mixed dishes, static and mixed flasks, rotating vessels) on structure, biochemical composition and mechanical properties of engineered cartilage were studied using the chondrocyte-PGA model system (87). The IGF-I and flow modulated tissue properties independently in a manner consistent with previous studies, and interacted to produce tissues superior to those obtained by utilizing the two factors independently. The study also confirmed that there is a positive correlation between tissue composition and mechanical properties. After 4 weeks of culture, the best constructs had wet weight fractions of GAG and collagen and equlibrium moduli that were approximately 50% of values measured for the middle zone of native articular cartilage.

In separate related studies, growth factors supplemented sequentially to culture medium (TGF-•/FGF-2 early, IGF-I later during culture) in hydrodynamically active bioreactor environment markedly and significantly improved the compositions and mechanical properties of engineered cartilage (198). After 4 weeks of culture, constructs contained up to 4.5% ww GAG, up to 4.5% ww collagen, and had equilibrium moduli of up to 400 kPa. Likewise, hydrodynamically active environment present in rotating bioreactors amplified the beneficial effects of polymer scaffolds on construct compositions and mechanical properties (199). Bioreactor hydrodynamics and scaffold structure acted in concert to yield engineered cartilage that contained high fractions of GAG and type II collagen and had equilibrium moduli of 400–540 kPa after only 4 weeks of bioreactor cultivation. Taken together, these recent studies demonstrated that engineered cartilage with the composition and mechanical behavior within the range of values measured for immature (fetal-like) native cartilage can be grown in bioreactors within approximately 4 weeks.

Gene transfer of the human IGF-I was recently utilized for cartilage tissue engineering in an attempt to further enhance construct compositions and functional properties (150). Calf articular chondrocytes (unmodified, genetically modified to overexpress the *Escherichia coli* β-galactosidase gene or the human IGF-I gene) were cultured on PGA scaffolds in bioreactors and evaluated structurally and functionally, *in vitro* and *in vivo*. Transgene expression was maintained both *in vitro* and *in vivo* and resulted in rapid and progressive chondrogenesis. After

4 weeks of culture, IGF-I constructs contained markedly larger amounts of GAGs and collagen, both total and per unit DNA, and had four-fold higher equilibrium moduli as compared with nontransfected or *lacZ* constructs. The observed enhancement of *in vitro* chondrogenesis by spatially defined overexpression of human IGF-I suggested that cartilage tissue engineering based on genetically modified chondrocytes may be advantageous compared with either gene transfer or tissue engineering alone.

Integration of engineered and native cartilage was studied under controlled *in vitro* conditions, using bioreactors (189). Disc-shaped constructs cultured for 5 days or 5 weeks, or cartilage explants (intact or trypsin treated) were sutured into cartilage rings made of cartilage (intact or trypsin treated), cultured for 1 to 8 weeks and evaluated structurally and functionally (compressive stiffness of the central disk, adhesive strength of the integration interface). Immature constructs integrated better than either mature constructs or cartilage explants. Bonding of engineered cartilage and bone *in vitro* was also better for immature constructs (229). Integration of immature constructs involved cell proliferation and the progressive formation of cartilaginous tissue, in contrast to the integration of more mature constructs or native cartilage that involved only the secretion of ECM components. Integration patterns correlated with the adhesive strength of the disc-ring interface, which was markedly higher for immature constructs than for either more mature constructs or cartilage explants. Trypsin treatment of the adjacent cartilage further enhanced the integration of immature constructs (189), as previously shown for the repair *in vivo* (114). Integration of two cartilage blocks *in vitro* by isolated chondrocytes was enhanced by viable cells and serum components (45,211), and depended on applied compression (143). The adhesive strength of the interface correlated with collagen biosynthesis and deposition (60).

2.3 Bone Engineered *In Vivo*

The field of bone tissue engineering is relatively mature because numerous substitute materials as well as autogenous bone grafts have been used

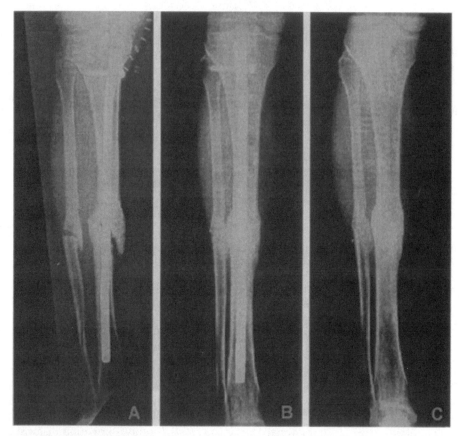

FIGURE 8-2. Scaffold delivery of an osteoinducing protein stimulates bone repair. In a prospective randomized clinical study published by Friedlaender (79), patients with established non-unions were treated with rhOP-1 delivered on a bovine type I collagen sponge. This patient demonstrated successful bone formation in the defect. **(A)** Postoperative, **(B)** 9 months after treatment, **(C)** 24 months after treatment. (From Friedlaender GE, Perry CR, Cole JD, et al. Osteogenic protein-1 (bone morphogenetic protein = 7) in the treatment of tibial nonunious. *J Bone Joint Surg Am* 2001;83-A[Suppl 1]:S151–S158, with permission.)

for many years in orthopaedic and related clinical practices. Autogenous bone grafts have been considered the gold standard for augmenting repair or regeneration of bone, but the limited volume and potential donor site morbidity have provided significant incentives for finding alternative techniques to promote consistent and robust bone formation. The majority of bone tissue engineering studies have been carried out *in vivo*, both in clinical applications and in preclinical animal models. For example, Friedlaender (79) presented the results of a prospective randomized clinical trial evaluating the use of rhOP-1 delivered with a collagen type I scaffold to treat non-unions. As illustrated in Fig. 8-2,

the delivery of the recombinant protein resulted in healing of the non-union defect.

One of the simplest forms of bone tissue engineering has been the augmentation of precursor cells and associated biofactors (55). Ten patients with established tibial delayed unions were treated by injection of marrow aspirate that was obtained from the patient's iliac wing. Aliquots of approximately 15 to 20 mL bone marrow aspirate were delivered to the fracture site after application of internal fixation hardware. Nine of the 10 delayed unions progressed toward healing by 4 months, and sufficient mechanical integrity was obtained to allow the patients to function without a cast or any fixation device (55). It might be inferred that the progenitor cells or osteoinductive factors contained within the marrow, delivered to a stabilized fracture site, enhanced the regenerative capability of the bone.

The field of orthopaedic surgery continues to use autograft and allograft materials to enhance bone repair. As noted in the early studies of Urist and colleagues (227,243–245), the osteogenic capacity of bone grafts appear to be related to incorporated factors such as the bone morphogenetic proteins (BMPs). Based on these early successes, the majority of bone tissue engineering research conducted over the last decade has involved the identification and delivery of recombinant proteins that were demonstrated to promote cell recruitment, proliferation or matrix expression, and thereby support bone formation.

Johnson and colleagues (119) treated four patients with established non-unions of the tibia. All patients received 50 to 100 mg of human BMP in PGA strips or capsules. Each of the fractures was augmented with internal fixation devices to provide mechanical stabilization. Three out of the four patients did well, demonstrating the potential of the approach. However, the specific factors (cells, biofactors, mechanical conditions) that could optimize the bone regenerative response were unknown.

Subsequent studies focused on specific BMPs that could be replicated through recombinant technology and delivered with carrier matrices ranging from polymers to biological materials such as demineralized bone matrix. Cook and colleagues (56) studied the delivery of recombinant human osteogenic protein 1 (analogous to BMP-7) in 1.5 cm defects in rabbit ulna. In a group of animals studied for 8 weeks, delivery of the OP-1 in a demineralized bone matrix stimulated healing in all defects and the attainment of 95% of the torsional strength of the contralateral control.

Similarly successful results were found when other recombinant proteins were delivered by a variety of matrices in bony defects. Sandhu (226) induced 100% solid fusions in a canine transverse process fusion model. Human recombinant BMP-2 was delivered by an open-cell PLA polymer applied to L4-5 posterior lateral fusions without the use of instrumentation. Biomechan-

ical as well as radiographic and tomographic data demonstrated exuberant bone formation (226). Kirker-Head (127) and colleagues found similar results in a large animal model with the implantation of recombinant human bone morphogenic protein 2 (rhBMP-2). Using a combination of a copolymer mixed with autogenous blood, the investigators delivered rhBMP-2 to 2.5 cm mid-diaphyseal segmental defects in the femora of sheep. A majority of these critical defects healed, progressing through a normal combined endochondral and membranous bone formation sequence. Many studies have demonstrated that the response to the delivery of recombinant proteins is dose dependent, and the numerous factors that have been discovered may play very different roles within the bone-promoting cascade (15).

Successful application of growth factors in promoting bone formation will also be dependent on the strategic selection of a carrier. For example, the use of an osteoconductive matrix may enhance the recruitment and attachment of bone cells to the carrier surfaces. Scaffolds made from a variety of materials have been used in bone defect studies for many years. Most of these have been utilized without the inclusion of growth factors or cultured cells and have demonstrated substantial success. For example, Chapman and colleagues (43) reported the results of a multicenter study to evaluate the efficacy of a collagen-calcium phosphate graft substitute material in long bone fractures. The material was a composite of type I collagen and a biphasic ceramic composed of hydroxyapatite and tricalcium phosphate. This prospective study included patients with traumatic long bone fractures treated with either internal or external fixation. Autogenous bone marrow aspirate was used with the implants, and the control group used autogenous bone graft. The authors found no significant differences between the graft substitute material and autogenous bone graft (43). Approximately 95% of the fractures healed in both groups by 3 months, with 100% healing at 2 years.

In an attempt to better characterize the repair dynamics of a similar collagen/ceramic composite as a carrier for BMP-2, Kusumoto (132) implanted scaffolds composed of type

I collagen and osteoconductive hydroxyapatite in pellets implanted into calf muscle pouches in rats. These investigators, as well as many others, hypothesized that using a delivery scaffold that had both osteoconductive properties and the ability to deliver a growth factor might further enhance bone formation and repair. The use of this composite to deliver rhBMP-2 demonstrated evidence of a dose response by the end of the 3-week sampling period. These data also demonstrated that the architecture of the carrier matrix might play a significant role in guiding or promoting specific patterns of bone formation.

Clearly, the chemistry as well as the architecture of the scaffolds may influence not only the delivery dynamics of any included biofactors, but also the pattern of induced bone formation. Numerous laboratories and investigators, as well as commercial entities, have specific research programs focused on discovering and optimizing the components of a carrier scaffold in an effort to enhance the promotion of bone formation under clinical circumstances. Several examples of these chemical and constituent modifications include the studies of Märtson et al. (161), Liljensten et al. (145), and Lee et al. (142). Märtson et al. (161) implanted cellulose sponges in femoral defects in male rats. Although unfilled defects in this rat model demonstrated more rapid bone infiltration and filling when compared with the cellulose sponges, bony infiltration and densification did finally occur in these sponges. It would be difficult to conclude that these cellulose sponges could enhance bone formation, even though they did demonstrate a compatibility with bony on-growth. In contrast, Liljensten et al. (145) demonstrated that composite scaffolds made of hydroxyapatite along with phospholipid polymers and/or sodium hyaluronan promoted greater bone formation than the controls. There were marked differences between the various composites, further underscoring the importance of choosing specific compositions for the scaffolds. Finally, Lee et al. (142) investigated the use of injectable hydrogels as scaffolds and as delivery vehicles for biofactors and cells. The initial mechanical properties of the hydrogels could be substantially altered by controlling the composition of the polymers, which also influenced the rate in which they are degraded *in vivo*. Poly(aldehyde guluronate) hydrogels mixed with osteoblasts induced the formation of mineralized tissue in a subcutaneous location in mice.

The delivery of cells alone or in conjunction with biofactors can create great opportunities for directing the reparative processes. The type or maturity of the cells may substantially influence the robustness of the regenerative response, and determine the degree of complexity and possibly regulatory hurdles associated with moving the technology into the clinic. Furthermore, the delivery of cells can be conceptualized in either three-dimensional scaffold applications or even on implant surfaces. For example, De Bruijn et al. (59) coated the surface of implants with calcium phosphate and demonstrated that bone marrow cells, and others, could adhere on the surface, enhancing the integration with natural tissue.

Although most investigators have relied on delivery of recovered or recombinant proteins or exogenously cultured cells, an alternative strategy utilizing a gene therapy approach has been proposed by several groups. The premise behind gene therapy approaches is the provision of local gene processing activity to induce the expression of appropriate stimulatory factors. It is hypothesized that this method may be more efficient and perhaps less costly.

Lieberman et al. (144) used a gene therapy approach to deliver BMP-2 to sites of bone formation. Their strategy included the *ex vivo* transfection of a bone marrow stromal cell line infected with an adenovirus, expressing recombinant bone morphogenetic protein cDNA that was delivered *in vivo* to bone defect sites in nude rats. The transfected cells synthesized and expressed sufficient levels of BMP-2 to stimulate a robust bone formation cascade.

A different localized gene therapy approach that avoided the need for delivering transfected cells was presented by Bonadio and colleagues (17). These investigators developed a technology for delivering the DNA from a matrix termed a "gene-activated matrix" (GAM). These studies demonstrated that it was possible to deliver

DNA within a bone repair site, and that DNA was taken up by resident repair cells that in turn synthesize and express the encoded protein. In a sense, this technology induces the patient to become the bioreactor. Utilizing plasmid for PTH_{1-34}, the investigators demonstrated that sufficient *in vivo* transfection and subsequent protein expression could be induced to promote robust bone formation in a critically sized defect in large animals. It was estimated that picograms of protein were produced, and the result demonstrated the potential power of this localized *in vivo* transfection. Although this study demonstrated that sufficient bone formation could occur, there may be many opportunities for further improvements, for example, by increasing the transfection efficiency, as well as strategically selecting optimal genes to deliver.

In a related study, Baltzer and colleagues (12) utilized local adenoviral delivery of the BMP-2 gene to treat fracture defects in rabbits. It was proposed that adenoviral delivery would substantially enhance the *in vivo* transfection efficiency, thereby increasing the amount of synthesized growth factor and subsequently increasing the rate of bone formation. The results of their study demonstrated robust bone formation and rapid attainment of biomechanical competence within the healing defect. Common to all gene therapy approaches is the ability to deliver biofactors such as transcription factors, as well as combinations of genes that would likely be difficult or impossible to provide using recombinant protein technology. Similar to most tissue engineering approaches, optimization would depend on strategic selection of the gene or gene sequences, the chemistry of the delivery matrix, and timing of the delivery.

2.4 Bone Engineered *In Vitro*

In contrast to tissue engineering of cartilage, bone tissue engineering research and practice has had a significantly reduced focus on *in vitro* formation of bone constructs. Most *in vitro* studies have been dedicated to screening new scaffold designs or experimentally exploring the response dynamics, between cells and matrices, thereby forming a basis for the use of scaffolds *in vivo* to guide the infiltration of host cells, and enhance and modulate bone regeneration.

Garcia and colleagues (83) investigated the effect of altering the surface of bioactive glasses by coating them with fibronectin. The ability for osteoblast-like cells to adhere to the surface of this biomaterial was dependent on the RGD binding site of the fibronectin and the thickness of the adsorbed fibronectin. Other investigators used *in vitro* systems to evaluate the effects of cell seeding density, culture period, scaffold architecture, and scaffold composition and cell source on matrix deposition and mineralization (112,148,155,261). Although all of these investigators were able to isolate important features of the scaffold design and cell seeding dynamics that led to enhanced matrix formation, the aggregate of their studies suggest there is a large number of controllable variables that can substantially effect the targeted properties of the constructs.

Little work has been done in bone tissue engineering involving the introduction of mechanical stimulation within bioreactors. Ma and colleagues (148) cultured cell scaffold constructs while on an orbital shaker moving at 75 rpm. Although these authors did not make any specific recommendations concerning this biomechanical stimulus, Botchwey et al. (20) suggested that the shear stress imparted to the cells within their rotating bioreactor influenced their activity and subsequently may be an important component of a strategy to enhance cell phenotypic expression and matrix organization. However, it is unclear whether a viable strategy will be developed to grow bone constructs to maturity in culture for transplantation, or if there will be a clinical need for such preformed bone constructs.

3 MODULATION OF ENGINEERED TISSUE PROPERTIES

Cells, biomaterial scaffolds, and biochemical and physical regulatory signals can be utilized in a variety of ways to engineer cartilage and bone, *in vitro* (using bioreactors) and *in vivo* (following implantation). In all cases, the goal of tissue engineering is to recapitulate some aspects of the environment present *in vivo* during tissue development and thereby stimulate the cells to regenerate functional tissues. This generally involves the presence of reparative cells, facilitated transport of chemical species, and the use of physical regulatory signals. Cartilage tissue engineering has been done both *in vitro* and *in vivo*, and it requires the addition of new cells. In contrast, bone tissue engineering has been done mostly *in vivo*, and in most cases involved the use of biomaterials and biofactors without added cells. We discuss here the modulation of the development and functionality of engineered cartilage and bone, *in vitro* and *in vivo*.

3.1 Cell-related Factors

Cell requirements for tissue engineering of cartilage and bone are quite different, as a result of the different healing capacities of these two tissues. High density of new, biosynthetically active cells is critical for cartilage regeneration, whereas bone regeneration can be based on the use of scaffold alone and the guided infiltration of the host cells (183). As compared with adult cartilage, which contains low concentration of differentiated chondrocytes and has limited capacity to heal, embryonic and young tissue contain blood vessels, high concentration of progenitor cells and high cell-to-matrix ratio (118). In fact, surgical techniques for cartilage repair are in most cases designed to induce bleeding or to penetrate the subchondral bone down to the marrow cavity and thereby facilitate the access to progenitor cells. Likewise, the only FDA-approved cell-based approach to cartilage repair (Carticel™) involves transplantation of isolated chondrocytes expanded in culture. These methods demonstrate that intrinsic cartilage repair can be enhanced if new cells and factors are introduced, normally present in young and developing cartilage but not in mature tissue.

In contrast to cartilage, bone tissue can regenerate in situ, due to access to bone forming cells (e.g., from vasculature, periosteum, bone marrow). The progression and outcome of bone regeneration depends on the availability of progenitor cells, a variety of molecular signaling

cascades, nutritional support, and an appropriate mechanical environment (81,167,202). To date, tissue engineering of bone is largely based on the utilization of cell-free biomaterial scaffolds that stimulate the mobilization of reparative cells from the host to its surface and may deliver bioactive factors that promote regeneration. However, several investigators have hypothesized that the delivery of bone cells or their precursors may enhance or hasten the regeneration (37,38,59,144).

The cells used thus far to engineer cartilage that has been functionally characterized have varied with respect to donor age (embryonic, neonatal, immature, or adult), differentiation state (precursor or phenotypically mature), and the method of preparation (selection, expansion, gene transfer). *In vitro* studies were done using bovine chondrocytes (34,75), rabbit chondrocytes (68), equine chondrocytes (105), embryonic chick limb bud cells (66), and human chondrocytes (236); *in vivo* studies were done using rabbit chondrocytes (228,252), perichondrocytes (48), periosteum (173) and precursor cells from periosteum or bone marrow (251), dog chondrocytes (181), and human chondrocytes (26,28,206). Scaffolds used alone (70,93) or in conjunction with growth factors (11) improved the repair of critically sized osteochondral defects compared with natural healing, but were inferior to treatments involving transplanted cells or engineered cartilage (251,252).

The choice of cell type can affect *in vitro* culture requirements (e.g., medium supplements, scaffold structure, and degradation rate), and *in vivo* function (e.g., potential for integration) of engineered cartilage constructs. Articular chondrocytes are phenotypically stable if cultured under appropriate conditions (e.g., up to 7 to 8 months *in vitro* (74,102)) and can be used to engineer mechanically functional cartilaginous constructs (35,74,189,230,248). However, chondrocytes are not easily harvested, cells from younger donors tend to be more responsive to environmental stimuli (105), and cell expansion involves the use of growth factors (158,160). In contrast, precursor cells from the bone marrow are relatively easier to harvest and expand in culture, remain metabolically active in older donors (103) and can recapitulate some aspects of skeletal tissue development (38).

High initial cell densities in engineered constructs were critical for rapid synthesis and functional assembly of ECM components in differentiated chondrocytes (75,247) and the induction of chondrogenesis in bone marrow derived precursor cells (36). It is possible that the cell responses to phenotypic induction were enhanced by (or even depended on) the presence of neighboring cells differentiating in the same way at the same time (77). *In vitro* integration of engineered and native cartilage (187), two cartilage explants (211), and engineered cartilage and bone (229) also depended on the presence of biosynthetically active cells capable of the progressive formation of cartilaginous tissue bond. In general, the choice of cells and cell density can largely determine the mechanical properties of engineered cartilage at the time of implantation (and thereby graft handling and survival) and the capacity for further development and integration (and thereby, as assumed in our hypothesis, the long-term success of tissue regeneration).

Bone formation and regeneration depend on two fundamental requirements: appropriate nutritional support (blood supply) and a stable surface for bone deposition (63,231). The nutritional supply is required due to the dependence of osteoblasts on capillary support. A stable surface can be provided by the preformation of the calcified cartilage matrix during endochondral bone formation or the condensation of a fibrous matrix that mineralizes during intramembranous bone formation (64,215,231). The cells involved in these pathways include multipotential precursor cells (mesenchymal stem cells) and differentiated populations of chondrocytes, fibroblasts, osteoblasts, macrophages, and osteoclasts (64,82,167,215,231). Tissue engineering strategies for bone regeneration must thus be capable of providing or inducing the formation of a stable surface (such as a scaffold) as well as delivering or attracting cell populations.

3.2 Biomaterial Scaffolds

Cartilage has been engineered without the use of a scaffold, both *in vitro* (68) and *in vivo* (26,27,

90,190). However, most studies suggest that the scaffold is essential for promoting orderly tissue regeneration within the defect (38,49,115,230). Scaffolds vary with respect to material chemistry (e.g., collagen, agarose, or synthetic polymers with and without coatings), geometry (e.g., gels, fibrous meshes, porous sponges), structure (e.g., porosity, pore size distribution, orientation and connectivity of the polymer phase), mechanical properties (e.g., tension, compression and shear stiffnesses, permeability, etc.; see Chapter 5 for more details), and degradation (degradation rate, degradation product) (77). A variety of different scaffolds have been used to engineer cartilage, including gels of agarose (35,141,163) and collagen (251,252), meshes of collagen (92) and PGA (42,74,75,92,186,228,248), and sponges of PLA (48).

In bone tissue engineering, the use of scaffolds alone or as delivery devices for biofactors or isolated cells has shown great promise. In contrast to cartilage, few studies have been devoted to establishing *in vitro* methods for forming bone tissue for subsequent transplantation (20,112,261). Most *in vitro* studies have been designed to serve as screening assays to qualify osteoinductive or osteoconductive constructs (65,83,112,203,204,208,261). These studies demonstrated the potential of optimizing *in vitro* conditions (including scaffold choice) to create a construct with a mineralized matrix for subsequent transplantation into bone defects. Importantly, there are no data available on the mechanical properties of bone tissue engineered *in vitro*. In addition, data are not available to evaluate whether there are distinct advantages to using cell seeded scaffolds and their cultivation in bioreactors in comparison to cell-free biomaterial scaffolds. It may be possible that a transplanted mineralized bone construct may induce faster healing and incorporation with the native tissue in the defect being treated.

A biomaterial scaffold provides a structural and "informational" template for cell attachment and tissue development, and biodegrades in parallel with the accumulation of tissue components. Scaffold structure determines the transport of nutrients, metabolites, and regulatory molecules to and from the cells. Scaffolds should be made of biocompatible, biodegradable materials to minimize immunogenicity *in vivo*. Materials such as PGA, PLA, and collagen are currently used in products approved by the FDA (e.g., Dexon® from Davis & Geck, UK; Ultrafoam® from Davol, Cranston, RI), whereas agarose is mainly used as an *in vitro* research tool. The rate of scaffold degradation should match the rate of ECM deposition by a specific cell type under specific conditions (76), and this rate can depend on scaffold material and structure, the seeding density, and metabolic activity of the cells. The maintenance of mechanical properties of the scaffold, and its rate of decline, may be critical for its efficacy, as well as for the modulation of the stress-strain environment at the cellular and tissue levels.

The patterns of chondrogenesis were quite different for cells embedded in gels (formation of cell clusters that accumulated matrix over time but remained separated with matrix-free regions after 6 weeks of culture (34)) and cells seeded onto meshes or sponges (initiation of chondrogenesis in the high-cell density region at the construct surface, with the progressive apositional development of continuously cartilaginous matrix over 6 weeks of culture (75)). These differences between the developmental patterns and matrix compositions in the two types of constructs may be important for their mechanical properties (including the scale dependence of mechanical behavior), as well as for the transduction of mechanical signals. For free-swelling cultures, construct compositions and mechanical properties were generally better for fibrous meshes (248) than agarose gels (34,163), which may be due to the spatial continuity of the cartilaginous matrix in constructs based on fibrous meshes. For constructs cultured with mechanical stimulation, the only report of improved construct compositions was for chondrocytes cultured in agarose gel (163), which may be due to the enhanced signal transduction and fluid flow through the gel between the cell clusters (for more details, see Chapter 6).

The structure and composition of scaffolds can also significantly affect the dynamics of bone regeneration. Many polymer and ceramic scaffolds were shown to act as osteoconductive surfaces, i.e., to support the ingrowth of osteoprogenitor cells onto a surface leading to the formation of bone (31). Materials with demonstrated osteoconductive properties include calcium phosphates, hydroxyapatite, calcium/collagen composites, and a variety of polymers and bioglasses (31,43,65,142,145,148,155,203,208,261). These materials can be fabricated with variations in chemistry, micro- and macroporosity, degradation properties, and mechanical integrity. Each of these properties can significantly alter the bone formation cascade by influencing cell chemotaxis, attachment, morphology, and subsequent matrix synthesis. In addition, these materials may be used to deliver biofactors ranging from cytokines, growth factors (such as recombinant proteins), cells, and genes. Optimizing the design of tissue-engineered bone constructs involves choosing or prioritizing one or more of these properties.

3.3 Bioreactor Hydrodynamics

Ideally, a bioreactor should provide an *in vitro* environment for rapid and orderly development of functional tissue structures by isolated cells on three-dimensional scaffolds. Bioreactors are designed to perform one or more of the following functions: (a) establish spatially uniform concentrations of cells within clinically sized biomaterial scaffolds, (b) control conditions in culture medium (e.g., temperature, pH, osmolality, levels of oxygen, nutrients, metabolites, regulatory molecules), (c) facilitate mass transfer between the cells and the culture environment, and (d) provide physiologically relevant physical signals (e.g., interstitial fluid flow, shear, pressure, mechanical compression) (76). Hydrodynamic factors present during *in vitro* culture can modulate chondrogenesis in at least two ways: by enhanced *mass transport* between the developing tissue and culture medium (e.g., oxygen, nutrients, growth factors), and by direct *physical stimulation* of the cells (e.g., shear, pressure). *In vivo*, mass transfer within articular cartilage involves a combination of diffusion and convective flow driven by gradients in concentrations of chemical and ionic species, hydrodynamic pressure and fluid content, that are associated with tissue loading.

In vitro, mass transfer between the forming tissue and its environment can determine the size and composition of engineered constructs and cartilage explants (249).

Three representative culture vessels that are frequently used for cartilage tissue engineering (static flasks, mixed flasks, rotating vessels) are compared in Fig. 8-3. All culture vessels are operated in incubators (to maintain the temperature and pH), with continuous gas exchange and periodic medium replacement. Flasks contain constructs that are fixed in place and cultured either statically or with magnetic stirring. Rotating vessels contain constructs that are freely suspended in culture medium between two concentric cylinders, the inner of which serves as a gas exchange membrane. The rotation rate is adjusted to maintain each construct settling at a stationary point within the vessel relative to an observer on the ground. After 6 weeks of culture in static flasks, cartilaginous matrix accumulated mostly at the periphery, in contrast to mixed flasks where cartilaginous matrix accumulated in the inner tissue phase but was surrounded by a thick fibrous capsule. Only in rotating vessels, constructs were uniformly cartilaginous throughout their entire cross sections (Fig. 8-3A). These differences in tissue morphology could be related to the respective differences in flow and mass transport conditions in the three culture vessels. In static flasks, mass transport in culture medium occurs by molecular diffusion only (therefore, tissue for-

mation on the construct periphery), and there is no hydrodynamic shear at construct surfaces. In mixed flasks, mechanical stirring generates convective flow that enhances mass transport in bulk medium, but also generates turbulent shear (therefore, capsule formation at construct surfaces). In rotating vessels, construct settling generates laminar fluid flow with dynamic fluctuations in fluid velocity, shear, and pressure that enhance mass transport at construct surfaces without adverse hydrodynamic effects (therefore, spatially uniform chondrogenesis throughout the construct volume) (Table 8-4).

The composition, morphology, and mechanical properties of engineered cartilage grown in mechanically active environments were generally better than in static environments. Studies of *in vitro* chondrogenesis in mixed flasks showed that the presence or absence of mixing, rather than the intensity of mixing, was the primary determinant of construct composition, and suggested the "all-or-none" nature of chondrocyte response to turbulent mixing (88). For cultivations in vessels described in Table 8-4, construct compositions (wet weight fractions of GAGs and total collagen) and some mechanical properties (equilibrium aggregate modulus, hydraulic permeability, dynamic stiffness, streaming potential) improved from static flasks to mixed flasks and rotating vessels (Fig. 8-4). In particular, the hydrodynamic stresses acting at the surfaces of constructs cultured in dynamic laminar flow of rotating bioreactors

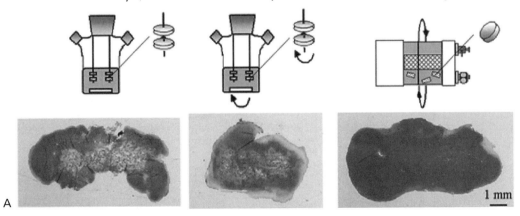

FIGURE 8-3. Representative bioreactors: Schematic presentation of construct cultivation in static flasks, mixed flasks, and rotating vessels with the respective full cross sections of tissue constructs cultured for 6 weeks. Stain: safranin-O/fast green. Scale bar: 1 mm.

TABLE 8-4. OVERVIEW OF THE OPERATING CONDITIONS FOR EACH VESSEL TYPE (47,52,73,76,182,246)

Cultivation Vessel	Static Flask	Mixed Flask	Rotating Vessel
Vessel diameter (cm)	6.5	6.5	14.6/5.1
Medium volume (cm3)	120	120	110
Tissue constructs or explants (5 mm diameter x 2 mm thick discs)	Fixed in place; n ≤ 12 per vessel	Fixed in place; n ≤ 12 per vessel	Freely settling; n ≤ 12 per vessel
Medium exchange	Batch-wise (3 cm3 per construct per day)	Batch-wise (3 cm3 per construct per day)	Batch-wise (3 cm3 per construct per day)
Gas exchange	Continuous, via surface aeration	Continuous, via surface aeration	Continuous, via an internal membrane
Stirring/rotation rate (s⁻¹)	0	0.83–1.25	0.25–0.67
Flow conditions	Static fluid	Turbulent[1]	Laminar[2]
Mixing mechanism	None	Magnetic stirring	Settling in rotational flow
Mass transfer in bulk medium	Molecular diffusion	Convection (due to medium stirring)	Convection (due to tissue settling)
Fluid shear at construct surfaces	None	Steady, turbulent	Dynamic, laminar
References	(70, 72, 75–77, 248, 249)	(75–77, 88, 157, 159, 246–249)	(71, 74–77, 88, 151, 188, 189, 198, 199, 213, 248–250)

[1]The smallest turbulent eddies had a diameter of 250 μm and velocity of 0.4 cm/s; estimated according to Cherry and Papoutsakis (47) by Vunjak-Novakovic et al. (246).
[2] Tissues were settling in a laminar tumble-slide regimen in a rotational field; estimated according to Clift et al. (52) by Freed and Vunjak-Novakovic (73) and Neitzel et al. (182).

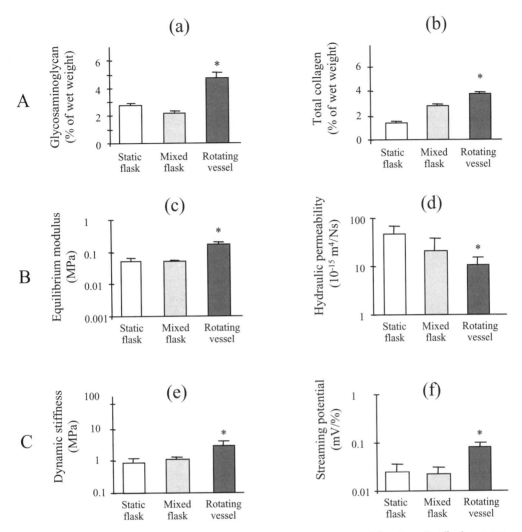

FIGURE 8-4. Effects of hydrodynamic factors on constructs structure and function. Cartilaginous constructs based on bovine articular chondrocytes and fibrous scaffolds were cultured for 6 weeks in static flasks, mixed flasks, or rotating bioreactors (see **Fig. 8-3**). **(A)** Biochemical compositions (% wet weight) at different times of bioreactor cultivation: **(a)** glycosaminoglycan, and **(b)** total collagen (hydroxyproline). **(B)** Mechanical behavior in confined compression: **(c)** equilibrium modulus determined in static confined compression from the slopes of stress-strain curves at 10%–40% strain (MPa) and **(d)** hydraulic permeability (10^{-15} m^4/Ns) determined from the static and dynamic compression data at 30% strain and 1 Hz frequency (based on data reported in (159,248)). **(C)** Mechanical behavior in confined compression: **(e)** dynamic stiffness calculated from the ratio of dynamic stress and applied strain, at 30% strain, as a function of frequency and **(f)** streaming potential normalized by the amplitude of applied strain, at 30% strain, as a function of frequency. Data represent average ± SD (n = 3–4) for 6-week constructs from static flasks, mixed flasks, and rotating bioreactors, and freshly explanted bovine articular cartilage (based on data reported in 159,248).

(approximately 1 dyn/cm^2(73)), yielded cartilaginous constructs with markedly improved compositions and mechanical properties as compared with constructs cultured either statically or in mixed flasks (75,248).

Direct perfusion through cultured tissue constructs also stimulated chondrogenesis, presumably due to combined effects of enhanced mass transport, pH regulation, and fluid shear in the cell microenvironment (62,197,236), in particular at physiological interstitial flow velocities (~1 μm/s) (153,171,173); also, for more details, see Chapter 5. It is possible that the observed effects of dynamic mechanical compression *in vitro* (35,163) and *in vivo* (242) were also due in part to the increased fluid flow within cultured tissue constructs. Physical stimuli (pressure, shear) conveyed by the flow of culture medium, although different in nature and intensity from physical signals associated with joint loading, can be utilized to promote *in vitro* synthesis and functional assembly of cartilaginous matrix (140).

3.4 Regulatory Molecules

Oxygen plays a particularly important role in engineering functional tissues. The synthesis and deposition of cartilaginous tissue components were significantly improved in constructs cultured at an oxygen tension in culture medium, P_{O_2}, of ~80 mm Hg (a value normally found at the cellular level in vascularized tissues (194) as compared with ~40 mm Hg (186). For comparison, the P_{O_2} in native adult cartilage ranges from approximately 50 mm Hg at the articular surface to less than 7 mm Hg in the deep zone (25); higher values are likely to be present in immature cartilage due to the presence of blood vessels. The finding that higher than physiological P_{O_2} increased the proteoglycan content in engineered cartilage is consistent with results reported for explant cultures of cartilage and periosteum (194,262) and cartilage regeneration *in vivo* (99), and is significant because proteoglycan content correlated positively with mechanical properties (248).

Growth factors (e.g., FGF-2, TGF-β1) are generally required to engineer cartilaginous tissues starting from bone marrow-derived mesenchymal stem cells (120,156) and expanded chondrocytes (158,160). Specific combinations of bioactive factors were shown to promote chondrocyte cells to first dedifferentiate during expansion in monolayers, and then redifferentiate and regenerate cartilaginous tissues during subsequent cultivation on biomaterial scaffolds (198). The growth factor IGF-I is known to have anabolic effects both in engineered and native cartilage (14,150,220,223). However, the concentration of IGF-I in adult cartilage is only 0.1–0.3 of that in serum, largely due to its exclusion by proteoglycan molecules acting as a selectively permeable barrier (the average pore size of the ECM is only 40–60 Å (154,171); see Chapter 5 for more details). The presence of blood vessels in immature cartilage and loading-induced fluid flow can each increase the local concentrations of growth factors and thereby modulate ECM synthesis and breakdown. This can explain the enhanced responsiveness to IGF-I observed in mechanically active environments, involving either hydrodynamic forces (87) or direct compression (18). Importantly, the mechanical environment and supplemental growth factors independently modulate the growth and mechanical properties of engineered cartilage, interact to produce results not suggested by the independent responses, and in certain combinations can produce tissues superior to those obtained by utilizing these factors individually (87). Recently, gene transfer of human IGF-I was shown to augment the structural and functional properties cartilaginous constructs grown in bioreactors, suggesting that spatially defined overexpression of growth factors may be advantageous for cartilage tissue engineering (150). One intriguing possibility is that the effects of growth factors overexpressed by the cells can be enhanced by physical regulatory signals in a manner similar to that observed for growth factors.

The cascade of bone induction during repair and regeneration is mediated by specific cytokines, growth factors, and transcription factors. A significant body of work has emerged to implicate members of the TGFβ super-family in these processes. TGFβ1 expression has been shown to be upregulated following fracture (7,21,122,162), particularly during endochondral ossification with much lower expression during intramembranous formation (16). Several bone morphogenic proteins (BMP2, BMP4, BMP7, BMP6) have been shown to induce bone formation *in vivo* (15,180,214,225,258) and therefore are considered to be some of the most viable targets for therapeutic intervention. Additional growth factors including FGF, PDGF, and IGF-1 have also been shown to play important roles in the promotion or support of bone formation (15,16,64). All of these factors, as well as several other regulatory factors and hormones, including PTH, VEGF, LMP-1, and GDF, have been shown to promote bone formation (15,63).

3.5 Duration of Culture

The progression of chondrogenesis in constructs based on articular chondrocytes cultured on fibrous scaffolds has been associated with temporal and spatial changes in local concentrations of the cells and cartilaginous matrix shown in Fig. 8-5A,B. Cells at the construct periphery proliferated more rapidly during the first 3 days of culture (Fig. 8-5d) and initiated chondrogenesis (Fig. 8-5a), which progressed apositionally, both inward toward the construct center and outward from its surface (Fig. 8-5a–c). By 6 weeks of culture, self-regulated cell proliferation and ECM deposition yielded constructs that had physiological cell densities and appeared uniformly cartilaginous (Fig. 8-5c and f). Quantitatively, the development of tissue-engineered cartilage has been modeled using a spatially varying, deterministic continuum model (188). The model accounted for the deposition and diffusion of oxygen and GAG as a function of the spatial position within the construct and the duration of tissue cultivation. Here, GAG was taken as a marker of chondrogenesis in light of prior association of its deposition with that of collagen type II (75). Oxygen consumption due to energy metabolism and matrix biosynthesis resulted in a gradual decrease of oxygen concentration from the construct surface toward its center (Fig. 8-5C). Model predictions for concentration profiles of GAGs (Fig. 5D, lines) were qualitatively and quantitatively consistent with those measured via high-resolution (40 μm) image processing of tissue samples (157) (Fig. 8-5D, data points).

Models of this kind can be used to rationalize experimental data for chondrogenesis in engineered constructs, and to relate these data to earlier observations of the dependence of global construct properties on cultivation conditions (the domain of focus in each case being limited by available analytical tools). Construct function has been correlated with overall construct composition, which itself depended on the conditions of bioreactor cultivation (248). Empirical relationships like these are fundamentally instructive. However, Fig. 8-5a–h shows clearly that the spatial distributions of cells and ECM are highly nonuniform during most of the cultivation period. Therefore, the spatial averaging intrinsic to measurement of overall construct properties can filter out potentially significant information regarding internal gradients and associated mass transfer limitations upon cell metabolism and tissue growth. Additional quantitative models are needed to describe structure-function relationships for engineered constructs and the repair tissue, and obtain predictive tools for the design of tissue-engineered cartilage repair (131,222).

For engineered cartilage, the optimal duration of *in vitro* cultivation (or even the need for *in vitro* cultivation) has not yet been determined. Implantations were done as early as within 2 hours of cell seeding, with functional tissue development required to occur *in vivo* (48,251,252), and using cartilaginous constructs engineered *in vitro* that appeared to be functional to some extent at the time of implantation (228). With time in culture, the constructs more closely approximated articular cartilage, structurally (Fig. 8-6A) and functionally (Fig. 8-6B) (74,248). The wet weight fraction of GAGs increased progressively from very low at 3 days to significantly higher than physiological at 7 months (Fig. 8-6a), whereas the fraction of total collagen increased during the first 6 weeks but remained at this level for the duration of culture (Fig. 8-6b). Compared with adult native cartilage, 6-week constructs had subnormal fractions of GAG and collagen (Fig. 8-6a and b), four-fold higher hydraulic permeability (Fig. 8-6c), and subnormal equilibrium modulus, dynamic stiffness, and streaming potential (Fig. 8-6d–f). After 7 months of culture, the equilibrium modulus and hydraulic permeability came into the range of values measured for adult cartilage (Fig. 8-6c, d), whereas dynamic stiffness and streaming potential remained subnormal (Fig. 8-6e,f) (for more details, see Chapter 5).

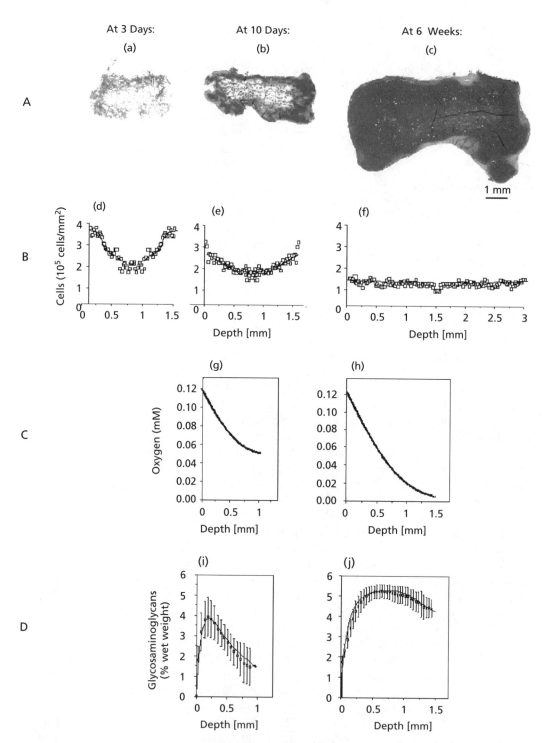

FIGURE 8-5. *In vitro* chondrogenesis: **(A)** Full cross sections of tissue constructs after **(a)** 3 days, **(b)** 10 days, and **(c)** 6 weeks of culture. Stain: safranin-O/fast green. Scale bar: 1 mm. **(B)** Spatial profiles of cell distribution after **(d)** 3 days, **(e)** 10 days, and **(f)** 6 weeks of culture (measured by image processing). **(C)** Spatial profiles of oxygen distribution after **(g)** 10 days and **(h)** 6 weeks of culture (model predictions). **(D)** Spatial profiles of glycosaminoglycan distribution after **(i)** 10 days and **(j)** 6 weeks of culture (data points: measured by image processing; lines: model predictions). (From Obradovic B, Meldon JH, Freed LE, et al. Glycosaminoglycan deposition in engineered cartilage: experiments and mathematical model. *AIChE J* 2000;46:1860–1871, with permission.)

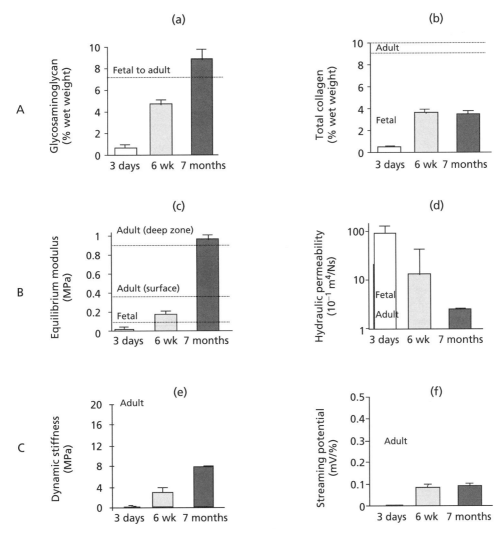

FIGURE 8-6. Effects of cultivation time on construct structure and function. Cartilaginous constructs based on bovine articular chondrocytes and fibrous scaffolds were cultured in rotating bioreactors for 3 days, 6 weeks, or 7 months. (**A**) Biochemical compositions (% wet weight) at different times of bioreactor cultivation. (**a**) glycosaminoglycan, and (**b**) total collagen (hydroxyproline). (**B**) Mechanical behavior in confined compression: (**c**) equilibrium modulus determined in static confined compression from the slopes of stress-strain curves at 10–40% strain (MPa) and (**d**) hydraulic permeability (10^{-15} m^4/Ns) determined from the static and dynamic compression data at 30% strain and 1 Hz frequency (based on data reported in (74,248); additional native cartilage data are from (46,256).

Importantly, the compositions and mechanical properties of 6-week constructs were in the range of values measured for fetal cartilage (Fig. 8-6A,B), suggesting that bioreactors yield engineered constructs resembling immature rather than mature native cartilage, even after prolonged cultivation. It is likely that the functional deficiencies present in engineered cartilage grown *in vitro* are due to the absence of specific biochemical and physical factors normally present *in vivo*. Following implantation, engineered cartilage remodeled into physiologically stiff cartilage and new subchondral bone (230,251), in response to local and systemic regulatory factors (38,235). Notably, columnar cells and a tidemark at an appropriate depth were observed in engineered cartilage following *in vivo* exposure to physiological loading (230), but not *in vitro*.

The lack of bonding between cultured constructs and host cartilage suggests that mature constructs may not have sufficient capacity for integration (94). Controlled bioreactor studies demonstrated a trade-off between the stiffness of engineered cartilage and its integration potential. Immature constructs integrated better than either more mature constructs or cartilage explants. Integration of immature constructs involved cell proliferation and the progressive formation of cartilaginous tissue (Fig. 8-7a–d), in contrast to the integration of more mature constructs or native cartilage that involved only the secretion of ECM components. Biomechanical properties improved from immature to more mature construct and cartilage explants (Fig. 8-7e), whereas the adhesive stiffness at disc-ring interface was markedly higher for immature constructs than for either more mature constructs or cartilage explants (Fig. 8-7f) (187). Ideally, the duration of *in vitro* cultivation should be selected for each specific application such that constructs have certain minimal construct stiffness along with certain minimal capacity for integration.

3.6 Physical Signals

Physical factors have been utilized to improve development *in vitro* and remodeling *in vivo* of native and engineered cartilage using a variety of physical signals, including fluid flow (197,259), dynamic fluctuations in hydrodynamic shear and pressure (74,248), cyclic hydrostatic pressure (42), cyclic mechanical compression (35,163), and cyclic stretch (260). *In vitro*, dynamic but not static compression enhanced synthesis of proteoglycans in cartilage explants (223), improved the mechanical function of engineered cartilage (34,35,42,141,163), and enhanced chondrogenesis of chick limb bud cells (66,67). *In vivo*, cyclic loading caused the mesenchymal cells to differentiate into cartilage overlaying bone (241).

Loading can cause changes to the extracellular environment of native and engineered cartilage:

(a) by direct effects on cell shape and interfibrillar spacing; (b) by increase in hydrostatic pressure; (c) by fluid flow, which can enhance mass transport to and from the cells, and generate streaming potentials; or (d) by change in fluid volume, which can cause changes in concentrations of chemical and ionic species (177) (also see Chapters 5 and 6 for more details). All these effects can modulate the synthesis, breakdown, and structural adaptations of the ECM, which in turn serves as a transducer of mechanical and electrochemical signals associated with joint loading, and thereby mediate the catabolic and anabolic changes in chondrocyte metabolism. The mechanotransduction will therefore also depend on material properties of the ECM. For example, fibrocartilaginous repair tissue in many cases reduces joint disability, but does not necessarily provide a long-term solution, due to the structural and functional properties that are different from those of articular cartilage. In a canine model (weight-bearing condyles of adult dogs), native healing of untreated large defects over a period of 10 months generated fibrocartilage that had five-fold lower aggregate modulus, two-fold lower Poisson ratios, and significantly higher hydraulic permeability as compared with normal cartilage (100). Under the same load, the extent of deformation, the increase in fluid flow or hydrostatic pressure, the change in the fluid content, and chondrocyte metabolism can be different for fibrocartilage and hyaline cartilage (183).

Since the observations of the 19th-century anatomists and engineers (39,257), mechanical forces have been assumed to exert a powerful influence on bone formation, repair, and adaptation (for more details, see Chapters 4, 5, and 6). Although strong evidence supporting a relationship between physical forces and patterns of bone formation continues to be produced, the mathematical laws relating bone response to the stress, strain, or mechanobiologic systems that mediate these processes remain incompletely characterized. Some of the proposed mechanical signaling mechanisms have included microfatigue damage, stress-generated currents and potentials, hydrostatic pressure on the extracellular fluids under load, alterations

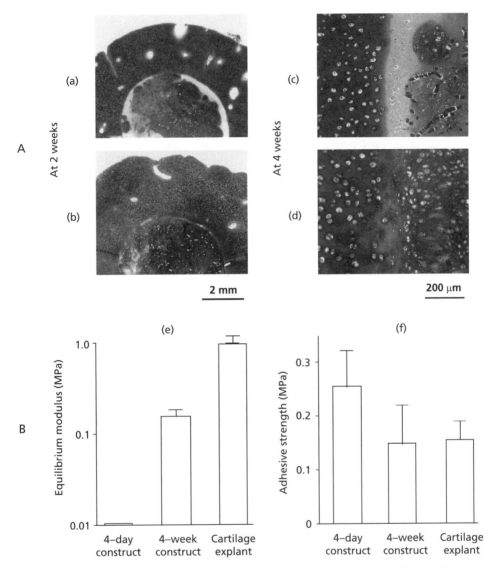

FIGURE 8-7. Integration of engineered cartilage. Discs of engineered cartilage (5 mm diameter x 2 mm thick) were sutured into rings of native cartilage (10/5 mm diameter x 2 mm thick) and cultured in bioreactors for 1–8 weeks. (**A**) Face sections of composites are shown after (**a, b**) 2 weeks of culture and (**c, d**) 4 weeks of culture; disc is in the center (a, c) and on the right (b, d). Stain: safranin-O/fast green. (**B**) Functional evaluation: (**e**) confined-compression equilibrium modulus of the discs at the time of construct preparation, and (**f**) adhesive strength of the integration interface (From Obradovic B, Martin I, Padera RF, et al. Integration of engineered cartilage. *J Orthop Res* 2001;19:1089–1097, with permission.)

in cell membrane diffusion due to direct load, stretch-activated membrane potentials, and the direct transduction of physical stresses via transmembrane proteins (32,39,44,50,57,108,116, 121,139,149,207,216,217,237,254).

Bone cells in various stages of differentiation have been shown to be highly responsive to mechanical stimulation *in vitro* and *in vivo*. Cyclic mechanical strains enhanced proliferation of *in vitro* cultured osteoblast cells and increased the production of type I collagen, but decreased the expression of osteocalcin and alkaline phosphatase (123,240), indicating delayed progression to a more mature osteoblastic phenotype.

Osteoblasts have also been shown to remodel their cytoskeleton, focal adhesions, and ECM—presumably in an effort to adapt to their perceived mechanical environment by altering the matrix attachment or orientation (168). Both osteoblasts and osteocytes responded to fluid shear *in vitro* by increasing production of nitric oxide (129,166), TGF$_\beta$1 (224), and prostaglandins (130). Even osteoclasts, whose response to various stimuli is often mediated by osteoblasts, have some degree of mechanoresponsiveness. Cyclic mechanical strain has been shown to either enhance or inhibit osteoclastogenesis in bone marrow cultures (218,219). Like articular cartilage, the mechanisms by which mechanical signals are perceived by bone cells, transduced into biochemical signaling cascades, and translated into specific patterns of gene expression remain a topic of intense investigation. It is clear, however, that successful tissue engineering of bone and cartilage will be dependent on an appropriate mechanical environment (*in vivo* or *in vitro*). It is likely that a balance or synergy between biological and mechanical stimuli will further enhance the effectiveness of tissue engineering strategies.

Loading regimes utilized in experimental studies in most cases only remotely mimic the complexity of joint loading *in vivo*. Articular cartilage is deformed as a result of the "rolling and sliding motion" of the joint (see Chapters 3 and 10 for more details), involving a combination of compressive, tensile, and shear stresses generating the pressure gradients for fluid motion (104,172,175) (also see Chapters 5 and 10 for more details). Notably, enhanced synthesis of proteoglycans in dynamically loaded cartilage correlated with the regions of physiologically high interstitial fluid flow (210). In a recent study, *in vitro* application of multidimensional strain that was designed to resemble the mechanical environment normally present in a human anterior cruciate ligament-directed human bone marrow cells to form ligament-like structures (4,5).

In addition, much of the information currently available on chondrocyte response to mechanical stress has been obtained either in explant cultures with fully developed cartilaginous matrix or in monolayer cultures of isolated cells, neither of which can adequately represent the cellular environment in the repair tissue. The lack of pericellular matrix during early stages of culture may have a particularly important influence on physical signals acting at the individual chondrocytes (98). Static and dynamic compression had little effect on chondrocytes in agarose gels early in culture, but affected synthesis rates of ECM by amounts that increased as more matrix deposited around the cells (35). The effects of the same load can thus be different for different areas of the same joint, young and old, healthy and damaged cartilage (255), and for different types and developmental stages of engineered tissues.

Studies of mechanical factors in tissue-engineered regeneration of cartilage and bone require utilization of physiologically relevant experimental models and loading regimes. These studies can be carried out on a variety of levels: from molecules to the cells, tissues, and whole joints (95), and there is generally a trade-off between the physiological relevance of the experimental situation and our ability to control the individual factors (95–98) (also see Chapter 6 for more details). Studies *in vivo* have the advantage of providing relevant loading conditions, local and systemic regulatory signals, but do not generally enable control of specific factors (e.g., loading history, levels of cytokines). As a result, it is difficult to eliminate confounding variables and to correlate specific aspects of loading to cell responses. *At the tissue level* (e.g., *in vitro* studies of native and engineered tissues), the loading conditions can be controlled but not necessarily in a way that enables distinguishing the individual effects of biophysical phenomena, and relating the measured effects to the situation *in vivo*. *At the cell level*, the individual stimuli can be precisely controlled (e.g., pH, strain) and their effects on cell function can be measured, but the physiological relevance of these studies can be limited (98). Experimental design is further complicated by interactions between physical signals associated with joint loading, genetic factors, and the soluble and matrix-immobilized regulatory molecules. The experiments conducted more than 40 years ago already suggested that mechanical factors (compression and stretch) and oxygen tension, acting in concert, can determine the type of connective tissue that differentiates in a culture of cells arising from bone (13).

4 CASE STUDIES

Three representative approaches to tissue engineering of cartilage and bone are described. The first case: *Cartilage tissue engineering by an integrated use of cells, biomaterial scaffolds, and bioreactors* demonstrates that immature but functional cartilaginous constructs can be engineered *in vitro* and used to repair osteochondral defects in animals. The second case: *Bone tissue engineering with the use of calcium phosphate cement* demonstrates the successful use of an osteoconductive biomaterial with no cells or biofactor delivery for bone regeneration in humans. The third case: *Bone tissue engineering utilizing local gene delivery* represents an example of *in situ* tissue engineering through the use of a carrier to deliver DNA and thereby promote *in vivo* transfection and expression of an osteoinductive factor.

4.1 Cartilage Tissue Engineering Using Cells, Biomaterial Scaffolds, and Bioreactors

One paradigm of tissue-engineered repair of articular cartilage involves cartilaginous constructs engineered *in vitro* using chondrogenic cells, biomaterial scaffolds and bioreactors, and implanted *in vivo* to undergo structural and functional maturation, and integrate with adjacent cartilage and subchondral bone. The construct structure, composition, and mechanical properties are characteristic of immature cartilage. The constructs have certain functionality at the time of implantation, as well as the capacity to further develop following implantation. An essential part of this paradigm is that the regulatory signals and local and systemic factors associated with physiological loading *in vivo*, will mediate construct remodeling into a tissue with structure, composition, and mechanical properties characteristic of adult articular cartilage.

To test this concept, large osteochondral defects in adult rabbits were repaired using composite grafts based on *in vitro* engineered cartilage (230). Articular chondrocytes were expanded in monolayers, seeded on fibrous PGA meshes, cultured for 4 to 6 weeks *in vitro*, sutured to a subchondral support (Collagraft®, Neucoll, Campbell, CA), with or without adsorbed autologous bone marrow, and press-fitted into 7 mm long × 5 mm wide × 5 mm deep osteochondral defects in knee joints of skeletally mature rabbits that were allowed free cage activity. Defects left empty and defects treated with cell-free PGA-Collagraft® scaffolds served as controls. Engineered constructs and the repair tissue were evaluated histologically, biochemically, and biomechanically (Young's moduli measured by indentation in intact joints).

At the time of implantation, constructs had wet weight fractions of CAGS and collagen that were respectively two-thirds and one-third those in adult cartilage, and equilibrium moduli that were one-fifth that of adult cartilage. Engineered cartilage allowed handling, withstood physiological loading immediately following implantation, and remodeled into osteochondral tissue with characteristic architectural features (Fig. 8-8a,c) and physiological composition and mechanical properties. After 6 months, defects implanted with engineered constructs repaired cartilaginous surface that had normal thickness and appearance and columnar arrangement of chondrocytes (see Fig. 8-8b), a tidemark at an appropriate depth, and new subchondral bone (see Fig. 8-8c). Regenerated cartilage had high and uniform concentrations of GAG (see Fig. 8-8b) and type II collagen (see Fig. 8-8d), in contrast to defects implanted with cell-free scaffolds or left untreated, which repaired with irregularly shaped fibrocartilage.

Repair tissues based on engineered cartilage (with or without adsorbed bone marrow within the subchondral support) had a Young's modulus comparable to that measured for unoperated age-matched controls. Integration with subchondral bone was excellent, whereas integration with cartilage was not consistently good. These results suggest that cartilage constructs engineered *in vitro* can provide a mechanically stable template that remodels into an osteochondral tissue that had physiological architecture,

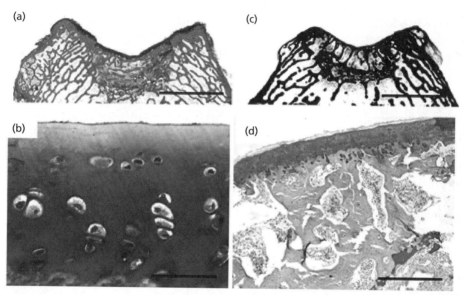

FIGURE 8-8. Tissue-engineered repair of large osteochondral defects in rabbits. Histological appearance of 6-month explants stained with **(a)** alcian blue and **(b)** toluidine blue; immunostained for **(c)** von Kossa and **(d)** type II collagen. The scale bars represent: (a, c) 5 mm; (b) 50 μm; (d) 200 μm. Engineered cartilage remodeled into osteochondral tissue with characteristic architectural features (a cartilaginous surface, a tidemark, new subchondral bone) and expressed characteristic molecular markers for hyaline cartilage and trabecular bone. (From Schaefer D, Martin I, Jundt G et al. Tissue engineered composites for the repair of large osteochondral defects. *Arthritis Rheum* 2002;46:2524–   ).

composition, and mechanical properties after 6 months *in vivo*. Further studies are needed to assess long-term results of this approach.

4.2 Bone Tissue Engineering with the Use of Calcium Phosphate Cement

A variety of calcium phosphate cements developed over the years have been shown to be osteoconductive and capable of obtaining substantial compressive strength (69). We conducted a study utilizing a calcium-deficient carbonated apatite originally produced by Norian Incorporated, Cupertino, California. This material had previously been demonstrated to have mechanical properties upon setting that were similar to those of human trabecular bone, and capable of being resorbed by osteoclasts and replaced by a newly formed bone.

This preclinical study was conducted using a large proximal tibial defect produced in adult mongrel male dogs. The defect was created by essentially resecting a 3.5-mm-thick slab of bone from the proximal tibial metaphyses. After removal of the bone, the calcium phosphate cement was injected until it completely filled the defect and the wounds closed. The cement sets at approximately 11 minutes and by 24 hours reaches 100% of its mechanical integrity. Because the inherent properties of the cement are equivalent to trabecular bone, no form of additional fixation was necessary postoperatively. The experimental design involved several groups of animals separated into times ranging from 24 hours to 16 weeks postoperative. Analysis included radiographic, biomechanical, and histologic analysis.

From a tissue engineering design perspective, this case represents the use of an osteoconductive material, which has initial mechanical properties similar to bone. The material is relatively easy to handle or sculpt surgically, and its biologic behavior was hypothesized to elicit a remodeling response over time with the expectation of being completely replaced by normal bone in the long term. Given these design and utilization parameters, the measures of success include rapid return of function of the animal,

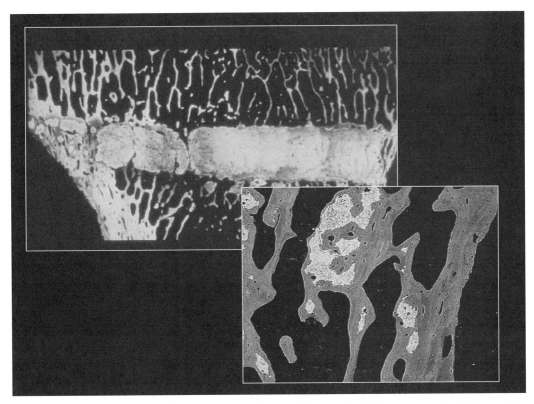

FIGURE 8-9. The efficacy of the calcium phosphate cement bone graft substitute was evaluated in a canine defect model. A 3.5-mm-thick slab of bone was removed from the proximal tibia and filled with the bone substitute. As demonstrated from this SEM image at low magnification 16 weeks postsurgery, the material was well incorporated with significant remodeling and replacement occurring in some regions (large image). At higher magnification (small image), the intimate relationship between the cement (white) and the bone (gray) can be visualized. Because this region was once completely filled with cement, the result of remodeling is illustrated (replacement of the cement with normal bone).

radiographic, and histologic evidence of integration with native bone tissue, resorption of the cement and subsequent replacement of normal bone over time, and biomechanical stability.

The results of the study demonstrated excellent biomechanical function throughout the life of the animals. By 2 weeks, significant integration with surrounding bone was observed as evidenced by bone formation on all exposed surfaces. By 16 weeks, as illustrated in Fig. 8-9, substantial regions of the material had been resorbed and replaced with the new bone, thereby forming an integrated composite of native bone tissue with the calcium phosphate cement.

These data strongly supported the efficacy of this material and, in fact, led to an eventual approval of the FDA for commercialization.

4.3 Bone Tissue Engineering Utilizing Local Gene Delivery

Numerous investigators successfully achieved bone healing of critical defects in animal studies, through the delivery of recombinant proteins that had previously been demonstrated to have osteoinductive properties. Despite these preclinical successes, a number of hurdles have delayed the introduction of these technologies into the clinic. An alternative approach to bone tissue engineering investigated by our research group involved delivering the DNA into a bone defect. The objective was to enable *in vivo* cell transfection that would result in the expression of bone-promoting factors by endogenous wound repair cells and promote robust bone formation.

The critical principles for this tissue engineering approach involve DNA delivery, *in vivo* transfection of the cells, production of the stimulatory proteins, bone formation, and integration with surrounding native tissue, at levels and with interactions sufficient to create biomechanically competent functional constructs.

A series of earlier studies demonstrated that the *in vivo* transfection could occur through delivery of the DNA with a number of carriers including type I collagen, various polymers and even calcium phosphate. For the purpose of demonstration, we present one of these studies that was focused on the clinical problem related to spine fusion procedures.

Spine fusions are performed each year for a variety of clinical conditions ranging from degenerative to traumatic injury. The use of bone grafts has been demonstrated to be critical in support of successful fusion. Unfortunately, the morbidity associated with acquiring autogenous bone graft and its limited volume has led to the need for bone graft substitute materials. This study was designed to test the efficacy of gene delivery from a bone graft substitute to augment spinal fusion. Specifically, lyophilized type I collagen was used as the carrier matrix for delivering plasmid DNA encoding several bone-promoting factors. The animal model involved a three-level fusion in sheep utilizing interbody fusion cages. The cages used in this study were cylindrical shells filled with the tissue-engineered constructs and laterally implanted between the prepared vertebral bodies. Because the cages provided stability by interlocking between adjacent vertebral bodies, no additional hardware was necessary to stabilize the spines of the animals. After surgical insertion, the animals were observed for a period of 12 weeks. The assessment included radiographs, biomechanical testing, and histologic analysis.

The study demonstrated that the collagen sponges with incorporated DNA were easily placed within the cages and implanted in the animals. Throughout the course of the study, all animals were stable and were observed to ambulate normally and with no restrictions. For the purposes of discussion, results from one of the groups will be demonstrated, involving the delivery of plasmid encoding a PTH_{1-34} hypothesized to be a moderately effective stimulant for bone formation. Biomechanical tests demonstrated solid fusions in all animals and the histologic results showed that greater than 95% of these constructs promoted substantial bone formation with complete integration with the surrounding bone and substantial bone throughout the cages. As illustrated in Fig. 8-10, the tissue-engineered constructs stimulated the formation of new bone that extended through the cage and integrated with the surrounding bone. Both the SEM imaging and biomechanical data demonstrated successful bone formation. Although the choice of the promoting factor was not evaluated for its optimality, this study demonstrated the potential for delivering biofactors through a local gene therapy approach. In this case, endogenous cells became "bioreactors" producing the protein of interest.

Although this approach to tissue engineering appears to be much more complicated than the use of a single biomaterial, it is expected that the rate and volume of bone produced, in particular in the more demanding and highly loaded circumstances, can be substantially increased by utilizing one or more carefully selected biofactors.

5   SUMMARY

The clinical demand for tissue-engineered cartilage and bone is already great, and continues to grow, reflecting our aging population with a demand for an increased quality of life and standard of care. The primary functions of these two tissues, which are biomechanical in nature, drive tissue engineering toward the restoration of the biomechanical function inherent for the tissue being replaced. The complex hierarchical organization of cartilage and bone, which varies with source, anatomical location, developmental stage, and pathology of the tissue, prescribes the functional properties at various scales, and at the same time can be altered in response to physical signals associated with loading. The current

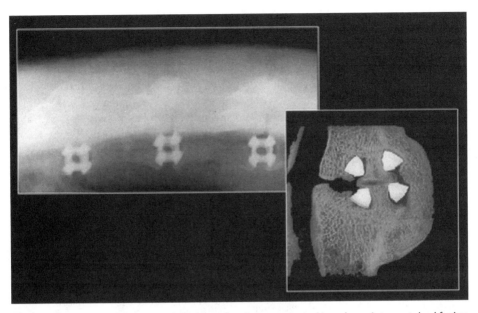

FIGURE 8-10. The Gene Activated Matrix technology was tested in a sheep intervertebral fusion model. As depicted in the radiograph, three levels of interbody fusions were performed in adult sheep using cylindrical interbody fusion cages. At 12 weeks, there was substantial infiltration of new bone formation within the cage as well as substantial anterior formation of bone outside the cage. This example demonstrates the potential of using localized delivery of a gene therapy for tissue engineering of bone (71,72).

paradigm is that the restoration of normal tissue function can be best achieved by using *in vitro* or *in vivo* engineered constructs that can regenerate the exact site-specific properties (molecular, structural, functional) of native cartilage and bone across different size scales.

Cells, biomaterial scaffolds, and regulatory factors (biochemical and physical) have been utilized in a variety of ways, *in vitro* (using bioreactors) and *in vivo* (implantation), to engineer functional cartilage and bone. At this time, there is no single optimal path for tissue-engineered repair of bone or cartilage. In a general case, the tissue engineering systems tend to recapitulate some aspects of the environment present *in vivo* during tissue development and thereby stimulate the cells to regenerate functional tissue structures. The presence of reparative cells, facilitated transport of chemical species, tissue regeneration template (scaffold), and physical regulatory signals are among common requirements for rapid and orderly tissue regeneration. However, cartilage tissue engineering has been

done both *in vitro* and *in vivo*, and it requires the addition of new cells, whereas bone tissue engineering has been done mostly *in vivo*, and in most cases has involved the use of biomaterials and biofactors without added cells.

To demonstrate the clinical value of a new therapeutic modality based on tissue-engineered cartilage or bone, one would need to document improved long-term clinical results as compared with natural healing and current treatment methods. For both tissues, the efforts are focused on promoting rapid, predictable, and mechanically competent repair. However, the specific criteria, experimental models, and evaluation methods for use in preclinical and clinical studies still need to be established. An evolving discipline called *functional tissue engineering* (FTE) is focused on the role of biomechanical factors in tissue regeneration, with an overall goal to develop rational design principles that can be used to guide orthopaedic tissue engineering. Some of the key principles identified so far include (a) definition of the functional properties of native tissues (for normal and pathological situations, and at various developmental stages); (b) selection and prioritization of the important requirements for engineered constructs and tissue regeneration; and (c) establishing standards for the evaluation of engineered constructs and tissue repair. The overview of representative tissue engineering studies, and the three case studies described in this chapter illustrate the current state of the art in FTE of cartilage and bone.

A chapter like this one, at this early stage of the development of orthopaedic tissue engineering, raises more questions than we can answer. Much more work needs to be done before tissue engineering can respond to all challenges of cartilage and bone loss, and offer new solutions to the problem. Some of the current research needs fall into three important categories: (a) experimental and modeling studies of tissue development (e.g., mechanotransduction in native and engineered tissues, mathematical models of tissue development, structure-function correlations, coordinated *in vitro*, animal and clinical studies), (b) new technologies (e.g., minimally invasive testing/monitoring methods, "custom-designed" scaffolds with incorporated genes and regulatory molecules, bioreactors with mechanical stimulation *in situ*, improved methods for autologous cell sourcing), and (c) methods and criteria for FTE (e.g., is the regeneration of exact tissue structure necessary, how much is enough, clinically relevant animal models, testing and evaluation methods).

It is hoped that the biomechanical principles of cartilage and bone tissue engineering discussed in this chapter in the context of clinical needs and the state of the art of FTE will help identify standards of success, assess progress in the field, and outline some of the scientific, engineering, and clinical research priorities in the field.

ACKNOWLEDGMENTS

Much of the work presented in this chapter has been supported by the National Aeronautics and Space Administration and the National Institutes of Health. One of the studies was funded by Selective Genetics Inc. (S.A. Goldstein is a founder and member of the Board of Directors of Selective Genetics and as such may benefit from the results of material presented). The authors would like to thank Dr. Farshid Guilak for his insightful comments and critical reading of the manuscript, and Sue Kangiser and Peggy Piech for their help with the manuscript preparation.

REFERENCES

1. Ahmad CS, Cohen ZA, Levine WN, et al. Biomechanical and topographic consideration for autologous osteochondral grafting in the knee. *Am J Sports Med* 2001;29:201–206.
2. Ahsan T, Sah RL. Biomechanics of integrative cartilage repair. *Osteoarthritis Cartilage* 1999;7:29–40.
3. Akizuki S, Mow VC, Muller F, et al. Tensile properties of human knee joint cartilage: I. Influence of ionic conditions, weight bearing, and fibrillation on the tensile modulus. *J Orthop Res* 1986;4:379–392.
4. Altman GH, Horan R, Martin I, et al. Cell differentiation by mechanical stress. *FASEB J* 2001;15:(10.1096/fj.01-0656fje).
5. Altman GH, Lu HH, Horan RL, et al. Advanced bioreactor with controlled application of multi-dimensional strain for tissue engineering. *J Biomech Eng* 2002;124:742–749.
6. An YH, Draughn RA, eds. *Mechanical testing of bone and the bone-implant interface.* Boca Raton: CRC Press; 1999:41–63.
7. Andrew JG, Hoyland J, Andrew SM, et al. Demonstration of TGF-beta 1 mRNA by in situ hybridization in normal human fracture healing. *Calcif Tissue Int* 1993;52:74–78.
8. Armstrong CG, Mow VC. Variations in the intrinsic mechanical properties of human articular cartilage with age, degeneration, and water content. *J Bone Joint Surg Am* 1982;44A:88–94.
9. Armstrong CG, Mow VC. Biomechanics of normal and osteoarthritic articular cartilage. In: Wilson PD, Straub LR, eds. *Clinical trends in orthopaedics.* New York: Thieme-Stratton, 1982:189–197.
10. Ateshian GA, Warden WH, Kim JJ, et al. Finite deformation biphasic material properties of bovine articular cartilage from confined compression experiments. *J Biomech* 1997;30:1157–1164.
11. Athanasiou K, Korvick D, Schenck R. Biodegradable implants for the treatment of osteochondral

defects in a goat model. *Tissue Eng* 1997;3:363–373.

12. Baltzer AWA, Lattermann C, Whalen JD, et al. Genetic enhancement of fracture repair: healing of an experimental segmental defect by adenoviral transfer of the BMP-2 gene. *Gene Ther* 2000;7:734–739.

13. Bassett CAL, Herrmann I. Influence of oxygen concentration and mechanical factors on differentiation of connective tissues in vitro. *Nature* 1961;190:460–461.

14. Blunk T, Sieminski AL, Gooch KJ, et al. Differential effects of growth factors on tissue-engineered cartilage. *Tissue Eng* 2002;8:73–84.

15. Boden SD. Bioactive factors for bone tissue engineering. *Clin Orthop* 1999;367S:S84–S94.

16. Bolander ME. Regulation of fracture repair and synthesis of matrix macromolecules. In: Brighton CT, Friedlaender GE, Lane JM, eds. *Bone formation and repair.* Rosemont, IL: AAOS, 1994:185–196.

17. Bonadio J, Smiley E, Patil P, et al. Localized, direct plasmid gene delivery in vivo: prolonged therapy results in reproducible tissue regeneration. *Nat Med* 1999;5:753–759.

18. Bonassar LJ, Grodzinsky AJ, Frank EH, et al. The effect of dynamic compression on the response of articular cartilage to insulin-like growth factor-I. *J Orthop Res* 2001;19:11–17.

19. Bostrom MPG, Boskey A, Kaufman JK, et al. Form and function of bone. In: Buckwalter JA, Einhorn TA, Simon SR, eds. *Orthopaedic basic science.* Rosemont, IL: American Academy of Orthopaedic Surgeons, 2000:319–369.

20. Botchwey EA, Pollack SR, Levine EM, et al. Bone tissue engineering in a rotating bioreactor using a microcarrier matrix system. *J Biomed Mater Res* 2001;55:242–253.

21. Bourque WT, Gross M, Hall BK. Expression of four growth factors during fracture repair. *Int J Dev Biol* 1993;37:573–579.

22. Braunstein EM, Goldstein SA, Kuhn JL, et al. Computed tomography and plain radiograph in experimental fracture healing. *Skeletal Radiol* 1986;15:27–31.

23. Breinan HA, Minas T, Hsu HP, et al. Effect of cultured autologous chondrocytes on repair of chondral defects in a canine model. *J Bone Joint Surg Am* 1997;79:1439–1451.

24. Breinan HA, Minas T, Hsu HP, et al. Autologous chondrocyte implantation in a canine model: change in composition of reparative tissue with time. *J Orthop Res* 2001;19:482–492.

25. Brighton CT, Heppenstall RB. Oxygen tension in zones of the epiphyseal plate, the metaphysis and diaphysis. *J Bone Joint Surg Am* 1971;53A:719–728.

26. Brittberg M, Lindahl A, Nilsson A, et al. Treatment of deep cartilage defects in the knee with autologous chondrocyte transplantation. *N Engl J Med* 1994;331:889–895.

27. Brittberg M, Nilsson A, Lindahl A, et al. Rabbit articular cartilage defects treated with autologous cultured chondrocytes. *Clin Orthop* 1996;326:270–283.

28. Brittberg M, Tallheden T, Sjogren-Jansson B, et al. Autologous chondrocytes used for articular cartilage repair: an update. *Clin Orthop* 2001;391 [Suppl]:S337–S348.

29. Brown TD, Shaw DT. In vitro contact stress distributions in the natural human hip. *J Biomech* 1983;16:373–384.

30. Buckwalter JA, Mankin HJ. Articular cartilage: degeneration and osteoarthritis, repair, regeneration, and transplantation. *Instr Course Lect* 1998;47:487–504.

31. Burg KJL, Porter S, Kellam JF. Biomaterial developments for bone tissue engineering. *Biomaterials* 2000;21:2347–2359.

32. Burr DB, Schaffler MB, Yang KH, et al. Skeletal change in response to altered strain environments: is woven bone a response to elevated strain? *Bone* 1989;10:223–233.

33. Bursac PM. Collagen network contributions to structure-function relationships in cartilaginous tissues in compression. Ph.D. Thesis. Boston, MA: Boston University; 2001.

34. Buschmann MD, Gluzband YA, Grodzinsky AJ, et al. Chondrocytes in agarose culture synthesize a mechanically functional extracellular matrix. *J Orthop Res* 1992;10:745–758.

35. Buschmann MD, Gluzband YA, Grodzinsky AJ, et al. Mechanical compression modulates matrix biosynthesis in chondrocyte/agarose culture. *J Cell Sci* 1995;108:1497–1508.

36. Butnariu-Ephrat M, Robinson D, Mendes DG, et al. Resurfacing of goat articular cartilage from chondrocytes derived from bone marrow. *Clin Orthop* 1996;330:234–243.

37. Caplan AI, Bruder SP. Cell and molecular engineering of bone regeneration. In: Lanza R, Chick W, Langer R, eds. *Textbook of tissue engineering.* Springer, NY: Landes Co., 1996:599–614.

38. Caplan AI, Elyaderani M, Mochizuki Y, et al. Principles of cartilage repair and regeneration. *Clin Orthop* 1997;342:254–269.

39. Carter DR. Mechanical loading history and skeletal biology. *J Biomech* 1987;20:1095–1109.

40. Carver SE, Heath CA. Influence of intermittent pressure, fluid flow, and mixing on the regenerative properties of articular chondrocytes. *Biotechnol Bioeng* 1999;65:274–281.

41. Carver SE, Heath CA. Increasing extracellular matrix production in regenerating cartilage with intermittent physiological pressure. *Biotechnol Bioeng* 1999;62:166–174.

42. Carver SE, Heath CA. Semi-continuous perfusion system for delivering intermittent physiological pressure to regenerating cartilage. *Tissue Eng* 1999;5:1–11.

43. Chapman MW, Bucholz R, Cornell C. Treatment of acute fractures with a collagen-calcium phosphate graft material. *J Bone Joint Surg Am* 1997;79-A:495–502.

44. Cheal EJ, Snyder BD, Nunamker DM, et al. Trabecular bone remodeling around smooth and porous implants in an equine patellar model. *J Biomech* 1987;20:1121–1134.

45. Chen AC, Nagrampa JP, Schinagl RM, et al. Chondrocyte transplantation to articular cartilage explants in vitro. *J Orthop Res* 1997;15:791–802.

46. Chen AC, Bae WC, Schinagl RM, et al. Depth-and strain-dependent mechanical and electromechanical properties of full-thickness bovine articular cartilage in confined compression. *J Biomech* 2001;34:1–12.

47. Cherry RS, Papoutsakis T. Physical mechanisms of cell damage in microcarrier cell culture bioreactors. *Biotechnol Bioeng* 1988;32:1001–1014.

48. Chu C, Dounchis JS, Yoshioka M, et al. Osteochondral repair using perichondrial cells: a 1 year study in rabbits. *Clin Orthop* 1997;340:220–229.

49. Chu CR, Coutts RD, Yoshioka M, et al. Articular cartilage repair using allogeneic perichondrocyte-seeded biodegradable porous polylactic acid (PLA): a tissue-engineering study. *J Biomed Mater Res* 1995;29:1147–1154.

50. Churches AE, Howlett CR, Waldron KS, et al. The response of living bone to controlled time varying loading: method and preliminary results. *J Biomech* 1979;12:35–45.

51. Ciarelli MJ, Goldstein S, Kuhn JL, et al. The orthogonal mechanical properties and density of human trabecular bone from the major metaphyseal regions utilizing materials testing and computed tomography. *J Orthop Res* 1991;9:674–682.

52. Clift R, Grace JR, Weber MF. *Bubbles, drops, and particles.* New York: Academic Press; 1978:16–29, 97–105,142–148.

53. Cody DD, Goldstein SA, Flynn MJ. Correlations between vertebral regional bone mineral density and whole bone fracture load. *Spine* 1991;16:146–154.

54. Cody DD, McCubbrey DA, Divine GW, et al. Predictive value of proximal femoral bone densitometry in determining local orthogonal material properties. *J Biomech* 1996;29:753–762.

55. Connolly JF, Guse R, Tiedeman J, et al. Autologous marrow injection for delayed unions of the tibia: a preliminary report. *J Orthop Trauma* 1989;3:276–282.

56. Cook SD, Baffes GC, Wolfe MW, et al. The effect of recombinant human osteogenic protein-1 on healing of large segmental bone defects. *J Bone Joint Surg Am* 1994;76-A:827–838.

57. Cowin SC, Moss-Salentijn L, Moss ML. Candidates for the mechanosensory system in bone. *J Biomech Eng* 1991;113:191–197.

58. Davisson T, Kunig S, Chen A, et al. Static and dynamic compression modulate matrix metabolism in tissue engineered cartilage. *J Orthop Res* 2002;20:842–848.

59. De Bruijn JD, Van Den Brink I, Menders S, et al. Bone induction by implants coated with cultured osteogenic bone marrow cells. *Adv Dent Res* 1999;13:74–81.

60. DiMicco MA, Sah RL. Integrative cartilage repair: adhesive strength correlates with collagen deposition. *J Orthop Res* 2001;19:1105–1112.

61. Duda GN, Haisch A, Endres M, et al. Mechanical quality of tissue engineered cartilage: results after 6 and 12 weeks in vivo. *J Biomed Mater Res* 2000;53:673–677.

62. Dunkelman NS, Zimber MP, Lebaron RG, et al. Cartilage production by rabbit articular chondrocytes on polyglycolic acid scaffolds in a closed bioreactor system. *Biotechnol Bioeng* 1995;46:299–305.

63. Einhorn TA. Enhancement of fracture healing by molecular or physical means: an overview. In: Brighton CT, Friedlaender G, Lane JM, eds. *Bone formation and repair.* Rosemont, IL: American Academy of Orthopaedic Surgeons, 1994:223–238.

64. Einhorn TA. The cell and molecular biology of fracture healing. *Clin Orthop* 1998;355S:S7–S21.

65. El-Amin SF, Attawia M, Lu HH, et al. Integrin expression by human osteoblasts cultured on degradable polymeric materials applicable for tissue engineered bone. *J Orthop Res* 2002;20:20–28.

66. Elder SH, Kimura JH, Soslowsky LJ, et al. Effect of compressive loading on chondrocyte differentiation in agarose cultures of chick limb-bud cells. *J Orthop Res* 2000;18:78–86.

67. Elder SH, Goldstein SA, Kimura JH, et al. Chondrocyte differentiation is modulated by frequency and duration of cyclic compressive loading. *Ann Biomed Eng* 2001;29:476–482.

68. Fedewa MM, Oegema TR Jr, Schwartz MH, et al. Chondrocytes in culture produce a mechanically functional tissue. *J Orthop Res* 1998;16:227–236.

69. Frankenburg EP, Goldstein SA, Bauer TW, et al. Biomechanical and histological evaluation of a calcium phosphate cement. *J Bone Joint Surg Am* 1998;80:1112–1124.

70. Freed LE, Grande DA, Lingbin Z, et al. Joint resurfacing using allograft chondrocytes and synthetic biodegradable polymer scaffolds. *J Biomed Mater Res* 1994;28:891–899.

71. Freed LE, Marquis JC, Vunjak-Novakovic G, et al. Composition of cell-polymer cartilage implants. *Biotechnol Bioeng* 1994;43:605–614.

72. Freed LE, Vunjak-Novakovic G, Biron R, et al. Biodegradable polymer scaffolds for tissue engineering. *Biotechnol* 1994;12:689–693.

73. Freed LE, Vunjak-Novakovic G. Cultivation of cell-polymer constructs in simulated microgravity. *Biotechnol Bioeng* 1995;46:306–313.

74. Freed LE, Langer R, Martin I, et al. Tissue engineering of cartilage in space. *Proc Natl Acad Sci U S A* 1997;94:13885–13890.

75. Freed LE, Hollander AP, Martin I, et al. Chondrogenesis in a cell-polymer-bioreactor system. *Exp Cell Res* 1998;240:58–65.

76. Freed LE, Vunjak-Novakovic G. Tissue engineering bioreactors. In: Lanza RP, Langer R, Vacanti J, eds. *Principles of tissue engineering,* 2nd ed. San Diego: Academic Press, 2000:143–156.

77. Freed LE, Vunjak-Novakovic G. Tissue engineering of cartilage. In: Bronzino JD, ed. *The biomedical engineering handbook,* 2nd ed. Boca Raton: CRC Press, 2000:124–126.

78. Frenkel SR, Toolan B, Menche D, et al. Chondrocyte transplantation using a collagen bilayer matrix for cartilage repair. *J Bone Joint Surg Br* 1997;79:831–836.

79. Friedlaender GE, Perry CR, Cole JD, et al. Osteogenic protein-1 (bone morphogenetic protein-7) in the treatment of tibial nonunions. *J Bone Joint Surg Am* 2001;83-A [Suppl 1]:S151–S158.

80. Froimson MI, Ratcliffe A, Gardner TR, et al. Differences in patellofemoral joint cartilage material properties and their significance in the etiology of cartilage surface fibrillations. *Osteoarthritis Cartilage* 1997;5:377–386.

81. Frost HM. The biology of fracture healing. An overview for clinicians. Part I. *Clin Orthop* 1989; 248:283–293.

82. Frost HM. The biology of fracture healing. An overview for clinicians. Part II. *Clin Orthop* 1989;248:294–309.

83. Garcia AJ, Ducheyne P, Boettiger D. Effect of surface reaction stage on fibronectin-mediated adhesion of osteoblast-like cells to bioactive glass. *J Biomed Mater Res* 1998;40:48–56.

84. Glüer C-C, Wu CY, Jergas M, et al. Three quantitative ultrasound parameters reflect bone structure. *Calcif Tissue Int* 1994;55:46–52.

85. Goldstein SA. The mechanical properties of trabecular bone: dependence on anatomic location and function. *J Biomech* 1987;20:1055–1061.

86. Goldstein SA, Bonadio J. Potential role for direct gene transfer in the enhancement of fracture healing. *Clin Orthop* 1998;355S:S154–S162.

87. Gooch KJ, Blunk T, Courter DL, et al. IGF-I and mechanical environment interact to modulate engineered cartilage development. *Biochem Biophys Res Commun* 2001;286:909–915.

88. Gooch KJ, Kwon JH, Blunk T, et al. Effects of mixing intensity on tissue-engineered cartilage. *Biotechnol Bioeng* 2001;72:402–407.

89. Gorski JP. Is all bone the same? Distinctive distributions and properties of non-collagenous matrix proteins in lamellar vs. woven bone imply the existence of different underlying osteogenic mechanisms. *Crit Rev Oral Biol Med* 1998;9:201.

90. Grande DA, Pitman MI, Peterson L, et al. The repair of experimentally produced defects in rabbit articular cartilage by autologous chondrocyte transplantation. *J Orthop Res* 1989;7:208–218.

91. Grande DA, Southerland SS, Manji R, et al. Repair of articular cartilage defects using mesenchymal stem cells. *Tissue Eng* 1995;1:345–353.

92. Grande DA, Halberstadt C, Naughton G, et al. Evaluation of matrix scaffolds for tissue engineering of articular cartilage grafts. *J Biomed Mater Res* 1997;34:211–220.

93. Grande DA, Athanasiou K, Schwartz R. Matrix engineering for repair of articular cartilage defects. *Trans Orthop Res Soc.* New Orleans, LA: 1998;23:801.

94. Grande DA, Breitbart AS, Mason J, et al. Cartilage tissue engineering: current limitations and solutions. *Clin Orthop* 1999;367 Suppl:S176–S185.

95. Guilak F, Sah RL, Setton LA. Physical regulation of cartilage metabolism. In: Mow VC, Hayes WC, eds. *Basic orthopaedic biomechanics.* Philadelphia: Lippincott-Raven Publishers, 1997:179–207.

96. Guilak F, Mow VC. The mechanical environment of the chondrocyte: a biphasic finite element model of cell-matrix interactions in articular cartilage. *J Biomech* 2000;33:1663–1673.

97. Guilak F, Butler DL, Goldstein SA. Functional tissue engineering: the role of biomechanics in articular cartilage repair. *Clin Orthop* 2001;391 [Suppl]:S295–S305.

98. Guilak F, Setton LA. Functional tissue engineering and the role of biomechanical signaling in articular cartilage repair. In: Guilak F, Butler D, Mooney D, et al., eds. *Functional tissue engineering: the role of biomechanics.* New York: Springer-Verlag, 2003:277–290.

99. Hadhazy C, Varga S. Studies on cartilage formation XIX. Oxygen and glucose supply of the regenerating articular surface. *Acta Biologica* 1976;27:215–230.

100. Hale JE, Rudert MJ, Brown TD. Indentation assessment of biphasic mechanical property deficit in size-dependent osteochondral defect repair. *J Biomech* 1993;26:1319–1325.

101. Hansen U, Schunke M, Domm C, et al. Combination of reduced oxygen tension and intermittent hydrostatic pressure: a useful tool in articular cartilage tissue engineering. *J Biomech* 2001;34:941–949.

102. Hauselmann HJ, Fernandes RJ, Mok SS et al. Phenotypic stability of bovine articular chondrocytes after long-term culture in alginate beads. *J Cell Sci* 1994;107:17–27.

103. Haynesworth SE, Reuben D, Caplan AI. Cell-based tissue engineering therapies: the influence of whole body physiology. *Adv Drug Deliv Rev* 1998;33:3–14.

104. Heath CA, Magari R. Mini-review: mechanical factors affecting cartilage regeneration in vitro. *Biotechnol Bioeng* 1996;50:430–437.

105. Heath CA. The effects of physical forces on cartilage tissue engineering. *Biotechnol Genet Eng Rev* 2000;17:533–551.

106. Hendrickson DA, Nixon AJ, Grande DA, et al. Chondrocyte-fibrin matrix transplants for resurfacing extensive articular cartilage defects. *J Orthop Res* 1994;12:485–497.

107. Herbage D, Bouillet J, Bernengo JC. Biochemical and physiochemical characterization of pepsin-solubilized type-II collagen from bovine articular cartilage. *Biochem J* 1977;161:303–312.

108. Hert J, Pribylova E, Liskova M. Reaction of bone to mechanical stimuli. *Acta Anat (Basel)* 1972;82:218–230.

109. Hodge WA, Carlson KL, Fijan RS, et al. Contact pressures from an instrumented hip endoprosthesis. *J Bone Joint Surg Am* 1989;71:1378–1386.

110. Hoffler CE, McCreadie BR, Smith EA, et al. A hierarchical approach to exploring bone mechanical properties. In: An YH, Draughn RA, eds. *Mechanical testing of bone and the bone-implant interface*. Boca Raton: CRC Press, 2000:133–149.

111. Hollander AP, Heathfield TF, Webber C, et al. Increased damage to type II collagen in osteoarthritic articular cartilage detected by a new immunoassay. *J Clin Invest* 1994;93:1722–1732.

112. Holy CE, Shoichet MS, Davies JE. Engineering three-dimensional bone tissue in vitro using biodegradable scaffolds: investigating initial cell-seeding density and culture period. *J Biomed Mater Res* 2000;51:376–382.

113. Hung CT, Lima EG, Mauck RL, et al. Anatomically shaped osteochondral constructs for articular cartilage repair. *J Biomech* (in press).

114. Hunziker EB, Kapfinger E. Removal of proteoglycans from the surface of defects in articular cartilage transiently enhances coverage by repair cells. *J Bone Joint Surg Br* 1998;80B:144–150.

115. Hunziker EB. Biologic repair of articular cartilage. Defect models in experimental animals and matrix requirements. *Clin Orthop* 1999;367[S]:S135–S146.

116. Ingber DE, Dike L, Hansen L, et al. Cellular tensegrity: exploring how mechanical changes in the cytoskeleton regulate cell growth, migration, and tissue pattern during morphogenesis. *Int Rev Cytol* 1994;150:173–224.

117. International Cartilage Repair Society. Injury Evaluation Package. In: http://www.cartilage.org/; 2000.

118. Jackson DW, Simon TM. Tissue engineering principles in orthopaedic surgery. *Clin Orthop* 1999;367 [Suppl]:S31–S45.

119. Johnson EE, Urist MR, Finerman GAM. Distal metaphyseal tibial nonunion: deformity and bone loss treated by open reduction, internal fixation, and human bone morphogenetic protein (hBMP). *Clin Orthop* 1990;250:234–240.

120. Johnstone B, Hering TM, Caplan AI, et al. In vitro chondrogenesis of bone marrow-derived mesenchymal progenitor cells. *Exp Cell Res* 1998; 238:265–272.

121. Jones DB, Holte H, Scholubbers J-G, et al. Biochemical signal transduction of mechanical strain in osteoblast-like cells. *Biomaterials* 1991;12:101–110.

122. Joyce ME, Terek RM, Jingushi S, et al. Role of transforming growth factor-beta in fracture repair. *Ann N Y Acad Sci* 1990;593:107–123.

123. Kaspar D, Seidl W, Neidlinger-Wilke C, et al. Dynamic cell stretching increases human osteoblast proliferation of CICP synthesis but decreases osteocalcin synthesis and alkaline phosphatase activity. *J Biomech* 2000;33:45–51.

124. Kawamura S, Wakitani S, Kimura T, et al. Articular cartilage repair-rabbit experiments with a collagen gel-biomatrix and chondrocytes cultured in it. *Acta Orthop Scand* 1998;69:56–62.

125. Kempson GE. Mechanical properties of articular cartilage. In: Freeman MAR, ed. *Adult articular cartilage*. Kent, England: Pitman Medical, 1979:333–414.

126. Kempson GE. Age-related changes in the tensile properties of human articular cartilage: a comparative study between the femoral head of the hip joint and the talus of the ankle joint. *Biochim Biophys Acta* 1991;1075:223–230.

127. Kirker-Head CA, Gerhart TN, Armstrong R, et al. Healing bone using recombinant human bone morphogenetic protein 2 and copolymer. *Clin Orthop* 1998;349:205–217.

128. Kitano T, Ateshian GA, Mow VC, et al. Constituents and pH changes in protein rich hyaluronan solution affect the biotribological properties of artificial articular joints. *J Biomech* 2001;34:1031–1037.

129. Klein-Nulend J, Van Der Plas A, Semeins CM, et al. Sensitivity of osteocytes to biomechanical stress in vitro. *FASEB J* 1995;9:441–445.

130. Klein-Nulend J, Burger EH, Semeins CM, et al. Pulsating fluid flow stimulated prostaglandin release and inducible prostaglandin G/H synthase mRNA expression in primary mouse bone cells. *J Bone Miner Res* 1997;12:45–51.

131. Klisch SM, diMicco MA, Hoger A, et al. Bioengineering the growth of articular cartilage. In: Guilak F, Butler D, Mooney D, eds. *Functional tissue engineering: the role of biomechanics*. New York: Springer-Verlag, 2003:194–210.

132. Kusumoto K, Bessho K, Fujimura K, et al. Self-regenerating bone implant: ectopic osteoinduction following intramuscular implantation of a combination of rhBMP-2, atelopeptide type I collagen

and porous hydroxyapatite. *J Craniomaxillofac Surg* 1996;24:360–365.

133. Kwan MK, Coutts RD, Woo SL, et al. Morphological and biomechanical evaluations of neocartilage from the repair of full-thickness articular cartilage defects using rib perichondrium autografts: a long-term study. *J Biomech* 1989;22:921–930.

134. Kwan MK, Lai WM, Mow VC. A finite deformation theory for cartilage and other soft hydrated connective tissues–I. Equilibrium results. *J Biomech* 1990;23:145–155.

135. Lai WM, Mow VC. Drag-induced compression of articular cartilage during a permeation experiment. *Biorheology* 1980;17:111–123.

136. Lai WM, Mow VC, Roth V. Effects of nonlinear strain-dependent permeability and rate of compression on the stress behavior of articular cartilage. *J Biomech Eng* 1981;103:61–66.

137. Lai WM, Hou JS, Mow VC. A triphasic theory for the swelling and deformation behaviors of articular cartilage. *J Biomech Eng* 1991;113:245–258.

138. Lai WM, Mow VC, Sun DD, et al. On the electric potentials inside a charged soft hydrated biological tissue: streaming potential vs. diffusion potential. *J Biomech Eng* 2000;122:336–346.

139. Lanyon LE. Functional strain in bone tissue as an objective, and controlling stimulus for adaptive bone remodelling. *J Biomech* 1987;20:1083–1093.

140. LeBaron RG, Athanasiou KA. Ex vivo synthesis of articular cartilage. *Biomaterials* 2000;21:2575–2587.

141. Lee DA, Bader DL. Compressive strains at physiological frequencies influence the metabolism of chondrocytes seeded in agarose. *J Orthop Res* 1997;15:181–188.

142. Lee KY, Alsberg E, Mooney DJ. Degradable and injectable poly(aldehyde glucuronate) hydrogels for bone tissue engineering. *J Biomed Mater Res* 2001;56:228–233.

143. Li R-K, Yau TM, Weisel RD, et al. Construction of a bioengineered cardiac graft. *J Thorac Cardiovasc Surg* 2000;119:368–375.

144. Lieberman JR, Le LQ, Wu L, et al. Regional gene therapy with a BMP-2 producing murine stromal cell line induces hetrotopic and orthotopic bone formation in rodents. *J Orthop Res* 1998;16:330–339.

145. Liljensten EL, Attaelmanan AG, Larsson C, et al. Hydroxyapatite granule/carrier composites promote new bone formation in cortical defects. *Clin Implant Dent Relat Res* 2000;2:50–59.

146. Lipshitz H, Etheredge R, III Glimcher MJ. Changes in the hexosamine content and swelling ratio of articular cartilage as functions of depth from the surface. *J Bone Joint Surg Am* 1976; 58:1149–1153.

147. Ma PX, Schloo B, Mooney D, et al. Development of biomechanical properties and morphogenesis of

in vitro tissue engineered cartilage. *J Biomed Mater Res* 1995;29:1587–1595.

148. Ma PX, Zhang R, Xiao G, et al. Engineering new bone tissue in vitro on highly porous poly (a-hydroxyl acids)/hydroxyapatite composite scaffolds. *J Biomed Mater Res* 2001;54:284–293.

149. MacGinitie LA, Seiz KG, Otter MW, et al. Streaming potential measurements at low ionic concentrations reflect bone microstructure. *J Biomech* 1994;27:969–978.

150. Madry H, Padera R, Seidel J, et al. Tissue engineering of cartilage enhanced by the transfer of a human insulin-like growth factor-I gene. *Transactions of the annual meeting of the Orthopaedic Research Society*, San Francisco, 2001;26:289.

151. Madry H, Padera R, Seidel J, et al. Gene transfer of a human insulin-like growth factor I cDNA enhances tissue engineering of cartilage. *Hum Gene Ther* 2002;13:1621–1630.

152. Majumdar S, Bay BK, eds. Noninvasive assessment of trabecular bone architecture and the competence of bone. *Adv Exp Med Biol 496.* 2001;63–83, 95–97.

153. Maroudas A. Physiochemical properties of articular cartilage. In: Freeman MAR, ed. *Adult articular cartilage, 2nd ed.* London: Pitman Medical, 1979:215–290.

154. Maroudas AI. Balance between swelling pressure and collagen tension in normal and degenerate cartilage. *Nature* 1976;260:808–809.

155. Marra KG, Szem JW, Kumta PN, et al. In vitro analysis of biodegradable polymer blend/ hydroxyapatite composites for bone tissue engineering. *J Biomed Mater Res* 1999;47:324–335.

156. Martin I, Padera RF, Vunjak-Novakovic G, et al. In vitro differentiation of chick embryo bone marrow stromal cells into cartilaginous and bone-like tissues. *J Orthop Res* 1998;16:181–189.

157. Martin I, Obradovic B, Freed LE, et al. A method for quantitative analysis of glycosaminoglycan distribution in cultured natural and engineered cartilage. *Ann Biomed Eng* 1999;27:656–662.

158. Martin I, Vunjak-Novakovic G, Yang J, et al. Mammalian chondrocytes expanded in the presence of fibroblast growth factor-2 maintain the ability to differentiate and regenerate three-dimensional cartilaginous tissue. *Exp Cell Res* 1999;253:681–688.

159. Martin I, Obradovic B, Treppo S, et al. Modulation of the mechanical properties of tissue engineered cartilage. *Biorheology* 2000;37:141–147.

160. Martin I, Suetterlin R, Baschong W, et al. Enhanced cartilage tissue engineering by sequential exposure of chondrocytes to FGF-2 during 2D expansion and BMP-2 during 3D cultivation. *J Cell Biochem* 2001;83:121–128.

161. Märtson M, Viljanto J, Hurme T, et al. Biocompatibility of cellulose sponge with bone. *Eur Surg Res* 1998;30:426–432.

162. Matsumoto K, Matsunaga S, Imamura T, et al. Expression and distribution of transforming growth factor-beta and decorin during fracture healing. *In Vivo* 1994;8:215–219.

163. Mauck RL, Soltz MA, Wang CCB, et al. Functional tissue engineering of articular cartilage through dynamic loading of chondrocyte-seeded agarose gels. *J Biomech Eng* 2000;122:252–260.

164. Mauck RL, Seyhan SL, Ateshian GA, et al. Influence of seeding density and dynamic deformational loading on the developing structure/function relationships of chondrocyte-seeded agarose hydrogels. *Ann Biomed Eng* 2002;30:1046–1056.

165. Mauck RL, Nicoll SB, Seyhan SL, et al. Synergistic action of growth factors and dynamic loading for articular cartilage tissue engineering. *Tissue Eng* 2003;9:597–611.

166. McAllister TN, Frangos JA. Steady and transient fluid shear stress stimulate NO release in osteoblasts through distinct biochemical pathways. *J Bone Miner Res* 1999;14:930–936.

167. McKibbin B. The biology of fracture healing in long bones. *J Bone Joint Surg Br* 1978;60B:150–162.

168. Meazzini MC, Toma CS, Schaffer JL, et al. Osteoblast cytoskeletal modulation in response to mechanical strain in vitro. *J Orthop Res* 1998;16:170–180.

169. Messner K, Gillquist J. Cartilage repair: a critical review. *Acta Orthop Scand* 1996;67:523–529.

170. Messner K, Maletius W. The long-term prognosis for severe damage to weight-bearing cartilage in the knee: a 14-year clinical and radiographic follow-up in 28 young athletes. *Acta Orthop Scand* 1996;67:165–168.

171. Mow VC, Kuei SC, Lai WM, et al. Biphasic creep and stress relaxation of articular cartilage in compression: theory and experiments. *J Biomech Eng* 1980;102:73–84.

172. Mow VC, Holmes MH, Lai WM. Fluid transport and mechanical properties of articular cartilage. *J Biomech* 1984;17:377–394.

173. Mow VC, Ratcliffe A, Rosenwasser MP, et al. Experimental studies on the repair of large osteochondral defects at a high weight bearing area of the knee joint: a tissue engineering study. *Trans Am Soc Mech Eng* 1991;113:198–207.

174. Mow VC, Ratcliffe A, Poole AR. Cartilage and diarthrodial joints as paradigms for hierarchical materials and structures. *Biomaterials* 1992;13:67–97.

175. Mow VC, Ratcliffe A. Structure and function of articular cartilage and meniscus. In: Mow VC, Hayes WC, eds. *Basic orthopaedic biomechanics*, 2nd ed. Philadelphia: Lippincott-Raven, 1997:113–177.

176. Mow VC, Ateshian GA, Lai WM, et al. Effects of fixed charges on the stress-relaxation behavior of hydrated soft tissues in a confined compression problem. *Int J Solids Struct* 1998;35:4945–4962.

177. Mow VC, Wang CB, Hung CT. The extracellular matrix, interstitial fluid and ions as a mechanical signal transducer in articular cartilage. *Osteoarthritis Cartilage* 1999;7:41–58.

178. Mow VC, Wang CC. Some bioengineering considerations for tissue engineering of articular cartilage. *Clin Orthop* 1999;367 [Suppl]:S204–S223.

179. Mow VC, Guo XE. Mechano-electrochemical properties of articular cartilage: their inhomogenieties and anisotropics. *Annu Rev Biomed Eng* 2002;4:175–209.

180. Nakase T, Nomura S, Yoshikawa H, et al. Transient and localized expression of bone morphogenetic protein 4 messenger RNA during fracture healing. *J Bone Miner Res* 1994;9:651–659.

181. Nehrer S, Breinan HA, Ramappa A, et al. Chondrocyte-seeded collagen matrices implanted in a chondral defect in a canine model. *Biomaterials* 1998;19:2313–2328.

182. Neitzel GP, Nerem RM, Sambanis A, et al. Cell function and tissue growth in bioreactors: fluid mechanical and chemical environments. *J Jpn Soc Microgr Appl* 1998;15:602–607.

183. Newman AP. Articular cartilage repair. *Am J Sports Med* 1998;26:309–324.

184. Niederauer GG, Slivka MA, Leatherbury NC, et al. Evaluation of multiphase implants for repair of focal osteochondral defects in goats. *Biomaterials* 2000;21:2561–2574.

185. Nixon AJ, Fortier LA, Williams J, et al. Enhanced repair of extensive articular defects by insulin-like growth factor-I-laden fibrin composites. *J Orthop Res* 1999;17:475–487.

186. Obradovic B, Carrier RL, Vunjak-Novakovic G, et al. Gas exchange is essential for bioreactor cultivation of tissue engineered cartilage. *Biotechnol Bioeng* 1999;63:197–205.

187. Obradovic B, Martin I, Padera RF, et al. Integrative potential of tissue engineered cartilage: bioreactor studies. *46th Transactions of the Orthopaedic Research Society,* Orlando, FL, 2000;25:616.

188. Obradovic B, Meldon JH, Freed LE, et al. Glycosaminoglycan deposition in engineered cartilage: Experiments and mathematical model. *AIChE J* 2000;46:1860–1871.

189. Obradovic B, Martin I, Padera RF, et al. Integration of engineered cartilage. *J Orthop Res* 2001;19:1089–1097.

190. O'Driscoll S. The healing and regeneration of articular cartilage. *J Bone Joint Surg Am* 1998;80-A:1795–1812.

191. O'Driscoll SW, Kumar A, Salter RB. The effect of the volume of effusion, joint position and continuous passive motion on intraarticular pressure in the rabbit knee. *J Rheumatol* 1983;10:360–363.

192. O'Driscoll SW, Salter RB. The induction of neochondrogenesis in free intra-articular periosteal autografts under the influence of continuous passive motion: an experimental study in the rabbit. *J Bone Joint Surg Am* 1984;66A:1248–1257.

193. O'Driscoll SW, Salter RB. The repair of major osteochondral defects in joint surfaces by neochondrogenesis with autogenous osteoperiosteal grafts stimulated by continuous passive motion. An experimental investigation in the rabbit. *Clin Orthop* 1986;208:131–140.

194. O'Driscoll SW, Fitsimmons JS, Commisso CN. Role of oxygen tension during cartilage formation by periosteum. *J Orthop Res* 1997;15:682–687.

195. O'Driscoll SW. Articular cartilage regeneration using periosteum. *Clin Orthop* 1999;367S:S186–S203.

196. O'Driscoll SW. Preclinical cartilage repair: current status and future perspectives. *Clin Orthop* 2001;391 Suppl:S397–S401.

197. Pazzano D, Mercier KA, Moran JM, et al. Comparison of chondrogenesis in static and perfused bioreactor culture. *Biotechnol Prog* 2000;16:893–896.

198. Pei M, Seidel J, Vunjak-Novakovic G, et al. Growth factors for sequential cellular de- and redifferentiation in tissue engineering. *Biochem Biophys Res Commun* 2002;294:149–154.

199. Pei M, Solchaga LA, Seidel J, et al. Bioreactors mediate the effectiveness of tissue engineering scaffolds. *FASEB J* 2002;16:1691–1694.

200. Peretti GM, Bonassar LJ, Caruso EM, et al. Biomechanical analysis of a chondrocyte-based repair model of articular cartilage. *Tissue Eng* 1999;5:317–326.

201. Peretti GM, Randolph MA, Zaporojan V, et al. A biomechanical analysis of an engineered cell-scaffold implant for cartilage repair. *Ann Plast Surg* 2001;46:533–537.

202. Perry CR. Bone repair techniques, bone graft, and bone graft substitutes. *Clin Orthop* 1999;360:71–86.

203. Peter SJ, Miller MJ, Yasko AW, et al. Polymer concepts in tissue engineering. *J Biomed Mater Res* 1998;43:422–427.

204. Peter SJ, Lu L, Kim DJ, et al. Marrow stromal osteoblast function on a poly(propylene fumarate)/beta-tricalcium phosphate biodegradable orthopaedic composite. *Biomaterials* 2000;21:1207–1213.

205. Peterson L, Minas T, Brittberg M, et al. Two- to 9-year outcome after autologous chondrocyte transplantation of the knee. *Clin Orthop* 2000;374:212–234.

206. Peterson L, Brittberg M, Kiviranta I, et al. Autologous chondrocyte transplantation. Biomechanics and long-term durability. *Am J Sports Med* 2002;30:2–12.

207. Pollack SR, Salzstein R, Pienkowski D. The electric double layer in bone and its influence on stress generated potentials. *Calcif Tissue Int* 1984;36:577–581.

208. Porter BD, Oldham JB, He SL, et al. Mechanical properties of a biodegradable bone regeneration scaffold. *J Biomech Eng* 2000;122:286–288.

209. Praemer A, Furner S, Rice DP. *Musculoskeletal conditions in the United States.* Rosemont, IL: American Academy of Orthopaedic Surgeons; 1999.

210. Quinn TM, Grodzinsky AJ, Buschmann MD, et al. Mechanical compression alters proteoglycan deposition and matrix deformation around individual cells in cartilage explants. *J Cell Sci* 1998;111:573–583.

211. Reindel ES, Ayroso AM, Chen AC, et al. Integrative repair of articular cartilage in vitro: adhesive strength of the interface region. *J Orthop Res* 1995;13:751–760.

212. Richardson JB, Caterson B, Evans EH, et al. Repair of human articular cartilage after implantation of autologous chondrocytes. *J Bone Joint Surg Br* 1999;81:1064–1068.

213. Riesle J, Hollander AP, Langer R, et al. Collagen in tissue-engineered cartilage: types, structure and crosslinks. *J Cell Biochem* 1998;71:313–327.

214. Ripamonti U, Reddi AH. Tissue engineering, morphogenesis, and regeneration of the periodontal tissues by bone morphogenetic proteins. *Crit Rev Oral Biol Med* 1997;8:154–163.

215. Robey PG. Normal bone formation: structure. In: Brighton CT, Friedlaender GE, Lane JM, eds. *Bone formation and repair.* Rosemont, IL: AAOS, 1994:3–12.

216. Rubin CT, Lanyon LE. Regulation of bone formation by applied dynamic loads. *J Bone Joint Surg Am* 1984;66A:397–402.

217. Rubin CT, McLeod KJ, Bain SD. Functional strains and cortical bone adaptation: epigenetic assurance of skeletal integrity. *J Biomech* 1990;23:43–54.

218. Rubin J, Fan X, Biskobring DM, et al. Osteoclastogenesis is repressed by mechanical strain in an in vitro model. *J Orthop Res* 1999;17:639–645.

219. Rubin J, Murphy T, Nanes MS, et al. Mechanical strain inhibits expression of osteoclast differentiation factor by murine stromal cells. *Am J Physiol* 2000;278:C1126–C1132.

220. Sah RL, Chen AC, Grodzinsky AJ, et al. Differential effects of bFGF and IGF-I on matrix metabolism in calf and adult bovine cartilage explants. *Arch Biochem Biophys* 1994;308:137–147.

221. Sah RL, Trippel SB, Grodzinsky AJ. Differential effects of serum, insulin-like growth factor-I, and fibroblast growth factor-2 on the maintenance of cartilage physical properties during long-term culture. *J Orthop Res* 1996;14:44–52.

222. Sah RL. The biomechanical faces of articular cartilage. In: Krall AM, Kuettner KE, Hascall VC, eds. *The many faces of osteoarthritis.* Basel, Switzerland: Birkhauser Verlag, 2003:409–422.

223. Sah RLY, Kim YJ, Doong JYH, et al. Biosynthetic response of cartilage explants to dynamic compression. *J Orthop Res* 1989;7:619–636.

224. Sakai K, Mohtai M, Iwamoto Y. Fluid shear stress increases transforming growth factor beta 1 expression in human osteoblast-like cells: modulation by cation channel blockade. *Calcif Tissue Int* 1998;63:515–520.

225. Sampath TK, Maliakal JC, Hauschka PV, et al. Recombinant human osteogenic protein-1 (hOP-1) induces new bone formation in vivo with a specific activity comparable with natural bovine osteogenic protein and stimulates proliferation and differentiation in vitro. *J Biol Chem* 1992;267:20352–20362.

226. Sandhu HS, Kanim LEA, Kabo JM, et al. Evaluation of rhBMP-2 with a OPLA carrier in a canine posterolateral (transverse process) spinal fusion model. *Spine* 1995;20:2669–2682.

227. Sato K, Urist MR. Induced regeneration of calvaria by bone morphogenetic protein (BMP) in dogs. *Clin Orthop* 1985;197:301.

228. Schaefer D, Martin I, Heberer M, et al. Tissue engineered composites for the repair of large osteochondral defects. *46th Transactions of the Orthopaedic Research Society,* Orlando, FL, 2000;25:619.

229. Schaefer D, Martin I, Shastri VP, et al. In vitro generation of osteochondral composites. *Biomaterials* 2000;21:2599–2606.

230. Schaefer D, Martin I, Jundt G, et al. Tissue engineered composites for the repair of large osteochondral defects. *Arthritis Rheum* 2002;46:2524–2534.

231. Schenk RK, Hunziker EB. Histologic and ultrastructural fractures of fracture healing. In: Brighton CT, Friedlaender GE, Lane JM, eds. *Bone formation and repair.* Rosemont, IL: AAOS, 1994:117–146.

232. Schinagl RM, Gurskis D, Chen AC, et al. Depth-dependent confined compression modulus of full-thickness bovine articular cartilage. *J Orthop Res* 1997;15:499–506.

233. Schreiber RE, Ilten-Kirby BM, Dunkelman NS, et al. Repair of osteochondral defects with allogeneic tissue-engineered cartilage implants. *Clin Orthop* 1999;367S:S382–S395.

234. Seidel JO, Pei M, Gray ML, et al. Long-term culture of tissue engineered cartilage in a perfused chamber with mechanical stimulation. *Biorheology* 2004;41:445–458.

235. Sellers RS, Zhang R, Glasson SS, et al. Repair of articular cartilage defects one year after treatment with recombinant human bone morphogenetic protein-2 (rhBMP-2). *J Bone Joint Surg Am* 2000;82:151–160.

236. Sittinger M, Bujia J, Minuth WW, et al. Engineering of cartilage tissue using bioresorbable polymer carriers in perfusion culture. *Biomaterials* 1994;15:451–456.

237. Skerry TM, Pitensky L, Chayen J, et al. Strain memory in bone tissue: is proteoglycan-based persistence of strain history a cue for the control of adaptive bone remodeling? *Trans Orthop Res Soc* San Francisco, 1987;75.

238. Soltz MA, Ateshian GA. A conewise linear elasticity mixture model for the analysis of tension-compression nonlinearity in articular cartilage. *J Biomech Eng* 2000;122:576–586.

239. Stading M, Langer R. Mechanical shear properties of cell-polymer cartilage constructs. *Tissue Eng* 1999;5:241–250.

240. Stanford CM, Morcuende JA, Brand RA. Proliferative and phenotypical responses of bone-like cells to mechanical deformation. *J Orthop Res* 1995;13:664–670.

241. Tagil M, Aspenberg P. Cartilage induction by controlled mechanical stimulation in vivo. *J Orthop Res* 1999;17:200–204.

242. Takahashi I, Nuckolis GH, Takahashi K, et al. Compressive force promotes Sox9, type II collagen and aggrecan and inhibits IL-1b expression resulting in chondrogenesis in mouse embryonic limb bud mesenchymal cells. *J Cell Sci* 1998;111:2067–2076.

243. Urist MR. Bone formation by autoinduction. *Science* 1965;150:893–899.

244. Urist MR, Sato K, Brownell AG, et al. Human bone morphogenetic protein (hBMP). *Proc Soc Exp Biol Med* 1983;173:194–199.

245. Urist MR, Huo YK, Brownell AG, et al. Purification of bovine bone morphogenetic protein by hydroxyapatite chromatography. *Proc Natl Acad Sci U S A* 1984;81:371–375.

246. Vunjak-Novakovic G, Freed LE, Biron RJ, et al. Effects of mixing on the composition and morphology of tissue-engineered cartilage. *AIChE Journal, the journal of the American Institute of* 1996;42:850–860.

247. Vunjak-Novakovic G, Obradovic B, Bursac P, et al. Dynamic cell seeding of polymer scaffolds for cartilage tissue engineering. *Biotechnol Prog* 1998;14:193–202.

248. Vunjak-Novakovic G, Martin I, Obradovic B, et al. Bioreactor cultivation conditions modulate the composition and mechanical properties of tissue engineered cartilage. *J Orthop Res* 1999;17:130–138.

249. Vunjak-Novakovic G, Obradovic B, Martin I, et al. Bioreactor studies of native and tissue engineered cartilage. *Biorheology* 2002;39:259–268.

250. Vunjak-Novakovic G. Fundamentals of tissue engineering: scaffolds and bioreactors. In: Caplan AI, ed. *Tissue engineering of cartilage and bone.* London: John Wiley, 2003:34–51.

251. Wakitani S, Goto T, Pineda SJ, et al. Mesenchymal cell-based repair of large, full-thickness defects of articular cartilage. *J Bone Joint Surg Am* 1994;76A:579–592.

252. Wakitani S, Goto T, Young RG, et al. Repair of large full-thickness articular cartilage defects with allograft articular chondrocytes embedded in a collagen gel. *Tissue Eng* 1998;4:429–444.

253. Wei X, Messner K. Maturation-dependent repair of untreated osteochondral defects in the rabbit knee. *J Biomed Mater Res* 1997;34:63–72.

254. Weibaum S, Cowin SC, Zeng Y. A model for the excitation of osteocytes by mechanical loading-induced bone fluid shear stresses. *J Biomech* 1994;27:339–360.

255. Wilkins RJ, Browning JA, Urban JP. Chondrocyte regulation by mechanical load. *Biorheology* 2000;37:67–74.

256. Williamson AK, Chen AC, Sah RL. Compressive properties and function-composition relationships of developing bovine articular cartilage. *J Orthop Res* 2001;19:1113–1121.

257. Wolff J. *Das Gaesetz der Transformation der Knochen.* Berlin: A. Hirchwild; 1882.

258. Wozney JM. The potential role of morphogenetic proteins in periodontal reconstruction. *J Periodontol* 1995;66:506–510.

259. Wu F, Dunkelman N, Peterson A, et al. Bioreactor development for tissue-engineered cartilage. *Ann N Y Acad Sci* 1999;875:405–411.

260. Wu Q-Q, Chen Q. Mechanoregulation of chondrocyte proliferation, maturation and hypertrophy: ion-channel dependent transduction of matrix deformation signals. *Exp Cell Res* 2000;256:383–391.

261. Xynos ID, Hukkanen MVJ, Batten JJ, et al. Bioglass ®45S5 stimulates osteoblast turnover and enhances bone formation in vitro: implications and applications for bone tissue engineering. *Calcif Tissue Int* 2000;67:321–329.

262. Ysart GE, Mason RM. Responses of articular cartilage explant cultures to different oxygen tensions. *Biochim Biophys Acta* 1994;1221:15–20.

QUANTITATIVE ANATOMY AND IMAGING OF DIARTHRODIAL JOINT ARTICULAR LAYERS

GERARD A. ATESHIAN
FELIX ECKSTEIN

The development of powerful medical imaging tools has recently brought a new and exciting perspective to the study of diarthrodial joint anatomy. Quantitation of topographic features and the thickness of articular cartilage layers is made possible by a combination of imaging technologies and geometric modeling tools that can now also be applied *in vivo* in a clinical environment and are not restricted to the laboratory setting. The ability to mathematically describe the three-dimensional (3D) geometry of articular layers is valuable in several respects: Quantitative representations can be used for basic anatomic and biomechanical studies, to describe the generic (fundamental) and individual features of joint surfaces. They permit one to generate finite element models of joints for computing contact and stresses of articular cartilage layers. Such models can eventually be used to optimize and plan the outcome of surgical procedures that aim to alter the stress distribution by parametric computer simulation. Mapping the proximity of two articulating surfaces, for instance, makes it possible to infer the location of contact areas in the joint for different positions (flexion angles), and open magnetic resonance imaging (MR) permits study of the kinematics and stability of joints under external loading and normal neuromuscular control. The clinical applications of these tools offer tremendous potential in the areas of diagnosis, monitoring of disease progression, or assessment of outcome. Patients with risk of joint and/or cartilage disease can be identified early, closely followed, and the time point and type of therapeutic intervention can be selected more specifically. In particular, the advent of new therapeutic strategies, such as chondrocyte or cartilage tissue transplantation, gene therapy, and matrix enzyme inhibitors requires objective methods for evaluating the structure-modifying capacity of these methods. Because clinical symptoms and structural status of diseased joints are only moderately correlated, such methods are required to select appropriate patients for clinical studies and to judge the long-term outcome of patients with joint disease.

In this chapter, we provide an overview of the methods for imaging and quantifying the anatomy of diarthrodial joint articular layers, along with selected recent applications of these methods in the study of human joints.

1 FUNCTION, DEFINITION, AND TYPES OF JOINTS

Joints can be viewed as the essential organs of the locomotion system. They allow for locomotion, spatial positioning relative to the environment, and active manipulation of the surroundings. They also ensure, under normal situations, that the loads and bending moments acting on long bones remain within physiologically acceptable limits. Their function is thus to allow ease of movement in certain directions, and to limit it in others, in order to provide stability to body segments.

There exist continuous joints (juncturae, synarthroses, solid joints) and discontinuous joints (articulations, diarthroses, synovial joints, cavitated joints) between skeletal elements. In continuous joints these elements are connected by tissue, fibrous tissue (juncturae fibrosae; syndesmoses, fibrous joints; e.g., interosseous membrane), cartilage tissue (juncturae cartilagineae;

synchondroses, cartilaginous joints; e.g., pubic symphysis or intervertebral disc), or bone tissue (juncturae osseae; synostoses, bony joints; e.g., sutures of the skull, after cessation of growth). Diarthrodial joints, on which this chapter focuses, are defined by (a) two or more articular surfaces/layers (Fig. 9-1), (b) a joint cavity, and (c) a joint capsule. "Movement" is not part of the definition of diarthrodial joints, as this also occurs in continuous joints, and may be minimal in some diarthrodial joints (so-called amphiarthroses; e.g., sacroiliac joint). Other elements that are frequently—if not always—found in diarthrodial joints are the synovial membrane, synovial fluid, ligaments (usually not a separate anatomical entity, but simply stronger parts of the joint capsule), intraarticular ligaments (e.g., the cruciate ligaments of the knee) or tendons (e.g., long biceps tendon in the shoulder), discs (e.g., sternoclavicular joint, wrist joint), menisci (knee joint), or a labrum

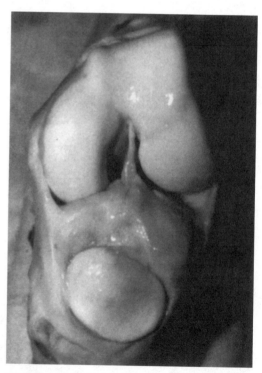

FIGURE 9-1. Typical femoral and patellar articular cartilage layers from a human knee joint. The patella has been reflected down to permit simultaneous visualization of the femoral surface (trochlea and condyles).

TABLE 9-1. CLASSIFICATION OF JOINTS BY SHAPE

Shape	Example
Plane joints	Intermetatarsal joints
Hinge joints (ginglymi)	Humeroulnar joint
Pivot (trochoid) joints	Radioulnar joints
Bicondylar joints	Femorotibial joint
Ellipsoid joints	Radiocarpal joint or metacarpophalangeal joints
Sellar (saddle) joints	Carpometacarpal joint of the thumb, ankle joint
Spheroidal joints	Hip and shoulder joint

(hip and shoulder joints). Joints can be classified according to several aspects, one being their shape as described in Table 9-1.

Joints occur between the 8th and 13th week of embryonic development in a proximal-to-distal time sequence throughout the limb. The position of presumptive joints is controlled by hox a and d gene complexes, which are able to modify cell adhesion and cell proliferation. This process is also influenced by BMP (bone morphogenetic protein) -2 and -4 and their antagonists (noggin, chordin), potentially also by GDF (growth and differentiation factors) -5 and -6. It has been shown that elimination of mechanical stimuli (muscle contraction) prevents joint cavitation, or induces refusion of skeletal elements after cavitation (221). Carter and Wong (43) and Carter et al. (44) proposed that hydrostatic pressure prevents the enchondral ossification process from progressing to the joint surface, and that the magnitude of the pressure determines the thickness of the cartilage layer in joint development. It has frequently been assumed that the inhomogeneity of cartilage thickness throughout joint surfaces and the differences in mean cartilage thickness between different joints (3) are explained by different mechanical "loading histories" (44,177).

2 GEOMETRIC MODELS OF ARTICULAR LAYERS

One of the aims of this chapter is to demonstrate how the application of quantitative techniques

can bring valuable insights to the study of the anatomy and biomechanics of diarthrodial joints and articular cartilage layers. Various measures can be extracted from anatomical data, given a suitable mathematical representation or geometric model. Mathematical representations of articular layers have been obtained using various surface-fitting methods. One such method was employed by Scherrer and Hillberry (191), who used the piecewise continuous parametric bicubic patch representation of Coons (53) to interpolate surface data obtained from the canine glenohumeral joint. The general equation of a bicubic patch is given by:

$$\mathbf{x}(u,v) = \sum_{i=0}^{3}\sum_{j=0}^{3} \mathbf{c}_{ij} u^i v^j \qquad (1)$$

where $\mathbf{x}$ is the position vector of a point on the bicubic patch at the parametric coordinates (u,v), and $\mathbf{c}_{ij}$ are vector coefficients. For highly curved articular surfaces, a large number of small patches are necessary to accurately represent the entire surface, and certain mathematical requirements are needed to guarantee continuity at the boundaries of adjoining patches. In the piecewise continuous implementation of Coons, continuity of the surface tangents was enforced (C^1 continuity). This technique, which is well adapted for gridded wireframes in which each grid cell represents a patch (Fig. 9-2), was later used by Huiskes et al. (132), Ateshian et al. (13), and Hefzy and Yang (120) for accurately representing knee joint articular surfaces and by Wood et al. (226) for modeling muscle surfaces. One immediate application of the bicubic representation is to evaluate surface normals, which are used for displaying shaded models of the articular surfaces (Fig. 9-3). The surface normal is obtained from the normalized cross product of the tangent vectors along each of the two parametric coordinates:

$$\mathbf{n} = \frac{\mathbf{x}_u \times \mathbf{x}_v}{|\mathbf{x}_u \times \mathbf{x}_v|} \qquad (2)$$

where $\mathbf{x}_u = \partial\mathbf{x}/\partial u$ and $\mathbf{x}_v = \partial\mathbf{x}/\partial v$ are the surface tangent vectors along the parametric coordinate directions u and v.

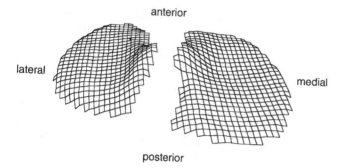

FIGURE 9-2. Wireframe representation of a tibial plateau surface, showing surface patches.

Despite their versatility, piecewise continuous bicubic patches have two drawbacks. First, they do not provide continuity of surface curvatures, which are needed in many applications that are described below. Second, they are fitted to the experimental data by interpolation, i.e., the mathematical representation passes exactly through every experimental surface data point. This interpolation becomes problematic because of the inevitable presence of measurement errors, which can lead to the creation of ripples in the mathematical representation of the articular surfaces.

Though the effect of small ripples may be neglected in some applications, these can be reduced or eliminated by surface approximation. In this approach, the mathematical surface need not pass exactly through every data point but may sufficiently deviate from the data such that it remains smooth up to at least two continuous partial derivatives that are needed to define surface curvatures. Surface approximation

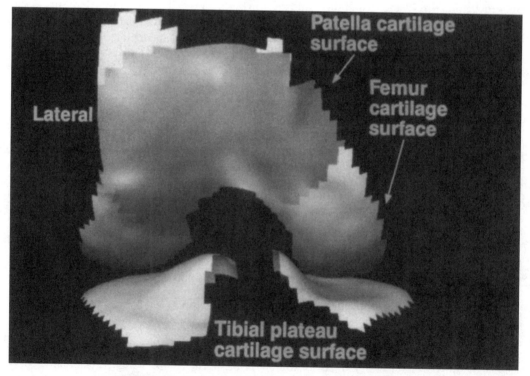

FIGURE 9-3. Shaded models of knee joint articular surfaces.

is generally achieved using the method of least squares, in which the root-mean-square (rms) of the residual error between the data points and the mathematical surface is minimized. Rushfeldt et al. (190) used this method to fit the mathematical equation of a sphere,

$$(x - x_0)^2 + (y - y_0)^2 + (z - z_0)^2 = R^2 \quad (3)$$

to articular surface data from the hip joint. In this equation, R is the sphere radius, (x_0, y_0, z_0) are the coordinates of its origin, and (x, y, z) are the coordinates of points on the sphere, relative to some laboratory-fixed coordinate system. Similarly, Soslowsky et al. (205) fitted spherical surfaces to surface data from the glenohumeral joint; they found that the rms residual error was on the order of 200 μm, or less than 1% of the surface radius, and concluded that this joint is well approximated by a spherically shaped geometry. Wismans et al. (224) and Blankevoort et al. (26) used surface approximation to represent the tibial plateau with algebraic surfaces of the form $z = f(x, y)$, where z values measured elevations of surface points relative to the xy plane, and $f(x, y)$ consisted of a bivariate polynomial of degree 6 or 7. These authors reported rms residual errors on the order of 300 μm to 500 μm. Although successful in many respects, algebraic representations of this form are not particularly suited for computer implementations because surface slopes parallel to the z-axis will be infinity. This difficulty can be avoided with the use of parametric surface representations akin to the bicubic patch of Eq. 1. For example, Ateshian et al. (14) employed least-squares surface fitting of biquintic parametric patches to represent the articular surfaces of the thumb carpometacarpal joint, with rms residual errors on the order of 70 μm. The equation of a parametric biquintic patch is given by

$$\mathbf{x}(u, v) = \sum_{i=0}^{5} \sum_{j=0}^{5} \mathbf{c}_{ij} u^i v^j \quad (4)$$

where, similar to bicubic patches, the $\mathbf{c}_{ij}$ s are vector coefficients. In their study, a single patch was used to represent the entire articular surface, providing continuous higher-order derivatives everywhere within the patch. Although a single biquintic patch could successfully represent the trapezial and metacarpal surfaces with small residual errors, not all articular surfaces of diarthrodial joints could be well approximated by Eq. 4. In order to combine the usefulness of parametric representations of surfaces with the versatility of piecewise C^2 continuous representations, some authors (15,57) used bicubic B-spline surfaces to approximate a wide variety of diarthrodial joint surfaces. The equation of a B-spline is given by

$$\mathbf{x}(u, v) = \sum_{i=1}^{n_u} \sum_{j=1}^{n_v} B_i^{k_u}(u) B_j^{k_v}(v) \mathbf{d}_{ij} \quad (5)$$

where $\mathbf{d}_{ij}$ s are B-spline coefficients or control points, n_u and n_v are the number of coefficients along each parametric coordinate direction, k_u and k_v are the B-spline orders along those directions ($k_u = k_v = 4$ for bicubic splines), and $B_i^{k_u}(u)$ and $B_i^{k_v}(v)$ are B-spline blending functions. Parametric surfaces, and in particular B-spline surfaces, can be "trimmed" to provide a more realistic smooth boundary, rather than the irregular boundary of a gridded wireframe, as illustrated in Fig. 9-4 for typical knee articular surfaces. The smooth boundary of a trimmed surface is better suited for finite element modeling of articular layers (207). Figure 9-5A shows

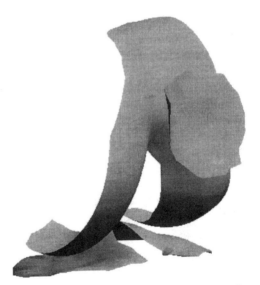

FIGURE 9-4. Shaded models of trimmed B-spline surface representations of knee joint surfaces.

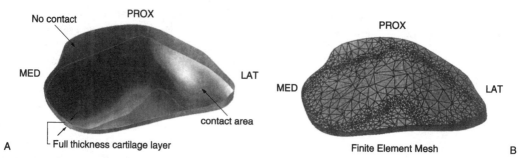

FIGURE 9-5. (A) Solid model of a patellar articular layer with contact area imprint superimposed. **(B)** Finite element mesh of the articular layer with mesh adaptation around the contact area periphery.

a solid model of the articular layer of a human patella, generated by combining the *B*-spline representations of its cartilage and subchondral bone surfaces (18), and Fig. 9-5B shows a finite element mesh of the same layer (86,175). In these figures, a representative contact area contour for a particular joint position is employed as a guide for refining the finite element mesh.

Other surface-fitting methods also exist that can provide further advantages to the methods described here. For example, thin-plate splines have been proposed by Boyd et al. (29), which are easily adapted to scattered data points and can provide suitable smoothing.

The curvature characteristics of any surface are intrinsic properties that provide quantitative measures of their shape (81). In biomechanics, there are many applications that motivate the calculation of these surface properties. The most straightforward application is the characterization of anatomic features, such as the presence and location of ridges and grooves, as well as their shapes, e.g., sellar (saddle-shaped), ovoid, and flat regions. In their simplest form, these measures provide a snapshot of such features in a joint: For example, they can be easily used to identify normal features and differentiate dysplastic joint surfaces from a normative database. Moreover, by use of noninvasive imaging methods such as MRI, changes in these anatomic features can be tracked in patients as a function of time to study joint growth and remodeling, and indeed they can be assessed in large-scale epidemiologic studies, to determine their relevance to the development of osteoarthritis (OA). For example, topographical

changes of subchondral bone are known to occur in arthritic joints as well as in congenital dysplasia. Characterizing early changes in the shapes and surface curvature of afflicted joints may provide a useful diagnostic tool in a clinical setting; such tools will undoubtedly become more useful as the accuracy of noninvasive imaging modalities increases.

Surface curvatures are also useful in the study of diarthrodial joint congruence and contact mechanics (e.g., 97,127,135,158). From basic principles of mechanics, it is recognized that under the same contact load a lesser degree of joint congruence leads to higher cartilage stresses. In canonical contact problems that analyze the mechanics of joint articulations (i.e., using cylindrical, spherical, or ellipsoidal geometries), the stresses in the cartilage are directly related to differences in the surface curvatures (i.e., the congruence) of the layers at the point of initial contact (e.g., 12,16,58,61–63,135,142, 158). Indeed, changes in hip joint congruence with age has been implicated as a primary etiological factor in hip OA (38). Furthermore, in recent studies, it has been shown that cartilage interstitial fluid pressurization, which shields the collagen-proteoglycan matrix from excessive stresses, is promoted by higher congruence of the contacting surfaces (19,58,142). Hence, an analysis of the curvature characteristics of diarthrodial joint surfaces can lead to a better understanding of the contact mechanics in joints.

The curvature characteristics at each point of a surface is most conveniently defined by the principal curvatures, κ_{min} and κ_{max}, and their corresponding mutually orthogonal principal directions (81). The inverses of the curvatures are the radii of curvature. A surface that is locally flat has zero curvature along both principal directions ($\kappa_{\min} = 0, \kappa_{\max} = 0$, at any point on a plane); a convex ovoid surface has positive principal curvatures ($\kappa_{\min} > 0, \kappa_{\max} > 0$, as on the outer surface of an egg); a concave ovoid surface has negative principal curvatures ($\kappa_{\min} < 0, \kappa_{\max} < 0$; e.g., on the inner surface of a bowl); a sellar surface has curvatures of opposite signs ($\kappa_{\min} < 0, \kappa_{\max} > 0$; e.g., on a saddle). A sphere has uniform curvatures ($\kappa_{\min} = \kappa_{\max} = 1/radius$), and at each surface point every great circle defines a principal direction. A ridge is characterized by a band of locally high maximum curvatures that follows directions of minimum curvature; similarly, a groove is characterized by a band of locally large negative minimum curvatures that follows directions of maximum curvature. These bands can be seen on maps of the minimum or maximum curvature. Similarly, by starting at arbitrary points on a surface and tracing lines that follow the principal minimum or maximum directions of curvature everywhere, one can produce a map of the lines of curvature, which can facilitate the identification of ridges and grooves. At any surface point of parametric coordinates (u,v), the principal curvatures are the roots of the quadratic equation

$$(EG - F^2)\kappa^2 - (EN + GL - 2FM)\kappa$$
$$+ (LN - M^2) = 0 \qquad (6)$$

where $E = \mathbf{x}_u \cdot \mathbf{x}_u$, $F = \mathbf{x}_u \cdot \mathbf{x}_v$, $G = \mathbf{x}_v \cdot \mathbf{x}_v$, $L = \mathbf{x}_{uu} \cdot \mathbf{n}$, $M = \mathbf{x}_{uv} \cdot \mathbf{n}$, $N = \mathbf{x}_{vv} \cdot \mathbf{n}$, and $\mathbf{x}_{uu} = \partial^2\mathbf{x}/\partial u^2$, etc. Similarly, the principal directions at that point are the roots of

$$(FN - GM)h^2 + (EN - GL)h$$
$$+ (EM - FL) = 0 \qquad (7)$$

where $h = dv/du$. These equations can easily be solved, given a parametric representation of the articular surface such as those in Eqs. 1, 4, or 5 (14,24).

MacConaill (160) was one of the earliest investigators to employ curvature theory for understanding the kinematics of diarthrodial joints from the topography of their articular surfaces.

He investigated the conjunct rotation of the bones of a joint during diadochal displacements and noted the opposite conjunct rotations occurring in ovoid versus sellar joints. Ateshian et al. (14) used curvature analysis to describe the anatomy and congruence of the thumb carpometacarpal (CMC) joint. These authors described the common features that characterize the predominantly saddle-shaped trapezium and metacarpal surfaces; in particular, they observed that lines of curvature were consistently aligned with the dorsovolar and radioulnar directions of the joint (Fig. 9-6), i.e., along the primary motions of flexion-extension and abduction-adduction. Perhaps more significant clinically, differences were found in the shape of the trapezial articular surface between men and women, with a subset of female joints exhibiting convex ovoid regions on the trapezium rather than the more common sellar topography (Fig. 9-7). It was also determined that female joints were less congruent than male joints, using a curvature-based global congruence index. These results led to the hypothesis that female CMC joints experience higher cartilage

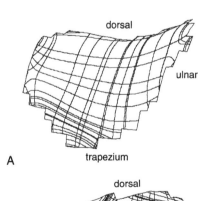

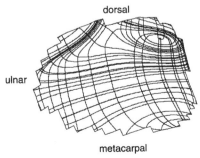

FIGURE 9-6. Lines of curvature on a carpometacarpal joint (14). **(A)** Trapezium. **(B)** Metacarpal.

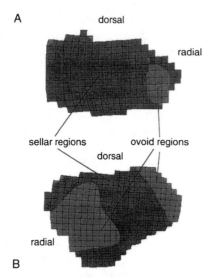

FIGURE 9-7. Gaussian curvature maps of female trapezial surfaces. The Gaussian curvature K is the product of the principal curvatures; i.e., $K = \kappa_{min}\kappa_{max}$. When K is negative, the surface is locally sellar; when it is positive, the surface is ovoid, and its concavity or convexity can be determined from the sign of κ_{min} or κ_{max}. **(A)** Typical sellar trapezial surface. **(B)** Trapezial surface with large convex ovoid region.

stresses than male joints during light to moderate activities of daily living that involve similar loads for men and women (14,230). Such higher stresses may help explain the greater prevalence of OA in the female population older than the age of 45 (143,154).

The curvature characteristics of the patello-femoral joint articular surfaces have also been determined in recent studies (151). Patellar maps of the maximum principal curvatures and the lines of minimum curvature have provided an unequivocal determination of the existence and location of patellar ridges (Fig. 9-8). These include a proximal median ridge that extends distally in some specimens, a lateral transverse ridge that extends medially in some specimens, and a secondary ridge that appears in most specimens. No more than one transverse ridge was observed in these studies, which included 31 patellae from 22 cadavers. Paired specimens exhibited remarkable symmetry, as shown in Fig. 9-9. On the opposing femoral surface, curvature maps confirmed that the trochlea is predominantly sellar within a band centered on the mid-sagittal plane, with ridges flanking it along its medial and lateral sides (Fig. 9-10). In all 12 femoral specimens, grooves were observed where the trochlea merges with the condyles, which were more pronounced on the lateral side. It has been suggested that the knee menisci rest against these grooves at full extension (91,169).

Recently, it has also been shown that curvature analysis can be performed on high-resolution MRI data sets of the human knee (48). Based on the work of Ateshian et al. (13,14,15, 18), Hohe et al. (127) analyzed surface curvature and the congruity/incongruity of the human knee from MRI. An algorithm for surface curvature analysis was validated in geometric test objects, by comparing results with the analytic solution. All knee joint surfaces displayed predominantly convex ovoid shapes (positive Gaussian curvature and positive mean curvature), except for the central aspect of the medial tibia (mean principal curvature $= -0.9 \pm$

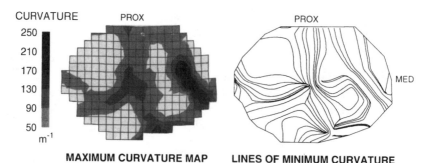

FIGURE 9-8. Maximum curvature map and lines of minimum curvature of a patellar cartilage surface, indicating the presence and location of ridges (151).

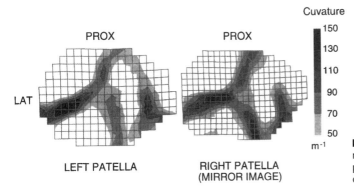

FIGURE 9-9. Maximum curvature maps of matched left and right patellae, demonstrating symmetry of curvature characteristics (151).

3.8 m^{-1}). Of all knee joint surfaces, the patella displayed the highest degree of convexity (mean principal curvature = 41 ± 6.0 m^{-1}), and none of the surfaces showed saddle-like properties (negative Gaussian curvature). Using the curvature-based global congruence index mentioned previously (14), the authors found the incongruity to be largest in the patellofemoral joint (80 ± 6.6 m^{-1}) and smallest in the medial femorotibial joint (29 ± 3.8 m^{-1}). Values of 42 ± 7.4 m^{-1} were found in the lateral femorotibial joint. The precision errors of the surface curvature analysis (2.9 – 5.7 m^{-1}) and congruence indices (4.1 – 7.4 m^{-1}) were lower than differences between joint surfaces, but only marginally lower than differences between healthy people.

Geometric models of articular layers can be used beyond their application to curvature analysis. Ateshian et al. (13) demonstrated the use of stereophotogrammetry (SPG) to calculate cartilage thickness maps *in vitro,* in the human knee. In their approach, the cartilage surface was first quantified with SPG, then the cartilage layer was dissolved using a mild solution of sodium hypochloride to expose the underlying subchondral bone. After quantifying the bone surface with SPG, geometric models of the two surfaces were obtained and realigned in a common coordinate system using data from optical targets rigidly fixed to the bone. From these geometric models, they calculated the cartilage layer thickness at various points on the subchondral bone, along directions perpendicular to the bone surface. Using the perpendicular direction to the subchondral bone surface as a geometric reference for measuring cartilage thickness allows for a more precise method than in-plane thickness measurement methods (e.g., sectioning) because it is not possible to obtain planes in a consistent manner that are perpendicular to the underlying bony surface. Mathematically,

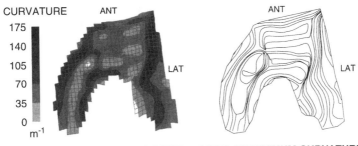

FIGURE 9-10. Maximum curvature map and lines of minimum curvature of the trochlea (151).

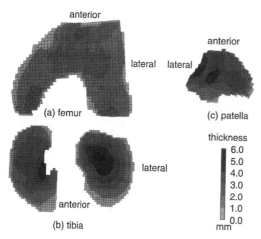

FIGURE 9-11. Thickness maps of the articular layers of a typical knee joint: **(a)** femur, **(b)** tibia, **(c)** patella. Thickness measurements are calculated along a direction perpendicular to the bone surface at every point.

this calculation consists of solving the following vector equation:

$$\mathbf{x}_{bone} + t\mathbf{n}_{bone} = \mathbf{x}(u, v) \qquad (8)$$

where $\mathbf{x}_{bone}$ is the position of a point on the subchondral bone surface where the cartilage thickness t is desired, $\mathbf{n}_{bone}$ is the unit normal to the bone surface at that point, and $\mathbf{x}(u,v)$ is the corresponding point on the cartilage surface. Equation 8 has three scalar component equations that can be solved for the three unknowns u, v, and t. The results of this analysis can be displayed as cartilage thickness maps, as shown in Fig. 9-11 for a representative knee joint. Similar studies have been conducted on the articular layers of the glenohumeral joint (206) and the thumb CMC joint (20), and this technique has been equally successful with data acquired from high-resolution MRI (48).

3 METHODS FOR MEASURING JOINT SURFACE GEOMETRY AND CARTILAGE THICKNESS

Several methods have been used to quantify diarthrodial joint surfaces. Mechanical techniques include the production of plastic mold-ings (194), the production of a silicone rubber mold used to make a plaster casting (191,192), and the use of a mechanical measuring pin attached to a dial gauge (224). Other methods such as slicing (200) and ultrasound have also been described (190). In some instances, casting techniques have been used to directly quantify the incongruity between articular surfaces rather than to quantify absolute surface topographies (66,82). Non-contacting *in vitro* methods include photogrammetery, SPG, multistation digital photogrammetry (13,14,94,95,132,187, 205), and laser scanning (116,117).

Similarly, several *in vitro* methods have been used for the determination of articular cartilage thickness, such as optical evaluation of punched or drilled specimens (149,172), analysis of sliced specimens (64,138,162–165,201), A-mode ultrasound (2,3,138,166,190), needle probe testing (125,138,170), and SPG (13,205).

To provide a surface-wide representation, thickness maps can be reconstructed from anatomical sections (64,67,68,162,165). However, this method is prone to errors in highly curved surfaces because results are dependent on the orientation of the sectioning plane. With the needle-probe method (127,138,170), a load cell is connected to a probe, which is aligned perpendicular to the surface. This sensor records a spike as the needle pierces the cartilage surface and another spike when the needle touches the subchondral bone: The thickness is derived from recordings of the needle displacement between these spikes. This method is practical only when a few measurements are needed. Optical methods have been used to measure the thickness of small plugs of articular cartilage; typically, several measurements are made around the plug periphery and averaged (138,166). A-mode ultrasound (2,3,166,190) can also measure the thickness of cartilage by recording the time required for an ultrasound wave to travel from the cartilage to the subchondral bone surface and be reflected back. The cartilage thickness is derived from the knowledge of the speed of sound in cartilage, and thickness maps for all major joint surfaces of the lower limb have been produced with this methodology (3). It is noted, however, that the speed of sound in cartilage depends not only on water, but also on the amount of extracellular solid matrix present (e.g., collagen and proteoglycan contents); because the extracellular composition and organization vary with age and disease (e.g., OA), the speed of sound in such tissues may not necessarily be known with precision or confidence. This may explain why when Jurvelin et al. (138) compared needle-probe, optical, and ultrasound methods for measuring cartilage thickness, they found a good correlation between optical and needle-probe methods, and greater scatter with the ultrasound method. Eckstein et al. (68) compared anatomical section, A-mode ultrasound, CT-arthrography, and MRI in the human patella and found reasonable agreement between cartilage thickness maps obtained by these four methods. *In vivo* methods for quantifying cartilage thickness include the measurement of joint space width on radiographs (11,28,35,36,37,114,219), arthrography (28,114), CT arthrography (28,134), B-mode ultrasound (6,136), and MRI (see below). It should be noted that plain x-ray radiography provides only an indirect measured of cartilage thickness (distance from one bone cartilage interface to another) and is generally confined to a one-point measurement per compartment. However, radiography has been shown to yield reproducible results if great care is taken in adequate joint positioning (semi-flexed, weight-bearing—37,219); it is the recommended technique for structural evaluation of joint status by the Food and Drug Administration (FDA) in clinical trials.

Two of the methods mentioned above have been shown to be particularly versatile and display distinct advantages: SPG, which can reach high accuracy *in vitro*, and MRI, which is applicable *in vivo*. These two methods are covered in more detail below.

3.1 Stereophotogrammetry

SPG has been in existence almost since the advent of photography. By capturing planar images of a 3D object from two or more directions in space, it is possible to reconstruct the 3D coordinates of that object using only the planar image data. This reconstruction can be achieved using basic principles of projective and perspective geometry. Photogrammetric tools are widely used in constructing 3D geographic maps from aerial or satellite photography. The SPG technique is not limited to the use of the visible light spectrum but can also use radar waves, x-rays, etc. In the medical field, the earliest use of roentgenphotogrammetry (using x-rays) was that by Davidson (56), though its modern application was pioneered by Selvik (197), who used the method to study the kinematics of the skeletal system. In 1975, Clark et al. (47) employed close-range SPG in the development of prosthetic devices, in particular, human aortic valves. Stokes and Greenapple (213) measured 3D soft tissue deformation with SPG, where the noncontacting nature of this method proved to be a distinctive advantage. In gait analysis, photogrammetry has been a standard tool for measuring limb kinematics since the early 1980s.

The first use of photogrammetry for articular surface measurements, however, was by Ghosh (95), who applied standard tools of cartography to reconstructing the 3D topography of the human femoral head and distal femoral surface. In his apparatus, Ghosh projected a fine grid on the articular surfaces, using a slide projector. The grid intersections provided recognizable landmarks on the photographic pair (the stereogram), which were necessary for completing the 3D reconstruction of the articular surface topography. The accuracy reported in these measurements was 200 μm. Huiskes et al. (132) and later Ateshian et al. (13) developed similar SPG systems for characterizing the topography of knee joint articular surfaces, with accuracies on the order of 200 μm and 90 μm, respectively, at a 95% confidence level. Using multistation digital photogrammetry, Ronsky et al. (187) achieved even better accuracies, on the order of 25 μm.

The basic apparatus of an SPG system consists of two cameras (or one camera that can be moved to two distinct positions if the measured object is stationary), a calibration frame, a slide projector (or optical spotlight) with a gridded slide (Fig. 9-12), and a two-dimensional (2D) digitizer. The calibration frame, which has

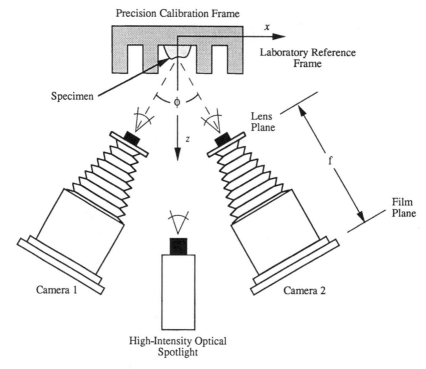

FIGURE 9-12. Schematic of the basic components of a stereophotogrammetry apparatus: cameras, calibration frame, slide projector/optical spotlight, and two-dimensional digitizer (not shown).

a workspace for inserting the object to be measured, is fitted with markers (calibration targets) whose 3D coordinates are accurately known a priori. When a stereogram of the object and calibration frame is obtained (Fig. 9-13), the planar image coordinates of these calibration targets are digitized with the 2D digitizer. From the knowledge of these 2D image coordinates and of the corresponding 3D calibration coordinates, the camera parameters can be determined for each camera position. Various procedures exist for performing this camera calibration, based on the collinearity condition (e.g., 94); these procedures can be elaborate, as they aim to compensate for many potential sources of error such as linear and nonlinear lens distortions. Once the camera parameters have been obtained, the digitized stereogram image coordinates of the grid intersections that appear on the articular surfaces (Fig. 9-13) can be used to reconstruct their corresponding 3D coordinates. By simply connecting these grid points together, it is pos-

sible to visualize the resulting wireframe model on a computer graphics workstation (Fig. 9-2). From these wireframe models, mathematical equations can be generated to represent the articular surfaces, producing geometric models as described above.

3.2 Magnetic Resonance Imaging

MRI is now the method of choice if measures on cartilage thickness are to be obtained *in vivo*. MR image generation is based on a strong magnetic field and high-frequency radio waves (rather than ionizing radiation). The technique has shown no adverse effects on health, other important advantages being its multiplanar capabilities and its superior soft tissue contrast. With MRI, tissue signals can be substantially modulated by choosing different types of pulse sequences and by changing specific parameters, such as repetition time, echo time, flip angle, etc. Hence, a variety of sequences can be selected for

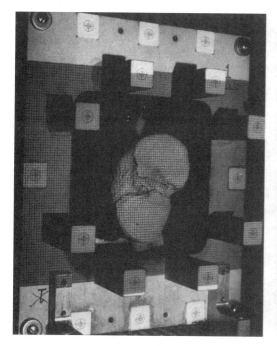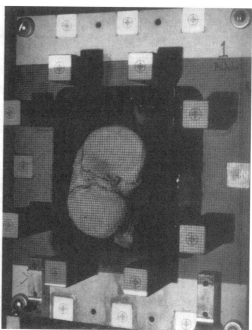

FIGURE 9-13. Typical stereogram of a tibial plateau, corresponding to the surface of Fig. 9-2.

optimal delineation of specific tissues, or even for specific aspects of this tissue. However, cartilage presents an imaging challenge due to its relatively short transverse relaxation time (T2) and to various sources of artifacts at the bone interface.

3.2.1 MR Sequences

For qualitatively evaluating cartilage and joints for diagnostic purposes, proton density-weighted and/or T2-weighted spin echo sequences with fat suppression have been recommended. These allow the detection of bone changes (bone marrow edema, osteophytes), general thinning of the cartilage, focal cartilage lesions, signal alterations in the cartilage, and osteochondral defects (31). Qualitative scoring systems of multiple tissues in OA have been developed, but these depend on the experience of the examiner and may therefore be less reliable in longitudinal studies. In particular, qualitative scores are only of limited usefulness in a scientific context, when addressing fundamental questions concerning the morphology, physiology, and functional adaptation of cartilage tissue

statistically. For these reasons, there has been increasing interest in deriving quantitative parameters from MR image data.

For the analysis of cartilage macromorphology (volume, thickness, surface areas), the bone cartilage interface and the articular surface need to be delineated accurately. In particular, the spatial resolution must be sufficient to permit quantitative measurements throughout the thickness. Today, it is widely accepted that T1-weighted gradient echo sequences with spectral fat suppression or water excitation are best suited for this purpose (67,178,179,183,203). These sequences produce images in which the cartilage appears bright (hyperintense) compared with all other tissues (Fig. 9-14), and in which artifacts at the bone cartilage interface are eliminated. Spectral fat-suppression techniques require high field systems (>1 T) and can be achieved by applying a prepulse, preventing the fat-bound protons from creating a signal during subsequent data acquisition (183). However, sequences with selective excitation of only the water-bound protons have been introduced recently, in which fat-signal elimination can be achieved with much shorter acquisition times (39,98,103,115,133).

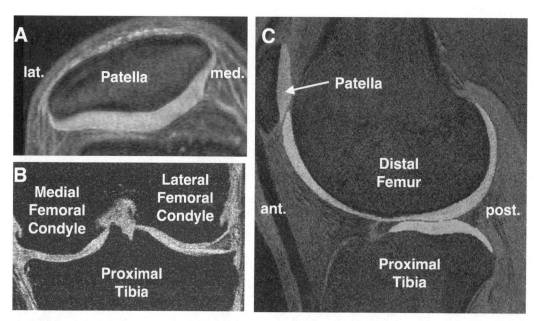

FIGURE 9-14. High resolution T1-weighted gradient echo sequences with spectral fat suppression or selective water excitation are best suited for imaging articular cartilage morphology. The figure shows **(A)** a transverse section through the patella, **(B)** a coronal section through the femorotibial joint, and **(C)** a sagittal section through the knee. Part **(B)** shows a case of severe osteoarthritis in the medial femorotibial compartment.

This technique can produce a data set of the human knee joint (about 60 slices of 1.5 mm thickness) at an in-plane resolution of 0.3 × 0.3 mm² in less than 10 min. It is noted that in MRI an improvement in resolution by a factor of 2 (in all three dimensions) requires a prolongation of the image time by a factor of 64, if an identical signal-to-noise ratio is to be achieved. Water-excitation sequences therefore also have the advantage that the spatial resolution can be improved without requiring excessive imaging time. In the elbow and foot (7,103), it has become possible to obtain image data at a resolution of 1 × 0.25 × 0.25 mm³ with acquisition times that are tolerable *in vivo* (<20 min) by the subject.

Several MR sequences have been proposed for compositional (biochemical/structural) analysis of articular cartilage (42,110). A "layering" of the cartilage has been observed with many pulse sequences (100,113,145,155,167,188, 189,228,229), and there is great interest in relating the signal intensity gradients to the microstructural variation of the cartilage (e.g., histologic zones) and its biochemical composition.

Such methods may also prove useful to indirectly assess mechanical properties of articular cartilage *in vivo*. Due to the anisotropic arrangement of collagen fibrils and the "magic angle" effect, however, cartilage appearance and "layering" is dependent on the relative orientation to the static magnetic field (100,113,145,228,229).

Recent work indicates that gadolinium-diethylene triamine pentaacetic acid (Gd-DTPA)-enhanced MR imaging can potentially be used to evaluate the proteoglycan (PG) content of normal and degenerated articular cartilage *in vivo* (9,21,22,23,42,110,216). Gd-DTPA is a negatively charged contrast agent that distributes inversely to the concentration of glycosaminoglycans in cartilage. Other investigators have also employed T1rho relaxation (60) and sodium imaging for measuring PGs (184,185), but these techniques require specific hardware that is not generally available with clinical MRI scanners.

Wolff et al. (225) employed magnetization transfer (MT) to evaluate cartilage macromolecules. This technique uses a low-power, off-resonance radio-frequency field, resulting in a decreased signal intensity in regions with tight magnetic coupling between the fluid and the macromolecules. It has been shown that the MT is dominantly influenced by collagen (10,144,198), but some investigators have also found contributing influences from the PGs (109,220). Magic angle imaging (113,229) and measurement of the transverse relaxation time (T2) (174) have also been advocated for assessing collagen content and microstructure. Attempts to evaluate the interstitial water content in cartilage have also been based on measurement of T2 (55,88,159). Alternatively, proton density images have been used for this purpose (196,199).

These approaches may eventually allow diagnosis of ultrastructural and biochemical alterations of the cartilage at an earlier stage of progression, and initiate preventive measures or treatment before macromorphological changes occur. However, the *in vivo* precision (reproducibility) and accuracy of quantitative compositional measurements remains to be established.

3.2.2 Image Segmentation

Segmentation is the process by which image points (voxels) are assigned to a specific anatomic structure, such as articular cartilage. To date, MRI provides insufficient contrast for fully automated segmentation of articular cartilage based on the gray value distribution alone. It may appear surprising that modern computer algorithms are not able to detect automatically what is evident to the human eye. However, this problem is comparable to that of speech recognition, which is still at its infancy, despite intense commercial interest. Nevertheless, current semi-automated segmentation algorithms can accelerate the segmentation process and improve consistency between users. Volume-growing (67,71,182) and edge detection algorithms (147,186) are sensitive to irregularities at the cartilage surface and often fail in regions where contrast is low. Several groups have therefore developed approaches with model-based components, such as active shape models (204),

fitting *B*-spline surfaces to segmented data from points either digitized manually or using a semi-automated snake algorithm (48), immersion-based watershed segmentation (96), and live wires (212). Stammberger et al. (209) presented a deformable contour (*B*-spline snake) algorithm that relies on the interaction of "image forces" (gray value gradients), "model forces" (stiffness of a parameterized *B*-spline curve), and "coupling forces" (segmentation of previous sections). This algorithm has been shown to provide a higher inter-observer precision than manual segmentation in experienced users. Representative segmented surfaces of the knee are presented in Fig. 9-15.

3.2.3 3D Analysis, Visualization, and Image Registration

Based on sectional images alone, the comparison between individuals or the longitudinal study of tissue alterations are unreliable because corresponding section locations and orientations cannot be reproduced consistently. In this context, 3D digital post-processing techniques are required to provide measurements that are independent of the specific section location and orientation.

An initial approach has been to determine the cartilage volume (65,178,181). This is easily achieved by numerical integration (multiplication of the voxel number assigned to a cartilage plate with the voxel size). Changes in cartilage volume can be used as direct parameters of cartilage growth, adaptation, and tissue loss in OA. However, they lack focal and region-specific information on the quantitative distribution of the tissue within a joint surface, and are determined both by changes in cartilage thickness as well as the size of the articular surface.

The size of the joint surface area can be quantified based on surface triangulation (127). Because the angle between the MR images and the surface can vary throughout the joint surface and from acquisition to acquisition, the computation of cartilage thickness should take into account the local out-of-plane deviations of the normal or minimal distance vectors. This is achieved by

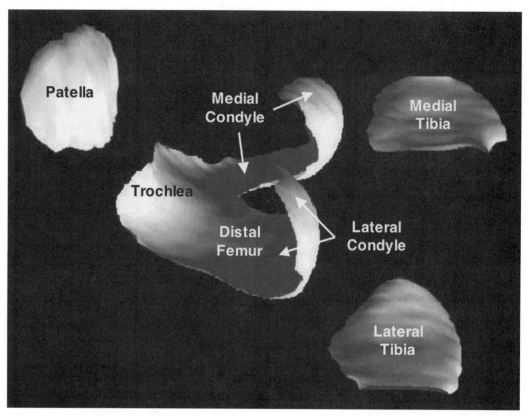

FIGURE 9-15. 3D reconstruction of the knee articular cartilage layers from segmentation of MRI data.

computing normal vectors of the bone cartilage interface, usually a fitted *B*-spline function (48), or minimal distances between the articular surface and the interface (157). Both implementations are mathematically identical, but can lead to slightly different results when being applied to discrete voxel objects (157). Stammberger et al. (210) developed a computational method that is based on 3D Euclidean distance transformation, avoiding the explicit calculation of surface normals. Comparison of thickness computations from sectional images with different spatial orientation relative to the knee joint surfaces (transverse versus sagittal for the patella and coronal versus sagittal for the tibia) have produced consistent results, showing that the algorithm works independent of the specific section orientation (73).

If a particular articular layer has been imaged more than once, such as would occur in a longitudinal study of a patient's joint or in a comparison of imaging modalities on the same joint, it is necessary to register the two data sets into a common reference frame prior to performing quantitative comparisons between them. To estimate the accuracy of MR-generated articular layer topography and thickness against corresponding SPG-generated data in a cadaver population, Cohen et al. (48) used least-squares minimization to find the optimal 3D rigid-body transformation that registers pairs of surfaces by finding the smallest rms Euclidian distance over all surface points. In order to depict local/regional cartilage thickness changes directly, Stammberger et al. (211) developed a 3D matching algorithm, in which the bone cartilage interfaces of two data sets are registered. First, a principal axis decomposition is used to align the surfaces, and in a second step corresponding image points are identified by elastically deforming the surfaces based on local geometric similarity measures (Euclidean distance and orientation compatibility). Kshirsagar et al. (147) proposed a rigid 3D registration algorithm and observed a higher precision of localized cartilage volume versus total cartilage volume measurements (2.0% versus 3.8%). Registration methods can be used to depict the spatial pattern of cartilage deformation during compression (see above) and are particularly useful in longitudinal studies that aim to monitor local changes of thickness, for instance, in epidemiological studies on disease progression, or in animal models of OA. However, in more advanced stages of OA, macromorphological changes are common and significantly afflict both bone and cartilage of the joint, thus rendering precise registration of image data challenging.

Not only morphological, but also compositional imaging of articular cartilage requires adequate 3D, post-processing tools. Hohe et al. (126) presented a technique by which the segmentation of the cartilage boundaries is first performed on a T1-weighted, fat-suppressed MR sequence. This topographic information was then transferred to data sets obtained with pulse-sequences that carried compositional information. The signal intensity was then analyzed throughout the entire cartilage layer (126) and,

in case of motion artifacts between acquisitions, the image data were registered with a 3D least-squares fit algorithm. Because biochemical and structural parameters are known to vary topographically by layer and region throughout cartilage, Hohe et al. (128) extended this computational technique to analyze the signal intensity characteristics both vertically throughout the depth of the tissue and horizontally throughout the joint surface. This technique can be used to quantify the MR signal distribution of any given MR sequence (or combination of sequences) throughout the cartilage, independent of the specific section orientation.

3.2.4 Validation

Because artifacts in MRI do not only depend on the equipment used, but on the specific composition of the tissue under investigation, validation studies must be performed directly on the biological object of interest (Table 9-2). Knee joint cartilage volume measurements (obtained with T1-weighted, fat-suppressed gradient echo sequence) have been shown to deviate not more than 5% to 10% on average from water displacement of surgically retrieved

TABLE 9-2. VALIDATION STUDIES OF QUANTITATIVE CARTILAGE IMAGING WITH MAGNETIC RESONANCE

Authors	Ref. No.	Joint	Technique of Validation[b]
Peterfy et al. 1994	(178)	Knee	WD of surgically removed tissue
Peterfy et al. 1995	(180)	Metacarpo-phalangeal	WD of surgically removed tissue
Piplani et al. 1996	(182)	Knee	WD of surgically removed tissue
Cicutini et al. 1999	(45)	Knee	WD of surgically removed tissue
Graichen et al. 2003a[a]	(107)	Shoulder	WD of surgically removed tissue
Graichen et al. 2003b[a]	(108)	Patella, tibia	WD of surgically removed tissue
Sittek et al. 1996	(203)	Patella	Anatomical sections
Eckstein et al. 1996	(67)	Knee	Anatomical sections
Kladny et al. 1996	(146)	Tibia	Anatomical sections
Eckstein et al. 1997	(68)	Patella	Anatomical sections
Graichen et al. 2003b[a]	(108)	Patella, tibia	Anatomical sections
Graichen et al. 2000[a]	(103)	Elbow	A-mode ultrasound
Graichen et al. 2003a[a]	(107)	Shoulder	A-mode ultrasound
Eckstein et al. 1997	(68)	Patella	A-mode ultrasound
Eckstein et al. 1998	(71)	Knee	CT arthrography
Graichen et al. 2000[a]	(103)	Elbow	CT arthrography
Cohen et al. 1999	(48)	Knee	Stereophotogrammetry

[a]Studies performed using a water excitation technique.
[b]WD, water displacement; CT, computed tomography.

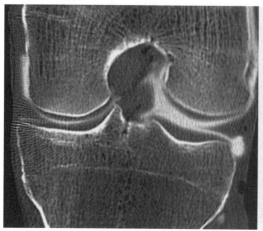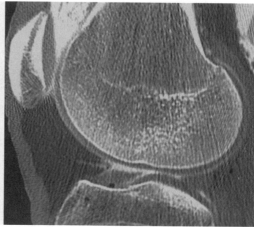

FIGURE 9-16. CT arthrography has been used to validate MRI measurements of cartilage topography and volume (71,75,103). See Fig. 9-14 for description of anatomical features.

tissue (45,59,107,108,178,180,182), anatomical sectioning (67,68,108,203), and CT arthrography as shown in Fig. 9-16 (68,71,73). *In vivo* preoperative MRI data of tibial cartilage with severe OA (obtained with a water excitation sequence) has been recently compared with volume displacement of surgically removed cartilage tissue of the resected tibial plateau during total knee replacement (39,108). Accurate volume measurements were obtained in these patients, with only little deviation from surgically removed tissue and a high linear relationship between methods (r = 0.98).

Regional distribution patterns of cartilage thickness were also found to be consistent with those derived from sectioning (67,68,146,203), A-mode ultrasound (68), and SPG (48). By exchanging frequency- and phase-encoding directions, it has been excluded that inhomogeneities of the magnetic field (introduced by susceptibility artifact) lead to relevant geometric distortion of the MR images (73). Glaser et al. (98) directly compared knee joint cartilage measurements with a frequency selective fat saturation (prepulse) versus water excitation technique and found deviations of only 1% to 4%, with slightly higher values for the water excitation sequence. These were attributed to a shorter echo time (TE) and higher signal intensity of the deeper cartilage layers.

Because other joints of the human body display significantly thinner cartilage than the knee,

spatial resolution is a critical issue in quantitative imaging of these articulations (156). Peterfy et al. (180) reported a satisfactory accuracy and precision of volume measurements in the metacarpophalangeal articulation. In elbow joint specimens (average cartilage thickness around 1 mm), Graichen et al. (103) found good agreement of cartilage measurements with a water excitation sequence (resolution $1 \times 0.25 \times 0.25$ mm^3, interpolated to an in-plane resolution of 0.125×0.125 mm^2), in relation to CT arthrography and A-mode ultrasound.

3.2.5 Precision (Reproducibility)

Measurement precision is particularly important in the context of reliably monitoring changes in longitudinal studies. The *in vivo* reproducibility of quantitative MR cartilage imaging has been studied in healthy volunteers and patients, by repeating measurements after joint repositioning and reshimming of the magnet. As a rule, the minimal interval of change that can be detected with 95% confidence in a single individual is 2.8 times the precision error (CV% = standard deviation/mean of repeated measurements $\times$ 100), and the minimal detectable difference in a group of 10 individuals is in the range of the precision error (54). The precision errors of cartilage volume and thickness measurements were found to be relatively low and in the range of most current densitometric measurement techniques for the diagnosis of osteoporosis. The highest precision (around 1%) was obtained for the patella with a transverse section orientation (water excitation sequence—74). In other knee joint surfaces, the precision ranged from 2% to 4%, this error being substantially lower than the intersubject variation (79,99). The long-term precision error (imaging sessions several weeks apart) was somewhat higher than that obtained for short-term conditions (40), but differences in coefficients were relatively small and not statistically significant. This suggests that factors such as scanner drift, changes in imaging conditions (temperature, humidity), and changes in patient conditions are not a critical problem in quantitative cartilage imaging. In patients with severe OA (prior to knee arthroplasty), the relative precision error (CV%) was higher than in healthy volunteers, but not the absolute error (SD), which is in the range of 50 mm^3 (39,46). In view of an estimated tissue loss of more than 1000 mm^3 in tibial cartilage volume before knee arthroplasty (39), these data suggest that reliable staging and monitoring of OA progression can be performed with quantitative MRI.

Computations of the mean cartilage thickness and joint surface areas have been shown to yield a similar precision to that of the cartilage volume, whereas the reproducibility of the maximal cartilage thickness value was found to be somewhat lower (128,133,210). With digital image analysis it has also been demonstrated that regional distribution patterns of articular cartilage throughout joint surfaces also display satisfactory precision (67,215).

When determining the *in vivo* precision of this imaging protocol in joints of the hind foot (average cartilage thickness 0.5 to 1 mm), precision errors of 2% to 11% were observed for single joint surfaces, but smaller errors (<3%) for cumulative measures of several joints (7). These results demonstrate that quantitative cartilage imaging is not confined to the knee, but can also be employed in other joints. In the hip and shoulder, however, circular extremity coils cannot be used, and total body coils do not provide adequate resolution. Advances will therefore depend on the design of more efficient surface coils to permit measurements in all major joints of the human body.

4 DETERMINANTS OF CARTILAGE VOLUME AND THICKNESS IN HUMAN JOINTS

Using invasive methods, Werner (223) and Adam et al. (3) described the patella to display the highest cartilage thickness of all human joint surfaces, with values up to 7 mm. The average values in the knee were 2.0 ± 0.3 mm, in the hip 1.4 ± 0.2 mm, and in the ankle 1.0 ± 0.2 mm in elderly individuals (3). The use of high-resolution MRI has recently produced a wealth of novel data on the morphology of human articular layers under physiological and pathophysiological conditions. This likely represents only a first step to a more complete understanding of cartilage morphology and (patho-) physiology, as these methods are now introduced to larger-scale population-based epidemiologic studies.

4.1 Intersubject Variability, Side Differences, and Correlation Between Different Joint Surfaces

Several studies reported a surprising degree of intersubject variability of the cartilage volume, thickness, and surface areas of the knee and other joints (7,45,69,75,76,103,137), and relatively low correlations with the body weight and height (45,69,75,76). A large database of knee joint cartilage with more than 100 young healthy volunteers has been presented recently (41,76,130), the high intersubject variability having been confirmed. When evaluating side differences in the knee, no significant differences were found between the left and right in volunteers with dominance of one of the lower limbs (78). The absolute deviations were substantially lower in all surfaces (~ 5%) than the intersubject variability (~ 20%).

Quantitative parameters displayed low correlations among the cartilage layers of the knee (patella, femur, medial, and lateral tibia), the coefficients (r) ranging from 0.16 to 0.70 for the volume, 0.24 to 0.62 for the surface areas, and 0.31 to 0.78 for the thickness (75). The tissue thus appears to be distributed inhomogeneously onto the various cartilage layers, and high or low values in one knee joint surface are not necessarily associated with high or low values in another. The patellar cartilage, for instance, can take up between 11% and 27% of the knee volume.

Within the hind foot (talocrural joint, subtalar joint, and talocalcaneonavicular joint), the correlation among different cartilage layers tended to be higher than within the knee (76). The correlation between the talocrural joint and talotarsal joint was r = 0.92 for cartilage volume, 0.80 for the surface areas, and 0.62 for the mean thickness, but there was no significant correlation with the cartilage thickness in the knee (r = −0.63 to +0.47). Thus, cartilage thickness values in different joints in the body appear not to be determined by identical factors.

4.2 Correlation with Gender, Age, and Anthropometric Variables

Cicuttini et al. (45) reported gender differences of cartilage volume in adults, and Jones et al. (137) in children and adolescents; these remained significant after adjusting for age, body weight, height, and femoral (condylar) bone volume. Faber et al. (85) also reported significant gender difference for cartilage volume in the medial (+43%) and lateral tibia (+47%), and smaller (albeit significant) differences in the patella (+20%) and femur (+27%). It was shown (85) that the gender differences in cartilage volume originated primarily from differences in the joint surface area size (total knee +23%; p < 0.01), but to a lesser extent from differences in cartilage thickness (+8%; difference not statistically significant). In a larger sample (n = 95), gender differences of cartilage thickness became significant, but were still considerably smaller than those of joint surface areas (76). When matching men and women with identical body weight or height, interestingly, the joint surfaces were still significantly larger in men. Cartilage thickness values showed a trend

to be larger in the men, but the differences did not reach statistical significance (76).

It has been controversial whether cartilage thinning occurs during the normal aging process (possibly as a result of reduction in mechanical loading) or whether the decrease only affects people with OA. In cadaver studies, Meachim (163) found no significant decrease of cartilage thickness in the shoulder with age, whereas in the patella Meachim et al. (164) described thinning of the cartilage, in particular in women older than the age of 50. These changes were, however, attributed to OA rather than to "matrix shrinkage." Karvonen et al. (140) concluded from local measurements in MR images that age accounted for a significant linear decrease in cartilage thickness in the absence and presence of OA. This observation was, however, confined to the site of frequent femorotibial contact of the lateral and medial femoral condyle and did not apply to the patella, the tibia, or the posterior aspects of the femoral condyles. Hudelmaier et al. (130,131) examined elderly men and women with no history of knee pain, trauma, or surgery (age 50 to 75 yr). They found no significant difference in cartilage thickness between elderly and young men (− 6%), but a significantly lower thickness (−12%; p < 0.05) in elderly women. In the other joint surfaces, age-dependent differences (old versus young) were similar in women and men, and amounted to approximately −4% per decade (131).

A relatively weak correlation was observed between the cartilage volume of the knee and elbow versus body weight or height (69,75,76,208). In a sample of only men (75), the correlations between cartilage volume and body weight/height were r = 0.06 to 0.27/0.28 to 0.45 for the various cartilage layers, whereas the size of the bone cartilage interface displayed higher correlation coefficients with the cartilage volume (r = 0.39 to 0.67). Interestingly, however, the size of the joint surface area and the mean cartilage thickness were not significantly associated (r = 0.02 to 0.34), showing that individuals with larger joints do not necessarily display thicker cartilage (75). It thus remains to be established which specific factors are responsible for the heterogeneity of cartilage thickness in different joints and different skeletal regions of the same individual.

4.3 Functional Adaptation to Mechanical Stimuli

Mechanical stimuli are known to be potent regulators of muscle and bone tissue mass. Animal studies have suggested that cartilage thickness decreases during immobilization (121), but investigations with increased levels of exercise have produced inconclusive and partly contradictory results (121,173). Jones et al. (137) observed an association between cartilage volume and self-reported level of exercise in children. Mühlbauer et al. (171) and later Eckstein et al. (77) examined adult triathletes, who had been training for at least 10 hours per week over the last 3 years and had been physically active also throughout childhood and adolescence. These were compared with individuals who had never been physically active (<1 hour sport per week throughout life), had no job that involved physical activity, and had a normal body mass index. Surprisingly, male or female thriathletes did not display significant differences in cartilage thickness compared with physically inactive volunteers. This suggests that substantial increases in mechanical stimulation do not increase the thickness of the cartilage, and that the natural variation in cartilage thickness is not explained by different levels of physical exercise. Interestingly, however, triathletes displayed larger knee joint surface areas (+9%/$p < 0.01$ in men; +7%/$p = 0.08$ in women; see reference 77). The data indicate that the biological mechanism to reduce high stress at the articular surface may be by an increase in the bearing surface rather than an increase in cartilage thickness. The reason for this may be that beyond a certain thickness the nutritive situation of the cartilage becomes critical, and/or that the stress distribution and load partitioning between the interstitial water and extracellular matrix (see Chapter 5) within the cartilage becomes unfavorable with thicker cartilage (16,227). With thicker cartilage, there is more space for the interstitial fluid to escape from the site of contact, the mechanism of hydrostatic pressurization being

impaired (e.g., 15,160). With larger contact areas, in contrast, interstitial fluid pressurization is enhanced and thus supports a greater share of the load at the articular surface.

Vanwanseele et al. (217) reported the cartilage thickness to be reduced in paraplegic patients, indicating that cartilage may undergo atrophy in the absence of mechanical stimulation. These findings have been confirmed in a recent longitudinal study (218) and have implications for the clinical management of the postoperative period in bone and joint surgery, and also for long-term space flight.

4.4 Quantitative Assessment of Cartilage Lesions from Thickness Maps

The ability to generate accurate cartilage thickness maps for a particular patient may be valuable for a clinical assessment of the tissue's integrity. However, a purely visual interpretation of such maps may be subjective because it would rely on the accuracy of the observer's knowledge of the pattern of normal thickness distribution in that specific articular layer, and his ability to differentiate the patient-specific map from the normative pattern in that joint. Because quantitative data are available from the generation of thickness maps, it follows that a quantitative assessment of localized or surface-wide regions of cartilage thinning should be possible. Regions of thinning may then be interpreted as potential cartilage lesions, within a statistical confidence level. In a recent study (51), a methodological approach was proposed to achieve the goal of quantifying regions of cartilage lesions in the patellofemoral joint.

The first step toward the assessment of lesions in a patient-specific joint is to create a template of the expected normal topography and cartilage thickness distribution in a target population. For example, a normal topography and thickness template could be created for the patellar and femoral cartilage of normal subjects, segregated by age and gender, and other categories if necessary, such as weight, height, ethnicity, etc. Examples of such templates are presented in

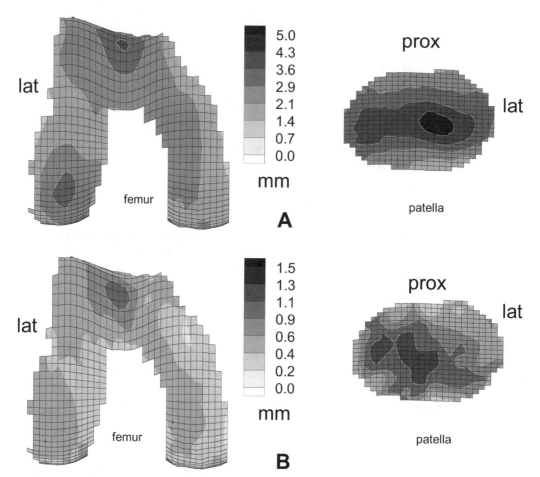

FIGURE 9-17. **(A)** Average cartilage thickness map, projected onto the average surface topography, for femur *(left)* and patella *(right)*. **(B)** Corresponding maps of standard deviations in thickness. Average data obtained from 14 normal subjects, 6 females, 8 males, ages 21–70 (51).

Fig. 9-17A, which show the average topography and thickness distribution in the femoral and patellar articular layers of human adults, generated from a population of 14 normal subjects (6 females, 8 males, ages 21–70). Furthermore, to assess the variability in cartilage thickness across the articular surfaces of the patellofemoral joint, a map of the local standard deviation in thickness can also be provided (Fig. 9-17B). The average thickness map represents the normal template of cartilage thickness distribution in that joint, whereas the standard deviation map indicates the extent by which the thickness varies across normal subjects.

When the 3D articular layer topography and corresponding thickness map of a particular patient are quantified, as shown for example in Fig. 9-18A, they first need to be aligned to the normal template; this may be achieved by aligning the body-fixed anatomical coordinate system of the patient's patella or femur with the corresponding coordinate system of the normal template (see below). The patient's topography and thickness map are then properly scaled to the size of the average template, to reduce differences arising from size alone. The patient's thickness map is then projected onto the topography of the normal template so that a

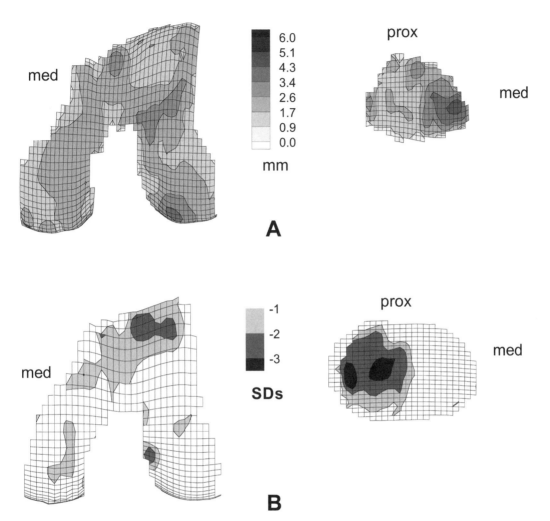

FIGURE 9-18. (A) Cartilage thickness maps for a 51-year-old female patient diagnosed with patellofemoral joint osteoarthritis. **(B)** Normalized difference maps for the same subject, showing regions most likely to represent cartilage lesions (51).

point-by-point difference can be calculated between the patient's thickness map and the normal template. Finally, the difference in thickness can be normalized by the local standard deviation and the result can be mapped onto the normal average topography as shown in Fig. 9-18B. This normalized difference distribution, which shows only the regions where deficits are observed, is a topographical map of cartilage lesions. For example, differences in excess of two standard deviations are unlikely to represent a normal variation across subjects, and may be interpreted as lesions with a 95% confidence level,

whereas higher deficits may provide greater confidence in that assessment.

Methodologies that take advantage of the quantitative measurement of cartilage thickness from MRI, such as the one described above, are still under developmental refinements. Clinical usage is predicated on the demonstration that such measures can provide a significantly better assessment of joint degeneration than current radiological practice, at a comparatively reasonable cost to the patient. Validation of such techniques also requires that normal templates be generated from large populations of normal subjects.

5 JOINT MECHANICS

5.1 *In Situ* Measurement of Cartilage Deformation

Although the mechanical properties of articular cartilage have been extensively investigated *in vitro*, see Chapter 5, there have—until recently—been no data on the amount of *in situ* cartilage deformation in the intact joint under *in vivo* loading conditions. These data cannot be easily extrapolated from *in vitro* studies, because the magnitudes of joint loads occurring during normal (in particular dynamic) exercise are uncertain, see Chapters 2 and 3. This also applies for the effect of the boundary conditions (e.g., nonlinear contact conditions between two incongruous joint surfaces, presence of a thin layer of synovial fluid). Data on the *in vivo* deformation of articular cartilage are, however, required for estimating the strain (and stress) to which the cartilage is subjected under normal conditions (e.g., as input data for experiments in cell biology and studies of mechanically loaded cartilage explants—see Chapters 6 and 8), and to characterize the mechanical target environment for tissue-engineered cartilage.

5.1.1 In Vivo Deformation

Eckstein et al. (70) reported a quantitative study on the changes of cartilage volume of healthy volunteers after 1 hour of physical rest and again 3 to 7 minutes after 50 knee bends. They observed a consistent change in volume (deformation) of approximately 6%. In a further study it was demonstrated that multiple sets of 50 knee bends (at 15-min intervals) did not lead to higher cartilage deformation, and that the time required for the cartilage volume to regain its preexercise levels may be as much as 90 minutes (72); this slow rate is likely to be due to a relatively low fluid flux through the surface (approximately 0.027 μm/s—see Chapter 5 and references 15,160). Comparing static (90° squatting for 20 s) versus dynamic loading (30 deep knee bends to 120° flexion), differences were found both in the amount and in the pattern of cartilage deformation throughout the joint surface (74). In elderly subjects without symptoms, Hudelmaier et al. (130) recently found a considerably smaller degree of patellar cartilage deformation than in younger individuals. A potential explanation for the reduced deformation was that elderly individuals present different motor strategies (176) and subject their knee joints to smaller loads during knee bending. It has, however, also been demonstrated that certain collagen cross links increase with aging (pentosidine), both in animals and in humans (30,214). This may render the cartilage matrix stiffer than in the young. Standardized *in vivo* loading protocols may be used clinically to evaluate functional properties of articular cartilage in the course of joint disease, and to study the effects of different types of therapy on cartilage biomechanical quality.

Waterton et al. (222) investigated volunteers in the morning and after a day of mainly standing activity. They reported no change in overall femoral cartilage volume and thickness, but they observed cartilage thinning in the femoropatellar and femorotibial contact zones. They found an increase in thickness in areas not subjected to loading during standing and hypothesized that this resulted from negative intraarticular pressure during joint extension by the quadriceps. However, it was alternatively suggested that interstitial fluid is displaced from load-bearing to non-load-bearing areas within cartilage.

5.1.2 In Vitro Deformation

Cartilage deformation during (rather than shortly after) loading cannot be easily investigated *in vivo* because it is difficult to apply relevant loads to the joint of a living person within the MRI scanner and—at the same time—keep the joint in a constant position relative to the coil. To overcome this limitation, Herberhold et al. (122) constructed a non-metallic compression apparatus for use in an MRI scanner. The pressure piston was capable of generating loads of up to 1500 N and the entire apparatus fitted into the extremity coil of a clinical MRI scanner. The time-dependent deformation of the femoropatellar cartilage was then studied in situ for 4 hours under continuous static loading with 150% body weight, the joint capsule being fully intact. A maximal thickness reduction of 57% ± 15% was observed for patellar cartilage and a volume change of >30%. The data suggest that more than 50% of the interstitial fluid had been displaced from the porous-permeable extracellular matrix. However, only very little deformation occurred during the first few minutes of loading (3% after 1 min, and 11% after 8 min). It was concluded that under in situ conditions the cartilage requires several hours to reach equilibrium under physiologically realistic load magnitudes, suggesting that the state in which the entire load is borne by the solid matrix is likely never reached *in vivo*. However, in OA tissues, where there is an increased permeability and decreased compressive stiffness of the solid matrix, the time required for interstitial fluid depressurization decreases significantly (89; also see Chapter 5). This process mandates the support of the applied load be transferred to the solid matrix more rapidly, thus increasing its duty cycle. Secondly, because cartilage deformed relatively little during the first minutes of loading, it was concluded that there is little time for the interstitial fluid to escape initially. The mechanism of load transmission in articular cartilage is thus by hydrostatic compression. In combination with biphasic finite element analysis (58), these experiments can be used to specifically calculate the load partitioning between the fluid phase (hydrostatic pressurization) and the proteoglycan-collagen matrix, the stresses in the latter eventually causing tissue failure.

Other investigators have constructed compression devices for subjecting cartilage probes to uniaxial compression and have observed cartilage properties with high-field MR systems (141,189). These experiments have shown that MR relaxation parameters and signal intensity values of the cartilage change during compression in a depth-dependent fashion, the apparent layering of the cartilage in MR images being modulated by loading.

5.2 Joint Contact Studies from Proximity Maps

Determination of contact areas in diarthrodial joints is a first step toward understanding the stress-strain environment and the effects of joint loading on articular cartilage. Although the goal

of many rehabilitation and surgical procedures is restoration of normal articular mechanics, little is known regarding the normal or abnormal contact mechanics of many joints. Historically, a variety of techniques have been utilized to measure diarthrodial joint contact areas, including dye staining (111), rubber or dental casting (66,82,148,195), piezoresistive transducers (33,34), and Fuji and other pressure-sensitive films (e.g., 5,52,82,90,129,202).

Another method, based on evaluating the proximity of articular surfaces to estimate contact areas using experimentally derived geometric models of the joint, has been developed (191,192). In this approach, kinematic data representing relative motion of opposing articular surfaces during a specific motion, or with the joint in a series of specified positions, are obtained. Subsequently, articular surfaces are exposed, and their geometry is quantified to create models of the joints. Next, spatial transformations that realign the articular surfaces into the relative positions that they assumed during the motion in question are performed. Finally, by calculating the points of closest proximity between opposing surfaces in this realigned position, contact areas can be estimated. This last step can be accomplished only with the availability of geometric models of the articular surfaces.

In 1994, Ateshian et al. reported a comparison of contact methods that included dye staining, silicone rubber casting, Fuji film, and an SPG method that utilizes a proximity criterion similar to that described above (17). In this comparison study, both congruent joints (modeled by bovine glenohumeral joints) and incongruent joints (modeled by bovine lateral tibiofemoral articulations without the menisci) were investigated. All methods provided consistent contact results for the incongruent articulation. However, for the congruent joint, the proximity and Fuji film methods yielded similar results, but the other two methods yielded significantly different contact regions. Some advantages of the proximity method are that it can be used in intact joints and that it can be used repeatedly and quickly through a range of motions. This contact method has been used to quantify contact in human joints such as the thumb CMC (20), the glenohumeral (shoulder) (206), and

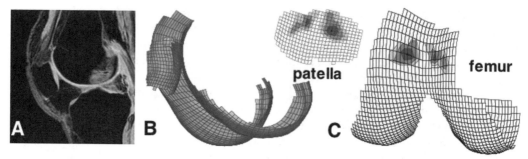

FIGURE 9-19. Proximity-based contact area maps obtained from MRI-generated patellofemoral joint articular surfaces. **(A)** Representative MR image; **(B)** 3D surface reconstructions of the femoral and patellar surfaces; **(C)** proximity maps representing likely areas of contact.

the knee tibiofemoral and patellofemoral joints (153). Current studies are beginning to apply the concepts developed through the SPG method for use with MRI, whereby proximity of MRI-generated articular surfaces can be used to assess contact areas in situ and *in vivo* (48,124). An illustration of this approach is shown in Fig. 9-19, which displays the proximity-based contact area map for MRI-generated patellofemoral joint articular layers.

5.3 Studies Using Open MRI Methods

Open MRI systems permit doctors to directly obtain 3D data on various anatomical articular structures (joint bodies, muscles, menisci, etc.) in various joint positions. This method has, for instance, been used to determine the acromio-humeral distance (101) and motion patterns of the glenoid (scapula) during elevation of the arm (105). Graichen et al. applied external loads during open MRI, analyzing the effect of normal (and pathologic) neuromuscular control on the subacromial space (102), on joint stability in the shoulder (104), and on skeletal motion patterns (106). These techniques have recently been applied to study patients with shoulder instability (83) and cruciate ligament deficiency of the knee (32). The cross-registration of high-resolution morphological data on articular cartilage with either open MRI (including the application of external forces) or kinematic/gait analysis (8) may be developed into an efficient tool for assessing joint mechanics during normal neuromuscular

control, and to analyze the specific mechanical factors that initiate or promote cartilage degeneration.

5.4 Anatomically Based Coordinate Systems

The development of quantitative tools for measuring joint kinematics, contact areas, cartilage thickness, and cartilage stresses has brought with it the necessity to describe these measurements in meaningful and reproducible body-fixed coordinate systems. For example, in a patient with patellar malalignment, the success of a corrective surgical procedure can be determined in part by measuring the shift in patellofemoral joint contact areas from pre- and postoperative MRIs. A precise measurement of this spatial shift can be achieved only if a body-fixed coordinate system is defined consistently in both sets of images. Similarly, joint kinematic measurements are best interpreted when they are referred to anatomically based coordinate systems.

Body-fixed coordinate systems can be associated with various bones of a joint by employing topographic measurements of the bone contours as well as the articular surfaces (25,112, 139,150,153). In the case of the knee, for example, Blankevoort et al. (25) defined coordinate axes for the femur and tibia, which are aligned with each other in full extension. The origins of these coordinate systems were determined relative to specific bony landmarks. A similar approach was followed by van Kampen and Huiskes (139) in the case of the patellofemoral

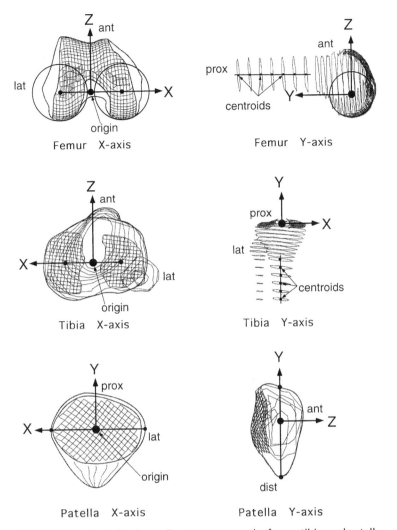

FIGURE 9-20. Body-fixed coordinate systems on the femur, tibia, and patella (150).

joint. However, Blankevoort et al. (25) demonstrated from a parametric analysis that relatively small misalignments in the choice of these coordinate systems may lead to large variations in some of the kinematic measurements. These variations could lead to inconsistent kinematic results among various specimens. Kwak et al. (150) proposed a set of body-fixed coordinate systems for the femur, tibia, and patella, which are derived from 3D geometric data of the bones and their articular surfaces. The articular surface data were derived from SPG, and bone contours were digitized with a coordinate-measurement machine (CMM) (Fig. 9-20). In this approach, the coordinate axes of the femur, tibia, and patella are no longer necessarily aligned in full extension: Thus, for example, the varus-valgus angle of the tibia relative to the femur is derived from the orientation of the femoral and tibial coordinate systems rather than prescribed arbitrarily to be zero when the flexion angle is zero. Blankevoort et al. (27) conducted a kinematic study on seven knee joints, where they compared outcomes using the coordinate systems of Blankevoort et al. (25) and van Kampen and Huiskes (139) against those of Kwak et al.

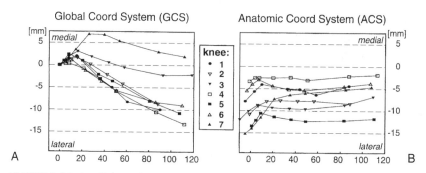

FIGURE 9-21. Mediolateral translation of the patella during flexion from 0° to 120° in six cadaver specimens, using two sets of coordinate systems: **(A)** coordinate axes that are globally aligned with bony landmarks of the knee joint, but which become parallel at full extension; **(B)** body-fixed coordinate systems that are derived from articular and bone surface geometry.

(150). They confirmed that for certain motions, such as mediolateral translation and rotation of the patella as well as internal-external and varus-valgus rotations of the tibia, the differences in the results were very significant (Fig. 9-21).

5.5 Computer Simulations and Multibody Modeling of Joints

Quantitative representations of bones and articular surfaces can be used for mathematically modeling diarthrodial joints to predict the normal mechanics and the outcome of simulated injuries, surgical repair procedures, or other pathologic conditions. Generally, these models are created from experimental data and are validated by predicting the outcome of experiments that have actually been performed. If the agreement between the model and experiment is found to be good it is possible to employ the mathematical model to predict the outcomes of other configurations that have not been tested experimentally. Such computer simulations are becoming more common in orthopaedic research (e.g., 46, 50,84,87,93,118–120,152), and may have potential applications for computer-assisted surgical planning.

In addition to finite element analysis, which is generally computationally intensive, joint modeling has been performed using the classical engineering approach of multibody modeling in which bones are assumed to be rigid bod-

ies, while cartilage, ligaments, muscles, tendons, and other soft tissue structures are often modeled using springs. For example, models of the wrist (193) and knee joint (e.g., 1,26,84, 93,118,119,123,152,224) have been described by several authors. A computer rendition of a knee joint model (152) that employs quantitative geometric data for representing bones, cartilage, ligament insertions, and muscle lines of action, is presented in Fig. 9-22A. By comparing their model predictions with actual experiments simulating open-chain knee exercises in a cadaver knee joint, Kwak et al. (152) have shown that predicted displacements and rotations of the patella were within 1 mm and 4°, respectively, of the experimental data over a range of 0° to 90° of knee flexion.

The potential clinical application of multibody models of diarthrodial joints in surgical planning may be illustrated in the example of Fig. 9-22A, which displays a patient-specific model for a 45-year-old woman diagnosed with OA of the patellofemoral joint. The model was generated from two MRI data sets; high-resolution images were employed for cartilage layer reconstruction and low-resolution images were used to determine joint kinematics in a flexed position (49). Muscle insertion points were determined from the MR images, but muscle lines of action and force magnitudes were based on an independent cadaveric study; similarly, representative soft tissue properties were

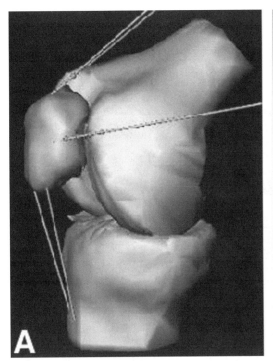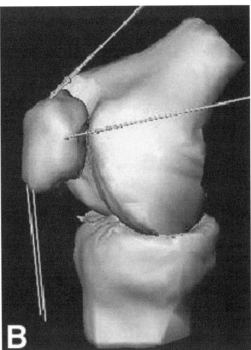

FIGURE 9-22. (A) Multibody model of the knee joint of a 45-year-old female patient with patellofemoral joint osteoarthritis, showing bone and articular surfaces, ligaments, and muscle lines of action, as determined from MRI data. **(B)** Simulation of tibial tuberosity anteriorization (49).

employed, based on literature data. Given the muscle loading conditions, the model can predict articular contact stresses, taking into account the patient-specific variation in cartilage thickness, including full thickness defects that may result in bone-to-bone contact. A patient such as this one may be a candidate for tibial tuberosity transfer surgery, a procedure whose aim is to reduce the contact stresses by shifting the contact area to less degenerated regions and by reducing the contact force across the joint. A variety of such surgical procedures have been proposed in the literature, including anteriorization (the Maquet procedure) and anteromedialization (the Fulkerson procedure) (92,161). Clinically, no single procedure has been shown to be superior for all patients, suggesting that the surgical outcome is specific to both the patient and the procedure, not the procedure alone. It would therefore be useful to develop a tool that may predict which procedure is most likely to succeed in a particular patient. Tuberosity trans-

fers are relatively straightforward to model in a multibody analysis, by translating the patellar tendon insertion points on the tuberosity medially and/or anteriorly, as shown in Fig. 9-22B. For various magnitudes of translation, the resulting contact stress distribution is displayed in Fig. 9-23, showing that, for this particular patient, 15 mm of anteriorization and 8 mm of medialization reduced the contact stress the most (by 18% for the mean stress and 25% for the peak stress) among the various tested procedures. In a patient population of 20 individuals diagnosed with patellofemoral joint OA, only in 12 of the patients did all simulated procedures result in a decrease in peak contact stress; in the other eight, at least one of the procedures led to an increase in peak contact stress. It is thus apparent that the ability to predict surgical outcome on a patient-specific basis could become very valuable.

Many of these surgical planning tools are still under development today, and they require

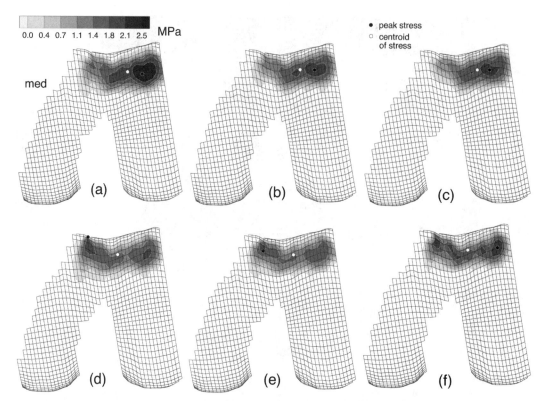

FIGURE 9-23. Patellofemoral contact stress maps for the female patient of Fig. 9-22 at 53° flexion, displayed on femoral surface: **(a)** pre-surgery; **(b)** 15 mm anteriorization; **(c)** 20 mm anteriorization; **(d)** 8 mm anteriorization and 8 mm medialization; **(e)** 15 mm anteriorization and 8 mm medialization; **(f)** same as **(e)** but using uniform thickness distribution and linear strain law instead of patient-specific cartilage thickness distribution and nonlinear law (49).

further validation. To verify that the predictions of a multibody model analysis are reasonably accurate would require double-blinded patient studies where surgical simulations are compared with actual outcome. If it is confirmed that such simulations have a reasonable predictive ability, computer-assisted orthopaedic surgical planning will likely serve as a useful clinical tool in the future.

6 SUMMARY

In this chapter, various applications of imaging, quantitative measurement and modeling of the articular layers of diarthrodial joints have been reviewed. Because of the rapidly advancing and continuing introduction of imaging and computer modeling tools into orthopaedic biomechanics, the review presented in this chapter does not purport to be exhaustive. Its primary aim is to provide the reader with some insights into the exciting potential of quantitative imaging and computer modeling in orthopaedic applications. Advances in noninvasive imaging tools offer the opportunity to transfer these techniques from the lab to the bedside. When they fulfill their full potential, these tools can be used in the areas of diagnosis, monitoring of disease progression in conditions such as OA, and assessing surgical outcomes as well as efficacy of structure modifying therapies for cartilage degeneration.

7 ACKNOWLEDGMENTS

This review chapter covers the work of many investigators. The material derived from the authors' own studies was supported by grants from the National Institutes of Health (AR41020, AR42850), and grants from the German Research Society DFG EC 159 2-1/DFG EC 159 2-2/ DFG EC 159 7-1.

REFERENCES

1. Abdel-Rahman E, Hefzy MS. A two-dimensional dynamic anatomical model of the human knee joint. *J Biomech Eng* 1993;115:357–365.
2. Adam C, Eckstein F, Milz S, et al. The distribution of cartilage thickness in the knee joint of old-aged individuals—measurement by A-mode ultrasound. *Clin Biomech* 1998;13:1–10.
3. Adam C, Eckstein F, Milz S, et al. The distribution of cartilage thickness within the joints of the lower limb of elderly individuals. *J Anat* 1998;193:203–214.
4. Ahmad CS, Cohen ZA, Levine WN, et al. Biomechanical and topographic considerations for autologous osteochondral grafting in the knee. *Am J Sports Med* 2001;29:201–206.
5. Ahmed AM, Burke DL. In-vitro measurement of static pressure distribution in synovial joints—part I: tibial surface of the knee. *J Biomech Eng* 1983;105:216–225.
6. Aisen AM, McCune WJ, MacGuire A. Sonographic evaluation of the cartilage of the knee. *Radiology* 1984;153:781–4.
7. Al-Ali D, Graichen H, Faber S. Quantitative cartilage imaging of the human hind foot: normal values and precision. *J Orthop Res* 2002;20:249–256.
8. Alexander EJ, Lang PK, Andriacchi TP. Dynamic functional imaging. In: Lemke HU, Vannier MW, Inamura K, et al., eds. *Proc. of Computer Assisted Radiology and Surgery, 14th International Congress,* Excerpta Medica Series 1214. Amsterdam: Elsevier Science, 2000:303–308.
9. Allen RG, Burstein D, Gray ML. Monitoring glycosaminoglycan replenishment in cartilage explants with gadolinium enhanced magnetic resonance imaging. *J Orthop Res* 1999;17:430–436.
10. Aoki J, Hiraki Y, Seo GS. Effect of collagen on magnetization transfer contrast assessed in cultured cartilage. *Nippon Igaku Hoshasen Gakkai Zashi* 1996;56:877–879.
11. Armstrong CG, Gardner DL. Thickness and distribution of human femoral head articular cartilage. *Ann Rheum Dis* 1977;36:407–412.
12. Armstrong CG. An analysis of the stresses in a thin layer of articular cartilage in a synovial joint. *Eng Med* 1986;15:55–61.
13. Ateshian GA, Soslowsky LJ, Mow VC. Quantitation of articular surface topography and cartilage thickness in knee joints using stereophotogrammetry. *J Biomech* 1991;24:761–776.
14. Ateshian GA, Rosenwasser MP, Mow VC. Curvature characteristics and congruence of the thumb carpometacarpal joint. *J Biomech* 1992;25:591–608.
15. Ateshian GA. A least-squares 5-spline surface-fitting method for articular surfaces of diarthrodial joints. *J Biomech Eng* 1993;115:366–373.
16. Ateshian GA, Lai WM, Zhu WB, et al. An asymptotic solution for the contact of two biphasic cartilage layers. *J Biomech* 1994;27:1347–1360.
17. Ateshian GA, Kwak SD, Soslowsky LJ, et al. A stereophotogrammetric method for determining *in situ* contact areas in diarthrodial joints, and a comparison with other methods. *J Biomech* 1994;21:11 1–124.
18. Ateshian GA. Generating trimmed B-spline models of articular cartilage layers from unordered 3D surface data points. *1995 Bioengineering Conference. ASME* 1995;BED-29:217–218.
19. Ateshian GA, Wang H. A theoretical solution for the frictionless rolling contact of cylindrical biphasic articular cartilage layers. *J Biomech* 1995;28:1341–1355.
20. Ateshian GA, Ark JW, Rosenwasser MP, et al. *In situ* contact areas in the thumb carpometacarpal joint. *J Orthop Res* 1995;13:450–458.
21. Bashir A, Gray ML, Burstein D. Gd DTPA2- as a measure of cartilage degradation. *Magn Reson Med* 1996;36:665–673.
22. Bashir A, Gray ML, Boutin RD. Glycosaminoglycan in articular cartilage: *in vivo* assessment with delayed Gd(DTPA)(2-) enhanced MR imaging. *Radiology* 1997;205:551–558.
23. Bashir A, Gray ML, Hartke J, et al. Nondestructive imaging of human cartilage glycosaminoglycan concentration by MRI. *Magn Reson Med* 1999;41:857–865.
24. Beck JM, Farouki RT, Hinds JK. Surface analysis methods. *IEEE CG&A* 1986;December:18–36.
25. Blankevoort L, Huiskes R, de Lange A. The envelope of passive knee joint motion. *J Biomech* 1988;21:705–720.
26. Blankevoort L, Kuiper JH, Huiskes R, et al. Articular contact in a three-dimensional model of the knee. *J Biomech* 1991;24:1019–1031.
27. Blankevoort L, Kwak SD, Ahmad CS, et al. Effects of global and anatomic coordinate systems on knee joint kinematics. *Proc Eur Soc Biomech* 1996;10:260.
28. Boven F, Bellemans MA, Geurts J, et al. A comparative study of the patello-femoral joint on axial roentgenogram, axial arthrogram, and computed tomography following arthrography. *Skeletal Radiol* 1982;8:179–181.
29. Boyd SK, Ronsky JL, Lichti DD, et al. Joint surface modeling with thin-plate splines. *J Biomech Eng* 1999;121:525–532.

30. Brama PA, TeKoppele JM, Bank RA, et al. Influence of site and age on biochemical characteristics of the collagen network of equine articular cartilage. *Am J Vet Res* 1999;60:341–345.

31. Bredella MA, Tirman PF, Peterfy CG, et al. Accuracy of T2-weighted fast spin echo MR imaging with fat saturation in detecting cartilage defects in the knee: comparison with arthroscopy in 130 patients. *Am J Roentgenol* 2000;172:1073–1080.

32. Bringmann C, Eckstein F, Bonel H, et al. Eine neue In-vivo-Technik zur dreidimensionalen Analyse der Translation der Femurkondylen und der menisken unter dem Einfluß antagonistischer Muskelkräfte. *Biomedizinisache Technik* 2000;45:258–265.

33. Brown TD, Shaw DT. *In vitro* contact stress distributions in the natural human hip. *J Biomech* 1983;16:373–384.

34. Brown TD, Shaw DT. *In vitro* contact stress distribution on the femoral condyles. *J Orthop Res* 1984;2:190–199.

35. Buckland-Wright JC, Macfarlane DG, Lynch JA, et al. Joint space width measures cartilage thickness in osteoarthritis of the knee: high resolution plain film and double contrast macroradiographic investigation. *Ann Rheum Dis* 1995a;54:263–268.

36. Buckland-Wright JC, Macfarlane DG, Williams SA, et al. Accuracy and precision of joint space width measurements in standard and macroradiographs of osteoarthritic knees. *Ann Rheum Dis* 1995b;54:872–880.

37. Buckland-Wright JC, Wolfe F, Ward RJ, et al. Substantial superiority of semiflexed (MTP) views in knee osteoarthritis: a comparative radiographic study, without fluoroscopy, of standing extended, semiflexed (MTP), and Schuss view. *J Rheumatol* 1999;26:2664–2674.

38. Bullough P, Goodfellow J, Greenwald AS, et al. Incongruent surfaces in the human hip joint. *Nature* 1968;217:1290.

39. Burgkart R, Glaser C, Hyhlik-Durr A, et al. Magnetic resonance imaging-based assessment of cartilage loss in severe osteoarthritis: accuracy, precision, and diagnostic value. *Arthritis Rheum* 2001;44:2072–2077.

40. Burgkart R, Glaser C, Heudorfer L, et al. Long-term precision of quantitative cartilage analysis in the knee with MR imaging vs interindividual variability in 100 healthy volunteers and tissue loss in OA patients. San Francisco: *47th Transactions of the annual meeting of the Orthopaedic Research Society* 2001; Vol. 26:232.

41. Burgkart R, Glaser C, Hinterwimmer S, et al. Feasibility of T and Z scores from magnetic resonance imaging data for quantification of cartilage loss in osteoarthritis. *Arthritis Rheum* 2003;48(10):2829–2835.

42. Burstein D, Bashir A, Gray ML. MRI techniques in early stages of cartilage disease. *Invest Radiol* 2000;3:622–638.

43. Carter DR, Wong M. The role of mechanical loading histories in the development of diarthrodial joints. *J Orthop Res* 1988;6:804–816.

44. Carter DR, Wong M, Orr TE. Musculoskeletal ontogeny, phylogeny, and functional adaptation. *J Biomech* 1991;24 [Suppl]1:3–16.

45. Cicuttini F, Forbes A, Morris K, et al. Gender differences in knee cartilage volume as measured by magnetic resonance imaging. *Osteoarthritis Cartilage* 1999;7:265–271.

46. Cicuttini F, Forbes A, Asbeutah A, et al. Comparison and reproducibility of fast and conventional spoiled gradient-echo magnetic resonance sequences in the determination of knee cartilage volume. *J Orthop Res* 2000;18:580–584.

47. Clark RE, Karara HM, Catalogu A, et al. Close-range photogrammetry and coupled stress analysis as tools in the development of prosthetic devices. *Trans Am Soc Artif Intern Organs* 1975;21:71–78.

48. Cohen ZA, McCarthy DM, Kwak, SD, et al. Knee cartilage topography, thickness, and contact areas from MRI: *in vitro* calibration and *in vivo* measurements. *Osteoarthritis Cartilage* 1999;7:95–109.

49. Cohen ZA, Henry JH, McCarthy DM. Computer simulations of patellofemoral joint surgery: tuberosity transfers on patient-specific models. *Am J Sports Med* 2003;31:87–98.

50. Cohen ZA, Roglic H, Grelsamer RP. Patellofemoral stresses during open and closed kinetic chain exercises: an analysis using computer simulation. *Am J Sports Med* 2001;29:480–487.

51. Cohen ZA, Mow VC, Henry JH, et al. Templates of the cartilage layers of the patellofemoral joint and their use in the assessment of osteoarthritic cartilage damage. *Osteoarthritis Cartilage* 2003;11:569–579.

52. Conzen A, Eckstein F. Quantitative determination of articular pressure in the human shoulder joint. *J Shoulder Elbow Surg* 2000;9:196–204.

53. Coons SA. *Surfaces for computer-aided design and space forms.* Cambridge, MA: Massachusetts Institute of Technology, Publication AD-663, 1967:504.

54. Cummings SR, Black D. Should perimenopausal women be screened for osteoporosis? *Ann Intern Med* 1986;104:817–823.

55. Dardzinski BJ, Mosher TJ, Li S, et al. Spatial variation of T2 in human articular cartilage. *Radiology* 1997;205:546–550.

56. Davidson M. Roentgen rays and localisation. An apparatus for exact measurement and localisation by means of roentgen rays. *Br Med J* 1898;10–14.

57. Dhaher YY, Delp SL, Rymer WZ. The use of basis functions in modelling joint articular

surfaces: application to the knee joint. *J Biomech* 2000;33:901–907.

58. Donzelli PS, Spilker RL, Ateshian GA. A finite element investigation of contact between transversely isotropic layers of biphasic cartilage. *J Biomech* 1999;32:1037–1047.

59. Dupuy DE, Spillane RM, Rosol MS, et al. Quantification of articular cartilage in the knee with three dimensional MR imaging. *Acad Radiol* 1996;3:919–924.

60. Duvvuri U, Charagundla SR, Kudchodkar SB, et al. Human knee: *in vivo* T1(rho)-weighted MR imaging at 1.5 T–preliminary experience. *Radiology* 2001;220:822–826.

61. Eberhardt AW, Keer LM, Lewis JL, et al. An analytical model of joint contact. *J Biomech Eng* 1990;112:407–413.

62. Eberhardt AW, Lewis JL, Keer LM. Contact of layered elastic spheres as a model of joint contact: effect of tangential load and friction. *J Biomech Eng* 1991;113:107–108.

63. Eberhardt AW, Lewis JL, Keer LM. Normal contact of elastic spheres with two elastic layers as a model of joint articulation. *J Biomech Eng* 1991;113:410–417.

64. Eckstein P, Müller-Gerbl M, Putz R. Distribution of subchondral bone density and cartilage thickness in the human patella. *J Anat* 1992;180:425–433.

65. Eckstein F, Sittek H, Milz S. The morphology of articular cartilage assessed by magnetic resonance imaging (MRI). Reproducibility and anatomical correlation. *Surg Radiol Anat* 1994;16:429–438.

66. Eckstein F, Löhe F, Hillebrand S, et al. Morphomechanics of the humero ulnar joint: I. Joint space width and contact areas as a function of load and flexion angle. *Anat Rec* 1995;243:318–326.

67. Eckstein F, Gavazzeni A, Sittek H, et al. Determination of knee joint cartilage thickness using three dimensional magnetic resonance chondrocrassometry (3D-MR-CCM). *Magn Reson Med* 1996;36:256–265.

68. Eckstein F, Adam C, Sittek H, et al. Non-invasive determination of topographical cartilage thickness maps using magnetic resonance imaging (MRI) optimization and comparison with other techniques. *J Biomech* 1997;30:285–289.

69. Eckstein F, Winzheimer M, Westhoff J, et al. Quantitative relathionships of normal cartilage volumes of the human knee joint—assessment by magnetic resonance imaging. *Anat Embryol* 1998;197:383–390.

70. Eckstein F, Tieschky M, Faber S, et al. Effects of physical exercise on cartilage volume and thickness *in vivo*—an MR imaging study. *Radiology* 1998;207:243–248.

71. Eckstein F, Schnier M, Haubner M, et al. Accuracy of three-dimensional knee joint cartilage volume and thickness mesurements with MRI. *Clin Orthop* 1998;352:137–148.

72. Eckstein F, Tieschky M, Faber S, et al. Functional analysis of articular cartilage deformation, recovery, and fluid flow following dynamic exercise *in vivo*. *Anat Embryol* 1999;200:419–424.

73. Eckstein F, Stammberger T, Priebsch J, et al. Effect of gradient and section orientation on quantitative analyses of knee joint cartilage. *J Magn Reson Imaging* 2000;11:161–167.

74. Eckstein F, Lemberger B, Stammberger T, et al. Effect of static versus dynamic *in vivo* loading exercises on human patellar cartilage. *J Biomech* 2000;33:819–825.

75. Eckstein F, Winzheimer M, Hohe J, et al. Interindividual variability and correlation among morphological parameters of knee joint cartilage plates:analysis with three-dimensional MR imaging. *Osteoarthritis Cartilage* 2001;9:101–111.

76. Eckstein F, Reiser M, Englmeier KH. *In vivo* morphometry and functional analysis of human articular cartilage with quantitative magnetic resonance imaging—from image to data, from data to theory. *Anat Embryol* 2001;203:147–173.

77. Eckstein F, Faber S, Muhlbauer R, et al. Functional adaptation of human joints to mechanical stimuli. *Osteoarthritis Cartilage* 2002;10:44–50.

78. Eckstein F, Müller S, Faber SC. Side differences of knee joint cartilage volume, thickness, and surface area, and correlation with lower limb dominance - an MRI-based study. *Osteoarthritis Cartilage* 2002;10:914–921.

79. Eckstein F, Heudorfer L, Faber SC, et al. Long-term and resegmentation precision of quantitative cartilage MR imaging (qMRI). *Osteoarthritis Cartilage* 2002;10(12):922–928.

80. Eckstein F, Muller S, Faber SC, et al. Side differences of knee joint cartilage volume, thickness, and surface area, and correlation with lower limb dominance-an MRI-based study. *Osteoarthritis Cartilage* 2002;10(12):914–921.

81. Eisenhart LP. *A treatise on the differential geometry of curves and surfaces.* New York: Dover, 1909.

82. Eisenhart-Rothe R, Adam C, Steinlechner M. Quantitative determination of joint incongruity and pressure distribution during simulated gait, and cartilage thickness in the human hip joint. *J Orthop Res* 1999;17:532–539.

83. Eisenhart-Rothe R, Wiedemann E, Bonel H, et al. MR-basierte 3D Analyse der glenohumeralen Translation bei Patienten mit Schulterinstabilität. *Z Orthop* 2000;138:481–486.

84. Essinger JR, Leyvraz PF, Heegard JH, et al. A mathematical model for the evaluations of the behaviour during flexion of condylar-type knee prostheses. *J Biomech* 1989;22:1229–1241.

85. Faber SC, Eckstein F, Lukasz S, et al. Gender differences in knee joint cartilage thickness, volume

and articular surface areas: assessment with quantitative three-dimensional MR imaging. *Skeletal Radiol* 2001;30:144–150.

86. Flaherty JE, Frachioni M, lluang L, et al. Parallel adaptive computations for soft tissue analysis. *1995 Bioengineering Conference, ASME Adv Bioeng* 1995;BED-29:165–166.

87. Flatow EL, Ateshian GA, Soslowsky LJ, et al. Computer simulation of glenohumeral and patellofemoral subluxation: estimating pathological articular contact. *Clin Orthop* 1994;306:28–33.

88. Frank LR, Wong EC, Luh WM, et al. Articular cartilage in the knee: mapping of the physiologic parameters at MR imaging with a local gradient coil-preliminary results. *Radiology* 1999;210:241–246.

89. Froimson MI, Ratcliffe A, Gardner TR, et al. Differences in patellofemoral joint cartilage material properties and their significance to the etiology of cartilage surface fibrillation. *Osteoarthritis Cartilage* 1997;5:377–386.

90. Fukubayashi T, Kurosawa H. The contact area and pressure distribution pattern of the knee. *Acta Orthop Scand* 1980;51:871–879.

91. Fulkerson JP, Hungerford DS. *Disorders of the patellofemoral joint.* Baltimore: Williams & Wilkins, 1990:7–12.

92. Fulkerson JP, Becker GJ, Meaney JA. Anteromedial tibial tubercle transfer without bone graft. *Am J Sports Med* 1991;18:490–496.

93. Garg A, Walker PS. Prediction of knee joint motion using a three-dimensional computer graphics model. *J Biomech* 1990;23:45–58.

94. Ghosh SK. *Analytical photogrammetry.* New York: Pergamon Press, 1979.

95. Ghosh SK. A close-range photogrammetric system for 3-D measurements and perspective diagramming in biomechanics. *J Biomech* 1983;16:667–674.

96. Ghosh S, Ries M, Lane N, et al. Segmentation of high resolution articular cartilage MR images. *46th Transactions of the annual meeting of the Orthopaedic Research Society,* Orlando, FL, 2000;25:246.

97. Gladwell GML. *Contact problems in the classical theory of elasticity.* Germantown, MD: Sijthoff Noorhoff, 1980.

98. Glaser C, Faber S, Eckstein F, et al. Optimization and validation of a rapid high-resolution T1-w 3D FLASH water excitation MRI sequence for the quantitative assessment of articular cartilage volume and thickness. *Magn Reson Imaging* 2001;19:177–185.

99. Glaser C, Burgkart R, Kutschera A, Englmeier KH, Reiser M, Eckstein F. Femoro-tibial cartilage metrics from coronal MR image data: technique, test-retest reproducibility and findings in osteoarthritis. *Magn Reson Med* 2003;50:1229–1236.

100. Goodwin DW, Zhu H, and Dunn JF. *In vitro* MR imaging of hyaline cartilage: correlation with scanning electron microscopy. *Am J Roentgenol* 2000;174:405–409.

101. Graichen H, Bonel H, Stammberger T, et al. A technique for determining the spatial relationship between the rotator cuff and the subacromial space in arm abduction using MRI and 3D image processing. *Magn Reson Med* 1998;40:640–643.

102. Graichen H, Bonel H, Stammberger T, et al. Three-dimensional analysis of the width of the subacromial space in healthy subjects and patients with impingement syndrome. *Am J Roentgenol* 1999;172:1081–1086.

103. Graichen H, Springer V, Flamann T, et al. High-resolution, selective water-excitation MR imaging for quantitative assessment of thin cartilage layers: validation with CT-arthrography and A-mode ultrasound. *Osteoarthritis Cartilage* 2000;8:106–114.

104. Graichen H, Stammberger T, Bonel H, et al. Glenohumeral translation during active and passive elevation of the shoulder—a 3D open MRI study. *J Biomech* 2000;33:609–613.

105. Graichen H, Stammberger T, Bonel H, et al. 3D MR based motion analysis of the supraspinatus muscle and adjacent shoulder bones during passive elevation. *Clin Orthop* 2000;370:154–163.

106. Graichen H, Bonel H, Stammberger T, et al. Changes of shoulder girdle and supraspinatus motion patterns in patients with impingement syndrome—analysis with open MRI and 3D postprocessing. *J Orthop Res* 2001;19:1192–1198.

107. Graichen H, Jakob J, Eisenhart-Rothe R, et al. Validation of cartilage volume and thickness measurements in the human shoulder with quantitative magnetic resonance imaging. *Osteoarthritis Cartilage* 2003;11(7):475–482.

108. Graichen H, v. Eisenhart-Rothe R, Vogl T, Englmeier KH, Eckstein F. Quantitative assessment of cartilage status in osteoarthritis by quantitative magnetic resonance imaging: technical validation for use in analysis of cartilage volume and further morphologic parameters. *Arthritis Rheum* 2004;50(3):811–816.

109. Gray ML, Burstein D, Lesperance LM, et al. Magnetization transfer in cartilage and its constituent macromolecules. *Magn Reson Med* 1995;34:319–325.

110. Gray ML, Burstein D, Xia Y. Biochemical (and functional) imaging of articular cartilage. *Semin Musculoskelet Radiol* 2001;5:329–343.

111. Greenwald AS, O'Connor JJ. The transmission of load through the human hip joint. *J Biomech* 1971;4:507–528.

112. Grood ES, Suntay WJ. A joint coordinate system for the clinical description of three-dimensional motions: application to the knee. *J Biomech Eng* 1983;105:136–144.

113. Gründer W, Wagner M, Werner W. MR-microscopic visualization of anisotropic internal

cartilage structure using the magic angle technique. *Magn Reson Med* 1998;39:376–382.

114. Hall FM, Wyshak G. Thickness of articular cartilage in the normal knee. *J Bone Joint Surg* 1980;62A:408–413.
115. Hardy PA, Recht MP, Piraino DW. Fat suppressed MRI of articular cartilage with a spatial-spectral excitation pulse. *J Magn Reson Imaging* 1998;8:1279–1287.
116. Haut TL, Hull ML, Howell SM. A high-accuracy three-dimensional coordinate digitizing system for reconstructing the geometry of diarthrodial joints. *J Biomech* 1998;31:571–577.
117. Haut TL, Hull ML, Howell SM. Use of roentgenography and magnetic resonance imaging to predict meniscal geometry determined with a three-dimensional coordinate digitizing system. *J Orthop Res* 2000;18:228–237.
118. Heegaard JH, Leyvraz PF, Curnier A, et al. The biomechanics of the human patella during passive knee flexion. *J Biomech* 1995;28(11):1265–79.
119. Heegaard JH, Leyvraz PF. Computer aided surgery: application to the Maquet procedure. 1995 Bioengineering Conference. *ASME, BED-*29:221–222.
120. Hefzy MS, Yang H. A three-dimensional anatomical model of the human patello-femoral joint, for the determination of patello-femoral motions and contact characteristics. *J Biomed Eng* 1993;15:289–302.
121. Helminen HJ, Kiviranta I, Säämänen AM, et al. Effect of motion and load on articular cartilage in animal models. In: Kuettner KE, Schleyerbach R, Peyron JG, et al., eds. *Articular cartilage and osteoarthritis.* New York: Raven Press, 1992:501–510.
122. Herberhold C, Faber S, Stammberger T, et al. *In situ* measurement of articular cartilage deformation in intact femoropatellar joints under static loading. *J Biomech* 1999;32:1287–1295.
123. Hirokawa S. Three-dimensional mathematical model analysis of the patellofemoral joint. *J Biomech* 1991;24:659–671.
124. Hobatho MC, Couteau B, Darmana R, et al. Contact surfaces of tibio-femoral joints *in vivo*. In: *Proceedings of the 2nd World Congress of Biomechanics.* Nijmegen, The Netherlands: Stichting World Biomechanics, 1994:300.
125. Hoch DH, Grodzinsky AJ, Koob TJ, et al. Early changes in the material properties of rabbit articular cartilage after meniscectomy. *J Orthop Res* 1983;1:4–12.
126. Hohe J, Faber S, Stammberger T, et al. A technique for 3D *in vivo* quantification of proton density and magnetization transfer coefficients of knee joint cartilage. *Osteoarthritis Cartilage* 2000;8:426–433.
127. Hohe J, Ateshian GA, Reiser M, et al. Surface size, curvature analysis, and quantitative assessment of knee joint incongruity with MR imaging *in vivo*. *Magn Reson Med* 2002;47:554–561.
128. Hohe J, Faber S, Mühlbauer R, et al. Three-dimensional analysis and visualization of regional MR signal intensity distribution of articular cartilage. *Med Eng Phys* 2002;24:219–224.
129. Huberti HH, Hayes WC. Patellofemoral contact pressures. *J Bone Joint Surg* 1984;66A:715–724.
130. Hudelmaier M, Glaser C, Hohe J, et al. Age-related changes in the morphology and deformational behavior of knee joint cartilage. *Arthritis Rheum* 2001;44:2556–2561.
131. Hudelmaier M, Glaser C, Englmeier KH, et al. Correlation of knee-joint cartilage morphology with muscle cross-sectional areas vs. anthropometric variables. *Anat Rec* 2003;270A(2):175–184.
132. Huiskes R, Kremers J, de Lange A, et al. Analytical stereophotogrammetric determination of three-dimensional knee-joint geometry. *J Biomech* 1985;18:559–170.
133. Hyhlik-Dürr A, Faber S, Burgkart R, et al. Precision of tibial cartilage morphometry with a coronal water-excitation MR-sequence. *Eur Radiol* 2000;10:297–303.
134. Ihara H. Double contrast CT arthrography of the cartilage of the patellofemoral joint. *Clin Orthop* 1985;198:50–55.
135. Johnson KL. *Contact mechanics.* Cambridge, MA: Cambridge University Press, 1985.
136. Johnsson K, Buckwalter K, Helvie M, et al. Precision of hyaline cartilage thickness measurements. *Acta Radiol* 1992;33:234–239.
137. Jones G, Glisson M, Hynes K, et al. Sex and site differences in cartilage development: a possible explanation for variations in knee osteoarthritis in later life. *Arthritis Rheum* 2000;43:2543–2549.
138. Jurvelin JS, Rasanen T, Kolmonen P, et al. Comparison of optical, needle probe and ultrasonic techniques for the measurement of articular cartilage thickness. *J Biomech* 1995;28:231–235.
139. van Kampen A, Huiskes R. The three-dimensional tracking pattern of the human patella. *J Orthop Res* 1990;8:372–382.
140. Karvonen RL, Negendank WG, Teitge RA, et al. Factors affecting articular cartilage thickness in osteoarthritis and aging. *J Rheumatol* 1994;21:1310–1318.
141. Kaufman JH, Regatte RR, Bolinger L, et al. A novel approach to observing articular cartilage deformation *in vitro* via magnetic resonance imaging. *J Magn Reson Imaging* 1999;9:653–662.
142. Kelkar R, Ateshian GA. Contact creep of biphasic cartilage layers: identical layers. *J Appl Mech* 1999;66:137–145.
143. Kelsey JL. *Epidemiology of musculoskeletal disorders.* New York: Oxford University Press, 1982.
144. Kim DK, Ceckler TL, Hascall VC, et al. Analysis of water macromolecule proton magnetization

transfer in articular cartilage. *Magn Reson Med* 1993;29:211–215.

145. Kim DJ, Suh JS, Jeong EK, et al. Correlation of laminated MR appearance of articular cartilage with histology, ascertained by artificial landmarks on the cartilage. *J Magn Reson Imaging* 1999;10:57–64.

146. Kladny B, Bail H, Swoboda B, et al. Cartilage thickness measurement in magnetic resonance imaging. *Osteoarthritis Cartilage* 1996;4:181–186.

147. Kshirsagar AA, Watson PJ, Tyler JA, et al. Measurement of localized cartilage volume and thickness of human knee joints by computer analysis of three dimensional magnetic resonance images. *Invest Radiol* 1998;33:289–299.

148. Kurosawa H, Fukubayashi T, Nakajima H. Load-bearing mode of the knee joint, physical behavior of the knee joint with or without menisci. *Clin Orthop* 1980;149:283–290.

149. Kurrat HJ, Oberländer W. The thickness of the cartilage in the hip joint. *J Anat* 1978;126:145–455.

150. Kwak SD, Blankevoort L, Ahmad CS, et al. An anatomically based 3-D coordinate system for the knee joint. *Adv Bioeng* ASME, 1995;BED 31: 309–310.

151. Kwak SD, Colman WW, Ateshian GA, et al. Anatomy of the human patellofemoral joint articular cartilage: a surface curvature analysis. *J Orthop Res* 1997;15:468–472.

152. Kwak SD, Blankevoort L, Ateshian GA. A mathematical formulation for 3D quasi-static multibody models of diarthrodial joints. *Comput Methods Biomech Biomed Engin* 2000;3:41–64.

153. Kwak SD, Ahmad CS, Gardner TR, et al. Hamstrings and iliotibial band forces affect knee kinematics and contact pattern. *J Orthop Res* 2000;18:101–108.

154. Lawrence JS, Bremner JM, Bier F. Osteoarthrosis: prevalence in the population and relationship between symptoms and X-ray changes. *Ann. Rheum Dis* 1966;25:1–23.

155. Lehner KB, Rechl HP, Gmeinwieser JK, et al. Structure, function, and degeneration of bovine hyaline cartilage: assessment with MR imaging *in vitro*. *Radiology* 1989;170:495–499.

156. Link TM, Majumdar S, Peterfy C, et al. High resolution MRI of small joints: impact of spatial resolution on diagnostic performance and SNR. *Magn Reson Imaging* 1998;16:147–155.

157. Lösch A, Eckstein F, Haubner M. A non invasive technique for 3 dimensional assessment of articular cartilage thickness based on MRI. Part I: development of a computational method. *Magn Reson Imaging* 1997;15:795–804.

158. Lur'e AI, Radok JRM, eds. *Three-dimensional problems of the theory of elasticity.* New York: Interscience, 1964.

159. Lüsse S, Claassen H, Gehrke T, et al. Evaluation of water content by spatially resolved transverse relaxation times of human articular cartilage. *Magn Reson Imaging* 2000;18:423–430.

160. MacConaill MA. Studies in the mechanics of synovial joints. *Ir J Med Sci* 1946;6:223–235.

161. Maquet P. Advancement of the tibial tuberosity. *Clin Orthop* 1976;115:225–230.

162. McLeod WD, Moschi A, Andrews JR, et al. Tibial plateau topography. *Am J Sports Med* 1977;5:13–18.

163. Meachim G. Effect of age on the thickness of adult articular cartilage at the shoulder joint. *Ann Rheum Dis* 1971;30:43–46.

164. Meachim G, Bentley G, Baker R. Effect of age on thickness of adult patellar articular cartilage. *Ann Rheum Dis* 1977;36:563–568.

165. Milz S, Eckstein F, Putz R. The thickness distribution of the subchondral mineralization zone of the trochlear notch and its correlation with the cartilage thickness:an expression of functional adaptation to mechanical stress acting on the humero ulnar joint. *Anat Rec* 1997;248:189–197.

166. Modest VE, Murphy MC, Mann RW. Optical verification of a technique for in situ ultrasonic measurement of articular cartilage thickness. *J Biomech* 1989;22:171–176.

167. Modl JM, Sether LA, Haughton VM, et al. Articular cartilage: correlation of histologic zones with signal intensity at MR imaging. *Radiology* 1991;181:853–855.

168. Moon KL Jr, Genant HK, Davis PL. Nuclear magnetic resonance imaging in orthopaedics: principles and applications. *J Orthop Res* 1983;1:101–114.

169. Moore KL. *Clinically oriented anatomy.* Baltimore: Williams & Wilkins, 1985:533.

170. Mow VC, Gibbs MC, Lai WM, et al. Biphasic indentation of articular cartilage-II. A numerical algorithm and an experimental study. *J Biomech* 1989;22:853–861.

171. Mühlbauer R, Lukasz S, Faber S, et al. Comparison of knee joint cartilage thickness in triathletes and physically inactive volunteers—3D analysis with magnetic imaging. *Am J Sports Med* 2000;28:541–546.

172. Müller-Gerbl M, Schulte E, Putz R. The thickness of the calcified layer of articular cartilage: a function of the load supported? *J Anat* 1987;154:103–111.

173. Newton PM, Mow VC, Gardner T, et al. The effect of lifelong exercise on canine articular cartilage. *Am J Sports Med* 1997;25:282–287.

174. Nieminen MT, Rieppo J, Toyras J, et al. T2 relaxation reveals spatial collagen architecture in articular cartilage: a comparative quantitative MRI and polarized light microscopic study. *Magn Reson Med* 2001;46:487–493.

175. O'Bara RM, Shephard MS, Ateshian GA. Geometric model construction and mesh generation for soft tissues in joints. 1995 Bioengineering Conference. American Society of Mechanical Engineers. BED-29:215–216.

176. Papa E, Cappozzo A. Sit-to-stand motor strategies investigated in able-bodied young and elderly subjects. *J Biomech* 2000;33:1113–1122.

177. Pauwels F. *Biomechanics of the locomotor apparatus.* New York: Springer-Verlag, 1980.

178. Peterfy CG, van Dijke CF, Janzen DL, et al. Quantification of articular cartilage in the knee with pulsed saturation transfer subtraction and fat-suppressed MR imaging: optimization and validation. *Radiology* 1994;192:485–491.

179. Peterfy CG, Majumdar S, Lang R, et al. MR imaging of the arthritic knee: improved discrimination of cartilage, synovium, and effusion with pulsed saturation transfer and fat-suppressed Ti-weighted sequences. *Radiology* 1994;191:413–419.

180. Peterfy CG, van Dijke CF, Lu Y, et al. Quantification of the volume of articular cartilage in the metacarpophalangeal joints of the hand: accuracy and precision of three dimensional MR imaging. *Am J Roentgenol* 1995;165:371–375.

181. Pilch L, Stewart C, Gordon D, et al. Assessment of cartilage volume in the femorotibial joint with magnetic resonance imaging and 3D computer reconstruction. *J Rheumatol* 1994;21:2307–2321.

182. Piplani MA, Disler DG, McCauley TR. Articular cartilage volume in the knee: semiautomatic determination from three-dimensional reformations of MR images. *Radiology* 1996;198:855–859.

183. Recht MP, Kramer J, Marcelis S. Abnormalities of articular cartilage in the knee: analysis of available MR techniques. *Radiology* 1993;187:473–478.

184. Reddy R, Insko EK, Noyszewski EA. Sodium MRI of human articular cartilage *in vivo*. *Magn Reson Med* 1998;39:697–701.

185. Regatte RR, Kaufman JH, Noyszewski EA. Sodium and proton MR properties of cartilage during compression. *J Magn Reson Imaging* 1999;10:961–967.

186. Robson MD, Hodgson RJ, Herrod NJ, et al. A combined analysis and magnetic resonance imaging technique for computerised automatic measurement of cartilage thickness in the distal interphalangeal joint. *Magn Reson Imaging* 1995;13:709–718.

187. Ronsky JL, Boyd SK, Lichti DD. Precise measurement of cat patellofemoral joint surface geometry with multistation digital photogrammetry. *J Biomech Eng* 1999;121:196–205.

188. Rubenstein JD, Kim JK, Morova-Protzner I. Effects of collagen orientation on MR imaging characteristics of bovine articular cartilage. *Radiology* 1993;188:219–226.

189. Rubenstein JD, Kim JK, Henkelman RM. Effects of compression and recovery on bovine articular cartilage: appearance on MR images. *Radiology* 1996;201:843–850.

190. Rushfeldt PD, Mann RW, Harris WH. Improved techniques for measuring I'M *vitro* the geometry and pressure distribution in the human acetabulum—I. Ultrasonic measurement of acetabular surfaces, sphericity and cartilage thickness. *J Biomech* 1981;14:253–260.

191. Scherrer PK, Hillberry BM. Piecewise mathematical representation of articular surfaces. *J Biomech* 1979;12:301–311.

192. Scherrer PK, Hillberry BM, Sickle DV. Determining the *in-vivo* areas of contact in the canine shoulder. *J Biomech Eng* 1979;101:271–278.

193. Schuind F, Cooney WP, Linscheid RL, et al. Force and pressure transmission through the normal wrist. A theoretical two-dimensional study in the postcroantcrior plane. *J Biomech* 1995;28:587–601.

194. Seedhom BB, Longton EB, Wright V, et al. Dimensions of the knee. *Ann Rheum Dis* 1972;31:54–58.

195. Seedhom BB, Tsubuku M. A technique for the study of contact between viscoelastic bodies with special reference to the patello-femoral joint. *J Biomech* 1977;10:253–260.

196. Selby K, Peterfy CG, Cohen ZA, et al. *In vivo* MR quantification of articular cartilage water content: a potential early indicator of osteoarthritis. In: *Book of abstracts: Society of Magnetic Resonance.* Berkeley, CA: Society of Magnetic Resonance. 1995:204.

197. Selvik G. *A roentgen stereophotogrammetric method for the study of the kinematics of the skeletal system.* Ph.D. Thesis, University of Lund, Sweden, 1974. Reprinted in *Acta Orthop Scand* 1989; 60[Suppl.]:232.

198. Seo GS, Aoki J, Moriya H, et al. Hyaline cartilage: *in vivo* and *in vitro* assessment with magnetization transfer imaging. *Radiology* 1996;201:525–530.

199. Shapiro EM, Borthakur A, Kaufman JH, et al. Water distribution patterns inside bovine articular cartilage as visualized by 1H magnetic resonance imaging. *Osteoarthritis Cartilage* 2001;9:533–538.

200. Shiba R, Sorbie C, Siu DW, et al. Geometry of the humero-ulnar joint. *J Orthop Res* 1988;6:897–906.

201. Simon WH. Scale effects in animal jonts I. Articular cartilage thickness and compressive stress. *Arthritis Rheum* 1970;13:244–255.

202. Singerman RJ, Pedersen DR, Brown TD. Quantitation of pressure-sensitive film using digital image scanning. *Exp Mech* 1987;March:99–105.

203. Sittek H, Eckstein F, Gavazzeni A, et al. Assessment of normal patellar cartilage volume and thickness with MRI an analysis of currently available sequences. *Skeletal Radiol* 1996;25:55–62.

204. Solloway S, Hutchinson CE, Waterton JC, et al. The use of active shape models for making

thickness measurements of articular cartilage from MR images. *Magn Reson Med* 1997;37:943–952.

205. Soslowsky LJ, Flatow EL, Bigliani LU, et al. Articular geometry of the glenohumeral joint. *Clin Orthop* 1992;288:181–190.

206. Soslowsky LJ, Flatow EL, Bigliani LU, et al. Quantitation of in situ contact areas at the glenohumeral joint: a biomechanical study. *J Orthop Res* 1992;10:524–534.

207. Spilker RL, Almeida ES, Clutz C, et al. Three dimensional automated biphasic finite element analysis of soft tissues from stereophotogrammetric data. *Adv Bioeng ASME* 1993;BED-26:15–18.

208. Springer V, Graichen H, Stammberger T, et al. Nichtinvasive Analyse des Knorpelvolumens und der Knorpeldicke im menschlichen Ellbogengelenk mittels MRT. *Ann Anat* 1998;180:331–333.

209. Stammberger T, Eckstein F, Michaelis M, et al. Interobserver reproducibility of quantitative cartilage measurements: comparison between B-spline snakes and manual segmentation. *Magn Reson Imaging* 1999a;17:1033–1042.

210. Stammberger T, Eckstein F, Englmeier K-H, et al. Determination of 3D cartilage thickness data from MR imaging—computational method and reproducibility in the living. *Magn Reson Med* 1999b;41:529–536.

211. Stammberger T, Hohe J, Englmeier K-H, et al. Elastic registration of 3D cartilage surfaces from MR image data for detecting local changes of the cartilage thickness. *Magn Reson Med* 2000;44:592–601.

212. Steines D, Cheng C, Wong A. Segmentation of osteoarthritic femoral cartilage from MR images. In: Lemke HU, Vannier MW, Inamura K, et al., eds. *Proc. of Computer Assisted Radiology and Surgery, 14th International Congress,* Excerpta Medica Series 1214. Amsterdam: Elsevier Science, pp. 303–308.

213. Stokes I, Greenapple DM. Measurement of surface deformation of soft tissue. *J Biomech* 1985;18:1–7.

214. Takahashi M, Hoshino H, Kushida K, et al. Direct measurement of crosslinks, pyridinoline, deoxypyridinoline, and pentosidine, in the hydrolysate of tissues using high performance liquid chromatography. *Anal Biochem* 1995;232:158–162.

215. Tieschky M, Faber S, Haubner M, et al. Repeatability of patellar cartilage thickness patterns in the living, using a fat-suppressed MRI sequence with short acquisition time and 3D data processing. *J Orthop Res* 1997;15:808–813.

216. Trattnig S, Mlynarik V, Breitenseher M, et al. MRI visualization of proteoglycan depletion in articular cartilage via intravenous administration of Gd DTPA. *Magn Reson Imaging* 1999;17:577–583.

217. Vanwanseele B, Eckstein F, Knecht H, Stüssi E, Spaepen A. Knee cartilage of spinal cord injured patients displays progressive thinning in the absence of normal joint loading and movement. *Arthritis Rheum* 2002;46:2073–2078.

218. Vanwanseele B, Eckstein F, Knecht H, Spaepen A., Stüssi E. Longitudinal analysis of cartilage atrophy in the knees of spinal cord injured patients. *Arthritis Rheum* 2003;48:3377–3381.

219. Vignon E, Conrozier T, Piperno M, et al. Radiographic assessment of hip and knee osteoarthritis. Recommendations: recommended guidelines. *Osteoarthritis Cartilage* 1999;7:434–436.

220. Wachsmuth L, Juretschke HP, Raiss RX. Can magnetization transfer magnetic resonance imaging follow proteoglycan depletion in articular cartilage? *MAGMA* 1997;5:71–78.

221. Ward AC, Pitsillides AA. Developmental immobilization induces failure of joint cavity formation by a progress involving selective changes in glycosaminoglycans synthesis. *44th Transactions of the annual meeting of the Orthopaedic Research Society,* New Orleans, 1998;23:199.

222. Waterton JC, Solloway S, Foster JE. Diurnal variation in the femoral articular cartilage of the knee in young adult humans. *Magn Reson Med* 2000;43:126–132.

223. Werner. *Die Dicke der menschlichen Gelenkknorpel.* Berlin:[Dissertation] 1897.

224. Wismans J, Veldpaus F, Janssen J. A three-dimensional mathematical model of the knee-joint. *J Biomech* 1980;13:677–686.

225. Wolff SD, Chesnick S, Frank JA, et al. Magnetization transfer: MR imaging of the knee. *Radiology* 1991;179:245–249.

226. Wood JE, Meek SG, Jacobsen SC. Quantitation of human shoulder anatomy for prosthetic arm control—I. Surface modelling. *J Biomech* 1989;22:273–292.

227. Wu JZ, Herzog W, Ronsky J. Modeling axisymmetrical joint contact with biphasic cartilage layers—an asymptotic solution. *J Biomech* 1996;29:1263–1281.

228. Xia Y. Relaxation anisotropy in cartilage by NMR microscopy (muMRI) at 14 micron resolution. *Magn Reson Med* 1998;39:941–949.

229. Xia Y. Magic-angle effect in magnetic resonance imaging of articular cartilage: a review. *Invest Radiol* 2000;3:602–21.

230. Xu L, Strauch RJ, Ateshian GA, et al. Topography of the osteoarthritic carpometacarpal joint and its variations with gender, age, site, and osteoarthritic stage. *J Hand Surg* 1998;23A:454–464.

FRICTION, LUBRICATION, AND WEAR OF ARTICULAR CARTILAGE AND DIARTHRODIAL JOINTS

GERARD A. ATESHIAN
VAN C. MOW

1   INTRODUCTION

The three types of joints that exist in the human body are fibrous, cartilaginous, and synovial. Synarthroses, or fibrous joints, are those in which the bony surfaces have very little movement relative to each other. Amphiarthroses, or cartilaginous joints, are those in which the bony surfaces may have some relative movement. Examples of fibrous joints are the junctions of bones in the skull, while examples of cartilaginous joints are those between the two pubic bones or joints between two vertebral bodies of the spine. Only synovial, or diarthrodial joints, will be discussed in this chapter. These joints are different from fibrous or cartilaginous joints in that they allow for a large range of relative motion between the opposing bones. Some examples of this type of joint are the shoulder, elbow, hip, knee, and ankle.

Diarthrodial joints have some common features. First, they are all enclosed by a strong fibrous capsule (Fig. 10-1A). Second, the inner surfaces of the joint capsules are lined with a metabolically active tissue, the synovium, which secretes the synovial fluid and the nutrients required by the tissues within the joint. The synovium also absorbs the normal metabolic waste products of cellular activities from these intraarticular tissues. For the human knee shown in Figs. 10-1A and 10-1B, the intraarticular tissues include anterior and posterior cruciate

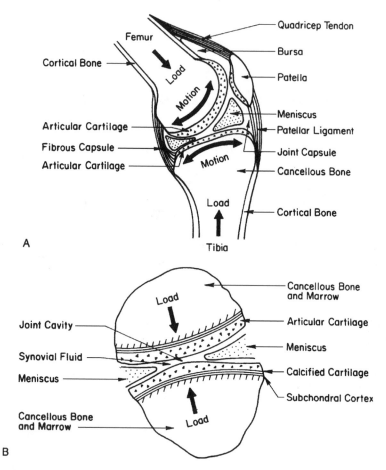

FIGURE 10-1. **(A)** Schematic representation of the human knee joint showing important anatomical features for mechanical function [171]. **(B)** Enlargement of the load-bearing region in the knee, depicting a thin layer of synovial fluid (<50 μm) and two layers of articular cartilage (each <7 mm) [9,171]. Each layer of articular cartilage contains approximately 80% fluid.

ligaments (not shown), the meniscus, and articular cartilage. The third common feature of diarthrodial joints is that the bone ends are lined with a thin layer of articular cartilage (see Chapter 5 for detailed discussions of articular cartilage structure-function relationships, and Chapter 9 for detailed descriptions of the geometric forms of the articular cartilage anatomy). These two linings, i.e., the synovium and the articular cartilage, form the joint cavity that contains the synovial fluid (see (23,24,82, 83,125,176,177,202) and references therein for detailed descriptions of synovial fluid composition and rheology). The synovial fluid, articular cartilage, and supporting bone form the di-

arthrodial joints that provide (in normal health) the smooth, nearly frictionless bearing systems of the mammalian body.

Other tissues, such as ligaments and tendons, are also important in providing stability for the joint, maintaining the proper relative positions of the bone ends during motion, and transmitting muscle forces (see Chapters 2 and 3 for detailed discussions of forces and moments on joints, Chapter 4 for bone, and Chapter 7 for tendons and ligaments).

Although diarthrodial joints are subjected to an enormous range of loading conditions, the cartilage surfaces undergo little wear and tear under normal circumstances. For example, the human hip joint sustains a variety of loading conditions (see Chapters 2 and 3). Under high-speed motion, such as during the swing phase of walking or running, loads of slightly more than body weight are sustained. However, heel strike and toe-off may generate forces three to six times body weight across the hip and knee joints (5,47,82,83,189,190). In the hip these forces may yield compressive stresses as high as 18 MPa *in vivo* (101) in the case of an elderly patient with an instrumented prosthesis, rising from the sitting position in a chair. During prolonged standing, or when a joint is held in a fixed loaded position, moderate loads are also generated (see Chapters 2 and 3).

Human diarthrodial joints must be capable of functioning effectively under these very high loads and stresses (1,2,29,30,47,82,83,101, 193–197,216), and at generally very low operating speeds (5,146,163,189) (also see Chapter 3) for seven or eight decades. This demands efficient lubrication processes to minimize friction and wear of cartilage in the joint (139,140,143). Breakdown in cartilage by either biochemical or biomechanical means may lead to arthritis ((32,85,106,219), and Chapters 5 and 6).

Tribology is defined as the mechanical engineering science that deals with the friction, lubrication, and wear of interacting surfaces in relative motion. Tribology is also an interdisciplinary science involving physics and chemistry of the bearing surfaces, and fluid and solid mechanics and applied mathematics. Biotribology is that branch of tribology that focuses on the understanding of the friction, lubrication, and wear phenomena found in diarthrodial joints. Over the past 50 years, many investigators have studied the friction, lubrication, and wear processes in diarthrodial joints. Precise and meticulous measurements have been made on the frictional properties of joints (38,54,111, 133,136,150,156,238,244,245) and wear properties of cartilage (72,77,139,140). Novel lubrication theories have been proposed to describe these extraordinarily efficient frictional and wear properties (20,21,39,40,48–50,57,64,67, 105,133–136,242). In recent times, our understanding of the many components of the synovial joint, i.e., articular cartilage, the biochemical and

biorheological properties of synovial fluid, the anatomy of the articulating surfaces of the joint (see Chapter 9), and the kinematics and load-bearing characteristics of these joints have greatly advanced, and these advances have provided us with the information necessary to improve our understanding of diarthrodial joint lubrication. The interactions between the various surfaces within the knee joint are schematically illustrated in Fig. 10-1B. This chapter presents the current state of understanding of the biotribological characteristics (friction, lubrication, and wear properties) of diarthrodial joints.

2 MATERIALS OF NATURAL JOINTS

2.1 Articular Cartilage

Details of articular cartilage are presented in Chapter 4. For the present purpose, it is sufficient to know that this tissue covers the ends of the articulating bones in the synovial joint. Its thickness varies among species, among joints, and with location within a specific joint (9,10,12,33,42,60–62,221,228,229). Typically, it ranges in thickness from 0.1–0.5 mm in rabbit knee joints to 1.0–6.0 mm in the human knee (9,42,60,61,62,221). The variation in thickness of this cartilage layer over the joint surface has been quantified using various methods, including stereophotogrammetry and magnetic resonance imaging (see (12,42,228,229) and Chapter 9). The main functions of this compliant biphasic viscoelastic layer of articular cartilage are to spread the applied load over a large area of the joint (1,2,12,29,30,62, 124,182,213,214,215) and to minimize the friction and wear of bearing surfaces that result from the continual sliding and rolling movements of the highly loaded, intermittently moving opposing joint surfaces. These functional properties must necessarily result from the properties of articular cartilage and synovial fluid.

The multiphasic nature of articular cartilage is essential to its function. The tissue is composed of a porous-permeable solid matrix, interstitial water, and dissolved electrolytes (see Chapter 5 for details). The solid phase accounts for approximately 15% to 32% of the wet weight of the tissue, depending on its health (3,4,6,135, 139,153,169,176,177,181,219), and decreases during disease to approximately 10% (i.e., tissue porosity of 90%) before total tissue disintegration occurs. Average water content (or porosity) of normal tissue usually ranges from 65% to 80%; severely diseased osteoarthritic (OA) tissue may range to 90%. Water content increases from the deep zone to the superficial zone (139).

The mechanical behavior of articular cartilage has been described by multiphasic theories, which take these overall compositional characteristics into consideration. A biphasic model has been developed to describe the deformational behavior of cartilage in terms of two immiscible phases: an elastic, porous-permeable solid matrix phase and an incompressible liquid phase (124,148,165,167–170) (see Chapter 5 for more details). Interaction between these two phases is modeled by a frictional diffusive drag resulting from the relative velocity between the solid phase and the fluid phase, and forms the basis for most of the observed compressive viscoelastic behaviors (e.g., 6,63,102,107,112,116,124,156,167–179,188,218,219,248). A triphasic model has also been developed, which describes the interactions between the two immiscible solid-fluid phases, as well as with a third miscible ion phase (cations, e.g., Na^+ or Ca^{2+}, and anions, e.g., Cl^-) (78,128,180). The ions modulate and dictate the swelling behavior of articular cartilage through changes in the Donnan osmotic pressure (128,153,176,180). For more details on articular cartilage deformational and swelling behaviors, see Chapter 5 and the references contained therein.

The solid phase is a charged, porous-permeable, fiber-reinforced composite, Fig. 10-2. In general, because of the complex microorganizational arrangements of the collagen network and proteoglycans, the inhomogeneous solid phase exhibits anisotropic, inhomogeneous, and nonlinear behaviors in tension, compression, and shear. In confined compression, the tissue appears to be isotropic (35,102,112,117,124, 149,168,169,175,176). Although permeability does not appear to be direction dependent, there does exist a variation with depth (153,156), and

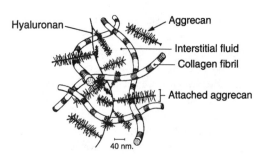

FIGURE 10-2. Schematic representation of the molecular organization of the solid matrix of cartilage. The molecular structural components, collagen, aggrecans, and proteoglycan aggregates, interact to form a porous-permeable, fiber-reinforced, composite solid matrix. The interstices of this porous solid matrix are filled with water and dissolved ions [168,172].

it does depend on the amount of compressive strain—either directly applied or caused by the drag of permeation (84,102,107,108,112,127, 153,168; see Chapter 5 for more details). These varying deformational characteristics make cartilage a highly nonlinear material and challenging to describe using a theoretical model (127,128,176). In uniaxial confined compression, the solid matrix of articular cartilage obeys the linear isotropic biphasic theory well (22,102,149,167–169,175,176). This theory has been used extensively to describe the compressive creep and stress-relaxation behaviors of the tissue and to determine its three material coefficients: permeability, aggregate modulus, and Poisson's ratio. From the predictions of this theory and supportive experimental data, it is known that the compressive viscoelastic creep and stress-relaxation behaviors of normal articular cartilage are primarily governed by interstitial fluid flow and exudation, though intrinsic viscoelasticity of the solid matrix is also believed to play a role (107,148,176,218). When a compressive load is applied to the surface of cartilage via a free-draining, porous platen, viscoelastic creep will occur; however, for cartilage, this is caused by the frictional drag associated with interstitial fluid flow through the angstrom size pores, not by the viscous dissipation within the fluid (Fig. 10-3) (84,104,168). This fluid transport, as well as pressurization, is essential for normal synovial joint lubrication and load support

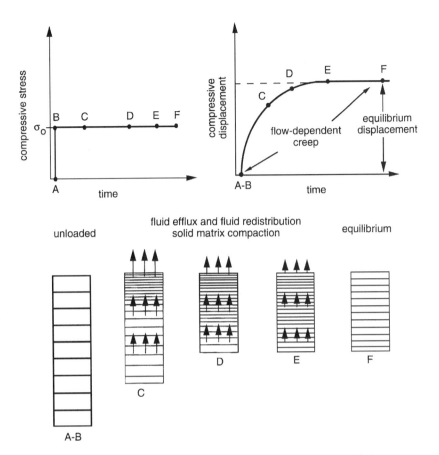

FIGURE 10-3. A constant stress σ_0 (load/area) applied to a sample of the porous-permeable articular cartilage (*top left*); creep response of the sample under the constant applied stress (*top right*). The boxes below the loading and creep curves illustrate that creep is accompanied by fluid exudation from the tissue. At equilibrium ($t \rightarrow \infty$), fluid flow ceases, and the load is borne entirely by the solid matrix **(F)**.

functions, as well as nutrient and waste product transport to and from the chondrocytes.

2.2 Synovial Fluid

Synovial fluid is a clear, or sometimes slightly yellowish, highly viscous liquid secreted into the joint cavity by the synovium. Small amounts of this fluid are contained in all human and animal synovial joints. The name derives from "syn" "ovial" like egg white. Approximately 1 to 5 mL of fluid is contained in a healthy human knee joint. Synovial fluid is a dialysate of blood plasma, without clotting factors, erythrocytes, or hemoglobin (e.g., 44,50,202), but containing hyaluronate, an extended glycosaminoglycan chain (23,24,86,186,202,204,230,233), as well as a lubricating glycoprotein (231–235) and wear-retarding phospholipids (92–96,246). Hyaluronic acid is an unbranched macromolecule whose basic dimer is a disaccharide composed of glucuronic acid linked with N-acetylglucosamine (23,24) (Fig. 10-4). A typical hyaluronate chain has a molecular mass from 0.5 to 2 million daltons.

Synovial fluid, like all polymeric fluids, exhibits non-Newtonian flow properties that include an elastic effect, a shear thinning effect, and a normal stress effect (24,26,37,44,45,50,65,80, 125,184,210,217). These flow properties are similar to those found for other biomacromolecular solutions such as proteoglycans (e.g.,

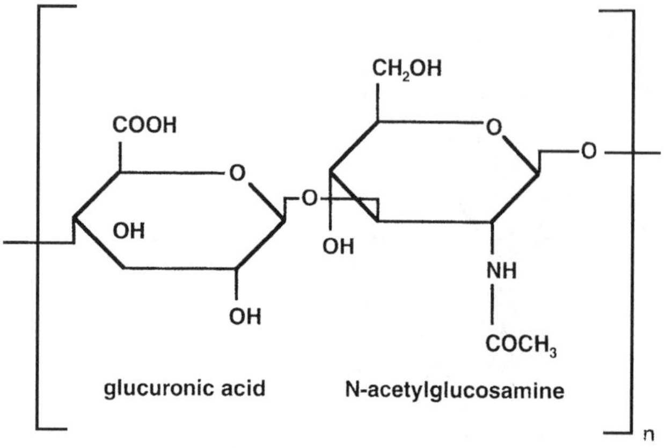

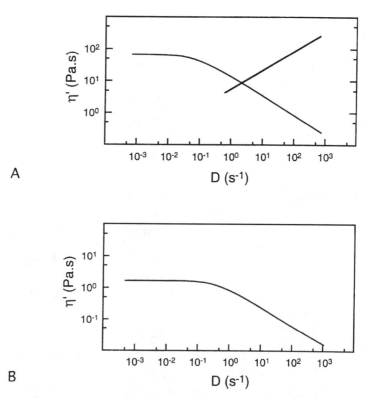

FIGURE 10-4. The repeating disaccharide unit of hyaluronic acid in synovial fluid. This is a nonsulfated dimer of glucuronic acid with N-acetylglucosamine. Hyaluronan is polymerized into long chains consisting of approximately 2,500 of these repeating units with molecular weight ranging from 500,000 to 2,000,000 daltons.

89,174,223,250,251). For example, in bovine knee joints, the apparent viscosity of synovial fluid has been shown to decrease nonlinearly from 10 to 0.02 N-sec/m^2 as the shear rate increased from 0.1 to 1000 s^{-1} (118). Synovial fluids obtained from degenerative joints show reduced apparent viscosity properties compared with those exhibited by normal synovial fluid (23,24,45,65,125,210). Figure 10-5 demonstrates the variations in apparent viscosity

FIGURE 10-5. (A) Shear-rate-dependent viscosity η' and normal stress σ_1 versus shear rate for normal synovial fluid. **(B)** Shear-rate-dependent viscosity η' versus shear rate for pathological synovial fluid (adapted from [210] with permission).

and normal stress due to varying shear rates for both normal and pathological synovial fluids. Many coefficients of assumed rheological equations of state, used to model the rheologic data in the literature, have been calculated (125). These fluid properties play an important role in understanding the lubrication mechanisms in diarthrodial joints (50,56,125,163,165, 167,171,184). Synovial fluid not only aids in lubrication, but also provides the necessary nutrients for cartilage (131,132,201,202,220). Furthermore, synovial fluid acts as a medium for osmosis between the joint and the blood supply, and as protection for cartilage against enzyme activity (43,86,131,132,186).

2.3 Bone

Bone is a supporting structural element of the body that is more rigid than cartilage and other soft tissues. It consists of an abundant matrix of type I collagen fibers impregnated with minerals, primarily calcium and phosphate compounds. Joints are junctures between the bony segments that permit motion. Detailed descriptions of cortical and cancellous bone are provided in Chapter 4.

Under the uncalcified cartilage layer, there is a very thin layer of calcified cartilage (Fig. 10-1B). The wavy line in the figure demarcating the uncalcified cartilage from calcified cartilage is the *tidemark* (31,34,198), which provides a gradual transition between the two dissimilar regions of cartilage and appears to have significant biomechanical functions (159,198). It is remodeled during life in response to microinjuries (34,79,81,196) and advances into the uncalcified cartilage. Postmortem studies show that the number of tidemarks is well correlated with age in humans (34,129). This remodeling process causes significant thinning of cartilage and alters the state of stress in the tissue (31,159). The subchondral cortex lies immediately below the thin layer of calcified cartilage. It is a layer of dense, stiff, cortical bone. In the mature animal, it forms a closed cap supporting the cartilage on one side and supported by the cancellous bone on the other. A sparse distribution of microperforations is sometimes seen on this subchondral cortex, which may have a significant effect on the interstitial fluid pressurization in the overlaying uncalcified cartilage (179). The apparent elastic modulus of the subchondral cortex ranges from 1.0 to 1.5 GPa (31). For cortical bone, the modulus is approximately 15 GPa. The cancellous bone is softer, less dense, and makes up the bulk of the bone end in the joint capsule (79,81). Cancellous bone is highly porous and contains the well-vascularized marrow within its intricate trabecular structure. Its stiffness ranges from 0.1 to 0.5 GPa (31,36,81). One possible mechanism for the initiation of cartilage damage may be the steep stiffness gradient in the subchondral bone caused by healing of trabecular bone fractures (79,115,195,196). According to this hypothesis, large shear stresses are developed at the cartilage-calcified cartilage-subchondral bone juncture causing deep horizontal splits in the tissue, thus damaging the layer of cartilage. Histologic sections of articular cartilage and bone often reveal the existence of blisters in the deep layers of cartilage, presumably caused by the mechanism described above (7,11,34,129,179,195,196,237,240). For a more detailed description of bone, see Chapter 4.

3 ANATOMIC FORMS OF DIARTHRODIAL JOINTS

A major consideration in determining the frictional characteristics between two surfaces sliding over each other is the topography of the given surfaces. Changes in topographic form affect the way in which loads are transmitted across joints, altering the mode of lubrication in that joint and thus the physiologic state of cartilage (32,33,72–75,141–143,158,164,176,197,242).

Macroscopically, approximations are made to simplify the mathematical analyses of these complex anatomic features for studies of joint lubrication (9,11–13,21,22,56,57,82,97–100,120, 163,167,176,225,226,238,239). In two dimensions, articulating surfaces are commonly approximated by a cylindrical surface interacting with a plane. In three dimensions, the simplest approximation used is a sphere in association with a half space. With the three-dimensional

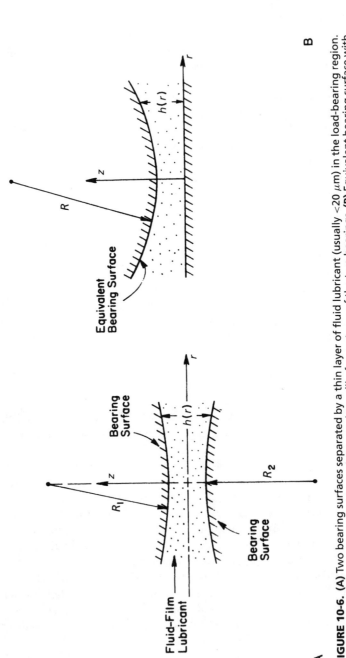

FIGURE 10-6. (A) Two bearing surfaces separated by a thin layer of fluid lubricant (usually <20 μm) in the load-bearing region. The thin film geometry is $h(r)$ and R_1 and R_2 are the radii of curvatures of the two bearings. **(B)** Equivalent bearing surface with curved surface of equivalent radius of curvature R and flat surface.

approximation, it has been estimated that the radius of an equivalent sphere near a plane can be as high as 1.0 m for hip joints or as low as 0.02 to 0.1 m for the knee joint (53,82,83,91,163,203). This radius of curvature is important in assessing the feasibility of fluid-film lubrication mechanisms in a given joint—Figs. 10-6A and 10-6B.

Microscopically, articular surfaces are relatively rough as demonstrated from Talysurf tracings and various microscopic methods (41, 53,74,75,119,120,142,143,164,197,206,241). These surfaces are much rougher than typical engineering bearings or joint replacement prostheses (55). A quantity called the arithmetic mean deviation, R_a, is used to define surface roughness. It is defined as the average value of the difference of the microscopic surface profile above and below a given reference line (Fig. 10-7). For example, values for articular cartilage range from 1 to 6 μm, while the metal femoral head of a typical artificial hip has a value of approximately 0.025 μm; i.e., the metal femoral head is much smoother (Table 10-1). A common terminology is used to describe the levels of topographic roughness of joint surfaces (74,143):

1. Primary anatomic contours
2. Secondary roughness less than 0.5 mm in diameter and less than 50 μm deep
3. Tertiary hollows on the order of 20 to 45 μm deep
4. Quaternary ridges 1 to 4 μm in diameter and 0.1 to 0.3 μm deep

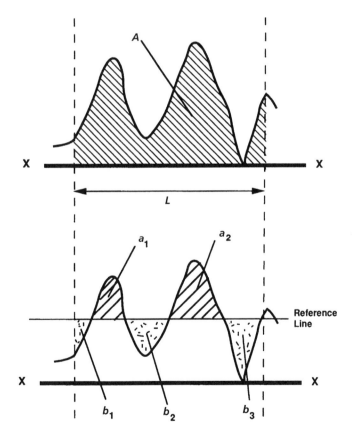

$$R_a = \frac{\text{Sum of areas } (a) + \text{Sum of areas } (b)}{L}$$

FIGURE 10-7. Illustration of the concept of the arithmetical mean deviation R_a of a rough surface. (Adapted from Dowson D. Basic tribology. In: Dowson D, Wright V, eds. *Introduction to the biomechanics of Joints and Joint Replacement.* London: Mechanical Engineering Publications Ltd., 1981:49–60, with permission).

TABLE 10-1. TYPICAL VALUES OF R_a FOR VARIOUS SURFACES

Components	R_a (μm)
Plain bearings	
bearing (bush or pad)	0.25–1.2
journal or runner	0.12–0.5
Rolling bearings	
tracks	0.2–0.3
rolling element	0.05–0.12
Gears	0.25–1.0
Articular cartilage	1.0–6.0
Endoprostheses	
metal (e.g., femoral head)	0.025
plastic (e.g., acetabulum)	0.25–2.5

Data from Dowson [55].

Topographic features are important in determining the causes of friction associated with the articulation, not only when actual contact between two surfaces occurs, but also under fluid-film lubrication conditions, where the surface roughness dictates the minimum fluid-film thickness necessary to keep the two moving surfaces completely separated. Scanning electron micrographs of arthritic cartilage depict a large degree of surface irregularity (Fig. 10-8A—C). Figure 10-8D shows three Talysurf tracings of surface roughness for fetal, young normal, and aging human femoral and condylar articular surfaces (241). Normal articular surface texture is shown in Fig. 10-8A, which depicts a tightly woven texture with fine pores. Degenerative tissues often exhibit tears (see Fig. 10-8B) and peeling (see Fig. 10-8C), on their surface. These surface irregularities may have profound effects on the lubrication mechanism involved, and thus, on the friction and the rate of degradation of the articular cartilage.

On the macroscopic level, the types of surface interactions occurring between different joints in the body vary greatly. For example, the hip joint is a deep congruent ball-and-socket joint (33,82,83,101,203,228,229,238); this differs from the glenohumeral joint of the shoulder, which is often described as a shallow ball-and-socket or a minimally constrained articulation (228). Furthermore, these joint shapes differ greatly from that of the distal femur in the knee joint, which is bicondylar in nature, or from the saddle shape of the thumb carpometacarpal or the ankle joints (9,12,16,33,42). These anatomic forms can also vary with age and disease (33,197,203). The degree of matching between the various bones and articulating cartilage surfaces comprising a joint is a major factor affecting the distribution of stresses in the cartilage and subchondral bone (1,2,10–13,29, 30,33,82,83,116). Thus, the precise methods to quantify joint anatomy is essential. A description of quantitative methods for characterizing the three-dimensional anatomy of articular surfaces is provided in Chapter 9. These methodologies include the calculation of surface radii of curvature and joint congruence, which are necessary for tribological analyses.

4 MOTION AND FORCES ON DIARTHRODIAL JOINTS

In vivo experimental measurements on the relative motions between articulating surfaces of a joint corresponding to daily activities are limited. Most quantitative information is obtained from gait studies (see Chapters 2 and 3 for more details), which do not provide the detailed information required for lubrication studies (5,59,71,82,145,189,190,216,243). Simple calculations show that peak translational speeds between two articulating surfaces can range from approximately 0.06 m/s between the femoral head surface and the acetabulum surface during normal walking to approximately 0.6 m/s between the humeral head surface and the glenoid cavity of the shoulder for a baseball pitcher during the throwing motion for a 100-mph pitch (163). Assuming, roughly, that synovial fluid film thicknesses are on the order of, or greater than the surface roughness, e.g., 6 μm, it is estimated that the shear rate found within joints may reach or exceed 10^5 s^{-1} (49,53,163,210).

The loads transmitted across a joint may be carried by the opposing joint surfaces via solid-to-solid contact, through a fluid-film layer, or a mixture of both. As in joint motion, the load on the joint is dependent on the type of activity; i.e., the loading sites change continuously as

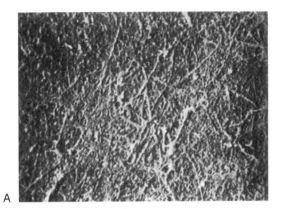

A

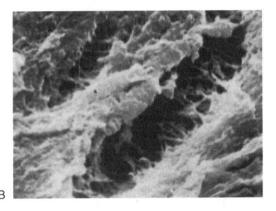

B

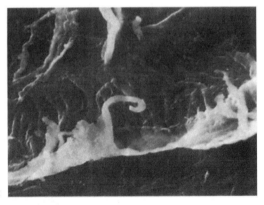

C

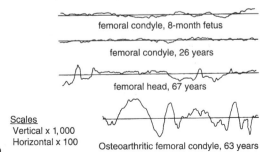

femoral condyle, 8-month fetus

femoral condyle, 26 years

femoral head, 67 years

Scales
Vertical x 1,000
Horizontal x 100

Osteoarthritic femoral condyle, 63 years

D

FIGURE 10-8. (A) Scanning electron microscopic view of the texture of normal human articular cartilage surface, showing a dense-pack random arrangement of collagen fibrils at the surface; specimen is a 21-year-old male femoral head retrieved from autopsy and magnified x3,000 [171]. **(B)** Typical appearance of articular cartilage surface from an osteoarthritic human specimen showing deep fissures forming, x3,000 [171]. **(C)** Scanning electron micrograph of an aging femoral head surface retrieved from the fracture neck of a femur; no OA was detected in this hip joint, x1,000 [171]. **(D)** Talysurf tracing of surface roughness for normal young and aging and osteoarthritic cartilage samples [241].

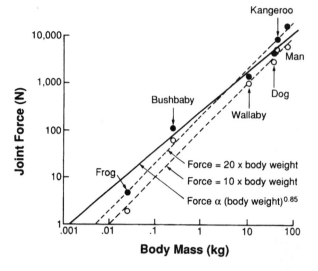

FIGURE 10-9. Maximum joint forces during jumping in the knee (*solid symbols*) and ankle (*open symbols*) of various animals versus body weight. (Adapted from Dowson D. Basic tribology. In: Dowson D, Wright V, eds. *Introduction to the biomechanics of joints and joint replacement.* London: Mechanical Engineering Publications Ltd., 1981:49–60, with permission.)

the articulating surfaces move relative to each other (1,2,12,16,29,59,77,155,203,207,213–215,229). During a normal walking cycle, the human hip, knee, and ankle joints can be subject to loads ranging up to 10 times body weight, thus causing very high stresses (1,2,42,82,83,101,147,151,160,161,189,190). In the lower extremity, the peak loads at the knee and ankle are attained at heel strike and toe-off and, at the hip, when rising from a seat. The average load on the joint is approximately three times body weight, which lasts maybe as high as 60% of the walking cycle. During the swing phase of walking, only light loads (one to three times body weight) are carried. During this phase, the articular surfaces move rapidly over each other. In addition, extremely high forces occur across the joints in the leg during jumping. Figure 10-9 illustrates the levels of force that can exist in the knees and ankles of different species. For these reasons, the magnitude and duration of the joint loading, as well as the relative motion between the two articulating surfaces, must be considered when lubrication mechanisms are discussed.

5 FRICTION

5.1 Basic Concepts

Friction is defined as the resistance to motion between two bodies in contact. The first type

of friction, called surface friction, comes either from adhesion of one surface to another because of roughness of the two surfaces or from the viscosity of the sheared lubricant film between the two surfaces, Fig. 10-10. In the case of *dry friction*, i.e., surface friction without a lubricant, three laws have been postulated by Amonton (1699) and Coulomb (1785):

1. Frictional force (F) is directly proportional to the applied load (W).
2. F is independent of the apparent area of contact.
3. The kinetic F is independent of the sliding speed (V).

These laws help to define a coefficient of friction μ by the simple, well-known equation $F = \mu W$. The second type of friction, called bulk friction, occurs from the internal energy dissipation mechanisms within the bulk material or within the viscous lubricant. For cartilage, an internal friction is produced by the frictional drag caused when interstitial fluid flows through the porous-permeable solid matrix (13,124,136,137,168,169,171,177), though this frictional component is negligible according to the theoretical calculations of (18). Plowing friction is a specific form of internal friction and occurs in diarthrodial joints when a load moves across a joint surface, causing interstitial fluid flow (136,137,176). Interstitial fluid flow patterns

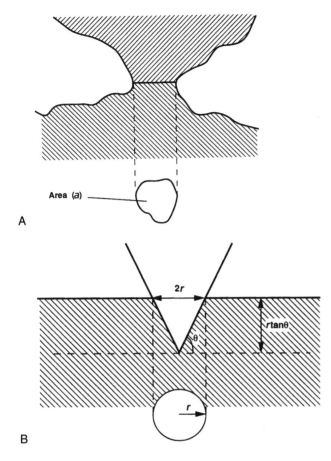

A

B

FIGURE 10-10. (A) Interaction between two asperities of two rough surfaces with similar hardness. For metals, adhesion by welding occurs at these junction sites. Adhesive friction is caused by the energy required to fracture these microwelds. **(B)** Penetration of a hard conical microasperity on one surface into a softer material of the other surface. A form of plowing friction occurs when the hard asperity is forced to cut through the softer surface. (Adapted from Dowson D. Basic tribology. In: Dowson D, Wright V, eds. *Introduction to the biomechanics of joints and joint replacement.* London: Mechanical Engineering Publications Ltd., 1981:49–60, with permission.)

throughout the tissue have been calculated (11,13,166,167). The dissipation related to interstitial fluid flow has been calculated and confirmed experimentally using a material testing protocol for the determination of hysteretic behavior of cartilage in uniaxial compression (170,176,177).

5.2 Measurements of Coefficients of Friction

For friction between articular surfaces, μ has remarkably low values in comparison to other engineering materials, Tables 10-2 and 10-3. This friction coefficient μ for articular surfaces of joints has been measured in two ways. First, specially designed "arthrotripsometers" or pendulum devices have been used on intact joints (55,111,136,137,138, 238,239). The second method involves sliding

TABLE 10-2. COEFFICIENTS OF FRICTION FOR TYPICAL MATERIALS

Material Combination	Coefficient of Friction
Gold on gold	2.8
Aluminum on aluminum	1.9
Silver on silver	1.5
Steel on steel	0.6–0.8
Brass on steel	0.35
Glass on glass	0.9
Wood on wood	0.25–0.5
Nylon on nylon	0.2
Graphite on steel	0.1
Ice on ice at 0°C	0.1
UHMWPE on cobalt chrome (artificial joints)	0.01–0.05

(Adapted from Dowson D. Basic tribology. In: Dowson D, Wright V, eds. *Introduction to the biomechanics of joints and joint replacement.* London: Mechanical Engineering Publications Ltd., 1981:49–60, with permission.)

excised pieces of cartilage over another surface (20,21,67,68,150,156,157,191,192,231–235, 241,242,244,245).

The pendulum-type experimental configuration uses a diarthrodial joint, e.g., the hip, as the fulcrum of a simple pendulum in which one of the joint surfaces rocks freely over the other, Fig. 10-11A. Such studies have produced coef-

ficients of friction from 0.003 to 0.06 for the combination of both plowing friction and surface friction, e.g., Fig. 10-11B. Unsworth and co-workers (238,239) demonstrated that when a load is applied to the hip joint suddenly, and synovial fluid is present in the joint cavity, the opposing surfaces approach each other under squeeze-film lubrication conditions. The

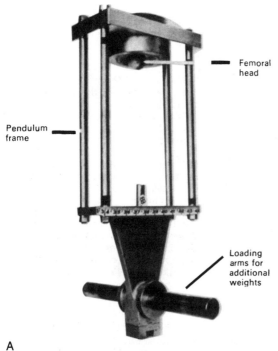

A

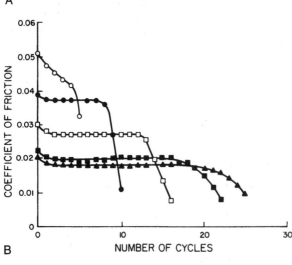

B

FIGURE 10-11. (A) A compound pendulum device with the human hip joint as its fulcrum; this device is used to measure the coefficient of friction between femoral head (*shown*) and the acetabulum (*not shown*) by the decay of the amplitude of the pendulum motion [238]. **(B)** A typical set of curves for the coefficient of friction versus the number of cycles from a hip specimen under suddenly loaded, unlubricated conditions (i.e., no synovial fluid). Results show a longer period of swing and a lower coefficient of friction with increasing load (*open circle*, 133.5 N; *solid circle*, 213 N; *open square*, 375 N; *solid square*, 577 N; *solid triangle*, 1,020 N) [238]. **(C)** Differences of the coefficient of friction between unlubricated and lubricated (with synovial fluid) hip joints at varying applied loads. At a load >90 N, no differences in coefficients of friction were observed [238].

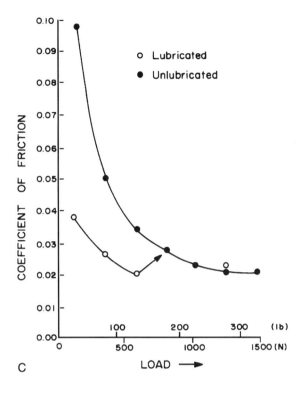

C

FIGURE 10-11. (Continued).

evidence presented in support of this mechanism was frictional resistance increased and then decreased with increasing cycles of oscillation because of the decrease of fluid film thickness with time. They also attempted to prevent squeeze-film action by pre-loading the joint before the first oscillation, and they observed that the friction coefficient monotonically decreased with increasing oscillations under this configuration; they observed a similar response after wiping away the synovial fluid and applying a sudden

load, thus confirming that squeeze-film lubrication occurs only in the presence of an external supply of lubricant, Fig. 10-11B. The maximum friction coefficients recorded for their tests with and without synovial fluid, as a function of joint load are shown in Fig. 10-11C. These results indicate that the friction coefficient of cartilage decreases with increasing load. Above a threshold of load, synovial fluid causes no difference in the frictional properties of joints. These authors hypothesized that in the absence of squeeze-film action, lubrication must have been generated from the interstitial fluid in articular cartilage or from boundary lubrication, Fig. 10-11C.

The second type of experimental configuration involves the sliding of a small piece of cartilage over another surface (e.g., glass, rubber, another piece of cartilage) (20,67,68,142,150, 156,157,191,192,231–235,241,242,244–246). This technique has the advantage that the effects of surface friction can be measured directly, as compared with measuring the combination of surface and plowing friction, as was done using the first configuration (176). When a flat

TABLE 10-3. COEFFICIENTS OF FRICTION FOR ARTICULAR CARTILAGE IN SYNOVIAL JOINTS

Investigator	Coefficient of Friction	Joint Tested
Charnley (40)	0.005–0.02	Human knee
McCutchen (156)	0.02–0.35	Porcine shoulder
Linn (136,137)	0.005–0.01	Canine ankle
Unsworth et al. (238,239)	0.01–0.04	Human hip
Malcom (150)	0.002–0.03	Bovine shoulder

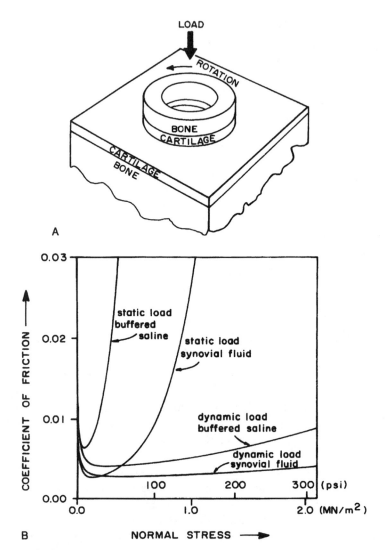

FIGURE 10-12. (A) Specimens cut from the bovine humeral head and glenoid surface provide conforming surfaces for studies on interfacial friction. This configuration is effective in preventing plowing friction [150]. **(B)** Variation of the coefficient of friction corresponding to the test configuration depicted in Fig. 10-14A under various lubrication and loading conditions: with and without synovial fluid; static and dynamic [150].

specimen is loaded, no plowing can occur (hypothetically). Malcom (150) tested excised annular plugs from a bovine humeral head against the apposing glenoid surface under a continuously rotating articulation, Fig. 10-12A. The coefficient of friction μ from his experiments ranged from 0.002 to 0.03. It was determined from this experimental study that the interfacial μ had the following characteristics:

1. μ increased with time after application of the load.
2. μ increased with magnitude of the load.
3. μ was lower when synovial fluid was used as the lubricant than with buffered saline.
4. μ was very sensitive to small vertical oscillations of the annular plug of cartilage and actually decreased in magnitude under such motions, Fig. 10-12B.

This last observation is likely related to pressurization of interstitial fluid caused by the applied dynamic compressive load (124,150). This topic is addressed further below.

5.3 Role of Synovial Fluid

Many experiments have been performed in an attempt to assess the role of synovial fluid or its components in joint lubrication (23,26,37,45, 49,50,118,125,217,231–235,241,242). This role has been difficult to quantify because it differs under varying kinematic and loading circumstances and with different material properties of cartilage and synovial fluid.

A series of experiments, in which synovial fluid was passed through filters with various pore sizes and/or treated with various enzymes, were performed. The components separated from filtration were subsequently tested for lubrication efficiency. McCutchen passed synovial fluid through filters with pore sizes of 0.22 μm in an attempt to sieve out the lubricating component of synovial fluid (157). He observed that the residue provided better lubrication than the filtrate. Filters with larger pore sizes of 0.65 μm were also used. In this case, the filtrate was the better lubricant. Thus, he concluded that a macromolecule, presumably a hyaluronate, whose size was between 0.22 μm and 0.65 μm, is a key component responsible for boundary lubrication; nevertheless, this boundary lubricant was observed to be weak and failed to lubricate under high loads. Malcom (150) also noted that above a threshold of applied pressure, frictional properties of cartilage became erratic and nonrepeatable.

Little and co-workers measured an average coefficient of friction of 0.008 in articular cartilage (141). They observed that treating the articular surfaces with a fat solvent increased the coefficient of friction to an average of 0.022. They concluded that boundary lubrication prevailed in joints and was aided by a lipid present in the articular cartilage. Maroudas (152) demonstrated the formation of hyaluronan gels by performing *in vitro* filtration experiments on synovial fluid. Walker and co-workers performed electron micrograph studies of cartilage surfaces

where they believed to observe aggregates of hyaluronic acid (242). However, Linn showed that purified hyaluronic acid "lacked lubricating ability" (137) and subsequent studies confirmed this finding (95,123,138,157,193,232).

In several studies throughout the 1970s and 1980s, Radin and co-workers (193) and Swann and co-workers (233–235) analyzed a glycoprotein isolated from bovine and human synovial fluid that they found to provide boundary lubricating ability. They called this synovial fluid constituent LGP-I (lubricating glycoprotein) or lubricin. Using LGP-I at a concentration between 65 μg/mL and 100 μg/mL (235), these investigators observed frictional responses identical to normal synovial fluid. More recently, Jay and Hong tested the boundary lubrication ability of a synovial fluid retentrate that they believed to be identical to lubricin (109). From latex-on-glass experiments under a 0.03-MPa stress, they observed that the friction coefficient decreased from 0.11 with a 0.9% NaCl solution to a modest 0.07 with lubricin at 260 μg/mL in 0.9% NaCl.

Schumacher (208,209) discovered a novel proteoglycan, of molecular weight 315 kDa, synthesized and secreted by chondrocytes of the superficial zone of articular cartilage, which they also found in synovial fluid. This superficial zone protein (SZP) could be degraded by enzymes that are known to degrade other proteoglycans, such as papain, trypsin, and pronase. Flannery et al. (66) demonstrated that SZP was homologous to a previously identified glycoprotein described as a precursor protein to a megakaryocyte stimulating factor (MSF). These authors showed that SZP contains large and small mucin-like repeat domains likely to be substituted by O-linked oligosaccharides, which may impart lubricating ability to this protein. Following these studies, Jay et al. (110) found a homology between lubricin, SZP and MSF, thus confirming the suggestion that SZP may serve as a boundary lubricant and possibly explaining its expression near the surface zone. They proposed that SZP and lubricin be categorized in a new class of biomolecules termed tribonectins.

Hills and Butler suggested that phospholipids were the major ingredients responsible for the lubricating ability of synovial fluid, in analogy to their previous findings in pleural movement (92). They indicated that the extraction procedure of Swann and co-workers was unlikely to have excluded phospholipids as contaminants in their lubricin, and subsequently Schwarz and Hills demonstrated that 12% of lubricin in normal synovial fluid is phospholipid (212). Hills and Butler demonstrated that these phospholipids were readily adsorbed to hydrophilic solids whose surfaces then became hydrophobic (92). In a subsequent study, Hills showed that dipalmitoyl phosphatidylcholine (DPPC) could rapidly adsorb on glass surfaces, making them hydrophobic (93). The DPPC could not be removed from glass by rinsing with saline but required the use of the same fat solvent as the one employed by Little and co-workers (141), and this was cited as evidence that DPPC is the active boundary lubricant in synovial fluid. Hills also argued that DPPC formed oligolamellar deposits on cartilage rather than monolayers. Williams et al. (246) performed friction tests with and without DPPC using borosilicate surfaces in a reciprocating apparatus. These authors observed that the friction coefficient in the presence of DPPC was velocity dependent. Under dry friction, static friction coefficients varied from 0.65 to 0.88 and scratches appeared on the sliding surfaces; with DPPC, average static coefficients of friction were in the range of 0.123 to 0.158, and no scratches were apparent. In a follow-up study, Foy et al. (69) tested bovine articular cartilage against glass ($\mu = 0.37 - 0.60$) and against polyurethane ($\mu = 0.18 - 0.36$) and found that the addition of DPPC significantly decreased the friction coefficient for both materials ($\mu = 0.14 - 0.39$ and $\mu = 0.05 - 0.10$, respectively), whereas the friction coefficient of delipidized cartilage against glass ($\mu = 0.38 - 0.76$) was greater than that of normal cartilage against glass. In the study of Higaki et al. (90), the addition of DPPC reduced the friction coefficient of pig cartilage from 0.015 to 0.010. Hills has also confirmed the wear-resistant properties of DPPC when used in engineering bearings (94). Subsequently, Hills and Monds (95) also showed that selective enzymatic degradation of synovial fluid and cartilage with hyaluronidase

(to degrade hyaluronic acid), trypsin (to degrade lubricin) and phospholipase (to degrade surface-active phospholipid, or SAPL) showed a significant dose-dependent increase in friction coefficient with phospholipase only (up to 43% above control), confirming that SAPL is the "active ingredient" of synovial fluid. These authors did note that trypsin decreased the friction coefficient of cartilage, and suggested that the destruction of lubricin as a carrier of phospholipid (212) may have led to the deposition of additional layers on the articular surface, thus enhancing lubrication. Hills has proposed that a unifying interpretation of boundary lubrication by synovial fluid can be achieved by recognizing that lubricin and hyaluronic acid have carrier functions for the highly insoluble SAPL, while hyaluronic acid may also act as a fluid-film lubricant under the special circumstances when this latter mode of lubrication prevails (96). Recently, Sarma et al. (205) have confirmed the existence of phospholipids at the articular surface of bovine articular cartilage and have quantitatively identified the distribution of the main classes into phosphatidylcholine (41%), phosphatidylethanolamine (27%), and sphingomyelin (32%). They also determined that the most abundant fatty acid within these lipids was oleic acid.

These recent developments provide strong evidence that some constituents of synovial fluid act as boundary lubricants. The effectiveness of this lubricant appears to be load dependent as well as velocity dependent. Under the best experimental configurations, however, this boundary lubricant appears to improve the friction coefficient only by a factor of 2 to 6, approximately. These observations are consistent with the previously reported differences in friction coefficient when using saline instead of synovial fluid (150,156), which may be attributed to the presence of boundary lubricant in the latter. Hence, it is necessary to further explore the mechanisms that may also contribute to reducing the friction coefficient of cartilage in order to explain the wide variations of frictional properties reported in the literature (Table 10-3).

Synovial fluid may also play the role of lubricant in fluid-film lubrication, though the viability of this mode of lubrication has not been established unequivocally for diarthrodial joints, as further discussed below. Several studies (95,123,137,138,157,193,232) have shown that hyaluronidase-treated synovial fluid lubricates almost as well as untreated fluid, even though hyaluronidase depolymerizes hyaluronic acid and decreases the viscosity of synovial fluid to that of saline. Such a result suggests that fluid-film lubrication, which is highly dependent on lubricant viscosity, cannot be the primary mechanism responsible for the low frictional coefficient of joints. When trypsin was used to treat synovial fluid (trypsin degrades proteins and glycoproteins, but not phospholipids), the coefficient of friction rose significantly while the viscosity remained similar to that of normal synovial fluid (193,232). It remains to be seen whether trypsin could indirectly degrade the ability of DPPC to adsorb to the cartilage surface as well. Interestingly, O'Kelly and coworkers (187) obtained results that contradicted the previous work; they used a static loading pendulum and a dynamic oscillator designed to reproduce physiologic loading patterns and observed that the lubrication properties of synovial fluid treated with hyaluronidase differed significantly from untreated synovial fluid. Furthermore, they found no evidence that lubrication efficacy was affected if synovial fluid was treated with trypsin to remove glycoproteins. These results suggest that additional mechanisms might be at work that have not yet been described appropriately.

In summary, very low friction appears to exist within diarthrodial joints even in the absence of synovial fluid or hyaluronate, though synovial fluid contributes to further decrease the friction coefficient. Furthermore, dynamically applied loads, oscillations, or sliding tends to lower the coefficient of friction. However, higher loads may decrease the friction coefficient (see Fig. 10-11C) or increase it (see Fig. 10-12B).

6 WEAR

Wear of bearings is a universal phenomenon of boundary degradation involving progressive loss of bearing substance from the body as a result of mechanical action. The two conventional types of wear are fatigue wear and interfacial wear. Fatigue wear is independent of the lubrication phenomenon occurring at the surfaces of bearings. It occurs because of the cyclic stresses and strains generated within the cartilage due to the application of repetitive loads caused by joint motion. It is estimated that a typical human joint may experience 1 million cycles of loading in a year. These large cyclical stresses and strains may cause fatigue failure within the bulk material and may grow by an accumulation of microscopic damage within the material. These internal failures within diseased tissues have been observed in the form of collagen fiber scission, and loosening of the normally tight collagen network (27,28). Eventually, the internal failures can extend to the material surface causing cracks and fissures (27,28,41,176,197). In time, if the rate of damage exceeds that by which the cartilage cells may regenerate the tissue, an accumulation of fatigue microdamage will occur that may lead to bulk tissue failure (176,197). Thus, *in vivo* wear is a balance of mechanical attrition and biological synthesis (106).

Interfacial wear results from solid-solid contact at the surface of bearing materials. There are two basic types of interfacial wear. Adhesive wear is the most common and occurs when a junction is formed between the two opposing surfaces as they come into contact (see Fig. 10-10A). If this junction is stronger than the cohesive strength of the individual materials, fragments of the weaker material may be torn off and may adhere to the stronger material (8,55). Abrasive wear occurs when a soft material comes into contact with a significantly harder material (see Fig. 10-10B). Under these circumstances, the asperities of the harder material surface may cut into the softer counterpart, causing abrasive wear. This harder material may be either the opposing bearing surface or loose particles between the bearing surfaces. When loose particles between the surfaces cause abrasive wear, the process is termed three-body wear. Wear is measured either as the mass of material removed from interacting surfaces per unit of time or as the volume lost. At present, wear analysis is mostly an empirical science. In general, it is difficult to predict either wear rates or their dependency on other physical parameters (8). For biological materials, little quantitative information exists on wear mechanisms or wear rates (140). Different types of wear produce different wear rates; for example, fatigue wear depends on the frequency and magnitude of the applied loads and on the intrinsic material properties of the bulk material. However, interfacial wear depends on the roughness of the bearing surfaces, the true size of the contact area of the two surfaces, and the magnitude of the applied load (8,55). However, some general rules on wear have been observed:

1. Wear rates increase with increasing applied normal load.
2. Wear rates increase with increasing sliding contact area between the two opposing bearing surfaces.
3. Wear rate of the softer bearing surface is higher than that of the harder bearing surface.

The function of typical engineering bearings is often impaired if even a relatively small amount of the bearing volume is lost. This is because minute changes of bearing surface geometry affect the hydrodynamics of the thin lubricant film, usually no more than 25 μm thick, in the worn bearing. For hydrated tissues such as cartilage, it is very difficult to quantify either mass loss or volume loss due to the phenomenon of swelling (see Chapter 5). In the 1970s, Lipshitz and co-workers, in a tedious set of experiments, measured wear and wear rates for cartilage using hydroxyproline (collagen) and hexosamine as markers (Fig. 10-13) (139,140), and found them to be extremely low. In these *in vitro* experiments, excised cartilage plugs were equilibrated in a buffered saline bath and loaded against a polished stainless steel surface. A steady harmonic sliding motion was imposed for long periods of time (140). Wear was measured by the hydroxyproline and hexosamine contents in the bathing solution and wear rates determined. In both the 4.62 MPa and 1.66 MPa cases, the initial *wear rate* was high, gradually decreasing to a steady state of wear rate. Removal of load to allow the tissue to recover its interstitial fluid

content (located by the arrow in Fig. 10-13) did not alter the wear rate. This figure shows that even at high pressures, similar to those found *in vivo* under physiological conditions, wear rate was extremely small. This may be because of the large number of redundant, "fail-safe" lubrication mechanisms that exist at the articular surface preventing wear. However, it is likely that once the ultrastructure of the articular surface is damaged and/or proteoglycans are lost, the cartilage becomes softer and more permeable (see Figs. 10-8B and 10-8C) (3,4,6,73,85,218,219). Under these conditions, cartilage loses its ability to support load by *hydrostatic* pressure and may not be as efficient in lubrication (167,173,224,225). In these cases, fluid-film lubrication is not likely to prevail, and adhesive and abrasive wear may occur (8,41,197).

Some general conclusions were drawn from the wear studies of cartilage-against-steel plate by Lipshitz and Glimcher (140):

1. Wear rates decrease with time until they reach a constant value; this value is dependent on the applied pressure and the roughness of the opposing stainless steel surface.
2. Wear rates increase with applied normal pressure and with increased relative speed of the opposing surfaces.
3. Wear rates decrease 5-fold if the tissue is fixed and stiffened by formaldehyde, which retards abrasive wear.
4. Wear rates may decrease 10-fold if synovial fluid is used as a lubricant.

Thus, though the role of synovial fluid in fluid-film lubrication may be questionable, its role in reducing the wear rate of articular cartilage against a stainless steel plate is remarkable. This fact may be very important clinically when a femoral head endoprosthesis articulates with the cartilage of the acetabulum. The wear rates determined by Lipshitz and co-workers (140) exhibit large variability and are very sensitive to the laboratory environment, the nature of the test, and the mechanical and chemical nature of the bearing materials. For these reasons, information regarding wear mechanisms is minimal despite the wide body of knowledge concerning changes in tissue composition.

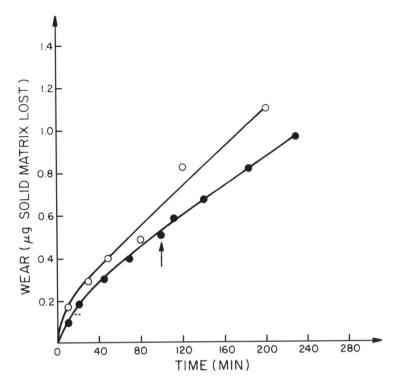

FIGURE 10-13. Variation of wear rate as a function of time (*open circle*, 4.62 MPa; *solid circle*, 1.66 MPa). At the point indicated by the *arrow*, the cartilage plugs were allowed to imbibe fluid overnight. No drop in wear rate was seen, and the wear rate continues without the initial "toe region" [140].

Repetitive joint motion and loading could cause cartilage damage and wear (72). Another cause of cartilage damage and wear is high-impact loading (7,51,194,195,199,237,240). As normal cartilage is compressed, its interstitial fluid pressurizes and contributes to support more than 90% of the applied load (11,13,147,176, 177,224,225,227), thus shielding the collagen-proteoglycan matrix from excessive and potentially damaging stresses. However, above a threshold level of stress, the cartilage matrix will fail, creating vertical fissures at the surface as well as horizontal splits at the cartilage-bone interface (7,11,193–197,199,237,240). For example, a single impact on the patellofemoral joint has been observed to cause cartilage damage at the surface and the tidemark (7) and biological remodeling of cartilage in the region surrounding the tidemark (51,129). Loss of fluid pressurization near these defects may lead to progressive

increases of stress on the solid matrix and enhanced rate of degeneration of the tissue (179), thereby accelerating the release of wear particles into the joint cavity under *in vivo* conditions. In other experiments, Radin and Paul (194) tested bovine metacarpal-phalangeal joints lubricated with veronate saline in the arthrotripsometer built by Linn (136,137). When a static load of 1,000 pounds was applied for 5,000 hours, no significant wear was evident. However, when a 500-pound static load was combined with a 500-pound periodic impact load, wear was observed in 200 hours. A similar study was repeated and indicated severe cartilage damage because of impact loading (195). Repo and Finlay (199) showed that an impact load larger than a critical value would cause surface fractures on cartilage plugs, and Armstrong and co-workers showed that an impact load greater than 6 kN will cause shear failure at the tidemark of porcine knee joints *in vivo* (7); radiologists often refer to these as occult lesions in the cartilage because they are not visible to observation from the surface.

7 HYPOTHESES FOR DIARTHRODIAL JOINT LUBRICATION

Many possible modes of lubrication have been proposed in attempts to explain the minimal friction and wear characteristics of cartilage found in diarthrodial joints. To be acceptable, each proposed mode of lubrication must be able to account for the friction and wear characteristics of these joints under a variety of loading and motion conditions. For fluid-film lubrication, the minimum fluid-film thickness predicted by a specific lubrication theory must exceed three times the combined statistical surface roughness of cartilage (e.g., 4 to 25 μm) (88). If the predicted fluid-film gap is too thin to produce the separation of the two bearing surfaces required for fluid-film lubrication under a given set of loading and motion conditions, then boundary lubrication must be present.

7.1 Fluid-film Lubrication

7.1.1 Hydrodynamic Lubrication

In 1932, MacConaill [146] proposed that the two articulating surfaces do not actually come into contact and that the load is transmitted via a thin layer of fluid lubricant. This hypothesis found early support in the low friction coefficients measured in synovial joints by Jones in 1936 [111]. MacConaill hypothesized that the high viscosity of synovial fluid and the relative motion of the joint surfaces can create the thin wedge-shaped fluid layer required for the hydrodynamic mode of lubrication to operate within the knee. The basic mechanism of hydrodynamic lubrication is shown in Fig. 10-14. A high-speed transversely moving surface is required to drag a layer of viscous fluid through a narrowing wedge-shaped gap. This action creates a hydrodynamic pressure in the fluid, generating lift, which forces the two surfaces apart (200). However, this conventional hydro-

dynamic lubrication theory generally requires a continuous high-speed relative motion between the two opposing bearing surfaces to provide a substantial load-carrying pressure. Although high-speed motion and lighter loads are occasionally present (e.g., the articulation at the glenohumeral joint of the shoulder of a baseball pitcher), many more activities of daily living involve intermittent and low-speed motions in various joints (38,39,163). Because of this argument, hydrodynamic lubrication is not likely to be a primary mechanism operating in the joint. Other factors such as deformation of cartilage and interstitial fluid flow may play important roles in determining the modes of joint lubrication.

To quantitatively examine the plausibility of the hydrodynamic mode of lubrication, let us use the mathematical results for the minimum film thickness and some salient approximations for diarthrodial joint operating conditions. Martin derived the formula for estimating the minimum film thickness for the hydrodynamic lubrication of a rigid cylinder on a plane (154). His equation for minimum film thickness expression is given by:

$$h/R = 4.9\, \eta u L/W \qquad (1)$$

Kapitza derived a similar relationship considering the hydrodynamic lubrication of a sphere on a plane (114). This expression is given by:

$$h/R = 113.7(\eta u R/W)^2 \qquad (2)$$

In both expressions, h is the minimum film thickness, R is the radius of the cylinder or sphere, L is the axial length of the cylinder, η is the constant viscosity of a Newtonian fluid, u is the entraining velocity, which is equal to one-half the sum of the velocities of the interacting surfaces, and W is the load on the bearing, Fig. 10-15. If the articulating surfaces can be approximated by either a rigid cylinder interacting with a plane, or by a rigid sphere on a plane, and if the synovial fluid is considered to be Newtonian with a known constant viscosity, these simplified approximations can be used to assess whether hydrodynamic lubrication can work in diarthrodial joints. The calculation of the fluid-film thickness under hydrodynamic conditions

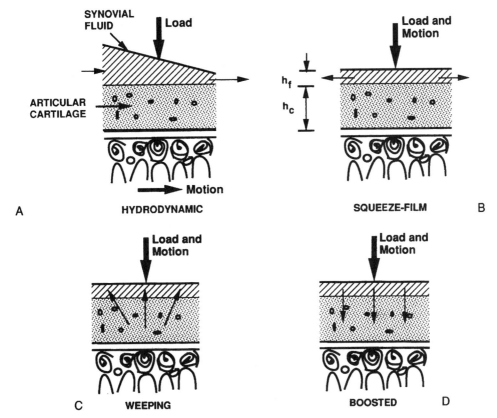

FIGURE 10-14. **(A)** Schematic representation of hydrodynamic lubrication. Viscous fluid is dragged into a convergent channel, causing a pressure field to be generated in the lubricant. Fluid viscosity, gap geometry, and relative sliding speed determine the load-carrying capacity. **(B)** As the bearing surfaces are squeezed together, the viscous fluid is forced from the gap in the transverse direction. This squeeze action generates a hydrodynamic pressure in the fluid for load support. The load-carrying capacity depends on the size of the surfaces, velocity of approach, and fluid viscosity. **(C)** Weeping lubrication hypothesis for the uniform exudation of interstitial fluid from the cartilage. The driving mechanism is a self-pressurization of the interstitial fluid when the tissue is compressed. **(D)** Direction of fluid flow under squeeze-film lubrication in the boosted mode for joint lubrication.

can be performed with some specific diarthrodial joint examples.

Example 1

For the knee joint during the stance phase of walking, the following values are taken to calculate the minimum fluid-film thickness: $R = 0.1$ m, $L/W = 2 \times 10^{-5}$ m/N, $u = 0.3$ m/s, and $\eta = 10^{-2}$ N.s/m^2.

Using Eq. 1 and multiplying through by R yields: $h = (0.1 \text{ m}) \times (4.9) \times (10^{-2} \text{ N.s/m}^2) \times (0.3 \text{ m/s}) \times (2 \times 10^{-5} \text{ m/N})$; the fluid-film thickness prediction is $h = 0.029 \ \mu$m. This value is much too low in comparison with the cartilage

surface roughness for an effective fluid lubricant film to be formed between the bearing surfaces.

Example 2

For the hip joint during the swing phase of walking, the following values are taken to calculate the approximate fluid-film thickness: $R = 1.0$ m, $W = 75$ kg, $u = 0.1$ m/s, and $\eta = 10^{-2}$ N.s/m^2.

Using Eq. 2 and multiplying through yields:

$$h = (1.0 \text{ m}) \times (113.7) \times [(10^{-2} \text{ N.s/m}^2)]$$
$$\times (0.1 \text{ m/s}) \times (1.0 \text{ m})/(75 \text{ kgf})]^2$$

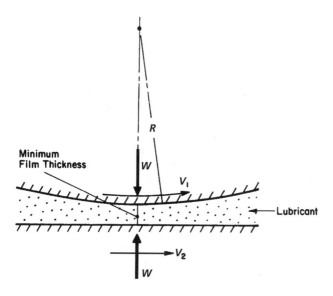

FIGURE 10-15. Cylinder-on-plane bearing configuration; u = entraining velocity = $(V_1 + V_2)/2$, R = effective radius of curvature; W = bearing load supported by the lubricant.

The fluid-film thickness prediction is $h =$ 0.020 μm. This value for fluid-film thickness is also much smaller than the articular cartilage surface roughness.

It is thus evident that hydrodynamic lubrication cannot operate in these joints under these loading conditions. However, under smaller loads, and during faster motions such as in the swing phase of walking, this mechanism of lubrication may possibly be responsible for lubrication. One should, however, remember that synovial fluid is non-Newtonian and exhibits a shear thinning effect (see Fig. 10-5) (210). Thus, these joint "model" assumptions may be far from reality.

Dintenfass included cartilage deformation in his theory (48,49). This would act to spread the joint load over a larger surface area and would decrease the velocity gradient between the two surfaces. In engineering terminology, this lubrication mode, in which both the viscous resistance of the lubricant as well as the elastic deformation of the bearing surfaces play a prominent role, is called elastohydrodynamic lubrication. For the hip and knee joints, film thickness provided by this mechanism has been calculated to be as high as 1.3 and 1.25 μm, respectively (56,87,91).

While Dintenfass allowed for cartilage deformability, he assumed a simplified deformation field to occur in a homogeneous, linearly elastic half-space. In reality, this deformation occurs in a soft cartilage layer backed by much stiffer subchondral bone. A layered structure with a rigid backing was studied by Hooke and O'Donoghue (103), who calculated the minimum film thickness for the cylinder and plane approximation using:

$$h/R = [L^{0.2}(\eta u)^{0.6}]/[W^{0.2}(E' R)^{0.4}] \quad (3)$$

where h, R, L, η, u, and W are as defined previously and E' is the "effective elastic modulus" given by:

$$1/E' = (1/2)\left[\left(1 - v_1^2\right)/E_1 + \left(1 - v_2^2\right)/E_2\right] \quad (4)$$

where E_1, v_1, E_2, and v_2 are the elastic moduli and Poisson ratio for the two-layer model (103). To see how the deformation of the cartilage might influence the minimum fluid-film predictions, let us use these two equations in an example.

Example 3

For the knee joint during the stance phase of walking, the following values are taken (as in Example 1) to calculate the approximate fluid-film thickness: $R = 0.1$ m, $L/W = 2 \times 10^{-5}$ m/N, $u = 0.3$ m/s, $\eta = 10^{-2}$ N.s/m^2, $E' = 10^7$ N/m^2.

Using Eq. 3 and multiplying through by R gives:

$$h = (0.1 \text{ m}) \times (2 \times 10^{-5} \text{ m/N})^{0.2} \times [(10^{-2} \text{N.s/m}^2)$$
$$\times (0.3 \text{ m/s})]^{0.6}/[(10^7 \text{ N/m}^2) \times (0.1 \text{ m})]^{0.4}$$

The fluid-film thickness prediction is $h = 1.4 \ \mu m$.

If cartilage is more compliant, the fluid-film thickness will be greater. Thus, the elastohydrodynamic mode appears more plausible than hydrodynamic lubrication for conditions observed in diarthrodial joints. Nevertheless, the film thicknesses reported for this lubrication mode are still smaller than the combined surface roughness of contacting cartilage layers.

Addressing this issue, Dowson and Jin (57,58) argued that the surface asperities of articular cartilage would be flattened out under the physiological pressures experienced in joints. They called this mechanism micro-elastohydrodynamic lubrication (micro-EHL) and they calculated a minimum film thickness on the order of 0.7 μm, but where the ratio of this thickness to the flattened composite surface roughness could be as great as 19 to 1. However, despite providing a possible theoretical mechanism for maintaining full-thickness fluid films between the surfaces, the predictions of the micro-EHL theory yielded smaller friction coefficients than experimental results (58).

More recently, Kirk et al. (119) used environmental scanning electron microscopy (ESEM) to demonstrate that cartilage surfaces are smooth under normal condition, and that the roughness reported in previous EM studies (e.g., 164, 197,241,249) was due to drying of specimens. Kirk et al. (120) also imaged a groove formed by Talysurf instrumentation on the cartilage surface, suggesting that such measurements (e.g., 236,249) reveal the topography of the collagen ultrastructure underneath the most superficial zone of cartilage. Similarly, using atomic force microscopy (AFM), Jurvelin et al. (113) and Kumar et al. (123) reported that the surface irregularities observed in EM studies were not apparent under AFM. If indeed cartilage is found to be a lot smoother than earlier reported, one of the major obstacles for accepting the viability of EHL will have been overcome. It will then remain to be demonstrated that the frictional properties, and their dependence on joint load, congruence, and material properties behave according to EHL theory. For example, to date, EHL theory has not been able to explain the time-dependent variation in the friction coefficient of cartilage (e.g., 142,150, 156,241).

It is generally accepted today that fluid film lubrication is likely to exist only under certain conditions of loading that are optimal for this mode of lubrication (high speed and low loads). Authors who have advocated fluid-film mechanisms for articular cartilage have also suggested that multiple modes of lubrication must coexist in diarthrodial joints (53,183,238,241).

7.1.2 Self-generating Mechanism

In a study by Mow and Lai, articular cartilage was modeled as a thin-layer biphasic medium supported by a hard bony substrate. In this formulation, normal cartilage was subjected to a constant-width, parabolically distributed normal load sliding over its surface at physiologic speeds V (127,167); a related analysis was also performed by Kwan and co-workers (124). The load distributions in these studies are representative of the hydrodynamic pressure in the synovial fluid film acting on the articular surface; the authors investigated whether under this prescribed traction, cartilage could yield its interstitial fluid for use as a fluid-film lubricant. In their original study, these authors employed a parametric analysis where they varied the load partition factor, which determines the load fractions applied to the solid and fluid phases of the tissue, respectively. Since that study, however, Hou and co-workers (104) demonstrated mathematically that the load is partitioned according to the solid and fluid fractions (or solidity and porosity) of cartilage at the surface. For this configuration, the formulation of Mow and Lai yielded a "self-generating mechanism" in which fluid was observed to exude under the leading and trailing edges of the load distribution, while it was resorbed into the tissue near the center, Fig. 10-16A (167). The exuded fluid at the

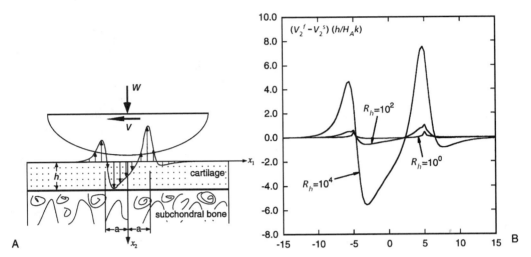

FIGURE 10-16. (A) Pattern of predicted fluid exudation and imbibition over the articular surface resulting from a hydrodynamic pressure distribution acting between a biphasic layer of thickness $h(r)$ and a moving indenter. Here V is the speed of the horizontal translation. **(B)** Fluid efflux from the tissue for various values of the nondimensional parameter $R_h = Vh/H_A k$.

leading edge could potentially provide a continuous supply of lubricant to maintain a fluid film between the surfaces, thus reducing the friction coefficient.

In the sliding load configuration, the effect of cartilage material properties and sliding speed is manifested through the non-dimensional parameter $R_h = Vh/H_A k$, where V is the sliding speed, k is the permeability coefficient of the tissue (assumed constant; see Chapter 5), H_A is the aggregate modulus of the solid matrix of cartilage, and h is the thickness of the cartilage layer. For normal tissues, R_h ranges from 10^3 to 10^5 and for pathologic tissues (with decreasing H_A and increasing k; see Chapter 5 for more details), and R_h in general decreases. Thus, the amount of fluid expelled into the joint space is a function of the characteristics of the applied sliding load and the properties of the solid matrix of cartilage, Fig. 10-16B. In this figure, it is assumed that $R_h = 10^4$ for normal cartilage, $R_h = 10^2$ for mildly degenerate cartilage, and $R_h = 1$ for highly degenerate cartilage (167). As degeneration proceeds, a decrease of interstitial fluid flow occurs, thus defeating the self-generating mechanism. This effect may have significant consequences on boundary lubrication, and on the inexorable wear-and-tear degeneration process in cartilage during osteoarthritis.

This self-generating mechanism was studied using an optical sliding-contact analytic rheometer (OSCAR), which produced a cinematographic record of the flow pattern (166). In this experiment, strips of cartilage were mounted on a glass slide and loaded normally by a sliding optical glass lens. The flow patterns provided visual evidence for this self-generating lubrication mechanism and supported the theory that articular cartilage can generate a fluid film under slow, moderate loading conditions.

This self-generating mechanism may not only contribute significantly to fluid-film lubrication, but may also create a mechanically generated circulation system required for the nutrition of chondrocytes in the tissue (131,132,202,220).

7.1.3 Squeeze-film Lubrication

In squeeze-film lubrication, two bearing surfaces simply approach each other along a normal direction, Fig. 10-14B. Because a viscous lubricant cannot be instantaneously squeezed out from the gap between the surfaces, a time-varying pressure field is built up as a result of the viscous resistance offered by the lubricant as it is being squeezed from the gap. The pressure field in the fluid film formed in this manner is capable of supporting large loads. Because the bearing surfaces are deformable layers of articular cartilage, the large pressure generated may cause localized depressions where the lubricant film can be trapped (122).

In 1967, Fein noted the importance of squeeze-film lubrication and derived expressions for the calculation of film thickness for various parameters using the sphere-on-plane configuration for his mathematical approximation of diarthrodial joints (64). Later, Higginson and Unsworth (91) demonstrated that for two compliant bearing surfaces, squeeze-film lubrication could yield physiologically meaningful squeeze-film times of approximately 60 s. The squeeze-film time is defined as the theoretical time required to reduce a lubricant film thickness down to a small prescribed minimum film thickness (Fig. 10-15), usually of the order of the surface roughness. Also, Dowson and co-workers (56) demonstrated that during lightly loaded portions of the swing phase of walking, a film thickness of 2.5 μm would decrease by only 0.06 μm in 0.5 s after heel strike. Mow (162,163) addressed the question of the non-Newtonian effects of synovial fluid in squeeze-film lubrication. He demonstrated that these non-Newtonian effects require a larger surface area to support a given load because of the lower peak hydrodynamic pressures that exist during squeeze film for the sphere-on-plane configuration. Thus, these non-Newtonian effects of the lubricant act to increase the squeeze-film time.

The viability of squeeze-film lubrication can be assessed from the squeeze-film time, which should be on the order of, or greater than, physiologic loading times and film thickness, as well as film replenishment. In lower extremity joints, where loading is intermittent and inertial effects during the swing phase of a gait cycle may contribute to separating the joint surfaces, squeeze-film action may be viable if it occurs in conjunction with other lubrication modes. In a study of transient EHL using thin-layer elastic models for cartilage, Medley et al. (158) and Smith and Medley (222) demonstrated theoretically that a minimum fluid-film thickness of 0.7 to 1.0 μm could be maintained during cyclical loading of a joint. This result is significant because it addresses the concern about film depletion

in fluid-film lubrication, over several cycles of loading, combining both the effects of squeeze-film and EHL actions. Assuming that the concerns about fluid-film thickness in relation to surface roughness can be addressed properly by micro-EHL or another related mechanism, it appears that squeeze-film lubrication does occur in lower-extremity joints (ankles, knees, and hips) under certain load configurations. This theoretical framework provides a cogent interpretation of the experimental results of Unsworth and co-workers (238,239). Further discussion of theoretical squeeze-film analyses is provided below, in the section on boosted lubrication.

7.2 Self-pressurized Hydrostatic Lubrication

A classical engineering lubrication theory, hydrostatic lubrication, exists in which a pressurized fluid film is maintained between two bearing surfaces via an external pump. In 1959, Lewis and McCutchen postulated a similar *self-pressurized hydrostatic lubrication* or *weeping lubrication* mechanism for diarthrodial joints (133,134,156) that functions in the absence of an external pump. According to this theory, lubricant fluid film between the two articulating surfaces is generated by compressing together the two layers of articular cartilage. Furthermore, a uniform exudation was hypothesized to occur over the entire articulating surface under compaction of the tissue, Fig. 10-14C. In a recent finite element study of a poroelastic spherical cartilage layer against an impermeable steel spherical endoprosthesis, Macirowski and co-workers reported numerical results that support this weeping phenomenon at the contact interface (147). McCutchen's weeping lubrication theory is the first to suggest a link between the time-dependent fluid pressurization and frictional response of articular cartilage, a mechanism that is addressed in greater detail below. In his study of the frictional response of pig articular cartilage against glass (156), the author observed that the friction coefficient under a constant load increased concurrently with the increasing creep deformation, which accompanies the exudation of fluid from cartilage. He also demonstrated that unloading and reloading the cartilage after a 10-second pause produced a higher friction coefficient than the initial response, and that squeeze-film lubrication could not explain this behavior because the bearing surfaces would have had ample time to be replenished by a fluid-film lubricant during the unloading period.

7.3 Boosted Lubrication

Another possible mechanism of lubrication of diarthrodial joints was proposed by Walker and co-workers in 1968 (241–243) and Maroudas in 1967 (152). This theory, termed *boosted lubrication*, hypothesizes that as the articulating surfaces approach each other, the solvent component of synovial fluid, i.e., water, passes into the articular cartilage over the contact region during squeeze-film conditions, thus leaving a concentrated pool of hyaluronic acid protein complex behind to lubricate the surfaces. It is reasoned that as the size of the gap between articulating surfaces decreases, the resistance of sideways efflux of the lubricant will eventually become greater than the resistance of flow into the articular cartilage, Fig. 10-14D. Furthermore, because of the small size (20 to 70 Å) of the pores in normal articular cartilage, Fig. 10-8A, the hyaluronate, with a diameter of its solution domain on the order of 4,000 Å (23,24) would be unable to penetrate the cartilage surface and is left behind in the gap. Thus, with the normal articulating surface acting as an ultrafiltration membrane, only water and small electrolytes are able to pass into the tissue.

Scanning electron microscopic observations indicating the presence of a hyaluronate-protein complex layer under squeeze-film conditions were made by Seller and co-workers (217), Fig. 10-17. Walker and co-workers noted that this concentrated hyaluronate and protein gel layer might be capable of supporting larger loads for longer periods of time than synovial fluid containing normal hyaluronate and protein concentrations (241). They postulated that this gel could become trapped in the normal roughness present in articular cartilage, forming micro-

pockets of concentrated gel on the articulating surfaces that aid in the lubrication process.

Lai and Mow (126) studied this ultrafiltration at the articular surface using a one-dimensional convection-diffusion model for the transport of macromolecules. They obtained quantitative information on the build-up rate of this gel near the articular surface. The rate and the extent of such a build-up depends on the Peclet number $(=VH_o/K)$, which characterizes the relative contribution of the diffusion (described by the diffusion coefficient K of hyaluronate in the fluid) versus the convection (with speed V, the rate of descent of the upper surface). Here H_o denotes the original thickness of the fluid. Because the concentration of hyaluronate and large protein molecules cannot increase indefinitely in the fluid, at a certain critical concentration C_{cr}, a three-dimensional molecular network will be formed creating a gel where C_{cr} is a nondimensional concentration given by C/C_o with C_o as the starting concentration in the fluid and C as the dimensional critical concentration. For hyaluronate, the concentration C_o in synovial fluid ranges from 2 to 5 mg/mL, and the critical concentration C may range from 10 to 20 mg/mL, though no firm data exist on this point (167). Thus, estimates of C_{cr} may range from 2 to 10.

Figure 10-18 shows that during ultrafiltration, as the upper surface descends, a height will be reached at which the gel begins to form at the lower surface. This gel or molecular network allows the complete passage of the solvent but is impermeable to the macromolecular solutes. Subsequent squeezing results in the growth of the thickness of this gel layer until the remaining gap is filled with the gel at a concentration C_{cr}. Figure 10-18 demonstrates the growth of the gel layer for various C_{cr} at a Peclet number of 2.5 and with the articular surface being entirely impermeable to large hyaluronate and protein molecules found in the fluid, i.e., N = 1. From Fig. 10-18, the final thickness h_f of the gel in boosted lubrication may be computed. The final thickness h_f is given by the expression $h_f = H_o\delta(t)$, where $\delta(t)$ is given by the curves for different C_{cr} in Fig. 10-18. For example, if

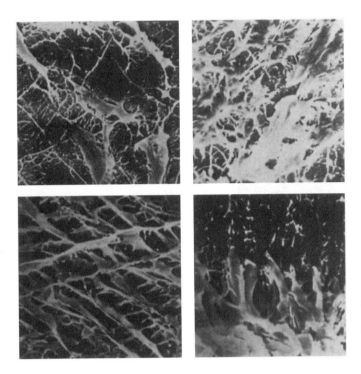

FIGURE 10-17. Scanning electron microscopy showing surface aggregation of dried hyaluronic acid-protein complexes on cartilage surfaces [217].

$H_o = 20 \ \mu$m and $C_{cr} = 3.07$, the final thickness of the gel is $h_f = 6.4 \ \mu$m.

In 1989, Hou and co-workers formulated the boundary conditions at the cartilage-synovial fluid interface (104). These boundary conditions are required for theoretical modeling of fluid exchanges between synovial fluid and articular cartilage interstitial fluid, in the cavity

of diarthrodial joints. This general formulation considers cartilage to be biphasic (168) and synovial fluid to be viscous Newtonian or viscoelastic non-Newtonian; a *pseudo-no-slip* kinematic boundary condition was proposed based on the principle that the conditions at the interface between a multiphasic mixture and a fluid must reduce to those boundary conditions in

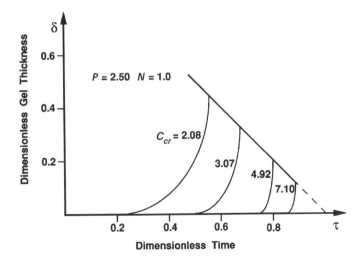

FIGURE 10-18. Predicted rate of growth of the thickness of the hyaluronic acid-protein gel for various critical concentrations [126]. The *upper line* represents the instantaneous position of the upper moving surface. Gelling stops when the whole gap is filled with the gel at C_{cr} and $\tau = Vt/H_0$.

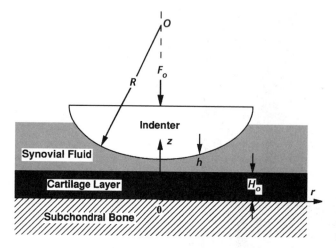

FIGURE 10-19. A model for joint squeeze-film lubrication between a viscous fluid and a thin layer of biphasic material attached to the impervious subchondral bone.

single-phase fluid mechanics. These relations have been used to solve the problem of squeeze-film lubrication of a spherical, rigid, impermeable indenter on a cartilage layer supported by a rigid bony substrate Fig. 10-19 (105). In this study, Hou and co-workers assumed that synovial fluid may be modeled as a viscous Newto-nian fluid. Their theoretical results demonstrate that fluid-film viscosity is dominant in affecting the fluid flow pattern just after loading when the fluid film is large; when the gap reduces in size, however, the effect of cartilage permeability becomes more significant. Figure 10-20A shows the location of the indenter surface, pressure

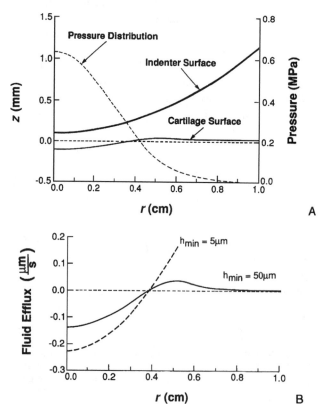

FIGURE 10-20. **(A)** Theoretical prediction of the squeeze-film problem illustrated in Fig. 10-19 for pressure distribution, indenter surface, and articular surface deformation. **(B)** Theoretical prediction of fluid efflux pattern at the articular surface for a minimum film thickness of 50 μm and 5 μm.

distribution, and deformed cartilage surface during squeeze film. It is seen that the cartilage surface deformation does promote the formation of the fluid-film gap. Figure 10-20B shows the fluid efflux patterns when the minimum film thickness h_{min} is 50 μm and 5 μm. These results indicate that fluid exudation and imbibition occur *simultaneously* across the cartilage surface, a situation in-between the weeping lubrication hypothesis (133,134,156,157) and boosted lubrication hypothesis (241,242). In general, the fluid lubricant is forced into the cartilage at the high-pressure central region and out of the cartilage in the peripheral region of the squeeze-film gap within the load support area. Furthermore, assuming typical values for loads, geometries, and biphasic material properties, calculations show that it takes approximately 2.4 seconds to close the gap from 100 μm to 1 μm. If the tissue permeability is increased by one order of magnitude as for diseased cartilage, the squeeze-film time is decreased to 0.9 s, whereas if the synovial fluid viscosity is increased by two orders of magnitude, the squeeze-film time is increased to 24 s. Thus, synovial fluid viscosity and cartilage permeability are the two dominant parameters governing the behavior of joints when operating under squeeze-film action. Because the synovial fluid was observed to filter into the cartilage layer in the high-pressure central region of the fluid film, Hou and co-workers conjectured that their mathematical predictions supported the premise of boosted lubrication.

In 1993, Hlaváček (97,98) elaborated considerably upon the biphasic squeeze-film model of Hou and co-workers. He first developed a biphasic model for synovial fluid in which one phase represents the low-molecular-weight substances and is assumed ideal and the other represents the hyaluronic acid protein complex and is assumed viscous and non-Newtonian, obeying a power law. He then employed this theory along with the cartilage biphasic theory of Mow et al. (168) to solve the problem of gel formation during squeeze-film lubrication of cartilage disks, similar to the ultrafiltration problem solved by Lai and Mow (126). He observed that for normal synovial fluid with a hyaluronic acid concentration of 50 mg/mL, a stable gel layer formed as

a result of homogeneous filtration in a model of the hip joint. The typical thickness of this gel layer was found to be 0.1 μm and was observed to be almost independent of the applied load. Models of inflammatory synovial fluid demonstrated significantly smaller gel thicknesses. In 1999 and 2000, Hlaváček (99,100) also showed that the time required for the formation of this gel and reduction in fluid-film thickness was less than 1 second, suggesting that any benefit of boosted lubrication would be much shorter than originally anticipated by the proponents of this lubrication mode, and that this mode could not easily explain the time-dependent frictional response of cartilage that is observed over much longer durations. Furthermore, there is now considerable evidence that hyaluronidase-treated synovial fluid lubricates almost as well as untreated fluid (95,137,138,157,193,232), which suggests that hyaluronic acid gel formation at the articular surface may not contribute to the lubrication of articular surfaces.

7.4 Boundary Lubrication

Charnley suggested that a monolayer of lubricant might serve to separate the two articulating surfaces during normal joint function (38–40). Davis and co-workers suggested a variation of this theme in which a thin layer of "structured water" (several water molecules thick) is absorbed into the articular surface, thus providing the required boundary lubricant (46). Such mechanisms fall into the category of boundary lubrication (Fig. 10-21A). In a series of investigations, Swann, Radin, and co-workers (231–235) isolated a single polypeptide chain from synovial fluid that is believed to be the boundary lubricant of cartilage. This molecule, called lubricin, is a protein-carbohydrate complex comprised of oligosaccharides distributed along the length of a protein core. Its molecular weight is approximately 250,000 daltons (233), and it can be adsorbed to each articulating surface of the cartilage. This monolayer on each surface has a thickness on the order of 10 to 1,000 Å and has the ability to carry weight and reduce friction (235). Hills and Butler suggested that the boundary

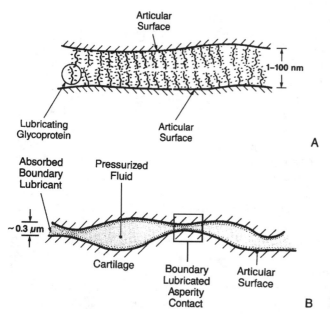

FIGURE 10-21. (A) Boundary lubrication of articular cartilage. In this mode, the load is carried by a monolayer of the lubricating glycoprotein, which is adsorbed onto the articular surfaces [171]. **(B)** Depiction of mixed lubrication. Boundary lubrication occurs where the thickness of the fluid film is on the same order as the roughness of the bearing surfaces. Fluid-film lubrication takes place in areas with more widely separated surfaces [171].

lubricant found in synovial fluid was more likely to be dipalmitoyl phosphatidylcholine (DPPC), a phospholipid (92,93), or what Hills and co-workers later called a surface-active phospholipid (SAPL) (95,96,211,212). Whether SAPL was present as a contaminant in lubricin or not, the evidence that these compounds act as effective boundary lubricants is very strong. However, it should be noted that experiments demonstrate that a boundary lubricant can account for a reduction in the friction coefficient by a factor of only 2 to 6 (109,141,235,246). Although this is a remarkable effect, it remains that the friction coefficient of cartilage has been shown to vary over a much greater range, e.g., by a factor of 60 or greater (67,68,156) within the same cartilage sample as a function of time. For example, over a period of 120 minutes under a constant load, Forster and Fisher (68) have reported that the friction coefficient of bovine cartilage against stainless steel increases from 0.005 to 0.6. Mabuchi et al. (145) showed that if sliding is initiated after a stationary period of loading, the startup friction coefficient of cartilage against cartilage increased from $\mu = 0.01$ at 0 s of stationary loading to $\mu = 0.31$ at 1,800 s; for cartilage against glass, the corresponding values of the friction coefficient were $\mu = 0.005$ and $\mu = 0.46$. Hence, boundary lubrication, which

is certain to occur, must be complemented by one or more mechanisms that can explain these observed phenomena. Figure 10-21B shows a proposed mixed mode of lubrication in which boundary lubrication and fluid-film lubrication coexist (53). In this mode, with limited solid-solid contact, the frictional coefficient may be minimized, providing an attractive alternative mechanism for joint lubrication.

8 INTERSTITIAL FLUID PRESSURIZATION AND DIARTHRODIAL JOINT LUBRICATION

Although a considerable amount of research has been done on various possible lubrication mechanisms in diarthrodial joints, there remain many experimental results that have not been successfully explained within a mathematically tractable theoretical framework. Perhaps the most notable of these is the observed time dependence of the friction coefficient of cartilage during creep or stress-relaxation experiments (20,67,68,150,156,192,249). It has been proposed that this time dependence is directly related to the exudation of cartilage interstitial water during tissue creep (150,156).

When the tissue has reached its equilibrium creep deformation, i.e., when the interstitial fluid pressure has reduced to zero (168,176,177), the friction coefficient has been shown experimentally to also achieve an equilibrium value (19,67,68,150,249). According to McCutchen's self-pressurized-hydrostatic-bearing weeping mechanism (156), the interstitial fluid pressure of cartilage supports the majority of the normal load transmitted across the cartilage layers, thus reducing the friction at the articular surfaces. Although it has long been recognized that the interstitial water of cartilage pressurizes under loading, one of the important achievements of cartilage biomechanics has been the ability to model this pressurization using porous media theories, such as the biphasic and triphasic theories of Mow, Lai, and co-workers (78,128,168) and the related porous media electromechanical theory of Frank and Grodzinsky (70) and Huyghe and Janssen (108). These mixture theories account for the presence of a solid matrix, representing primarily the collagen-proteoglycan network of cartilage, a fluid phase representing primarily the interstitial water, and when necessary, dissolved ion phases such as sodium, chloride, calcium, potassium, etc. The biphasic theory has been shown to describe the pressurization and flow of interstitial water in the porous-permeable solid matrix upon loading and it has been shown experimentally that this theory can describe the confined compression creep, stress-relaxation, and dynamic responses of articular cartilage accurately (102,130,168,224,225).

Based on these studies, Ateshian and co-workers (14,15,17,20) proposed a mathematical formulation of a boundary friction model for articular cartilage that uses the theoretical framework of the biphasic theory (167,168). The biphasic theory accounts for the fluid stress in the tissue, given by the stress tensor $\sigma^f = -\varphi^f p\mathbf{I}$, where p is the interstitial fluid pressure, φ^f is the porosity, and $\mathbf{I}$ is the identity tensor; it also accounts for the solid stress $\sigma^s = -\varphi^s p\mathbf{I} + \sigma^e$, where $\varphi^s = 1 - \varphi^f$ is the solid volumetric (and area) fraction, and σ^e is the effective (or elastic) stress, which results from the state of strain in the solid collagen-proteoglycan matrix. The total

stress in the tissue is given by $\sigma = \sigma^s + \sigma^f = -p\mathbf{I} + \sigma^e$, which is the combination of the isotropic interstitial fluid pressure and the effective stress. Given a constitutive equation relating σ^e to the solid matrix strain (for example, the classical linear isotropic elasticity relation), the biphasic theory can predict the temporal and spatial variation of the interstitial fluid pressure p throughout the tissue. The experimental measurement of p as a function of time has been reported by Oloyede and Broom (188) under confined compression creep loading, and by Soltz and Ateshian (224–226) under creep, stress-relaxation, and dynamic loading in confined or unconfined compression (Fig. 10-22A). The latter authors have also shown that these experimental measurements are well predicted by the biphasic theory (Fig. 10-22B), lending support to the predictions of this theory for more complex loading configurations such as contact creep loading (11,52,116), and rolling and sliding contact (13,18). At the interfacial contact surface between two biphasic articular layers, the surface traction vector is given by $\sigma\mathbf{n}$, where $\mathbf{n}$ is the unit surface normal at the interface. This traction vector can be resolved into a normal traction component $\mathbf{n} \cdot \sigma\mathbf{n}$, and a tangential component $\tau \cdot \sigma\mathbf{n}$ along the direction of relative motion of the surfaces, where τ is a unit vector orthogonal to $\mathbf{n}$. By integrating these traction components over the area A of the contact interface, the normal load W across the articular surfaces and the friction force F tangential to the surfaces are produced:

$$W = \int \mathbf{n} \cdot \sigma\mathbf{n} dA \quad F = \int \tau \cdot \sigma\mathbf{n} dA. \quad (5)$$

The effective (measured) friction coefficient at the surfaces is then given by $\mu_{eff} = F/W$. By substituting the expression for σ in the above integrals, the normal load W can be separated into a component contributed by interstitial fluid pressure, $W^p = \int -p\, dA$, and another contributed by the effective stress, $W^e = \int \mathbf{n} \cdot \sigma^e\mathbf{n} dA$, such that $W = W^p + W^e$; because the interstitial fluid pressure is isotropic, the friction force F is found to depend on the effective stress alone, $F = \int \tau \cdot \sigma^e\mathbf{n} dA$.

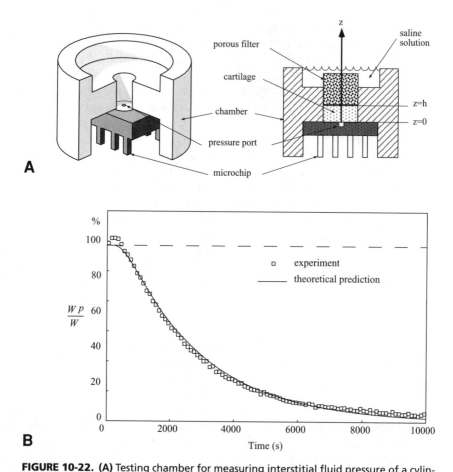

FIGURE 10-22. **(A)** Testing chamber for measuring interstitial fluid pressure of a cylindrical cartilage plug under confined compression. The tissue sample is loaded using a free-draining porous filter and the fluid pressure is measured at the center of the opposite specimen face using a microchip pressure transducer. **(B)** Under a constant creep load W, the interstitial fluid pressure p varies as a function of time; assuming for this one-dimensional configuration that p is uniform over the specimen cross-sectional area A, the load supported by interstitial fluid pressurization is $W^p = pA$ and the interstitial fluid load support W^p/W varies as shown here for a typical bovine cartilage specimen. The biphasic (168) material properties can be determined from curve-fitting of the creep response (*not shown*) and used to predict the interstitial fluid pressure from theory, which agrees with the experimental response of p. (From Soltz MA, Ateshian GA. Experimental verification and theoretical prediction of cartilage interstitial fluid pressurization at an impermeable contact interface in confined compression. *J Biomech* 1998;31:927–934, with permission.)

When two porous-permeable articular surfaces are in direct contact (in the absence of a fluid film separating the articular surfaces), the solid matrix of one surface contacts the solid matrix of the other surface over a fraction φ of the contact area A given by $\varphi = \varphi^{s0}\varphi^{s1}$, where φ^{s0} and φ^{s1} are the solid area fractions of the opposing articular surfaces. This estimation of φ is based on the idealized assumption that the articular surfaces are perfectly smooth; when taking into account that undulating surface topography and roughness might produce asperity contact (e.g., in a mixed lubrication mode), then solid-to-solid contact occurs over an even smaller fraction, $\varphi < \varphi^{s0}\varphi^{s1}$, of the apparent contact area A, as shown for example in the experimental study of Kobayashi et al. (122). Over the remaining contact area fraction

$1 - \varphi$, fluid is in contact with fluid or with solid, thus the component of W supported by this pressurized fluid is $(1 - \varphi) W^p$. The remainder, $W^s = W - (1 - \varphi) W^p$, represents that component of the normal load that is transmitted by solid-to-solid contact.

The model proposed by Ateshian et al. (14, 15,17,20) embodies the hypothesis that most of the frictional force results from the solid phase of one articular layer sliding against the solid phase of the opposing articular layer (the solid-to-solid interactions), whereas viscous shear stresses in the interstitial fluid and synovial fluid produce a negligible contribution; a similar hypothesis was proposed by Forster and Fisher (67). Thus, the friction force F should depend primarily on the component W^s, as may be represented in a Coulomb-like relation, $F = \mu_{eq} W^s$ (20). Accordingly, the effective friction coefficient would depend on interstitial fluid pressurization as

$$\mu_{eff} = \mu_{eq} W^s / W = \mu_{eq}[1 - (1 - \varphi) W^p / W]. \quad (6)$$

To understand the meaning of μ_{eq}, consider the limiting condition when the interstitial fluid pressure reduces to zero (as observed for example in Fig. 10-22B), in which case $W^p = 0$, $W^s = W$, and $\mu_{eff} = \mu_{eq}$; thus, μ_{eq} is the friction coefficient achieved at creep or stress-relaxation equilibrium when the interstitial fluid pressure has subsided. The above expression satisfies the interface continuity requirements derived by Hou and co-workers (104). The ratio W^p / W is the interstitial fluid load support, and it can be determined from theory for various biphasic contact configurations (13,52,116), or measured experimentally under certain conditions as reported above (188,224–226) (Figs. 10-22A and 10-22B). The value of μ_{eq} need not be constant but may vary with the magnitude of surface roughness or the amount of boundary lubricant present on the articular surfaces (lubricin, SAPL, etc., see above); μ_{eq} may even be velocity dependent (150,244–246), load dependent (150), and strain dependent (21,244).

In the simplest model, where μ_{eq} is assumed to be constant, Eq. 6 demonstrates that the measured friction coefficient μ_{eff} may be time dependent through the time dependence of the interstitial fluid load support, W^p / W, as shown

in Fig. 10-22B. In most physiologically relevant loading configurations, biphasic theory predicts that the peak value of W^p / W is in excess of 95% at the initiation of contact (13,116,147,226). Consider for example that $W^p / W|_{max} = 0.98$ and $\varphi^{s0} = \varphi^{s1} = 0.2$ (cartilage water content of 80%), thus for an idealized contact of two smooth articular surfaces ($\varphi = 0.04$), the minimum friction coefficient would be approximately 16 times smaller than its equilibrium value according to Eq. 6. If the surfaces are not smooth, and fluid is initially trapped between the surfaces (122), the initial value of φ would be smaller, for example, $\varphi = 0.01$, producing a ratio $\mu_{eff} : \mu_{eq}$ of 1:34. In contrast, as W^p / W decreases toward zero, this ratio would approach unity, i.e., the effective coefficient of friction μ_{eff} is given by the "dry" friction μ_{eq}. The model also suggests that lubrication of cartilage by interstitial fluid pressurization will be effective regardless of whether synovial fluid or Ringer's solution is used in an experiment because the primary mechanism for reducing friction is hydrostatic fluid load support, W^p / W, which is virtually independent of fluid viscosity. Where the nature of the lubricant can influence the frictional response is through μ_{eq}, which may depend on the presence of a boundary lubricant in synovial fluid, e.g., lubricin, DPPC or other. Indeed, experimental studies have shown that testing cartilage friction in Ringer's solution can produce very low friction coefficients, and that synovial fluid may reduce this friction coefficient by a factor of 2 to 6 (68,136,150,156) (Fig. 10-12B).

This model also predicts that in the limiting case of pure fluid-film lubrication, when all the load is supported by synovial fluid pressurization ($W^p / W = 1$), i.e., with no solid-to-solid contact ($\varphi = 0$), the friction coefficient becomes vanishingly small, $\mu_{eff} = 0$, consistent with the model's assumption that viscous shear stresses in synovial fluid are negligible. As a result, this model formulation is able to accommodate the primary modes of lubrication advocated in the literature, ranging from fluid-film lubrication to mixed lubrication, boundary lubrication, and interstitial fluid load support. This can be achieved by recognizing that each of the

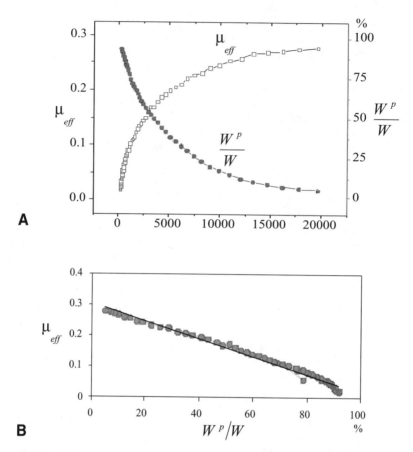

FIGURE 10-23. Frictional response of a bovine articular cartilage cylindrical plug against glass, under unconfined compression creep loading, using a frictional apparatus with reciprocating sliding motion. **(A)** The time-dependent friction coefficient μ_{eff} steadily increases to an equilibrium value μ_{eq} while the interstitial fluid load support W_p/W steadily decreases toward zero. **(B)** A plot of the same data as μ_{eff} versus W_p/W demonstrates a nearly linear relationship, in agreement with Eq. 6 and in support of the hypothesis that the frictional response is governed by interstitial fluid pressurization. (Data from Krishnan R, Ateshian GA. Experimental verification of the role of interstitial fluid pressurization in the frictional response of bovine articular cartilage. In: *Proceedings of the IVth World Congress Biomech.* Calgary, August 4–9, 2002, with permission.)

parameters appearing in Eq. 6, namely, W^p/W, φ, and μ_{eq}, are variable; the biphasic theory can predict the variation in W^p/W with time after onset of loading, and provide an estimate of the temporal variation in φ (given an initial surface roughness profile, as described by Soltz and Ateshian (227)); however, the dependence of μ_{eq} on the nature of the boundary lubricant in synovial fluid, the applied load, the sliding velocity, or the surface roughness, must be provided from experiments.

To verify that the model agrees with experimental measurements, Krishnan and Ateshian (121) recently reported a study where the friction coefficient and interstitial fluid load support were measured simultaneously in unconfined compression creep loading (Fig. 10-23A). They observed a time-increasing frictional coefficient in good agreement with previous studies (19,67,68,150,156,192,249), as well as a time-decreasing interstitial fluid load support consistent with prior fluid pressure measurements

(188,224). By plotting the friction coefficient μ_{eff} against the interstitial fluid load support W^p / W, they observed a nearly linear response (Fig. 10-23B), as predicted by the model of Eq. 6 given a constant μ_{eq} and constant φ. These novel results strongly support the underlying hypothesis of the model, indicating that interstitial fluid pressurization is a dominant factor in the regulation of the frictional response of articular cartilage. Furthermore, theoretical studies of contacting biphasic layers (13,116) have shown that the peak value of W^p / W increases with increasing applied load, because higher loads produce larger contact areas, increasing the pathway (thus the resistance) for interstitial fluid to escape the loaded region. Consequently, Eq. 6 would predict a decrease of the friction coefficient with increasing load, consistent with some of the experimental findings in the earlier joint lubrication literature, as illustrated in Figs. 10-11B and 10-11C.

It should be appreciated that equilibrium conditions where W^p / W reduces to zero, while achievable under laboratory testing conditions, are not likely to occur in situ under physiological loading (17,225). In diarthrodial joints, the friction coefficient is not expected to approach the equilibrium values reported in the literature, which may be as high as $\mu_{eq} \sim 0.5$ with synovial fluid and $\mu_{eq} \sim 0.6$ with Ringer's solution (68). Nevertheless, factors that affect interstitial fluid pressurization and the equilibrium friction coefficient will alter its frictional response. For example, Wright and Dowson (249) and Ateshian and co-workers (21) showed that alterations in the ionic environment of cartilage can change the temporal and equilibrium responses of the friction coefficient (Fig. 10-24); changes in interstitial fluid pressure as a function of ionic environment can be predicted from the triphasic theory of Lai et al. (128); however, the mechanism by which the ionic environment affects

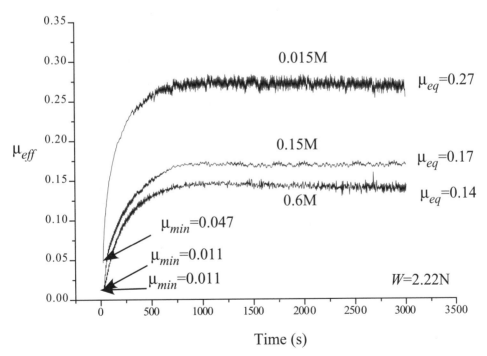

FIGURE 10-24. Frictional response of bovine articular cartilage cylindrical plugs ($\varnothing$2mm) against glass under unconfined compression creep loading, using bathing solutions with various NaCl concentrations. The friction coefficient increases with decreasing bathing solution concentration, which is also known to cause an increase in osmotic pressure. (From Ateshian GA, Soltz MA, Mauck RL, et al. The role of osmotic pressure and tension-compression nonlinearity in the frictional response of articular cartilage. *Transport in Porous Media* 2003;50:5–23, with permission.)

μ_{eq} remains unclear. Nishida and co-workers have proposed that chondroitin sulphates in the lamina splendens may act as a charge barrier, which can influence the frictional response, thus changes in the ionic environment could alter that mechanism (185). Pathological conditions that may affect interstitial fluid pressurization, such as the softening and increased permeability of osteoarthritic cartilage, may also potentially alter its frictional response. Hills and Monds (95) attributed their measured changes in cartilage friction coefficient to their enzymatic degradation of synovial fluid (alteration of μ_{eq}), though the tested cartilage samples were also digested in their protocol, which could have affected W^p / W. Kumar et al. (123) found that the friction coefficient between articular cartilage and Pyrex glass increased when cartilage was digested with chondroitinase ABC or alkaline protease, but not with hyaluronidase. However, in the studies of Pickard et al. (191,192), where the temporal frictional response of bovine articular cartilage was investigated prior and subsequent to enzymatic digestion with chondroitinase or trypsin, no significant changes were observed in the friction coefficient or in the creep deformation. These results suggest that further investigation of the influence of cartilage enzymatic degradation on fluid load support is required.

9 SUMMARY OF DIARTHRODIAL JOINT LUBRICATION

Lubrication acts to keep wear of articular cartilage in diarthrodial joints to a minimum. Under normal circumstances, with proper lubrication, together with repair responses by chondrocytes in the tissue, diarthrodial joints can function normally for many decades. However, in pathological cases, or under conditions of abnormally severe loading, both fatigue and interfacial wear become evident. As the wear process initiates, the tissue becomes more susceptible to both surface and interior damage, thus leading to a progressive degeneration process. Failure of cartilage as a bearing surface results from the loss of balance between the wear rate and the ability of chondrocytes to repair the microdamage.

For many decades, a considerable amount of work has been done in the field of diarthrodial joint friction, lubrication, and wear with various theories proposed to explain the vast body of experimental data. All of these theories are based on conceptually attractive arguments and are often complementary. From a theoretical perspective, fluid-film lubrication theories, whether using elastic or mixture models for cartilage, have been arguably analyzed more thoroughly than any other. This is because of the availability of historically well-understood equations for fluid-film lubrication in engineering bearings, developed originally by Reynolds (200). From these studies, and later developments accounting for the elastic deformation of the bearing surfaces, e.g., Dowson and Jin (57), it appears that micro-EHL and squeeze-film lubrication may be viable mechanisms under favorable conditions of loading, but are unlikely to be sustained under high loads and slow velocities. Boundary lubrication by lubricin (193,231,235) or SAPL (92,96) appears to be well supported by experimental data, though a boundary lubricant alone cannot account for the remarkably low friction coefficients measured in cartilage because cartilage has been shown to produce elevated friction coefficients after prolonged loading, only to return to very low values upon allowing sufficient time for recovery, without the addition of fresh boundary lubricant.

Based on this review of the biotribology of cartilage and diarthrodial joints, it appears that a dominant mechanism for regulating the frictional response of articular layers is interstitial fluid pressurization (15,17,19,67,150,156). The experimental and theoretical evidence in support of this mode of lubrication is strong. It is able to explain the fundamental experimental findings reported in the literature over the last several decades, particularly the time dependence of the friction coefficient, and the ability to produce low friction at high loads and at any sliding velocity, including quasi-stationary loading. Because it is premised on the hypothesis that pressurized interstitial fluid, and possibly a temporarily trapped lubricant pool, supports the majority of the load at the articular surfaces, this mode of lubrication could also explain the low wear characteristics of articular cartilage. It is compatible with fluid-film lubrication, mixed lubrication, and boundary lubrication, to the extent that all of these modes of lubrication may serve to enhance the role of interstitial fluid pressurization. It intimately ties the frictional response at the articular surfaces to the mechanics of cartilage because interstitial fluid pressurization is primarily regulated by the porous-permeable nature and intrinsic properties of the tissue. For example, the magnitude of interstitial fluid pressurization has been shown to depend on the tension-compression nonlinearity of the cartilage solid matrix (e.g., 21,107,126,169,226), which is most significant in the surface zone and is enhanced with increasing loads. Thus, it would be insufficient to investigate the frictional response of cartilage as a purely interfacial mechanism, as much benefit and insight in cartilage biotribology may be gained from the fundamentals of cartilage mechanics.

Over the last few decades, the field of lubrication and wear of natural cartilage has attracted much attention and some measure of controversy, as competing theories have been proposed and challenged in the literature. In more recent years, investigators have continued to focus on this field, guided principally by a basic science interest in elucidating the fundamental mechanism of joint lubrication as well as the opportunity to develop therapeutic modalities to counter the effects of joint degenerative diseases. We view cartilage biotribology as an integral part of the study of articular cartilage mechanics and biology; progress in any one of these areas yields insight into the others and a greater understanding of structure-function relationships in diarthrodial joints.

10 PROBLEMS

1. From Table 10-3 and Fig. 10-9, what is the typical range of friction forces acting on a joint surface?

2. From Fig. 10-13, determine the wear rate of cartilage for the two applied pressures at early times (<40 min) and at late times (>120 min). Explain why it is difficult to measure wear of any bearing surface.

3. What are typical R_a values for articular cartilage versus those for the surfaces of artificial implants? Read the papers by Sayles et al. (206) and Walker et al. (242).

4. Does it seem reasonable that no single lubrication theory can explain the process of lubrication of diarthrodial joints? Why? Provide three important deformation effects each for synovial fluid and articular cartilage that must be considered in understanding joint lubrication.

5. Jones (111) and Charnley (40) used the outcome of pendulum experiments to investigate whether joints were lubricated by a fluid film or by boundary friction. By reading these papers, determine the specific experimental observation these authors used to justify their conclusions. How did Barnett and Cobbold (25) address the contradictory interpretations of these previous authors? What was the corresponding explanation provided by Unsworth et al. (238)?

6. Fluid-film lubrication theories require the knowledge of the lubricant viscosity η in order to calculate the minimum film thickness (e.g., Eqs. 1-3). By estimating the shear rate D of a lubricant film in a joint, can you determine an appropriate value for η from Fig. 10-5? Are the values used in Examples 1 to 3 appropriate, a little too low, or a little too high?

7. Synovial fluid is non-Newtonian and exhibits a characteristic normal stress σ_1, as shown in Fig. 10-5A. Can this normal stress contribute significantly to load support in a typical joint? (Hint: Use Fig. 10-9 to estimate loads in human joints, and assume a typical joint contact area of 5 cm^2.)

8. The "flat-on-flat" experimental configuration of the frictional tests by Malcom (150) (Fig. 10-12A) precluded the formation of a wedge-shaped gap necessary for fluid-film lubrication. His results demonstrated that synovial fluid yields a lower friction coefficient than buffered saline (Fig. 10-12B). What is a likely explanation of that result?

9. McCutchen (156) conducted an experiment in which he observed that the friction coefficient of cartilage against glass increases

with time when the surfaces are subjected to a step constant load. He also demonstrated that separating the contacting surfaces for a few seconds then loading them again in an identical fashion does not produce identical frictional coefficients. He concluded that squeeze-film lubrication is not responsible for this observed behavior. What explanation can you provide to support this claim?

10. Describe the process of squeeze-film lubrication. How do the permeability and elastic moduli of the solid matrix of cartilage and the viscosity of synovial fluid affect squeeze-film lubrication?

11. Describe the fluid-film lubrication hypotheses proposed by MacConaill, Jones, Dintenfass, McCutchen, and Walker and co-workers.

12. Define elastohydrodynamic lubrication. How does it differ from hydrodynamic lubrication? What is elastorheodynamic lubrication?

13. Describe the "self-lubrication mechanism" of articular cartilage for joint lubrication.

14. Other than lubrication, describe the functions for the synovial fluid.

15. What are the main types of wear? Briefly describe how these mechanisms work.

16. In general terms, how do the material properties of articular cartilage change following rupture of the anterior cruciate ligament of the knee (85,219)? How would these material property changes affect cartilage lubrication, wear, and load support?

17. Describe the "stress-shielding effect" in normal articular cartilage.

18. How would changes of the biphasic properties (elastic moduli and permeability) of articular cartilage during the osteoarthritic process (e.g., 73; Chapter 5) affect its frictional properties?

ACKNOWLEDGMENTS

This review chapter covers the work of many investigators in the field of cartilage lubrication and wear, and the authors are grateful to those who have authorized reproduction of material from their publications. The material derived from the authors' own studies was supported by grants from the National Institutes of Health (GAA: AR43628, AR46532; VCM: AR38733, AR41020, AR41913).

REFERENCES

1. Ahmed AM, Burke DL. In-vitro measurement of static pressure distribution in synovial joints—part I: tibial surface of the knee. *J Biomech Eng* 1983;105:216–225.

2. Ahmed AM, Burke DL. In-vitro measurement of static pressure distribution in synovial joints—part II: retropatellar surface. *J Biomech Eng* 1983;105:226–236.

3. Akizuki S, Mow VC, Muller F, et al. Tensile properties of knee joint cartilage: I. Influence of ionic condition, weight bearing, and fibrillation on the tensile modulus. *J Orthop Res* 1986;4:379–392.

4. Akizuki S, Mow VC, Muller F, et al. The tensile properties of human knee joint cartilage II: the influence of weight bearing, and tissue pathology on the kinetics of swelling. *J Orthop Res* 1987;5:173–186.

5. Andriacchi TP, Ogle JA, Galante JO. Walking speed as a basis for normal and abnormal gait measurements. *J Biomech* 1977;10:261–268.

6. Armstrong CG, Mow VC. Variations in the intrinsic mechanical properties of human articular cartilage with age, degeneration, and water content. *J Bone Joint Surg* 1982;64A:88–94.

7. Armstrong CG, Mow VC, Wirth CR. Biomechanics of impact-induced microdamage to articular surface—a possible genesis for chondromalacia patella. In: Finerman G, ed. *AAOS symposium sports medicine: the knee.* St. Louis: C.V. Mosby Co., 1985:54–69.

8. Archard JF. Wear theory and mechanisms. In: Peterson MB Winder WO, eds. *Wear control handbook.* New York: ASME Publications, 1980:35–80.

9. Ateshian GA, Soslowsky LJ, Mow VC. Quantitation of articular surface topography and cartilage thickness in knee joints using stereophotogrammetry. *J Biomech* 1991;24:761–776.

10. Ateshian GA, Rosenwasser MP, Mow VC. Curvature characteristics and congruence of the thumb carpometacarpal joint: differences between male and female joints. *J Biomech* 1992;25:591–607.

11. Ateshian GA, Lai WM, Zhu WB, et al. An asymptotic solution for the contact of two biphasic cartilage layers. *J Biomech* 1994;27:1347–1360.

12. Ateshian GA, Kwak SD, Soslowsky LJ, et al. A new stereophotogrammetry method for determining in situ contact areas in diarthrodial joints: a comparison study. *J Biomech* 1994;27:111–124.

13. Ateshian GA, Wang H. A theoretical solution for the frictionless rolling contact of cylindrical biphasic articular cartilage layers. *J Biomech* 1995;28:1341–1355.

14. Ateshian GA. Continuity requirements across a contact interface in the formulation of a boundary friction model for biphasic articular cartilage. 1995 Bioengineering Conference, ASME, Bioengineering Divison 1995;29:147–148.

15. Ateshian GA. A theoretical model for boundary friction in articular cartilage. In: Yang K, Hayashi K, Woo SL-Y, et al., eds. *Proceedings of the 4th China-Japan-U.S.A.-Singapore Conference on Biomechanics.* International Academic Publishers, 1995:142–145.

16. Ateshian GA, Ark JW, Rosenwasser MP, et al. Contact areas in the thumb carpometacarpal joint. *J Orthop Res* 1995;13:450–458.

17. Ateshian GA. A theoretical formulation for boundary friction in articular cartilage. *J Biomech Eng* 1997;119:81–86.

18. Ateshian GA, Wang H. Rolling resistance of articular cartilage due to interstitial fluid flow. *Proc Inst Mech Eng[H],* 1997;211:419–424.

19. Ateshian GA, Wang X. Sliding tractions on a porous deformable layer. *J Tribology* 1998;120: 89–96.

20. Ateshian GA, Wang H, Lai WM. The role of interstitial fluid pressurization and surface porosities on the boundary friction of articular cartilage. *J Tribology* 1998;120:241–251.

21. Ateshian GA, Soltz MA, Mauck RL, et al. The role of osmotic pressure and tension-compression nonlinearity in the frictional response of articular cartilage. *Transport in Porous Media,* 2003;50:5–33.

22. Athanasiou KA, Rosenwasser MP, Buckwalter JA, et al. Interspecies comparison of in situ intrinsic mechanical properties of distal femoral cartilage. *J Orthop Res* 1991;9:330–340.

23. Balazs EA, Watson C, Duff IF, et al. Hyaluronic acid in synovial fluid: I. Molecular parameters of hyaluronic acid in normal and arthritic human fluids. *Arthritis Rheum* 1967;10:357–376.

24. Balazs EA, Gibbs DA. The rheological properties and biological function of hyaluronic acid. In: Balazs EA, ed. *Chemistry and molecular biology of the intercellular matrix,* Vol. 3 New York: Academic Press, 1970:1241–1253.

25. Barnett CH, Cobbold AF. Lubrication within living joints. *J Bone Joint Surg* 1962;44B:662.

26. Bloch B, Dintenfass L. Rheological study of human synovial fluid. *Aust N Z J Surg* 1963;33:108–113.

27. Broom ND. Structural consequences of traumatising articular cartilage. *Ann Rheum Dis* 1986;45:225–234.

28. Broom ND. The collagen framework of articular cartilage: its profound influence on normal and abnormal load-bearing function. In: Nimni ME, ed. *Collagen: chemistry, biology and biotechnology,* Vol. II. Boca Raton: CRC Press, 1988:243–265.

29. Brown TD, Shaw DT. In vitro contact stress distributions in the natural hip. *J Biomech* 1983;16:373–384.

30. Brown TD, Shaw DT. In vitro contact stress distribution on the femoral condyles. *J Orthop Res* 1984;2:190–199.

31. Brown TD, Vrahas MS. The apparent elastic modulus of the juxtarticular subchondral bone of the femoral head. *J Orthop Res* 1984;2:32–38.

32. Buckwalter JA, Rosenberg LC, Coutts R, et al. Articular cartilage: injury and repair. In: Woo SL-Y, Buckwalter JA, eds. *Injury and repair of the musculoskeletal soft tissues.* Chicago: Am. Acad. Orthop. Surg. Press, 1988.

33. Bullough PG. The geometry of diarthrodial joints, its physiologic maintenance, and the possible significance of age-related changes in geometry-to-load distribution and the development of osteoarthritis. *Clin Orthop Rel Res* 1981;156:61–66.

34. Bullough P, Jagannath P. The morphology of the calcification front in articular cartilage: its significance in joint function. *J Bone Joint Surg* 1983;65B:72–78.

35. Buschmann MD, Jurvelin JS, Hunziker EB. Confined compression of articular cartilage: small-amplitude linear and nonlinear stress responses and the effect of the porous compression platen. *Advances in Bioengineering, ASME, Bioengineering Divison* 1995;31:307–398.

36. Carter DR, Hayes WC. The compressive behavior of bone as a two phase porous structure. *J Bone Joint Surg* 1977;59A:965–967.

37. Caygill JC, West GH. The rheological behavior of synovial fluid and its possible relation to joint lubrication. *Med Biol Eng* 1969;7:507–516.

38. Charnley J. The lubrication of animal joints. In: *Symposium on biomechanics.* London: Institution of Mechanical Engineers, 1959:12–22.

39. Charnley J. How our joints are lubricated. *Triangle* 1960;4:175.

40. Charnley J. The lubrication of animal joints in relation to surgical reconstruction by arthroplasty. *Ann Rheum Dis* 1960;19:10–19.

41. Clarke IC. The microevaluation of articular surface contours. *Ann Biomed Eng* 1972;1:31–43.

42. Crowninshield RD, Johnston RC, Andrews JG, et al. A biomechanical investigation of the human hip. *J Biomech* 1978;11:75–85.

43. Davies DV. Synovial fluid as a lubricant. *Fed Proc* 1966;25:1069.

44. Davies DV. Properties of synovial fluid. *Proc Inst Mech Eng* 1967;181:25.

45. Davies DV, Palfrey AJ. Some of the physical properties of normal and pathological synovial fluids. *J Biomech* 1968;1:79–88.

46. Davis WH Jr, Lee SL, Sokoloff L. A proposed model of boundary lubrication by synovial fluid: structuring of boundary water. *J Biomech Eng* 1979;101:185–192.

47. Dickinson JA, Cook SD, Leinhardt TM. The measurement of shock waves following heel strike while running. *J Biomech* 1985;18:415–422.

48. Dintenfass L. Lubrication in synovial joints. *Nature* 1963;197:496–497.

49. Dintenfass L. Lubrication in synovial joints: a theoretical analysis. *J Bone Joint Surg* 1963;45A:1241–1256.

50. Dintenfass L. Rheology of complex fluids and some observations on joint lubrication. *Fed Proc* 1966;25:1054–1060.

51. Donohue JM, Buss D, Oegema TR Jr, et al. The effects of indirect blunt trauma on adult canine articular cartilage. *J Bone Joint Surg* 1983;65A:948–957.

52. Donzelli PS, Spilker RL, Ateshian GA, et al. A finite element investigation of contact between transversely isotropic layers of biphasic cartilage. *J Biomech* 1999;32:1037–1047.

53. Dowson D. Modes of lubrication in human joints. *Proc Inst Mech Eng* 1967;181:45–54.

54. Dowson D, Longfield MD, Walker PS, et al. An investigation of the friction and lubrication in human joints. *Proc Inst Mech Eng* 1968;182:68–76.

55. Dowson D. Basic tribology. In: Dowson D Wright V, eds. *Introduction to the biomechanics of joints and joint replacement.* London: Mechanical Engineering Publications Ltd., 1981:49–60.

56. Dowson D, Unsworth A, Cooke AF, et al. Lubrication of joints. In: Dowson D Wright V, eds. *An introduction to the biomechanics of joints and joint replacement.* London: Mechanical Engineering Publications Ltd., 1981:120–145.

57. Dowson D, Jin Z-M. Micro-elastohydrodynamic lubrication of synovial joints. *Eng Med* 1986;15:63–65.

58. Dowson D, Jin ZM. An analysis of micro-elastohydrodynamic lubrication in synovial joints considering cyclic loading and entraining velocities. *Proceedings of the 13th Leeds-Lyon Symposium on Tribology,* 1987;pp. 375–386.

59. Eberhart HD, Inman VT, Saunders JB de C. *Fundamental studies of human locomotion and other information relating to design of artificial limbs.* Berkeley: University of California Press 1947.

60. Eckstein F, Muller-Gerbl M, Putz R. Distribution of subchondral bone density and cartilage thickness in the human patella. *J Anat* 1992;180:425–433.

61. Eckstein F, Sittek H, Milz E, et al. The potential of magnetic resonance imaging (MRI) for quantifying articular cartilage thickness 3/4 a methodological study. *Clin Biomech* 1995;8:4434–4440.

62. Eckstein F, Lohe F, Hillebrand S. Morphomechanics of the humero-ulnar joint: I. Joint space width

63. and contact areas as a function of load and flexion angle. *Anat Rec* 1995;243:318–326.

63. Eisenfeld J, Mow VC, Lipshitz H. The mathematical analysis of stress relaxation in articular cartilage during compression. *Math Biosci* 1978;39:97–111.

64. Fein RS. Are synovial joints squeeze film lubricated? *Proc Inst Mech Eng* 1967;181:125–128.

65. Ferguson J, Boyle JA, McSween RNM, et al. Observations on the flow properties of the synovial fluid from patients with rheumatoid arthritis. *Biorheology* 1968;5:119–131.

66. Flannery CR, Hughes CE, Schumacher BL. Articular cartilage superficial zone protein (SZP) is homologous to megakaryocyte stimulating factor precursor and is a multifunctional proteoglycan with potential growth-promoting, cytoprotective, and lubricating properties in cartilage metabolism. *Biochem Biophys Res Commun* 1999;254:535–541.

67. Forster H, Fisher J. The influence of loading time and lubricant on the friction of articular cartilage. *Proc Inst Mech Eng[H]* 1996;210:109–119.

68. Forster H, Fisher J. The influence of continuous sliding and subsequent surface wear on the friction of articular cartilage. *Proc Inst Mech Eng[H]* 1999;213:329–345.

69. Foy JR, Williams PF, Powell GL, et al. Effect of phospholipidic boundary lubrication in rigid and compliant hemiarthroplasty models. *Proc Inst Mech Eng[H]* 1999;213:5–18.

70. Frank EH, Grodzinsky AJ. Cartilage electromechanics–II. A continuum model of cartilage electrokinetics and correlation with experiments. *J Biomech* 1987;20:629–639.

71. Frankel VH, Burstein AH. *Orthopaedic biomechanics.* Philadelphia: Lea & Febiger, 1971.

72. Freeman MAR, Meachim G. Ageing and degeneration. In: Freeman MAR, ed. *Adult articular cartilage,* 2nd ed. Kent: Pitman Medical Publishing, 1979:487–543.

73. Froimson MI, Ratcliffe A, Gardner TR, et al. Differences in patellofemoral joint cartilage material properties and their significance in the etiology of cartilage surface fibrillations. *Osteoarthritis Cartilage* 1997;5:377–386.

74. Gardner DL. The influence of microscopic technology on knowledge of cartilage surface structure. *Ann Rheum Dis* 1972;31:235–258.

75. Ghadially FN, Moshurchak EM, Thomas I. Humps on young human and rabbit articular cartilage. *J Anat* 1977;124:425–435.

76. Ghosh SK. A close-range photogrammetric system for 3-D measurements and perspective diagramming in biomechanics. *J Biomech* 1983;16:667–674.

77. Goodfellow J, Hungerford DS, Zindel M. Patello-femoral joint mechanics and pathology. 1.

Functional anatomy of the patello-femoral joint. *J Bone Joint Surg* 1976;58B:287–290.

78. Gu WY, Lai WM, Mow VC. Transport of fluid and ions through a porous-permeable charged-hydrated tissue, and streaming potential data on normal bovine articular cartilage. *J Biomech* 1993;26:709–723.

79. Guo XE, Gibson LJ, McMahon TA, et al. Finite element modeling of damage accumulation in trabecular bone under cyclic loading. *J Biomech* 1994;27:145–155.

80. Gibbs DA, Merrill EW, Smith KA. Rheology of hyaluronic acid. *Biopolymers* 1968;6:777–791.

81. Goldstein SA, Wilson DL, Sonstegard DS, et al. The mechanical properties of human tibial trabecular bone as a function of metaphyseal location. *J Biomech* 1983;16:965–969.

82. Greenwald AS, Haynes DW. Weight bearing areas in human hip joint. *J Bone Joint Surg* 1972;54B:157–163.

83. Greenwald AS. Joint congruence—a dynamic concept. In: Harris WH, ed. *The hip.* St. Louis: Mosby, 1974:3–22.

84. Gu WY, Lai WM, Mow VC. A mixture theory for charged-hydrated soft tissues containing multi-electrolytes: passive transport and swelling behaviors. *J Biomech Eng* 1998;120:169–180.

85. Guilak F, Ratcliffe A, Lane N, et al. Mechanical and biochemical changes in the superficial zone of articular cartilage in a canine model of osteoarthritis. *J Orthop Res* 1994;12:474–484.

86. Hamerman D, Schuster H. Hyaluronate in normal human synovial fluid. *J Clin Invest* 1958;37:57–64.

87. Hamrock BJ, Dowson D. Elastohydrodynamic lubrication of elliptical contacts for materials of low elastic modulus: I. Fully flooded conjunction. *J. Lubric Technol, Trans. ASME* 1978;100:236–245.

88. Hamrock BJ. *Fundamentals of fluid film lubrication.* New York: McGraw-Hill, 1994.

89. Hardingham TE, Muir H, Kwan MK, et al. Viscoelastic properties of proteoglycan solutions with varying proportions present as aggregates. *J Orthop Res* 1987;5:36–46.

90. Higaki H, Murakami T, Nakanishi Y, et al. The lubricating ability of biomembrane models with dipalmitoyl phosphatidylcholine and γ-globulin. *J Eng Med I Mech E* 1998;212:337–346.

91. Higginson GR, Unsworth A. The lubrication of natural joints. In: Dumbleton JH, ed. *Tribology of natural and artificial joints.* Amsterdam: Elsevier Science, 1981:47–73.

92. Hills BA, Butler BD. Surfactants identified in synovial fluid and their ability to act as boundary lubricants. *Ann Rheum Dis* 1984;43:641–648.

93. Hills BA. Oligolamellar lubrication of joints by surface active phospholipid. *J Rheum* 1989;16:82–91.

94. Hills BA. Remarkable anti-wear properties of joint surfactant. *Ann Biomed Eng* 1995;23:112–115.

95. Hills BA, Monds MK. Enzymatic identification of the load-bearing boundary lubricant in the joint. *Br J Rheumatol* 1998;37:137–142.

96. Hills BA. Boundary lubrication in vivo. *Proc Inst Mech Eng[H]* 2000;214:83–94.

97. Hlaváček M. The role of synovial fluid filtration by cartilage in lubrication of synovial joints. I. Mixture model of synovial fluid. *J Biomech* 1993;26:1145–1150.

98. Hlaváček M. The role of synovial fluid filtration by cartilage in lubrication of synovial joints II. Squeeze-film lubrication: homogeneous filtration. *J Biomech* 1993;26:1151–1160.

99. Hlaváček M. Lubrication of the human ankle joint in walking with the synovial fluid filtrated by the cartilage with the surface zone worn out: steady pure sliding motion. *J Biomech* 1999;32:1059–1069.

100. Hlaváček, M. Squeeze-film lubrication of the human ankle joint with synovial fluid filtrated by articular cartilage with the superficial zone worn out. *J Biomech* 2000;33:1415–1422.

101. Hodge WA, Fijan RS, Carlson KL, et al. Contact pressure in the human hip joint measured in vivo. *Proc Nat Acad Sci* 1986;83:2879–2883.

102. Holmes MH, Lai WM, Mow VC. Singular perturbation analysis of the nonlinear, flow-dependent, compressive stress-relaxation behavior of articular cartilage. *J Biomech Eng* 1985;107:206–218.

103. Hooke CJ, O'Donoghue JP. Elasticohydrodynamic lubrication of soft, highly deformed contacts. *J Mech Eng Sci* 1972;14:34–48.

104. Hou JS, Holmes MH, Lai WM, et al. Boundary conditions at the cartilage-synovial fluid interface for joint lubrication and theoretical verifications. *J Biomech Eng* 1989;111:78–87.

105. Hou JS, Mow VC, Lai WM, et al. Squeeze film lubrication for articular cartilage with synovial fluid. *J Biomech* 1992;25:247–259.

106. Howell DS, Treadwell BV, Trippel SB. Etiopathogenesis of osteoarthritis. In: Moskowitz et al., eds. *Osteoarthritis: diagnosis and medical/surgical management,* 2nd ed. Philadelphia: WB Saunders, 1992:233–252.

107. Huang C-Y, Mow VC, Ateshian GA. The role of flow-independent viscoelasticity in the biphasic tensile and compressive responses of articular cartilage. *J Biomech Eng* 2001;123:410–417.

108. Huyghe JM, Janssen JD. Quadriphasic mechanics of swelling incompressible porous media. *Int J Eng Sci* 1997;35:793–802.

109. Jay GD, Hong B-S. Characterization of a bovine synovial fluid lubricating factor. *Connect Tissue Res* 1992;28:71–98.

110. Jay GD, Tantravahi U, Britt DE, et al. Homology of lubricin and superficial zone protein (SZP): products of megakaryocyte stimulating factor

(MSF) gene expression by human synovial fibroblasts and articular chondrocytes localized to chromosome 1q25. *J Orthop Res* 2001;19:677–687.

111. Jones ES. Joint lubrication. *Lancet* 1936;230: 1043–1044.

112. Jurvelin JS, Buschmann MD, Hunziker EB. Characterization of the equilibrium response of bovine humeral cartilage in confined and unconfined compression. *Trans Orthop Res Soc* 1995;20: 512.

113. Jurvelin JS, Muller D, Wong M, et al. Surface and subsurface morphology of bovine humeral articular cartilage as assessed by atomic force and transmission electron microscopy. *J Struct Biol* 1996;117:45–54.

114. Kapitza PL. Hydrodynamic theory of lubrication during rolling. *Zh Tekh Fiz* 1955;25:747–762.

115. Keaveny TM, Watchtel EF, Guo XE, et al. The mechanical properties of damaged trabecular bone. *J Biomech* 1994;27:1309–1318.

116. Kelkar R, Ateshian GA. Contact creep of biphasic cartilage layers: identical layers. *J Appl Mech* 1999;66:137–145.

117. Khalsa PS, Eisenberg SR. Direct measurement of axial and radial confining stresses in articular cartilage during uniaxial confined compression. *Trans Orthop Res Soc* 1995;20:519.

118. King RG. A rheological measurement of three synovial fluids. *Rheological Acta* 5:41.

119. Kirk TB, O'Neill PL, Stachowiak GA. The effects of dehydration on the surface morphology of articular cartilage. *J Orthop Rheum* 1993;6.2:75–80.

120. Kirk TB, Stachowiak GA, Wilson AS. The morphology of the surface of articular cartilage. *Proc. 2nd World Cong. Biomech.*, Amsterdam, 1994;I:208a.

121. Krishnan R, Kopacz M, and Ateshian GA. Experimental verification of the role of interstitial fluid pressurization in cartilage lubrication. *J Orthop Res* 2004;33:565–570.

122. Kobayashi M, Toguchida J, Oka M. Study on the lubrication mechanism of natural joints by confocal laser scanning microscopy. *J Biomed Mater Res* 2001;55:645–651.

123. Kumar P, Oka M, Toguchida J, et al. Role of uppermost superficial surface layer of articular cartilage in the lubrication mechanism of joints. *J Anat* 2001;199:241–250.

124. Kwan MK, Lai WM, Mow VC. Fundamentals of fluid transport through cartilage in compression. *Ann Biomed Eng* 1984;12:537–558.

125. Lai WM, Kuei SC, Mow VC. Rheological equations for synovial fluids. *J Biomech Trans ASME* 1978;100:169–186.

126. Lai WM, Mow VC. Ultrafiltration of synovial fluid by cartilage. *ASCE J Eng Mech Div* 1978;104:79–96.

127. Lai WM, Mow VC. Flow fields in a single layer model of articular cartilage created by a sliding load. *Adv Bioeng Trans ASME* 1979;101:101–104.

128. Lai WM, Hou JS, Mow VC. A triphasic theory for the swelling and deformation behaviors of articular cartilage. *J Biomech Eng* 1991;113:245–258.

129. Lane LB, Bullought PG. Age-related changes in the thickness of the calcified zone and the number of tidemarks in adult human articular cartilage. *J Bone Joint Surg* 1980;62B:372–375, 1980.

130. Lee RC, Frank EH, Grodzinsky AJ, et al. Oscillatory compressional behavior of articular cartilage and its associated electromechanical properties. *J Biomech Eng* 1981;103:280–292.

131. Levick JR. The influence of hydrostatic pressure on trans-synovial fluid movement and on capsular expansion in the rabbit knee. *J Physiol* 1979;331:1–15.

132. Levick JR. Synovial fluid and trans-synovial flow in stationary and moving normal joints. In: Helmien HJ et al., eds. *Joint loading*. Bristol, UK: Wright, 1987:149–186.

133. Lewis PR, McCutchen CW. Experimental evidence for weeping lubrication in mammalian joints. *Nature* 1959;184:1284–1285.

134. Lewis PR, McCutchen CW. Lubrication of mammalian joints. *Nature* 1960;185:920–921.

135. Linn FC, Sokoloff L. Movement and composition of interstitial fluid of cartilage. *Arthritis Rheum* 1965;8:481–494.

136. Linn FC. Lubrication of animal joints: I. The arthrotrip-someter. *J Bone Joint Surg* 1967;49A: 1079–1098.

137. Linn FC. Lubrication of animal joints: II. The mechanism. *J Biomech* 1968;1:193–205.

138. Linn FC, Radin EL. Lubrication of animal joints: III. The effect of certain chemical alterations of the cartilage and lubricant. *Arth Rheum* 1968;11:674–682.

139. Lipshitz H, Etheredge R, Glimcher MJ. In vitro wear of articular cartilage. I. Hydroxyproline, hexosamine, and amino acid composition of bovine articular cartilage as a function of depth from the surface; hydroxyproline content of the lubricant and the wear debris as a measure of wear. *J Bone Joint Surg* 1975;57A:527–534.

140. Lipshitz H, Glimcher MJ. In vitro studies of the wear of articular cartilage. II. Characteristics of the wear of articular cartilage when worn against stainless steel plates having characterized surfaces. *Wear* 1979;52:297–339.

141. Little T, Freeman M, Swanson SAV. Experiments on friction in the human hip joint. In: Wright V, ed. *Lubrication and wear in joints*. Sector Pub., 1969:110.

142. Longfield MD, Dowson D, Walker PS, et al. "Boosted lubrication" of human joints by fluid enrichment and entrapment. *Biomed Eng* 1969;4: 517–522.

143. Longmore RB, Gardner MJ. Development with age of human articular cartilage surface structure. *Ann Rheum Dis* 1975;34:26–37.

144. Lu TW, O'Connor JJ, Taylor SJG, et al. Validation of a lower limb model with in vivo femoral forces telemetered from two subjects. *J Biomech* 1998;31:63–69.

145. Mabuchi K, Ujihira M, Sasada T. Influence of loading duration on start-up friction in synovial joints: measurements using a robotic system. *Clin Biomech* 13:492–494.

146. MacConaill MA. The function of intra-articular fibrocartilages, with special references to the knee and inferior radio-ulnar joints. *J Anat* 1932; 66:210–227.

147. Macirowski T, Tepic S, Mann RW. Cartilage stresses in the human hip joint. *J Biomech Eng* 1994;116:11–18.

148. Mak AF. The apparent viscoelastic behavior of articular cartilage—the contributions from the intrinsic matrix viscoelasticity and interstitial fluid flows. *J Biomech Eng* 108:123–130.

149. Mak AF, Lai WM, Mow VC. Biphasic indentation of articular cartilage: part I. Theoretical analysis. *J Biomech* 1987;20:703–714.

150. Malcom LL. *An experimental investigation of the frictional and deformational responses of articular cartilage interfaces to static and dynamic loading.* University of California, San Diego, 1976, [dissertation].

151. Maquet PG, van de Berg AJ, Simone JC. Femorotibial weight-bearing areas. *J Bone Joint Surg* 1975;57A:766–771.

152. Maroudas A. Hyaluronic acid films. *Proc Inst Mech Eng* 1967;181:122–124.

153. Maroudas A. Physicochemical properties of articular cartilage. In: Freeman MAR, ed. *Adult articular cartilage,* Chapter 4, 2nd edition. Kent, UK: Pitman Medical Publishing, 1979:215–290.

154. Martin HM. Lubrication of gear teeth. *Engineering* 1916;102:199.

155. Mattews LS, Sonstegard DA, Henke JA. Load bearing characteristics of the patellofemoral joint. *Acta Orthop Scand* 1977;48:511–516.

156. McCutchen CW. The frictional properties of animal joints. *Wear* 1962;5:1.

157. McCutchen CW. Boundary lubrication by synovial fluid: demonstration and possible osmotic explanation. *Fed Proc* 1966;25:1061.

158. Medley JB, Dowson D, Wright V. Transient elastohydrodynamic lubrication models for the human ankle joint. *Eng Med* 1984;13:137–151.

159. Mente PL, Lewis JL. Elastic modulus of calcified cartilage is an order of magnitude less than that of subchondral bone. *J Orthop Res* 1994;12:637–647.

160. Morrison JB. Bioengineering analysis of force actions transmitted by the knee. *Biomed Eng* 1968;3:154–170.

161. Morrison JB. The mechanics of the knee joint in relation to normal working. *J Biomech* 1970;3:51–61.

162. Mow VC. Effects of viscoelastic lubricant on squeeze film lubrication between impinging spheres. *J Lubric Tech Trans ASME* 1968;90:113–116.

163. Mow VC. The role of lubrication in biomechanical joints. *J Lubric Tech Trans ASME* 1969;91:320–329.

164. Mow VC, Lai WM, Redler I. Some surface characteristics of articular cartilage, part I. *J Biomech* 1974;7:449–456.

165. Mow VC, Lai WM. Mechanics of animal joints. *Ann Rev Fluid Mech* 1979;11:247–288.

166. Mow VC, Lai WM. The optical sliding contact analytical rheometer (OSCAR) for flow visualization at the articular surface. *Adv Bioeng Trans ASME* 97–99.

167. Mow VC, Lai WM. Recent developments in synovial joint biomechanics. *SIAM Rev* 1980;22:275–317.

168. Mow VC, Kuei SC, Lai WM, et al. Biphasic creep and stressrelaxation of articular cartilage in compression: theory and experiments. *J Biomech Eng* 1980;102:73–84.

169. Mow VC, Holmes MH, Lai WM. Fluid transport and mechanical properties of articular cartilage: a review. *J Biomech* 1984;17:377–394.

170. Mow VC, Kwan MK, Lai WM, et al. A finite deformation theory for nonlinearly permeable soft hydrated biological tissues. In: Schmid-Schonbein GW, Woo SL-Y, Zweifach BW, eds. *Frontiers in biomechanics.* New York: Springer-Verlag, 1986:153–179.

171. Mow VC, Mak AF. Lubrication of diarthrodial joints. In: Skalak R, Chien S, eds. *Handbook of bioengineering.* New York: McGraw-Hill, 1987:5.1–5.34.

172. Mow VC. Molecular structure and function relationships for articular cartilage. *J Educ Inform Rheum* 1988;17:9–13.

173. Mow VC, Rosenwasser MP. Articular cartilage: Biomechanics. In: Woo SL-Y, Buckwalter JA, eds. *Injury and repair of the musculoskeletal soft tissues.* Chicago: Am. Acad. Orthop. Surg. Press, 1988:427–463.

174. Mow VC, Zhu W, Lai WM, et al. The influence of link protein stabilization on the viscometric properties of proteoglycan solutions. *Biochim Biophys Acta* 1989;112:201–208.

175. Mow VC, Gibbs MC, Lai WM, et al. Biphasic indentation of articular cartilage—part II. A numerical algorithm and an experimental study. *J Biomech* 1989;22:853–861.

176. Mow VC, Ratcliffe A, Poole AR. Cartilage and diarthrodial joints as paradigms for hierarchical materials and structures. *Biomaterials* 1992;13:67–97.

177. Mow VC, Ateshian GA, Ratcliffe A. Anatomic form and biomechanical properties of articular cartilage of the knee joint. In: Finerman GAM, Noyes FR, eds. *Biology and biomechanics of the traumatized synovial joint: the knee as a model.* Rosemont, IL: American Academy of Orthopaedic Surgery, 1992:55–81.

178. Mow VC, Ateshian GA, Spilker RL. Biomechanics of diarthrodial joints: a review of twenty years of progress. *J Biomech Eng* 1993;115:460–467.

179. Mow VC, Bachrach NM, Ateshian GA. The effects of a subchondral bone perforation on the load support mechanism within articular cartilage. *Wear* 1994;175:167–175.

180. Mow VC., Ateshian GA, Lai WM, et al. Effects of fixed charges on the stress-relaxation behavior of hydrated soft tissues in a confined compression problem. *Int J Solids Struct* 1998;35:4945–4962.

181. Muir H. Proteoglycans as organizers of the intercellular matrix. *Biochem Soc Trans* 1983;11:613–622.

182. Muller-Gerbl MR, Putz R, Kenn R, et al. People in different age groups show different hip joint morphology. *Clin Biomech* 1993;8:66–72.

183. Murakami T, Higaki H, Sawae Y, et al. Adaptive multimode lubrication in natural synovial joints and artificial joints. *Proc Inst Mech Eng[H]* 1998;212:23–35.

184. Myers RR, Negami S, White RK. Dynamic mechanical properties of synovial fluid. *Biorheology* 1966;3:197–209.

185. Nishida K, Inoue H, Murakami T. Immunohistochemical demonstration of fibronectin in the most superficial layer of normal rabbit articular cartilage. *Ann Rheum Dis* 1995;54:995–998.

186. Ogston AG, Stanier JE. On the state of hyaluronic acid in the synovial fluid. *J Biochem* 1950;46:364–376.

187. O'Kelly J, Unsworth A, Dowson D, et al. A study of the role of synovial fluid and its constituents in the friction and lubrication of human hip joints. *Eng Med* 1978;7:72–83.

188. Oloyede A, Broom ND. Is classical consolidation theory applicable to articular cartilage deformation? *Clin Biomech* 1991;6:206–212.

189. Paul JP. Joint kinetics. In: Sokoloff L, ed. *The joints and synovial fluid,* Vol. II. New York: Academic Press, 1980:139–176.

190. Pandy MG, Berme N. Quantitative assessment of gait determinants during single stance via a 3-dimensional model: 1. Normal gait. *J Biomech* 1989;22:717–724.

191. Pickard JE, Fisher J, Ingham E, et al. Investigation into the effects of proteins and lipids on the frictional properties of articular cartilage. *Biomaterials* 1998;19:1807–1812.

192. Pickard J, Ingham E, Fisher J. Investigation into

193. Radin EL, Swann DA, Weisser PA. Separation of a hyaluronate-free lubricating fraction from synovial fluid. *Nature* 1970;228:377–378.

194. Radin EL, Paul IL. Response of joints to impact loading. I: in vitro wear. *Arthritis Rheum* 1971;14:356–362.

195. Radin EL, Martin RB, Burr DB, et al. Effects of mechanical loading on the tissue of rabbit knee. *J Orthop Res* 1984;2:221–234.

196. Radin EL, Rose RM. Role of subchondral bone in the initiation and progression of cartilage damage. *Clin Orthop Rel Res* 1986;213:34–40.

197. Redler I, Mow VC. Biomechanical theories of ultrastructural alterations of articular surfaces of the femoral head. In: Harris WH, ed. *The hip.* St. Louis: Mosby, 1974:23–59.

198. Redler I, Zimny M, Mansell J, et al. The ultrastructure and biomechanical significance of the tidemark of articular cartilage. *Clin Orthop Rel Res* 1975;112:357–362.

199. Repo RU, Finlay JB. Survival of articular cartilage after controlled impact. *J Bone Joint Surg* 1977;59A:1068–1076.

200. Reynolds O. On the theory of lubrication and its application to Mr. Beauchamp Tower's experiment, including an experimental determination of the viscosity of olive oil. *Philos Trans R Soc Lond B Biol Sci* 1886;177:157–234.

201. Rhinelander FW, Bennett GA, Bauer W. Exchange of substances in aqueous solutions between joints and the vascular system. *J Clin Invest* 1939;18:1–13.

202. Ropes MW, Bauer W. *Synovial fluid changes in joint disease.* Cambridge, MA: Harvard University Press, 1953.

203. Rushfeldt PD, Mann RW, Harris WH. Improved techniques for measuring in vitro the geometry and pressure distribution in the human acetabulum: I. Ultrasonic measurement of acetabular surfaces, sphericity and cartilage thickness. *J Biomech* 1981;14:253–260.

204. Sandson J. Human synovial fluid: detection of a new component. *Science* 1967;155:839–841.

205. Sarma AV, Powell GL, LaBerge M. Phospholipid composition of articular cartilage boundary lubricant. *J Orthop Res* 2001;19:671–676.

206. Sayles RS, Thomas TR, Anderson J. Measurement of the surface microgeometry of articular cartilage. *J Biomech* 1979;12:257–267.

207. Scherrer PK, Hillberry BM, Van Sickle DC. Determining the in vivo areas of contact in the canine shoulder. *J Biomech Eng* 1979;101:271–278.

208. Schumacher BL, Block JA, Schmid TM, et al. A novel proteoglycan synthesized and secreted by chondrocytes of the superficial zone of articular

the effect of proteoglycan molecules on the tribological properties of cartilage joint tissues. *Proc Inst Mech Eng[H]* 1998;212:177–182.

cartilage. *Arch Biochem Biophys* 1994;111:144–152.

209. Schumacher BL, Hughes CE, Kuettner KE, et al. Immunodetection and partial cDNA sequence of the proteoglycan, superficial zone protein, synthesized by cells lining synovial joints. *J Orthop Res* 1999;17:110–120.

210. Schurz J, Ribitsch V. Rheology of synovial fluid. *Biorheology* 1987;24:385–399.

211. Schwarz IM, Hills BA. Synovial surfactant: Lamellar bodies in type B synoviocytes and proteolipid in synovial fluid and the articular lining. *Br J Rheumatol* 1996;35:821–827.

212. Schwarz IM, Hills BA. Surface-active phospholipid as the lubricating component of lubricin. *Br J Rheumatol* 1998;37:21–26.

213. Seedhom BB, Tsubuku M. A technique for the study of contact between visco-elastic bodies with special reference to the patello-femoral joint. *J Biomech* 1977;10:253–260.

214. Seedhom BB. Transmission of the load in the knee joint with special reference to the role of the menisci: I. Anatomy, analysis and apparatus. *Eng Med* 1979;8:207–219.

215. Seedhom BB, Hargreaves DJ. Transmission of the load in the knee joint with special reference to the role of the menisci: II. Experimental results, discussion and conclusions. *Eng Med* 1979;8:220–228.

216. Seireg A, Arvikar RJ. The prediction of muscular load sharing and joint forces in the lower extremities during walking. *J Biomech* 1975;8:89–102.

217. Seller PC, Dowson D, Wright V. The rheology of synovial fluid. *Rheol Acta* 1971;10:2–7.

218. Setton LA, Zhu WB, Mow VC. The biphasic poroviscoelastic behavior of articular cartilage in compression: role of surface zone. *J Biomech* 1993;26:581–592.

219. Setton LA, Mow VC, Muller FJ, et al. Mechanical properties of canine articular cartilage are significantly altered following transection of the anterior cruciate ligament. *J Orthop Res* 1994;12:451–463.

220. Simkin PA, Nilson KL. Trans-synovial exchange of large and small molecules. *Clin Rheum Dis* 1981;7:99–129.

221. Simon WH. Scale effects in animal joints. I. Articular cartilage thickness and compressive stress. *Arth Rheum* 1970;13:244–256.

222. Smith TJ, Medley JB. Development of transient elasto-hydrodynamic models for synovial joint lubrication. *Proceedings of 13th Leeds-Lyon Symposium on Tribology,* 1987;369–374.

223. Soby L., Jamieson AM, Blackwell J, et al. Viscoelastic and rheological properties of concentrated solutions of proteoglycan subunit and proteoglycan aggregates. *Biopolymers* 1990;29:1587–1592.

224. Soltz MA, Ateshian GA. Experimental verification and theoretical prediction of cartilage interstitial fluid pressurization at an impermeable contact interface in confined compression. *J Biomech* 1998;31:927–934.

225. Soltz MA, Ateshian GA. Interstitial fluid pressurization during confined compression cyclical loading of articular cartilage. *Ann Biomed Eng* 2000;28:150–159.

226. Soltz MA, Ateshian GA. A conewise linear elasticity mixture model for the analysis of tension-compression nonlinearity in articular cartilage. *J Biomech Eng* 2000;122:576–586.

227. Soltz MA, Ateshian GA. Hydrostatic pressurization and depletion of trapped lubricant pool during creep and sliding of a rippled indenter against a biphasic articular cartilage layer. In: Casey J, Bao G, eds. *Mechanics in biology,* ASME AMD-Vol. 242/BED-Vol. 46, pp. 243–253.

228. Soslowsky LJ, Flatow EL, Bigliani LU. Articular geometry of the glenohumeral joint. *Clin Orthop* 1992;288:181–190.

229. Soslowsky LJ, Flatow EL, Bigliani LU, et al. Quantitation of in situ contact areas at the glenohumeral joint: a biomechanical study. *J Orthop Res* 1992;10:524–534.

230. Sundblad L. Glycosaminoglycans and glycoproteins in synovial fluid. In: Balazs EA, Jeanloz RW, eds. *The amino sugars,* Vol. 2A. New York: Academic Press, 1965:229–250.

231. Swann DA, Radin EL. The molecular basis of articular lubrication: I. Purification and properties of a lubricating fraction from bovine synovial fluid. *J Biol Chem* 1972;247:8069–8073.

232. Swann DA, Radin EL, Nazimiec M, et al. Role of hyaluronic acid in joint lubrication. *Ann Rheum Dis* 1974;33:318–326.

233. Swann DA. Macromolecules of synovial fluid. In: Sokoloff L, ed. *The joints and synovial fluid,* Vol. 1. New York: Academic Press, 1978:407–435.

234. Swann DA, Radin EL, Hendren RB. The lubrication of articular cartilage by synovial fluid glycoproteins. *Arthritis Rheum* 1979;22:665–666.

235. Swann DA, Silver FH, Slayter HS, et al. The molecular structure and lubricating activity of lubricin from bovine and human synovial fluids. *J Biochem* 1985;225:195–201.

236. Thomas TR, Sayles RS, Haslock I. Human joint performance and the roughness of articular cartilage. *J Biomech Eng* 1980;102:50–56.

237. Thompson RC, Oegema TR, Lewis JL, et al. Osteoarthritic changes after acute transarticular load. *J Bone Joint Surg* 1991;73-A,990–1001.

238. Unsworth A, Dowson D, Wright V. The frictional behavior of human synovial joints: I. Natural joints. *J Lubr Tech Trans ASME* 1975;97:360–376.

239. Unsworth A, Dowson D, Wright V. Some new evidence on human joint lubrication. *Ann Rheum Dis* 1975;34:277.

240. Vener JM, Thompson RC, Lewis JL, et al. Subchondral damage after acute transarticular loading: an in vitro model of joint injury. *J Orthop Res* 1992;10:759–765.

241. Walker PS, Dowson D, Longfield MD, et al. "Boosted lubrication" in synovial joints by fluid entrapment and enrichment. *Ann Rheum Dis* 1968;27:512–520.

242. Walker PS, Unsworth A, Dowson D, et al. Mode of aggregation of hyaluronic acid protein complex on the surface of articular cartilage. *Ann Rheum Dis* 1970;29:591–602.

243. Walker PS. *Human joints and their artificial replacements.* Springfield, IL: Thomas, 1977.

244. Wang H, Ateshian GA. The normal stress effect and equilibrium friction coefficient of articular cartilage under steady frictional shear. *J Biomech* 1997;30:771–776.

245. Wang H, Ateshian GA. The normal stress effect of articular cartilage under steady frictional shear persists after removal of the surface zone. *Trans Orthop Res Soc* 1996;21:8.

246. Williams PF, Powell GL, Laberge M. Sliding friction analysis of phosphatidylcholine as a boundary lubricant for articular cartilage. *Proc Inst Mech Eng* 1993;207:59–66.

247. Wismans J, Veldpaus F, Janssen J, et al. A three-dimensional mathematical model of the knee-joint. *J Biomech* 1980;13:677–685.

248. Woo SL-Y, Mow VC, Lai WM. Biomechanical properties of articular cartilage. In: Skalak R, Chien S, eds. *Handbook of bioengineering.* New York: McGraw-Hill, 1987:4.1–4.44.

249. Wright V, Dowson D. Lubrication and cartilage. *J Anat* 1976;121:107–118.

250. Zhu W, Lai WM, Mow VC. The density and strength of proteoglycan-proteoglycan interaction sites in concentrated solutions. *J Biomech* 1991;24:1007–1018.

251. Zhu W, Mow VC, Rosenberg LC, et al. Determination of kinetic changes of aggrecan-hyaluronan interactions in solution from its rheological properties. *J Biomech* 1994;27:571–579.

BIOMATERIALS

AHMED EL-GHANNAM
PAUL DUCHEYNE

1 THE MATERIALS SCIENCE TRIAD

Biomaterials including ceramics, metals, and polymers have been widely used in surgery. Some biomaterials with relatively high mechanical strength such as the titanium alloy Ti-6Al-4V, the Co-Cr alloys, alumina, or zirconia have been used in joint replacement devices. Others with bioactivity and bone bonding ability such as calcium phosphate ceramics and bioactive glasses have been used as artificial bone grafts.

The principle that is of most value with respect to assessing properties of a material originates from the internal structure of that material. At an ultramicroscopic and light microscopic level, materials are made up of atoms that are associated with their neighbors in crystals, molecules, multiphase arrangements, and microstructures. In this chapter we will focus extensively on structures and how they affect the behavior of the biomaterial.

Biomaterials must be processed to meet the requirements of a specific biological application. The most familiar processing steps simply change the shape of the materials by machining or forging. However, processing commonly involves more than simply changing the shape of the material. For example, thermal processing is required to coat metallic implants with a calcium phosphate surface intended to enhance fixation and hence longevity of the implant. During coating the internal structure of the material may be altered, in its turn resulting in a change of biological properties. It is obvious then that the processing-induced structural changes must be understood, lest it be impossible to formulate appropriate processing steps.

The relationship among structure, properties, and processing is called the materials science triad. This concept is all important in biomaterial science, no matter which material is considered. Thus, in this chapter we will always indicate properties as a function of structure and processing.

2 CLASSES OF MATERIALS

As is the case for materials, biomaterials can be conveniently grouped into three classes: metals, polymers, and ceramics. This scheme is based primarily on the chemical makeup and atomic structure of the various materials. Composites, representing another group of materials, consist of combinations of two or more metals, polymers, or ceramics. An alternative classification scheme relates to the biological properties of biomaterials, including bioinert or bioactive. In this chapter we do not use this method to organize material classes.

2.1 Metals

Metal atoms are held together in a crystal lattice by the interaction of the valence electrons (outermost electrons) with the positive metallic ions. These nonlocalized electrons are free to move throughout the solid because the valence electrons are not tightly bound to the metal ions. Such an arrangement is called the metallic bond. This distinguishes it from the covalent and ionic bonds present in polymers and ceramics, respectively. In these other configurations, electrons are not free to roam (Fig. 11-1). In what follows, some illustrations of the importance of the type of bond vis-à-vis biomaterials behavior are given.

The independent electrons in the metallic bonds can quickly transfer electric charge and thermal energy. As a result of the different binding states of the electrons, there is a difference in thermal expansion coefficient between met-

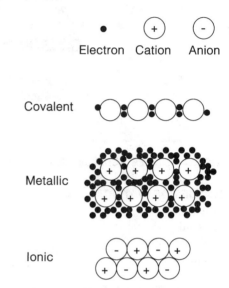

FIGURE 11-1. Schematic representation of covalent, metallic, and ionic bonding.

als and ceramics. Because it is often desirable to coat metallic implants with a bioactive ceramic film in order to improve implant fixation, the difference in thermal properties between metals and ceramics is an important issue, as this difference may be at the basis of destabilization of the coating. Specifically, the difference in the thermal expansion coefficient between metals and ceramics results in interfacial shear stresses that can create microcracks at the interface during cooling subsequent to plasma-spraying a calcium phosphate coating onto a metallic implant. After implantation, preferential degradation of the ceramic at the ceramic–metal interface can result in removal of the coating layer, and hence, poor fixation.

As the electrons can move easily in metals, neighboring atoms are weakly bonded, making metals easily deformable. This facilitates wear, except if special processing techniques are employed with the intent to enhance bonding in the metallic structure. Wear of a metallic implant can result from micromotion and friction in the implantation bed against a counterpart that has the same or higher hardness. Accumulation of wear debris has been related to aseptic loosening and implant failure.

As the number of valence electrons increases down the periodic table, they become more localized and the metallic bonds become more directional, resulting in more brittle metals. This property is also related to the high melting temperature of such brittle metals as tungsten. As the mechanical properties (and also the chemical and physical properties) of metals can be improved by alloying, most metals used in orthopedic surgery are alloyed. Obvious examples are the alloys based either on titanium or on cobalt.

2.2 Ceramics

Ceramics are composed of compounds made of metallic and nonmetallic elements. With nonmetallic elements typically oxygen, nitrogen, or carbon, ceramics are frequently oxides, nitrides, or carbides. Ceramic biomaterials include calcium phosphate ceramics, bioactive glasses, bioactive glass ceramics, alumina, and zirconia. Each of these materials is relatively hard and brittle. In fact, hardness and brittleness are typical properties of ceramics, as are excellent resistance to high temperatures and corrosive environments. The basis of these characteristics is again related to the type of atomic bonds. The metallic elements release their outermost electrons to the nonmetallic atoms. This directional bond produces electrons that are localized in the structure. Thus, typical ceramic materials are good insulators, both electrically and thermally. Considerable energy is usually required to separate the atoms that have lost electrons (cations) from the atoms that have gained electrons (anions). As a corollary, wear is low with ceramic implant materials.

Glasses and carbon materials are commonly regarded as ceramic materials, as they are composed of ionically bonded components and display the characteristic properties of ceramics, such as great hardness, lack of permanent deformability, and excellent chemical inertness. These materials, however, do not have the long-range order typical of crystalline materials. Their atomic arrangement is one of short order. Bioactive glass is a family of glass compositions with the ability to bond to bone and enhance bone tissue formation. Collectively, bone bonding and bone tissue growth enhancement are termed bone bioactive behavior. Bioactive glasses are composed of silicon oxide, which is the network former in the glass structure, and calcium oxide and sodium oxide, which are the network modifiers. Figure 11-2 shows the schematic structure of a random glass network composed of a network former (SiO_2) and network modifiers (Na_2O and CaO). Some of the Si are bonded to each other by bridging oxygen bonds, and others are coordinated with nonbridging oxygen bonds to network modifying ions in SiO_2-Na_2O-CaO glass. Other additives such as phosphorus pentoxide (P_2O_5) can be added to modulate bone bioactivity reactions. With decreasing SiO_2 concentration, the instability and, hence, the bioactivity of the bioactive glasses increase. Bioactive glass granules with a SiO_2 concentration as low as 45% by weight can be used as a resorbable bone graft material.

2.3 Polymers

Unlike metals, which have migrant electrons, the nonmetallic atoms of polymers are covalently bonded. That is, elements such as C, N, and O have an affinity for attracting or sharing

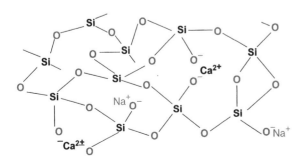

FIGURE 11-2. Schematic structure of a random glass network composed of a network former (SiO_2) and network modifiers (Na_2O and CaO).

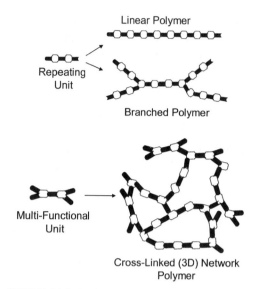

Linear Polymer

Repeating Unit

Branched Polymer

Multi-Functional Unit

Cross-Linked (3D) Network Polymer

FIGURE 11-3. Various polymer chains. (From Park JB. *Biomaterials science and engineering.* New York: Plenum Press, 1984.)

additional electrons. Thus, in covalently bonded elements, each electron is associated with a pair of atoms. Materials that contain only nonmetallic elements share electrons to build up large molecules, often called macromolecules. These large molecules contain many repeating units, or mers, from which comes the word *polymers*. The polymeric molecular arrangements can be linear, branched, or cross-linked (Fig. 11-3). The simplest example is polyethylene, which is derived from ethylene ($CH_2 = CH_2$), in which the carbon atoms share electrons with two other hydrogen and carbon atoms $-CH_2(CH_2-CH_2)_nCH_2-$, where *n* indicates the number of repeat units. To make a strong solid, *n* should be well over 10,000, making the molecular weight of the polymer more than 1 million grams/mole. Polymers bear a close resemblance to natural tissue components such as

collagen. This makes it possible to incorporate other substances by direct bonding. An example is a heparin coating on polymer surfaces in an effort to prevent blood clotting. During polymer processing additives such as antioxidants, antidiscoloring agents, and plasticizers are added to facilitate the polymerization reaction and enhance processability. Some of these additives are toxic; therefore, pure medical-grade polymers are not readily available, except in very limited cases.

2.4 Composites

Composite materials are solids that contain two or more distinct constituent materials or phases, on a scale larger than the atomic. The term *composite* is usually reserved for those materials in which the distinct phases are separated on a scale larger than the atomic and in which properties such as the elastic modulus are significantly altered in comparison to those of a homogenous material. Accordingly, reinforced plastics such as fiberglass as well as bone are viewed as composite materials, but alloys are not. The properties of a composite material depend on the shape, volume fraction, and interface between the constituent phases. The shape of the phases in a composite material is classified into three categories as shown in Fig. 11-4. Most composite biomaterials have been developed to enhance mechanical and biocompatibility behavior. The strength of composites derives in part from the fact that fine fibers or whiskers of a material can be made nearly defect free for greatly increased strength, as is shown in Table 11-1. Carbon fibers have been incorporated in high-density polyethylene tibial plateaus of total knee replacements. Although strength was greatly enhanced, wear behavior was fully unsatisfactory.

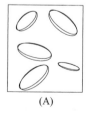
(A)

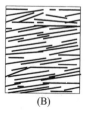
(B)

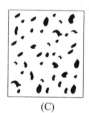
(C)

FIGURE 11-4. Morphology of basic composite inclusions: **(A)** platelet; **(B)** fiber; **(C)** particle.

TABLE 11-1. PROPERTIES OF FIBERS USED FOR COMPOSITE MATERIALS

Class	Material	Tensile Strength (GPa)	Young's Modulus (GPa)
Whisker	Graphite	20.7	675.7
	Al_2O_3	15.2	524.0
	Iron	12.4	193.1
	Si_3N_4	13.8	379.2
	SiC	20.7	689.5
	Boron	—	441.3
Glass, ceramic	Asbestos	5.9	186.2
	Drawn silica	5.9	72.4
	Boron glass	2.4	379.2
Polymer fibers	High-tenacity nylon 66	0.8	4.8
Metal wire	Carbon steel	3.9	206.9
	Molybdenum	2.1	365.4
	Tungsten	2.9	344.8

3 CRYSTAL STRUCTURE

3.1 Metals and Ceramics

Analyzing the atomic arrangements within a solid considerably facilitates studying the effect of bond type on resulting material properties. All metals, most ceramics, and some polymers crystallize when they solidify. A crystalline material is characterized by long-range order and an infinitely repeating unit cell of atoms/ions. For example, metals can have their atoms arranged in an orderly three-dimensional lattice, of which a two-dimensional section is shown in Fig. 11-5. In this two-dimensional lattice any square can be repeated by moving one lattice spacing "a" in any direction. If this is extended into three dimensions, the spatial structure so defined is a simple cube, and the crystal structure is called a cubic crystal system. The unit cell is the smallest three-dimensional structure that can be repeated within the lattice. The unit cell

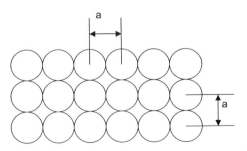

FIGURE 11-5. Two-dimensional section of a simple cubic lattice structure (a, lattice space).

of stainless steel is a cube with atoms located at the corners and middle of each side. This crystal structure is called a face-centered cubic (FCC) crystal. A cubic crystal with atoms located at corners and in the center of the cube is called a body-centered cubic crystals lattice (BCC).

In addition to a cubic structure, there are six other structures (Fig. 11-6). Apart from the face-centered location of atoms, several other so-called space lattices are possible; we indicate these only as they specifically relate to the biomaterials analysis. Figure 11-7 shows the arrangements of the atoms in an FCC and a hexagonal structure, specifically the hexagonal close-packed (HCP) structure. As this figure shows, these two lattice systems have the closest packing of atoms. In the FCC structure, the plane of closest packing runs through the three corners indicated by 1, 1', and 1''. Neighboring planes run through corners 2 or 3. Closest-packed planes of the HCP lattice are parallel with the base of the hexagonal prism. It is apparent that there is considerable configurational symmetry in these structures. This allows deformation of the structure in a great variety of ways. Thus, because the cubic and hexagonal lattices are very common metal lattices, it further substantiates the easy deformability of metals. The crystal structures, at room temperature, of some of the materials used in hip surgery are summarized in Table 11-2.

Figure 11-8 shows the HCP structure of hydroxyapatite (HA), a bone bioactive ceramic.

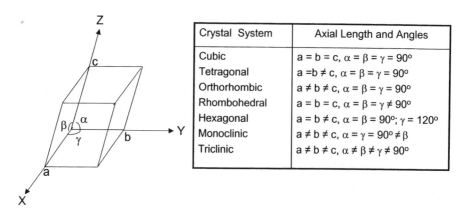

Crystal System	Axial Length and Angles
Cubic	$a = b = c,\ \alpha = \beta = \gamma = 90°$
Tetragonal	$a = b \neq c,\ \alpha = \beta = \gamma = 90°$
Orthorhombic	$a \neq b \neq c,\ \alpha = \beta = \gamma = 90°$
Rhombohedral	$a = b = c,\ \alpha = \beta = \gamma \neq 90°$
Hexagonal	$a = b \neq c,\ \alpha = \beta = 90°;\ \gamma = 120°$
Monoclinic	$a \neq b \neq c,\ \alpha = \gamma = 90° \neq \beta$
Triclinic	$a \neq b \neq c,\ \alpha \neq \beta \neq \gamma \neq 90°$

FIGURE 11-6. Geometric representation of the seven atomic lattices.

Comparison of the titanium HCP structure with this structure reveals that the HA structure is considerably more complex, as a result of which, displacement of atoms within the lattice is difficult. Thus the structure is resistant to deformation and, when overloaded, fractures rather than deforming permanently.

3.2 Polymers

Polymers are the result of chain reactions that give rise to linear, branched, or cross-linked polymeric molecular arrangements (Fig. 11-3). As the extent of polymerization increases and the molecular chains become longer, the relative mobility of the chains in the structure decreases (Fig. 11-9). As a result, alignment of the chains and formation of long-range order, i.e., crystallinity, is difficult. Polymers such as polyethylene and polyamide cannot be crystallized easily because the individual chains are long. Alignment is further rendered difficult by the variability of the chain length. As the chain ends act as defects, this repeatedly interrupts the regular continuity in the structure. Nevertheless, under optimal conditions, some crystallization is possible: Various multimolecular structures are shown in Fig. 11-10.

The chain mobility, which is directly proportional to the molecular weight, is related not only to crystallinity, but also to mechanical strength. Thus, the molecular and microstructural arrangements have a profound influence on resulting properties. Factors affecting the strength of polymers further include chemical composition, side groups, cross-linking, copolymerization, and blending. By way of example we can consider the very strong aromatic polyamid fibers, better known by their trade name Kevlar. These fibers are made up of highly directional molecular chains, which confer on the fibers great strength. This structure, however, cannot be obtained in thick sections. Thus, in order to make optimal use of the excellent strength, these

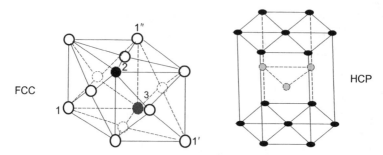

FIGURE 11-7. FCC and HCP crystal lattices.

Material	Structure
Cobalt–chromium alloy	FCC
Stainless steel AISI 316L	FCC
Titanium (Ti)	HCP
Titanium alloy (Ti-6Al-4V annealed)	Two-phase material: α–HCP β–BCC
Tantalum (Ta)	BCC
Niobium (Nb)	BCC
Gold (Au)	FCC
Alumina (Al_2O_3)	HCP
Hydroxyapatite [$Ca_{10}(PO_4)_6(OH)_2$]	HCP

fibers are usually embedded in a matrix, i.e., used in composites.

4 MECHANICAL BEHAVIOR

4.1 Mechanical Properties

Mechanical properties including elasticity and strength are important properties to consider in the selection of a material for a specific implant design. In this section we describe the various mechanical properties relevant to biomaterials.

Many of the mechanical properties of a material take into account how it behaves under load. If a load, F, is applied to a material of cross section area A, it is subjected to a stress, σ,

$$\sigma = F/A \qquad (1)$$

The units of σ ($N/m^2 = Pa$) show that stress and pressure are similar concepts. Under this force, there also will be a strain, ϵ, due to change from the original length (l_0).

$$\varepsilon = \Delta l/l_0 \qquad (2)$$

At low stress and low strain, stress is proportional to strain, i.e.,

$$\sigma = E\varepsilon \qquad (3)$$

E is constant for a material at low σ. It is called Young's modulus or modulus of elasticity of the material. E is a measure of stiffness (i.e., resistance to strain) of a material, and is quite distinct from strength. A small value of E means that a small stress gives a large extension (as in rubber); a large value of E indicates that the material is very stiff (as in diamond). The E values are 7 MPa and 1.2×10^6 MPa for rubber and diamond, respectively.

Whereas Eq. 3 describes the mechanical behavior of a material at low stress, a more extensive graphical representation of materials deformation is given in Fig. 11-11. This figure shows the proportionality of stress to strain at low stress, as well as the deviation from linearity at higher stress. The stress at which elongation is no longer reversible is called the limit of elasticity. For metallic and ceramic materials, the elastic region shows a linear relationship between stress and strain, but for polymers the relationship can be nonlinear. The yield strength is defined as the value of the stress when the strain is 0.2% more than the elastic region will allow, i.e., the stress

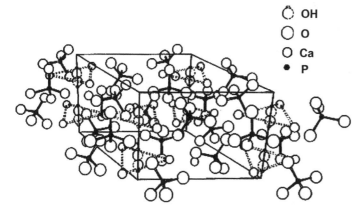

○ OH
○ O
○ Ca
● P

FIGURE 11-8. The HCP structure of hydroxyapatite.

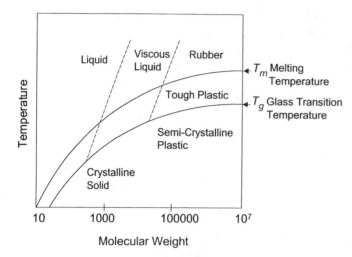

FIGURE 11-9. Approximate relation among molecular weight, T_g, T_m, and polymer properties.

level at which 0.2% permanent deformation occurs; this value is also referred to as the 0.2% proof stress. As it is very difficult to determine the onset of permanent or plastic deformation, the yield strength is a more practical property than the limit of elasticity. Plastic deformation (plastic strain) is permanent strain and it occurs beyond the yield strength, as removal of stress leaves the material deformed. The ultimate tensile strength (UTS) is the maximum technical stress (load divided by the original section) the material can sustain in tension. Ductility is the strain at failure (usually expressed as percent). Fracture toughness is the measure of the energy required to break a material (the area under the stress-strain curve at failure). Fracture toughness varies with the material: it is 0.75 MPa.m$^{1/2}$ for silica glass, 4 MPa.m$^{1/2}$ for diamond, and up to 100 MPa.m$^{1/2}$ for steel.

Hardness is another mechanical property. It is the resistance of a material to the penetration of its surface. The fatigue strength is the maximum stress a material can withstand for either an infinite or an arbitrary large number of

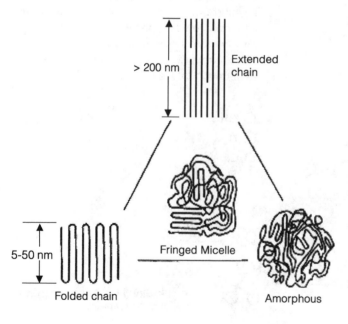

FIGURE 11-10. Two-dimensional representation of multimolecular polymer structures: extended chain fibers; folded-chain single crystals; glassy polymer amorphous structure; and semicrystalline "fringed micelle" combination structure. (Reprinted with permission from Wunderlich, B. in *Crystals of linear macromolecules*, ACS Audio Course, American Chemical Society, Washington DC, 1973. Copyright © 1973, American Chemical Society.)

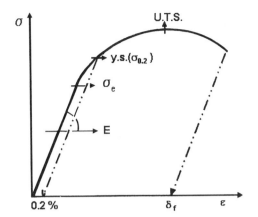

FIGURE 11-11. Stress deformation curve for a simple tensile test. *E*, elastic modulus; σ_e, proportionality limit; y.s., 0.02% offset yield stress; U.T.S., ultimate tensile stress; δ_f, total plastic deformation at fracture.

cycles. Usually the number of cycles selected is 10 million. This represents about 10 years of loading a hip prosthesis for a patient with limited activity. As any device is subjected to cyclic loading, designing against fatigue is essential for most orthopaedic implants.

Typical mechanical property values of some materials are given in Tables 11-3 and 11-4. Table 11-5 summarizes Young's modulus for some of the commonly used materials.

TABLE 11-3. TYPICAL VALUES OF TENSILE STRENGTH FOR VARIOUS MATERIALS AT ROOM TEMPERATURE

Material	Tensile Strength (MPa)
Diamond	1.05×10^6
Kevlar	4,000
High-strength carbon fiber	4,500
High-tensile steel	2,000
Superalloy	1,300
Spider webs (drag line)	1,000
Ti-6Al-4V	860
CoCr alloy (F75)	655
Aluminum	570
Titanium (grade 4)	550
316L SS (F745, annealed)	485
(Cold forged)	1,351
Bone	200
Nylon	100
Rubber	100

4.2 Fracture Mechanics of Ceramics

Biomaterials made of glass or ceramic (e.g., bioactive glass or alumina) fail in a brittle manner. This is a process in which fracture occurs with little or no plastic deformation. Brittle fracture generally occurs by cleavage over particular crystallographic planes (in crystalline structures). Although not applicable here, it is useful to know that at high temperatures, the crystalline component of the ceramic can fail intergranularly. This occurs when grain-boundary shearing takes place and cracks open between the grains, causing a local stress concentration and ultimate fracture.

Fatigue fracture occurs in metals under cyclic stressing by the nucleation and extension of a crack within an extensively deformed area at or near the surface. Such a phenomenon is unlikely in ceramics. However, "static fatigue" or delayed fracture is common in ceramics. In this case, stress corrosion occurs preferentially at the tip of preexisting defects under the influence of a static stress. This leads to subcritical crack progression prorated to the time at which the part is stressed. Eventually fracture occurs some time after the load was first applied. This kind of fracture, called fatigue in ceramics, is particularly sensitive to environmental conditions.

The static fatigue is dependent on the total time during which the load is applied, plus the loading rate and the total number of loading cycles. The relationship between the time to failure *t* and the fracture stress σ_f of a material can be described by the equation

$$\log t = A/\sigma_f + B \qquad (4)$$

where *A* and *B* are constants. This relationship is not valid at very short times but provides a useful description over a long time period.

The fatigue process has been associated with two phenomena: (a) a stress corrosion process, in which a sufficiently large stress enhances the rate of corrosion at the crack tip relative to that at the site, leading to a sharpening and deepening of the crack and eventually resulting in failure; and (b) a lowering of the surface energy, γ, by the adsorption of an active species. This leads to

TABLE 11-4. FATIGUE PROPERTIES OF IMPLANT METALS

Material	ASTM Designation	Condition	Fatigue Endurance Limit (at 10^7 Cycles, $R = -1$) (MPa)
Stainless steel	F745	Annealed	221–280
	F55, F56, F138, F139	Annealed	241–276
		30% Cold worked	310–448
		Cold forged	820
Co-Cr alloys	F75	As-cast/annealed	207–310
		P/M HIP[a]	725–950
	F799	Hot forged	600–896
	F90	Annealed	Not available
		44% Cold worked	586
	F562	Hot forged	500
		Cold worked, aged	689–793 (axial tension $R = 0.05$, 30 Hz)
Ti alloys	F67	30% Cold-worked grade	300
	F136	Forged annealed	620
		Forged, heat treated	620–689

[a]P/M HIP, Powder metallurgy produced, hot-isostatically pressed.

a decrease in the surface energy contribution to the fracture surface work. However, as the estimated surface energies only represent about 30% of the total fracture surface work, changes in surface energy would not be sufficient to account for the observed long exposure to loads. For this reason, as well as for its generally satisfactory description of many experimental data, the stress corrosion model is preferred. Although static fatigue is closely related to a corrosion process, the dissolution must be of a particular type that leads to slow crack growth, increasing the stress concentration at the crack tip until it grows to a size that causes fracture. Such phenomena have been reported for alumina and zirconia heads of hip prostheses. Growth of subcritical crack-like defects until they reach a critical size can be prevented by designing for surface stresses significantly lower than those for which failure would occur during the life of the device.

4.3 Elastic Properties of Composites

It is often useful to stiffen or harden a material, commonly a polymer, by the incorporation of

TABLE 11-5. ELASTIC PROPERTIES OF SOME TYPICAL MATERIALS

Materials	Directionality Properties	Modulus of Elasticity (MPa)
Cortical bone	Anisotropic	Longitudinal axis, 17,000
Trabecular bone	Anisotropic	Longitudinal axis of femur intertrochanteric 316 $\pm$ 293
High-density polyethylene	Isotropic	410–1,240
PMMA	Isotropic	3,000–10,000
Stainless steel AISI 316L	Isotropic	200,000
Cobalt–chromium alloy	Isotropic	220,000
Titanium	Isotropic	107,000
Ti-6A1–4V	Isotropic	110,000
Carbon fiber-reinforced graphite fibers	Anisotropic	Parallel to unidirectional 140,000
Alumina	Isotropic	Single crystal, 362,700 Polycrystal, 408,900

particulate inclusions. The shape of the particle is important. In isotropic systems, stiff platelet inclusions are the most effective in creating a stiff composite, followed by fiber inclusions. The least effective geometry is a spherical particle. A dilute concentration of spherical particulate inclusions of stiffness E_i and volume fraction V_i, in a matrix, denoted by the subscript m, with a Poisson's ratio of 0.5, gives rise to a composite with a stiffness E:

$$E = [5(E_i - E_m) V_i/(3 + 2 E_i/E_m)] + E_m \tag{5}$$

Even if the particles are perfectly rigid compared with the matrix, their stiffening effect at low concentrations is modest.

Fibers incorporated in a polymer matrix increase strength and fatigue life, in addition to the stiffness (2). Unidirectional fiber composites, when loaded along the fibers, can have a strength and stiffness comparable to that of steel, but with much less weight. However, if unidirectional fiber composites are loaded transverse to the fibers, such a composite will be compliant, with stiffness not much greater than that of the matrix alone. If stiffness and strength is needed in all directions, the fibers must be oriented randomly. For such a three-dimensional isotropic composite,

$$E = (E_i V_i/6) + E_m \tag{6}$$

Thus, the stiffness is reduced by a factor of about 6 in comparison with a unidirectional composite. However, if the fibers are aligned randomly in a plane, the reduction in stiffness is only a factor of 3.

Conversely, when inclusions are used to reduce the stiffness and the inclusions are more compliant than the matrix, spherical ones reduce the stiffness the least and platelets reduce it the most. In this case, platelets resemble cracklike defects, and soft spherical inclusions are used intentionally as crack stoppers to enhance the toughness of polymers, with only a small sacrifice in stiffness.

5 WEAR RESISTANCE

5.1 Ultrahigh-molecular-weight Polyethylene

Ultrahigh-molecular-weight polyethylene (UHMWPE) (MW above 2×10^6 g/mol) has long been used for the acetabular cup of total hip prostheses and the tibial plateau and patellar surface of knee prostheses. The success of UHMWPE in these applications is due to its favorable properties, including abrasion resistance, impact strength, low coefficient of friction, chemical inertness, and resistance to stress cracking. Table 11-6 summarizes the mechanical and physical properties of four different medical grades of UHMWPE: compression molded sheet (1020 CMS); ram extruded bar (1020 REB); partially crystallized 1050 CMS (Poly Hi); and partially crystallized 1050 REB (Poly Hi) (70).

In the majority of contemporary total joint replacements, a metallic component articulates against UHMWPE. As a patient may be expected to take an average of 1,200 steps per day, the joint replacement is expected to withstand millions of loading cycles during its service lifetime (148). In total hip replacements, where the articulating geometries consist of conforming spherical surfaces, the wear occurs at a microscopic length scale (μm or less). Wear resistance has been related to its resistance to

TABLE 11-6. MECHANICAL AND PHYSICAL PROPERTIES OF MEDICAL GRADES OF UHMWPE ($\pm$ STANDARD DEVIATION)

	1020 CMS	1020 REB	1050 CMS	1050 REB
Yield stress (MPa)	23.6 ± 0.1	23.6 ± 0.1	22.6 ± 0.1	22.3 ± 0.4
UTS (MPa)	42.1 ± 2.6	37.2 ± 6.4	43.8 ± 3.5	39.9 ± 5.0
% Elongation	396 ± 20	376 ± 52	359 ± 20	354 ± 33
Impact strength (kJ/m^2)	161 ± 1.9	140 ± 1.4	93.7 ± 3.4	97.9 ± 2.9
Density (g/cm^3)	0.9366 ± 0.0001	0.9357 ± 0.0001	0.9308 ± 0.0003	0.9332 ± 0.0001

multidirectional stresses (13,16,25,62,90,119, 120,137,161–165). In total knee replacements, where the articulating surfaces consist of non-conforming cylindrical, toroidal, or flat surfaces, the wear process includes various surface damage mechanisms ranging from pitting and delamination to burnishing and adhesive wear (5,161, 172,174,175).

Focusing on acetabular components and the analysis of retrieved devices, it is evident that there are three different mechanisms of wear. Adhesive wear is a process in which surface asperities of the polymer adhere to the metal surface and subsequently are torn off. As a result, either a polymer film is formed on the metal surface or polymer particles are released and entrapped in the joint. Such particles as well as remaining cement fragments can generate abrasive wear, a second mode of wear. This process can also be generated by asperities on the gliding metal partner. A third mechanism is fatigue wear; as a result of creep or plastic flow, folds or cracks are formed that cause small polymer particles to break off.

It is generally accepted that particulate debris generated by mechanical wear (adhesion, abrasion, and fatigue) of prosthetic components stimulates the generation of a pseudosynovial membrane at the interface between implant and bone and the infiltration of fibrocytes and macrophages. In the presence of debris, these cells release various cytokines and mediators (such as IL-1β, TNFα, collagenase, and prostaglandin E$_2$) (69,85,89,155). These cytokines have been shown to be involved in bone resorption by activating osteoclasts (110). A recent study showed a positive correlation between cytokine concentration in the loosening membrane and the degree of underlying osteolysis (153). Many reports have investigated the size of wear debris retrieved from failed total joint arthroplasty (TJA) and demonstrated that phagocytosis and cell mortality increase with particle size and concentration (18). The mechanism that results in this cell death remains unknown, although a potential role for apoptosis in the pathogenesis of wear debris-associated osteolysis has recently been suggested (19). Aseptic loosening, which is the single most common cause for long-term failure of TJA, is associated with periprosthetic osteolysis with the incidence of up to 25% of implant recipients (59,91,93).

The analysis of wear mechanisms *in vivo* readily points out the importance of the test conditions for the usefulness of wear data collected *in vitro*. As loading controls the fatigue wear, both the loading cycle and the size and shape of the contact area influence the wear behavior. Choosing the test solution is no less important, as this also affects the adhesive wear process. It is widely recognized, however, that wear rates produced in hip simulator studies are often lower than those generated *in vivo* (6,12,22), and this has been explained by a lack of abrasive wear due to roughened heads, third-body particles, and polymer degradation. Although these parameters are clearly influential in wear debris production, the influence of alternative gait activities must also be considered.

Hip simulator validation studies have correlated the mechanical behavior and surface morphology of polymeric biomaterials with the wear performance (49,50,101). Because of the multidirectional motion prevalent at the articulating surface of total hip prostheses, the mechanical behavior of UHMWPE under multiaxial loading conditions has been shown to provide important insight into the wear resistance (102). Based on equibiaxial tension testing performed on miniature 0.5-mm thick, 6.4-mm diameter disk specimens obtained from the surface of wear-tested cups, work to failure has been significantly correlated with the wear performance in a hip simulator for a wide range of virgin and cross-linked semicrystalline polymers (49,50). Furthermore, the surface morphology of the wear-tested acetabular components has been related to the mechanical behavior of semicrystalline polymers, in that materials with greater toughness (work to failure) under multiaxial loading conditions were associated with lower surface roughness during hip simulator testing (101). Figure 11-12 shows an eight-station hip joint simulator used in some of these studies.

Multiple factors can affect polyethylene wear and the production of wear debris *in vivo* after joint arthroplasty. Such factors include the roughness and material of the femoral head, the method of polyethylene sterilization, and

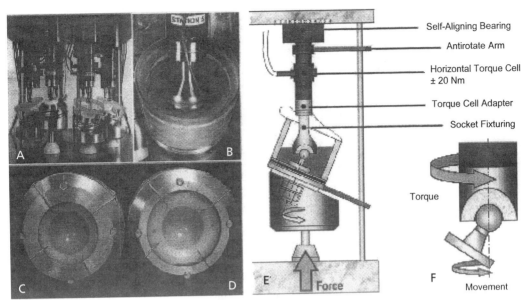

FIGURE 11-12. Photographs and schematics showing **(A)** MTS eight-station hip joint simulator, **(B)** physiological test setup, **(C)** fully constraining socket fixture, **(D)** partially constraining socket fixture, **(E)** location of horizontal torque cells, and **(F)** direction of torque measured.

the mechanical properties of the polyethylene itself (149). The alterations of the mechanical properties of polyethylene associated with gamma irradiation in air and shelf life have been demonstrated in the laboratory (24,26,169). Recent laboratory studies have confirmed that the wear resistance of UHMWPE can be significantly increased when applying additives or high-dose irradiation (21,68,105,121,125,176), with many studies reporting extremely low quantities of wear, typically as low as 2.0 mm³ per million cycles for highly cross-linked polyethylenes. A study undertaken by Laurent et al. (105) reported no measurable wear after 20 million cycles of normal walking and highlights the potential of such materials. Radiographic measurements are also evidencing extremely low *in vivo* wear rates of cross-linked polyethylene (176), with recent retrieval studies undertaken by Oonishi et al. (130) showing little evidence of *in vivo* scratching and delamination on sockets irradiated at 100 Mrad. As these materials continue to maintain an acceptable biocompatibility, the overall success of polyethylene hip arthroplasty should greatly increase, thereby offering a highly cost-effective treatment.

5.2 Alumina

High-density, high-purity alumina is used in load-bearing hip prostheses because of its outstanding wear resistance and excellent corrosion resistance. It has a high Young's modulus and a hardness second only to that of diamond. These properties have made the alumina-on-alumina couple for femoral heads and acetabular cups a materials combination of considerable importance. Most alumina devices are very fine-grained polycrystalline α-Al$_2$O$_3$ produced by pressing and sintering at high temperature (1600°C to 1700°C). A very small amount of MgO (less than 0.5%) is used to aid sintering and limit grain growth during sintering. Static and fatigue strength and fracture toughness are a function of grain size and percentage of sintering aid (i.e., purity). Alumina with an average grain size below 4 μm and a purity greater than 99.7% exhibits excellent flexural and compressive strength. Table 11-7 summarizes these properties.

Studies have reported excellent performance of the alumina-on-alumina bearing in terms of low annual wear (<5 μm) (10,11,124, 128,160,170). The long-term friction of an

TABLE 11-7. PHYSICAL CHARACTERISTICS OF Al_2O_3 BIOCERAMIC

	High-alumina Ceramics	ISO Standard 6474
Alumina content (% by weight)	>99.8	$\geq$99.50
Density (g/cm³)	>3.93	$\geq$3.90
Average grain size (μm)	3–6	<7
Surface roughness, Ra (μm)	0.02	
Hardness (Vickers hardness number, VHN)	2,300	>2,000
Compressive strength (MPa)	4,500	
Bending strength (MPa)	550	400
Young's modulus (GPa)	380	
Fracture toughness	5–6	
(K_1c) (MPa)	5–6	

alumina–alumina joint prosthesis decreases with time and approaches the value of a normal joint. This lead to wear on alumina articulating surfaces being nearly 10 times lower than on polyethylene surfaces gliding against metallic heads (Fig. 11-13).

Careful operative technique with correct positioning of the prosthesis is necessary to avoid excessive wear (37,83,113). Impingement between the femoral neck and the rim of the acetabular cup has been associated with massive wear and osteolysis (173) and high wear rates have been associated with "stripe" and severe wear of Mittelmeier prostheses (127). Nevertheless, given good surgical technique it is possible to achieve very low volumes of wear with ceramic-on-ceramic prostheses.

Histological studies of the pseudosynovial tissue obtained from around retrieved uncemented ceramic–ceramic prostheses have identified numerous alumina ceramic particles with a mean size of 5 μm (100). In addition, Henssge et al. (79) observed particles up to 5 μm in diameter in the periprosthetic tissues from around cemented alumina–alumina prostheses. More recently, very small alumina wear particles in the

size range 5 to 90 nm were revealed by transmission electron microscopy (TEM), whereas scanning electron microscopy (SEM) (lower resolution) revealed particles in the 0.05 to 3.2 μm size range (72). The bimodal size range of alumina ceramic wear debris overlapped with the size ranges commonly observed with metal particles (10 to 30 nm) and particles of UHMWPE (0.1 to 1000 μm). It is possible that the two types of ceramic wear debris are generated by two different wear mechanisms *in vivo*; under normal articulating conditions, relief polishing wear and very small wear debris is produced, while under conditions of microseparation of the head and cup and rim contact, intergranular and intragranular fracture and larger wear particles are generated.

The *in vivo* wear rate of the ceramic–ceramic joint couple is reported to be up to 200 times less than that of the metal–PE joint couple (37). Although ceramics are considered more bioinert than PE ceramic particles generated *in vivo*, when present in large concentrations, they can initiate an inflammatory response in periprosthetic tissue (107,108). Moreover, alumina ceramic particles could induce macrophage

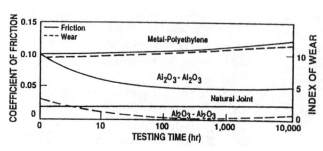

FIGURE 11-13. Time dependence of (solid line) coefficient of friction and (dashed line) index of wear of alumina–alumina versus metal–PE hip joint (*in vitro* testing). (Reprinted from Hench LL. Bioceramics: from concept to clinic. *J Am Ceram Soc* 1991;74(7):1487–1510, by permission of the American Ceramic Society.)

TNF-α release (18,20) and apoptosis (19). Petit et al. (135) compared the macrophage response with identically sized particles of alumina ceramic (Al_2O_3) and UHMWPE in terms of TNF-α release and induction of apoptosis of J774 mouse macrophages. The stimulation of TNF-α release was much greater (8 to 10 times higher) with UHMWPE than with Al_2O_3. However, the induction of apoptosis as measured by activation of caspase-3, PARP cleavage, and DNA laddering was different for these two particle compositions, being faster and more important with Al_2O_3 than with UHMWPE. One of the highlights of apoptotic cell death, as it applies to periprosthetic osteolysis, is that the whole process terminates in the elimination of dead macrophages without the induction of a significant inflammatory reaction (23). Therefore, it could be possible that the ability of Al_2O_3 particles to induce macrophage apoptosis may explain the lower TNF-α release observed with these particles and explain the differences seen in osteolysis patterns of ceramic–ceramic versus metal–PE articulations (107). The induction of macrophage apoptosis may therefore be a desirable therapeutic endpoint.

6 METALLIC BIOMATERIALS— CORROSION RESISTANCE AND RELATED PROPERTIES

Corrosion is the unwanted chemical reaction of a metal with its environment, resulting in its continued degradation to oxides, hydroxides, or other compounds. Biological fluids in the human body contains water, salt, dissolved oxygen, bacteria, proteins, and various ions such as chloride and hydroxide. As a result, the human body is a very aggressive environment for metals. Consequently, corrosion resistance of a metallic implant material is an important aspect of its biocompatibility. Metallic biomaterials are normally considered to be highly corrosion resistant because of the presence of an extremely thin passive oxide film that spontaneously forms on their surfaces. These films serve as a barrier to corrosion processes in alloy systems that would otherwise experience very high cor-

rosion rates. That is, in the absence of passive films, the driving force for corrosion for typical implant alloys [e.g., titanium-based, cobalt-chromium (Co-Cro)-based, and stainless-steel alloys] is very high, and corrosion rates would also be high. The properties of these passive oxide films depend to a large extent on their structure and chemistry, which are themselves dependent on the substrate's prior thermal, mechanical, and electrochemical history. In this section, the basis for the excellent corrosion resistance of currently used implant metals is explained.

There are two Co-Cr alloys extensively used in implant fabrications such as artificial joints, or stems of prostheses for heavily loaded joints such as knees and hips: the castable Co-Cr-Mo alloy and the Co-Ni-Cr-Mo alloy, which is usually wrought by (hot) forging. The chromium is a reactive element and is added to produce a stable firmly adherent protective chromium oxide surface layer. Chromium also enhances the solid solution strengthening of the alloy. The molybdenum is added to produce finer grains, which results in higher strengths after casting or forging. As with stainless steel, molybdenum also enhances the corrosion resistance of Co-Cro alloys (136). The inhomogeneous microstructure of the cast Co-Cr-Mo alloy renders it more susceptible to corrosion than the forged alloy (36), presumably due to the presence of chromium-depleted dendritic regions acting as the more anodic sites in a galvanic reaction. Wrought Co-Cr-Mo has lower carbon content than cast Co-Cr-Mo and, as a result, a lower corrosion resistance when tested in physiologic solution (36,82). The metallic products released from the prosthesis because of wear, corrosion, and fretting may impair organs and local tissues, and moreover, some alloys with certain amount of Co can be toxic in the body. Low wear has been recognized as an advantage of metal-on-metal hip articulations because of their hardness and toughness.

Both c.p. Ti and Ti-6Al-4V possess excellent corrosion resistance for a full range of titanium oxide states and pH levels. Titanium is a base metal in the context of the electrochemical series; however, it derives its resistance to corrosion by the formation of a solid oxide layer to a depth of 10 nm. Under *in vivo* conditions the oxide, TiO_2, is a very stable reaction product. Corrosion currents in normal saline are very low ($10^{-8}\ Acm^{-2}$). The low dissolution rate and near chemical inertness of titanium dissolution products allow bone to thrive and therefore osseointegrate with titanium.

Titanium implants remain virtually unchanged in appearance; however, even in their passive condition, metals, including titanium, are not inert. It is established beyond doubt, by both *in vitro* and *in vivo* experiments (60,73,103, 104,168), that there is a passive dissolution from the metal. Thus, linked to the issue of electrochemical behavior are several questions: (a) What material is released? (b) How much material is released under static conditions? (c) How is the release modified by wear conditions? (d) What subsequent reactions do the release products get involved in? (e) What percentage of the release products is excreted and what percentage is retained? (f) Of the percentage that is retained, where does it accumulate? (g) What biological response(s) will result from the retained fraction (14,15,44,48,96,122,166)?

Stainless steel contains enough chromium to confer corrosion resistance by passivity. The passive layer (chromium oxide) is not as robust as in the case of titanium or the Co-Cro alloys. The relatively resistant varieties of stainless steel are the austinitic types 316, 316L, and 317, which contain molybdenum (2.5% to 3.5%). Even these types of stainless steels are vulnerable to pitting and to crevice corrosion around screws, under certain circumstances such as in a highly stressed and oxygen-depleted region (4). The corrosion resistance can be enhanced by increasing the thickness of the protective oxide using concentrated nitric acid ("passivation"), by boiling in distilled water, or by electrochemical means (anodization) (87). The reduction of carbon to less than 0.03% has virtually eliminated the risk of intercrystalline corrosion, which can occur when there is precipitation of chromium carbide at the grain boundary in stainless steel with a carbon content above this value (133). Unfortunately, lowering the carbon content results in lowering the ultimate tensile strength of stainless steel.

Corrosion of an implant in the clinical setting can result in symptoms such as local pain and swelling in the region of the implant, with no evidence of infection; only cracking or flaking of the implant (seen on roentgenograms), and excretion of excess metal ions. At surgery, gray or black discoloration of the surrounding tissues may be seen and flakes of metals may be found in the tissue. Corrosion also plays a role in the mechanical failures of orthopaedic implants. Most of these failures are due to fatigue, and the presence of a saline environment certainly exacerbates fatigue. The extent to which corrosion influences fatigue in the body is not precisely known, although once an initial crack has formed, crack propagation will be faster than in air or vacuum. Other mechanisms of corrosion such as fretting may also be involved at point of contact such as in the countersink of hip nails.

Different parts of the body undergo different types and rates of corrosion. Wounds and infections can significantly change pH. *In vivo*, the equilibrium state between a metal and its reaction products (oxide, hydroxide, etc.), which causes passivation, may not occur if the reaction products are removed by the tissue fluid turnover. The replenishment of ions accumulated at the implant–tissue interface may cause an adverse increase in the rate of ion release that may cause damage on the cellular level. Focusing on the major alloying elements in cobalt-based materials (Co, Cr, and Ni), Co and Ni ions bind to serum albumin, and Cr^{6+} binds to red blood cells (14). Chemical analyses of urine from animals subjected to metal salts indicated that most Co and Ni is rapidly excreted, while less than 50% of the Cr is excreted, and this occurs at a slower rate than Co or Ni (15,123). Furthermore, organ levels of Co and Ni are not significantly elevated, whereas they are for Cr. Serum and urine analyses of patients with total joint replacements have also indicated a dose–response relationship (154,127). Koegel and Black (96), using a cast Co-Cr-Mo microsphere model, found dose-related elevations in serum Co and Cr, with peak concentrations achieved 3 days after implantation. Scaling for the implant surface area to animal body weight ratio (300×), the Co and Cr elevations were 20 and 12, respectively. In a related study (166), it was determined that the form of the released chromium was Cr^{6+}, a more biologically active form of Cr than Cr^{3+}. Black et al. (7) found that when a pyrolytic carbon coating was applied to cast Co-Cr-Mo, the carbon-coated implants released more Co and Cr than the uncoated implants. Relative motion between the implant and tissue may have caused the release of additional debris, possibly in the form of metal carbides. Ducheyne and Healy (44) determined that hydroxyapatite coatings reduce the Ti and Al passive dissolution rate from porous coated Ti-6Al-4V. Hydroxyapatite, however, did not produce a change in the release kinetics of Co and Cr from Co-Cr alloys. Other studies on Ti and Ti-6A1-4V have shown that titanium is preferentially accumulated locally, with elevated levels of Ti detected in adjacent soft tissue and bone (48). Healy and Ducheyne (74) further determined that serum proteins increase the release rate kinetics of titanium compared with solutions containing only serum electrolytes.

7 BONE BIOACTIVE CERAMICS

7.1 Calcium Phosphates—Structure, Mechanical Properties, and Processing

Bioactive materials including calcium phosphate ceramics and bioactive glasses bond to bone and enhance bone tissue formation. The forms of calcium phosphate ceramics most widely used are tricalcium phosphate [$Ca_3(PO_4)_2$, whitlockite], tetracalcium phosphate ($Ca_4P_2O_9$), and hydroxyapatite [$Ca_{10}(PO_4)_6(OH)_2$] (HA). There is a wide variation of mechanical properties of synthetic calcium phosphates as given in Table 11-8. This variation of properties is the result of variation of density and crystalline structure of calcium phosphates, in turn the result of differences in processing methods. Sintering of calcium phosphate ceramics is usually carried out in the range of 1,000°C to 1,500°C. Depending on the final firing conditions, the calcium phosphate can be hydroxyapatite or β-whitlockite. In many instances, however, both types of chemistries exist in the same final product.

The phases formed at high temperature depend not only on the sintering temperature but also on the partial pressure of water in the sintering atmosphere. This is because with water present, HA can be formed and is a stable phase up to 1,360°C as shown in the phase equilibrium diagram for CaO and P_2O_5 with 500 mm Hg partial pressure of water (Fig. 11-14). The temperature range of stability of HA increases with the partial pressure of water, as does the rate of phase transition of tricalcium phosphate or tetracalcium phosphate to HA. The ideal Ca/P ratio of HA is 10:6 and the calculated density is 3.219 g/cm^3. HA has a high elastic modulus (40 to 117 GPa), whereas the elastic modulus of compact bone is 12 to 18 GPa. Poisson's ratio for HA is about 0.27, which is close to that of bone (approximately 0.3).

At body temperature only two calcium phosphates are stable when in contact with aqueous media such as body fluids. At pH less than 4.2, the stable phase is $CaHPO_4 \cdot 2H_2O$ (dicalcium phosphate or brushite), whereas at pH greater than 4.2 the stable phase is HA.

7.2 Calcium Phosphates—Biological Behavior

Daculsi et al. used TEM to determine the *in vivo* degradation of biphasic implant materials, which were various mixtures of HA and tricalcium phosphate (27). Implants were inserted in surgically created periodontal defects. At 6 months, a direct correlation was established between the rate of dissolution of the material and the quantity of newly formed microcrystals with Ca/P ratios similar to those of bone apatite. The TEM studies carried out by Jarcho et al. (88) and Tracy and Doremus (156), who each used dense, stoichiometric HA, showed direct apposition of bone crystals onto the synthetic apatite lattice. Whereas in these studies solid-solution ion exchange was not addressed, Davies et al. (32) documented in a more recent study a limited *in vivo* reactivity of this material.

A similar result of limited reactivity of dense, stoichiometric HA was also found by Schepers et al. (145), who implanted granules of this material in various bone tissue sites of the

TABLE 11-8. MECHANICAL PROPERTIES AND STRENGTH OF CALCIUM PHOSPHATE CERAMICS

Material	Porosity (%)	Density (mg/m³)	Young's Modulus (GPa)	Microhardness (GPa)	Compressive Strength (MPa)	Tensile Strength (MPa)	Flexural Strength (MPa)
Hydroxyapalite	0.1–3	3.05–3.15	7–13	4.2–4.5	350–450	38–48	100–120
	10	2.7	—	4.2	—	—	—
	30	—	—	—	120–170	—	—
	40	—	—	—	60–120	—	15–35
	2.8–19.4	2.55–3.07	44–88	—	310–510	—	60–115
	2.5–26.5	—	55–110	—	≤800	—	50–115
Tetracalcium phosphate	Dense	3.1	—	—	120–200	—	—
Triacalcium phosphate	Dense	3.14	—	—	120	—	—
	36	—	—	—	7–21	5	—
Other calcium phosphates	Dense	2.8–3.1	—	—	70–170	—	—

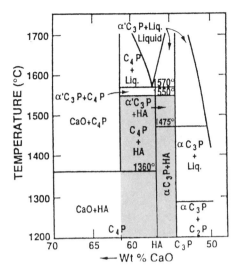

FIGURE 11-14. Phase equilibrium diagram of calcium phosphates in a water atmosphere. Shaded area is processing range to yield HA-containing implants.

beagle mandible. Bone tissue grew from the pre-existing bone along the particles that were closest to the defect wall. However, bone tissue did not grow further than about 1 mm into the defect after about 12 weeks. In addition, the presence of multinucleated cells was continuously observed from that time on, and the ceramic surface exhibited a moth-eaten appearance resulting from the local resorption of the material. In the areas where multinucleated cells were present, there was no new bone tissue formation. Osteoconduction and multinucleated cell-mediated resorption frequently had taken place on separate sides of a single particle. These phenomena are shown in Fig. 11-15A and B.

This experiment showed beyond doubt that dense, stoichiometric HA is osteoconductive *in vivo*. However, it also revealed that this material displays only a limited bone bioactivity. If a key element for bone bioactive behavior is the development of a carbonated apatite surface, one might expect an excellent response by using a carbonated apatite as implant material. However, implantation data do not unequivocally support this hypothesis. The tissue response to a porous carbonated apatite material implanted in beagle mandibular bone was very similar to that with dense, stoichiometric

HA (145). Osteoconduction from the bone defect wall occurred over a limited distance, and bone tissue conduction into the center of the defects was not observed. In addition, a chronic, mild multinucleated cell resorption of the material started as early as 3 months after implantation. This limited osteoconductivity is attributed to the high stability of the HA ceramic in tissue fluids, which results in a considerable induction time for precipitation of a fresh apatite layer from the interfacial tissue fluids onto the material surface. Another factor that contributes significantly to the delay in the formation of the

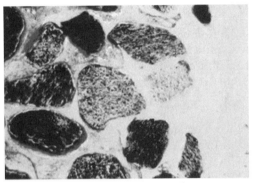

A

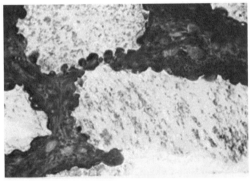

B

FIGURE 11-15. Histological section of dense, stoichiometric hydroxyapatite. **(A)** After 3 months, bone tissue has grown along the particle surface, but only over a distance of about 1 mm. **(B)** From 6 months on, the particle surfaces have a moth-eaten appearance caused by multinucleated cell resorption. The resorption is not paralleled by a bone formation process (Reprinted from Schepers E, Declercq M, Ducheyne P, et al. Bioactive glass particulate material as a filler for bone lesions. *J Oral Rehab* 1991;**18**:439–452, with permission.)

bioactive apatite surface layer is protein adsorption.

7.3 Calcium Phosphates—Coatings

Coating metallic prostheses with a calcium phosphate layer provides direct implant–bone bonding and better fixation and longevity. When a porous stainless-steel fiber network was coated with a slip-cast HA lining, a marked increase in bone ingrowth was observed in comparison to the ingrowth in the same porous metal without HA lining. This effect was pronounced at 2 and 4 weeks, but it disappeared at 12 weeks (45). This phenomenon provided the distinct therapeutic benefit of faster rehabilitation for patients with HA-coated devices. However, structural and compositional changes of the Ca-P ceramic occur as a result of processing the coatings. These variations of the material characteristics affect the rate of enhancement of the bioactive ceramic coating. Using an experimental protocol that extensively controlled factors such as animal model, pore size, pore morphology, and properties of the metallic substrate, it was found that there were statistically significant variations in bonding strength in the first few weeks after implantation arising from differences in ceramic characteristics (40). Figure 11-16 shows that calcium-phosphate coatings significantly enhanced bone tissue growth fixation, but that the effect differed among coatings. In addition, these data show that the intensity of the effect was consistent among the three early time points studied.

The clinical experience with HA coatings has been excellent. Most trials have focused on the performance of the femoral component. There has been variability in the implant design studied, the method and characteristics of the applied coatings, and the extent of the coating on the surface of femoral stems (64). There have been numerous cohort studies but few randomized clinical trials (29,30,65,66,143). Larger uncontrolled series have reported *valuable* results (17,29,65). D'Antonio et al. reported a multicenter study of 316 hips (280 patients) with proximally HA-coated titanium alloy

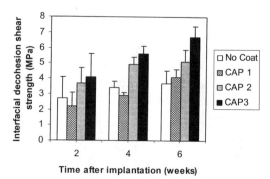

FIGURE 11-16. Shear strength as a function of implantation time for controls (porous-surfaced titanium) and porous specimens with various calcium phosphate coatings. Note that the greatest effect on bone tissue ingrowth fixation is associated with coating CAP3, which is the coating with the highest *in vitro* dissolution rate (Reprinted from Ducheyne P, Beight J, Cuckler J, et al. Effect of calcium-phosphate coating characteristics on early post-operative bone tissue ingrowth. *Biomaterials* 1990;11:531–540, with permission.)

stems that were implanted in a young and active patient population from 1987 through 1990 (31). Clinically, these patients had early pain relief and rapid restoration of function. The results show excellent lasting fixation of this tapered titanium alloy stem coated proximally with a thin, dense layer of HA. Another report by Hernandez et al. described the 11-year follow-up results of 52 unilateral primary hip arthroplasties performed with HA-coated stems (80). The femoral prosthesis used was a collarless titanium alloy implant, with proximal circumferential HA coating and increased distal thickness to fit the proximal diaphyseal region of the femur. At the end of the follow-up period, excellent clinical results were recorded in 40 arthroplasties (77%). The 11-year survival rate was 92.3%. Geesink and Hoefnagels (66) reported their 6-year results of 118 primary total hip arthroplasties using a metaphysis filling Ti stem that had a 50-μm-thick air plasma-sprayed coating of HA on the proximal third of its surface. The study's reported survival rate of the prosthesis at 6 years was 100% for the 118 HA-coated stems and 99% for the HA-coated cups. Vidalain reported a 0.97 survival rate of the Corail femoral stem at 10 years of implantation (158). This survival rate is considered to be even higher than that of many series of Charnley prostheses, which remain the absolute standard in this respect. During that period (10 years), more than 6,700 implantations have been performed and analyzed by the surgeons of the ARTRO Group, with a consistent annual rate of about 700 replacements. Functional results have been rated as excellent using the Postel Merle d'Aubigné or Harris hip scores. According to the PMA hip scale, the preoperative score was 11.29; it was 17.01 at 1 year, 17.21 at 5 years, and 17.20 at 10 years. Actually, scores are very similar to those achieved with the best cemented prostheses, particularly for pain, with the absence of significant thigh pain, which is typical of the CORAIL hip prosthesis. Altogether, 63% of patients are totally pain free and have recovered normal motion and function. Based on these clinical results it is concluded that osteo-conductive coatings have established an excellent performance record in primary and revision hip arthroplasty.

In view of all the advantages of HA coating, are there drawbacks or at least concerns or questions? It is now well established that HA is not toxic, does not produce inflammatory or allergic reactions, and is not carcinogenic. Still, four problems can be discussed: HA resorption and long-term stability, osteolysis that is occasionally observed, polyethylene wear and potential risk of granuloma, and the difficulty of extracting an HA-coated stem, particularly when it is perfectly ingrown.

Resorption of HA is more or less inescapable, due to both chemical dissolution and cell-mediated degradation. However, the kinetics of this degradation process are influenced by a number of factors that are still not clearly understood, and consequently, are not all well known. Aebli et al. carried out a histological study of a proximally HA-coated femoral component, retrieved after 9.5 years of good function (1). The HA coating had completely degraded. Bone was in direct contact with the titanium surface in all the areas which had been coated, with no interposing fibrous tissue. There were no signs of particles, third-body wear, adverse tissue reactions, or osteolysis. Bone remodeling was evident by the presence of resorption lacunae; tetracycline

labeling showed bone laid down 6 years after implantation. The loss of the HA coating had no negative effect on the osseointegration of the stem. It was concluded that the HA coating contributes to the fixation of the implant and that its degradation does not adversely affect the long-term fixation.

HA, when first used as a hip stem coating more than 10 years ago, was considered sufficiently insoluble at neutral pH not to be degraded after implantation. However, it then became apparent that the HA was decomposed during plasma spraying. Several phases (α- or β-TCP, CaO, TTCP, oxyapatite, and amorphous calcium phosphate) can be evidenced in the HA coating after spraying. These different phases occur in various amounts and at preferential locations in the coating, depending on plasma-spray parameters and powder characteristics. CaO, for example, is found at the interface with the metal, whereas the contaminating calcium phosphate phases occur around the crystalline phase of the coating grains. Most of the contaminating phases are more soluble than HA at neutral pH and their presence in the HA coating increases its degradability.

The coating environment is also determinant in coating degradation. The dielectric constant and pH of the extracellular fluids are key factors and can be modified by cell activity. The pH can, for example, be modified by osteoclast activity, the pH in the resorption chamber of osteoclasts being as low as 4.5 to 5. Similar low-pH compartments are found in cytoplasmic compartments such as lysosomes. These different factors explain the degradation of calcium phosphate coatings evidenced in contact with or in the close vicinity of osteoclasts, macrophage, or giant cells. Degradation of the calcium phosphate coatings constituted by the stacking of calcium phosphate grains occurs preferentially at the interface between the grains, where the most soluble phases facilitating the release of calcium phosphate particles are located. Particle release by a material implanted in bone is a cause of concern due to the osteolytic reactions that have been evidenced in the vicinity of metal or polymeric particles debris. Furthermore, Bloebaum et al. (8) suggested that the calcium particles emitted by acetabular coatings could migrate to the surface of polyethylene cups, thereby triggering third-body wear responsible for osteolysis and aseptic loosening.

When HA-coated metallic implants have been retrieved from humans and animals, evidence has been found of loose HA particles and osteolysis (3,9,28,42,63). Bloebaum et al. reported that histologic evaluation of 14 retrieved implants revealed HA particles, evidence of inflammatory reactions, and osteolysis (9). Furthermore, resorption of HA can create a void between the metal implant and the surrounding bone matrix (151), which may lead to mechanical instability and eventual failure. Reikeras et al. reported the outcome of 191 acetabular gritblasted titanium cups with a hemispherical design for press-fit insertion and coated with HA (139). The prosthesis was made of gritblasted titanium entirely coated with HA. The 155 patients, ages 15 to 78 years, were operated on during the years 1991 to 1993 and followed for 7 to 10 years. During this period, 39 cups were revised because of mechanical loosening, a further 9 had radiolucent lines, and 2 had focal osteolysis. None of these 11 patients had clinical symptoms. Failure was associated with age, wear, and radiolucency/osteolysis. At revision, it was found that the soft tissues were discolored, and that most of the coating had disappeared. It has been concluded that this design of HA-coated cups has a high rate of debonding and failure. Regardless of these reports, the overall clinical benefit of calcium phosphate coatings has been decidedly positive. Basic science studies proved that next-generation biomimetic HA coatings will expand the application range of osteoconductive coatings to three-dimensional ingrowth structures and combinations with antibi-

otics, growth factors, or other achievements of modern biotechnology.

7.4 Bioactive Glasses

Bioactive glasses are silica-based glasses in which silica (SiO_2) is the network former and alkali metals, e.g., Na and K, or alkaline earth metals, e.g., Ca and Mg, are the network modifier. The ratio of network former to network modifier in the composition of bioactive glass determines its solubility in physiological solutions, and hence, its bioactivity and resorbability. Table 11-9 summarizes the chemical composition of selected bioactive glasses and glass ceramics with different degrees of bioactivity.

The amorphous structure of bioactive glass impairs its mechanical strength and lowers its fracture toughness. Tensile strength of most of the bioactive glass compositions in Table 11-9 is in the range 40 to 60 MPa, which makes them unsuitable for load-bearing applications. For some applications low strength is offset by the glasses low modulus of elasticity of 30 to 35 GPa, which is close to that of cortical bone (7 to 25 GPa).

A unique characteristic of bioactive glass is its ability to form a strong interfacial bond with adjacent tissues in the host, and it has been used successfully as a bone-substitute material in orthopedic and dental surgery (131,147, 150,152,171). To understand the basic mechanisms of the formation of the bone–biomaterials bond, two main approaches were considered. One focused on studying the bone–biomaterials interface that developed *in vivo*. The examination of bonding zone revealed the consistent presence of an interfacial HA layer (78,126). The other approach used *in vitro*

TABLE 11-9. COMPOSITION OF BIOACTIVE GLASSES AND GLASS CERAMICS (IN WEIGHT PERCENT)

Type	Code	SiO_2	CaO	Na_2O	P_2O_5	MgO	K_2O	CaF_2
Bioactive glass	45S5	45	24.5	24.5	6	—	—	—
	45S5F	45	12.5	24.5	6	—	—	12.5
	55S4.3	55	19.5	19.5	6	—	—	—
Bioactive glass ceramic	Ceravital	40–50	30–35	5–10	10–15	2.5–5	0.5–3	—
	A-W GC	34.2	44.9	—	16.3	4.6	—	0.5

immersions in simulated physiological fluids or cell-containing media (99,77,53). Upon immersion of bioactive glass in acellular, simulated body fluids (with ionic concentration and pH similar to the interstitial fluid) the following reactions take place (77):

Leaching of Na^+ (or K^+) into solution (i.e., exchange with H^+ or H_3O^+ from solution) and formation of SiOH (silanol):

$$-Si-O-Na + H^+ + OH \rightarrow -Si-O-H + Na^+ \text{ (solution)} + OH^-$$

Loss of soluble silica (SiO_2) and formation of SiOH:

$$-Si-O-Si- + H_2O \rightarrow -Si-OH + HO-Si-$$

Polycondensation of silanols to form hydrated silica gel:

$$O-Si-OH + HO-Si-O \rightarrow O-Si-O -Si-O + H_2O$$

Formation of amorphous calcium phosphate layer: Ca^{2+} and PO_4^{3-} migrate to the surface through the SiO_2-rich layer, forming a $CaO-P_2O_5$-rich layer on top of the SiO_2 gel layer (the $CaO-P_2O_5$ layer proceeds to grow by incorporation of soluble Ca^{2+} and PO_4^{3-} from solution).

In the absence of proteins and bone cells the amorphous calcium phosphate layer crystallizes into apatite on surface [either hydroxycarbonate apatite (HCA) or fluorapatite—CO_3^{2-} or F^-— from solution].

These reactions, however, do not occur as such *in vivo* or *in vitro* in the presence of proteins, the HA layer does not form on the glass surface. Only when osteoblasts are present on the bioactive glass surface does the HA surface form again, evidently as a result of cellular activity (53–57).

There is a good correlation between the ability of a biomaterial to develop an HA surface layer in acellular SBF and its ability to bond to bone. Therefore, the degree of bioactivity of biomaterials is evaluated based on their ability to develop an HA surface layer *in vitro*. As already stated, this does not necessarily imply that the above dissolution–precipitation reactions take place at the material–tissue fluid interface *in vivo*. In addition to the major difference in composition between tissue fluid and SBF as shown in Table 11-10, there is a considerable difference in the parametric conditions under which the above reactions take place *in vivo* and *in vitro*.

It is obvious from Table 11-10 that one cannot expect that the material behavior *in vitro* is similar to that *in vivo,* especially in the first few days after implantation where the wound healing mechanism is in effect. Figure 11-17 schematically shows a variety of events that were reported to occur at the bioactive ceramic–tissue interface (41). The list does not imply a ranking in terms of time sequence or importance: (a) dissolution from the ceramic (35,47,78,94,106,126,134);

TABLE 11-10. DIFFERENCES IN MEDIUM COMPOSITION AND PARAMETRIC CONDITIONS UNDER WHICH THE BIOACTIVITY REACTIONS AT THE BIOMATERIAL SURFACE TAKE PLACE *IN VIVO* AND *IN VITRO*

Parameter	SBF (Simulated Body Fluid)	Tissue Fluid
Cellularity	Acellular	Highly cellular
Protein content	No protein	Protein-rich
Replenishment	Non	Fluid turnover (blood circulation)
Variation in solution composition during contact	Limited to dissolution–precipitation	Unlimited, due to chemotaxis and macrophage activity
pH	7.4	Could reach 9 due to wound healing mechanism
Temperature	37°C	Could reach 40°C due to wound healing processes

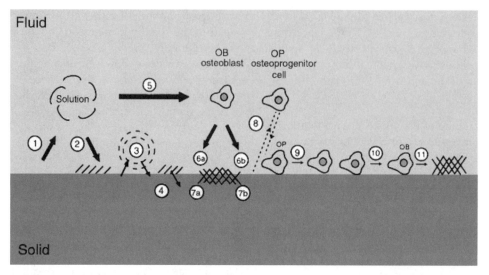

FIGURE 11-17. Schematic diagram representing the events that take place at the interface between bioactive ceramics and the surrounding biological environment (Reprinted from Ducheyne P, Bianco P, Radin S, et al. Bioactive materials: mechanisms and bioengineering considerations. In: Ducheyne P, Kokubo T, van Blitterswijk CA, eds. *Bone-bioactive biomaterials*. Leiderdorp, The Netherlands: Reed Healthcare Communications, 1993:1–12, with permission.)

(b) precipitation from solution onto the ceramic (27,34,106,126,134); (c) ion exchange and structural rearrangement at the ceramic-tissue interface (3,27,34,78,126,145); (d) interdiffusion from the surface boundary layer into the ceramic (46); (e) solution-mediated effects on cellular activity (71,86,129,145,159); (f) deposition of either the mineral phase or the organic phase, without integration into the ceramic surface (27,33,34,55,106); (g) deposition with integration into the ceramic (27, 106,145); (h) chemotaxis to the ceramic surface (145); (i) cell attachment and proliferation (33,71,86,92,118); (j) cell differentiation (145); and (k) extracellular matrix formation (33,55,118).

The observation of what transpires at the interface, however, does not represent a mechanistic explanation for the effect that bioceramics have on bone tissue formation. We can focus on mechanisms by relying on an increasing body of evidence that suggests that bone bonding and bone tissue ingrowth enhancement are the result of multiple, parallel, and sequential reactions at the material–tissue interface. These interactions either are related to physicochemical phenomena that occur in the presence or absence of cells, or are related to reactions affected by cellular activity. An important aspect of the overall reaction sequence between these materials and tissues is that, in the absence of a biologically equivalent, calcium-deficient, carbonate-containing hydroxyapatite (HCA) surface upon implantation, dissolution, precipitation, and ion-exchange reactions lead to a biologically equivalent apatitic surface on the implanted material. This reaction does not proceed by itself, but is accompanied by parallel reactions, such as adsorption and incorporation of biological molecules and attachment of surrounding cells. Furthermore, cells that have adhered to the ever-reacting material surface interact with the material and produce some of the surface changes. In the inverse direction, i.e., from material to environment, there is both a solution-mediated and a surface-controlled effect on cellular activity, organic matrix deposition, and mineralization. The gradual change of the ceramic surface to become a biologically equivalent HA with small crystal dimensions is a rate-determining step in the cascade of events underlying bioactive behavior. All phenomena, collectively, lead to the gradual incorporation of the bioactive implant into developing bone tissue.

7.5 Bioactive Glass Ceramics

Approaches to achieving enhanced mechanical and biochemical properties included transformation of bioactive glass into glass-ceramic, and using bioactive glass as a coating on a substrate or as a second phase in a composite combining the characteristics of both into a new material (77). In these techniques, bioactive glass is subjected to thermal treatments that alter the material's microstructure and limit its biological activity. Thermal treatment of bioactive glass (45S5) in the temperature range 550°C to 680°C resulted in the formation of $Na_2Ca_2Si_3O_9$ crystals (61). Raising the treatment temperature to 800°C led to the development of calcium phosphate crystals similar to the structure of HA (78). Other investigators showed that when bioactive glass in the system $MgO-CaO-SiO_2-P_2O_5$ was thermally treated, the glass transformed into apatite/wollastonite (A-W) glass ceramic (97). According to powder x-ray diffraction, the crystallized glass consisted of 38% apatite, 34% wollastonite, and 28 wt% residual glassy phase (97). The resulting bioactive A-W glass ceramic is characterized by a high mechanical strength (Table 11-11) and has been used successfully for load-bearing prostheses (75, 98,177). However, *in vivo* studies showed that the improved mechanical strength of bioactive glass ceramic is at the expense of the rate of bone bonding to the material (98,109).

An important change in the glass microstructure, which usually precedes crystallization, is the

TABLE 11-11. PHYSICAL PROPERTIES OF A-W BIOACTIVE GLASS CERAMIC

Density (g/cm^3)	3.07
Bending strength (MPa)	215
Compressive strength (MPa)	1,080
Young's modulus (GPa)	118
Vickers hardness (HV)	680
Fracture toughness (MPa $^1\!/_2$)	2.0

glass-in-glass phase separation (112). After separation, the glass no longer has a homogeneous composition, but rather, consists of two or more immiscible glassy phases of different chemical constituents. Unlike crystallization, phase separation in glass might not be visible by optical microscopy and in most cases can be detected only by electron microscopy. Previous work revealed that thermal treatment of bioactive glass at 550°C resulted in glass-in-glass phase separation and minor crystallization (58). These changes in bioactive glass microstructure altered the corrosion behavior and led to a significant increase in the negative ZP of the material. In conjunction with the increase in negative ZP there was a significant decrease in the amount of serum protein adsorption onto the material surface. The inhibition of protein adsorption could be responsible for the slow rate of bone bonding to bioactive glass ceramic. It is also possible that conformation changes inhibited the activity of the protein adsorbed onto thermally treated bioactive glass. Moreover, alteration of corrosion behavior after bioactive glass crystallization delayed the formation of the HA surface layer necessary for bone bonding.

8 TISSUE ENGINEERING AND RECENT DEVELOPMENTS

8.1 Bone Tissue Engineering

The field of tissue engineering has recently emerged as a result of growing understanding of the mechanism of action of biomaterials *in vitro* and *in vivo* combined with latest advances in cell isolation, culture procedures, molecular biology, and biochemistry techniques. Tissue engineering offers a promising new approach to repair fractures that do not heal, major bone loss, and fractures associated with bone tumors. In this approach, a porous scaffold that seeds the cells can serve as a vehicle to deliver cells necessary for tissue regeneration. With this approach, it is possible to use the patient's own cells so that immunosuppression is not needed. The design of a scaffolding material can significantly affect the cell seeding and growth both *in vitro* and *in vivo* (111). Scaffolding materials should be biocompatible and biodegradable. The degradation products should be nontoxic and easily excreted by metabolic pathways. The scaffold material should be mechanically strong to maintain structural integrity during culture. The ideal scaffolding materials also should be easy to fabricate into a desired shape and have a controlled porous architecture to allow for cell growth, tissue regeneration, and vascularization. The scaffolding materials should be osteoconductive so that osteoblasts and osteoprogenitor cells can adhere, migrate on the scaffolds, differentiate, and synthesize new bone matrix. The new tissue should also have the potential to grow and remodel, which is especially important for pediatric patients.

Use of degradable scaffolds to support cell proliferation and extracellular matrix synthesis implies a transient microenvironment that may influence cell behavior. Poly(α-hydroxyl acids), such as poly(L-lactic acid) (PLLA), poly(glycolic acid) (PGA), and poly(D,L-lactic acid-*co*-glycolic acid) (PLGA), satisfy many of these material requirements and already have been fabricated into scaffolds for cell transplantation and tissue engineering (81,84,178,179). One of the disadvantages of these materials is that the degradation products reduce the local pH value, which, in turn, may accelerate the polyesters' degradation rates (157) and induce an inflammatory reaction. Another disadvantage is that the mechanical properties of the highly porous scaffolds made from poly(α-hydroxyl acids) are relatively weak, which limits their use for bone tissue regeneration, especially in the *in vivo* implant site. Incorporation of HA with PLLA resulted in a compact composite with little porosity and improved mechanical strength. By monitoring for 24 weeks the pH value variations during their incubation in phosphate-buffered saline (PBS), it has been found that the pH value of PLLA/HA composite is more stable than that of pure PLLA and pure HA (142,167).

HA ceramic and its composites are composed of the same ions as bone and are considered to be suitable candidate materials for the synthesis of bone tissue engineering scaffold. However, HA ceramic, which is stoichiometric HA, re-

sorbs very slowly or remains unchanged in bone sites (95,114,115). Bioactive glass (45S5) is an attractive scaffold material because it stimulates osteoprogenitor cell function and possesses controlled resorbability (39,43,52,55,76,146). The goal is to use the *in vitro* synthesized bone as a graft material to treat major bone loss in orthopedic or maxillofacial surgery. Modification of the bioactive glass surface before cell seeding serves two goals: (a) to minimize the adverse effect on medium pH due to the accumulation of the bioactive glass degradation products and (b) to create the bioactive HA surface layer, which otherwise will not form in the presence of serum. It was discovered that the calcium phosphate layer that forms on the surface of bioactive glass is highly selective toward adsorption of serum fibronectin, an attachment protein known to enhance osteoblast adhesion and activity (53,54). Other bioactive materials such as HA ceramic or unmodified bioactive glasses do not have any selectivity toward fibronectin. Thus, when bone cells were cultured on bioactive glass pretreated to be covered with a dual layer of calcium phosphate and serum protein, abundant and expeditious bone tissue was formed on and within the porous template. Figure 11-18 is an SEM of the cross section of porous BG showing the formation of extracellular matrix and bonelike tissue after 7 days in culture. The cells also exhibited a high alkaline phosphatase activity and synthesized collagen type I and osteocalcin (57).

8.2 Engineering Surfaces with Peptides

Adherence of osteoblasts to a biomaterial surface is dependent on topography, chemistry, and surface energy. Cell attachment activity is also related to a tripeptide sequence, arginine-glycine-aspartic acid (RGD), located in the cell-binding domain of many adhesion molecules (144). Following attachment, there is reorganization of cytoskeletal proteins, resulting in the flattening and spreading of the cell and formation of focal contacts, replete with clustered integrins. This form of cytoskeletal organization participates in cell signaling events and serves to regulate cell

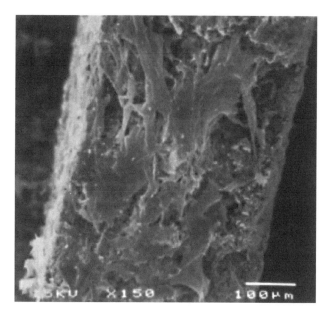

FIGURE 11-18. SEM micrograph of the fractured surface of the porous modified bioactive glass template seeded with neonatal rat calvaria osteoblasts for 7 days. Note the uniform formation of extracellular matrix and bonelike tissue throughout the porous disk. (With permission from El-Ghannom A, Ducheyne P, Shapiro IM. Bioactive material template for *in vitro* systhesis of bone. *J Biomed Mater Res* 1995;29:359–370.)

behavior (67). However, the adsorption of attachment proteins may not be successful in promoting long-term cell attachment to biomaterials *in vivo* because of several limitations. These include protein desorption and/or exchange and denaturation, the removal of the oligopeptide sequences due to proteolysis, difficulties in controlling the sequence presentation (i.e., C- or N-terminus binding), and specifically arranging a sequence or a series of sequences on the surface (117,138).

In order to derivatize in a stable manner the surfaces with RGD-sequence peptides, covalent immobilization of the active peptide is necessary. The use of covalently coupled small peptide mimics allows control over the density and orientation of ligand attachment. Many investigators have bound RGD peptides to polymeric surfaces and evaluated cell activity (116,132). These studies have shown that the chemistry of the surface layer can modify the conformation of the peptide and thereby change its interaction with cells. For example, Drumheller and Hubbell showed that complete cell spreading on poly(ethylene glycol) networks required a peptide density three orders of magnitude greater than that required for silanated glass (38). A 15-mer peptide containing the RGD motif grafted onto a quartz surface enhanced the strength of bone cell attachment and promoted spreading and focal contact formation (141). In a parallel investigation, the surface of quartz was engineered to contain different ratios of cell binding (–RGD–) and heparin binding (–FHRRIKA–) domains (140). It was found that heterogeneous peptides containing –RGD– and –FHRRIKA– in the ratio 75:25 or 50:50 enhanced cell spreading and mineralization compared with homogenous surfaces containing either –RGD– or –FHRRIKA–. Results of the studies discussed above provide evidence that the immobilized peptides containing the RGD sequence serve to enhance cell attachment to polymeric and ceramic surfaces. In most cases, the biomaterial exhibits a new topography, surface chemistry, and functionality depending on the modification strategy. Even the method chosen to activate the surface (e.g., wet versus dry chemistry) can alter the biomaterial surface properties.

Cell behavior on surfaces grafted with the minimal tripeptide RGD devoid of any flanking groups or spacers was investigated. Using an atomically smooth silicon substrate covered with a reproducible oxide layer, the oxide surface was activated using 3-aminopropyl triethoxysilane (APTS) (51). This layer exhibited nanoscale roughness and presented amine functional groups for grafting the RGD tripeptide. The attachment of RGD to the APTS surface was confirmed by time-of-flight secondary ion mass spectrometry analyses. Contact angle measurements indicated that the hydrophobicity of the APTS surface was significantly lower than that of the surface with grafted RGD (RGD-APTS). Atomic force microscopy roughness measurement values showed that surfaces covered with RGD-APTS were smoother (Ra = 0.71 nm) than those covered with APTS alone (Ra = 1.59 nm). MC3T3-E1 bone cells were seeded on these various substrates and incubated in a serum-free medium for different periods of time. Whereas attachment was similar on both APTS and RGD-APTS surfaces, cell spreading and cytoskeletal organization were clearly favored on the relatively smooth grafted peptide surface. Thus, neither surface roughness nor the amine group alone of the APTS layer account for improved cell–biomaterial interaction. These data suggest that the combination of surface roughness and RGD modification provides the most favorable surface for cell spreading and cytoskeletal organization. These events significantly enhanced downstream maturation-related activities such as those linked to cytodifferentiation and mineralization of the extracellular matrix.

REFERENCES

1. Aebli N, Krebs J, Schwenke D, et al. Degradation of hydroxyapatite coating on a well-functioning femoral component. *J Bone Joint Surg* 2003;85-B,4:499–503.
2. Agarwal AG, Broutman LJ. *Analysis and performance of fiber composites.* New York: John Wiley & Sons, 1980.
3. Andersson OH, Karlsson KH, Kangasniemi K. Calcium-phosphate formation at the surface of bioactive glass in vivo. *J Non-Cryst Solids* 1990;119:290–296.
4. Atkinson JR, Jobbins B. Properties of engineering materials for use in the body. In: Dowson D, Wright V, eds. *Introduction to the biomechanics of joints and joint replacement.* London: Mechanical Engineering Publications, 1981.
5. Bartel DL, Bicknell VL, Wright TM. The effect of conformity, thickness, and material on stresses in ultra-high molecular weight components for total joint replacement. *J Bone Joint Surg Am* 1986;68:1041–1051.
6. Bigsby RJA, Hardaker CS, Fisher J. Wear of ultra-high molecular weight polyethylene acetabular cups in a physiological hip joint simulator in the anatomical position using bovine serum as a lubricant. *Proc Inst Mech Eng* 1997;211H:265–269.
7. Black J, Oppenheimer P, Morris DM, et al. Release of corrosion products by F-75 cobalt base alloy in the rat III: effects of a carbon surface coating. *J Biomed Mater Res* 1987;21:1213–1230.
8. Bloebaum R, Beeks D, Dorr L, et al. Complications with hydroxyapatite particulate separation in total hip arthroplasty. *Clin Orthop* 1994;298:19–26.
9. Bloebaum RD, Dupont JA. Osteolysis from a pressfit hydroxyapatite implant: a case study. *J Arthroplasty* 1993;8:195–203.
10. Bohler M, Knahr K, Plenk H Jr, et al. Long-term results of uncemented alumina acetabular implants. *J Bone Joint Surg*, 1994;76B:53–59.
11. Boutin P, Christel PS, Dorlot JM, et al. The use of dense alumina–alumina combination in total hip replacement. *J Biomed Mater Res* 1988;22:1203–1209.
12. Bowsher JG, Shelton JC. The influence of stumbling on the wear of ultra-high molecular weight polyethylene. In: *Proceedings of the Sixth World Biomaterials Congress Transactions, Society for Biomaterials,* Hawaii, 2000;2:867.
13. Bragdon CR, O'Connor DO, Lowenstein JD, et al. The importance of multidirectional motion on the wear of polyethylene. *Proc Inst Mech Eng* 1996;210:157–165.
14. Brown SA, Farnsworth LJ, Merritt K, et al. Biological significance of metal ion release. *J Biomed Mater Res* 1988;22:321–338.
15. Brown SA, Merritt K, Farnsworth LJ, et al. In vitro and in vivo metal ion release. In: Lemons JE, ed. *ASTM STP 953—quantitative characterization and performance of porous implants for hard tissue applications.* Philadelphia: ASTM, 1987:163–181.
16. Bruckman H, Huttinger KJ. Carbon in endoprosthetics, Part I. *Biomaterials* 1980:1:67–72.
17. Capello WN. Hydroxyapatite in total hip arthroplasty: five-year clinical experience. *Orthopedics* 1994;17:781–792.
18. Catelas I, Huk OL, Petit A, et al. Flow cytometric analysis of macrophage response to ceramic and polyethylene particles: effects of size, concentration, and composition. *J Biomed Mater Res* 1998;41:600–607.
19. Catelas I, Petit A, Zukor DJ, et al. Induction of macrophage apoptosis by ceramic and polyethylene particles in vitro. *Biomaterials* 1999;20:625–630.

20. Catelas I, Petit A, Marchand D, et al. Cytotoxicity and macrophage cytokine release induced by ceramic and polyethylene particles in vitro. *J Bone Joint Surg Br* 1999;81:516–521.

21. Clarke IC, Good V, Williams P. Simulator wear study of high dose gamma irradiated UHMWPE cups. *Trans Soc Biomater* 1997;20:71.

22. Clarke IC, Good V, Anissian L, et al. Charnley wear model for validation of hip simulators: ball diameter versus polytetrafluoroethylene and polyethylene wear. *Proc Inst Mech Eng* 1997;211H:25–36.

23. Cohen JJ. Apoptosis. *Immunol Today* 1993;14: 126–130.

24. Collier JP, Sutula LC, Currier BH, et al. Overview of polyethylene as a bearing material: comparison of sterilization methods. *Clin Orthop* 1996;333:76–86.

25. Cooper JR, Dowson D, Fisher J. Macroscopic and microscopic wear mechanisms in ultra-high molecular weight polyethylene. *Wear* 1993;162–164:378–384.

26. Currier BH, Currier JH, Collier JP, et al. Effect of fabrication method and resin type on performance of tibial bearings. *J Biomed Mater Res* 2000;53:143–151.

27. Daculsi G, LeGeros RZ, Nery E, et al. Transformation of biphasic calcium phosphate ceramics in vivo: ultrastructural and physicochemical characterization. *J Biomed Mater Res* 1989;23:883–894.

28. Dalton JE, Cook SD. In vivo mechanical and histological characteristics of HA-coated implants vary with coating vendor. *J Biomed Mater Res* 1995;29:239–245.

29. D'Antonio JA, Capello WN, Crothers OD, et al. Early clinical experience with hydroxyapatite-coated femoral implants. *J Bone Joint Surg* 1992;74A:995–1007.

30. D'Antonio JA, Capello WN, Jaffe WL. Hydroxyapatite-coated hip implants. Multicenter three-year clinical and roentgenographic results. *Clin Orthop* 1992;285:102–115.

31. D'Antonio JA, Capello WN, Manley MT, et al. Hydroxyapatite femoral stems for total hip arthroplasty: 10- to 13-year followup. *Clin Orthop* 2001;393:101–111.

32. Davies JE, Pilliar RM, Smith DC, et al. Bone interfaces with retrieved alumina and hydroxyapatite ceramics. In: Bonfield W, Towner KE, Hastings G, eds. *Bioceramics.* Oxford: Butterworth, 1991;4:199–204.

33. de Bruijn JD, Davies JE, Klein CPAT, et al. Biological responses to calcium-phosphate ceramics. In: Ducheyne P, Kokubo T, van Blitterswijk CA, eds. *Bone-bonding biomaterials.* Leiderdorp, The Netherlands: Reed Healthcare Communications, 1993:57–72.

34. de Bruijn JD, Bovell YP, van Blitterswijk CA. Structural arrangements at the interface between plasma sprayed calcium-phosphates and bone. *Biomaterials* 1994;15:543–550.

35. de Bruijn JD, Flach TS, Leenders H, et al. Degradation and interface characteristics of plasma sprayed hydroxyapatite coatings with different crystallinities. In: Yamamuro T, Kokubo T, Nakamura T, eds. *Bioceramics.* Kyoto: Kobunshi Kankokai, 1992;5:291–298.

36. Devine TM, Wulff J. Cast vs. wrought cobalt-chromium surgical implant alloys. *J Biomed Mater Res* 1975;9:151–176.

37. Dorlot JM, Christel P, Meunier A. Wear analysis of retrieved alumina ceramic heads and sockets of hip prostheses. *J Biomed Mater Res* 1989;23:299–310.

38. Drumheller PD, Hubbell JA. Polymer networks with grafted cell adhesion peptides for highly biospecific cell adhesive substrates. *Anal Biochem* 1994;222:380–388.

39. Ducheyne P. Stimulation of biological function with bioactive glass. *MRS Bull* 1998;23:43–49.

40. Ducheyne P, Beight J, Cuckler J, et al. Effect of calcium-phosphate coating characteristics on early post-operative bone tissue ingrowth. *Biomaterials* 1990;11:531–540.

41. Ducheyne P, Bianco P, Radin S, et al. Bioactive materials: mechanisms and bioengineering considerations. In: Ducheyne P, Kokubo T, van Blitterswijk CA, eds. *Bone-bioactive biomaterials.* Leiderdorp, The Netherlands: Reed Healthcare Communications, 1993:1–12.

42. Ducheyne P, Cuckler JM. Bioactive ceramic prosthetic coatings. *Clin Orthop* 1992;276:102–112.

43. Ducheyne P, El-Ghannam A, Shapiro I. Effect of bioactive glass templates on osteoblast proliferation and in vitro synthesis of bone-like tissue. *J Cell Biochem* 1994;56:162–167.

44. Ducheyne P, Healy KE. The effect of plasma-sprayed calcium phosphate ceramic coatings on the metal ion release from porous titanium and cobalt-chromium alloys. *J Biomed Mater Res* 1988;22:1137–1163.

45. Ducheyne P, Hench LL, Kagan A, et al. Effect of hydroxyapatite impregnation on skeletal bonding of porous coated implants. *J Biomed Mater Res* 1980;14:225–237.

46. Ducheyne P, Kim CS, Pollack SR. The effect of phase differences on the time-dependent variation of the zeta potential of hydroxyapatite. *J Biomed Mater Res* 1992;26:147–168.

47. Ducheyne P, Radin S, King L. The effect of calcium-phosphate ceramic composition and structure on in vitro behavior. I. Dissolution. *J Biomed Mater Res* 1993;27:25–34.

48. Ducheyne P, Willems G, Martens M, et al. In vivo metal ion release from porous titanium fiber material. *J Biomed Mater Res* 1984;18:293–308.

49. Edidin AA, Pruitt L, Jewett CW, et al. Plasticity-induced damage layer is a precursor to wear in radiation-cross-linked UHMWPE acetabular components for total hip replacement. Ultra-high-molecular-weight polyethylene. *J Arthroplasty* 1999;14:616–627.

50. Edidin AA, Kurtz SM. Influence of mechanical behavior on the wear of 4 clinically relevant polymeric biomaterials in a hip simulator. *J Arthroplasty* 2000;15:321–331.

51. El-Ghannam A, Ducheyne P, Shapiro IM, et al. Engineering RGD peptide surface regulates adhesion, spreading and cytoskeletal organization of osteoblast-like cells. *Bioceramics* 2002;14:245–248.

52. El-Ghannam A, Ducheyne P, Shapiro IM. Bioactive material template for in vitro synthesis of bone tissue. In: *Proceedings of the 19th annual meeting, Society for Biomaterials.* 1993;XVI:9.

53. El-Ghannam A, Ducheyne P, Shapiro IM. Formation of surface reaction products on bioactive glass and their effects on the expression of the osteoblastic phenotype and the deposition of mineralized extracellular matrix. *Biomaterials* 1997;18:295–303.

54. El-Ghannam A, Ducheyne P, Shapiro IM. Effect of serum protein adsorption on osteoblast adhesion to bioactive glass and hydroxyapatite. *J Orthop Res* 1999;17:340–345.

55. El-Ghannam A, Ducheyne P, Shapiro IM. Bioactive material template for in vitro synthesis of bone. *J Biomed Mater Res* 1995;29:359–370.

56. El-Ghannam A, Ducheyne P, Shapiro I. Bioactive glass templates for the synthesis of bone-like tissue in vitro. In: Mikos AG, Murphy RM, Bernstein H, Peppas NA, eds. *Biomaterials for cell and drug delivery.* Pittsburgh: Materials Research Society, 1994:257–262.

57. El-Ghannam A, Ducheyne P, Shapiro IM. Porous bioactive glass and hydroxyapatite ceramic affect bone cell function in vitro along different time lines. *J Biomed Mater Res* 1997;36:167–180.

58. El-Ghannam A, Hamazawy E, Yehia A. Effect of thermal treatment on bioactive glass microstructure, corrosion behavior, potential, and protein adsorption. *J Biomed Mater Res* 2001;55:387–395.

59. Farizon F, de Lavison R, Azoulai JJ, et al. Results with a cementless alumina-coated cup with dual mobility. A twelve-year follow-up study. *Int Orthop* 1998;22:219–224.

60. Ferguson AB Jr, Laing PG, Hodge ES. The ionization of metal implants in living tissues. *J Bone Joint Surg* 1960;42A:77–90.

61. Filho OP, LaTorre GP, Hench LL. Effect of crystallization on apatite layer formation of bioactive glass 45S5. *J Biomed Mater Res* 1996;30:509–514.

62. Fisher J, Dowson D. Tribology of total artificial joints. *Proc Inst Mech Eng* 1991;205:73–79.

63. Frayssinet P, Vidalain JP, Ranz X, et al. Hydroxyapatite particle migration. *Eur J Orthop Surg Traumatol* 1999:9:95–109.

64. Geesink RG. Osteoconductive coatings for total joint arthroplasty. *Clin Orthop* 2002;395:53–65.

65. Geesink RG. Hydroxyapatite-coated total hip prostheses. *Clin Orthop* 1990;261:39–58.

66. Geesink RG, Hoefnagels NH. Six year results of hydroxyapatite-coated total hip replacement. *J Bone Joint Surg* 1995;77B:534–547.

67. Giancotti FG, Rouslahti E. Integrin signaling. *Science* 1999;285:1028–1032.

68. Goldman M, Pruitt L. Comparison of the effects of gamma radiation and low temperature hydrogen peroxide gas plasma sterilisation on the molecular structure, fatigue resistance, and wear behaviour of UHMWPE. *J Biomed Mater Res* 1998;40:378–384.

69. Goldring SR, Schiller AL, Roelke M, et al. The synovial-like membrane at the bone–cement interface in loose total hip replacements and its proposed role in bone lysis. *J Bone Joint Surg Am* 1983;65:575–584.

70. Greer K, Richard R, King R. The properties of UHMWPE following annealing above the melt. In: *47th annual meeting, Orthopedic Research Society* 2001:1016.

71. Gregoire M, Orly I, Manankau J. The influence of calcium-phosphate biomaterials on human bone cell activities. An in vitro approach. *J Biomed Mater Res* 1990;24:165–177.

72. Hatton A, Nevelos JE, Nevelos AA, et al. Alumina–alumina artificial hip joints. Part i: a histological analysis and characterisation of wear debris by laser capture microdissection of tissues retrieved at revision. *Biomaterials* 2000;23-16:3429–3440.

73. Healy KE, Ducheyne P. Oxidation kinetics of titanium thin films in model physiologic environment. *J Colloid Interface Sci* 1992;150(2):404–417.

74. Healy KE, Ducheyne P. The mechanisms of passive dissolution of titanium in a model physiological environment. *Trans Soc Biomater* 1989;15:147.

75. Hench LL. Bioceramics: from concept to clinics. *J Am Ceram Soc* 1991;74:1487–1510.

76. Hench LL. Bioactive ceramics. In: Ducheyne P, Lemons JE, eds. *Bioceramics: material characteristics versus in vivo behavior.* New York: The New York Academy of Sciences, 1988:54–71.

77. Hench LL, Andersson O. Bioactive glasses. In: Hench L, Wilson J, eds. *An introduction to bioceramics.* New Jersey: World Scientific, 1993:41–62.

78. Hench L, Splinter R, Greenlee T, et al. Bonding mechanisms at the interface of ceramic prosthetic materials. *J Biomed Eng* 1971;2:117–141.

79. Henssge EJ, Bos I, Willman G. Al_2O_3 against Al_2O_3 combination in hip endoprostheses. histologic investigations with semiquantitative grading of revision and autopsy cases and abrasion measures. *J Mater Sci Mater Med* 1994;5:657–661.

80. Hernandez CP, Najera SO, Mesa RF, et al. Hydroxyapatite-coated stems with metaphyseal and diaphyseal press-fit. Eleven-year follow-up results. *Acta Orthop Belg* 2002;68:24–32.

81. Heughebaert M, LeGeros RZ, Gineste M, et al. Physicochemical characterization of deposits associated with HA ceramics implanted in nonosseous sites. *J Biomed Mater Res* 1988;22(3 Suppl):257–268.

82. Hoar TP, Mears DC. Corrosion resistant alloys in chloride solutions: materials for surgical implants. *Proc R Soc London* 1966;A294:486.

83. Hoffinger SA, Keggi KJ, Zatorski LE. Primary ceramic hip replacement: a prospective study of 119 hips. *Orthopaedics* 1991;14:523–531.

84. Holmes RE. Osteoconduction in hydroxyapatite-based materials. In: Brighton CT, Friedlaender G, Lane JM, eds. *Bone formation and repair.* Rosemont: American Academy of Orthopedic Surgeons, 1994:355–365.

85. Howie DW, Haynes DR, Rogers SD, et al. The response to particulate debris. *Orthop Clin North Am* 1993;24:571–581.

86. Hyakuna K, Yamamuro T, Kotoura Y, et al. The influence of calcium-phosphate ceramics and glass–ceramics on cultured cells and their surrounding media. *J Biomed Mater Res* 1989;23:1049–1066.

87. Jacobs JJ, Gilbert JL, Urban RM. Corrosion of metal orthopaedic implants. *J Bone Joint Surg* 1998;8OA:268–282.

88. Jarcho M, Kay JF, Gumaer KI, et al. Tissue, cellular and subcellular events at a bone–ceramic hydroxylapatite interface. *J Bioeng* 1977;1:79–92.

89. Jasty M. Clinical reviews: particulate debris and failure of total hip replacements. *J Appl Biomater* 1993;4:273–276.

90. Jasty M, Goetz DD, Bragdon CR, et al. Wear of polyethylene acetabular components in total hip arthroplasty. An analysis of one hundred and twenty-eight components retrieved at autopsy or revision operations. *J Bone Joint Surg Am* 1997;79:349–358.

91. Kawamoto K, Hasegawa Y, Iwase T, et al. Failed cementless total hip arthroplasty for osteoarthrosis due to hip dysplasia. A minimum five-year follow-up study. *Bull Hosp Joint Dis* 1998;57:130–135.

92. Keeting PE, Oursler MJ, Weigand KE, et al. Zeolite A increases proliferation, differentiation, and transforming growth factor beta production in normal adult human osteoblast-like cells in vitro. *J Bone Miner Res* 1992;7:1281–1289.

93. Kim YH, Kim VE. Cementless porous-coated anatomic medullary locking total hip prostheses. *J Arthroplasty* 1994;9:243–252.

94. Klein CP, Driessen AA, de Groot K, et al. Biodegradation behavior of various calcium phosphate materials in bone tissue. *J Biomed Mater Res* 1983;17:769–784.

95. Klein C, Patka P, den Hollander W. Macroporous calcium phosphate bioceramics in dog femora: a histological study of interface and biodegradation. *Biomaterials* 1989;10:59–62.

96. Koegel A, Black I. Release of corrosion products by F-75 cobalt base alloy in the rat. I: acute serum elevations. *J Biomed Mater Res* 1984;18:513–522.

97. Kokubo T, Ito S, Sakka S, Yamamuro T. Formation of a high strength bioactive glass ceramic in the system $MgO-CaO-SiO_2-P_2O_5$. *J Mater Sci* 1986;21:536–540.

98. Kokubo T, Kushitani H, Ohtsuki C, et al. Chemical reaction of bioactive glass and glass ceramics with a simulated body fluid. *Mater Med* 1992;3:79–83.

99. Kokubo T, Kushitani H, Sakka S, et al. Solutions able to reproduce in vivo surface-structure changes in bioactive glass–ceramic A-W. *J Biomed Mater Res* 1990;24:721–734.

100. Kummer FJ, Stuchin SA, Frankel H. Analysis of removed autophor ceramic on ceramic components from mittelmeier total hip athroplasties. *J Arthroplasty* 1990;5:28–33.

101. Kurtz SM, Muhlstein C, Edidin AA. Surface morphology and wear mechanisms of four clinically relevant biomaterials after hip simulator testing. *J Biomed Mater Res* 2000;52:447–459.

102. Kurtz SM, Pruitt LA, Jewett CW, et al. Radiation and chemical cross-linking promote strain hardening behavior and molecular alignment in ultra high molecular weight polyethylene during multi-axial loading conditions. *Biomaterials* 1999;20:1449–1462.

103. Lacombe P. Corrosion and oxidation of Ti and Ti alloys. In: Williams JC, Belov AF, eds. *Titanium and titanium alloys.* New York: Plenum Press, 1982:847–880.

104. Laing PG, Ferguson AB Jr, Hodge ES. Tissue reaction in rabbit muscle exposed to metallic implants. *J Biomed Mater Res* 1967;1:135–149.

105. Laurent MP, Yao JQ, Bhambri SK, et al. High cycle wear of highly cross-linked UHMWPE acetabular liners evaluated in a hip simulator. In: *Proceedings of the Sixth World Biomaterials Congress Transactions, Society for Biomaterials,* Hawaii, 2000;2:851.

106. LeGeros RZ, Daculsi G, Orly I, et al. Formation of carbonate apatite on calcium phosphate materials: dissolution/precipitation processes. In: Ducheyne P, Kokubo T, van Blitterswijk CA, eds. *Bone-bonding biomaterials.* Leiderdorp, The

Netherlands: Reed Healthcare Communications, 1993:201–212.

107. Lerouge S, Huk O, Yahia LH, et al. Characterization of in vivo wear debris from ceramic-ceramic total hip arthroplasties. *J Biomed Mater Res* 1996;32:627–633.

108. Lerouge S, Huk O, Yahia L'H, et al. Ceramic-ceramic and metal-polyethylene total hip replacements. Comparison of pseudomembranes after loosening. *J Bone Joint Surg Br* 1997;79:135–139.

109. Li P, Yang Q, Zhang F, et al. The effect of residual glassy phase in a bioactive ceramic on the formation of its surface apatite layer *in vitro*. *J Biomed Mater Res* 1992;3:452–456.

110. Linder L. Implant stability, histology, RSA and wear: more critical questions are needed. *Acta Orthop Scand* 1994;65:654–658.

111. Ma PX, Langer R. Fabrication of biodegradable polymer foams for cell transplantation and tissue engineering. In: Yarmush M, Morgan J, eds. *Tissue engineering methods and protocols*. Totowa, NJ: Humana Press, 1999;1:15–28.

112. MacMillan PW. *Glass ceramics*. London: Academic Press, 1979:40.

113. Mahoney OM, Dimon JH. Unsatisfactory results with a ceramic total hip prosthesis. *J Bone Joint Surg* 1990;72A:663–665.

114. Martin RB, Chapman MW, Sharkey NA, et al. Bone ingrowth and mechanical properties of coralline hydroxyapatite 1 yr after implantation. *Biomaterials* 1993;14:341–348.

115. Martin RB, Chapman MW, Holmes RE, et al. Effects of bone ingrowth on the strength and non-invasive assessment of a coralline hydroxyapatite material. *Biomaterials* 1989;10:481–488.

116. Massia SP, Hubbell JA. Covalently attached GRGD on polymer surfaces promotes biospecific adhesion of mammalian cells. *Ann N Y Acad Sci* 1990;589:261–270.

117. Massia SP, Hubbell J. Covalent surface immobilization of Arg-Gly-Asp and Tyr-Ile-Gly-Ser-Arg containing peptides to obtain well-defined cell-adhesive substrates. *Anal Biochem* 1990;187:292–301.

118. Matsuda T, Davies JE. The in vitro response of osteoblasts to bioactive glass. *Biomaterials* 1987;8:275–284.

119. McKellop HA, Wear assessment. In: Callaghan JJ, Rosenberg AG, Rubash HE, eds. *The adult hip*. Philadelphia: Lippincott-Raven, 1998.

120. McKellop HA, Campbell P, Park SH, et al. The origin of submicron polyethylene wear debris in total hip arthroplasty. *Clin Orthop* 1995;311:3–20.

121. McKellop H, Shen F, Lu B, et al. Development of an extremely wear-resistant ultra-high molecular weight polyethylene for total hip replacements. *J Orthop Res* 1999;17:157–167.

122. Merritt K, Brown SA, Sharkey NA. The binding of metal salts and corrosion products to cells and proteins in vitro. *J Biomed Mater Res* 1984;18:1005–1015.

123. Merritt K, Crowe TD, Brown SA. Elimination of nickel, cobalt, and chromium following repeated injections of high dose metal salts. *J Biomed Mater Res* 1989;23:845–862.

124. Mittelmeier H, Heisel J. Sixteen-years experience with ceramichip prostheses. *Clin Orthop* 1992;282:64–74.

125. Muratoglu OK, Bragdon CR, O'Connor DO, et al. Unified wear model for highly cross-linked ultra-high molecular weight polyethylene (UHMWPE). *Biomaterials* 1999;20:1463–1470.

126. Neo M, Nakaruma T, Yamamuro T, et al. Transmission microscopic study of apatite formation on bioactive ceramics in vivo. In: Ducheyne P, Kokubo T, van Blitterswijk CA, eds. *Bone-bonding biomaterials*. Leiderdorp, The Netherlands: Reed Healthcare Communications, 1993:111–120.

127. Nevelos JE, Ingham E, Doyle C, et al. Analysis of retrieved alumina ceramic components from Mittelmeier total hip prostheses. *Biomaterials* 1999;20:1833–1840.

128. Nizard RS, Sedel L, Christel P, et al. Ten-year survivorship of cemented ceramic–ceramic total hip prostheses. *Clin Orthop* 1992;282:53–63.

129. Ohgushi H, Goldberg VM, Caplan AI. Heterotopic osteogenesis in porous ceramics induced by marrow cells. *J Orthop Res* 1989;7:568–578.

130. Oonishi H, Tsuji E, Kim YY. Retrieved total hip prostheses—Part II. Wear behaviour and structural changes. *J Mater Sci Mater Med* 1998;10:575–581.

131. Oonishi H, Kushitani S, Yasukawa E, et al. Particulate bioglass compared with hydroxyapatite as a bone graft substitute. *Clin Orthop Rel Res* 1997;334:316–325.

132. Pakalns T, Haverstick KL, Fields GB, et al. Cellular recognition of synthetic peptide amphiphiles in self-assembled monolayer films. *Biomaterials* 1999;20:2265–2279.

133. Park JB, Lakes RS. Metallic implant materials. In: *Biomaterials—an introduction*. New York: Plenum Publishing, 1992;75–115.

134. Patka P, den Hollander W, Klein CPAT, et al. Behavior of ceramics, hydroxyapatite, and tricalcium phosphate in bone. *Trans Soc Biomater* 1989;15:103.

135. Petit A, Catelas I, Antoniou J, et al. Differential apoptotic response of J774 macrophages to alumina and ultra-high-molecular-weight polyethylene particles. *J Orthop Res* 2002;20-1:9–15.

136. Pilliar RM, Weatherly GC. Developments in implant alloys. In: Williams DF, ed. *CRC critical reviews in biocompatibility*. Boca Raton, FL: CRC Press, 1986;1:371–403.

137. Ramamurti BS, Bragdon CR, Do OC, et al. Loci of movement of selected points on the femoral head during normal gait: three-dimensional computer simulation. *J Arthroplasty* 1996;11:845–852.

138. Ranieri JP, Bellamkonda R, Bekos EJ, et al. Neuronal cell attachment to fluorinated ethylene propylene films with covalently immobilized laminin oligo-peptides YIGSR and IKAV II. *J Biomed Mater Res* 1995;29:779–785.

139. Reikeras O, Gunderson RB. Failure of HA coating on a grit-blasted acetabular cup: 155 patients followed for 7–10 years. *Acta Orthop Scand* 2002;73:104–108.

140. Rezania A, Healy KE. Biomimetic peptide surfaces that regulate adhesion, spreading, cytoskeletal organization and minerlization of the matrix deposited by osteoblast-like cells. *Biotechnol Prog* 1999;15:19–32.

141. Rezania A, Thomas CH, Branger AB, et al. The detachment strength and morphology of bone cells containing materials modified with a peptide sequence found within bone sialoprotein. *J Biomed Mater Res* 1997;37:9–19.

142. Ribeiro AS, Malafaya PB, Reis RL. Two new routes for producing porous bioactive ceramics: polyurethane precursors microwave baking. In: LeGeros RZ, LeGeros JP, eds. *Bioceramics 11.* New York: World Scientific, 1998:735–738.

143. Rothman RH, Hozack WJ, Ranawat A, et al. Hydroxyapatite-coated femoral stems. *J Bone Joint Surg* 1996;78A:319–324.

144. Ruoslahti E. RGD and other recognition sequences for integrin. *Annu Rev Cell Dev Biol* 1996;12:697–715.

145. Schepers E, Declercq M, Ducheyne P, et al. Bioactive glass particulate material as a filler for bone lesions. *J Oral Rehab* 1991;18:439–452.

146. Schepers EJG, Ducheyne P. Bioactive glass particles of narrow size range for the treatment of oral bone defects: a 1–24 month experiment with several materials and particle sizes and size ranges. *J Oral Rehab* 1997;24:171–181.

147. Schepers EJG, Ducheyne P, Barbier L, et al. Bioactive glass particles of narrow size range: a new material for the repair of bone defects. *Implant Dent* 1993;2:151–156.

148. Schmalzried TP, Szuszczewicz ES, Northfield MR, et al. Quantitative assessment of walking activity after total hip or knee replacement. *J Bone Joint Surg Am* 1998;80:54–59.

149. Scott DL, Campbell PA, McClung CD, et al. Factors contributing to rapid wear and osteolysis in hips with modular acetabular bearings made of hylamer. *J Arthroplasty* 2000;15:35–46.

150. Shapoff CA, Alexander DC, Clark AE. Clinical use of bioactive glass particulate in the treatment of human osseous defects. *Compodium* 1997;18:352–363.

151. Soballe K. Hydroxyapatite ceramic coating for bone implant fixation. Mechanical and histological studies in dogs. *Acta Orthop Scand* 1993;255:1–58.

152. Stanley HR, Hall MB, Clark AE, et al. Using 45S5 bioglass cones as endosseous ridge maintenance implants to prevent alveolar ridge resorption: a 5-year evaluation. *Int J Oral Maxillofac Implants* 1997;12:95–105.

153. Stea S, Visentin M, Granchi D, et al. Cytokines and osteolysis around hip prostheses. *Cytokine* 2000;12:1575–1579.

154. Sunderman FW Jr, Hopfer SM, Swift T, et al. Cobalt, chromium, and nickel concentrations in body fluids of patients with porous-coated knee or hip prostheses. *J Orthop Res* 1989;7:307–315.

155. Thornhill TS, Ozuna RM, Shortkroff S, et al. Biochemical and histological evaluation of the synovial-like tissue around failed (loose) total joint replacement prostheses in human subjects and a canine model. *Biomaterials* 1990;11:69–72.

156. Tracy BM, Doremus RH. Direct electron microscopy studies of the bone-hydroxylapatite interface. *J Biomed Mater Res* 1984;18:719–726.

157. Vacanti CA, Bonassar LJ. An overview of tissue engineered bone. *Clin Orthop* 1999;367:S375–S381.

158. Vidalain JP. The corail system in primary THA: results, lessons and comments from the series performed by the ARTRO Group (12-year experience). *Eur J Orthop Surg Traumatol* 1999;9:87–90.

159. Vrouwenvelder WC, Groot CG, de Groot K. Histological and biochemical evaluation of osteoblasts cultured on bioactive glass, hydroxylapatite, titanium alloy, and stainless steel. *J Biomed Mater Res* 1993;27:465–475.

160. Walter A. On the material and the tribology of alumina-alumina couplings for hip joint prostheses. *Clin Orthop* 1992;282:31–46.

161. Wang A, Essner A, Polineni VK, et al. Lubrication and wear of ultra-high molecular weight polyethylene in total joint replacements. *Tribol Int* 1998;31:17–33.

162. Wang A, Essner A, Polineni VK, et al. Polyethylene wear in orthopaedic implants. *Workshop Soc Biomater* 1997;22:4–18.

163. Wang A, Essner A, Stark C, et al. Comparison of the size and morphology of UHMWPE wear debris produced by a hip joint simulator under serum and water lubricated conditions. *Biomaterials* 1996;17:865–871.

164. Wang A, Stark C, Dumbleton JH. Role of cyclic plastic deformation in the wear of UHMWPE acetabular cups. *J Biomed Mater Res* 1995;29:619–626.

165. Wang A, Stark C, Dumbleton JH. Mechanistic and morphological origins of ultra-high molecular weight polyethylene wear debris in total joint replacement prostheses. *Proc Inst Mech Eng* 1996;210:141–155.

166. Wapner KL, Morris DM, Black I. Release of corrosion products by F-75 cobalt based alloy in the rat II. Morbidity apparently associated with chromium release in vivo: a 120 day rat study. *J Biomed Mater Res* 1986;20:219–233.

167. White R, Weber J, White E. Replamineform: a new process for preparing porous ceramic, metal and polymer prosthetic materials. *Science* 1972;176:922–924.

168. Williams DF. Biocompatibility of clinical implant materials. In: Williams DF, ed. *Biocompatibility of clinical implant materials,* Vol. I. Boca Raton, FL: CRC Press, 1981:9–44.

169. Williams IR, Mayor MB, Collier JP. The impact of sterilization method on wear in knee arthroplasty. *Clin Orthop* 1998;356:170–180.

170. Willman G. Oxide ceramics for articulating components of total hip replacements. In: Sedel L, Rey C, eds. *Bioceramics, Proceedings of the 10th International Symposium on Ceramics in Medicine.* Paris: Elsevier Science, 1997;10:123–126.

171. Wilson J. Bioactive glass: clinical applications. In: Hench LL, Wilson J, eds. *An introduction to bioceramics.* River Edge, NJ: World Scientific, 1993:63–73.

172. Wimmer MA, Andriacchi TP, Natarajan RN, et al. A striated pattern of wear in ultrahigh-molecular-weight polyethylene components of Miller-Galante total knee arthroplasty. *J Arthroplasty* 1998;13:8–16.

173. Wirganowicz PZ, Thomas BJ. Massive osteolysis after ceramic on ceramic total hip arthroplasty. *Clin Orthop* 1997;338:100–104.

174. Wright TM, Bartel DL. The problem of surface damage in polyethylene total knee components. *Clin Orthop* 1986;205:67–74.

175. Wright TM, Rimnac CM, Stulberg SD, et al. Wear of polyethylene in total joint replacements. Observations from retrieved PCA knee implants. *Clin Orthop* 1992;276:126–134.

176. Wroblewski BM, Siney PD, Dowson D, et al. Prospective clinical and joint simulator studies of a new total arthroplasty using alumina ceramic heads and cross-linked polyethylene cups. *J Bone Joint Surg Br* 1996;78:280–285.

177. Yamamuro T. Replacement of the spine with bioactive glass ceramic prostheses. In: Yamamuro T, Hench L, Wilson J, eds. *Handbook of bioactive glass ceramics.* Boca Raton, FL: CRC Press, 1990:335–342.

178. Yuan HP, Kurashina K, de Bruijn JD, et al. A preliminary study on osteoinduction of two kinds of calcium phosphate ceramics. *Biomaterials* 1999;20:1799–1806.

179. Zhang X, Zhou P, Zhang J, et al. A study of HA ceramics and its osteogenesis. In: Ravaglioli A, Krahewsky A, eds. *Bioceramics and the human body.* London: Elsevier Science, 1991;408–416.

BIOMECHANICS OF THE SPINE

IAN A.F. STOKES
JAMES C. IATRIDIS

1 INTRODUCTION

The biomechanics of the spine is unusual because of the large number of articulations, and unique because the intervertebral joints are flexible in all six degrees of freedom. As a result, muscle function must be coordinated to control motion in each degree of freedom. The intervertebral disc has an intricate mi-crostructure and unique mechanical properties that are central to these flexible articulations. The disc is also the largest avascular structure in the human body with very slow tissue turnover and repair rates, and largely devoid of innervation. The muscular anatomy is also unusual compared with other joint systems. Whereas most of the dorsal musculature is multi-layered and highly redundant, with numerous muscle attachments at each vertebral level, the ventral musculature consists almost entirely of "global" muscles that cross multiple anatomical levels, without intermediate connections to the vertebrae.

The components of the spine that must be considered in a biomechanical analysis include the vertebrae, intervertebral discs, ligaments, and spinal musculature. Each of these functions *in vivo* in a complex way, interacting with its blood supply and innervation. In the thoracic region the spine also articulates with the ribs. The spine is commonly considered to consist of a series of motion segments. Each motion segment is a structural unit consisting of two vertebrae and the intervening soft tissues.

The biomechanics of the spine can be viewed from different scale perspectives: whole trunk biomechanics, the spine and motion segment, and structures such as the facet joints and intervertebral disc, as well as the tissues and the cells that populate them. Spinal biomechanics also involves a wide range of organ systems, including bone, muscle, soft connective tissue, blood supply, and nerves. This chapter starts by examining the large-scale trunk biomechanics, and then proceeds to increasingly smaller scales, while attempting to demonstrate how these different scales and perspectives are interdependent.

2 TRUNK BIOMECHANICS

The forces that act on the components of the spine are calculated by considering the statics and dynamics of the trunk as it interacts with external forces, including gravity. These analyses are commonly used in ergonomic studies and studies of injury mechanisms, as well as in basic biomechanical studies.

2.1 Equilibrium Analyses of Muscle Force Distribution and Spinal Loads

The number of muscles crossing just the lumbar spine exceeds 180 (184), and this is much greater than the number of degrees of freedom (six per vertebra). In a static analysis of the lumbar spine, this means that there is a highly redundant number of muscle activation patterns that could be used to satisfy equilibrium. In indeterminate biomechanical analyses, it is usually assumed that the central nervous system (CNS) control of trunk muscle activation strategy is in some way optimal (45) compatible with equilibrium and other constraints, as discussed in Chapter 2. Optimization methods are therefore used to calculate the forces that not only satisfy equilibrium and other constraints, but also minimize a supposed physiological cost function. Several different physiological cost functions have been proposed to represent differing supposed strategies of muscle activation. Among these are cost functions to minimize intervertebral forces, to minimize muscle forces (14,41,81,162,202), to minimize the total of muscle and intervertebral forces (214), to maximize the external effort (185), or to optimize spinal displacements (175,213). If more than one variable is entered into the cost function, then weighting factors must be assigned to each component (186). Alternatively, the components of the optimization can be analyzed sequentially (14).

The optimization approach, although intuitively attractive, may not provide a perfect match to physiological muscle activations. For example, models that minimize the spinal compression force predict that as the amount of effort increases in any particular task or loading direction, advantageously placed muscles are activated first and are augmented by other muscles at larger efforts. Thus the number of muscles activated and the level of activation in each muscle increase discontinuously with effort. This is contradicted by experimental electromyography (EMG) recordings of EMG versus effort (110) that report small changes in the relative activations of trunk muscles with increasing effort, as if muscles were recruited in a pattern that did not vary with the magnitude of the external effort. The idea of a preprogrammed pattern of synergies that remains constant with changing effort is attractive because of its simplicity, but this would not always produce biomechanically optimal strategies.

Optimization models of the spine consider the physiological costs of activating muscles and loading the skeleton. These physiological costs have generally been considered singly or as competing objectives, whereas in reality several costs may be taken into account in establishing an efficient muscle activation strategy. Stokes and Gardner-Morse (186) predicted muscle force distributions analytically by minimizing a cost function that was the weighted sum of several biomechanical variables in an anatomically complex biomechanical model. These predictions were compared with EMG data from subjects performing isometric tasks. They found that simulations with single-component cost functions did not agree with experimental data as well as the simulations in which a combination of the muscle stresses and either intervertebral forces or intervertebral displacements was minimized.

It is interesting to consider the extent to which the coordination of muscle synergies are preprogrammed, relative to the amount of "real-time" automatic control in response to sensory and mechano-transduction of signals from muscle spindles, ligaments, etc. If the central nervous system (CNS) were continuously evaluating cost functions to control muscles optimally, then more complex relationships between muscle activation and external force might be generated, but this seems unlikely because of the large "computational" efforts that are required of the CNS.

When the intent is just to calculate spinal forces, such as in ergonomic analyses, EMG-driven models (68,123) present a pragmatic alternative to the optimization approach to solving the redundancy problem. In EMG-driven models the muscle forces are specified by estimates from EMG recordings of subjects performing the task under consideration. Certain synergies are assumed, so that muscle force values can be assigned to those muscles lacking EMG data. In general the resulting forces are not in equilibrium, so subsequently adjustments must be made to satisfy the equilibrium constraint (32). A variation of this approach is the neural network (136) method in which a model is "trained" using one set of EMG data, and subsequently used to predict muscle activation patterns under different sets of conditions, but using the rules "learned" in the first step.

In static or quasistatic analyses the forces included in the calculations are muscle forces, intervertebral forces, and external loads, but not the inertial forces associated with accelerations. For many real-life activities involving the trunk this seems to be adequate. If the accelerations of masses such as that of a lifted weight are significant, then these effects can be included in a quasistatic analysis by considering the inertial forces as additional external forces whose values are estimated typically from an inverse dynamic analysis (see Chapters 2 and 3). True dynamic analyses may be required in situations where rapid trauma occurs and the accelerations of trunk segments themselves must be taken into account, e.g., whiplash or impacts.

2.2 Static Analyses (Slow Lifting Tasks, etc.)

The equilibrium of the spine and trunk can be analyzed using a "free-body" analysis for each degree of freedom. Many simplified models have considered only rotational degrees of freedom and have included only a single anatomical level, thereby specifying three equilibrium equations (162). A more generalized approach was introduced by Stokes and Gardner-Morse (185) in which the lumbar spine was considered as a system of five lumbar vertebrae together with a lumped body representing the thorax, with each component having six degrees of freedom, providing a total of 36 equilibrium equations. The forces acting on each vertebra consisted of the forces in muscles that attached to it, and of the intervertebral forces that were considered to be the end reactions of beam elements joining adjacent vertebrae. This analysis required that the stiffness properties of the intervertebral joints first be identified and simplified as "equivalent" shear beams with linear elastic properties (61). The equilibrium of one vertebra is shown in Fig. 12-1.

The resulting underspecified system of equations has unknown muscle forces. Other variables include intervertebral forces (or corresponding intervertebral displacements) that are generally a linear function of the muscle forces F_m and the external forces F_e and M_e. The

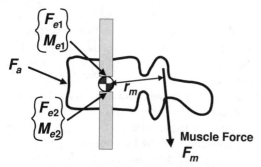

FIGURE 12-1. Equilibrium of a vertebra acted on by forces from muscle attachments (F_m), forces (F_e) and moments (M_e) from interactions with adjacent vertebrae, and an externally applied force (F_a). The forces between each vertebra and its neighbor are related to their relative displacements by the stiffness matrix of the motion segment, here simplified as a beam element.

solution is found after first specifying physiological upper and lower bounds on muscle forces and intervertebral displacements. Then a cost function objective C is specified (as a function of unknown forces and/or displacements) and a solution is obtained using linear or nonlinear programming (depending on the form of the cost function) by solving:

$$\text{Min } C, \quad \text{subject to} \quad 0 < F_m < \sigma A;$$
$$\text{(muscle force constraints)}$$

$$F_{min} < F_e < F_{max}; M_{min} < M_e < M_{max}$$
(bounds on intervertebral forces and moments)

$$\sum F_m + \sum F_e = F_a; \quad \text{(equilibrium of three}$$
force components acting on each vertebra)

$$\sum F_m \times r_m + \sum M_e = M_a \quad \text{(equilibrium of}$$
three moments acting on each vertebra)

where

σ = maximum muscle stress per unit area
A = muscle cross-sectional area
F_m = muscle forces
r_m = vector from muscle attachment to vertebra center
M_e = intervertebral moment
F_e = intervertebral forces
M_e = external moments
F_e = external forces

Here, the inertia in both the force and moment equations has been neglected. Note that intervertebral forces are the product of the intervertebral displacements and the corresponding motion segment's stiffness matrix (see Section 3.2).

McGill and Norman recognized that often the ligaments can become important contributors to spinal equilibrium, depending on the posture of the spine (and hence the ligaments' lengths and tensions). They developed a method to "partition" forces between ligaments and muscles, using data on the geometry of these structures from several sources, including *in vivo* studies (31,124). The ligaments can essentially replace the function of extensor muscles in extreme positions of trunk flexion, producing the "flexion–relaxation" phenomenon in which many extensor muscles become inactive (160). Other analyses have incorporated the variations in muscle force that depend on the muscle length (length–tension relationship) and the muscle shortening or lengthening velocity (e.g., by using a Hill model for the muscle).

2.3 Dynamic Analyses

The dynamic behavior of the spine is of great importance in potentially traumatic situations such as vehicle crashes or falls (especially of elderly and frail individuals) and specialized situations such as ejection from military aircraft. In a classic dynamic analysis of a nine-body structure with elastic and damping elements between the bodies, Tien and Huston (195) compared their analytic predictions of head and neck accelerations with experimental data. Many of the biomechanical investigation of spinal injuries are reported in the Proceedings of the Stapp Car Crash Conferences (http://www.stapp.org). Whiplash is a troubling clinical problem associated with car collision that is thought to have a biomechanical cause. A whiplash is thought to be an injury of the cervical spine after a forward acceleration (e.g., from a "rear-end" collision). However, to date, there is no general agreement about the specific structures that are injured. Empirical tests with dummies, cadavers, ligamentous spine specimens, and live volunteers have pointed to large intervertebral displacements (measured *in vivo* by cineradiography) (98), excessive facet joint capsule strains (measured *in vitro* by photogrammetry) (169), and ligamentous or vertebral artery overstretch (based on *in vitro* measures of ligamentous spines) (142).

2.4 Intraabdominal Pressure Effects

Abdominal muscle activation has presented an enigma in trunk biomechanics. Abdominal muscles are classically described in anatomy texts as flexors and rotators of the trunk, but paradoxical antagonistic activation of the abdominal musculature is observed during extension efforts. Also, the abdominal muscles are activated bilaterally when forces are generated by the trunk at other angles (lateral flexion, etc.). The reasons for this biomechanically inefficient antagonistic activation are unclear. However, pressurization of the abdominal cavity is observed in association with activation of the abdominal muscles during lifting and other activities (5,37,43,73,130). This pressure acts against the diaphragm and the pelvic floor to produce an extension moment that also tends to unload the lumbar spine. Thus the activation of the abdominal muscles may produce two competing mechanical effects: a flexion moment about the spine, and an extension moment generated by the associated intraabdominal pressure. The extension moment may exceed the flexion moment generated by activation of the abdominal muscles under certain circumstances (43). In a different biomechanical explanation of the paradoxical antagonistic activation of the abdominal musculature, the abdominal muscles are activated in order to increase the stability of the trunk by increasing muscle stiffness.

2.5 Stability Analyses

Antagonistic activation of abdominal muscles is thought to increase trunk stability. The fact that most optimization models do not predict antagonistic muscle coactivation has been seen as a limitation of these models. The vertebrae of the lumbar spine are like a series of inverted pendulums (Fig. 12-2), which may become unstable under load (39). A combination of muscle forces, muscle stiffness (15,33,39), and motion segment stiffness (144) is required to prevent buckling instability *in vivo*. Otherwise, a sudden excessive displacement could occur and result in tissue injury. Whether buckling episodes ever do

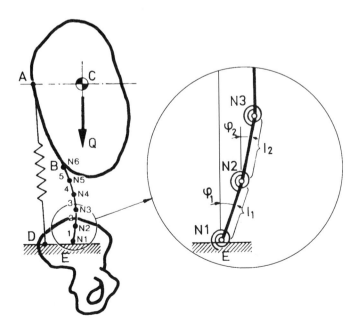

FIGURE 12-2. The lumbar spine, considered as a series of elastic links that may become unstable and buckle. The stiffness of the motion segments, along with the stiffness of muscles crossing the spine, may prevent buckling. (Reproduced from Bergmark A. Stability of the lumbar spine. A study in mechanical engineering. *Acta Orthop Scand* 1989;230(Suppl.):1–54, with permission.)

occur *in vivo* is a matter of conjecture, but the tissue injuries that might result from them provide a plausible explanation for the sudden onset of back pain under apparently benign external loading conditions. There is considerable debate as to what constitutes spinal instability in a clinical setting (9,144).

In general stability is defined as the ability of a system to return to its equilibrium position after a small perturbation. Stability can be analyzed by two equivalent approaches: (a) the sign of the net force resulting from a perturbation displacement (whether it increases or decreases the displacement), and (b) whether there is an increase or decrease in potential energy occurring with a perturbation.

For a single (rotational) degree of freedom (Fig. 12-3) of an inverted pendulum in equilibrium the net torque (T) acting about the lower joint is zero:

$$T = k_j\theta - F_j r_2 + (F_m + k_m \Delta L) r_1 = 0 \quad (1)$$

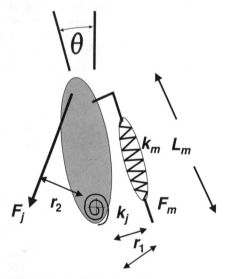

FIGURE 12-3. Equilibrium and stability analysis of a single idealized link in the spinal column in one degree of freedom, considering forces due to loading from an adjacent segment (F_j), muscle force (F_m), and the stiffness (k_j) of the motion segment and of the muscle (k_m). Alternatively (but equivalently) both equilibrium and stability are analyzed by derivatives of the potential energy (PE) with respect to angular perturbation. For stable equilibrium, PE must be at a minimum. For equilibrium the first derivative of PE is zero; for stable equilibrium the second derivative PE must be positive.

where k_j is the stiffness of the joint; F_j is the joint force vector; r_2 is the moment arm of F_j; F_m is the muscle force; r_1 is the moment arm of F_m; k_m is the muscle stiffness; and ΔL is the muscle stretch, relative to resting length. If the link is rotated a small perturbation through angle $\delta\theta$ from the equilibrium position, the net torque becomes

$$\delta T = k_j(\theta + \delta\theta) - F_j(r_2 + \delta r_2)$$
$$+ (F_m + k_m(\Delta L + \delta L))(r_1 + \delta r_1), \quad (2)$$

with δr_2, δL, and δr_1 being the length changes associated with $\delta\theta$ by geometric relationships.

For stability (in the limiting case as $\delta\theta$ vanishes):

$$dT/d\theta > 0. \quad (3)$$

This stability analysis can also be performed by considering the potential energy changes associated with the perturbation $\delta\theta$. The potential energy consists of work done against forces, and elastic energy storage in muscles and joints. If δPE is the potential energy change associated with the perturbation, then for equilibrium the first derivative of PE dPE $/d\theta = 0$ and for stability the second derivative is positive (i.e., at the equilibrium position PE is a minimum, not a maximum).

The stiffness of the muscle increases with activation. The relationship $k_m = qF/L$ is given by Bergmark (15). Here k_m is the value of the muscle stiffness at a muscle-generated force F, for a muscle with resting length L. The nondimensional parameter q has a value about 40 (40).

2.5.1 Spinal Buckling Analyses

It has been shown analytically that muscle stiffness (which increases with intensity of muscle activation) can prevent lumbar spine buckling that could occur spontaneously under certain loading conditions or in response to a perturbation. Stability analyses have predicted that antagonistic muscle coactivation would increase stability (57), and the existence of such antagonistic activity has been confirmed in electromyographic studies of muscle activation (110,191). Therefore, the patterns of human trunk muscle recruitment must not only provide static equilibrium and appropriate response to changes in loading and displacement perturbations, but must also provide sufficient stiffness to ensure stability of the vertebral column (15,57). Coactivation of antagonistic muscles is a part of a strategy that can increase the muscular stiffness and hence stability, but at the cost of increased spinal loads (67,81,191).

The concept that muscle stiffness together with motion segment stiffness stabilize the trunk (i.e., prevent buckling episodes of the spine) was introduced by Bergmark (15), who presented the analytical framework for multi-degree-of-freedom stability analyses of the lumbar spine. For a single degree of freedom, the stability is based on a calculation of scalar quantities, as shown above for a single degree-of-freedom inverted pendulum. For the spinal column, which is a multi-degree-of-freedom system, the buckling modes are not a priori known.

Again, considerations of the restoring force after a virtual perturbation of the spine can be used to determine whether the spine is stable (Fig. 12-4) (58). The restoring force is the net of the forces associated with elastic stiffness of the spine and muscles, together with incremental forces associated with the geometric stiffness (e.g., the additional tension in a muscle produced by a displacement transverse to its line of action).

Thus, the following matrix equation describes the net forces:

$$(\boldsymbol{K}_S + \boldsymbol{K}_M)v - \lambda(\boldsymbol{G}_S + \boldsymbol{G}_M)v = 0 \quad (4)$$

where $\boldsymbol{K}_S$ and $\boldsymbol{K}_M$ are the elastic stiffness matrices for the spine and muscles, respectively, and $\boldsymbol{G}_S$ and $\boldsymbol{G}_M$ represent the geometric stiffness of the spine and muscles.

For nontrivial solutions of this equation, the displacement is given by the eigenvector v. At the critical buckling state, the two components of force are equal, i.e., the smallest eigenvalue λ is equal to 1.

Alternatively, the buckling conditions can be obtained by finding eigenvalues of the matrix of partial second derivatives of the trunk and lumbar spine potential energy with respect to each degree of freedom (the Hessian matrix) (15). The value of the smallest eigenvalue λ_1 must be greater than zero if the system is stable (i.e., all the eigenvalues of the Hessian matrix must be positive). The critical value is the value that produces a value of λ_1 equal to 0, thus the critical state for buckling. The degree of stability is indicated by the magnitude of the smallest eigenvalue. Alternatively, the degree of stability can be expressed as the critical value of a muscle stiffness parameter that gives rise to the critical buckling condition (15).

2.5.2 Muscle Stiffness and Passive Elastic Contributions to Stability

Although increases in muscle activation produce increased muscle stiffness, they also increase the forces acting on the spinal column. These two effects are counteractive in terms of the stability of the column. It is thought that coactivation

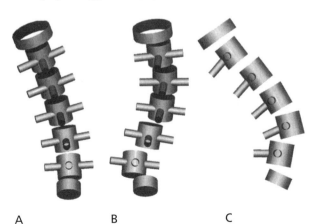

A   B   C

FIGURE 12-4. The first three buckling mode shapes of a lumbar spine model in a maximum extension effort. **(A)** The first buckling mode, with bending to the left. **(B)** The second mode, which occurred at 1.65 times the loading required for the first mode. **(C)** The third mode (lateral view), which also occurred at 1.65 times the load required for the first mode. (Reproduced from Gardner-Morse M, Stokes IA, Laible JP. Role of muscles in lumbar spine stability in maximum extension efforts. *J Orthop Res* 1995;13(5):802–808, with permission.)

of the abdominal and dorsal muscles produces a net increase in lumbar spinal column stability, with the beneficial (increased stability) effect exceeding the counterproductive (increased compressive load) effect. Gardner-Morse and Stokes (57) used an analytical model to predict that forcing abdominal muscle activation would increase trunk stability by a proportion generally greater than the increase in spinal compression, but with a comparable percentage increase in the cube of muscle stresses (a measure of muscle fatigue rate). Also from an analytical approach, Gardner-Morse et al. (58) reported simulations predicting that a reduction of motion segment stiffness of as little as 10% can compromise the stability of the spine.

It is expected that under more heavily loaded conditions the trunk would be stiffer because of increased muscle activation, and there is experimental evidence of this occurring. The amplitude of trunk motion in response to an added (dropped) weight was less in subjects who were already exerting a "preload" of 15% of maximum efforts than when the subjects were exerting a "preload" of 5% of their maximum (29). Stokes et al. (181) imposed a transient full-sinewave force perturbation on subjects who were exerting a preload of 20% or 40% of voluntary maximum to study the idea that a more heavily preloaded trunk would produce fewer muscular responses to these perturbations. Under the conditions of these experiments, a detectable muscle activation response to a perturbation was detected overall in 25% of trials at the higher preload, but 33% of trials at the lower preload.

2.5.3 Muscular Responses after Perturbations

Trunk stability has passive and active components, both controlled by the CNS. In passive (anticipatory) stabilization, the CNS has preactivated muscles to a preset level that provides sufficient muscle stiffness, together with motion segment stiffness, to stabilize the trunk. In the active mode the CNS responds to a perturbation by active muscle activation (e.g., reflexive,

or purposeful activation) to achieve a restoration of equilibrium. There are inherent neuromuscular delays from the time of the initiating stimulus to the time when muscular force is generated (193). The resulting muscle responses may occur as a result of triggering by muscle spindles, Golgi tendon organ, joint mechanoreceptors, or cutaneous sensory afferents, or a combination of these, based on the magnitude of perturbation applied and the displacements induced. The innervation of the facet joints includes strain sensitive mechanoreceptors and nociceptors (28) (the function was inferred from their conduction velocities and threshold of response to stretch), and similar nerve endings have been observed in the disc (152). Proprioceptive and mechanoreceptor-initiated responses in dorsal musculature have been demonstrated with stretching of the supraspinous ligament (176) and as a result of electrical stimulation of nerves in the facet joints and sacroiliac joint (90,91).

Most human experimental studies of trunk muscle responses to perturbations have used a sudden increase or decrease in load (drop or sudden release of a weight) or sudden translation or rotation of the support surface (74,75). These experimental conditions produce a step change in loading (in addition to an impulse in the case of a dropped weight) and require obligatory trunk muscle responses. In these experiments, EMG electrodes are used to record which muscles respond, as well as the relative timing (latency) and amplitude of the responses.

Lavender, Marras, and colleagues (111,120) found that if their subjects were expecting the sudden loading from a dropped weight there were anticipatory activations of trunk muscles, especially of abdominal muscles. They noted that the resulting muscular forces could cause large forces on the spine, but presumably they also increase the muscle stiffness and hence increase trunk stability. These anticipatory responses are apparently part of a coordinated movement planning requiring the trunk muscles to participate in the dynamic chain of body segments. Carlson et al. (27) and Cresswell et al.

(36) used a similar paradigm with weights suddenly added or removed from a harness over the shoulders. They observed that the abdominal muscles were usually the first to activate. Wilder et al. (208) reported the latency of responses to sudden perturbation from a dropped weight in the range 65 to 385 msec, with evidence that latency was increased with muscle fatigue. In subjects with low back pain the latency was longer than in other subjects, but after an exercise program the latency of the trunk muscle EMG responses was reduced. Alterations in muscle latencies have also been identified in the transversus abdominis (TA) muscle in persons with chronic low back pain (LBP). Hodges and Richardson (77) reported a delay in the activation of the left TA in subjects with LBP compared with healthy subjects. Subjects were asked to raise their right arm rapidly in response to a visual cue. The left TA was activated before the arm muscle (deltoid) in healthy subjects and after the arm muscle in LBP subjects. Whether such differences have a causal relationship to pain or are consequential or pain avoidance strategies is difficult to establish. Dynamic modeling of the control mechanisms involved might provide insights, but such modeling is challenging and has not yet been undertaken in detail.

2.6 EMG-based Experimental Data and Model "Validation"

Optimization and other models can be tested for realism by comparing predicted muscle forces with EMG recordings from muscles of living subjects. These model evaluations are at best semiquantitative because the EMG–force relationship is not well defined, and the number of EMG channels is limited by practical considerations including the inaccessibility of deep muscles. The "validation" of muscle force models against EMG data must be done carefully, to avoid the pitfall of "curve-fitting" the model parameters to fit the available data. In general, the model must be shown to be robust in the sense that the same model, when used to simulate quite differing external loading states or

other conditions, continues to provide a close match to experimental data.

Schultz et al. (161) evaluated a 10-muscle static equilibrium model of the third lumbar level by comparing its predictions of muscle and spinal forces in a wide range of sitting and standing activities with direct measurements of intradiscal pressure and of EMG activity at 12 locations. The model predictions of spinal compressive forces correlated ($r = 0.94$) with the average intradiscal pressures of four subjects. The regression relationship indicated that an intradiscal pressure of 1.5 MPa corresponded to a calculated spinal compression force of 2,000 N. Hughes et al. (81) compared the level of agreement between measured EMG amplitudes and predicted muscle forces in a 10-muscle model of the L3-4 level, using four different optimization models. They found that the model that minimized the sum of cubed muscle stresses provided the most acceptable match, with coefficients of determination (R^2) varying from 0.08 to 0.98 for different muscles. A similar approach was used to compare a 28-muscle static model of the C4 level of the cervical spine, with EMG recordings from eight locations (129).

Because the relationships between root mean square (RMS) EMG and the external force were observed to be nearly linear during the ramped voluntary increase of force, Stokes et al. (186) considered that a linear, monotonic increase of muscle activation with effort indicated a realistic performance of a model. They used the linear regression coefficients from a regression analysis of the muscle activation versus generated force to quantify muscle activation in both experimental data and model prediction. They then compared these gradients for different external loading directions.

A further difficulty in using EMG to validate trunk muscle models arises when the simulated activities involve forces that vary over time. The EMG–force relationship for trunk muscles differs at differing rates of change of force, even if the activity is nominally isometric (192,193). There also appear to be time delays in the range of 111 to 218 msec between the EMG signal and the generated force (193).

3 BIOMECHANICS OF THE SPINAL MOTION SEGMENT

3.1 General Principles: Six Degrees of Freedom, Nonlinearity, Time Dependence, Hysteresis, Preload Effects

The spinal motion segment is a structural unit of the spine consisting of two vertebrae and the intervening soft tissues (Fig. 12-5). It is a valuable tool in spinal biomechanics because it is the basic element of the spinal column. Once motion segment behavior is defined, the behavior of the whole spine can be represented by a series of fundamentally similar components. The motion segment can be considered as being symmetrical about the sagittal plane; thus, right and left lateral bends, axial rotation, and shear are theoretically symmetrical. The presence of the posterior elements (zygoapophyseal or facet joints and the ligaments) introduces differences between the flexion and extension behaviors. The presence of these posterior structures also produces a posterior displacement (relative to the disc center) of the effective structural axis of the motion segment.

The vertebrae have complex anatomy and geometry, whereas the intervertebral disc has an

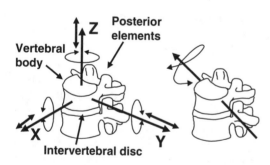

FIGURE 12-5. The motion segment, also called the functional spinal unit, is the basic mechanical element of the spine. It consists of two vertebrae and the intervening soft tissue. There are six degrees of freedom (three translations and three rotations), all of which have stiffness associated with them. An alternative way to consider the relative motion between vertebrae is to represent it as a translation along and a rotation about the helical axis of rotation.

apparently simple structure but very complex tissue properties that vary with water content, as described in Section 5 of this chapter (also, see Chapter 5 for more details). An appreciation of the intervertebral disc as a multiphasic material can facilitate understanding of its mechanical behavior (69,70,84–89,164) and its contributions to spinal mechanical behavior and failure mechanisms.

The intervertebral articulations have six degrees of freedom (three translations and three rotations), each of which has a measurable stiffness. Traditionally, the load–displacement characteristics of these joints have been described by a stiffness matrix (143). This stiffness matrix has off-diagonal terms as well as diagonal terms. This tendency of certain degrees of freedom to be associated with each other (especially axial rotation and lateral bending) has been referred to as coupling. Therefore, the pattern of motion that occurs between two vertebrae depends on the combination of forces applied, and the axis of rotation is not fixed. It is only possible to define an instantaneous axis of rotation. The helical axis of motion is an alternative to describing intervertebral motion as three rotations and three translations (Fig. 12-5). Using the helical axis of rotation, the motion is described by the position and direction of an axis of motion, together with a scalar translation along this axis and a scalar rotation around it.

Most experimental motion segment stiffness data are limited as they do not include all six degrees of freedom, were obtained by inverting flexibility data, and were obtained without physiological levels of axial compressive force. Physiological axial compression has been observed to increase lumbar motion segment stiffness by a factor of two or more (47,96). Janevic et al. (96) reported that the stiffening of the motion segment with preload was approximately linear with preload magnitude. With 2,200 N preload, rotational flexibility decreased on average 2.6 times, and shear flexibility 6.16 times, the effects being even greater at 4,400 N preload. Wilke et al. (209) used an apparatus with cables and deadweights to simulate muscle forces of 80 to 400 N. They also reported increased stiffness with increased applied "muscular" forces, but these forces also extended the spine, potentially confounding the results. Conversely, Panjabi et al. (141) reported some loss of stiffness with axial load, but this was probably an experimental artifact resulting from the displacement of the preload point of application accompanying the displacements used to measure the flexibilities in other degrees of freedom (38,47). This illustrates the methodological difficulties in simulating *in vivo* preload. Experimental systems that aim to simulate muscle actions using cables under tension (145,146,209) can produce confounding effects where the effects of forces in the cables may not be readily distinguishable from the intrinsic load–displacement behavior of the isolated motion segment.

The stiffening of the motion segment with preload appears to result from nonlinearities in the intrinsic material properties of the annulus fibers as well as the more easily visualized engagement of the facet joints. Analyses that have partitioned the preload effect between the disc and the posterior elements (59,96) indicate that both components are affected by preload, but overall the disc's contribution is larger. The facets are considered to engage as the motion segment is compressed, thereby explaining their altered contribution to stiffness. Broberg (22) analytically predicted a doubling in stiffness for rotational degrees of freedom with increased axial preload (700 N to 3,000 N) in a disc model that includes the geometric effects of disc compression and bulging as well as a nonlinear fiber stress–strain relationship (22). Axial preload may also stretch annular fibers so that their load–displacement behavior is more linear (and hence decrease the nonlinearity of the disc load–displacement behavior) and increase hysteresis (59,183).

The mechanical behavior of the spinal motion segment is nonlinear and is dependent on the loading history. The neutral zone concept (139) was introduced as a way to describe both the elastic nonlinearity (a region of low stiffness near the neutral position) and the hysteresis behavior (difference in the zero load position, dependent on the direction of prior displacement). Thus, it is an approximate description of nonlinear and time-dependent behavior of motion segment. The neutral zone has been shown to be larger with intersegmental injury and intervertebral disc degeneration (128,139) and smaller with simulated muscle force across a motion segment (139,209).

3.2 Experimental Considerations for Measuring Stiffness Properties of Motion Segments

In a linearized analysis the loads and displacements are considered to be related to each other by a symmetric stiffness matrix:

$$[K]\{\Delta\} = \{F\}, \tag{5}$$

where $[K]$ is a 6×6 stiffness matrix with 36 coefficients (21 independent coefficients because of matrix symmetry), $\{\Delta\}$ is a 6×1 displacement vector of three translations followed by the three rotations (using a zero-load state as the reference position), and $\{F\}$ is a 6×1 load vector of the three resulting forces and three resulting moments.

Experimentally, the force–deformation behavior can be obtained from a "stiffness experiment" in which each displacement is applied in turn to the specimen, and the resulting forces are recorded. The linear regression relationships of each force component with each displacement provide the columns of the linearized stiffness matrix. Alternatively, a flexibility matrix can be obtained by the analogous process of applying each of the six loads and recording the displacements. The flexibility matrix can be inverted to obtain the stiffness matrix (143). Either method provides initially 36 recordings (three moments and three forces for each the three rotations and three translations). The number of coefficients can initially be reduced to 21 by considerations of matrix symmetry and conservation of energy and by assuming linear load–displacement properties; hence, $k_{12} = k_{21}$, etc., in Fig. 12-6. Considerations of the sagittal plane symmetry and beamlike behavior of the motion segment permit further reduction of the number of coefficients to six diagonal terms and two "primary" off-diagonal terms as defined by Goel (64). (The beamlike behavior assumption requires that the axis system be aligned with the structural axis of the motion

MOTION SEGMENT STIFFNESS MATRIX
$$\{F\} = [K]\{\Delta\}$$

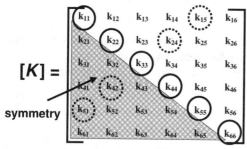

$$[K] = $$

symmetry

FIGURE 12-6. Layout of a motion segment stiffness matrix, indicating the diagonal terms (*solid circles*), "primary" off-diagonal terms (*broken circles*), matrix symmetry, and remaining terms that can be considered negligible because of geometrical symmetry of the spine about the sagittal plane.

segment, such that axial load produces only axial displacement, i.e., uncoupling.) The other terms are considered to be zero because no force is expected to be generated by that displacement (e.g., no lateral force associated with axial compression; hence, k_{13} and $k_{31} = 0$). The six diagonal terms are those stiffness terms that relate forces or moments to the colinear displacements or rotations (e.g., flexion moment associated with flexion rotation). The two primary off-diagonal terms relate the anterior–posterior (AP) shear forces to the applied flexion–extension rotations (or the complementary flexion–extension moments to AP shear displacements) and lateral shear forces to lateral bending rotations (or the complementary lateral bending moments to lateral shear displacements). The complementary pairing of off-diagonal terms is a result of stiffness matrix symmetry.

Realistic testing conditions should include physiological "preload" and the correct fluid and ionic environment. Discs tested mechanically in a physiological saline bath have greater hydration than discs that are just exposed to saline spray and wrap (148). This increased hydration presumably affects the mechanical properties.

3.3 Differences Associated with Degenerative Changes

With increased degeneration, compositional and geometric changes occur in both the nucleus

and annulus of the intervertebral disc (see Section 5.1). With advanced degeneration, the gross moment–rotation properties of the motion segment demonstrate some reduced range of motion, but also a tendency for the region of laxity (for smaller applied moments) to increase (128,132). For lesser degrees of degeneration the segmental motion may increase with increasing severity of disc degeneration (55). These changes in the mechanical behavior may result from a combination of arthritic changes in the facet joints and subchondral sclerosis, though apparently independent of the presence of osteophytes (55). However, the amount of variability between individual motion segments is large compared with the differences associated with degeneration (132).

3.4 Mechanically Induced Degeneration Mechanisms

Mechanical factors acting on the spine predispose to degeneration. The pathologic processes or the micromechanical disorders that give rise to disc degeneration and LBP remain obscure (125), but epidemiological studies point to a relationship. The apparently iatrogenic acceleration of degeneration in motion segments that are adjacent to a spinal fusion is often attributed to altered mechanics in the spinal column including increased intervertebral motion, facet loads, and stresses (66,71,112), which are affected by the length, location, and stiffness of the fusion mass (66,112,134). Furthermore, physically fit people have a decreased incidence of LBP, whereas sedentary posture is associated with back pain (52,125). Development of lumbar disc rupture is associated with activities generating higher disc stresses, including frequent bending and twisting, heavy physical work (52), and exposure to vibration (149,204).

Causal relationships are difficult to prove, but recent experimental studies in rodent tails point to possible mechanisms whereby altered mechanical conditions can produce altered composition or metabolic changes. Discs of the rodent tails subjected to chronic compressive load above physiological levels result in altered motion segment stiffness, compositional changes (84), and accelerated rate of disc cell apoptosis

(113,114). Coil springs attached to lumbar vertebrae of dogs for up to 1 year resulted in alterations in the amounts of proteoglycans and collagen in the disc but no apparent signs of degeneration (83). These experiments in which the mechanical environment of a disc can be closely controlled *in vivo* are still not completely unambiguous because the experimental conditions create disc hypomobility as well as abnormal forces.

4 MECHANICAL ASPECTS OF SPINAL DEFORMITY AND FRACTURE

4.1 Scoliosis: Mechanical Contribution to Etiology and Progression of Deformity

The exact biomechanical contributions to etiology and progression of scoliosis deformities are not well understood. Scoliosis consists of a lateral spinal curvature, together with transverse plane rotations of the spine and rib cage. A biomechanical analysis that explains the development of the deformity should explain all the geometric components. Several biomechanical factors have been invoked to explain the biomechanics of scoliosis. These include intervertebral motion coupling, spinal tethering and buckling, and mechanical influences on growth.

It has been noted that both lateral bending of the spine and scoliotic deformities involve transverse plane rotation, but it appears unlikely that coupling of rotational motion in intervertebral segments controls the development of vertebral rotation in scoliosis. The normal kinematic relationships between lateral bending and axial rotation produce a different spinal shape than that seen in scoliosis (182,203,206). In particular these changes do not explain the pattern of deformity that develops in scoliosis with maximal vertebral rotation at the curve apex. Spinal tethering by posterior structures of the spine (177) has also been invoked to explain the spinal shape in scoliosis and its etiology. There are several parts to this theory. First, tethering is thought to prevent flexion of the spine and lead to a hypokyphotic or lordotic shape, which then has a

greater tendency to instability. Second, the tether is thought to maintain a straighter alignment of the posterior elements than of the vertebral bodies, thus rotating the vertebrae in the curve. The fact that sagittal plane curvature of the spine is flattest in the early teen years supports the idea that this shape places the spine at risk for development of scoliosis. The shape of the spine in scoliosis is reminiscent of a buckled beam, but buckling may not explain the development of lateral curvatures because buckling of the ligamentous spine first occurs in the sagittal plane (157).

In the progression of a small deformity to a large one, it has been proposed that a small lateral curvature of the spine would load the vertebrae asymmetrically, leading to asymmetrical growth in the vertebral growth plates, and acceleration of the deformity in a vicious cycle (189). This would start after a certain threshold of spinal deformity has been reached. This theory of spinal growth sensitivity to loading asymmetry must however explain why the normal spinal curvatures (kyphosis and lordosis) in the sagittal plane do not progress into hyperkyphosis and hyperlordosis by the same mechanism, although progressive deformity in Scheuermann's kyphosis has been attributed to a similar mechanism. This concept of a biomechanical mechanism of progression of deformity is attractive intuitively and has been incorporated into the rationale for brace and other treatments. However, it cannot be quantified without better knowledge of the normal spinal loading and the alteration of loading in scoliosis, and better understanding of the sensitivity of growth to the time course of mechanical load and its magnitude.

4.2 Spondylolisthesis and Spondylolysis

Children who participate in certain sports are at risk for spondylolysis (unilateral or bilateral fracture of the part of the neural arch that lies between superior and inferior facet joints). Although usually asymptomatic in children, spondylolysis may develop into spondylolisthesis (forward slippage of the superior vertebrae) during the adolescent growth spurt. Spondylolysis is more common in gymnasts (95) and football players (122). The prevalence of spondylolysis is reported as 4.4% of the population at age 6, increasing to 6% in adulthood (50). Important epidemiological observations emerged from studies of skeletons removed from the graves of Alaskan natives (179). Four percent of the skeletons of 6-year-olds had this defect, which increased to 34% in adulthood. These observations led to the idea that spondylolysis is a fatigue fracture, resulting from repetitive loading. Cyron and Hutton (42) were able to reproduce a spondylolysis fracture in cadaver vertebrae subjected to repetitive loading of the posterior elements. Their experiments were complemented by a simplified mechanical model that showed how facet joint loading, combined with tension from the extensor musculature, produced bending moments in the neural arch. It has been reported (155) that spondylolysis is not seen in spine-paralyzed subjects, which provides further evidence for a mechanical etiology of spondylolysis.

4.3 Burst and Compression Fracture, and Loss of Strength Due to Osteoporosis and Osteolytic Tumors

Compression loading of the vertebral bodies may produce a failure of the end plate (Schmorl node) or crushing of the vertebra (compression fracture), and the injury may include bone fragments that displace into the neural canal (burst fracture). Loading rate as well as magnitude and direction of load are thought to determine the fracture pattern. Because of the clinical significance of vertebral body fractures associated with osteoporosis and pathological conditions (primarily osteolytic metastatic tumors), vertebrae have become a focus for biomechanical studies of the relationship between bone composition, bone structure and architecture, and vertebral strength. The vertebrae are composed principally of trabecular (cancellous) bone (171). The proportion of the vertebral bone that is mineralized can be estimated by single or dual energy x-ray absorptiometry (DEXA), or by quantitative computed tomography (QCT). The former provides a measure of the total mineral in the selected projection and is commonly referred to as bone mineral density (BMD), measured in grams per unit area of the projection. This is a potentially misleading term since it takes no account of the distance through which the absorbed x-ray beam has traveled (here "density" refers to the image density per unit area, not the tissue density per unit volume). QCT provides volumetric measurement of apparent bone mineral content, and regression relationships have been developed to convert the CT pixel density (Hounsfield number) into a bone modulus estimate. Windhagen et al. used these relationships to predict vertebral compressive rigidity (212). The rigidity estimates were found to correlate quite closely with vertebral compressive strength in intact vertebrae and in vertebrae with real or simulated internal defects. Silva et al. (170) reported a more detailed examination of the ability of CT images to predict failure loads as well as the mode of failure, using a finite element analysis having geometry and material properties derived from the CT images. They examined sagittal plane slab sections of vertebrae of a wide age range (32–102 years) and reported that predicted failure loads were typically within 25% of the values found experimentally. The observed regions of bone failure occurred close to regions of predicted high strain.

The properties of vertebral bone depend on its architecture as well as its density (as determined radiologically), but to a first approximation it seems likely that the apparent density would indicate the amount of tissue, and hence the mechanical properties. At the tissue level, Kopperdahl and Keaveny (104) demonstrated clear differences between tensile and compressive behavior of cancellous bone in the relationship between yield strain and apparent density. For tensile behavior the yield strain was independent of density, but in compression there was a positive correlation. It appeared that differences might result from buckling modes of failure predominating in compressed trabecular bone. The time-dependent behavior of bone tissue is probably also important in actual fractures and was incorporated into an analysis of potential failures of vertebral bodies having tumor erosions, using elastic properties, permeability, and geometric properties (including tumor size) as parameters (207).

4.4 Biomechanical Considerations in Treatment and Management of Spinal Problems

The spine has many articulations; therefore, arthrodesis (fusion) of one or more levels is a common surgical approach to injuries, painful degenerative problems, and deformity. In non-surgical management, biomechanical principles are helpful in design of braces, ergonomic analyses, and prescription of specific muscle exercises and strengthening regimens.

A surgeon planning surgical treatment of the spine has many variables to consider when using modern instrumentation. These variables include the design of instrumentation system, the number and location of vertebrae to be instrumented, rod shape (curvature), and interconnections between instrumentation components, as well as the amount of deformity correction to attempt with maneuvers of the instrumentation. In theory, if the mechanical properties of both the spine and the instrumentation were completely known, then biomechanical models could predict the outcome of surgery. There have been a number of attempts to develop and validate such models of surgery (60,97,159,180), and also the correction of deformity by electrical stimulation (158) and by braces (213). The large number of variables and unknowns in these models has been the probable cause of their limited success. Finite element modeling has been used to estimate the stresses in bone and instrumentation (63,174). More rigid fixation promotes more rapid fusion (121) and reduces the strains in the instrumentation as well as the bone. Despite concern that extremely rigid fixation techniques would also produce stress shielding and osteopenia of bone, this does not appear to be a problem in practice.

Information about *in vivo* loading of surgical implants has been provided by signals from force transducers built into the implanted devices (24,154). These show forces on the order of 250 N and moments on the order of 6 Nm transmitted through the instrumented surgical implants during walking, but this constitutes an unknown proportion of the total load carried by the spine and the instrumentation. For comparison, Cappozzo (25) calculated that the cyclic component of the compressive force in the spine during walking is typically 700 N (about body weight).

5 BIOMECHANICS OF THE INTERVERTEBRAL DISC

The intervertebral disc is the largest avascular structure in the body, with very low cellularity and largely without sensory innervation. It has a slow rate of tissue turnover, on the order of months for the glycosaminoglycans and on the order of decades for the collagen (199). Its viability depends primarily on transport of dissolved nutrients and metabolites through long diffusion pathways. The disc has been implicated in painful degenerative changes that affect a large proportion of the population. Many bioengineering studies in the past focused on acute injury mechanisms (e.g., to understand the role of stress concentrations in the postero-lateral region and their role in disc herniations). However, the epidemiological data suggest that acute overload injuries are probably less significant than progressive degenerative changes in the etiology of most painful and chronic conditions of the spine.

The mechanics and physiology of the disc are recognized as crucial to understanding how the avascular tissue of the disc receives its nutrition and retains its viability. Many aspects of these complex interactions, and their possible implications for disc degeneration, require an understanding of how the tissue properties interact with the 3D microstructure of the disc. Accurate models of these interactions are required to infer the consequences of a change in one parameter or component of the disc for other aspects of disc function. For instance, it is not yet clear how variations in mechanical loading within the physiological range can influence fluid flow and nutrition, and how the consequential changes are involved in signaling cellular responses and regulation of disc metabolism.

5.1 Tissue Structure and Composition

The intervertebral disc is composed of three major substructures: annulus fibrosus, nucleus pulposus, and cartilage end plate. The composition and structure of each component is distinct, suggesting that each component has a unique mechanical role. In the lumbar region of the spine, the intervertebral disc cross section has a kidney shape in the horizontal plane with the nucleus centered posteriorly (Fig. 12-7). The gelatinous nucleus pulposus is surrounded on its periphery by the highly organized annulus fibrosus; the annulus has discrete fibrous layers, or lamellae; and the cartilage end plate is a thin hyaline cartilaginous layer that lies between the intervertebral discs and the adjacent vertebrae.

5.1.1 Nucleus Pulposus

The healthy nucleus pulposus is highly gelatinous, composed almost 90% of water, and contains significant amounts of proteoglycans, collagen, and other matrix proteins (Table 12-1). The proteoglycans are predominantly the aggregating proteoglycan aggrecan, but versican, decorin, and other species are also found. The collagen fibers are organized in a loose, randomly organized network that yields isotropic material properties. The collagens of the nucleus are largely type II.

5.1.2 Annulus Fibrosus

The structure of the annulus fibrosus varies significantly in the radial direction from the inner

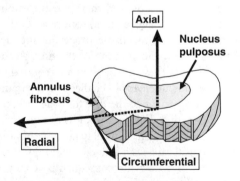

FIGURE 12-7. Schematic of a lumbar intervertebral disc with cylindrical polar coordinate system.

annulus (often termed the transition zone) to the outer annulus. The annulus fibrosus structure is comprised of successive plies of unidirectional lamina that can be considered a symmetric angle-ply laminate (Fig. 12-7). There are roughly 20 distinct plies ranging in thickness from 0.1 mm at the outer annulus to 0.4 mm in the innermost layers (26,118,196). Fiber angles have a similar radial variation ranging from approximately 60° (to the spinal axis) at the outer annulus to 45° in the innermost regions. The mechanisms of layer termination (or generation) are complex, involving sharp discontinuities in the laminate and suggesting that the strength of such a structure is lower than that of a regular laminate without these discontinuities. The frequency of these layer interruptions is maximal at the posterolateral part of the disc, and this may be due to the presence of higher stresses and strains in this location. The biochemical composition of the annulus is mostly water (about 70%) with significant amounts of collagen and proteoglycans (Table 12-1). The fibrocartilaginous annulus has mostly type I collagen fibers in the outer layers and fine type II fibers in the inner annulus (19).

5.1.3 End Plate

The cartilage end plate is a layer of hyaline cartilage approximately 0.6 mm thick, lying between the vertebral body and the intervertebral disc (151). The human cartilage end plate undergoes marked thinning and eventual calcification beginning in adolescence (194). The composition is similar to that of articular cartilage with water content of 70% to 80% and proteoglycans approximately 7% of the dry tissue weight (151,164). The composition is heterogeneous with regions above the outer annulus and nearer the bone having higher collagen but lower proteoglycan and water contents than the end plate nearest the disc at the nucleus (151). The blood supply of the vertebral body is a major pathway for nutrients to reach the nucleus pulposus by diffusion through this cartilage end plate. Similarly, the degree of accumulation of metabolic waste products and degraded matrix products in the disc is controlled by the permeability of the cartilaginous end plate (151).

TABLE 12-1. COMPOSITION OF INTERVERTEBRAL DISC

	Outer Annulus Fibrosus	Inner Annulus Fibrosus	Nucleus Pulposus
Water (per wet weight)	65–75%	75–80%	75–90%
Collagen (per dry weight)	75–90%	40–75%	25%
Proteoglycans (per dry weight)	10%	20–35%	20–60%
Other proteins (per dry weight)	5–15%	5–40%	15–55%

Data taken from Antoniou et al. (6).

5.1.4 Relationship Between Composition and Mechanics

The water content of the disc constitutes 65% to 90% by weight. This extrafibrillar fluid component is mobile but its motion is limited because of the low permeability of the disc tissue, which creates significant frictional drag between the solid and water phases. The solid-phase electric charges derive from the well-known fixed charges of the proteoglycan aggregate (119). The glycosaminoglycan chains contain fixed sulfate (SO_4^{2-}) and carboxyl $(COOH^-)$ groups that become ionized under physiological conditions (1.5 M NaCl, pH 7.4) and become negatively charged. This gives rise to the term fixed charge density (FCD). The tissue behaves like a semipermeable membrane, allowing the passage of water and ions but prohibiting the motion of the fixed negative charges of the proteoglycans. This selective transport generates an osmotic pressure that, along with charge-to-charge repulsion forces and hydraulic pressurization, makes up the high swelling pressures found in the tissue. The mobility of the water (126) results in diurnal variations in disc height and water content (117). Water (and hence nutrients and metabolites) may be transported into and out of the disc through the end-plate route and through the outer periphery of the annulus. The vertebral end plate provides an additional impediment to the mobility of the water, and recent evidence points to a nonlinear flow direction-dependent resistance to fluid flow (10,11,69). The water content in the disc then is related to the balance in forces between the swelling pressure in the nucleus, the collagen fiber tension in the annulus, and the applied load (see Section 5.6).

5.2 *In Vitro* Tissue Properties and Mechanical Behaviors in Swelling, Tension, Compression, and Shear

The intervertebral discs and the spine are very inaccessible to direct measurement. *In vivo* measures of intradiscal pressure (131,210) have given insights into the mechanism of disc function. *In vitro* experimental data on bulging (187), disc surface strain (188), and internal deformations (105,163) have been useful for quantitative verification of structural models of the disc. Isolated sections of annulus fibrosus (1,16,53,54,56,86,87), nucleus pulposus (85,89,138), and cartilage end plate (10,164) with measured geometry have been tested to quantify the heterogeneous, nonlinear, and anisotropic and viscoelastic material properties (Tables 12-2 to 12-4).

5.2.1 Nucleus Pulposus

Nucleus pulposus tissue (and also the annulus) increases in volume by more than 200% when placed in normal saline. If the volume is constrained, a swelling pressure is generated. Saline injection into the nucleus was found to increase the hydrostatic pressure and the motion

TABLE 12-2. AVERAGE MATERIAL PARAMETERS FOR ANNULUS AND NUCLEUS TISSUE

Material Parameter	Value	Reference
Annulus fibrosus properties		
Porosity[a]	$\phi^W = 0.70$	Antoniou et al. (6)
Aggregate modulus(compression)[a]	$H_A = 0.56$ MPa	Iatridis et al. (86)
Nonlinear stiffening coefficient	$\beta = 2.13$	Iatridis et al. (86)
Shear modulus	$\mu_s = 0.1$ MPa	Iatridis et al. (87)
Tensile modulus[a,b]	$E_s = 20$ MPa	Acaroglu et al. (1)
Poisson's ratio[a,b]	$\nu_s = 1$	Elliott and Setton (48)
Hydraulic permeability	$k = 0.20 \times 10^{-15}$ m⁴/Ns	Iatridis et al. (86)
Strain-dependent permeability coefficient	$M = 1.18$	Iatridis et al. (86)
Nucleus pulposus properties		
Porosity	$\phi^W = 0.75$	Antoniou et al. (6)
Aggregate modulus (compression)[c]	$H_A = 0.3$ MPa	Using isotropic assumption
Shear modulus	$\mu_s = 0.025$ MPa	Iatridis et al. (85)
Tensile modulus[c]	$E_s = 0.04$ MPa	Panagiotacopulos et al. (138)
Poisson's ratio[c]	$\nu_s = 0.47$	Using isotropic assumption
Hydraulic permeability	$k = 0.20 \times 10^{-15}$ m⁴/N-s	Same as for annulus

[a] Regional effects are reported in literature.
[b] Full set of anisotropic tensile properties for Young's modulus and Poisson's ratio can be found in Elliott and Setton (48).
[c] Estimated values for parameters taken from information found on shear modulus for nucleus pulposus, from properties of annulus fibrosus tissue, or from isotropic material assumption.

segment stiffness, suggesting that the disc hydration state is also an important determinant of swelling pressure and motion segment behavior (4). Chemical equilibration with polyethylene glycol (PEG) demonstrated that the equilibrium swelling pressure of intervertebral discs is due to the fixed charges of the proteoglycan molecules (197,198). The nucleus has therefore often been represented as an incompressible and inviscid fluid in finite element simulations (e.g., 167). More realistically, the nucleus pulposus may be represented as a biphasic or poroelastic material with low modulus and chemical (swelling) and electrical effects (108,109,172), yet there are few experimental data providing values of these properties.

Experimental measurements of the nucleus in shear (85,89) and tension indicate that the nucleus has an intrinsically viscoelastic solid matrix with a set of material constants given (Table 12-2). The instantaneous and dynamic shear moduli range from 0.005 to

TABLE 12-3. TENSILE MODULUS (MEAN ± SD) AT OUTER AND INNER ANNULUS SITES

Orientation		Outer (Mean ± SD)	Inner (Mean ± SD)
Circumferential	E_0 (MPa)	2.52 ± 2.27	1.70 ± 1.21
	E (MPa)	17.45 ± 14.29	5.60 ± 4.67
Axial	E_0 (MPa)	0.27 ± 0.28	0.34 ± 0.21
	E (MPa)	0.82 ± 0.71	0.96 ± 1.17
Radial	E_0 (MPa)	0.19 ± 0.04	—
	E (MPa)	0.45 ± 0.25	—

E_0, toe region modulus; E, modulus in the linear region of the stress–strain response.
Circumferentially oriented specimens are significantly different at outer versus inner sites.
Data taken from Elliott and Setton (48).

TABLE 12-4. FINITE DEFORMATION COMPRESSIVE PROPERTIES OF HUMAN ANNULUS FIBROSUS

Finite Deformation Properties	Healthy	Degenerate
H_{A0} (MPa)	0.56 ± 0.21[a]	1.10 ± 0.53[a]
β	2.7 ± 2.6[a]	0.44 ± 0.61[a]
k_0 ($\times 10^{-15} m^4/Ns$)	0.18 ± 0.07	0.16 ± 0.06
M	1.5 ± 1.6	1.4 ± 1.9

H_{A0}, zero-strain compressive aggregate modulus; β, nonlinear stiffening coefficient; k_0, reference hydraulic permeability; M, strain-dependent permeability coefficient.
[a] Healthy $\neq$ Degenerate ($p < 0.05$)
Values are the averages for radial and axial specimens (no significant difference by orientation was detected).
Data taken from Iatridis et al. (86). Note that values for these nonlinear parameters are dependent on initial state of hydration and reported values vary, e.g., Klisch and Lotz (99).

0.06 MPa and are strongly influenced by loading frequency and grade of degeneration. Under shear loading, nucleus tissue has strain rate-sensitive viscoelastic material properties. A model representation of nucleus tissue with variable amplitude and continuous relaxation spectrum demonstrates good agreement with experimentally measured stress relaxation behavior (89). Tensile moduli have magnitudes similar to those in shear (0.03 to 0.04 MPa) (138).

5.2.2 Annulus Fibrosus

The highly fibrous nature of the annulus is well suited to resist tensile stresses and strains in the disc resulting from motion of adjacent vertebrae and swelling pressure. The fiber angle of approximately 60° indicates that circumferential hoop stresses are greater than stresses in the axial direction. Galante (56) measured tensile properties of the annulus fibrosus and showed that this tissue behaves as a nonlinear, heterogeneous, anisotropic, and viscoelastic material whose properties are sensitive to its state of hydration. Skaggs et al. (173) characterized the tensile properties of single-layer specimens tested along the predominant fiber direction with values for E ranging from 60 to 140 MPa, depending on the region of the annulus. Galante tested multiple-layer specimens in the circumferential–axial plane and found that the elongation was lowest (i.e., the tissue was stiffest) along the fiber direction (i.e., 60° to the spinal axis), and the tis-

sue was least stiff perpendicular to the fiber direction. Young's modulus for multiple-layer samples is as high as 25 MPa in the circumferential direction (1) (Table 12-2) and as low as 0.5 MPa in the radial direction (53), but these measurement show substantial nonlinear behavior in the physiological strain range. Measured values for Poisson's ratio (1) are much larger than 0.5 (i.e., the theoretical limit for isotropic materials), and this further demonstrates the anisotropic behavior of the annulus.

A comprehensive set of bilinear, anisotropic, and heterogeneous tensile properties of annulus were measured in a combined theoretical and experimental study (48,49) (Table 12-3). Fiber-induced anisotropy was represented in a nine-parameter model using structural tensors and a hyperelastic formulation based on a linear strain energy function (49). The literature includes other variations on the form of the strain energy formulations used in hyperelastic fiber-reinforced models (46,102). In finite element models, fiber-induced anisotropy is represented by using tension-only cable elements, e.g., (135,168,178), but the required model parameters (e.g., fiber modulus, matrix modulus, fiber–matrix interactions) are difficult or impossible to measure directly.

Annulus fibrosus tissue material properties are further complicated by large variations with region, significant alterations with degeneration, and nonlinearities in tension, compression, and shear. Significant variations in tensile properties with degeneration include decreases in Poisson's ratio, tensile failure stress, and strain energy density to failure as well as a modest decrease in tensile modulus (1). Some, but not all, of the tensile properties are inhomogeneous. For example, the circumferential modulus decreases from outer to inner sites and from anterior to posterior sites (1,48), whereas the radial modulus does not (53). Nonlinear tensile stress–strain behavior has been modeled using linear, bilinear, exponential, and cubic functions (1,48,53,56). Uniaxial tensile tests with very slow strain rate (i.e., quasistatic) or static test conditions are used to minimize viscoelastic effects and obtain elastic properties. Viscoelastic behaviors of annulus in tension were described by Panagiotacopulos et al. (138), who presented a stress–relaxation curve for annulus tissue in which water content had a dominant effect.

Values for equilibrium compressive moduli (Table 12-4) are similar to values for the radial tensile modulus, suggesting that the marked tension–compression nonlinearity in the tissue is predominantly related to fiber-induced strengthening and not to nonlinearities in the nonfibrous ground substance (Fig. 12-8). This is confirmed by the isotropy reported for the compressive modulus in confined compression (86).

Shear loading on the annulus fibrosus requires fiber stretching. Consequently the shear modulus for the annulus is anisotropic with values ranging from 0.05 to 0.5 MPa, depending on orientation and level of compressive prestrain (54). Compressive stresses on the tissue (in an unconfined orientation) increase the stretch in the annulus fibers and also reduce the tissue volume (thereby decreasing tissue hydration and increasing fiber density). This change is consistent with observed increases in shear moduli with compressive stress (87). In torsional shear experiments the flow-independent viscoelastic effects are isolated from flow-dependent viscoelasticity and demonstrate that the annulus tissue does have intrinsic viscoelasticity (87).

Confined compression testing, however, indicates that fluid pressurization and viscoelasticity resulting from the biphasic mechanism dominate the viscoelastic response in the annulus tissue in compression. The value for hydraulic permeability (k) is in the region of 0.17×10^{-15} m^4/Nsec (16,44,86), which is approximately an order of magnitude lower than that of articular cartilage. Measured values of hydraulic permeability also depend on initial loading condition (and associated water content) as a result of the strain-dependent permeability of the tissue,

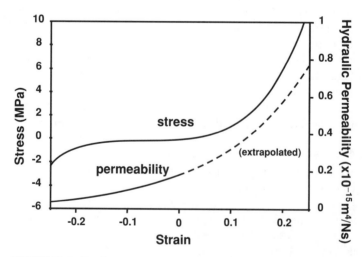

FIGURE 12-8. Nonlinear stress–strain relationship and strain-dependent hydraulic permeability of annulus fibrosus in tension and compression. Note that the annulus is much stiffer in tension than in compression. (Adapted from data (1,86) with permission.)

i.e., $M > 0$ (Table 12-4). Measurements of permeability have reported values as much as an order of magnitude greater ($k = 1.75 \times 10^{-15} \, \text{m}^4/\text{Nsec}$) (69,99), with the difference associated with differing water content or strain state (see Fig. 12-8). Because *in vivo* the strain and water content may be quite variable, material parameters for annulus tissue should specify the tissue reference state and should include measurements of water content.

5.2.3 Cartilage End Plate

Significant compressive deformations are generated in the cartilage and vertebral end plate *in situ*. End-plate deformation is comparable in magnitude with disc bulge and overall disc compression under compressive loading of a motion segment (20). Prolonged deformation of the cartilage end plate in compressive creep experiments *in vitro* was attributed to fluid flow and intrinsic viscoelastic effects for the solid matrix of the cartilage end plate (164). Accordingly, a biphasic poroviscoelastic model (i.e., both flow-dependent and flow-independent viscoelastic effects are present) was used to describe the compressive behavior of the cartilage end plate (164). The model parameters were the compressive modulus (H_A approximately 0.4 MPa), hydraulic permeability (k approximately $10^{-13} \, \text{m}^4/\text{Nsec}$), and parameters ($c, \tau_1, \tau_2$) describing the intrinsic viscoelastic effects. The permeability of the end plate is higher than that of the annulus, apparently because of rapid transport and pressurization of the interstitial fluid in response to loading and greater flow-independent viscoelastic effects. This fluid pressurization in the end plate is important in the maintenance of a uniform stress distribution across the boundary between vertebral body and intervertebral disc. The partial or complete loss of the end plate that occurs with degeneration (194) would lead to a nonuniform distribution of applied loads across the entire disc and contributes to the development of site-specific damage in the disc. Recent evidence points to a nonlinear flow direction-dependent resistance to fluid flow in the end plate *in situ* that has significant implications for load carriage and nutrition in the disc (10,11). This direction dependence may help explain how the fluid lost during daily loading (about 16 hours) is recovered during rest (about 8 hours) (11).

5.2.4 Intervertebral Disc Degeneration

There are significant changes in composition and color of the entire disc, increasing fiber content of the nucleus and an altered fiber network in the annulus (23,115,147,194). The hydration of the nucleus and annulus decreases, probably as a result of a decrease in proteoglycan content and the associated fixed charge density (6,34,62,198), that in turn changes the mechanical, chemical, and electrical fields in the tissue. There are also significant alterations in proteoglycan structure. The water content of the nucleus decreases to less than 75% with an associated loss of proteoglycans from 60% of the tissue dry weight to less than 20%. With degeneration, the thickness of the end plate becomes irregular and focal defects appear, followed by calcification (153,194).

The collagen content seems unaffected by mild or early disc degeneration, but alterations in the distribution of collagen type I and type II do occur. A decrease in the relative amount of type II collagen is found in the inner annulus with degeneration (6,7,19). Other degenerative changes include increases in the percentage of denatured type II collagen, slight decreases in the amount of newly synthesized aggrecan and type II collagen, decreases in the number of layers of the annulus, and an increase in layer thickness and interbundle spacing (6,19,118).

These compositional and microstructural changes in turn alter the macroscopic behaviors as seen in the disc flexibility (128) and intradiscal pressure (2,127,140,156). The shear modulus of the nucleus increases eightfold with degeneration, and the decrease in relative energy dissipation suggests that the nucleus pulposus undergoes a transition from "fluidlike" to "solidlike" behavior with aging and degeneration (85). In the annulus fibrosus there is a significant increase in compressive modulus (86) and decrease in radial permeability (69), as well as a moderate increase in shear modulus (87) of the tissue with grade of disc degeneration. These alterations may be explained by the loss of water content and increase in tissue density. Increases in the axial and circumferential permeability (69) as well as alterations in the Poisson's ratio (1) with degeneration are probably related to structural remodeling and perhaps microfailure resulting from the degenerative process. Alterations in the streaming potential response of annulus tissue with degeneration provide further evidence of the relationship between tissue FCD, water content, and material properties (70).

Aging and degeneration of the disc may be considered different processes, with degeneration having a more deleterious influence on the structure and function of the disc. Because these two processes frequently occur in parallel, it is difficult to distinguish between them. Separating these two effects may be a key step in understanding the process of disc degeneration.

5.3 *In Situ* Strains, Stresses, and Pressures: Experimental Data

5.3.1 *Intradiscal Pressure*

Intradiscal pressures have been reported to be nearly proportional to external applied loading (161) and therefore provide a measure of the stress state in the disc. The relative ease of inserting pressure transducers into the disc has provided a means of assessing relative pressures inside the intervertebral disc in situ. Discal pressures range from 0.1 to 0.3 MPa under resting and light loading conditions and from 1 to 3 MPa under extreme loading *in vitro* and *in vivo* (127,131,133,210). Intradiscal pressures are lowest when reclining and greater when standing and sitting, particularly when in the flexed-forward posture (131,210).

5.3.2 *Internal Deformations*

In a radiographic method to measure tissue deformations of intact and denucleated discs under different loading conditions in situ, metal beads were implanted into a mid-sagittal section of the disc, and plane radiographs were taken and digitized (105,163). Inward bulging of the denucleated specimens was observed to cause radial tensile stresses and disruption of adjacent layers of annulus (163). This suggests a potential annulus failure mechanism because low values of radial tensile modulus have been reported (48,53). Magnetic resonance imaging (MRI) shows promise as a minimally invasive method for obtaining internal disc deformations; however, these techniques are still being developed (18,100,106).

5.4 Nutrient Transport (Diffusion and Biosynthesis)

Intervertebral disc cells obtain nutrition through diffusion and convection from the end plate and outer annulus. Cells in the outer annulus are supplied by blood vessels in the surrounding tissue, but cells of the nucleus and inner annulus are likely to be supplied via the vertebral bodies (153,201). Capillaries arising from vertebral vessels penetrate the subchondral bone but not the cartilaginous end plate and supply nutrients that then diffuse into the disc. The end-plate route for nutrition, however, is precarious and is adversely affected by factors that include aging, or pathology, tobacco smoking, or vibrational loading (76,78,201).

The work of Urban and Holm (79,200) on diffusion and transport of nutrients and metabolites provided information from *in vivo* incorporation of radioactive tracers (labeled glucose, sulfate) on the nutritional pathways into the disc. Passive diffusion was found to be the predominant transport mechanism. The ionic charge and molecular weight of solutes were shown to be important variables. The annulus periphery was the major pathway for charged ions such as sulfate, and for uncharged solutes the annulus and end plate were of approximately equal importance. For small nutrients, passive diffusion is the primary mechanism for transport, whereas transport of larger nutrients such as growth factors is enhanced by convection associated with loading and deformations of the disc that cause volumetric changes.

Because of its size, the avascular disc provides an environment that is low in oxygen and high in lactate (12), but the cellularity and rate of tissue turnover (and hence the nutritional requirements) are low. Recent studies on disc cells in agarose gel in a diffusion chamber support the idea that cell viability and metabolism are affected by nutrient supply (80). The maximum cell density in the disc is regulated by nutritional constraints with both glucose concentration and pH being important factors. Another interesting finding is that the intervertebral disc cells remained viable at low oxygen concentrations but produce very little matrix (80). Decreased nutrient supply in the apical discs of scoliosis patients *in vivo* have been recorded using microelectrodes. This may result from altered mechanics or calcification of the end plates in these patients (201).

5.5 Biomechanical Contribution to Intervertebral Disc Degeneration

Mechanical factors may accelerate disc degeneration by three related mechanisms. In the first, alterations in the material properties of disc subcomponents may predispose the disc to failure. In the second, certain loading conditions may predispose the disc to failure, e.g., hyperflexion. Recent studies using animal models (84, 113,114) suggest a third pathway in which certain loading conditions applied chronically will cause tissue remodeling and altered material properties, which in turn can promote altered motion segment properties and cellular apoptosis and/or degenerative response.

Habitual long-distance running was shown to influence the proteoglycan content in canine intervertebral discs, with reductions in the cervical and thoracic regions, but increases in the lumbar discs (150). The differences with spinal region were attributed to different biomechanical demands on different regions, suggesting that the type of mechanical forces, loading frequency, and duration all influence composition. These compositional changes are also suggestive of changes in mechanical properties of the intervertebral disc. In a canine model of spine fusion,

a decrease in the aggregating capacity of proteoglycans in the intervertebral disc at the fused level as well as a decrease in proteoglycan content in the nucleus were found at the fused and adjacent levels (35). These changes were attributed to the altered mechanical environment. Region-specific reductions in collagen, water, and proteoglycans and alterations in collagen types occur with scoliosis, e.g., total collagen concentration and ratio of type I to type II collagen are greatest on the concave side of the curve (3,8,19,201). Although tissue remodeling resulting from scoliosis is apparently a response to altered mechanical environment, it is difficult to distinguish between primary (causative) and secondary (consequential) biological processes.

5.6 Analytical Models of the Intervertebral Disc and Motion Segment

Stresses in the disc (and other materials) cannot be measured directly without the use of invasive transducers that will interfere with the stresses being measured. Disc models therefore provide the necessary and valuable tools to calculate mechanical aspects of disc function that are inaccessible to direct measurement. The geometry of the disc permits the annulus to bulge, thereby providing flexibility in all six degrees of freedom. When loaded axially, the annulus contains the pressure generated within the nucleus, with a force equilibrium between tension in bulging fibers and internal (nuclear) pressure. The force equilibrium at the end plates includes the effects of hydraulic pressure, and the counteracting solid-phase tissue stress arising from the fiber tension. The difference between these two components produces the reaction forces and moments transmitted from the vertebra.

In Fig. 12-9, a simplified analysis of static equilibrium predicts that the stresses in the annulus are several times the average compressive stress imposed on the disc. Assuming that the section is circular, and the radius of the nucleus b is 70% of the outer annulus radius a (i.e., $b = 0.7a$), then by equilibrium, the stress in the annulus fibrosus σ_{af} multiplied by the cross section of the annulus must equal the pressure in the

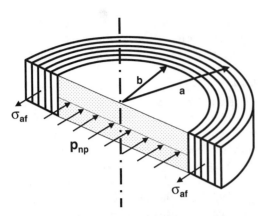

FIGURE 12-9. Estimation of annular tensile stress resulting from nucleus pulposus pressure based on a simplified balance of forces.

nucleus p_{np}, multiplied by its area. Hence

$$\sigma_{af} \times 2 \times 0.3a = p_{np} \times 2 \times 0.7a$$

i.e.,

$$\sigma_{af} = p_{np} \times 1.4/0.6 \approx 2.3 \times p_{np}$$

because it is observed (133) that the nucleus pressure p_{np} is approximately 1.5 times the mean end-plate load/unit area p,

$$\sigma_{af} \approx 3.45\,p$$

Analyses of a homogeneous and isotropic thick-walled vessel that is under internal pressure and with capped ends (215) yield similar results. The circumferential stress (σ_c) in the annulus ranges from approximately $3\,p_{np}$ at the inner annulus to $2\,p_{np}$ at the outer surface of the annulus. This analysis also yields values for radial compressive stress (σ_r) that equal the nucleus pressure at the inner annulus and is zero at the outer periphery of the annulus. The equilibrium of elastic stresses predicts a value for $\sigma_{axial} = 2\,p_{np}$, which is greater than that measured by Nachemson (133). The large radial variation in tensile and compressive moduli of the annulus (increasing toward the outer annulus), combined with observations from intradiscal pressure measurements, suggests that both of these stress components (σ_c and σ_r) may really be more uniform across the radius of the annulus than is suggested by these simplified analyses.

Broberg provided a comprehensive structural analysis of the static force equilibrium for discs that are deformed in each of the six principal directions (three translation directions and three angular) (22). The analyses also predicted that angular and shear stiffnesses of the disc increase with axial compressive preload. This model was further modified to describe time-dependent deformation resulting from viscoelastic deformation of the annulus fibers and fluid flow to and from the disc (21). This analysis suggested that the many daily short-duration fluctuations of disc axial load do not significantly affect the change of height or fluid content over a long time, but do increase the total flow through the end plate and outer annulus.

5.6.1 Elastic and Multiphasic Finite Element Representations

Elastic finite element models have provided insights into the flexibility as well as the mode of failure of the disc (e.g., 65,135,165,178). Effects of degeneration can be represented in finite element methods by parametrically varying material properties and geometry of the disc (135,166). The predictions made by these model simulations of pathology vary widely, but suggest changes in the loading pattern of the annulus. For example, it was reported that the presence of discrete peripheral tears in the annulus fibrosus may have a role in the formation of concentric annular tears and in accelerating the degenerating process of the disc (135). Continuum models may provide further useful insights into possible stimuli for tissue adaptation and causes of degeneration if they include spatial and temporal variations in the mechanical and electrochemical fields that are thought to influence cellular activity (17).

Finite element models have been extended to include solid-phase time-dependent behavior (or flow-independent viscoelasticity) (205) and the contributions of the fluid phase in contributing to time-dependent behaviors (biphasic viscoelasticity) (172). These analyses have been helpful in explaining the time-dependent disc behavior and possible roles of fluid transport in influencing disc nutrition. The most advanced constitutive models currently used for biological materials are multiphasic models that include contributions from electrically charged and permeable solid matrix, fluid pressure, and the electrochemical potential of mobile charged molecules (e.g., Na^+, K^+, Cl^-) (107). These approaches are based on methods initially developed to represent cartilage and meniscal mechanics, as described in Chapter 5. Multiphasic disc finite element models (51,88,108,109) allow more accurate prediction of physical fields in the tissue, including mechanical stresses and strains, fluid pressure, swelling pressure, and streaming potential (or current) (69,70). These factors, together with nutrient concentration, may influence the cellular response to externally applied loading. Modeling studies can be helpful in predicting the consequences of a change in composition for the disc behavior. In a simulation study a loss of proteoglycan content in the disc (as seen with degeneration) reduced hydrostatic pressure and electrical potential in the disc, increased solid matrix stresses, and had a profound effect on fluid transport (88).

5.6.2 End-plate Boundary Conditions

In addition to accurate material properties and geometry, boundary conditions are crucial components in models of the intervertebral disc because they determine the strains at the end plates and the annulus periphery, as well as the fluid flow exchange and hence the internal flows. For multiphasic models, these conditions must include force, deformation, pressure, chemical and electrical conditions. The permeability of cancellous and cortical bone is on the order of $10^{-10}\,m^4/Nsec$ and $10^{-16}\,m^4/Nsec$, respectively (103,116). Although the stiffness of even cancellous bone can be 100 times that of the annulus and cartilage end plate in compression, significant viscoelastic effects under high loading-rate conditions and observed vertebral endplate deformations call into question the assumption that these boundaries are rigid. Mechanical loading conditions are often simplified to a single force (e.g., compression) or bending moment (e.g., flexion) but are also reported for complex (i.e., combined) loading conditions (167,178).

5.7 Mechanical Influences on Disc and Chondrocytic Physiology

The mechanical environment of the disc can influence the behavior of its cells by direct mechanical stimulation of the cells themselves, as well as by influencing the transport of ions and molecules into and out of the extracellular matrix, and hence altering their concentrations.

It is expected that disc cells respond to mechanical stimuli, but they probably have a different response compared with chondrocytes from other tissues such as hyaline cartilage. The mechanobiology of cartilage cells is reviewed in Chapter 6 of this book. The disc cells exist in a very different environment compared with cartilage. In the disc, hydrostatic stress is habitually present (about 0.1 MPa), and activity can produce stress up to about 3 MPa. Thus, the resting stress is higher but that due to activity is lower than localized stresses that occur in articular cartilage. Whether the deformational strains differ is not known. The chemical conditions in the matrix differ between disc and cartilage because of differences in the nutritional pathways. It therefore seems likely that the *in situ* response of disc chondrocytes to mechanical stimulus differs from that in cartilage because the environment is different. Disc chondrocytes in culture have been shown to respond to hydrostatic pressure (72,82,94), as well as to axial loading (137,190), osmolality (93), and oxygen concentration (92,211) of the extracellular environment. At the organ level, Ohshima et al. (137) used bovine caudal discs in a perfusion chamber to show that mechanical load influences the rate of sulfate incorporation into the intact intervertebral disc.

Differences between cells in the annulus compared with the nucleus have been reported. In the nucleus, proteoglycan synthesis was stimulated by a pressure of 2.5 MPa and no response was observed in the annulus (94). Similar differences are reported for nucleus- and annulus-derived cells by Hutton et al. (82) with hydrostatic pressure of 1 MPa. It is tempting to infer that these differences relate to differing habitual mechanical conditions between these functionally different regions of the disc.

There is evidence of a "window" of stress (0.3 to 3 MPa) in which proteoglycan production in the nucleus and inner annulus is stimulated by hydrostatic pressure, and above which production of matrix degrading proteinases is increased (72) and proteoglycan synthesis may be inhibited (94). When short-term (20-second) compared with longer term (2-hour) pressures of 2.5 MPa were applied, Ishihara et al. (94) reported that proteoglycan synthesis in the inner regions of the disc was only stimulated by the short-term application of pressure.

These specific aspects of disc chondrocytic biomechanics and metabolism have implications for the emerging area of disc tissue engineering, as well as understanding of the mechanical influences on healthy disc metabolism and degeneration. Some insights into the conditions that support disc tissue homeostasis and cell viability have emerged from attempts to culture intervertebral discs. Because of the disc's strong tendency to swell, the culture medium must provide a counteracting stress, either chemically [e.g., by using polyethylene glycol (13)], or physically [e.g., in alginate (30)] or through mechanical pressure (99). These mechanical conditions are important, in addition to the choice of culture medium and oxygen concentration. The regulation of the cell phenotype and its biosynthetic activity probably depends on a complex interaction among mechanical stimuli, presence of growth factors, and cytokines, as well as other chemical signals from the extracellular matrix. A complete understanding of the mechanisms that control spinal function requires that these interactions be understood at a molecular, cellular, organ, and gross anatomical scales.

6   CONCLUSION

Biomechanics has made substantial contributions to knowledge about the causes of spinal problems, notably spinal trauma, spinal deformity (e.g., scoliosis), and low back pain. These clinical problems can be managed better with an understanding of spinal biomechanics, including how muscles are activated, how the spine is loaded, and how those loads are distributed between the anterior and posterior structures of the spine. Spinal pathologies are among the costliest of all orthopaedic problems, and they are becoming more prevalent in the population.

However, despite much recent progress, many questions remain to be fully resolved:

- How are the muscles activated, and according to which strategies under differing situations? What are the relative roles of muscle function and spinal column stiffness in preventing buckling instabilities and other abnormal motion in the spinal column?
- What are the effects of differing magnitude and frequency of spinal loading and motion on transport of nutrients and metabolites in the spinal tissues, on the stimulation of metabolic activity in cells, and on tissue remodeling? Which mechanical conditions cause (and prevent) acute and chronic tissue damage and degenerative changes? Is there a "safe window" of mechanical conditions that these tissues tolerate without damage?
- How is pre- and postnatal spinal growth influenced by mechanical environment, and does mechanical environment influence the initiation and progression of spinal deformities?
- Can information about the *in vivo* behavior of spinal tissues and their cells be applied to the engineering of tissues for implantation?

REFERENCES

1. Acaroglu ER, Iatridis JC, Setton LA, et al. Degeneration and aging affect the tensile behavior of human lumbar annulus fibrosus. *Spine* 1995;20(24):2690–2701.
2. Adams MA, McNally DS, Dolan P. 'Stress' distributions inside intervertebral discs. The effects of age and degeneration. *J Bone Joint Surg Br* 1996;78(6):965–967.
3. Aigner T, Greskotter KR, Fairbank JC, et al. Variation with age in the pattern of type X collagen expression in normal and scoliotic human intervertebral discs. *Calcif Tissue Int* 1998;63(3):263–268.
4. Andersson GBJ, Schultz AB. Effects of fluid injection on mechanical properties of intervertebral discs. *J Biomech* 1979;12:453–458.
5. Andersson GBJ. Posture and compressive spine loading: intradiscal pressures, trunk and

myoelectric activities, intra-abdominal pressures, and biochemical analysis. *Ergonomics* 1985;28(1):91–93.

6. Antoniou J, Steffen T, Nelson F, et al. The human lumbar intervertebral disc: evidence for changes in the biosynthesis and denaturation of the extracellular matrix with growth, maturation, ageing, and degeneration. *J Clin Invest* 1996;98(4):996–1003.

7. Antoniou J, Goudsouzian NM, Heathfield TF, et al. The human lumbar endplate. Evidence of changes in biosynthesis and denaturation of the extracellular matrix with growth, maturation, aging, and degeneration. *Spine* 1996;21(10):1153–1161.

8. Antoniou J, Arlet V, Goswami T, et al. Elevated synthetic activity in the convex side of scoliotic intervertebral discs and endplates compared with normal tissues. *Spine* 2001;26(10):E198–206.

9. Ashton-Miller JA, Schultz AB. Spine instability and segmental hypermobility biomechanics: a call for the definition and standard use of terms. *Semin Spine Surg* 1991;3:136–148.

10. Ayotte DC, Ito K, Tepic S. Direction-dependent resistance to flow in the endplate and intervertebral disc: an *ex vivo* study. *J Orthop Res* 2001; 19(6):1073–1077.

11. Ayotte DC, Ito K, Perren SM, et al. Direction-dependent constriction flow in a poroelastic solid: the intervertebral disc valve. *J Biomech Eng, Trans ASME* 2000;122(6):587–593.

12. Bartels EM, Fairbank JC, Winlove CP, et al. Oxygen and lactate concentrations measured *in vivo* in the intervertebral discs of patients with scoliosis and back pain. *Spine* 1998;23(1):1–7.

13. Bayliss MT, Urban JP, Johnstone B, et al. *In vitro* method for measuring synthesis rates in the intervertebral disc. *J Orthop Res* 1986;4(1):10–17.

14. Bean JC, Chaffin DB, Schultz AB. Biomechanical model calculation of muscle contraction forces: a double linear programming method. *J Biomech* 1998;21(1):59–66.

15. Bergmark A. Stability of the lumbar spine. A study in mechanical engineering. *Acta Orthop Scand (Suppl)* 1989;230:1–54.

16. Best BA, Guilak F, Setton LA, et al. Compressive mechanical properties of the human annulus fibrosus and their relationship to biochemical composition. *Spine* 1994;19(2):212–221.

17. Brand RA. What do tissues and cells know of mechanics? *Ann Med* 1997;29:267–269.

18. Brault JS, Driscoll DM, Laakso LL, et al. Quantification of lumbar intradiscal deformation during flexion and extension, by mathematical analysis of magnetic resonance imaging pixel intensity profiles. *Spine* 1997;22:2066–2072.

19. Brickley-Parsons D, Glimcher MJ. Is the chemistry of collagen in intervertebral discs an expression of Wolff's law? A study of the human lumbar spine. *Spine* 1984;9:148–163.

20. Brinckmann P, Frobin W, Hierholzer E, et al. Deformations of the vertebral endplate under axial loading of the spine. *Spine* 1983;8:851–856.

21. Broberg KB. Slow deformations of intervertebral discs. *J Biomech* 1983;26:501–512.

22. Broberg KB. On the mechanical behaviour of intervertebral discs. *Spine* 1983;8:151–165.

23. Buckwalter JA. Aging and degeneration of the human intervertebral disc. *Spine* 1995;20(11):1307–1314.

24. Calisse J, Rohlmann A, Bergmann G. Estimation of trunk muscle forces using the finite element method and *in vivo* loads measured by telemeterized internal spinal fixation devices. *J Biomech* 1999;32(7):727–731.

25. Cappozzo A. Compressive loads in the lumbar vertebral column during normal level walking. *J Orthop Res* 1984;1(3):292–301.

26. Cassidy JJ, Hiltner A, Baer E. Hierarchical structure of the intervertebral disc. *Connect Tissue Res* 1989;23(1):75–88.

27. Carlson H, Nilsson J, Thorstensson A, et al. Motor responses in the human trunk due to load perturbations. *Acta Physiol Scand* 1981;111:221–223.

28. Cavanaugh JM, Ozaktay AC, Yamashita HT, et al. Lumbar facet pain: biomechanics, neuroanatomy and neurophysiology. *J Biomech* 1996;29(9):1117–1129.

29. Chiang J, Potvin JR. The *in vivo* dynamic response of the human spine to rapid lateral bend perturbation: effects of preload and step input magnitude. *Spine* 2001;26(13):1457–1464.

30. Chiba K, Andersson GB, Masuda K, et al. A new culture system to study the metabolism of the intervertebral disc *in vitro*. *Spine* 1998;23:1821–1827.

31. Cholewicki J, McGill SM. Lumbar posterior ligament involvement during extremely heavy lifts estimated from fluoroscopic measurements. *J Biomech* 1992;25(1):17–28.

32. Cholewicki J, McGill SM. EMG assisted optimization: a hybrid approach for estimating muscle forces in an indeterminate biomechanical model. *J Biomech* 1994;27(10):1287–1289.

33. Cholewicki J, McGill SM. Mechanical stability of the *in vivo* lumbar spine: implications for injury and chronic low back pain. *Clin Biomech* 1996;11,1–15.

34. Cole TC, Ghosh P, Taylor TK. Variations of the proteoglycans of the canine intervertebral disc with ageing. *Biochim Biophys Acta* 1986;880(2–3):209–219.

35. Cole TC, Burkhardt D, Ghosh P, et al. Effects of spinal fusion on the proteoglycans of the canine intervertebral disc. *J Orthop Res* 1985;3:277–291.

36. Cresswell A, Oddsson L, Thorstensson A. The influence of sudden perturbations on trunk muscle activity and intra-abdominal pressure while standing. *Exp Brain Res* 1994;98:336–341.

37. Cresswell A, Grundstrom H, Thorstensson A. Observations on intra-abdominal pressure and

patterns of abdominal intra-muscular activity in man. *Acta Physiol Scand* 1992;144:409–418.

38. Cripton PA, Bruehlmann SB, Orr TE, et al. *In vitro* axial preload application during spine flexibility testing: towards reduced apparatus-related artefacts. *J Biomech* 2000;33(12):1559–1568.

39. Crisco JJ, Panjabi MM, Yamamoto I, et al. Euler stability of the human ligamentous lumbar spine. Part 2: experimental. *Clin Biomech* 1992;7:27–32.

40. Crisco JJ III, Panjabi MM. The inter-segmental and multisegmental muscles of the lumbar spine. A biomechanical model comparing lateral stabilizing potential. *Spine* 1991;16(7):793–799.

41. Crowninshield RD, Brand RA. A physiologically based criterion of muscle force prediction in locomotion. *J Biomech* 1981;14:793–801.

42. Cyron BM, Hutton WC. The fatigue strength of the lumbar neural arch in spondylolysis. *J Bone Joint Surg Br* 1978;60:234–238.

43. Daggfeldt K, Thorstensson A. The role of intra-abdominal pressure in spinal unloading. *J Biomech* 1997;30(11–12):1149–1155.

44. Drost MR, Willems P, Snijders H, et al. Confined compression of canine annulus fibrosus under chemical and mechanical load. *J Biomech Eng, Trans ASME* 1995;117:390–396.

45. Dul J, Johnson GE, Shiavi R, et al. Muscular synergism. II. A minimum fatigue criterion for load sharing between synergistic muscles. *J Biomech* 1984;17:675–684.

46. Eberlien R, Holzapfel GA, Schulze-Bauer CAJ. An anisotropic model for annulus tissue and enhanced finite element analyses of intact lumbar disc bodies. *Comput Methods Biomech Biomed Engin* 2001;4:209–229.

47. Edwards WT, Hayes WC, Posner I, et al. Variation of lumbar spine stiffness with load. *J Biomech Eng, Trans ASME* 1987;109:35–42.

48. Elliott DM, Setton LA. Anisotropic and inhomogeneous tensile behavior of the human annulus fibrosus: experimental measurement and material model predictions. *J Biomech Eng, Trans ASME* 2001;123(3):256–263.

49. Elliott DM, Setton LA. A linear material model for fiber-induced anisotropy of the annulus fibrosus. *J Biomech Eng, Trans ASME* 2000;122(2):173–179.

50. Fredrickson BE, Baker D, McHolick WJ, et al. The natural history of spondylolysis and spondylolisthesis. *J Bone Joint Surg Am* 1984;66:699–707.

51. Frijns AJ, Huyghe JM, Janssen JD. A validation of the quadriphasic mixture theory for intervertebral disc tissue. *Int J Eng Sci* 1997;35(15):1419–1429.

52. Frymoyer J. Epidemiology. In: Frymoyer JW, Gordon SL, eds. *New perspectives on low back pain*. Park Ridge, IL: American Academy of Orthopaedic Surgeons, 1989:19–34.

53. Fujita Y, Duncan NA, Lotz JC. Radial tensile properties of the lumbar annulus fibrosus are site and degeneration dependent. *J Orthop Res* 1997;15(6):814–819.

54. Fujita Y, Wagner DR, Biviji AA, et al. Anisotropic shear behavior of the annulus fibrosus: effect of harvest site and tissue prestrain. *Med Eng Phys* 2000;22(5):349–357.

55. Fujiwara A, Lim TH, An HS, et al. The effect of disc degeneration and facet joint osteoarthritis on the segmental flexibility of the lumbar spine. *Spine* 2000;25(23):3036–3044.

56. Galante JO. Tensile properties of the human lumbar annulus fibrosus. *Acta Orthop Scand* 1967;Suppl:1–91.

57. Gardner-Morse MG, Stokes IAF. The effects of abdominal muscle co-activation on lumbar spine stability. *Spine* 1998;23(1):86–92.

58. Gardner-Morse M, Stokes IA, Laible JP. Role of muscles in lumbar spine stability in maximum extension efforts. *J Orthop Res* 1995;13(5):802–808.

59. Gardner-Morse GM, Stokes IA. Physiological axial compressive preloads increase motion segment stiffness, linearity and hysteresis in all six degrees of freedom. *J Orthop Res* 2003;21(3):547–552.

60. Gardner-Morse M, Stokes IAF. Three-dimensional simulations of scoliosis derotation by Cotrel-Dubousset instrumentation. *J Biomech* 1993;27:177–181.

61. Gardner-Morse MG, Laible JP, Stokes IAF. Incorporation of spinal flexibility measurements into finite element analysis. *J Biomech Eng, Trans ASME* 1990;112:481–483.

62. Ghosh, P, Bushell GR, Taylor TKF, et al. Distribution of glycosaminoglycans across the normal and scoliotic disc. *Spine* 1980;5:310.

63. Goel VK, Pope MH. Biomechanics of fusion and stabilization. *Spine* 1995;15;20(24 Suppl):85S–99S.

64. Goel VK. Three-dimensional motion behavior of the human spine—a question of terminology. *J Biomech Eng, Trans ASME* 1987;109(4):353–355.

65. Goel VK, Monroe BT, Gilbertson LG, et al. Interlaminar shear stresses and laminae separation in a disc. Finite element analysis of the L3-L4 motion segment subjected to axial compressive loads. *Spine* 1995;20(6):689–698.

66. Goel V, Lim T, Gwon J, et al. Effects of rigidity of an internal fixation device. A comprehensive biomechanical investigation. *Spine* 1991;16(Suppl):S155–161.

67. Granata KP, Marras WS. Cost-benefit of muscle cocontraction in protecting against spinal instability. *Spine* 2000;25(11):1398–1404.

68. Granata KP, Marras WS. An EMG-assisted model of trunk loading during free-dynamic lifting. *J Biomech* 1995;28(11):1309–1317.

69. Gu WY, Mao XG, Foster RJ, et al. The anisotropic hydraulic permeability of human lumbar annulus

fibrosus. Influence of age, degeneration and water content. *Spine* 1999;24(23):2449–2455.

70. Gu WY, Mao XG, Rawlins BA, et al. Streaming potential of human lumbar annulus fibrosus is anisotropic and affected by disc degeneration. *J Biomech* 1999;32(11):1177–1182.

71. Ha K, Schendel M, Lewis J, et al. Effect of immobilization and configuration on lumbar adjacent-segment biomechanics. *J Spinal Disord* 1993;6:99–105.

72. Handa T, Ishihara H, Ohshima H, et al. Effects of hydrostatic pressure on matrix synthesis and matrix metalloproteinase production in the human lumbar intervertebral disc. *Spine* 1997;22(10):1085–1091.

73. Hemborg B, Moritz U, Lowing H. Intra-abdominal pressure and trunk muscle activity during lifting. IV. The causal factors of the intra-abdominal pressure rise. *Scand J Rehabil Med* 1985;17(1):25–38.

74. Henry SM, Fung J, Horak FB. Control of stance during lateral and anterior/posterior surface translations. *IEEE Trans Rehabil Eng* 1998;6(1):32–42.

75. Henry SM, Fung J, Horak FB. EMG responses to maintain stance during multidirectional surface translations. *J Neurophysiol* 1998;80:1939–1950.

76. Hirano N, Tsuji H, Ohshima H, et al. Analysis of rabbit intervertebral disc physiology based on water metabolism. II. Changes in normal intervertebral discs under axial vibratory load. *Spine* 1998;13(11):1297–1302.

77. Hodges P, Richardson C. Inefficient muscular stabilization of the lumbar spine associated with low back pain. *Spine* 1996;21:2640–2650.

78. Holm S, Nachemson A. Nutrition of the intervertebral disc: acute effects of cigarette smoking. An experimental animal study. *Ups J Med Sci* 1998;93:91–99.

79. Holm S, Nachemson A. Variations in the nutrition of the canine intervertebral disc induced by motion. *Spine* 1983;8:866–874.

80. Horner HA, Urban JP. 2001 Volvo Award Winner in Basic Science Studies: effect of nutrient supply on the viability of cells from the nucleus pulposus of the intervertebral disc. *Spine* 2001;26:2543–2549.

81. Hughes RE, Chaffin DB, Lavender SA, et al. Evaluation of muscle force prediction models of the lumbar trunk using surface electromyography. *J Orthop Res* 1994;12(5),689–698.

82. Hutton WC, Elmer WA, Boden SD, et al. The effect of hydrostatic pressure on intervertebral disc metabolism. *Spine* 1999;24(15):1507–1515.

83. Hutton WC, Ganey TM, Elmer WA, et al. Does long-term compressive loading on the intervertebral disc cause degeneration? *Spine* 2000;25(23):2993–3004.

84. Iatridis JC, Mente PL, Stokes IA, et al. Compression-induced changes in intervertebral disc properties in a rat tail model. *Spine* 1999;24(10):996–1002.

85. Iatridis JC, Setton LA, Weidenbaum M, et al. Alterations in the mechanical behavior of the human lumbar nucleus pulposus with degeneration and aging. *J Orthop Res* 1997;15(2):318–322.

86. Iatridis JC, Setton LA, Foster RJ, et al. Degeneration affects the anisotropic and nonlinear behaviors of human annulus fibrosus in compression. *J Biomech* 1998;31(6):535–544.

87. Iatridis JC, Kumar S, Foster RJ, et al. Shear mechanical properties of human lumbar annulus fibrosus. *J Orthop Res* 1999;17(5):732–737.

88. Iatridis JC, Laible JP, Krag MH. Influence of fixed charge density magnitude and distribution on the intervertebral disc: applications of a poroelastic and chemical electric (PEACE) model. *J Biomech Eng* 2003;125(1):12–24.

89. Iatridis JC, Setton LA, Weidenbaum M, et al. The viscoelastic behavior of the nondegenerate human lumbar nucleus pulposus in shear. *J Biomech* 1997;30(10):1005–1013.

90. Indahl A, Kaigle A, Reikeras O, et al. Electromyographic response of the porcine multifidus musculature after nerve stimulation. *Spine* 1995;20:2652–2658.

91. Indahl A, Kaigle A, Reikeras O, et al. Sacroiliac joint involvement in activation of the porcine spinal and gluteal musculature. *J Spinal Disord* 1999;12(4):325–330.

92. Ishihara H, Urban JP. Effects of low oxygen concentrations and metabolic inhibitors on proteoglycan and protein synthesis rates in the intervertebral disc. *J Orthop Res* 1999;17(6):829–835.

93. Ishihara H, Warensjo K, Roberts S, et al. Proteoglycan synthesis in the intervertebral disk nucleus: the role of extracellular osmolality. *Am J Physiol* 1997;272(5 Pt 1):C1499–1506.

94. Ishihara H, McNally DS, Urban JP, et al. Effects of hydrostatic pressure on matrix synthesis in different regions of the intervertebral disk. *J Appl Physiol* 1996;80(3):839–846.

95. Jackson DW, Wiltse LL, Cirincione RJ. Spondylolysis in the female gymnast. *Clin Orthop Rel Res* 1976;117:69–73.

96. Janevic, J, Ashton-Miller JA, Schultz AB. Large compressive preloads decrease lumbar motion segment flexibility. *J Orthop Res* 1991;9(2):228–236.

97. Jayaraman G, Zbib HM, Jacobs RR. Biomechanical analyses of surgical correction techniques in idiopathic scoliosis: significance of biplanar characteristics of scoliotic spines. *J Biomech* 1989;22:427–438.

98. Kaneoka K, Ono K, Inami S, et al. Motion analysis of cervical vertebrae during whiplash loading. *Spine* 1999;24(8):763–769.

99. Kim JG, Lim T, Kim KW, et al. A novel biomechanical culture system for the studies of the intervertebral disc. *Trans Orthop Res Soc* 2002;813.

100. Kingma I, van Dieen JH, Nicolay K, et al. Monitoring water content in deforming intervertebral disc tissue by finite element analysis of MRI data. *Magn Reson Med* 2000;44(4):650–654.

101. Klisch SM, Lotz JC. A special theory of biphasic mixtures and experimental results for human annulus fibrosus tested in confined compression. *J Biomech Eng, Trans ASME* 2000;122(2):180–188.

102. Klisch SM, Lotz JC. Application of a fiber-reinforced continuum theory to multiple deformations of the annulus fibrosus. *J Biomech* 1999;32(10):1027–1036.

103. Kohles SS, Roberts JB, Upton ML, et al. Direct perfusion measurements of cancellous bone anisotropic permeability. *J Biomech* 2001:34(9): 1197–1202.

104. Kopperdahl DL, Keaveny TM. Yield strain behavior of trabelcular bone. *J Biomech* 1998;31:601–608.

105. Krag MH, Seroussi RE, Wilder DG, et al. Internal displacement distribution from *in vitro* loading of human thoracic and lumbar spinal motion segments: experimental results and theoretical predictions. *Spine* 1987;12(10):1001–1007.

106. Kusaka Y, Nakajima SI, Uemura O, et al. Intradiscal solid phase displacement as a determinant of the centripetal fluid shift in the loaded intervertebral disc. *Spine* 2001;26(9):E174–E181.

107. Lai WM, Hou JS, Mow VC. A triphasic theory for the swelling and deformation behaviors of articular cartilage. *J Biomech Eng, Trans ASME* 1991;113(3):245–258.

108. Laible JP, Pflaster D, Krag MH, et al. A poroelastic-swelling finite element model with application to the intervertebral disc. *Spine* 1993;18(5):659–670.

109. Laible JP, Pflaster D, Simon BR, et al. A dynamic material parameter estimation procedure for soft tissue using a poroelastic finite element model. *J Biomech Eng, Trans ASME* 1994;116:19–29.

110. Lavender SA, Tsuang YH, Andersson GB, et al. Trunk muscle coactivation: the effects of moment direction and moment magnitude. *J Orthop Res* 11992;0,691–700.

111. Lavender SA, Mirka GA, Schoenmarklin RW, et al. The effects of preview and task symmetry on trunk muscle response to sudden loading. *Human Factors* 1989;31(1):101–115.

112. Lee C, Langrana N. Lumbosacral spinal fusion: a biomechanical study. *Spine* 1984;9:574–581.

113. Lotz JC, Colliou OK, Chin JR, et al. Compression-induced degeneration of the intervertebral disc: an *in vivo* mouse model and finite-element study. *Spine* 1998;23(23):2493–2506.

114. Lotz JC, Chin JR. Intervertebral disc cell death is dependent on the magnitude and dura-tion of spinal loading. *Spine* 2000;25(12):1477–1483.

115. Lyons G, Eisenstein SM, Sweet MB. Biochemical changes in intervertebral disc degeneration. *Biochim Biophys Acta* 1981;673(4):443–453.

116. Mak AF, Huang DT, Zhang JD, et al. Deformation-induced hierarchical flows and drag forces in bone canaliculi and matrix microporosity. *J Biomech* 1997;30:11–18.

117. Malko JA, Hutton WC, Fajman WA. An *in vivo* magnetic resonance imaging study of changes in the volume (and fluid content) of the lumbar intervertebral discs during a simulated diurnal load cycle. *Spine* 1999;24(10):1015–1022.

118. Marchand F, Ahmed AM. Investigation of the laminate structure of lumbar disc annulus fibrosus. *Spine* 1990;15(5):402–410.

119. Maroudas A, Muir H, Wingham J. The correlation of fixed negative charge with glycosaminoglycan content of human articular cartilage. *Biochim Biophys Acta* 1969;177(3):492–500.

120. Marras WS, Rangarajulu SL, Lavender SA. Trunk loading and expectation. *Ergonomics* 1987;30(3): 551–562.

121. McAfee PC, Farey ID, Sutterlin CE, et al. The effect of spinal implant rigidity on vertebral bone density. *Spine* 1991;16:S190–S197.

122. McCarroll JR, Miller JM, Ritter MA. Lumbar spondylolysis and spondylolisthesis in college football players. A prospective study. *Am J Sports Med* 1986;14:404–406.

123. McGill SM. A myoelectrically based dynamic three-dimensional model to predict loads on lumbar spine tissues during lateral bending. *J Biomech* 1992;25(4):395–414.

124. McGill SM, Norman RW. Partitioning of the L4–L5 dynamic moment into disc, ligamentous, and muscular components during lifting. *Spine* 1986;11(7):666–678.

125. McKenzie R, Donelson R. Mechanical diagnosis and therapy for low back pain. Toward a better understanding. In: Weisel SW, Weinstein JN, Herkowitz, H, et al., eds. The lumbar spine, 2nd ed., Vol. 2. Philadelphia: WB Saunders, 1996:998–1011.

126. McMillan DW, Garbutt G, Adams MA. Effect of sustained loading on the water content of intervertebral discs: implications for disc metabolism. *Ann Rheum Dis* 1996;55(12):880–887.

127. McNally D, Adams M. Internal intervertebral disc mechanics as revealed by stress profilometry. *Spine* 1992;17:66–73.

128. Mimura M, Panjabi M, Oxland T, et al. Disc degeneration affects the multidirectional flexibility of the lumbar spine. *Spine* 1994;19:1371–1380.

129. Moroney SP, Schultz AB, Miller JA. Analysis and measurement of neck loads. *J Orthop Res* 1988;6(5):713–720.

130. Morris JM, Lucas DB, Bresler MS. The role of the trunk in stability of the spine. *J Bone Joint Surg Am* 1961;43(3):327–351.

131. Nachemson A, Morris JM. *In vivo* measurement of intradiscal pressure. Discometry, a new method for the determination of pressure in the lower lumbar discs. *J Bone Joint Surg Am* 1964;46:1077–1092.

132. Nachemson AL, Schultz AB, Berkson MH. Mechanical properties of human lumbar spine motion segments; influences of age, sex, disc level, and degeneration. *Spine* 1979;4(1):1–8.

133. Nachemson AL. Lumbar intradiscal pressure. *Acta Orthop Scand Suppl* 1960;43:1–104.

134. Nagata H, Schendel M, Transfeldt E, et al. The effects of immobilization of long segments of the spine on the adjacent and distal facet force and lumbosacral motion. *Spine* 1993;18:2471–2479.

135. Natarajan RN, Ke JH, Andersson GB. A model to study the disc degeneration process. *Spine* 1994;19:259–265.

136. Nussbaum MA, Martin BJ, Chaffin DB. A neural network model for simulation of torso muscle coordination. *J Biomech* 1997;30(3):251–258.

137. Ohshima H, Urban JP, Bergel DH. Effect of static load on matrix synthesis rates in the intervertebral disc measured *in vitro* by a new perfusion technique. *J Orthop Res* 1995;13(1):22–29.

138. Panagiotacopulos ND, Pope MH, Krag MH, Bloch R. A mechanical model for the human intervertebral disc. *J Biomech* 1987;20(9):839–850.

139. Panjabi M, Abumi K, Duranceau J, et al. Spinal stability and inter-segmental muscle forces. A biomechanical model. *Spine* 1989;14:194–200.

140. Panjabi M, Brown M, Lindahl S, et al. Intrinsic disc pressure as a measure of integrity of the lumbar spine. *Spine* 1988;13(8):913–917.

141. Panjabi MM, Krag MH, White AA, et al. Effects of preload on load displacement curves of the lumbar spine. *Orthop Clin North Am* 1977;8:181–192.

142. Panjabi MM, Cholewicki J, Nibu K, et al. Simulation of whiplash trauma using whole cervical spine specimens. *Spine* 1998;23(1):17–24.

143. Panjabi MM, Brand RA, White AA. Three dimensional flexibility and stiffness properties of the human thoracic spine. *J Biomech* 1976;9:185–192.

144. Panjabi MM. The stabilizing system of the spine. Part I: function, dysfunction, adaptation, and enhancement. *J Spinal Disorders* 1992;5:383–389.

145. Patwardhan AG, Havey RM, Meade KP, et al. A follower load increases the load-carrying capacity of the lumbar spine in compression. *Spine* 1999;24(10):1003–1009.

146. Patwardhan AG, Havey RM, Ghanayem AJ, et al. Load-carrying capacity of the human cervical spine in compression is increased under a follower load. *Spine* 2000;25(12):1548–1554.

147. Pearce RH, Grimmer BJ, Adams ME. Degeneration and the chemical composition of the human lumbar intervertebral disc. *J Orthop Res* 1987;5(2):198–205.

148. Pflaster DS, Krag MH, Johnson CC, et al. Effect of test environment on intervertebral disc hydration. *Spine* 1997;22(2):133–139.

149. Pope MH, Magnusson M, Wilder DG. Kappa Delta Award. Low back pain and whole body vibration. *Clin Orthop Rel Res* 1998;354:241–248.

150. Puustjarvi K, Lammi M, Kiviranta I, et al. Proteoglycan synthesis in canine intervertebral discs after long-distance running training. *J Orthop Res* 1993;11(5):738–746.

151. Roberts S, Menage J, Urban JP. Biochemical and structural properties of the cartilage end-plate and its relation to the intervertebral disc. *Spine* 1989;14:166–174.

152. Roberts S, Eisenstein SM, Menage J, et al. Mechanoreceptors in intervertebral discs. Morphology, distribution, and neuropeptides. *Spine* 1995;20(24):2645–2651.

153. Roberts S, Urban JP, Evans H, et al. Transport properties of the human cartilage endplate in relation to its composition and calcification. *Spine* 1996;21(4):415–420.

154. Rohlmann A, Bergmann G, Graichen F. Loads on an internal spinal fixation device during walking. *J Biomech* 1997;30(1):41–47.

155. Rosenberg NJ, Bargar WL, Friedman B. The incidence of spondylolysis and spondylolisthesis in nonambulatory patients. *Spine* 1981;6:35–38.

156. Sato K, Kikuchi S, Yonezawa T. In vivo intradiscal pressure measurement in healthy individuals and in patients with ongoing back problems. *Spine* 1999;24(23):2468–2474.

157. Scholten PJM. *Idiopathic scoliosis. Some fundamental aspects of the mechanical behaviour of the human spine.* Thesis, Free University of Amsterdam. Amsterdam: Free University Press, 1986:88–101.

158. Schultz A, Haderspeck K, Takashima S. Correction of scoliosis by muscle stimulation. Biomechanical analyses. *Spine* 1981;6:468–476.

159. Schultz AB, Hirsch C. Mechanical analysis of techniques for improved correction of idiopathic scoliosis. *Clin Orthop Rel Res* 1974;100:66–73.

160. Schultz AB, Haderspeck-Grib K, Sinkora G, et al. Quantitative studies of the flexion-relaxation phenomenon in the back muscles. *J Orthop Res* 1985;3:189–197.

161. Schultz AB, Andersson GBJ, Ortengren R, et al. Loads on the lumbar spine. Validation of a biomechanical analysis by measurements of intradiscal pressures and myoelectric signals. *J Bone Joint Surg Am* 1982;64:713–720.

162. Schultz AB. Biomechanical analyses of loads on the lumbar spine. In: Weinstein JN, Wiesel SW, eds. *The lumbar spine.* Philadelphia: WB Saunders, 1990:160–171.

163. Seroussi RE, Krag MH, Muller DL, et al. Internal deformations of intact and denucleated human lumbar discs subjected to compression, flexion, and extension loads. *J Orthop Res* 1989;7(1):122–131.

164. Setton LA, Zhu W, Weidenbaum M, et al. Compressive properties of the cartilaginous endplate of the baboon lumbar spine. *J Orthop Res* 1993;11:228–239.

165. Shirazi-Adl A. Strain in fibers of a lumbar disc. Analysis of the role of lifting in producing disc prolapse. *Spine* 1989;14(1):96–103.

166. Shirazi-Adl A. Finite-element simulation of changes in the fluid content of human lumbar discs. Mechanical and clinical implications. *Spine* 1992;17(2):206–212.

167. Shirazi-Adl A, Ahmed AM, Shrivastava SC. Mechanical response of a lumbar motion segment in axial torque alone and combined with compression. *Spine* 1986;11:914–927.

168. Shirazi-Adl A. On the fibre composite material models of disc annulus—comparison of predicted stresses. *J Biomech* 1989;22:357–365.

169. Siegmund GP, Myers BS, Davis MB, et al. Mechanical evidence of cervical facet capsule injury during whiplash: a cadaveric study using combined shear, compression, and extension loading. *Spine* 2001;26(19):2095–2101.

170. Silva MJ, Keaveny TM, Hayes WC. Computed tomography–based finite element analysis predicts failure loads and fracture patterns for vertebral sections. *J Orthop Res* 1998;16(3):300–308.

171. Silva MJ, Keaveny TM, Hayes WC. Load sharing between the shell and centrum in the lumbar vertebral body. *Spine* 1997;22(2):140–150.

172. Simon BR, Wu JS, Carlton MW, et al. Structural models for human spinal motion segments based on a poroelastic view of the intervertebral disk. *J Biomech Eng, Trans ASME* 1985;107(4):327–335.

173. Skaggs DL, Weidenbaum M, Iatridis JC, et al. Regional variation in tensile properties and biochemical composition of the human lumbar annulus fibrosus. *Spine* 1994;19:1310–1319.

174. Skalli W, Lavaste F, Robin S, et al. A biomechanical analysis of short segment spinal fixation using a 3-D geometrical and mechanical model. *Spine* 1993;18(5):536–545.

175. Skogland LB, Miller JAA. On the importance of growth in idiopathic scoliosis: a biochemical, radiological and biomechanical study. PhD Dissertation, University of Oslo, Oslo, Norway, 1980.

176. Solomonow M, Zhou BH, Harris M, et al. The ligamento-muscular stabilizing system of the spine. *Spine* 1998;23(23):2552–2562.

177. Somerville EW. Rotational lordosis: the development of the single curve. *J Bone Joint Surg Br* 1987;34:421–427.

178. Spilker RL, Daugirda DM, Schultz AB. Mechanical response of a simple finite element model of the intervertebral disc under complex loading. *J Biomech* 1984;17:103–112.

179. Stewart TD. The age incidence of neural arch defects in Alaskan natives, considered from the standpoint of aetiology. *J Bone Joint Surg Am* 1953;35:937–950.

180. Stokes IAF, Gardner-Morse M. Three-dimensional simulation of Harrington distraction instrumentation for surgical correction of scoliosis. *Spine* 1993;18:2457–2464.

181. Stokes IAF, Gardner-Morse M, Henry S, et al. Trunk muscular response to perturbation with preactivation of lumbar spinal musculature. *Spine* 2000;25(15):1957–1964.

182. Stokes IAF, Gardner-Morse M. Analysis of the interaction between spinal lateral deviation and axial rotation in scoliosis. *J Biomech* 1991;24:753–759.

183. Stokes IAF, Gardner-Morse M, Churchill D, et al. Measurement of a spinal motion segment stiffness matrix. *J Biomech* 2002;35(4):517–521.

184. Stokes IAF, Gardner-Morse M. Quantitative anatomy of the lumbar musculature. *J Biomech* 1999;32:311–316.

185. Stokes IAF, Gardner-Morse M. Lumbar spine maximum efforts and muscle recruitment patterns predicted by a model with multijoint muscles and joints with stiffness. *J Biomech* 1995;28(2):173–186.

186. Stokes IAF, Gardner-Morse M. Lumbar spinal muscle activation synergies predicted by multicriteria cost function. *J Biomech* 2001;34(6):733–740.

187. Stokes IAF. Bulging of intervertebral discs: noncontacting measurements of anatomic specimens. *J Spinal Disord* 1988;1:189–193.

188. Stokes IAF. Surface strain on human intervertebral discs. *J Orthop Res* 1987;5:348–355.

189. Stokes IAF. Analysis of symmetry of vertebral body loading consequent to lateral spinal curvature. *Spine* 1997;22(21):2495–2503.

190. Terahata N, Ishihara H, Ohshima H, et al. Effects of axial traction stress on solute transport and proteoglycan synthesis in the porcine intervertebral disc *in vitro*. *Eur Spine J* 1994;3(6):325–330.

191. Thelen DG, Schultz AB, Ashton-Miller JA. Co-contraction of lumbar muscles during the development of time-varying triaxial moments. *J Orthop Res* 1995;13(3),390–398.

192. Thelen DG, Schultz AB, Fassois SD, et al. Identification of dynamic myoelectric signal-to-force models during isometric lumbar muscle contractions. *J Biomech* 1994;27(7):907–919.

193. Thelen DG, Schultz AB, Ashton-Miller JA. Quantitative interpretation of lumbar muscle myoelectric signals during rapid cyclic attempted trunk flexions and extensions. *J Biomech* 1994;27(2):157–167.

194. Thompson JP, Pearce RH, Schechter MT, et al. Preliminary evaluation of a scheme for grading the gross morphology of the human intervertebral disc. *Spine* 1990;15(5):411–415.

195. Tien CS, Huston RL. Numerical advances in gross-motion simulations of head/neck dynamics. *J Biomech Eng, Trans ASME* 1987;109(2):163–168.

196. Tsuji H, Hirano N, Ohshima H, et al. Structural variation of the anterior and posterior annulus fibrosus in the development of human lumbar intervertebral disc. A risk factor for intervertebral disc rupture. *Spine* 1993;18(2):204–210.

197. Urban JP, McMullin JF. Swelling pressure of the inervertebral disc: influence of proteoglycan and collagen contents. *Biorheology* 1985;22:145–157.

198. Urban JP, McMullin JF. Swelling pressure of the lumbar intervertebral discs: influence of age, spinal level, composition, and degeneration. *Spine* 1988;13:179–187.

199. Urban JP, Roberts S. Development and degeneration of the intervertebral discs. *Mol Med Today* 1995;1(7):329–335.

200. Urban JPG, Holm S, Maroudas A, et al. Nutrition of the intervertebral disc. Effect of fluid flow on solute transport. *Clin Orthop Rel Res* 1982;170:296–302.

201. Urban MR, Fairbank JC, Etherington PJ, et al. Electrochemical measurement of transport into scoliotic intervertebral discs *in vivo* using nitrous oxide as a tracer. *Spine* 2001;26(8):984–990.

202. van Dieën JH. Are recruitment patterns of the trunk musculature compatible with a synergy based on the maximization of endurance? *J Biomech* 1997;30:1095–1100.

203. Veldhuizen AG, Scholten PJM. Kinematics of the scoliotic spine as related to the normal spine. *Spine* 1987;12:852–858.

204. Videman T, Sarna S, Battie MC, et al. The long-term effects of physical loading and exercise lifestyles on back-related symptoms, disability, and spinal pathology among men. *Spine* 1995;20(6):699–709.

205. Wang JL, Parnianpour M, Shirazi-Adl A, et al. Viscoelastic finite-element analysis of a lumbar motion segment in combined compression and sagittal flexion. Effect of loading rate. *Spine* 2000;25(3):310–318.

206. White AA. Kinematics of the normal spine as related to scoliosis. *J Biomech* 1971;4:405–411.

207. Whyne CM, Hu SS, Lotz JC. Parametric finite element analysis of vertebral bodies affected by tumors. *J Biomech* 2001;34(10):1317–1324.

208. Wilder DG, Aleksiev AR, Magnusson ML, et al. Muscular response to sudden load. A tool to evaluate fatigue and rehabilitation. *Spine* 1996;21(22):2628–2639.

209. Wilke H, Wolf S, Claes L, et al. Stability increase of the lumbar spine with different muscle groups. *Spine* 1995;20:192–198.

210. Wilke HJ, Neef P, Caimi M, et al. New *in vivo* measurements of pressures in the intervertebral disc in daily life. *Spine* 1999;24(8):755–762.

211. Wilkins RJ, Browning JA, Urban JP. Chondrocyte regulation by mechanical load. *Biorheology* 2000;37(1–2):67–74.

212. Windhagen HJ, Hipp JA, Silva MJ, et al. Predicting failure of thoracic vertebrae with simulated and actual metastatic defects. *Clin Orthop Rel Res* 1997;(344):313–319.

213. Wynarsky GT, Schultz AB. Optimization of skeletal configuration: studies of scoliosis correction biomechanics. *J Biomech* 1991;24(8):721–732.

214. Yettram AL, Jackman MJ. Structural analysis for the forces in the human spinal column and its musculature. *J Biomed Eng* 1982;4(2):118–124.

215. Young WC, Budynas RG. *Roark's formulas for stress and strain.* New York: McGraw-Hill, 2002.

BIOMECHANICS OF FRACTURE FIXATION AND FRACTURE HEALING

LUTZ E. CLAES
KEITA ITO

1 INTRODUCTION

Up to the nineteenth century, fracture treatment was performed by external splinting to achieve an anatomical alignment of the broken bone, to relieve pain and stabilize the fragments so that bony union could follow. From a biomechanical point of view, fracture fixation must have sufficient stability, which means it has to reduce the interfragmentary movement that occurs under external loading and muscle activity to such a degree that bone healing may take place.

The key factor that guides bone healing is the interfragmentary movement, which determines the tissue strain and the cellular reaction in the fracture healing zone. Therefore, the methods of fracture fixation will be assessed with regard to their capability to reduce the interfragmentary movement.

Today, the majority of all fractures are still stabilized with plaster casts or braces. Complex fractures, fractures through joint surfaces, and fractures with extensive soft-tissue damage, as well as open and infected fractures, however, can hardly be treated successfully with plaster cast stabilization. As a consequence, the operative treatment of fractures, which involved new fixation systems and implants, was developed in the twentieth century. To achieve good healing results with these techniques, biomechanical principles should be known and taken into consideration, as described in the following sections.

2 MECHANICAL PRINCIPLES OF FRACTURE FIXATION

2.1 Splinting

2.1.1 External Fixation

2.1.1.1 Plaster Cast and Brace

The classical way to stabilize a fracture is plaster cast fixation. This external splinting produces an anatomical alignment of the fragments. Under partial loading or merely muscle contraction of the broken extremity, a relatively large interfragmentary movement occurs. Axial loading of splinted long bone fractures is possible for simple oblique fractures where fracture ends are supported and under compression. Instability due to bending movements and torque must be limited by a good fit between the plaster cast and the outer shape of the extremity (49). The stability of fixation is influenced by the circular compression of the plaster cast against the soft-tissue envelope around the bone (Fig. 13-1). Muscles and skin can act as an incompressible medium, and this soft-tissue compression helps to stabilize the fragments (49). In the early healing stage, an axial load of 150 N, for example, led to an axial displacement of 1 to 4 mm, depending on the type of fracture (49). The rotational and angular displacement was 1° and 3°, respectively. Because of the increasing stiffness of the callus, the displacement under load decreased steadily. After 8 weeks it was only about 0.5 mm (50). Because of the patients' reduced activity, an atrophy of the muscles occurs during the healing period, which leads to diminished soft-tissue compression. Consequently, the plaster cast must be adapted to these changes in order to maintain stability. This is easier to perform with a brace and adjustable fixations than with a plaster cast, which must be removed and replaced by a new one.

2.1.1.2 External Fixator

When a fracture is accompanied by an open soft-tissue wound, a plaster cast or brace is often not possible. In such cases, an external stabilization of the fracture can be performed by using an external fixator. An external fixator is a system that allows the stabilization of fragments away from the open wound with the aid of percutaneous screws or wires that are connected to one or more bars on the outside of the skin (Fig. 13-2). The stability of this fixation is mainly determined by the stiffness of the fixator construct and the quality of the connection between the screws and the bone. The stiffness is described by the interfragmentary movement occurring under external loads. The stiffness of the fixation device

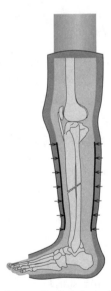

FIGURE 13-1. Schematic drawing of a plaster cast splinting of a tibial/fibula fracture. Compression of the soft-tissue envelope around the fractured bones contributes to the stability of the fixation.

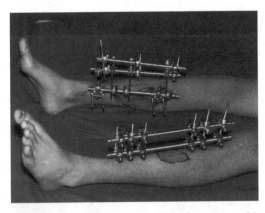

FIGURE 13-2. Bilateral open tibia fractures stabilized by two external fixators. Left leg: monolateral double tube fixator; right leg: biplanar external fixator.

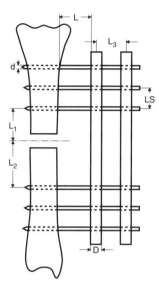

FIGURE 13-3. Geometric parameters influencing the stability of the fractures stabilized by external fixation. d, diameter of the screws; D, diameter of the connecting bar; L, free length between bar and bone; L₁, L₂: shortest distance between inner screw and fracture; L₃, distance between connecting bars; LS, distance between screws.

is mainly influenced by the following factors described in Fig. 13-3:

1. The free length (L) of the screw or wire between the bone surface and the connecting bar. The smaller the distance, the stiffer and more stable the fixation stiffness proportional to $3\pi d^4 E/64 L^3$.
2. The diameter (d) of the screw or wire. The greater the diameter the stiffer and more stable the system (see formula above).
3. The number of screws or wires. The more, the stiffer.
4. The distance (L_1, L_2) of screw or wire from the fracture line. The closer, the stiffer.
5. The size (D) and number of connecting bars. There are monolateral systems with large bar diameters (D) that provide a high stiffness and systems with one or two smaller bars at one site or in a biplanar arrangement (Fig. 13-2).
6. The distance between two connecting bars (L_3) and the distance between two screws in one fragment (LS). The greater the distance, the higher the stability.

The stiffness and stability of a fracture fixation can be modified over a wide range by the factors mentioned above (15,31). This technique is the only one that allows the surgeon to adapt the stability as needed not only preoperatively, but also intraoperatively and postoperatively. However, there are limitations. From a biological point of view, it cannot be proposed to increase the number or the diameter of the screws as much as possible to achieve maximal stability. Such a procedure would impair the blood supply in the fracture healing zone and diminish the biological healing capacity.

The interfragmentary movement of the stabilized fracture under loading depends on the amplitude and direction of loading and the stiffness characteristics of the fixator used. For most activities, the loading by forces and moments is complex and changes with the type of activity such as walking or stair climbing. In addition, the arrangement of the external fixator shows great variation. This multifactorial situation leads to a great variety of interfragmentary movements in all three directions in space (22,25). Our measurements on patients with tibial fractures that were stabilized by a monolateral ventromedial external fixator with four 5-mm screws (Fig. 13-4) showed interfragmentary movements of 1 to 3 mm under partial axial loading (300 N). The largest movement was found in the mediolateral direction (shear) followed by axial movement and movement in the plane of the screws (shear, anteroposterior).

The ratio between axial and shear movements in the fracture gap depends on the fixator stiffness and arrangement. Depending on the type of fixator, interfragmentary movements of up to 5 mm were reported (22). Smaller movements could be seen with stiff fixators using screws that were 6 mm in diameter and three screws in each fragment (25).

2.1.2 Internal Fixation

2.1.2.1 Intramedullary Nail

Intramedullary nailing is a generally accepted internal splinting technique (33). The conventional Küntscher nail is a longitudinally slotted tube that is inserted into a long bone under

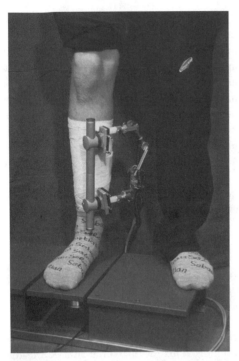

FIGURE 13-4. Measurement of fixator deformation under partial load bearing. The load is determined by a six-degree-of-freedom load cell underneath the foot and the deformation is measured with a six-degree-of-freedom goniometer system. The interfragmentary movement in the fracture gap can be calculated by coordinate transformation.

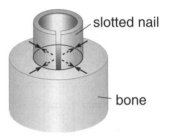

FIGURE 13-5. Radial stress between the slotted intramedullary nail and the reamed bone leads to increased friction in the interface and higher stability against rotational movements and axial forces.

prestress. The medullary cavity of the bone is reamed about 20 mm proximally and distally to the fracture in order to increase the area of contact between nail and bone. The inserted nail has a diameter that is 0.5 mm larger than the reamed bone diameter, which gives the nail a tight fit. The radial stress caused by this implantation leads to friction between nail and bone that secures the movement between the two nailed fragments (Fig. 13-5). However, as these frictional forces are limited, the application of this technique is restricted to simple midshaft diaphyseal fractures. To overcome these limitations, additional interlocking screws are introduced (29), thus avoiding movement of the fragments under higher loads and widening the range of indications to include complex fractures, defect fractures, and metaphyseal fractures.

The reaming of the bone can cause a considerable rise in intramedullary pressure and temporary damage to the bone's blood supply (48). This led to the development of solid nails

with a smaller diameter that could be implanted without reaming (Fig. 13-6). Most of the time, these nails require interlocking screws or bolts to achieve sufficient stability (48) (Fig. 13-7).

The stability of fracture fixation by nailing mainly depends on the mechanical properties of the nail, the nail's fit in the medullary space, and the mechanical properties of the locking screws or bolts. The bending and torsional stiffness of the nailed bone mainly depends on the diameter of the nail. Nails with a large diameter showed a significantly higher stiffness compared to implants with a small diameter (51). The torsional stiffness of unslotted nails is generally much higher than the stiffness of slotted nails.

Because the stiffness of the internal fixation with nails is mainly influenced by the nail

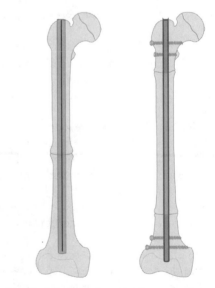

FIGURE 13-6. Splinting of a femur fracture with a reamed intramedullary nail (*left*) and with an unreamed interlocking nail (*right*).

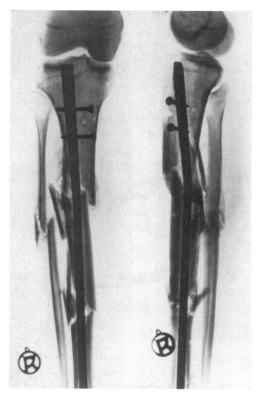

FIGURE 13-7. X-ray of a complex tibia fracture stabilized by an unreamed interlocking nail. (Adapted from ref. 48, Rüedi T, Murphy W. *AO principles of fracture management*. Stuttgart: Thieme, 2000.)

diameter, the bending stiffness can be estimated by $S_b = E \times I$ (E, modulus of elasticity; I, second moment of inertia), and the torsional stiffness can be calculated by $S_t = G \times I_t$ (G, shear modulus; I_t, second moment of inertia for rotation).

Measurements on a patient with an instrumented nail showed that because of muscle activities the axial load on the nail was about 20% higher than the ground reaction force (53). The bending moment under partial weight bearing of 250 N already reached 20 Nm, and the torsional

moment was about 40% of this. This torsional load led to rotations of about 6° to 30°, depending on the stiffness of the nail (51). For a bone with a diameter of 30 mm, this would cause a reversible shear movement of 1.5 to 7.5 mm at the outer diameter of the bone. Whereas deformations caused by the axial forces and bending moments seem to be noncritical, the low stiffness of most of the nails under torsional moments can reach critical values.

2.1.2.2 Internal Fixator

The fixateur interne is a plate that is fixed to the bone like an external fixator but is underneath the skin, close to the bone. The plate is rigidly fixed with screws or bolts locked into the plate hole and driven into the bone (48). In contrast to a conventional plate, the fixateur interne is not pressed against the underlying bone. As a positive biological effect, the blood supply of the periosteum underneath the plate might be reduced to a lesser degree than under a conventional plate.

2.2 Interfragmentary Compression

In order to achieve absolute stability, the compression over the whole cross section of a fracture must be sufficiently high to neutralize all forces and moments acting on the fracture site (Fig. 13-8). When this requirement is met, no interfragmentary movement occurs. Such an interfragmentary compression can be achieved by lag screws, compression plates, and tension band systems (48).

2.2.1 Lag Screws

Interfragmentary compression leads to increased stability through friction. Theoretically, the

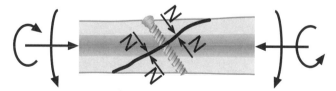

FIGURE 13-8. Interfragmentary compression (N) created by a lag screw, for example, has to neutralize external forces and moments to achieve stability of the fracture. (Adapted from ref. 48, Rüedi T, Murphy W. *AO principles of fracture management*. Stuttgart: Thieme, 2000.)

security against dislocation of two fragments that are fixed together by a lag screw depends on the screw force that is normally created on the fracture surface (N) and the coefficient of friction (μ). As long as the frictional force $F = N\mu$ is greater than the resultant force in the fracture plane, the construct is stable. The amount of force created by a lag screw mainly depends on the type of screw, the thread geometry, the length in the bony thread, and the mechanical quality of the bone.

In the cortex of large long bones such as the tibia and femur, forces of up to 2500 N per screw can be created. These originally applied forces are reduced by the viscoelastic properties of the bone and biological bone remodeling processes. However, the bone can keep about 50% of these forces in a diaphyseal area over a period of 6 weeks (48).

Fractures in metaphyseal and epiphyseal areas with lower bone density (spongy bone) can be stabilized with lag screws but need screws of larger diameter and a different thread design. To achieve sufficient holding power of the screws in the mechanically weaker bone, larger thread depths are necessary (Fig. 13-9). The interfragmentary compression that can be achieved by lag screw fixation in these areas is limited, especially for elderly patients with mechanically weak osteoporotic bones.

Therefore, an internal fixation of a fracture with lag screws alone is rarely stable enough to allow load bearing of the operated extremity. In most cases, a lag screw is used in combination with a plate.

2.2.2 Compression Plate

In transverse or short oblique fractures of the diaphysis, the placement of a lag screw is not always possible. In such cases, a stabilization can be performed with a compression plate. After the fixation of the plate on one main fragment, a tension device placed on the second fragment is used temporarily to pull both fragments together and create an interfragmentary compression (Fig. 13-10, top). Then the second fragment is fixed to the plate with additional screws (Fig. 13-10, bottom). Compression forces of more than 1,000 N can be achieved with this procedure (48). There are also plates available that allow the compression of two fragments without a tension device. These plates have a special hole design (48) with a slope on which the screw head slides. When the screw is inserted into the bone, it moves toward the bone cortex, which is only possible if the slope of the screw hole is pushed axially (Fig. 13-11). As with the tension device, this axial movement of the plate creates a compression between two fragments fixed by a compression plate (Fig. 13-12).

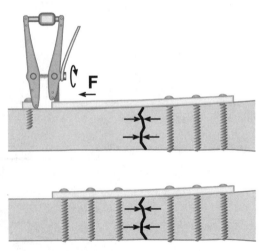

FIGURE 13-10. Application of interfragmentary compression by a tension device pulling on the plate. (Adapted from ref. 48, Rüedi T, Murphy W. *AO principles of fracture management.* Stuttgart: Thieme, 2000.)

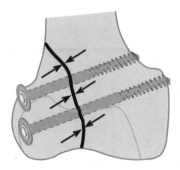

FIGURE 13-9. Interfragmentary compression created by two spongy bone lag screws in the epiphyseal fracture of the distal femur.

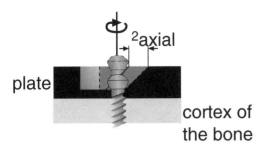

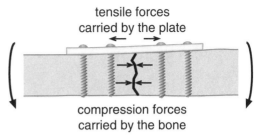

FIGURE 13-11. Compression hole principle. When the screw is inserted into the bone, the screw head moves toward the bone, sliding on the slope and pushing the plate in horizontal direction (Δ axial). (Adapted from ref. 48, Rüedi T, Murphy W. *AO principles of fracture management.* Stuttgart: Thieme, 2000.)

FIGURE 13-13. The application of the tension band principle by a plate fixed on the tensile force site of a fractured bone. (Adapted from ref. 48, Rüedi T, Murphy W. *AO principles of fracture management.* Stuttgart: Thieme, 2000.)

2.2.3 Interfragmentary Compression by Tension Band Principle

Bones are seldom loaded by axial forces alone. Depending on the external load phase and the muscle activity, bending and torsional moments can also occur. After a fracture, pure axial compression forces would lead to interfragmentary compression without the need for additional fixation. Tensile forces, however, would lead to dislocation of the fragments. Bending moments acting on a bone create tensile forces on one side and compression forces on the other side. When a fractured bone is loaded under bend-

ing moments, it is necessary to neutralize the tensile forces and allow the fracture surfaces to carry the compression forces. The neutralization of the tensile forces must be done by implants, whereas the compression forces can be carried by the fracture surfaces (48) when reduction of the fragments is possible (tension band principle, Fig. 13-13).

The tension band principle can be applied particularly well to bones on which muscle and tendons create large tensile forces. Tensile forces created by the quadriceps muscle and counteracted by the patella tendon pull on the patella. In a fractured patella, these tensile forces can be neutralized by a cerclage wire placed anteriorly to the patella (48). Upon knee flexion, the distraction forces are carried by the wire and create a compression force at the fracture surface (tension band principle, Fig. 13-14).

In contrast to interfragmentary compression forces applied by screws and compression plates (static compression), the compression forces achieved by the tension band principle change dynamically. Depending on the external loads and muscle activity, the compression forces change cyclically (dynamic compression).

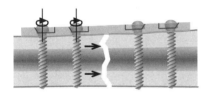

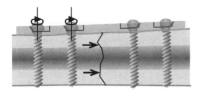

FIGURE 13-12. Compression holes can be used to close fracture gaps and create interfragmentary compression. (Adapted from ref. 48, Rüedi T, Murphy W. *AO principles of fracture management.* Stuttgart: Thieme, 2000.)

3 BIOMECHANICS OF FRACTURE HEALING

3.1 Bone Healing under Interfragmentary Movement

Fracture healing under interfragmentary movement occurs by callus formation that

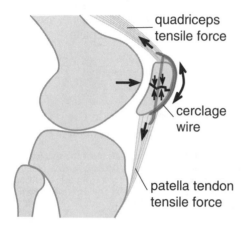

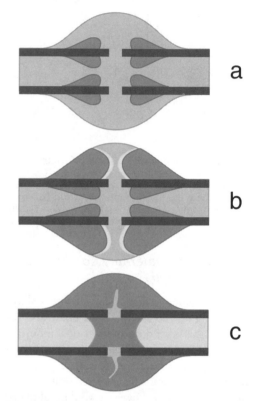

FIGURE 13-14. Tension band principle applied for the cerclage fixation of a patella fracture. (Adapted from Burny F, Donkerwolcke M, Bourgois R. Twenty years of experience in fracture healing measurements with strain gauges. *Orthopaedics* 1984;7:1823–1826.)

FIGURE 13-15. Schematic drawing of the callus healing process. Early intramembranous bone formation **(a)**, growing callus volume and diameter mainly by enchondral ossification **(b)**, and bridging of the fragments **(c)**.

mechanically unites the bony fragments. After trauma and fracture, a hematoma occurs that undergoes tissue differentiation. The sequence of fracture healing involves four stages: inflammation, soft callus, hard callus, and remodeling (40). The hard callus formation begins in areas remote from the fracture and progresses toward the fracture until the distal and proximal callus wedges unite (Fig. 13-15).

The callus formation starts with intramembranous bone formation at the surface of the periosteum and endosteum and changes to enchondral ossification later on, when the callus increases in diameter and grows toward the fracture (Figs. 13-15 and 13-16).

The flexural and torsional rigidity of a fracture depends on the material properties and the second moment of inertia (rigidity $= EI$) of the callus. Particularly the increase in callus diameter has a significant effect on the stabilization of the fracture. Whereas there is a linear relation to the mechanical quality of the callus tissue (E), the rigidity is proportional to the fourth power of the diameter ($I_{\text{Bending}} = \pi d^4/64$, $I_{\text{Torsion}} = \pi d^4/32$).

The interfragmentary movement under external loading decreases with healing time in relation to the rigidity of the callus. Finally, the hard callus bridges the bony fragments and re-

duces the interfragmentary movement to such a low level that a healing of the fracture in the cortex can take place (Fig. 13-17). When this has happened, the callus tissue is no longer required and is resorbed by osteoclasts. Finally, after a remodeling process, the shape and strength of the normal bone are reconstituted.

3.2 Fracture Healing under Interfragmentary Compression

Compression forces created by implants and external loads maintain compression and close contact between two fragments as long as the external traction forces do not exceed the internal compression preload at the fracture site. With the compression preload and friction between the fragments, relative movement between the fragments is avoided.

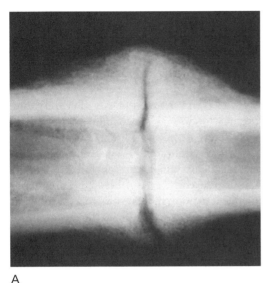

A

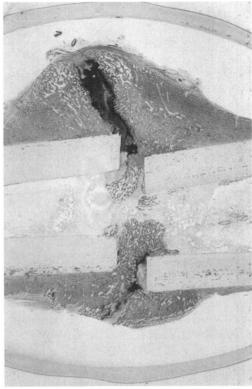

B

FIGURE 13-16. A: Roentgenogram of a callus healing in a sheep tibia with the osteotomy line still visible (6 weeks p.o.). **B**: Histological picture of a sheep tibia osteotomy (fracture model) after bone bridging by external and intramedullary callus formation. A few areas of fibrocartilage remain at the level of the former fracture line (dark areas).

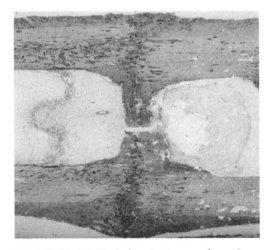

FIGURE 13-17. Healed osteotomy of a sheep metatarsal with bony bridging of the cortical osteotomy gap and only small remaining callus volume.

Under this absolutely stable fixation, bone healing can occur by direct osteonal bridging of the fracture line with minimally or no callus formation (52). However, in complex fractures the fragments are not ideally adapted and show areas of contact as well as areas of gaps between the fragments. In areas with direct contact, remodeling starts a few weeks after fracture fixation, which leads to bridging of the fragments by newly formed osteons (52). Haversian osteons with osteoclasts in their cutter heads resorb bone, create a tunnel that crosses the fracture line, and fill the tunnel with new bone in a process of osteoblastic activity (Figs. 13-18 and 13-19). In areas with a gap between the fragments, a filling of the gap by woven bone occurs as a first step before the Haversian osteons can cross the fracture area (Fig. 13-19). In

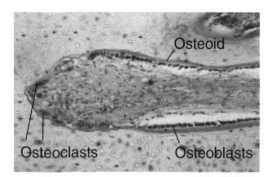

FIGURE 13-18. Osteon with bone-resorbing osteoclasts (*left*) that drill a tunnel into the bone and osteoblasts that lay down new bone (osteoid) and fill the tunnel with a new bone layer (original magnification 100×).

reality a mixture of contact and gap healing will occur.

An advantage of absolute stability is that the blood vessels may cross the fracture site more easily and lead to faster revascularization (48). In contrast to callus healing, there is no increased bone diameter under direct osteonal healing. This limits the load-bearing capacity of the healing bone, which consequently requires a longer period of protection by the implant.

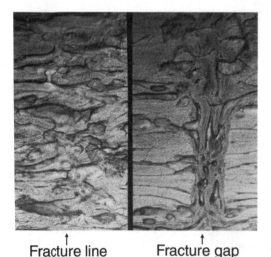

FIGURE 13-19. Contact healing with osteons crossing the fracture line (*left*). Healing of a fracture gap (*right*). Woven bone fills the gap before the osteons can bridge the fracture area.

3.3 Delayed Healing and Nonhealing under Unstable Fixation

When the interfragmentary movement is too large, the bony bridging of the fragments is delayed or even prevented (41). Callus formation begins with normal intramembranous bone formation remote from the fracture in areas of low mechanical strain and the callus grows in volume and diameter, but the bridging of the fracture line is delayed or even prevented. Large interfragmentary movements cause large tissue strains and hydrostatic pressures in the fracture that prevent the vascularization of the fracture zone. Without this vascularization bone cells cannot survive, bone cannot be built, and only fibrocartilage can be formed (46). Because the resisting fibrocartilage layer in between the two bony fragments looks like the image of a joint, the nonunion is also called pseudarthrosis (false joint).

4 MAIN FACTORS INFLUENCING THE BIOMECHANICS OF FRACTURE HEALING

4.1 Interfragmentary Movement

4.1.1 Axial Movement

Small interfragmentary movements (IFMs) stimulate callus formation in animal experimental models (14,20,23,30,37,59). With small fracture gaps, the stimulated callus volume seems to correlate with the amplitude of the cyclic axial movement (Fig. 13-20). When the fracture gap is too large, the callus formation seems to be limited and bridging of the fracture gap is delayed. For large gaps, a more stable fixation with smaller interfragmentary movements seems to be advantageous (14). Very stiff fixation of a fracture can suppress the callus formation and delay healing. In such cases, an externally applied interfragmentary movement can be used to stimulate callus healing (30). However, when the fracture fixation itself allows axial movements to a sufficient extent to stimulate callus formation, an additional external application of interfragmentary

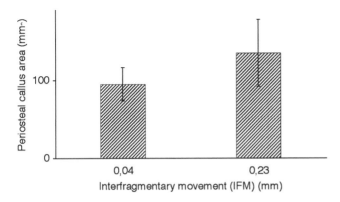

FIGURE 13-20. Periosteal callus area for the osteotomy healing of a sheep metatarsal with a 0.7-mm osteotomy gap and stable fixation (IFM; 0.04 mm) or axial flexible fixation (IFM; 0.23 mm).

movements does not lead to further improvement of the healing process (5).

4.1.2 Shear Movement

There is an ongoing controversial discussion whether a shear movement delays the fracture healing when compared with an axial movement of similar amplitude (3,42,60). It is assumed that shear movements impede vascularization and promote fibrous tissue differentiation (57). However, oblique tibial fractures treated with functional bracing show rapid natural healing (50) even though this type of fixation allows shear movements of up to 4 mm.

Experimental studies found shear movement to induce delayed unions and nonunions (3, 60), whereas other studies found no impairment of healing (42). However, these studies did not control the shear movement sufficiently (60) or

compared different osteotomies (osteotomy = standardized model fracture) of oblique and transverse type (3). In experiments conducted by Augat et al. (4), healing of a tibial osteotomy in sheep with an osteotomy gap of 3 mm and an axial or plane shear movement of 1.5 mm was compared (Fig. 13-21). The results showed significantly more callus formation and larger flexural rigidity of the bones healed under axial movement in comparison with the bones healed under plane shear movements. In contrast, Bishop et al. (7) conducted similar experiments and found different results. They compared healing of a 2.4-mm gap osteotomy in the sheep tibia with 25% axial compression (0.6 mm) or torsional shear (7.2°) interfragmentary strain (interfragmentary motion/gap size). These results showed denser callus formation and stiffer bending stiffness of the bones healed under torsional shear compared with those healed under axial motion (Fig. 13-22). In addition to differences in

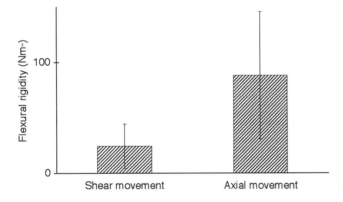

FIGURE 13-21. Flexural rigidity of sheep tibiae after external fixation and axial or shear movement of 1.5 mm in the 3-mm fracture gap.

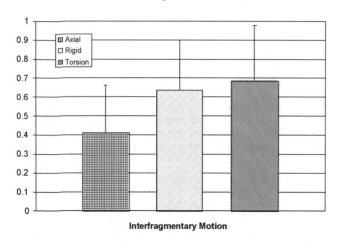

FIGURE 13-22. Four-point bending stiffness (pin-plane) of a 2.4-mm mid-diaphyseal transverse gap osteotomy in the ovine tibia after 8 weeks of healing with external fixation stimulated daily with 25% interfragmentary axial compression or torsional shear (mean ± SD).

gap size (3 mm versus 2.4 mm), another major difference in these experiments was the timing and magnitude of interfragmentary motion. In the experiment by Augat et al., interfragmentary motion was achieved by loading of the tibia during gait by the sheep themselves, whereas in the experiment by Bishop et al., the motion was produced by a displacement-controlled hydraulic actuator with a force limitation. Thus, because of pain-mediated biofeedback regulation, the actual interfragmentary motions in the former experiment were quite small initially and began to approach the full allowed magnitude only after several weeks. In the latter experiment, the interfragmentary motions were full scale for the first 4 weeks and then diminished with time as the callus became stiffer and the force cutoff in the actuator control was implemented. Hence, the effects of shear compared with axial interfragmentary motion appears to be sensitive to timing, magnitude, and/or gap size.

4.2 Fracture Type

There are various types of fractures that can be associated with various degrees of injuries: simple oblique, transverse, and spiral fractures or more severe fractures with one or more fragments. From a purely mechanical point of view, a fracture with several fragments and several fracture gaps might be less critical with regard to an unstable fixation than a simple oblique frac-

ture. The overall deformation of fracture fixation, which takes place in one fracture gap of a simple fracture, will be distributed and shared by several fracture gaps in a complex fracture. This can reduce large overall deformations of fixation to individual interfragmentary movements that are small enough for uncritical bone healing.

Besides this mechanical view, however, we should take into consideration that complex fractures with several fragments are mainly caused by high-energy injuries and are associated with severe damage to the blood supply and the surrounding periosteum and soft tissue. Therefore, fast revascularization is more important than stable fixation, and less invasive surgical intervention for stabilization of the fracture is the preferred technique (17,26).

4.3 Blood Supply

Fracture healing has two major prerequisites: mechanical stability and sufficient blood supply. Blood supply is necessary for the nutrition of the healing zone, and an insufficient blood supply is likely to result in a delayed union or even an atrophic nonunion (54). In addition to other reasons for a diminished blood supply such as trauma or smoking, there is a different pattern of vascularization under stable and unstable fixation conditions (46). It is speculated that under unstable fixation, capillaries required for osseous repair are constantly ruptured and delay the fracture healing process, resulting in the development of fibrocartilaginous tissue (46). However, there is only one study known that quantitatively correlates the revascularization and tissue transformation under well-defined biomechanical conditions (16). This study showed that greater interfragmentary movements in a 2-mm osteotomy gap of the sheep metatarsal led to significantly more fibrocartilage, less bone formation, and a smaller number of vessels close to the periosteum than under smaller interfragmentary movements (16). Large interfragmentary movement causes considerable tissue strains and hydrostatic pressure in the non-ossified callus tissue (18,19). Whereas large tissue strains may prevent revascularization, large hydrostatic pressures may cause a collapse of the blood vessels.

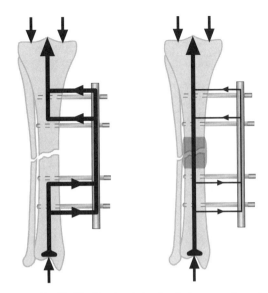

FIGURE 13-23. The load sharing between external fixator and repair tissue in the fracture at the beginning (*left site*) and with a loadable callus formation at a later stage of healing.

5 BIOMECHANICAL MONITORING OF FRACTURE HEALING

The interfragmentary movement can be used for the monitoring of the bone healing process for patients with fracture treatment by external fixation (9,22,25). External loads applied to the operated extremity by the activity of the patient are shared by the external fixator and the repair tissue. Directly after surgery, there is only hematoma in the fracture, and the external fixator has to carry the entire load. As the healing process progresses, the callus increases in size and rigidity and shares more and more of the external load. The load at the external fixator decreases, which leads to decreasing deformation of the fixateur frame (Fig. 13-23). Therefore, the measurement of fixator deformation allows an indirect determination of the interfragmentary movement and stiffness of the callus. By measuring the fixator deformation under constant loading conditions (scale), e.g., every 3 weeks (Fig. 13-24), the course of the fracture healing process can be seen and used as a criterion for the speed of healing. Whereas under normal healing conditions, for instance in tibia shaft fractures, the callus formation reduces the interfragmentary movement to zero in about 10 to 15 weeks (Fig. 13-25), delayed unions take more than

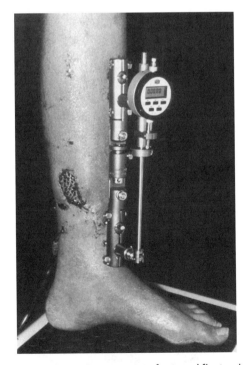

FIGURE 13-24. Measurement of external fixator deformation on an axially loaded tibia using an electromechanical measuring device and a conventional scale.

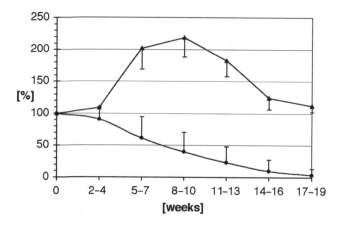

FIGURE 13-25. The course of inter-fragmentary movement monitored for human tibial fractures. The postoperative initial interfragmentary movements under an axial load of 300 N (normalized to 100% at the outset) decrease with a normal fracture healing but do not show a significant reduction for nonunions (*upper curve*).

20 weeks and nonunions do not show a significant reduction (Fig. 13-25).

6 MECHANOBIOLOGY OF FRACTURE HEALING

6.1 Mechanical Stimulation of Fracture Callus Cells

Callus formation and maturation that occur during fracture healing with interfragmentary motion are controlled and facilitated by the cells within the callus. In normal fracture healing, at the beginning of the soft callus phase, multipotential progenitor cells begin to invade the granulation tissue callus, developed during the inflammatory stage. The progenitor cells are believed to arise from the periosteum, endosteum, marrow, and surrounding extracortical soft tissue. Their migration into the callus is understood to be modulated by growth factors and cytokines released during the inflammatory stage. As they migrate into the callus, they differentiate into various cell phenotypes and proliferate within the callus. Away from the fracture gap and along the periosteum and endosteum, the cells differentiate into osteoblasts and begin to directly produce bone through intramembranous ossification. This allows the quick growth of bone toward the fracture gap. Within the callus and the gap, the progenitor cells differentiate into fibroblasts or chondrocytes, proliferate, and begin to produce a fibrous connective tissue or cartilage matrix, respectively. This soft tissue bridges the fragment ends and stabilizes the fracture to some degree.

In the hard callus stage, chondrocytes at the hard and soft tissue interface proliferate, hypertrophy, and calcify, forming bone through endochondral ossification. Elsewhere in the callus, fibroblasts and connective tissue are slowly replaced by chondrocytes and cartilage. Both of these processes allow creeping substitution of bone from the distal ends of the callus until an initial osseous bridge of the fracture gap is established at the periphery of the callus. Then the creeping substitution turns inward. When the gap is filled with woven bone, the fracture is considered healed. In the final remodeling stage and at the end of the hard callus stage, osteoclasts begin to resorb the woven bone in the extraperiosteal callus as osteonal remodeling occurs across the gap.

Throughout this healing process, the various cells found in the callus are modulated by the local mechanical environment of the tissue in which they are embedded. Cyclic hydrostatic pressure applied to *in vitro* cell cultures of bone marrow-derived mesenchymal stem cells were found to enhance differentiation into chondrocytes and stimulated cartilaginous matrix production (2). Mechanical compression was also found to regulate synthesis of distinct proteoglycan types by fibroblasts in tendon explants (32). When intermittent hydrostatic pressure was applied to embryonic bone organ cultures, hypertrophy of chondrocytes and mineralization were accelerated (56). Osteoblasts have also been demonstrated to be sensitive to mechanical stimuli. Cyclic tensile strain has been found to increase their proliferation and osteoid production (28). In contrast, biaxial stretch was found to regulate apoptosis and proliferation of osteoblasts in a differential fashion dependent on their state of differentiation (58).

Hence, the mechanoregulation of callus cells is a feedback loop where the signals are created by the applied load and modulated by the callus tissue. Mechanical loading applied to the callus tissue produces local biophysical stimuli sensed by the cells. This may regulate cell phenotype, proliferation/apoptosis, and anabolic and catabolic synthesis activities. With alteration of the extracellular matrix and the associated changes in material properties of the tissue, the biophysical stimuli produced by mechanical loading is modulated, producing different biophysical signals with even the same loads. In normal fracture healing this feedback process reaches steady state when the callus has ossified and the original cortex has regenerated. However, this feedback process may also explain some complications of fracture healing such as delayed or nonunions where the tissue properties combined with loading may promote the persistence of soft tissues. Thus, the mechanobiology of callus cells is integral to understanding the biomechanics of fracture healing.

6.2 Mechanoregulation of Fracture Healing

6.2.1 Mechanoregulation of Tissue Differentiation

The concept that biological processes at the cellular level can be regulated by mechanical loading dates back to the late 1800s when Roux introduced his theory of functional adaptation. He proposed that the mechanical environment or "irritations" actually stimulated the formation of particular types of connective tissue (47). Based on teleological understanding of anatomy, he postulated that compression stimulated the formation of bone, tension for connective tissue, and relative displacement, i.e., tissues moving relative to each other, in combination with compression or tension for cartilage (47). In modern times, Roux's basic premise of functional adaptation as it relates to tissue differentiation is widely accepted, but the identification of the mechanical parameters of importance and their mechanisms of actions, from multipotential progenitor cells to bone, are unresolved and continue to be investigated.

Almost a century later, Pauwels proposed a more rigorous mechanoregulation theory based on continuum mechanics (43). He analyzed the mechanical environment with a healing fracture callus and hypothesized that the invariants of the strain and stress tensors guided the differentiation pathway, whereby hydrostatic pressure resulted in cartilage, distortional strain, or elongation favored fibrous tissue, and with low magnitudes of strain and hydrostatic stress, the natural course was followed resulting in bone (Fig. 13-26). He also showed how this theory was consistent with different healing patterns including that of pseudarthrosis. About the same time, a much simpler idea, strain modulation, was postulated by Perren and Cordey (44). They believed that tissue differentiation was a result of tissue disruption. If stresses exceeded the tissue strength or tissue elongation resulted in rupturing, the tissue would change its phenotype such that tissue failure would not occur. Using finite-element analysis (FEA) to calculate the complex tissue strain in the callus at the beginning of healing, Cheal et al. (13) compared histology of the fracture callus with magnitudes of strain. Although they did not demonstrate tissue damage, they found an association of high strain levels with soft tissues and bone resorption and low strain levels with bone formation.

Based on the framework of Pauwels, Carter et al. proposed local stress or strain history as a method to allow a range of cyclically applied loads to influence tissue differentiation over time (10,11). They postulated that compressive hydrostatic stress history guides formation of cartilage, whereas tensile strain history guides synthesis of fibrous connective tissue and bone is formed in regions without significant levels of both (Fig. 13-27). However, unlike Pauwels, they also recognized the influence of vascular perfusion and proposed that low oxygen tension

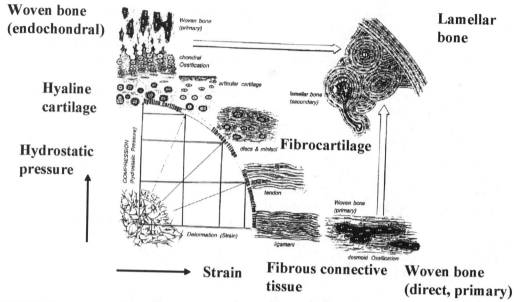

FIGURE 13-26. A schematic of the mechanoregulation concept stimulating differentiation of musculoskeletal connective tissue as proposed by F. Pauwels. (Adapted from Pauwels F. *Atlas zur Biomechanik der Gesunden und Kranken Hüfte.* Berlin: Springer-Verlag, 1973.)

diverts cells down the cartilaginous pathway. Using FE models, Carter and his co-workers showed that normal differentiation patterns in fracture healing (8,12) at various stages of healing were consistent with patterns of pressure and strain in the fracture callus. More recently, Loboa et al. demonstrated that this was also the case for a general oblique pseudarthrosis (38). Interestingly, the mechanoregulation concept of Carter

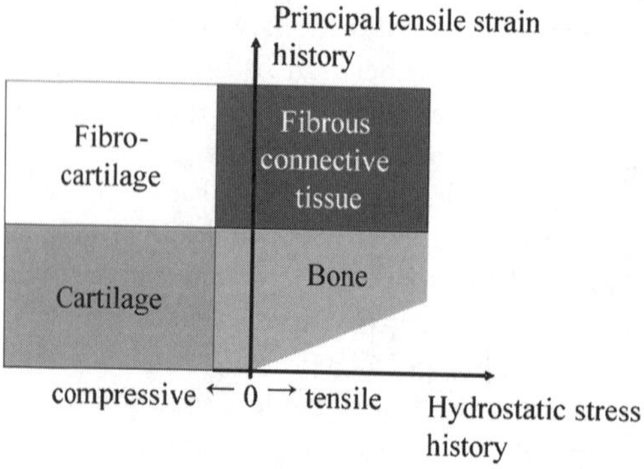

FIGURE 13-27. The mechanoregulation concept controlled by hydrostatic stress history and distorsional strain as proposed by Carter et al. (Adapted from ref. 11, Carter DR, Beaupre GS, Giori NJ, Helms, JA. Mechanobiology of skeletal regeneration. *Clin Orthop* 1998;S41–S55.)

et al. has been much discussed, but it has never been presented in quantitative terms.

In contrast, the mechanoregulation theory of Claes and Heigele (18) was initially presented in quantitative terms, and although the resulting concept is similar to that of Carter et al., they based their mechanoregulation theory on the observation that bone formation occurs mainly near calcified surfaces and that both intramembranous and endochondral ossification exist in fracture healing. Depending on the amount of tissue strain and hydrostatic pressure, different cellular reactions and tissue differentiation processes were predicted to occur (12,18,19). Very small tissue strains (less than approximately 5%) and hydrostatic pressures (below about −0.15 MPa) would allow direct intramembranous bone formation by bone cells (osteoblasts), larger values (less than about 15%, greater than −0.15 MPa) would allow endochondral ossification, and tissue strains above approximately 15% would lead to fibrocartilage and connective tissue preventing bone healing (18,19) (Fig. 13-28). Comparing FEA of fracture healing in the ovine tibia with histological findings from *in vivo* experiments, they were able to demonstrate that the quantitative formulation

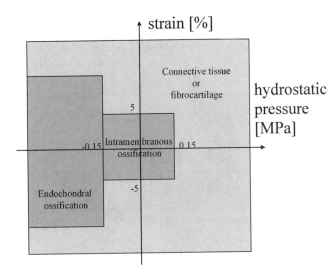

FIGURE 13-28. The mechanoregulation concept controlled by hydrostatic pressure and strain as proposed by Claes and Heigele. (Adapted from ref. 18, Claes LE, Heigele CA. Magnitudes of local stress and strain along bony surfaces predict the course and type of fracture healing. *J Biomech* 1999;32: 255–266.)

did indeed properly predict tissue differentiation events in the callus at three states of healing.

Finally, Prendergast, Huiskes, and colleagues have developed a different mechanoregulation concept taking into consideration that connective tissues are poroelastic and comprise both fluid and solid (27,45). They proposed a mechanoregulatory pathway composed of two biophysical stimuli, octahedral strain of the solid and interstitial fluid velocity relative to the solid. High magnitudes of either favored formation of fibrous tissue and less cartilage, and only when both were sufficiently small could ossification occur (Fig. 13-29). Based on *in vivo* experiments of motion-induced tissue differentiation at implant to bone interfaces, they quantified their regulatory model and demonstrated that it was consistent with observed temporal changes in implant motion.

Although different in their details, the proposed mechanoregulation theories are not that much different. They all propose that higher

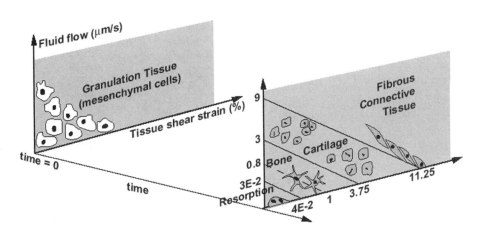

FIGURE 13-29. The mechanoregulation concept controlled by deviatoric strain and interstitial fluid velocity as proposed by Prendergast and Huiskes. (Adapted from ref. 45, Prendergast PJ, Huiskes R, Soballe K. ESB Research Award 1996. Biophysical stimuli on cells during tissue differentiation at implant interfaces. *J Biomech* 1997;30:539–548.)

magnitudes of tissue deformation result in the stimulation of softer fibrous connective tissue whereas cartilage and bone are formed in the presence of lower strains. In the more recent models, the two mechanical tissue parameters of importance are measures of volumetric (pressure or fluid flow) and deviatoric load or deformation (octahedral, shear, or principal strain). With low magnitudes of deviatoric strain, higher levels of volumetric parameters stimulate cartilage formation and lower levels, that of bone. Hence, it should not be too surprising that all of these proposed mechanisms are consistent with the temporal sequence and spatial distribution of resulting callus tissues in healing fractures, and it raises the question of how can we discriminate among the subtle difference between the theories, and whether other parameters may not be just as important in regulating tissue differentiation of musculoskeletal connective tissues.

6.2.2 Mechanoregulation Models of Fracture Healing

Mechanoregulation theories of tissue differentiation have been applied in particular to fracture healing because of several reasons. It is well known that fracture healing is modulated by mechanical loading and induced motion. Also the temporal variation in cellular events and tissue morphology are well characterized. However, more important, fracture healing has the potential to increase our understanding of mechanoregulation rules because of the vast knowledge already accumulated concerning the wide variety of conditions resulting in different healing responses, e.g., fracture geometry, loading magnitudes and rates, and loading directions. To learn from this body of data, models that are governed by mechanoregulation rules and that can predict tissue histomorphologies under various conditions should be compared and validated with experimental results.

Toward this goal, many of the mechanoregulation concepts have already been incorporated into numerical models that can simulate the biological process of fracture healing. The models are generally divided into two parts that are solved in an iterative fashion. In one part, the tis-

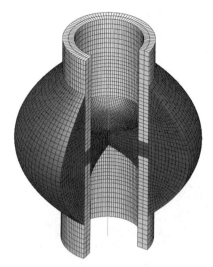

FIGURE 13-30. Three-dimensional finite-element model for the calculation of the strain and hydrostatic pressure in the bone healing zone.

sue deformations and stresses are calculated using FEM of the healing fracture with tissue morphology, material properties, and loading conditions as the input (Figs. 13-29 and 13-30). In the other part, the mechanoregulation algorithm is described by a set of mathematical or logical rules and used to predict changes in tissue material properties (Fig. 13-31). Although this may

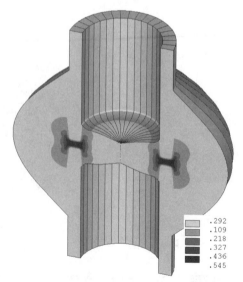

FIGURE 13-31. Strain distribution calculated for a fracture gap of 3 mm, an interfragmentary movement of 1.3 mm, and a healing time of 8 weeks.

appear straightforward, modeling of the biological aspects of healing can be quite complex, and a variety of approaches have been used.

It is well recognized that the callus tissue can be quite heterogeneous even at the length scale of well-refined FE meshes. To account for this, elemental material properties have been calculated as a biophysical stimuli–weighted mixture of different tissue types which slowly evolves with healing (34). Alternatively, others have tried to calculate material property changes based on matrix biochemical composition whose production and extracellular structural changes are directly related to the biophysical stimuli (39).

It is also clear that cell migration, proliferation, and apoptosis within the callus are likely to be modulated by the mechanical environment and must be modeled. In a first step, progenitor cell migration was described as a diffusive process but was not coupled to tissue deformation (36). Later, differential mass transport equations were used to describe cell density changes due to migration, proliferation, and apoptosis individually for each major cell type, i.e., stem cells, fibroblasts, chondrocytes, and osteoblasts (24). Although proliferation/apoptosis was also regulated by biophysical stimuli, there was no direct coupling between tissue deformation and transport. In both cases, matrix density and material properties were related to the density and population of the different cells. Also in the latter model, changes in matrix volume was modeled using thermoelastic analysis. In a very different approach, the effect of growth factors on cell phenotype, density, and matrix production was modeled first (6). Differential equations were formulated to describe the autocrine and paracrine effects of growth factors on cell phenotype, migration, proliferation/apoptosis,

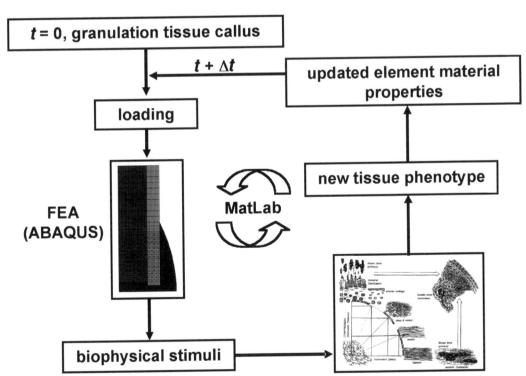

FIGURE 13-32. Flowchart diagram of an example iterative computer simulation. The tissue mechanical environment is calculated by the FEA. Based on the mechanical environment, the tissue phenotype is determined for each element using the mechanoregulation algorithm. Various methods are used to calculate new material properties of each element of the FE model, and a new iteration is simulated. (Adapted from ref. 35, Lacroix D, Prendergast PJ. A mechano-regulation model for tissue differentiation during fracture healing: analysis of gap size and loading. *J Biomech* 2002;35(9):1163–1171.)

and synthesis activities including production of growth factors themselves. Although this model did not include the effects of the mechanical environment, fascinatingly the uneventful course of normal fracture healing was simulated.

In addition to the callus tissue itself, other factors may also have significant influences on mechanoregulation of fracture healing. The most obvious of these is the vascularity, without which the chondrocytes would not mineralize and osteoblasts could not receive enough nutrition to produce bone. As observed in the case of histology, the proposed effect of mechanical environment on angiogenesis could be modeled such that the effect of gap size on temporospatial patterns of tissue differentiation and revascularization was correctly simulated (55).

Finally, it appears that currently the most significant factors and mechanoregulation hypotheses can be implemented in sophisticated structural and biological models. However, there are many parameter values that are unmeasured and must be assumed. Although parametric analyses can comfort us that any few assumptions are robust, the sheer number of parameters makes it difficult to determine if indeed there are no significant coupling effects. Furthermore, the number of biological rules are growing quickly and to order, weight, or resolve them can be daunting. Most models have overcome this by fixed deterministic algorithms (6,24,35,38) and other have used fuzzy logic (1,55). The benefit of the latter is that fuzzy rules are analogous to biological variations observed in nature, but in contrast these rules make it difficult to understand the relationship between basic physical parameters.

Now that these complex models have been developed, the next challenge will be to compare them with known *in vivo* results demonstrating the mechanosensitivity of tissue differentiation during fracture healing. With such comparisons, the most significant mechanobiological interaction can be resolved and mechanically guided tissue transformation functions defined (Fig. 13-32). These could then be combined with dramatically improving computer and imaging technology (computed tomography, nuclear magnetic resonance) and musculoskeletal loading simulations (21) to develop fracture healing models that would enable us to optimize fracture treatment for individual patients from a biomechanical point of view.

REFERENCES

1. Ament C, Hofer EP. A fuzzy logic model of fracture healing. *J Biomech* 2000;33:961–968.
2. Angele P, Yoo JU, Smith C, et al. Cyclic hydrostatic pressure enhances the chondrogenic phenotype of human mesenchymal progenitor cells differentiated in vitro. *J Orthop Res* 2003;21:451–457.
3. Aro HT, Wahner HT, Chao EY. Healing patterns of transverse and oblique osteotomies in the canine tibia under external fixation. *J Orthop Trauma* 1991;5:351–364.
4. Augat P, Burger J, Schorlemmer S, et al. Shear movement at the fracture site delays the healing of long bone fractures. In: 49th annual meeting of the Orthopaedic Research Society, New Orleans, 2003:0113.
5. Augat P, Merk J, Wolf S, et al. Mechanical stimulation by external application of cyclic tensile strains does not effectively enhance bone healing. *J Orthop Trauma* 2001;15:54–60.
6. Bailon-Plaza A, van der Meulen MC. A mathematical framework to study the effects of growth factor influences on fracture healing. *J Theor Biol* 2001;212:191–209.
7. Bishop NE, Tami I, van Rhijn MJ, et al. Effects of volumetric vs. shear deformation on tissue differentiation during secondary bone healing. In: 49th annual meeting of the Orthopaedic Research Society, New Orleans, 2003:0114.
8. Blenman PR, Carter DR, Beaupre GS. Role of mechanical loading in the progressive ossification of a fracture callus. *J Orthop Res* 1989;7:398–407.
9. Burny F, Donkerwolcke M, Bourgois R. Twenty years of experience in fracture healing measurements with strain gauges. *Orthopaedics* 1984;7:1823–1826.
10. Carter DR. Mechanical loading history and skeletal biology. *J Biomech* 1987;20:1095–1109.
11. Carter DR, Beaupre GS, Giori NJ, et al. Mechanobiology of skeletal regeneration. *Clin Orthop* 1998; S41–S55.
12. Carter DR, Blenman PR, Beaupre GS. Correlations between mechanical stress history and tissue differentiation in initial fracture healing. *J Orthop Res* 1988;6:736–748.
13. Cheal EJ, Mansmann KA, DiGioia AM III, et al. Role of interfragmentary strain in fracture healing: ovine model of a healing osteotomy. *J Orthop Res* 1991;9:131–142.

14. Claes L, Augat P, Suger G, et al. Influence of size and stability of the osteotomy gap on the success of fracture healing. *J Orthop Res* 1997;15:577–584.

15. Claes L, Burri C, Heckmann G, et al. Biomechanische Untersuchungen zur Stabilität von Tibiaosteosynthesen mit dem Fixateur externe und einer Minimalosteosynthese. *Akt Traumatol* 1979;9:185–189.

16. Claes L, Eckert-Hubner K, Augat P. The effect of mechanical stability on local vascularization and tissue differentiation in callus healing. *J Orthop Res* 2002;20:1099–1105.

17. Claes L, Heitemeyer U, Krischak G, et al. Fixation technique influences osteogenesis of comminuted fractures. *Clin Orthop* 1999;221–229.

18. Claes LE, Heigele CA. Magnitudes of local stress and strain along bony surfaces predict the course and type of fracture healing. *J Biomech* 1999;32:255–266.

19. Claes LE, Heigele CA, Neidlinger-Wilke C, et al. Effects of mechanical factors on the fracture healing process. *Clin Orthop* 1998;S132–S147.

20. Claes LE, Wilke HJ, Augat P, et al. Effect of dynamization on gap healing of diaphyseal fractures under external fixation. *Clin Biomech (Bristol, Avon)* 1995;10:227–234.

21. Duda GN, Heller M, Albinger J, et al. Influence of muscle forces on femoral strain distribution. *J Biomech* 1998;31:841–846.

22. Duda GN, Sollmann M, Sporrer S, et al. Interfragmentary motion in tibial osteotomies stabilized with ring fixators. *Clin Orthop* 2002;163–172.

23. Egger EL, Histand MB, Norrdin RW. An experimental comparison of canine osteotomy healing stabilized with constantly rigid fixation against decreasingly rigid fixation. *Trans Orthop Res Soc* 1986; 11:473 (Transactions of the 32nd Annual Meeting, February 17–20, 1986, New Orleans, LA).

24. Garcia JM, Kuiper JH, Doblaré M, et al. A numerical model to study the mechanical influence on bone fracture healing. *Acta Bioeng Biomech* 2002;4:394–395.

25. Gardner TN, Evans M, Hardy J, et al. Dynamic interfragmentary motion in fractures during routine patient activity. *Clin Orthop* 1997:216–225.

26. Heitemeyer U, Claes L, Hierholzer G. [The significance of postoperative stability for osseous repair of a multiple fragment fracture. Animal experiment studies]. *Unfallchirurg* 1990;93:49–55.

27. Huiskes R, van Driel WD, Prendergast PJ, et al. A biomechanical regulatory model for periprosthetic fibrous-tissue differentiation. *J Mater Sci Mat Med* 1997;8:785–788.

28. Kaspar D, Seidl W, Neidlinger-Wilke C, et al. Dynamic cell stretching increases human osteoblast proliferation and CICP synthesis but decreases osteocalcin synthesis and alkaline phosphatase activity. *J Biomech* 2000;33:45–51.

29. Kempf I, Grosse A, Beck G. Closed locked intramedullary nailing. Its application to comminuted fractures of the femur. *J Bone Joint Surg Am* 1985;67:709–720.

30. Kenwright J, Goodship AE. Controlled mechanical stimulation in the treatment of tibial fractures. *Clin Orthop* 1989:36–47.

31. Kleinig R, Hierholzer G. Biomechanische Untersuchungen zur Osteosynthese mit dem Fixateur externe. *Akt Traumatologie* 1976;81:71–76.

32. Koob TJ, Clark PE, Hernandez DJ, et al. Compression loading in vitro regulates proteoglycan synthesis by tendon fibrocartilage. *Arch Biochem Biophys* 1992;298:303–312.

33. Küntscher G. *Praxis der Marknagelung.* Stuttgart: Schattauer, 1962.

34. Lacroix D, Prendergast PJ. A homogenisation procedure to prevent numerical instabilities in poroelastic tissue differentiation models. In: 8th Annual Symposium, on Computational Methods in Orthopaedic Biomechanics, March 2000, Orlando, FL.

35. Lacroix D, Prendergast PJ. A mechano-regulation model for tissue differentiation during fracture healing: analysis of gap size and loading. *J Biomech* 2002;35:(9)1163–1171.

36. Lacroix D, Prendergast PJ, Li G, et al. Biomechanical model to simulate tissue differentiation and bone regeneration: application to fracture healing. *Med Biol Eng Comput* 2002;40:14–21.

37. Larsson S, Kim W, Egger EL. Effect of dynamization on healing of a transverse osteotomy in canine tibia under external fixation. *Trans Orthop Res Soc* 1993;18:132 (Transactions of the 39th Annual Meeting, February 15–18, 1993, San Francisco, CA).

38. Loboa EG, Beaupre GS, Carter DR. Mechanobiology of initial pseudarthrosis formation with oblique fractures. *J Orthop Res* 2001;19:1067–1072.

39. Loboa EG, Wren TAL, Carter DR. Mechanobiology of soft tissue regeneration. *Trans Orthop Res Soc* 2001;26:138 (Transactions of the 47th Annual Meeting, February 25–28, 2001, San Francisco, CA).

40. McKibbin B. The biology of fracture healing in long bones. *J Bone Joint Surg Br* 1978;60-B:150–162.

41. Muller J, Schenk R, Willenegger H. [Experimental studies on the development of reactive pseudarthroses on the canine radius]. *Helv Chir Acta* 1968;35:301–308.

42. Park SH, O'Connor K, McKellop H, et al. The influence of active shear or compressive motion on fracture-healing. *J Bone Joint Surg Am* 1998;80:868–878.

43. Pauwels F. *Biomechanics of the locomotor apparatus.* Berlin: Springer-Verlag, 1980.

44. Perren SM, Cordey J. The concept of interfragmentary strain. In: Uhtoff HK, ed. *Current concepts of internal fixation of fracture.* New York: Springer-Verlag, 1980:63–77.

45. Prendergast PJ, Huiskes R, Soballe K. ESB Research Award 1996. Biophysical stimuli on cells during tissue differentiation at implant interfaces. *J Biomech* 1997;30:539–548.

46. Rhinelander FW. Tibial blood supply in relation to fracture healing. *Clin Orthop* 1974;105:34–81.

47. Roux W. *Gesammelte Abhandlungen über Entwicklungsmechanik der Organismen.* Leipzig: Wilhelm Engelmann, 1895.

48. Rüedi T, Murphy W. *AO principles of fracture management.* Stuttgart: Thieme, 2000.

49. Sarmiento A, Latta LL. *Closed functional treatment of fractures.* Berlin: Springer-Verlag, 1981.

50. Sarmiento A, McKellop HA, Llinas A, et al. Effect of loading and fracture motions on diaphyseal tibial fractures. *J Orthop Res* 1996;14:80–84.

51. Schandelmaier P, Krettek C, Tscherne H. [Biomechanical studies of 9 tibial interlocking nails in a bone-implant unit]. *Unfallchirurg* 1994;97:600–608.

52. Schenk R, Willenegger H. Zum histologischen Bild der sogenannte Primärheilung der Knochenkompakta nach experimentellen Osteotomien am Hund. *Experimentia* 1963;19:593–595.

53. Schneider E, Michel MC, Genge M, et al. Loads acting in an intramedullary nail during fracture healing in the human femur. *J Biomech* 2001;34:849–857.

54. Schweiberer L, Schenk R. [Histomorphology and vascularization of secondary healing of bone fractures with emphasis on tibial shaft fractures (author's transl)]. *Unfallheilkunde* 1977;80:275–286.

55. Simon U, Augat P, Utz M, et al. Dynamical simulation of the fracture healing process including vascularity. In: Proceedings of the 13th conference of European Society of Biomechanics, Wroclawskiej, Poland, 2002:772–773.

56. van't Veen SJ, Hagen JW, van Ginkel FC, et al. Intermittent compression stimulates cartilage mineralization. *Bone* 1995;17:461–465.

57. Watson-Jones R, Wilson JN. *Fractures and joint injuries.* New York: Churchill Livingstone, 1982.

58. Weyts FA, Bosmans B, Niesing R, et al. Mechanical control of human osteoblast apoptosis and proliferation in relation to differentiation. *Calcif Tissue Int* 2003;72:505–512.

59. Wu JJ, Shyr HS, Chao EY, et al. Comparison of osteotomy healing under external fixation devices with different stiffness characteristics. *J Bone Joint Surg Am* 1984;66:1258–1264.

60. Yamagishi M, Yoshimura Y. The biomechanics of fracture healing. *J Bone Joint Surg Am* 1955;5:1035–1068.

BIOMECHANICS AND PRECLINICAL TESTING OF ARTIFICIAL JOINTS: THE HIP

RIK HUISKES
JAN STOLK

1 INTRODUCTION

1.1 Development of Hip Replacement

Total hip arthroplasty (THA) was one of the major surgical advances of the twentieth century (19). At an estimated occurrence of between 500,000 and 1 million operations per year (115), it is second only to dental reconstruction as an invasive treatment of body ailments. It is an effective treatment for serious forms of osteoarthrosis (OA) and for disabling effects of rheumatoid arthritis, congenital deformities, and particular kinds of posttraumatic conditions. OA is the most frequent indication for THA, comprising about 65% of the total volume. According to an Ameican study (2), it is responsible for the majority of cases involving musculoskeletal discom-

fort and, second to cardiovascular conditions, is an important cause of complete or partial disabilities. About 17% of Americans have some form of OA or arthritis (44,54,211). Ten percent of all Americans suffer from OA, half of them chronically.

The development and application of THA have achieved a tremendous reduction in disabilities, particularly in the older segment of the population. The economic effects of this surgical treatment on society as a whole, in terms of savings in medical care, drugs, and disability aids and the reduction in sickness-related absence from jobs, are significant (44,54,211). The personal effects on the happiness and life fulfillment of patients are overwhelming. The majority of patients receiving THA can hardly walk at all and suffer serious continuous pain, day and night. A few weeks after the operation they will, with few exceptions, be pain free, able to function normally, and resume jobs and sometimes even active sports. Complications will usually not recur until after 10 to 20 years. When they do, as a result of eventual wear or loosening, a revision operation is possible. At least 90% of the patients live normal, pain-free lives for at least 10 years after the operation (22,58,115).

The successful application of THA on a large scale, which essentially evolved during the past four decades, is an accomplishment of scientific and technological developments in orthopaedic surgery and bioengineering, in particular from biomaterials and biomechanics sciences. The proliferation of applications started around 1960 with the introduction of two inventions by Sir John Charnley (17,18). One was the adoption of the "low-friction" principle, whereby a relatively small metal femoral head was made to rotate against a polyethylene (PE) acetabular cup. Another was the introduction of acrylic cement [poly(methyl methacrylate) or PMMA] as a filling material to accommodate uniform load transfer between the smooth-shaped prosthesis and the irregular texture of bone. PMMA, when introduced in a doughy phase, interdigitates with the bone and cures to form a solid but relatively flexible mantle between bone and prosthesis (Fig. 14-1).

PMMA is a relatively weak material, however, and long-term loosening of prostheses was attributed to its mechanical disintegration. Although cemented fixation remained the standard method for the older, post-65-year-old population, alternative prosthetic designs were aimed at replacing acrylic cement with other means of fixation for younger generations. Early noncemented prostheses were of the press-fitted or screwed-in type. Porous-coated prostheses were introduced to provoke bony ingrowth for improved fixation (40). The more recent hydroxylapatite-coated hip prostheses (48–50,92,134) are meant to form a firm biological bond with bone (osseous integration); hydroxylapatite is the mineral substance of bone itself (Fig. 14-2). Their results are promising (see also Chapter 11), but definite conclusions about their ultimate clinical performance, and about

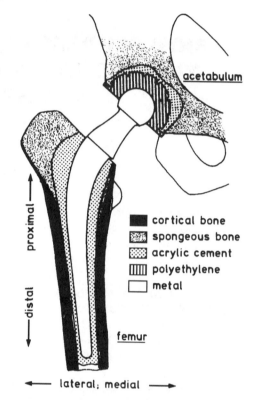

FIGURE 14-1. Schematic section of a cemented Charnley prosthesis. (From Huiskes R. Some fundamental aspects of human-joint replacement. *Acta Orthop Scand [Suppl]* 1980;185, with permission.)

the best fixation methods or designs, require longer-term studies than are presently available.

1.2   Success in Perspective

As a result of successful developments in joint replacement, a new hip has become a standard treatment in the Western world. Whereas in the beginning it was a last resort to reambulate the elderly, bedridden from pain in their grossly distorted joints, now it is a solution for those who undergo restrictions in their work, or sports, due to cartilage degeneration. The younger—and more active—the patient, the higher the probability of prosthetic loosening, but that does not deter those who want to live now. Still, time of service, intensity of mechanical use, young age at operation, and prior hip replacements are some of the most important risk factors for prosthetic loosening. "Given enough service time for the

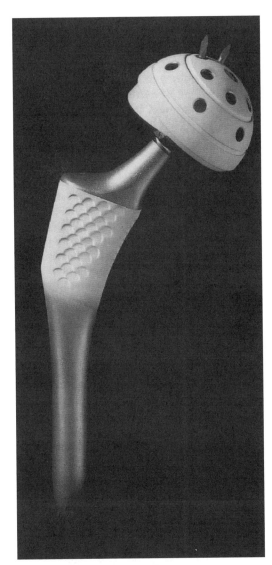

FIGURE 14-2. The ABG noncemented hip prosthesis (Stryker-Howmedica-Osteonics, Allendale, NJ) has a proximal hydroxylapatite (HA) coating on the stem and an anatomical shape to ensure a good proximal fit. Also, the cup is coated with HA.

patient, every hip prosthesis will loosen" is not an irrational prediction. The most frequent complication is long-term loosening, unrelated to infection, and usually called "aseptic" or "mechanical" loosening. Aseptic loosening is a gradual process whereby the mechanical integrity of the implant–bone interface is lost, and a fibrous tissue is formed between the two surfaces (38,52,96,149,161). A gradual increase

in thickness of the soft layer occurs with time. As a result, the patient develops pain and functional restrictions, until revision is the only option to restore functionality. Aseptic loosening is the predominant limiting factor for the functional life span of THA reconstructions. Although most revisions are successful, the expected endurance of a revised hip replacement is less than that of a primary one.

Although the final stage of the loosening process is well known, why and how it develops, and how it can be prevented—the main emphasis of this chapter—is not fully understood. Endurance is basically determined by *prosthetic, surgical,* and *patient factors* (Table 14-1).

In order to monitor the safety and efficacy of joint replacements and relate that to the various factors—as cited in Table 14-1—the European Nordic Registers were started, of which the Swedish Hip Register was the first (1979) (1,58–60,62,63,115,116,147). In the Nordic countries every patient has a national identification number for health care. Hence, every patient can be followed on a national level. For the hip registers, forms are filled out at operations and reported for virtually all hip replacements (more than 95%), specifying relevant implant, surgeon, and patient factors. Revisions are reported in the same way. Hence, the endurance of virtually every hip replacement can be related statistically to the factors. The Swedish Hip Register now contains two cohorts of hip replacements: 1979–1989 (55,839 hip replacements) and 1990–2000 (76,391 hip replacements), the latter reflecting improved cementing techniques and prosthetic designs. Owing to the large number of cases, the individual factors can be evaluated statistically relative to their effects on endurance, with years between operation and revision as an endurance criterion (Fig. 14-3).

In the latest publication from the Swedish Hip Register (116), for example, we find that 14,081 hip replacements out of 76,391 (1990–2000 cohort) had been revised after 10 years of service, of which 75.4% are due to aseptic loosening (or "mechanical loosening"). Considering only those patients operated for osteoarthritis as diagnosis, and aseptic loosening as cause for failure, the average endurance after 10 years in

TABLE 14-1. FACTORS AFFECTING SAFETY AND EFFICACY OF JOINT REPLACEMENT (ARBITRARY SELECTION)

Implant Factors	Surgeon Factors	Patient Factors
• Design concept	• Indication for operation	• Weight and dimensions
• Design details	• Prosthesis selection	• Age
• Materials	• Preplanning	• Activity level
• Production technology	• Reaming procedure	• Musculoskeletal condition
• Surgical guidelines	• Cementing procedure	• Health condition

the latest cohort was 94.8%. Of those patients operated in 1991, the cumulative frequency of revision for aseptic loosening after 10 years was about 3% for cemented and about 7% for noncemented prostheses. At 3 years postoperative the cumulative frequency was about 0.3% for cemented and 0.4% for noncemented prostheses. From the Finnish Hip Register it was reported for the years 1989–1999 that only 7% of cemented hip replacements were used for patients

Percentage not revised

Charnley
Exeter
Lubinus SPII
Mueller Curved

Years postoperatively

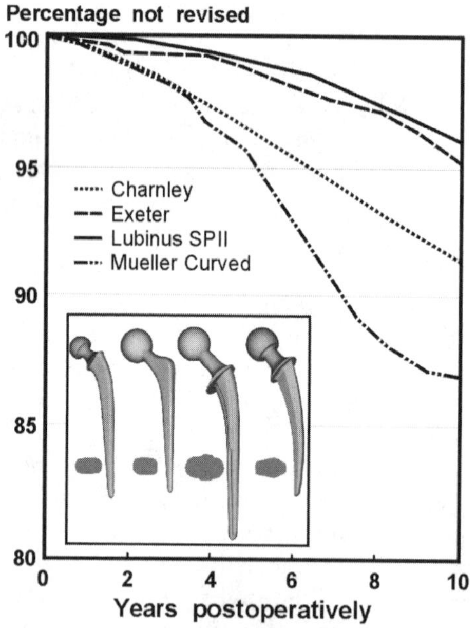

FIGURE 14-3. Probability of survival (percentage not revised) of four cemented total hip replacements. The stems of these replacements are shown on the inset; from left to right: Charnley, Exeter, Lubinus SPII, Mueller Curved. The data are taken from the Swedish Hip Register containing a total of 92,675 patients who received a THR between 1978 and 1990. (Adapted from Heberts P, Malchau H. Long-term registration has improved the quality of hip replacement: a review of the Swedish THR Register comparing 160,000 cases. *Acta Orthop Scand* 2000;71:111–121.)

younger than 60 years (147). As for surgeon-related factors, particularly cementing technique was evaluated in the registers. It was found from the Swedish Hip Register that the risk ratio for premature revision among the Swedish clinics varied between 0.60 and 1.72 (1.0 being the average), which indicates the importance of surgical factors. From the Norwegian Hip Register it was reported that the average 10-year fixation endurance of one particular cemented stem (Charnley type) varied between 75% and 99% among the Norwegian clinics; after 3 years the variation was between 96% and 100% (60). This again highlights the prominence of surgical technique as an individual risk factor.

Considering patient-related factors, diagnosis and age are usually evaluated. We can find that average endurance for all hip replacements at 9 years was estimated at 87.6% for those younger than 55 years at the time of surgery, at 94.3% for those between 54 and 76, and at 96.9% for those older than 75 (116).

Although the Nordic Hip Registers evaluate implant, surgeon, and patient factors relative to the associated risks for premature failure of the arthroplasty, they do so retrospectively. Many years can go by before the quality of a new prosthetic design can be assessed in this way. It was proposed that the quality assurance of new prostheses should be regulated (43). To accomplish that, preclinical tests of new designs are essential. Biomechanical preclinical testing methods are a prime subject of this chapter.

1.3 Biomechanics and Preclinical Testing

The hip joint has a biomechanical function, and also the failure processes for prosthetic loosening are caused or affected by dynamic load transfer from the articulation to the bone, causing excessive stresses and strains that may damage prosthetic components and cement and interface bonds, and promote a loosening process. It is important for orthopaedic surgeons and prosthetic designers to understand the origin and patterns of the stresses involved, and how these can lead to failure. These stresses can be evaluated using finite-element analysis (FEA), a computer method enabling calculations of stresses throughout a structure, using numerical descriptions of its geometry and loads, and mechanical properties of its materials, as input. A brief introduction to stress analysis in solid structures, and the application of FEA, is added as an appendix to this chapter. The next section deals with stresses in hip-prosthetic structures in general, informing the reader of the stress distributions to be expected and providing an explanation of why they are patterned in their particular ways. It is true that those who have experience in stress analysis of hip-prosthetic reconstructions, as we do, can usually predict roughly what to expect before analyses are concluded. That is because we understand the character of the load-transfer mechanisms. We want to share this understanding with our readers.

But understanding the stress patterns in hip reconstructions does not necessarily imply understanding clinical failure. The reason is that failure—clinical loosening—is the result of a process, hardly ever of an event. Although fracture of a THA component would clearly be registered as caused by mechanical loading, gradual loosening—the most common cause of failure—involves mechanical load-transfer and biological reactions in bone and at interfaces; the biological *fitness* of the patient plays a role as well. Failure can be from *biological, biomechanical,* or *mechanobiological* causes, but this chapter emphasizes biomechanics. Again, given enough time, all hip reconstructions would eventually fail. Optimization means postponing this moment past the lifetime of the patient. Hence, the real question is why, how, and when the stress patterns produce the failure mechanisms. For this purpose *failure scenarios* can be formulated (75) and simulated in the laboratory or the computer, which is the subject of Section 3 of this chapter. These methods are useful for preevaluations of new prosthetic design concepts (design confirmation studies), and for preclinically testing actual new prostheses before they are tried in patients.

2 PRINCIPLES OF STRESS TRANSFER IN COMPOSITE STRUCTURES

2.1 General Considerations

A bone–prosthesis structure is known as a composite structure. This implies that it consists of separate substructures with different elastic and geometric properties that are bonded to each other in some specified manner. The stress patterns in these composite structures depend on the bonding characteristics at the interfaces between the substructures, and on the relative magnitudes of their elastic moduli. This effect can be illustrated relative to the phenomenon of 'load sharing' in a composite bar (Fig. 14-4A,B). A tensile force *F* is transferred through a composite bar comprised of two bars bonded to each other. The two bars have different Young's moduli, E_1 and E_2, and cross-sectional areas A_1 and A_2. The quantity AE is known as the "axial stiffness." When the loading is applied as shown, the individual bars of the composite will share in the load transfer from one to the other such that $F_1 + F_2 = F$. The forces F_1 and F_2 are given by the ratio of axial stiffness:

$$F_1 / F_2 = A_1 E_1 / A_2 E_2 \qquad (1)$$

This formula shows that the bar with the higher axial stiffness will carry more load. We note that Eq. 1 is based on the assumption that the axial strains in the bars are equal, i.e., $\varepsilon_1 = \varepsilon_2 = \varepsilon$. Hence, from Hooke's law in uniaxial tension for the stresses, $\sigma_1 = E_1\varepsilon$ and $\sigma_2 = E_2\varepsilon$, it follows that

$$\sigma_1 / \sigma_2 = E_1 / E_2 \qquad (2)$$

Equation 2 states that when a deformation (ε) is imposed on a composite bar, the material

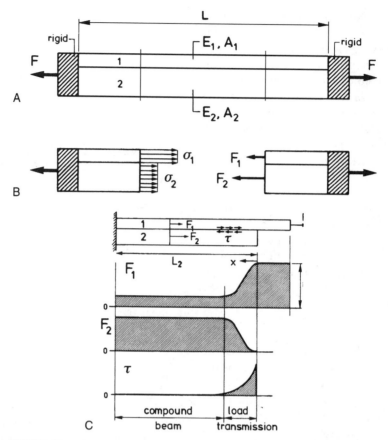

FIGURE 14-4. A: A composite structure consisting of two bonded bars with different elastic moduli and cross-sectional areas. The structure is uniformly stretched by an external axial force F. **B:** The internal forces F_1 and F_2 differ by virtue of the different elastic moduli; the internal stresses $\sigma_1 = F_1/A_1$ and $\sigma_2 = F_2/A_2$ are also different. **C:** Load transfer by means of shear stress τ at the interface between the two bars. The loads F_1 and F_2 inside the two bars and the shear-stress distribution τ at the interface are shown. (From Huiskes R. Principle and methods of solid biomechanics. In: Ducheyne P, Hastings G, eds. *Functional behavior of orthopaedic materials. Vol. I: fundamentals.* Boca Raton, FL: CRC Press, 1984:51–98, with permission.)

with higher elastic modulus experiences greater stresses. Similar formulas exist for the composite beam loaded transversely in bending and composite shafts loaded in torsion (69). For each case, the stiffer beam will carry the higher load.

The illustrative example of Fig. 14-4A and B is one of pure load sharing because the external force F is applied to both bars simultaneously. If the force were only applied to bar 1, then load sharing would not occur in the segment of bar 1 that is to the right of bar 2 (Fig. 14-4C). Obvi-

ously, load sharing would take place only where bar 1 and bar 2 are bonded together. In this example, load transfer is via the shear stress developed at the interface between bar 1 and bar 2. In bar 1, in going from right to left, the load F_1 reduces from $F_1 = F$ to $F_1 = A_1E_1F/(A_1E_1 + A_2E_2)$, and in bar 2 the load F_2 increases from $F_2 = 0$ to $F_2 = A_2E_2F/(A_1E_1 + A_2E_2)$.

This load-transfer mechanism between the two bars is important because the shear stresses it produces may cause the bond to fail at the interface. Clearly, the total amount of load F transferred from bar 1 to bar 2 must satisfy equilibrium conditions, hence

$$F_2 = A_2 E_2 F / (A_1 E_1 + A_2 E_2) \qquad (3)$$

This force must act over the available area for the bar, $L_2 d_2$, at the interface. Here, L_2 is the length of the bar, and d_2 its depth (in the perpendicular direction). Although the average shear stress over the length L_2 would be $\tau_{av} = F_2 / L_2 d_2$, the actual maximal stress is much higher because τ is far from uniform, with a peak value at L_2, where bar 2 begins to carry load. The actual shear-stress pattern $\tau(x)$ can be determined from a shear-lag distribution function given by

$$\tau(z) = \lambda F_2 e^{-\lambda x} / d_2, \qquad (4)$$

where λ is a structural parameter depending on the elastic moduli and on the cross-sectional areas of the two bars (68). Again, similar formulas exist for beams in bending and shafts in torsion (68–70).

To review some basic concepts of compressive load transfer in composite structures, we consider a simple model of a solid layer (prosthesis) fixed to a substrate (bone) (Fig. 14-5). We assume both materials, separately, to have uniform elastic properties and that the top layer is rigidly bonded to the substrate. Figures 14-5A and B present von Mises stress patterns (see appendix for definition) in the materials for the case where the prosthesis is loaded by a single force F. Figure 14-5A presents the case in which the prosthesis has the same elastic properties as bone ("isoelastic material"), whereas in Fig. 14-5B the prosthesis is made out of a metal, say titanium, that is much stiffer than bone. From these results, we note the following characteristics:

1. The stresses are essentially non-uniform, concentrated predominantly in a central band in the structure, directly under the applied load.
2. When the moduli of the two materials are equal (Fig. 14-5A), the stresses are continuous over the interface; when the materials are different (Fig. 14-5B), the stresses are discontinuous over the interface.
3. The stress patterns are more uniformly distributed for the case of the stiff prosthesis

(Fig. 14-5B) than in the case of the more flexible prosthesis (Fig. 14-5A). As a result, the stress magnitudes are higher for the case of the prosthesis made of flexible material.

The normal (compressive) stress in the (vertical) y-direction σ_y at the interfaces in Fig. 14-5 must balance the applied force F in the y direction. It would be immediately obvious from a free-body diagram of the prosthesis that the average compressive interface stress $\bar{\sigma}_y$ equals F/Ld, when L is the length and d the width of the elastic layer. The *actual* stress, σ_y, is nonuniform and must also satisfy the equilibrium condition. Thus, a simple relationship exists between the average stress, $\bar{\sigma}_y$, and the actual stress σ_y, as

$$\bar{\sigma}_y L d = d \int_0^L \sigma_y \, dx = F \qquad (5)$$

We note that the average stress should not be taken as representative of the maximal stress value. Equation 5 also shows that because the stress distribution σ_y must always balance the applied load F, a composite structure that leads to a narrower load distribution (Fig. 14-5A), when compared with that in Fig. 14-5B, has a higher maximal value. This demonstrates that our intuitive expectation that a material with similar elastic properties to bone would be ideal for implants in fact may not be true. In general, the stress patterns in a surface-fixation structure depend not only on the articular loading characteristics (magnitude, direction, contact location, and contact area size), but also the flexural rigidity (elastic moduli and dimensions) of the component, the elastic characteristics of the supporting bone, and the bonding characteristics.

This illustrates that the load-transfer and load-sharing mechanisms in composite structures can be complex, even in relatively simple, regular structures. In general, stresses within a structure cannot simply be determined by dividing the load to be transferred by the area available for load transfer. As a rule, the stresses are not uniform over a particular area, and peak values are bound to occur, depending on the geometry and the material characteristics of the separate components in the composite. High values of

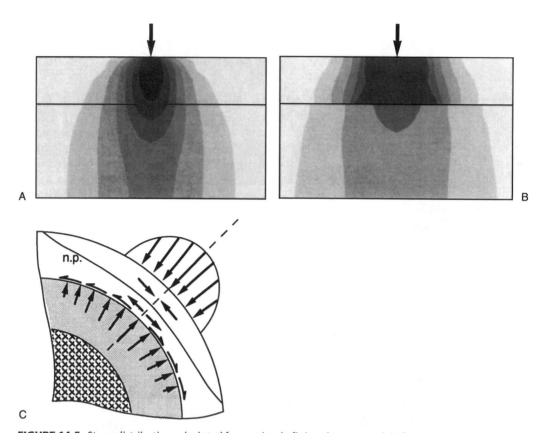

FIGURE 14-5. Stress distribution calculated from a simple finite-element model of an elastic layer resting on an elastic foundation subject to a force *F*. **A:** The von Mises stress distribution (see Chapter 4 for definition) is shown for the case in which the top layer (prosthesis) has the same elastic properties as the foundation (bone). **B:** The von Mises stress distribution for the case in which the prosthesis is made out of a material (e.g., titanium) much stiffer than the foundation (bone). **C:** Load transfer through a plate on a flexible foundation. In addition to compressive stress developed at the interface as a direct effect of load transfer, shear stresses also develop. The load also created bending of the plate, with compression on one side and tension on the other side of the neutral plane (n.p.). (Adapted from Huiskes R, Strens PHGE, van Heck J, et al. Interface stresses in the resurfaced hip. *Acta Orthop Scand* 1985;56:474–478, with permission.)

stress generally occur in structures with notches, sharp corners, and holes. These high values are known as stress concentrations.

Very often, stresses in composite structures are generated not as a direct effect of load sharing or load transfer but as an indirect effect of deformational variations caused by differences in elastic moduli (Fig. 14-5C). Because of the compressive force, compressive stresses arise at the interface as direct effects of the load-transfer mechanism. However, high shear stresses at the interface may also arise as an *indirect* effect. This is caused by the difference in lateral displacements of the plate and the foundation. If the elastic foundation has a lower elastic modulus than the plate, it would tend to expand more in the lateral direction. This expansion is resisted by the shear stresses developed at the interface. Another mechanism occurs as well: the external load causes the plate to deform in bending. Hence, we find a "neutral plane" (n.p.) where the bending stress in the plate is zero. Above it, compression occurs, and under it tension. These three mechanisms are, of course, interrelated and depend on the precise characteristics of the structure. For instance, if the plate is relatively stiff, it deforms less and would reduce the maximal interface stress.

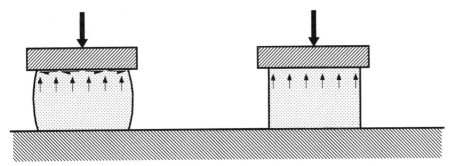

FIGURE 14-6. Compression of a material by a force applied onto an adhesive interface will create both compression and shear at the interface *(left)*. When the interface is unbonded and lubricated, it can slide without friction at the interface. In this case, only compressive stresses occur *(right)*.

Stress transfer in composite structures is very much affected by the bonding characteristics at the interface. The frictional and adhesive characteristics of the surfaces are important factors. The orientation of the interface relative to the dominant direction of loading is also important, as are surface microstructures and textures. If the interface is smooth, unbonded, and lubricated, then no shear stress will be developed no matter how large the disparity in the lateral displacement. The difference between bonded (adhesive) and unbonded (lubricated) interfaces can be most simply seen for uniaxial loading (Fig. 14-6). For the unbonded or lubricated case (right), only compressive stress is developed in the material; the material is in a state of uniaxial compression. For the bonded or perfectly adhesive case (left), shear stresses are developed at the interface in

addition. The compressive stresses at the interface are sufficient to balance the external force. The shear stresses merely develop as a secondary effect, and they must balance themselves.

This is no longer true when the interface is not perpendicular to the applied force. Figure 14-7 depicts a cone-shaped object (implant) inserted into a tubular structure (bone) where the interface is bonded by cement or by some other mechanism. In this case, the applied force will create compressive and shear stresses along the interface. If the cone angle is relatively small, as is the case with most hip prostheses, the magnitude of the shear stress developed will be much greater than the compressive stress. This load transfer would occur predominantly by the shear stress, as shown in Fig. 14-7. When the interface is unbonded and lubricated (e.g., by body fluids

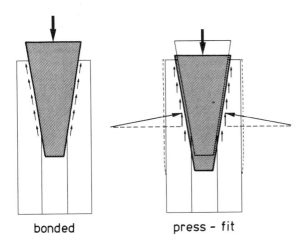

bonded   press - fit

FIGURE 14-7. Load transfer via a straight-tapered cone pushed into a cylindrical counterpart. *(Left)* The shear stress at the bonded interface can equilibrate the applied force. *(Right)* At a smooth, press-fitted interface, equilibrium relies on the vertical component of compressive interface stress. For slightly tapered cones, a significant amount of subsidence must occur in order for the compressive stress required for equilibrium to develop. (From Huiskes R. The various stress patterns of press-fit, ingrown and cemented femoral stems. *Clin Orthop* 1990;261:27–38, with permission.)

at the bone surface), shear stress at the interface can no longer exist or is minimal. To develop a significant reaction force to equilibrate the applied load (Fig. 14-7), the cone-shaped prosthesis must subside into the tubular bone to create a significant compressive stress at the interface. Again because of the small cone angle, a very large compressive stress must be developed at the interface to generate a sufficient amount of force to equilibrate the applied load. In this process, a tensile hoop stress must be developed in the bone to prevent expansion.

The basic concepts just discussed are of importance for any composite implant structure. In the next two sections, intramedullary stem fixation of the femoral component in THA and acetabular cup fixation are considered in more detail.

2.2 Intramedullary Stem Fixation

The principles of load transfer in intramedullary fixation are based on load sharing, similar to the principles in Fig. 14-4. As a simplified model,

we choose a metal rod (the stem) fixed in a tubular bone. An axial force (Fig. 14-8A) that must be transferred to the bone loads the stem. Again, the load transfer between the stem and the bone is realized by shear stresses at the interfaces. In fact, a free-body diagram of the stem would indicate that these shear stresses must balance the external load; hence, the average shear stress times the surface area of the stem equals the axial force. But again, these shear stresses are not uniformly distributed; rather, stress concentrations occur on the distal and the proximal sides. This is illustrated in Fig. 14-8A, together with the load-sharing patterns in the stem and the bone.

When the stem is loaded in bending (Fig. 14-8B), a very similar load-transfer mechanism occurs. This time, however, the bending moment is to be transferred from the stem to the bone via interface stresses (tension, compression, and tangential shear) to effectuate this moment transfer. These stresses are again nonuniform and are concentrated mainly at the proximal and distal sides.

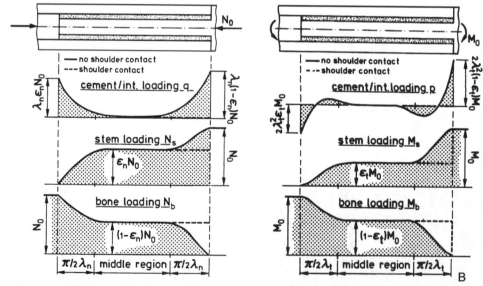

FIGURE 14-8. The load-transfer characteristics in a simple model of a straight stem cemented in tubular bone with and without shoulder contact. **A:** Axial loading. **B:** Bending. In both drawings, left is distal, right proximal. From top to bottom: **(A)** distributions of shear loading and **(B)** the bending moment in the stem; and **(A)** the axial force and **(B)** the bending moment in the bone. (From Huiskes R. Design, fixation, and stress analysis of permanent orthopedic implants: the hip joint. In: Ducheyne P, Hastings G, eds. *Functional behavior of biomaterials. Vol. II: applications.* Boca Raton, FL: CRC Press, 1984:121–162, with permission.)

The graphs of Fig. 14-8 illustrate the most important basic principles of load transfer in intramedullary fixation of artificial joints (68–70):

1. The structure can be divided into three regions, a middle region where load sharing occurs and two load-transfer regions on the proximal and distal sides.

2. In the middle region, pure load sharing occurs, whereby the stem carries $\varepsilon_n \times 100\%$ of the axial force or $\varepsilon_t \times 100\%$ of the bending moment. Here, ε_n and ε_t are relative axial and flexural rigidities defined as:

$$\varepsilon_n = A_s E_s / (A_s E_s + A_b E_b) \qquad (6)$$

and

$$\varepsilon_t = I_s E_s / (I_s E_s + I_b E_b) \qquad (7)$$

where E, A, and I are the elastic moduli, the cross-sectional areas, and the second moments of inertia of the stem (s) and the bone (b).

3. The load carried by the stem and the bone is normally carried by the bone alone; hence, the bone is stress-shielded by the stem. The higher ε_n and ε_t are, the higher is the percentage of load that is carried by the stem, and the more extensive the stress-shielding effect.

4. The higher the percentage of load carried by the stem in the middle region, the less is transferred proximally and the more distally, and vice versa. As can be seen in Fig. 14-8, the proximal load transfer is proportional to $(1 - \varepsilon_n)$ and $(1 - \varepsilon_t)$, and the distal load transfer to ε_n and ε_t, respectively. Hence, the stiffer the stem, the higher the distal interface stresses; the more flexible the stem, the higher the proximal interface stresses.

5. The length of the distal and proximal load-transfer regions and the peak interface loads on the distal and proximal sides depend on the parameters λ_n and λ_t, the fixation exponents for axial and transverse loading (68–70). These parameters depend not only on the axial and flexural rigidities of the stem and the bone but also, and most predominantly, on the elastic modulus and the thickness of an intermediate layer (e.g., acrylic ce-

ment or cancellous bone). A stiff intermediate layer (i.e., high modulus and/or thin layer) reduces the length of the load-transfer regions and thus increases the gradients in the interface loads.

6. The peak interface stresses do not necessarily decrease when the stem is made longer. Here again, the notion "stress is load per available area" is misleading. When the stem is made longer, the load-transfer regions merely shift further apart, and nothing else changes. It is only when the stem is made short (less than π / λ_n, or π / λ_t) (Fig. 14-8), which makes the middle region disappear, that a further reduction in length starts to affect the interface stresses.

7. If a collar on the proximal stem is bonded to the proximal bone (Fig. 14-8) it transfers some of the load directly, at least conceptually. However, lasting contact between collar and bone is rare.

The preceding considerations are basic principles derived from a simplified, generalized model (68) and in fact are very helpful as baseline information for prosthetic design. In reality, of course, the load-transfer mechanism and the stress patterns are much more complex. Loads do not occur as isolated axial compression or bending, stems are usually not straight, interfaces are not always rigidly bonded, and bone has more complex properties and shapes than in this model. However, awareness of these basic phenomena facilitates the interpretation of more realistic, and complicated, analyses. If we formulate the conceptual analytic model of Fig. 14-8 in an FEA model, we see the basic principles reflected in the results (68).

In the case of a more realistically tapered stem in an "anatomic" bone model, these basic principles are less obvious, but still recognizable, as illustrated in Figs. 14-9 and 14-10. The interface stress patterns in the two-dimensional (2D) (Fig. 14-9) and three-dimensional (3D) FE models (Fig. 14-10) clearly demonstrate the proximal and distal stress-concentration regions. The ratio between proximal and distal stresses in these "anatomic" cases is regulated not just by the stiffness of the stem, but also by the prominence

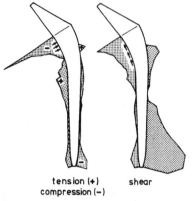

FIGURE 14-9. Distribution of tensile, compressive, and shear stresses at a stem–cement interface for a loaded cemented THA stem from a two-dimensional finite-element model. *(Left)* Stress normal to the interface (tension-compression). *(Right)* Shear stress. (From Huiskes R. The various stress patterns of press-fit, ingrown and cemented femoral stems. *Clin Orthop* 1990;261:27–38, with permission.)

of the taper shape. The stronger the distal taper of the stem, the more the distal stresses are reduced (68). Hence, although the principles of the load-transfer mechanism remain intact, the actual stress patterns are affected by stem design (83).

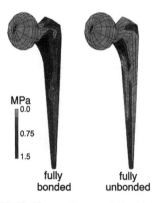

FIGURE 14-10. Shear stresses at the stem–cement interface generated by stems that are either fully bonded *(left)* or unbonded *(right)* to the cement mantle, calculated with a CT-based three-dimensional finite-element model. (From Verdonschot N, Huiskes R. Mechanical effects of stem–cement interface characteristics in total hip replacement. *Clin Orthop* 1996;329:326–336, with permission.)

The rigidity of the stem is an important design parameter, as it affects both the bone stresses (which may provoke bone resorption) and the interface stresses (which may provoke interface loosening). Using the same stem design, we obtain less abnormal bone stresses but higher proximal interface stresses when a flexible (isoelastic) material is used instead of a metal. We see that confirmed in a 3D FEA study (87). In view of the potential problems of bone resorption and interface loosening, this principle presents *incompatible design goals* for which a compromise must be sought: Noncemented stems tend to be medullary-canal filling and much thicker, hence stiffer, than cemented ones. This means that stress shielding is more of a problem in noncemented THA, whereas proximal cement and interface stresses are more of a concern in the cemented ones.

Many designers do not realize, however, that the governing parameter for the load-sharing ratio between stem and bone is not the stem rigidity but the ratio between stem rigidity and bone rigidity (10,68,78). The basis for this relationship was shown in Eqs. 8 and 9. It was found both clinically and analytically that long-term adaptive bone resorption around hip stems, as a result of stress shielding, is highly sensitive for initial bone rigidity (41,74,77,87). These results suggest that, in the foregoing relationship, the bone stiffness plays a more important role in load transfer than the stem stiffness because the former is more highly variable than the latter in a patient population. Hence, bone stiffness, as dependent on density and thickness, is a significant "design" parameter.

Another set of parameters that plays an important role for the load-transfer mechanism are the mechanical characteristics of bonds between the different materials. Earlier (Fig. 14-7), we saw that an unbonded, conically shaped stem has a different load-transfer mechanism than a bonded one. An unbonded, frictionless cone pushed in a tube must subside to create enough compressive interface stress for equilibrium, which also produces excessive tensile hoop stress in the tube. Cemented stems in THA tend to become debonded from the cement early postoperatively (95). Figure 14-11 illustrates the effects of debonding on cement stresses, as determined in a 3D FEA. We see dramatic increases in cement stresses from a bonded (Fig. 14-11, left) to a debonded, frictionless configuration (Fig. 14-11, right). If we do assume friction to occur (Fig. 14-11, middle), the cement stresses are still higher than those in the bonded case, but not that much higher. Evidently, the bonding and friction conditions are very important for the cement stresses and the probability of cement failure (55,119,195).

Two strategies are adopted in implant design to cope with the problems of stem–cement debonding. In one, the objective is to produce a lasting stem–cement bond with the aid of a rough surface finish, a precoating, a collar, or an anatomical shape, so that debonding of the stem is postponed. In the other, under the assumption that debonding can hardly be prevented, the objective is to neutralize negative effects of debonding, such as loss of stability and increased wear when the stems rub against the cement. Such stems are often straight tapered and polished. Both strategies are adopted in practice, and clinically successful stem designs are found in both categories.

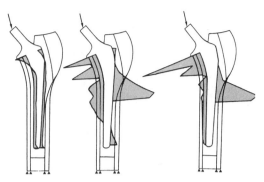

FIGURE 14-12. Normal stresses in the cement at the stem–cement interface assuming bonded interface conditions *(left)*, frictionless unbonded conditions *(middle)*, and frictionless unbonded conditions with fibrous-tissue interposition *(right)* at the cement–bone interface. (Adapted from Weinans H, Huiskes R, Grootenboer HJ. Trends of mechanical consequences and modeling of a fibrous membrane around femoral hip prostheses. *J Biomech* 1990;23:991–1000.)

Another effect of similar consequences is that of cement–bone interface loosening, bone resorption, and fibrous-tissue interposition. Figure 14-12 shows an example of that, as determined in a 2D FE model, applying nonlinear interface conditions to model the effects of loosening and a nonlinear constitutive description of a 1-mm-thick fibrous tissue membrane (204). As evident from Fig. 14-12, the stem–cement interface normal stresses (indicative for the character of the load-transfer mechanism) change drastically from a bonded to a (frictionless) debonded cement–bone interface and then again somewhat from a debonded interface to one with the fibrous membrane interposed. An example of the detrimental effect of a fibrous tissue membrane on the cement stresses is given in Fig. 14-13. Using 3D FE models of cemented reconstructions with and without a 1-mm fibrous membrane around the cement mantle, the cement stresses around a Mueller Curved stem were determined. The formation of a soft tissue layer dramatically increased the cement stresses, and hence the failure probability of the cement mantles.

The stem–bone bonding conditions also play important roles in the load-transfer mechanism of noncemented THA, particularly

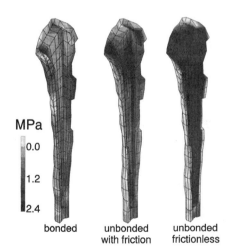

MPa

0.0

1.2

2.4

bonded   unbonded   unbonded
          with friction   frictionless

FIGURE 14-11. Tensile stress distribution in the cement mantle assuming bonded or unbonded (frictionless and frictional) stem–cement interface conditions. Only the anterior half of the cement mantle is shown. (Adapted from Verdonschot N, Huiskes R. Mechanical effects of stem–cement interface characteristics in total hip replacement. *Clin Orthop* 1996;329:326–336.)

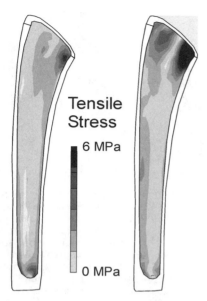

FIGURE 14-13. The tensile stress distribution in the cement mantle around a Lubinus SPII stem, with *(right)* and without *(left)* a 1-mm-thick fibrous tissue membrane present around the cement mantle. A view is presented on the inside of the anterior half of the mantle. With a soft tissue layer the stresses are higher in the proximal zone and along the lateral side of the stem.

concerning interface stresses and relative motions (12,51,100). These conditions depend largely on the precision of fit of the stem and on the extent and location of ingrowth coatings. Where debonding from the bone and friction are concerned, similar relationships occur in the load-transfer mechanism as for stem debonding from cement (119,195). An important difference is, of course, that cemented stems are bonded best in the beginning, whereas noncemented ones become bonded only later on. During the ingrowth period, stem design and interface-stress transfer play important roles in the ingrowth process (78). For noncoated, press-fitted stems, the interface coefficient of friction is very important for the eventual fixation characteristics, as these stems tend to sink in the bone and find fixation later. In this process, proximal load transfer may shift to distal, with stress shielding and bone resorption as a result (186).

Usually, a noncemented stem is not fully coated for bone ingrowth, but only proximally.

The reason for that is twofold. First, this is thought to promote proximal stress transfer rather than distal stress transfer, so stress shielding and adaptive bone resorption would be reduced. This can be confirmed in FEA, but the effect is not as pronounced as sometimes expected when the distal stem is still in (compressive stress transferring) contact with the bone (89,209). Second, it facilitates a possible revision operation. Full coatings are sometimes preferred because they are thought to enhance the extent of ingrowth, thereby reducing the probability of interface debonding. This thought is partly based on the idea that interface stresses are reduced when the contact area is increased. As we have seen, however, one must be very careful with the notion that stress is force per unit area. If we compare the interface stresses for the same prosthesis in the same bone, coated fully, proximally, and with five proximal bands, we find that the differences in maximal values are very small (89; Fig. 14-14). The reason, again, is that not all parts of the interfaces participate equally in stress transfer. So ingrowth at mechanically strategic locations is more important than the total area it occupies. An example of this concept is found for the ABG noncemented, hydroxylapatite-coated hip stem (Howmedica, Staines, UK) (187; Fig. 14-15). This hip stem has a proximal coating and an anatomical shape, ensuring a good proximal fit.

2.3 Acetabular Cup Fixation

The acetabulum is structurally more complex than the femur and does not easily lend itself for reduction to a simpler geometric model, which would make it accessible for conceptual analytical studies, in the same way as composite beam theory provided the basis for femoral reconstructions. In addition, in comparison to the femoral reconstruction, far fewer stress analyses were conducted. Some strain-gauge experiments were reported to study the effects of cup fixation on acetabular surface stress transfer (31,45,94,112,142,152). FEA of the acetabular reconstruction were conducted, using 2D (14,150,188), axisymmetric (71,136), or 3D models (33,108,151). In addition, the stresses

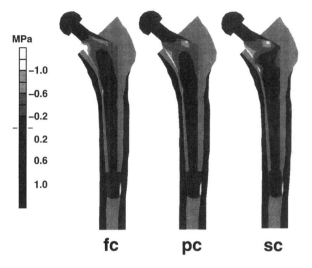

MPa

-1.0
-0.6
-0.2
0.2
0.6
1.0

fc   **pc**   **sc**

FIGURE 14-14. Normal stress distributions at the implant–bone interface for different coating configurations, shown as shades on the stem surface. High tensile stresses (positive) are white, and high compressive stresses black; zero stress is a medium gray shade. (fc, fully coated; pc, proximally coated; sc, proximally stripe coated.) (Adapted from Huiskes R, Van Rietbergen B. Preclinical testing of total hip stems; the effects of coating placement. *Clin Orthop* 1995;319:64–76.)

Bone density

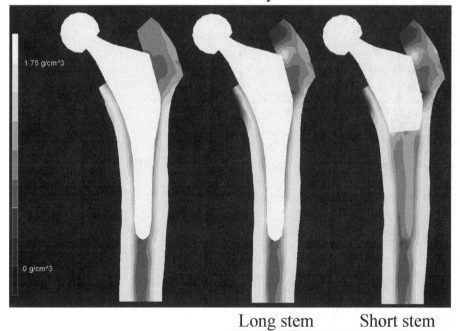

1.75 g/cm^3

0 g/cm^3

Long stem   Short stem
Pre-remodeling   Post-remodeling

FIGURE 14-15. Density distributions in the femur around the ABG stem (see Fig. 14-2) as predicted in a three-dimensional FEA simulation of strain-adaptive bone remodeling. Immediate postoperative situation on the left, as predicted for the normal AGB stem in the middle, and as predicted for a potential short stem on the right. Bone resorption around the proximal stem is clearly seen, but there is not much reduction when shortening the stem. (Adapted from Van Rietbergen B, Huiskes R. Load transfer and stress shielding of the hydroxyapatite-ABG hip. *J Arthroplasty* 2001;16(Suppl 1):55–63.)

in the PE liner were analyzed, particularly with regard to friction, wear, and PE failure prospects (6). Some generic information is discussed here, mostly as it resulted from our own 3D FEA model (30,32–34).

The hip joint force is introduced by the contact between femoral head and PE liner and varies greatly in magnitude and orientation during gait. The stresses in the pelvis reach a maximum at the beginning of the single-leg stance phase (32). The distribution of the stresses over the articulating surface of the PE liner depends on its stiffness characteristics, which are determined by the PE thickness and whether or not a metal backing is present (6,34). A thicker PE liner distributes stress better and reduces the peak value. This mechanism is similar to what was discussed relative to Fig. 14-5. At the time of heel strike, when the force is maximal, the superior-anterior rim is the high-stress location. From the liner the stress is then distributed to the bone, through the cement (if a cemented cup is used) and the metal backing (if present). The stress-transfer mechanism here again depends mostly on the rigidity of the structure. Metal backing, providing a higher stiffness, tends to distribute stress better over the cement and the subchondral bone. This was originally thought to be its greatest mechanical advantage (28). However, 3D FEA has shown that it does provide cement and interface stress concentrations at the rim of the fixation (Fig. 14-16). As an effect, the maximal cement and bone interface stress peaks of the metalbacked cup surpass those of a nonbacked one, providing higher failure

probabilities. This is a result of the fact that the bone rim and the metal backing are both stiff relative to their environments in the structure.

The stress transfer to the subchondral trabecular bone differs between the intact and the reconstructed case (Fig. 14-17). Whereas in the intact acetabulum the stresses are well distributed, in the reconstructed case they are concentrated in the anterior-superior region (30). It is also clear that stress shielding in the acetabular bone does occur, particularly in the dome region. This region is also the one where bone resorption is often seen (143), which is usually attributed to a loosening process. The stress patterns, however, do suggest that it might be a result of mechanical disuse, similar to what occurs in the femur (179; Fig. 14-18). Further away from the cup in the cortical shells, there is very little difference between the stress patterns of intact and reconstructed cases. The consequence of this is that little information about the local stresses in and around the implant can be obtained from experiments involving strain gauges on the external bone surfaces. The strains here are simply not very sensitive to the design and fixation characteristics of the cup.

3 DESIGN ASSESSMENT, CLINICAL AND PRECLINICAL TESTING

THA is a very successful treatment modality, and it became that owing to pioneering efforts of innovative surgeons and engineers. In the early

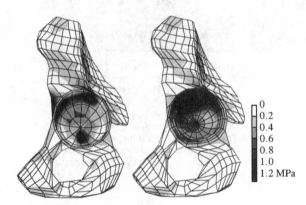

FIGURE 14-16. Distributions of the von Mises stresses in the trabecular bone of a normal bone *(left)* and a pelvic bone with a cemented nonbacked cup *(right)*. (Adapted from Dalstra M, Huiskes R. The effects of total hip replacement on pelvic load transfer. Chapter IV *Biomechanical aspects of the pelvic bone and design criteria for acetabular prostheses.* Dalstra M, Doct. Diss. University of Nijmegen, Netherlands. 15 November 1993)

0
0.2
0.4
0.6
0.8
1.0
1.2 MPa

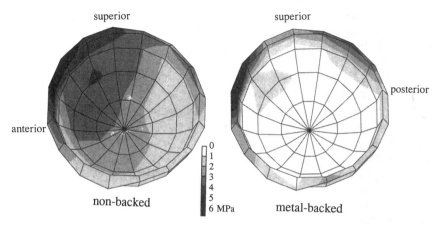

FIGURE 14-17. von Mises stresses in the cement mantle for a nonbacked polyethylene cup *(left)* and a metal-backed cup *(right)*. (From Dalstra *M. Biomechanical aspects of the pelvic bone and design criteria for acetabular prostheses.* Ph.D. thesis, Nijmegen University, The Netherlands, 1993, with permission.)

days, new ideas had to be tested in patients, in a trial-and-error way. Now, there are many good prostheses, proven in practice. Clinical monitoring systems, with revision as an endpoint, as in the Nordic National Registers, will detect unsafe prosthetic devices and surgical methods, but only after a large number of patients have been followed up and analyzed. However much more is known now about early signs of failure, and quantitative detection methods have been developed in the course of time. So new prosthetic designs, materials, and surgical tools should be preclinically tested in the laboratory before they are tried in patients. Many testing

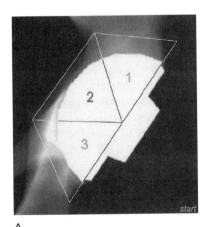

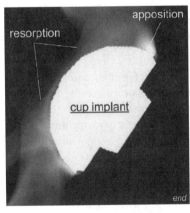

A   B

FIGURE 14-18. Bone resorption due to stress shielding around a noncemented titanium acetabular cup, as predicted by a computer simulation. **A:** A simulated DEXA scan, showing the bone density around the acetabular cup in the direct postoperative situation. The bone density changes were computed for three zones. **B:** Simulated DEXA scan with the bone density distribution at the end of the adaptation process. Bone resorption occurs primarily around the dome of the cup. (Adapted from Stolk J, Dormans KW, Sluimer J, et al. Is early bone resorption around non-cemented THA cups related to stress shielding? In: 50th annual meeting of the Orthopaedic Research Society, March 7–10, 2004, San Francisco, CA.)

modalities have been developed in recent years, in the forms of laboratory bench tests as well as computer-simulation analyses. It is also obvious that new devices must be tested in restricted clinical trials, before being freely sold on the market. For this purpose also new clinical measurement tools were developed, which allow quantitative detection of loosening in a much earlier stage than possible with the traditional evaluation of pain scores or conventional radiography. Examples are roentgen stereophotogrammetric analysis (RSA), allowing detection of prosthetic migration and inducible motions to a precision of 100 μm (166), dual-energy x-ray absorptiometry for monitoring bone density over time (10,21,42,146), and gait analysis (65,133,140).

In testing one has to know what to test for. In order to facilitate that, we proposed the application of "failure scenarios" to which testing methods can be tailored (75). A failure scenario is a paradigm of a failure mechanism. It is a course of events that does or does not occur but is always latent. Preclinical tests can be designed to establish how sensitive THA components are for a particular failure scenario.

3.1 Failure Scenarios and Design Assessment

It has become evident in recent years that stems do not stay put after implantation at operation. Because of the forces exerted in the hip they have been shown to migrate to at least some extent in the early postoperative phase, even those with a relatively rough surface finish. Conceptually, polished stems subside more than rough-textured ones. Stem subsidence promotes, again conceptually, stress elevation and *cement crack formation* and eventually loosening (compare discussion in relation to Fig. 14-11). However, acrylic cement is known to have viscoelastic properties and, hence, is subject to stress relaxation while loaded (200). This has motivated designers to promote polished stem surfaces (111). Debonded stems rub against the cement in hip loading and produce wear particles, which may invoke *cement–bone interface resorption*, soft tissue formation, pain, and loosening

(199,202). That is why other designers prefer rougher surface finish. Both these *failure scenarios* may cause premature clinical failure of the reconstruction. So what to choose from these two options? The answer is that the relationship between stem roughness and cement wear, and the one between stem subsidence and cement-crack propagation, both depend on stem shape (91). The likelihood of a stem design to be sensitive to either of these failure scenarios can be tested before actual production (in computer analyses), clinical trials (in laboratory bench tests), and introduction to the market (in clinical testing with Roentgen stereophotogrammetric analysis). These methods are discussed in the next sections of this chapter.

Generally speaking, when testing new prostheses, one has to know what to test for. In other words, failure scenarios are required. Six of those were proposed for hip prostheses (75). The first of these is the *accumulated-damage* scenario. This is based on gradual accumulation of mechanical damage in materials and interfaces from repetitive dynamic loading. The damaging process eventually proliferates to disruption of the implant from the bone, interface micromotion, bone resorption and fibrous interposition, and finally, gross loosening. As a generic scenario, it is certainly relevant not only for cemented stems, as in the preceding example, but also for cemented acetabular cups and for noncemented components of both sides (e.g., it may lead to disruption of prosthetic coatings). The fact that cemented stems are more sensitive than other types of components for this scenario is not the issue here. The whole point of failure scenarios is how easily they could be provoked by a new design.

The second, also involved in the example, is the *particulate-reaction* scenario. Wear particles from articulating surfaces, debonded interfaces, or modular-component connections can migrate into the cement–bone (cemented) or implant–bone (noncemented) interfaces. These small particles activate microphages at the interface into inflammatory responses of local bone resorption (lysis), thereby gradually debonding cement and bone (3,36,161). Eventually, this process produces relative interface motions and proliferates to gross loosening in much the same way as the final stage of the accumulated-damage scenario described earlier. This means that one usually cannot discriminate between these two scenarios by studying radiograms or retrieved specimens because the eventual results are the same. The elements of the particulate-reaction scenario include, besides wear-particle production, particle transport and biological bone reactions. Although the latter is a patient, rather than an implant design factor, the characteristics of wear particles in terms of material, size, and shape are certainly relevant for this scenario (118,167). This could be tested preclinically. The same is true for the potential of a design, and its inherent fixation method, to produce excessive wear particles and provoke transportation to the implant–bone interface.

The next, valid for noncemented components only, is the *failed-bonding* scenario. This implies that ingrowth or osseus integration does not occur because of gaps and relative motions at the implant–bone interface (40,159,169). The biological bonding or ingrowth processes require a certain quiescence at the interface to succeed. If relative motions occur beyond some 150 μm (144), ingrowth will be prevented, and motions will be enhanced, provoking bone resorption, fibrous tissue formation, and, eventually, loosening. The elements of this scenario are initial fit, osseus induction (the capacity of a coating material to induce bony adhesion and fill gaps), initial relative interface motions, and interface motion-induced bone resorption. Methods to test for these biomechanical interface phenomena are discussed later. Where fit is concerned, preclinical tests can be performed in series of postmortem bones (131,160). This seems rather trivial, but tests like this are hardly ever reported.

The *stress-shielding* scenario particularly involves the bone around the femoral stem. Because the bone is stress-shielded by the stem, the bone stresses are subnormal (see Figs. 14-8, 14-15). In accordance with Wolff's law (154,210), resorption develops. Although this does not automatically lead to prosthetic loosening, it may enhance bone or stem fracture and complicate a possible revision operation. The potential of a particular stem design to provoke excessive bone

resorption can now be preclinically tested with computer-simulation methods with good accuracy, as discussed later.

A fifth model is the *stress-bypass* scenario. This is similar to the stress-shielding scenario but develops through another route, when proximal load transfer in noncemented femoral THA is bypassed in favor of distal load transfer. As a result, the proximal bone is again understressed. Its cause can be inadequate proximal fit, either initially as an effect of inadequate fit or bone preparation, or gradually postoperatively as an effect of stem subsidence (186).

The final one proposed is the *destructive-wear* scenario. This implies that articulating surfaces or modular-component connections (e.g., cone connections between metal head and stem of the femoral component, or connections between PE liner and metal backing in the acetabulum) simply wear out, to the extent that mechanical integrity can no longer be maintained. The sensitivity of a design for this scenario can be preclinically tested in hip simulators (122,158).

It must be noted that whether or not an innovative design will be successful cannot be determined preclinically with certainty. This also depends on patient and surgical factors independent of design. In addition, new materials or shapes may introduce failure mechanisms hitherto unknown. In this respect, the scenarios just discussed may not be complete or sufficiently detailed. Further research will have to provide more certainty. In any case, preclinical testing can provide only a first sieve for unsafe devices.

3.2 Clinical Testing

3.2.1 Roentgen Stereophotogrammetric Analysis

RSA was developed by the late Dr. Goran Selvik (166). The method is based on the principle that 3D coordinates can be reconstructed from two radiographic images (Fig. 14-19A). To determine the 3D position of a point in space, the space has to be defined in the so-called laboratory coordinate system. When the positions of the two x-ray foci and the radiographic

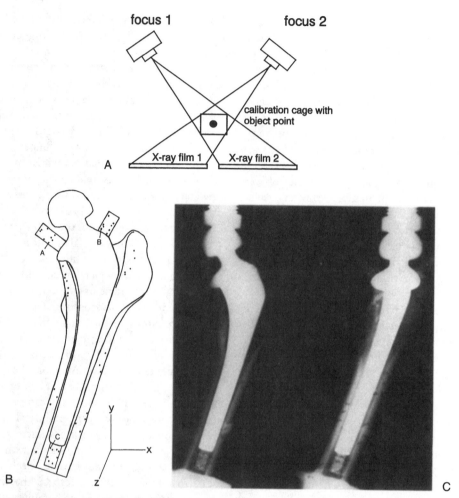

FIGURE 14-19. For the RSA analysis, the bone and stem with attached acrylic posts are provided with tantalum pellets. **A:** The projections of the calibration cage markers and object point on two radiographic films. **B:** Schematic. **C:** Stereo radiographs.

plates are known, the position of an object point can be reconstructed by calculating the intersection of the x-ray beams. A calibration cage determines the laboratory coordinate system. To this cage, markers made out of a high-density material (tantalum) have been attached, and their relative positions are accurately measured. Within the calibration cage, two planes with markers can be distinguished. The plane closer to the foci contains "control markers" and is called the "control plane." The plane closer to the radiographic films contains "fiducial markers" and is called the "fiducial plane." The fiducial markers are used to define the laboratory coordinate system, whereas the control points

are used to calculate the positions of the two foci.

To determine the 3D coordinates of an object point somewhere in the calibration cage, we create two images. Both images have a 2D local coordinate system (x',y'). The relationship between the global coordinates (x,y) of the fiducial markers and those on the images (x',y') can be determined using the Hallert transformation (166)

and

$$x = \frac{a_1 \cdot x' + b_1 \cdot y' + d_1}{a_4 \cdot x' + b_4 \cdot y' + 1}$$

$$y = \frac{a_2 \cdot x' + b_2 \cdot y' + d_2}{a_4 \cdot x' + b_4 \cdot y' + 1} \tag{8}$$

These relations have four unknown variables (a_1, b_1, d_1, a_2, b_2, d_2, a_4, b_4), which depend on the position and orientation of the fiducial plane relative to the radiographic films and on the positions of the two foci. If four fiducial markers of the calibration cage are projected on both x-ray films, the eight measuring points can be used to solve the eight unknown variables in Eq. 8. After this procedure, the (imaginary) projection of an object point in the fiducial plane can be calculated. Subsequently, the positions of the foci can now be reconstructed by using the control coordinates of the calibration cage and the calculated projections of these points in the fiducial plane. After this procedure, the 3D position of any point in space, provided that it is projected on both radiographic films, can be reconstructed by calculation of the intersection of the two lines between the foci and the projection of the object point on the (x,y) fiducial plane. Once the coordinates of the foci are determined and remain steady with respect to the fiducial plane, the control plane becomes redundant for the duration of a measurement session. For that reason, a "reference plate" with markers is commonly added to the configuration, to represent the fiducial plane after calibration (166). This implies that the calibration cage can be removed, and the object no longer needs to be positioned within its constraints. Because of measuring errors, the two lines do not usually intersect mathematically, which leads to inaccuracies in the results. The accuracy can be improved by using a redundant system of fiducial and control markers (for example, nine of each). A computer program (X-RAY; 166) is used to determine the most probable intersection point by mathematical optimization. In addition, the program provides information about the accuracy of the measurements, based on the standard deviations of the redundant system. With this technique, the 3D coordinates of an object point can be reconstructed with an accuracy of about 25 μm (166).

Usually, one is interested in the position of a rigid body (prosthesis) relative to another one (bone), and how this changes in time. The position of each of these rigid bodies can be determined from at least three marked points in the bodies. When two or more pairs of radiographs

in a particular time sequence are available, the migration of one rigid body relative to the other over time can be determined in terms of three rotations and three translations (166). To minimize errors, more than three markers should be used, particularly when it is expected that the bodies do not behave as ideally rigid. A computer program (KINEMA; 166) is used to determine the relative kinematics of the two rigid bodies. In addition to the information about measuring errors produced by X-RAY, the computer program KINEMA provides information about the rigidity of the bodies. For this purpose, the program calculates the distances between the marker points in the rigid body. If the body is ideally rigid, these distances are constant in time. If this is not the case, the body does not behave as a rigid one, meaning that the body is very flexible or that one marker may have come loose.

An experimental setup to measure relative motion (migration) of a femoral component of a THA requires, apart from a testing machine, two x-ray tubes, specially prepared x-ray cassettes with optimally flat films, tantalum pellets to mark the bone and the prosthesis, and a calibration cage. Figure 14-19B shows the arrangements of the tantalum pellets in bone, cement, and prosthesis. In order to minimize measurement errors, the scattering of the pellets should be optimal. The scattering can be quantified using a condition number as defined by Söderqvist and Wedin (170). It is possible to use clear markings on the prosthetic components for the RSA measurements, such as the metal ring in the PE cup, the prosthetic tip, the center of the prosthetic head, or the collar of the prosthesis. In an experimental setup one could come close to the optimal scattering of the pellets. However, under *in vivo* conditions the surgeon has a limited region where the pellets can be inserted (only the proximal femur). Some pellets may migrate as a result of bone remodeling and the images of the pellets may not always be visible on the radiograph, as they are obscured by the image of the metal implant. Standardizing pellet insertion and radiographic production can minimize this problem. Figure 14-19C shows the radiographic pair of the specimen. First, all markers must be identified and numbered, and then digitized. The digitizer must have a high resolution (about 5 μm). The identification and digitization procedures are time consuming but can be automated.

The RSA system was originally developed as a method to accurately determine 3D motion patterns between bone segments, such as in human joints. In addition to this application, the method has been used in studies concerning bone growth, the stability of joints, bone fractures and spinal segments, volume measurements, and fixation of prostheses (98). With respect to joint reconstructions, the method was applied to study permanent displacements (migration) and induced relative motions between prosthetic components and bone *in vivo* (99,124,156,168). These studies have shown that early excessive migration of components is correlated with early revision and that the RSA technique has appropriate sensitivity to detect these early micromotions (Fig. 14-20). Kärrholm et al. (99) could identify a migration threshold by 6 months, beyond which there was an increased risk of subsequent revision.

The advantage of RSA is that it can provide significant information about the quality of THA designs early postoperatively (6 to 24 months). The RSA technique is very precise and dependable, and it provides real 3D relative mo-

tions between two segments, which are impossible to obtain with other techniques. On the negative side, the evaluation tends to be rather tedious and time consuming. In addition, the technique is suitable for quasistatic loading only, because radiographs must be made after each load increment. In the near future, dynamic RSA studies will be possible as the techniques for synchronization of the Roentgen cameras are developed and high-speed film exchangers become available. Using this dynamic technique in addition to the quasistatic one will make the RSA technique even more effective as an *in vivo* tool to analyze failure processes in THA reconstructions.

3.2.2 DEXA Scanning

Dual energy x-ray absorptiometry (DEXA) is a method to measure bone density with some precision (Fig. 14-21). The method is 2D, hence not as precise as computed tomography (CT), but quite suitable for longitudinal studies on patients, for instance, in relation to "stress shielding" of bone around prostheses (18,35,41,146). It was developed for clinical use, but it is also quite useful to students in the postmortem laboratory, for example, to compare results of computational bone-remodeling simulations to reality (102). For this purpose

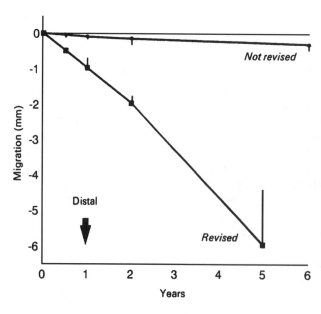

FIGURE 14-20. *In vivo* proximal/distal migration (mm) of the center of the femoral head (mean and standard error) determined with RSA techniques in a series of 80 cemented THR reconstructions. The reconstructions that were revised within 6 years because of failure, and those that were not, could be discriminated significantly within 1 year postoperatively by using RSA. (From Kärrholm J, Borssén B, Löwenhielm G, et al. Does early micromotion of femoral stem prostheses matter? *J Bone Joint Surg Br* 1994;76:912–917, with permission.)

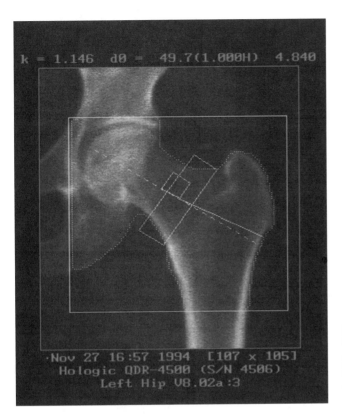

FIGURE 14-21. A dual energy x-ray absorptiometry (DEXA) scan of the hip joint. Regions of interest can be indicated to measure local bone density. The method is two dimensional; hence, the thickness of the bone in perpendicular direction provides a bias.

DEXA-simulating algorithms for FEA models can be applied (185).

3.3 Laboratory Tests

Laboratory experiments to investigate or preclinically test the mechanical behavior of THA reconstructions can grossly be divided into three types. The first type measures the relative motions of components under (dynamic) loading (12,117,162–164,181,183,203). The second type measures stresses in the bone–implant composite (33,37,45,47,67,79,97,109,132,153). The third type measures the wear properties of the components, for which the reader is referred to Chapter 15.

3.3.1 Relative Motions between THA Components

A distinction can be made between inducible displacements, which are recoverable movements between two components occurring within a single loading cycle, and migration—or subsidence, which is the permanent relative movement of components occurring on the long term. Investigation of inducible motions is particularly important for noncemented hip implants. The amount of inducible motion between implant and bone is a critical factor in the fixation of noncemented prostheses. These implants require minimal motions at the implant–bone interface, to allow bony ingrowth into porous surfaces or bonding to hydroxylapatite coatings (144). High relative motions may also cause bone to resorb at the interface and create a fibrous tissue membrane (85,138,207). Hence, it is important for noncemented stems to have adequate "initial stability," which can be tested in laboratory bench settings. Inducible motion analysis can also be applied to cemented THA (12,117,203). The detection of relative motion would indicate that the stems had debonded from the cement mantle, thereby giving rise to the accumulated-damage or particulate-reaction failure scenarios. However, in the case of cemented implants tests are more often aimed at investigating permanent migrations. Clinically, it has been shown that for stems of the same type, those with high migration rates are likely to fail early. Hence, it is important to know the typical migration characteristics of a new design. Some implants, such as smooth, straight tapered stems, may accommodate high migration rates better than others because of stress attenuation by creep. Some designs typically display continuous migration patterns, whereas others set over time.

In laboratory tests for relative motion, the stems are (dynamically) loaded, and their motions recorded. A complete evaluation of prosthetic motions is not trivial. The complete rigid-body motion of a prosthesis relative to bone must be described by three translations of a chosen base point (e.g., superior–inferior subsidence, anterior–posterior translation, and medial–lateral translation) and three rotations about mutually perpendicular axes (e.g., axial rotation, flexion, and varus–valgus rotation). In order to determine these six rigid-body motions, at least six relative displacements of three points must be determined (e.g., the x, y, and z displacements of one point, the x and y displacements of a second point, and the z displacement of a third point).

One technique to measure these relative motions experimentally is by providing the prosthesis with sensors that measure the displacements at one or more points of the prosthesis, relative to the bone (162,163,181,183,203). Often LVDTs (linear variable differential transducers) or extensometers are used. Both devices measure the relative displacement of two base points. If a full 3D description of the prosthetic motion is required, six LVDTs are required. Some prosthetic components undergo nonnegligible deformations when loaded, such as the bending of a hip stem. Then the prosthesis does not behave as a rigid body, and additional displacement sensors are required. Sometimes only particular motion components are measured, for instance subsidence in axial or rotation in torsional loading of femoral stems, in which case fewer sensors are needed. When tests of this kind are conducted, the displacements must be divided into permanent ones, representing a setting process or migration of the prosthesis, and recoverable ones, which are the true repetitive relative motions occurring under dynamic loading.

Figure 14-22A shows an example of an experimental setup (113,114) in which three rigid-body translations and three rotations of the prosthesis are measured relative to the bone. The load can be applied dynamically, and the sensors allow for continuous data sampling. The system was used to compare the migration patterns of two stem types with considerable differences in clinical performance. It was found that the two stems displayed substantial differences in migration patterns. The most striking difference was in the repetitive relative motions (inducible displacement), which decreased over time for the clinically superior stem and increased over time for the clinically inferior stem. The authors hypothesized that the development of the inducible displacement can be used to differentiate between stems with different clinical quality in laboratory preclinical tests.

Another technique that is can be used to measure relative motions in laboratory bench tests is RSA. This technique was discussed earlier. It is most suited to measure permanent migration of implants relative to the femur or the cement mantle (91,165). Although the technique has also been applied to measure inducible interface motions (213), RSA may not be suited for that purpose because they are generally of smaller magnitudes than permanent migrations, likely to approach the accuracy of the RSA system (213).

3.3.2 Experimental Stress Analysis of Bone–implant Composites

Stress analysis of bone–implant composites is usually applied on laboratory models of THA reconstructions, using postmortem bone specimens or synthetic bone substitutes (33,37,45, 47,67,79,97,109,132,153). In all cases, deformations are actually measured and then either visually interpreted or used to calculate stresses, utilizing elasticity theory. Methods used are strain-gauge analysis, holography, photoelastic analysis (with photoelastic coatings or films), and thermography.

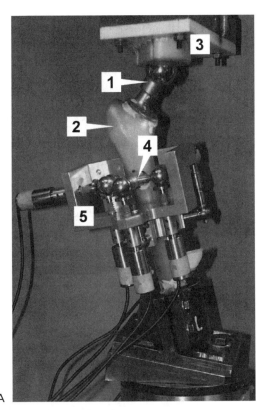

A

FIGURE 14-22A. An experimental setup for direct measurements of motion of a prosthesis implanted in bone. A prosthesis (*1*), cemented in a composite femur (*2*), is loaded cyclically through a nylon cup (*3*) mounted on the actuator of the testing machine. A cruciform structure with three spheres (*4*) is attached to the prosthesis through a hole in the cortex. During the test LVDTs are used to measure the displacement of the spheres relative to a box (*5*) mounted on the femur. (Adapted from Maher SA, Prendergast PJ, Lyons CG. Measurement of the migration of a cemented hip prosthesis in an in vitro test. *Clin Biomech* 2001;16:307–314, with permission.)

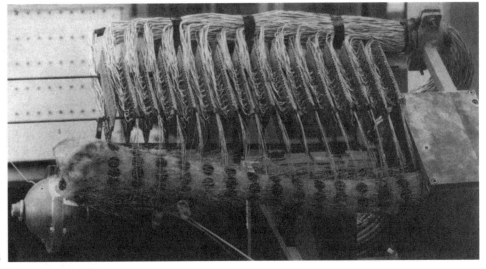

B

FIGURE 14-22B. Femur specimen with 100 strain-gauge rosettes for strain analysis on the periosteal bone. (Reprinted from Huiskes R, Janssen JD, Slooff TJ. A detailed comparison of experimental and theoretical stress-analyses of a human femur. In: Cowin SC, ed. *Mechanical properties of bone.* New York: The American Society of Mechanical Engineers, 1981:211–234, with permission.)

The most popular method is strain-gauge analysis whereby an electrical gauge is glued to the free surface of an object (29). The gauge contains one or more electrical filaments, which deform with the surface to which they are attached. A strain gauge works on the principle that the deformation of a filament is proportional to a change in its electrical resistance; thus, the strain of the material at the point where the gauge is applied can be measured by simply measuring the change in electrical resistance. Because the filament is a lineal element, it can only measure strain in one direction. To determine the complete strain state (two lineal strains and one shear strain) at a free surface, a strain-gauge rosette is used. A rosette contains three filaments (usually oriented at 30° or 45° to each other) that measure three lineal strains at the point of application. The three lineal strains are used to calculate the complete strain state, as well as the principal strain values and principal directions within the plane of measurement. When the elastic properties of the object are known, the stresses are calculated using generalized Hooke's law.

In biomechanics, strain gauges were applied mostly to assess deformation patterns at periosteal bone surfaces (37,45,47,79,109,132). In an example of this procedure (Fig. 14-22B), 100 rosette strain gauges were glued to the surface of the femur to assess strain patterns in the bone before and after prosthetic fixation. Strain gauges applied for this purpose have some limitations, however. First, the deformation patterns, and therefore stress patterns, at the outside bone surface are not very sensitive to the details of stress transfer far away within the structure at implant–bone interfaces. Second, no information can be derived from the surface measurements about the stress state within the structure. Hence, this method lacks the required sensitivity for most aspects of artificial joint design. Third, strains are obtained in a particular region of finite dimensions. The number of spots to be sampled is limited by space, instrumentation, and cost restrictions. Hence, to obtain a good representation of the stress patterns, one must know a priori where the values of interest might occur. A successful application of strain-gauge technology in preclinical testing is found in tests that determine the amount of stress shielding in the periprosthetic bone after implantation of a femoral stem (24). The loss in strain is determined by comparing the bone surface strains in the implanted femur with the strains in the intact femur, and is considered to be a measure for the amount of bone resorption that will occur in the long term.

Strain gauges have also been applied on the surface of prosthetic components (94) and have even been enclosed in acrylic cement (27). In the latter case, strain within the material is measured. Although the accuracy of this technique was limited in the past (46), recently a

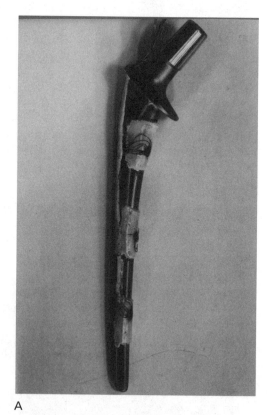

A

FIGURE 14-23A. A Lubinus SPII cemented hip prosthesis with strain-gauge rosettes mounted on a thin layer of bone cement on the medial aspect of the stem. The entire construct can be cemented in a femur, after which strains can be measured in the cement mantle. (Reproduced from Stolk J, Verdonschot N, Cristofolini L, et al. Finite element and experimental models of cemented hip joint reconstructions can produce similar bone and cement strains in pre-clinical tests. *J Biomech* 2002;35:499–510.)

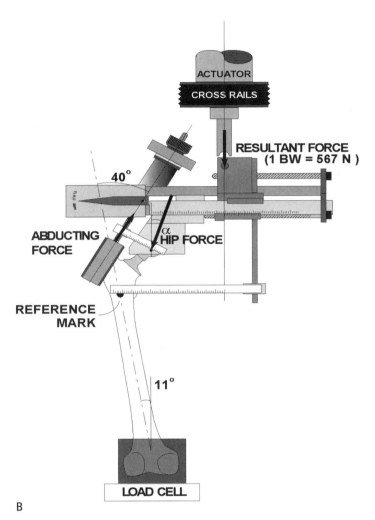

FIGURE 14-23B. Schematic representation of a loading device to reproducibly apply a hip joint force and an abductor force to a hip joint reconstruction in a laboratory bench test. Through a cantilever beam the compressive force of the machine actuator is converted to a compressive force on the prosthetic head and a tensile force on a lateral tension band attached to the greater trochanter. (Adapted from Cristofolini L. A critical analysis of stress shielding evaluation of hip prostheses. *Crit Rev Biomed Eng* 1997;25:409–483.)

method was presented to apply gauges for strain measurement inside the cement mantle with sufficient accuracy (26; Fig. 14-23). The problem was that pressure acting perpendicular to the gauge, likely to occur when it is used within cement, causes distortion of the signal. As the authors found a linear relation between the amount of pressure and the strain readout, they were able to correct the strain to produce the actual strain

value. A disadvantage is that the pressure acting normal to the gauge is often unknown and must be determined in alternative ways—for example, from stress analyses, using FEA.

A technique to visualize continuous strain patterns on the outside surface of bone specimens is the use of photoelastic coatings (215). The deformations in the coating, which is thin and flexible, follow precisely those of the bone surface and can be visualized as optical fringe patterns when viewed under polarized light. Photoelastic coatings have the same limitations as strain gauges because information is obtained only about the outside surface of the bone. They have an additional disadvantage of being difficult to quantify accurately. However, they do give continuous strain patterns that provide easy qualitative interpretation. Methods with similar results, advantages, and limitations are holography and thermography. These methods also display continuous deformation patterns on the outside surface of structures. Holography has been used to provide very accurate measurements of deformation, whereas thermography usually provides rough qualitative pictures of the deformation field. These methods have been occasionally used in this area of biomechanics (103).

3.3.3 General Considerations for Laboratory Bench Tests of Hip Reconstructions

The loading configurations in laboratory bench tests are usually simplified, as the complex muscle configuration around the hip joint cannot be adequately incorporated. As a result muscle forces are often absent (e.g., 162,203) or restricted to the representation of the abductor muscles only (e.g., 13,117). In the latter case, a strap can be attached to the greater trochanter and connected to a loading rig, such that a contact pressure is exerted on the prosthetic head and a tensile force to the greater trochanter (24). It was shown that such loading configurations provide sufficient detail and adequacy for several testing purposes (25,135,172). There is no standard loading configuration for bench testing of hip prostheses. This is partly due to a lack of knowledge about joint and muscle loads acting around the hip during all kinds of activities, and about the number of loading cycles that patients are subjected to on a daily basis. To overcome this problem, an extensive study was performed recently. Hip joint forces during several activities were measured with instrumented hip prostheses for four patients (9). With patient-specific models of the lower limb the corresponding muscle forces were determined using computer optimization strategies (61). Activity profiles were recorded for several patients, describing the type of activity and the number of repetitions performed on a monthly basis (125; Table 14-2). From this extensive database two simplified loading configurations were extracted for realistic testing of hip prostheses for walking and stair-climbing conditions. The latter activity was selected because it was shown to be detrimental to the fixation of stemmed hip implants in comparison with several other daily activities

TABLE 14-2. MONTHLY CYCLES OF HIP-JOINT LOADING FOR SEVEN MUSCULOSKELETAL TASKS THAT ARE FREQUENTLY PERFORMED AND GENERATE CHARACTERISTIC LOADING PATTERNS

| Activity | Force Rp for Normal Load | | | Force Rp for High Load | | |
| | Hip Contact Force | | Cycles | Hip Contact Force | | Cycles |
	[%BW]	[N]	[1]	[%BW]	[N]	[1]
Walking normal	238	1,785	240,000	390	3,900	450,000
Stairs up	251	1,883	3,400	470	4,700	12,000
Stairs down	260	1,950	3,400	460	4,600	12,000
Chair up	190	1,425	840	290	2,900	2,600
Chair down	156	1,170	840	260	2,600	2,600
Standing 2-1-2 legs	269	2,018	24,000	360	3,600	35,000
Stumbling	—	—	—	1,100	11,000	10

Note: The data were divided in values for 'normal' patients and for highly active ones. Force characteristics are shown as percentage body weight and in Newtons. The average monthly frequencies are also given (125).

(8,174). Four muscle loads were included in the two loading configurations, in addition to the hip joint contact force: the abductor load, the load of the iliotibial band, and the loads of the vastus medialis and lateralis. This implies a substantial reduction of the actual number of muscle forces active around the hip, but these were shown to provide most of the common loading modes.

Laboratory studies with series of postmortem femurs lose consistency through the variety in the geometric and mechanical properties of these femurs. To overcome this problem, synthetic composite femurs were developed consisting of a glass fiber-reinforced epoxy layer representing the cortex and a polyurethane foam core representing trabecular bone (Pacific Research Labs, Vashon Island, WA). It was shown that the mechanical properties of these femurs, such as their bending stiffness, are within the range of human femurs (123). This indicates that the cortical bone is adequately represented. However, this is not the case for the trabecular bone represented by the foam on the inner side of the femur, particularly where anisotropy of trabecular bone is concerned. Older femurs did not have intramedullary canals, but their design recently improved to overcome this problem. Although synthetic femurs may be adequate for a range of laboratory testing purposes, one should be aware of their weaknesses when selecting them for experiments.

Another problem may arise when different prosthetic designs are tested and mutually compared. Ideally, the positions of load are application should be the same in all cases. However, because of variable prosthetic shapes and implantation procedures, the position of load application may vary considerably (e.g., as a consequence of different offsets). This can affect the local loading conditions considerably (a smaller offset results in reduction of the bending moment) and obscures the interpretation of the results obtained with the various designs. Some authors therefore correct the loading magnitudes to account for differences in position of load application with different prostheses, such that the bending moments remain constant with respect to the femoral long axis (24).

3.4 Computer-simulation Tests

Computer-simulation methods are useful for the purpose of research in THA, preclinical testing, and design testing. Particularly in the last decade its applicability was improved tremendously, through research and developments in computer capacity (88,175). As tools for investigating failure processes, computer-simulation models are conceptually similar to others, such as laboratory, animal, and clinical models. In any investigation, one must consider closeness to reality of the model used versus experimental control. Patients are very real, but when one is used for investigative purposes as a clinical model, there is very little control over the experimental parameters. Conversely, a computer simulation provides virtually absolute experimental control but is remote from reality. Other models can be positioned between these two extremes. With computer-simulation models we can investigate pure cause–effect relationships for well-defined sets of parameters. A single parameter can be varied to estimate its role in a particular process. Another advantage is that computer simulation is relatively cheap. For example, THA designs can be tested directly from the drawing board; no prototypes are required. These advantages can be exploited and weighted against the limitations of remoteness from reality. A number of computer-simulation methods for analyzing mechanical processes in implant failure are described hereafter.

3.4.1 Interface Debonding and Micromotion

Debonding of stem–cement interfaces is rule rather than exception in cemented THA; all stems migrate to some extent after the operation (56,76,95). Not much is known about the (fatigue) strength of the bond, but if we assume that debonding does occur, we can at least determine where it is most likely to be initiated and how it progresses. For that purpose we need a failure criterion expressing the failure probability for different combinations of normal and shear stresses, such as the multiaxial Hoffman failure index (66). Weinans et al. incorporated this index in a finite-element model to investigate the process of noncemented prosthesis–bone disruption (207). Verdonschot and Huiskes (196) used the index to investigate stem debonding of cemented hip stems. The failure index (*FI*) can be defined as a function of the interface normal stress σ and the interface shear stress τ as

$$FI = \frac{\sigma^2}{S_t S_c} + \left(\frac{1}{S_t} - \frac{1}{S_c}\right)\sigma + \frac{\tau^2}{S_s^2}$$
$$\text{where bonded} \quad (9a)$$

$$FI = 0 \quad \text{where debonded} \quad (9b)$$

where $S_t = 8$ MPa is the tensile strength of the metal–cement interface (101), $S_c = 70$ MPa is the compressive strength of the interface [the compressive strength of acrylic cement according to Saha and Pal (157)], and $S_s = 6$ MPa is the shear strength of the interface (4,5,148,180). *FI* greater than 1.0 indicates immediate failure. A lower value indicates that no immediate static interface failure can be expected, although strength may deteriorates due to long-term cyclic loading.

Simulation of the debonding process requires an iterative FE simulation, starting with a completely bonded stem–cement interface. In every increment, the maximal *FI* is calculated, and the interface is debonded at that location. This change in local interface condition will affect the interface stresses elsewhere in the structure and requires a new FE iteration to calculate these changes. This procedure is repeated until the whole interface is debonded. Verdonschot and Huiskes (196) applied this method to a 3D FE model of a cemented femoral THR to simulate the stem–cement debonding process (Fig. 14-24). In this model, debonding started in the distal and proximal regions. These regions expanded until the whole interface was debonded.

Stem–cement debonding not only elevates the cement stresses, but it also allows the stem to move relative to the cement mantle. Depending on the roughness and the relative motions, this can lead to the production of metal and acrylic cement wear products, which promote the particulate-reaction failure scenario. Finite-element models can be used to determine the micromotions at the debonded inter-

Debonded sites at the stem-cement interface

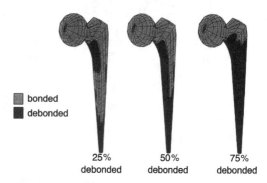

- bonded
- debonded

25% debonded   50% debonded   75% debonded

FIGURE 14-24. Sites of stem–cement debonding at various stages in a debonding process during dynamic loading. (Adapted from Verdonschot N, Huiskes R. Cement debonding process of THA stems. *Clin Orthop* 1997;336:297–307.)

face (195). A result of such an analysis is depicted in Fig. 14-25. The cyclic slip at the stem–cement interface is shown under dynamically loaded (stance-phase loading in walking) and unloaded (swing-phase) conditions. Obviously friction and surface roughness affect these motions. Assuming no friction at the interface, a cyclic slip in the range of 200 μm was generated in the FEA model (Fig. 14-25). After load release, the stem returned to its original position. In any consecutive load cycle, this behavior was repeated. When friction is assumed, the stem

Cyclic slip at the stem/cement interface

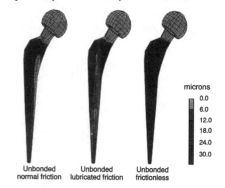

microns
0.0
6.0
12.0
18.0
24.0
30.0

Unbonded normal friction   Unbonded lubricated friction   Unbonded frictionless

FIGURE 14-25. Cyclic micromotion patterns between the stem and the cement, assuming friction coefficients of 0.25, 0.05, and 0.0 (from left to right). (From Verdonschot N, Huiskes R. Mechanical effects of stem–cement interface characteristics in total hip replacement. *Clin Orthop* 1996;329:326–336, with permission.)

dynamic interface motions (μm)

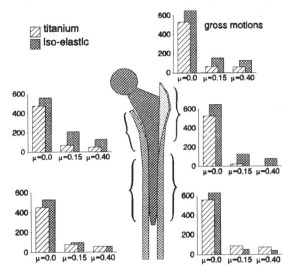

FIGURE 14-26. Amplitudes of the cyclic movements along the implant–bone interface for two values of the prosthetic Young's modulus and three values of the coefficient of friction between bone and implant. (Adapted from Kuiper JH, Huiskes R. Friction and stem stiffness affect dynamic interface motion in total hip replacement. *J Orthop Res* 1996;14:36–43.)

sticks to the cement mantle after the first loading cycle, which leads to a considerable reduction of the micromotions at the stem–cement interface (Fig. 14-25). Hence, due to friction the stem is clamped within the cement and puts it under pressure (194). The pressure may cause microcracks to develop and initiate a process of cement fatigue failure. The pressure might also relax due to cement creep. In that case the chances for cracks to develop are reduced, but the process of subsidence may continue, while motions may cause cement particles to be rubbed from the cement inner surface, causing particulate reactions in the tissues. So it seems that long-term stem fixation endurance follows a narrow pathway between the threats of the *accumulated-damage* and the *particulate-reaction* failure scenarios at either side. As shown in the next section, stem shape and surface finish particularly affect the chances for long-term endurance.

For noncemented components large gaps and relative motions between implant and bone play a dominant role in the failure process according to the *failed-bonding scenario* (75). High cyclic micromotions can be generated because of a lack of mechanical stability and prevent the bone from growing into the surface of the implant. Finite-element computer simulations have been utilized to analyze this problem (100,107,135,155,171,201,204). An example

of such an analysis is shown in Fig. 14-26. The analysis was performed with a 2D side-plated FEA model using three different loading modes (107). The analysis shows that implant–bone motions are clearly affected by interface friction and material stiffness properties. If the stem is made of a material with a similar stiffness as cortical bone (an "isoelastic" material) instead of much stiffer titanium, higher micromotions are produced.

A limitation of FEA micromotion studies is that they do not usually consider the mismatch between the implant shape and the bone cavity created by the surgeon. These studies only consider the stability of the implant assuming a perfect fit. Although this is a serious limitation, they can still provide important information about the inherent stability of the implant, depending on shape, material properties, and interface characteristics, and thus provide the possibility of testing this at a preclinical stage, before patients are put at risk.

3.4.2 Damage Accumulation and Creep in Acrylic Cement

The accumulated-damage failure scenario is one of the most prominent ones in cemented THA, particularly where the femoral component is concerned (75,95). According to this scenario

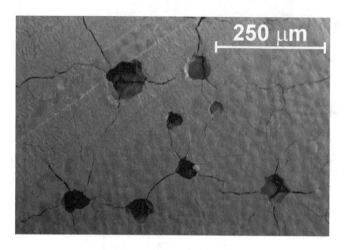

FIGURE 14-27. A piece of PMMA bone cement with microcracks emanating from pores in the cement mantle (Reproduced from Stolk J, Verdonschot N, Murphy BP, et al. Finite element simulation of anisotropic damage accumulation and creep in acrylic bone cement. *Eng Fract Mech* 2003;71:513–528.)

mechanical damage accumulates in the bulk cement and along the interfaces, leading to disintegration of the cement mantle and eventually to gross loosening of the implant. When subjected to cyclic loading, polymerized acrylic cement displays brittle failure behavior. Microcracks (damage) accumulate within the material and coalesce to form macroscopically visible cracks (Fig. 14-27).

Another time- and load-dependent process occurring in polymers such as acrylic cement is creep (175,178). Creep is defined as time-dependent deformation of a material under constant loading conditions. The material "flows," in a way, deforming while stresses in the cement mantle are attenuated, reducing the probability of crack formation. Hence, creep and damage accumulation are two interacting mechanical processes. Their combined effects should be considered when analyzing mechanical failure of the cement mantle. Within the framework of a large-scale European Union-sponsored research project ("PreClinTest"), FEA algorithms were developed to simulate these processes and validated for the purpose of preclinical testing hip prostheses against the accumulated-damage failure scenario. Next we first describe how damage accumulation and creep can be simulated separately with FEA, and then describe the formulation of the combined FEA simulation.

To simulate damage accumulation we use the theory of continuum damage mechanics (CDM) (177,178,193,194). The amount of damage ac-

cumulated in a material can be measured by a reduction in stiffness, strength, or residual lifetime (16,17). Assuming constant environmental conditions, the amount of actual damage depends on the load applied and on the number of prior loading cycles. Consider, for the sake of simplicity, the one-dimensional case, where damage can be described with a scalar variable. When only the load level is varied during the damage process, the amount of damage (D) becomes a function of the number of cycles (n) and the load level (σ), as in

$$D = F(n, \sigma) = f(n/N_f) \qquad (10)$$

with the restrictions $D = 0.0$ when $n = 0$ and $D = 1.0$ when $n = N_f$, where N_f is the number of cycles to failure for constant-amplitude loading in a fatigue bench test of the same material. In these tests, specimens are exposed to a dynamic load with a constant load level, and the number of cycles to failure is recorded. Repeating the tests with different load levels allows the relationship between load level (σ) and the number of cycles to failure (N_f) to be determined. Results of fatigue tests are often presented as S–N curves, or Woehler curves. The function $f(n/N_f)$ in Eq. 10, called the damage-growth equation, defines the relationship between the amount of damage and the ratio of the number of loading cycles to the number of cycles to failure. Murphy and Prendergast (128) determined the rate of microcrack development in fatigue experiments on Cemex RX bone cement (Tecres, Verona, Italy). They showed that the damage does not develop linearly, but exponentially, as

$$D = f(n/N_f) = (n/N_f)^{3.92} \qquad (11)$$

From fatigue bench tests they also determined the *S–N* curve for the same material (129,130) as

$$\sigma = -4.736 \log(N_f) + 37.8 \qquad (12)$$

By Eqs. 11 and 12 the damage accumulated in the cement is related to the stress levels acting in the cement. In reality, structures are often exposed to dynamic loads in which the load level varies in time. The total damage accumulated during fatigue loading at *m* different load levels σ_i, for a number of n_i cycles per load level, can be written as (93)

$$D = \sum_{i=1}^{m} \Delta D_i \qquad (13)$$

where ΔD_i represents the amount of damage accumulated during fatigue at load level σ_i. Using CDM it is assumed that the amount of damage *D* affects the elastic properties of the material. Often a coupled relationship is assumed, meaning that the Young's modulus diminishes gradually as a function of damage (110). However, when the material is brittle, as is the case for acrylic cement (128), it can be assumed that damage and stiffness are uncoupled. This means that the elastic properties of the cement are assumed constant until the damage is complete ($D = 1.0$). In the case of 2D or 3D FEA models, the damage (*D*) becomes a tensor instead of a scalar. This allows damage to grow anisotropically. In that case the material can be completely damaged in one direction, while unaffected in another direction. Perpendicular to the damage directions (the crack direction), the material loses its stiffness, resulting in anisotropic postdamage material behavior. After one crack is formed, the local stress state may reorient, such that damage growth occurs perpendicular to the first crack and a second crack, or even a third one, may form perpendicular to the first. In most FEA codes, the material anisotropy resulting from the damage accumulation can be accommodated. The stress patterns in the ce-

ment mantle change when it cracks locally. After creation of each cement crack a new FEA iteration is required to calculate the new stress distribution. Hence, iterative FEA simulation of the accumulation of damage over time in the cement mantle is required. We assumed that only tensile stresses cause accumulation of damage. Shear and compressive stresses were thought to leave the material intact.

The constitutive theory used to simulate creep of cement is based on a 3D Maxwell model (178,194,197). It is assumed that the total strain is composed of an elastic component and a creep component. The elastic component can be determined from Hookean relationships between stress and strain. The creep component is determined from empirical creep laws, relating creep strain to the loading time and the local stress levels. As the stress state in the cement mantle around femoral hip implants is typically 3D, three principal stress component values and orientations determine the local stress state. Experimental creep data are based on uniaxial tests, which consider the presence of only one stress component (20,191,192). For this reason, the uniaxial creep laws cannot be applied directly to structures with 3D stress states. The solution for this problem is to define an equivalent stress, which relates the 3D stress state to the uniaxial one and can be used in the creep laws. We selected the von Mises stress (σ_{vm}) as the equivalent stress, which is usual in creep simulations (80). To determine creep strain under dynamic loading conditions, we used an empirical relation from Verdonschot and Huiskes (191,192), as

$$\begin{aligned} \varepsilon^c &= 7.985 \times 10^{-7} \\ &\times n^{0.4113 - 0.116 \cdot \log \sigma_{vm}} \cdot \sigma_{vm}^{1.9063} \end{aligned} \qquad (14)$$

relating the creep strain ε^c to the number of loading cycles *n* and the von Mises stress amplitude (MPa). As the creep process develops the stress levels in the structure change. Hence, when this creep model is implemented in an FEA simulation an incremental procedure is required. Each time step represents a certain number of loading cycles. The creep strain increment $\Delta \varepsilon^c$ in each time step can be calculated from Eq. 14.

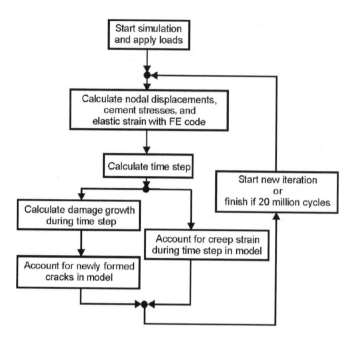

FIGURE 14-28. Iteration scheme of the finite-element computer simulation to model creep and damage accumulation in the cement mantle around a cemented hip implant. (Adapted from Stolk J, Maher SA, Verdonschot N, et al. Can finite element models detect clinically inferior cemented hip implants? *Clin Orthop* 2003;409:138–150.)

The creep-strain increment can then be used in the FEA code to calculate the various 3D creep-strain components $\Delta \varepsilon_{ij}^c$, using a flow rule that identifies how the von Mises stress is affected by the various stress components, as in

$$\Delta \varepsilon_{ij}^c = \Delta \varepsilon^c \cdot \partial \sigma_{vm} / \partial \sigma_{ij} \qquad (15)$$

From the creep-strain components and the stiffness matrix, a nodal force vector is calculated, which is subtracted from the force vector already present. Then a new FEA iteration is performed with the modified force vector.

Based on these models for creep and damage accumulation, an FEA simulation algorithm was developed that simulates both processes simultaneously. Figure 14-28 shows a conceptual flow scheme of the combined simulation. When applied to an FEA model of a THA reconstruction, the simulation monitors damage and creep for every integration point (eight per element) in the cement individually. Damage and creep strains are set to zero at the start of the simulation. The muscle and joint loads are represented by their maximal peak values during one loading cycle. Each iteration starts with calculating the nodal displacements, the cement stresses, and the elastic strains due to the loads applied.

Then an incremental time step is taken, representing a certain number of loading cycles. The stresses are assumed to remain constant during this increment. The time step is chosen such that the creep-strain increment is smaller than 5% of the elastic strain and that no more than one crack is formed in each of the cement integration points. These restrictions ensure that the time steps are small relative to the characteristic time scales of the failure processes. A loop is then started over all integration points to update the creep strain and the amount of damage at each integration point within the cement mantle. The creep-strain increment is calculated from Eqs. 14 and 15 and added to the creep strain already present. The damage accumulating during the increment is calculated from Eqs. 11 and 12 and added to the amount of damage already present, as given by Eq. 13. Once the damage is updated, an additional step is taken to check whether the total damage accumulated has locally reached a value of 1.0. In that case, a crack is included in the model by locally adapting the stiffness of the cement, such that the cement can no longer carry loads in the direction perpendicular to the crack. Once damage and creep strain are updated, a new iteration is started by recalculation of the stresses, strains, and nodal displacements, which are generally different from the ones in the former iteration, due to creep and newly formed cracks. The iterative procedure continues until the desired total number of loading cycles is reached.

The creep and damage formulations presented here are based on FEA algorithms derived in earlier studies, in which these processes were analyzed separately (193,197,198). To combine the two processes in one algorithm compromises had to be made to reduce the computational costs: (a) The algorithm used for creep simulation does not differentiate between creep under compressive and tensile loading conditions, and (b) the algorithm assumes stresses to cycle between zero and peak value. An earlier formulation could account for stresses cycling between a residual stress level and peak value, with the residual stress being the amount that remains present in the cement after unloading of the implant. The damage-development algorithm (c) does not include a "crack closure formulation," allowing cracks formed due to tension to close in compression. However, the damage algorithm was also improved by allowing nonlinear damage accumulation (Eq. 11), as opposed to linear damage accumulation.

The mechanical processes simulated in this way are likely to cause prosthetic subsidence in the cement mantle when the stem–cement interface is debonded (120). Creep and crack formation reduce the supportive properties of the cement mantle. As nodal displacements are calculated after each time step, the subsidence patterns of the prosthesis can be monitored as creep and damage accumulation proceed. This is a valuable feature of the simulation method, as long-term stability of cemented implants is an important issue. The current simulation process allows one to analyze the migration characteristics of prostheses, as caused by mechanical failure of the cement mantle.

Example: Testing the "Accumulated-damage" Failure Scenario on Cemented Hip Stems. Within an EU-sponsored research project (PreClinTest), the simulation scheme described above was applied to two femoral stems. The implants analyzed were (see Fig. 14-3) the Lubinus SPII

(Waldemar Link GmBH, Hamburg, Germany) and the Mueller Curved (JRI Ltd, London, UK) with revision rates of 4% and 13% at 10 years postop, respectively (63,115). The purpose was validation relative to experimental and clinical data.

FEA models of the reconstructions with both prostheses were developed (Fig. 14-29) and analyzed, evaluating the stresses in bone and cement. The same two prostheses were studied experimentally, using composite femur models in the loading device shown in Fig. 14-23A. Stresses both at the bone surface and in cement were measured, and then compared with the FEA stresses evaluated at the same locations (Fig. 14-30). The FEA models were able to reproduce experimental bone and cement strains within an overall agreement of less than 10% (173). In a second study (113), the migrations of the two prostheses in composite femurs under dynamic loading were measured, using the laboratory testing rig shown in Fig. 14-22A. This test was also simulated with the two FEA models (175), which produced similar migration patterns and values, not significantly different from the experimental ones (Fig. 14-31). After the migration tests the specimens were sectioned to inspect them for cement cracks. Again, their locations and extents coincided with those predicted by the FEA analyses (175; Fig. 14-32). The Mueller Curved stem produced more cracks, and higher migrated rates, than the Lubinus SPII stem in the FEA models and the experiments (175). This coincides with their rankings in the clinical results of the Swedish Hip Register (13% versus 4% revisions after 10 years, Fig. 14-3). However, the register did not differentiate at the time between causes of revision, nor did it differentiate between stem and cup loosening. Hence, the similarity between predictions and register results could be circumstantial.

In the next study within the PreClinTest project we used FEA models similar to those just discussed to evaluate all four stems shown in Fig. 14-3, relative to their tendencies to migrate and produce cement cracks (176). The results were compared with those in the Swedish Hip Register, relative to their revision-rate ranking (63,115; Fig. 14-3). The FEA simulations

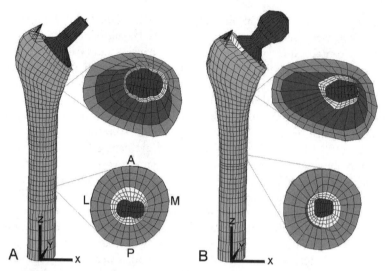

FIGURE 14-29. Finite-element models of two cemented hip reconstructions. The models represent the proximal part of a left femur with (*left*) a Lubinus SPII stem and (*right*) a Mueller curved stem. (Reproduced from Stolk J, Maher SA, Verdonschot N, et al. Can finite element models detect clinically inferior cemented hip implants? *Clin Orthop* 2003;409:138–150, with permission.)

predicted a similar ranking for cement-crack development (Fig. 14-33); more cement cracks were generated for clinically inferior stem types. The predicted subsidence patterns per stem, however, were not representative for the clinical ranking in the register. Particularly the Exeter design showed relatively high migration rates in FEA, without much crack formation. This is a striking example of what we discussed in the earlier section on interface debonding and micromotion relative to the interrelationships between stem design, stem subsidence, cement creep, and cement-damage accumulation. We conclude that the evaluation of cement-damage accumulation is the most relevant target in preclinical testing of stem designs.

3.4.3 Periprosthetic Fibrous Tissue Formation Induced by Micromotion

Bone resorption and fibrous tissue formation between implants and bone are important determinants for clinical loosening. They can be the result of reactions to wear particles but can also be induced by relative motions between implant and bone (11,53,137,139,145,169,214). A conceptual scheme for such a process is shown in Fig. 14-34. Relative motions in a local interface region are the effects of external joint and muscle loads in combination with the structural and bonding characteristics of the THA reconstruction as a whole. It is assumed that if these local motions exceed 150 μm, bone ingrowth or osseus integration does not occur, and fibrous tissue starts to develop (144,169). The motion-induced interface resorption paradigm now implies that the repetitive deformations in that fibrous membrane are the driving forces for its growth (Fig. 14-34). Which mechanical signal derived from the tissue deformation would in fact stimulate the cells in the tissues, we do not know.

For a first conceptual analysis of this process, we assumed that the growth rate of the tissue membrane is proportional to the strain in the tissue (207); hence,

$$db(t)/dt = c_{ij}\varepsilon_{ij} \qquad (16)$$

where $b(t)$ is the actual tissue thickness, and ε_{ij} is the strain tensor (Fig. 14-35A). For the purpose of computer simulation in conjunction with an FEA model, we reduced this feedback relationship to the iterative formula

$$\Delta b = (c'\Delta u_n/b + c''\Delta u_p/b)\Delta t \qquad (17)$$

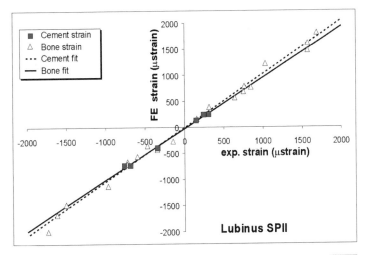

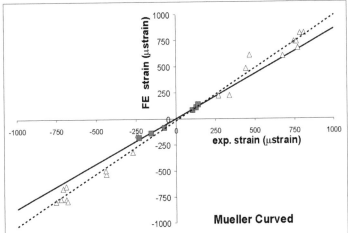

FIGURE 14-30. Comparison of experimental and computed bone and cement strains in hip reconstructions with *(top)* Lubinus SPII stems and *(bottom)* Mueller Curved stems. The experimental reconstructions were loaded with the device shown in Fig. 14-23B. Bone surface strains were measured at 10 locations on the cortical surface; internal cement strains were measured at three locations in the cement mantle (see Fig 14-23A). Computational strains were determined for these locations with the finiteelement models shown in Fig. 14-29. Regression analysis showed that overall agreement was within 10%. (Reproduced from Stolk J, Verdonschot N, Cristofolini L, et al. Finite element and experimental models of cemented hip joint reconstructions can produce similar bone and cement strains in pre-clinical tests. *J Biomech* 2002;35:499–510, with permission.)

where c' and c'' are constants, and Δu_n, and Δu_p are the overall elastic displacements of the implant relative to bone in normal and tangential directions (Fig. 14-35A). This relationship is for a plane-strain state and assumes that the fibrous layer is relatively thin (204). For the purpose of FEA, we modeled the fibrous tissue as a nonlinear elastic material with negligible resis-

tance against shear and tension (64,207). This model was used to simulate soft tissue formation processes of a number of implant configurations (207). It concerns a screw used in fracture fixation with bone plates, which gradually loosens as an effect of repetitive transverse forces (139). The simulation model is able to predict the typical resorption patterns around the screw

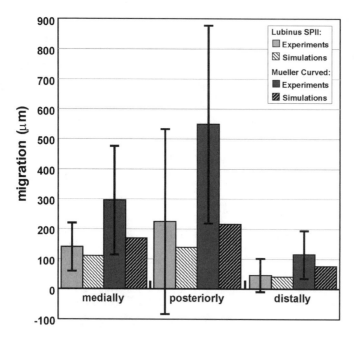

FIGURE 14-31. Migration values of Lubinus SPII and Mueller Curved stems. Experimental values were determined from reconstructions loaded with the device shown in Fig. 14-22A. Computed values were determined from the finite-element models shown in Fig. 14-29, simulating the experimental loading conditions. (Reproduced from Stolk J, Verdonschot N, Cristofolini L, et al. Finite element and experimental models of cemented hip joint reconstructions can produce similar bone and cement strains in pre-clinical tests. *J Biomech* 2002;35:499–510, with permission.)

in both bone-cortex regions it penetrated (Fig. 14-35B). Similarly, the typical resorption patterns of femoral-head surface replacements could be predicted in this way (85).

However, the foregoing model neglects the 3D viscoelastic properties of the fibrous tissue, important in relation to the dynamic character of the loads. It also neglects feedback from the residing mechanical stresses and strains in the fibrous layers to the actual bone-resorbing cells in the membrane (Fig. 14-34). The membrane can be considered as a biphasic tissue, with a fluid and a solid phase, for which analyses biphasic theory (126; see also Chapter 5) can be used in FEA. One can then apply the theories of mechanically driven tissue differentiation to investigate the influences of mechanical variables on implant integration (145). These theories are similar to those used for explaining bone-fracture healing, which are discussed in Chapter 13, and to those applied to explain the effects of mechanical forces on bone gestation, discussed in Chapter 4.

For instance, a mechanoregulation index (M) can formulated as (90,184)

$$M = \frac{\gamma}{a} + \frac{v}{b} \qquad (18)$$

where γ [-] is the maximal distortional (or octahedral shear) strain, v [μm/s] the interstitial fluid-flow velocity, $a = 0.0375$ and $b = 3$ [μm/s]. Based on experimental data (145,169) it was proposed that where M is greater than 3, fibrous tissue would prevail (characterized by a modulus of 2.0 MPa and a permeability of 1.0×10^{-14} m^{4}N^{-1}s^{-1}); where M is in the range from 1 to 3, cartilage would prevail (modulus 10.0, permeability 5.0×10^{-15}); and where M is less than 1, bone would form (modulus 4590, permeability 3.7×10^{-13}). In a well-controlled animal experimental model (169), the differentiation of tissue from fibrous to cartilaginous and eventually to bone could be explained as the effects of these mechanical stimuli (Fig. 14-36). Other theories were proposed as well, using hydrostatic pressure instead of interstitial fluid flow as a differentiation promoting variable (see also Chapter 13). The reason for our choice was that the hydrostatic pressure in the periprosthetic tissue model applied proved insensitive to differentiation, and hence, would not be suitable for a feedback variable (145). It is expected that these models can be used to explain and predict implant-loosening processes as effects of dynamic loads.

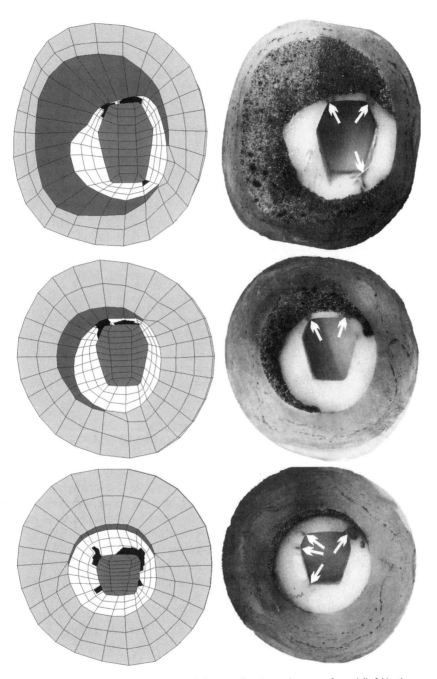

FIGURE 14-32. Crack patterns around the Mueller Curved stem as found *(left)* in three transverse sections of experimental reconstructions loaded with the device shown in Fig. 14-22A and *(right)* in a finite-element simulation of damage accumulation using the model shown in Fig. 14-29. (Reproduced from Stolk J, Verdonschot N, Cristofolini L, et al. Finite element and experimental models of cemented hip joint reconstructions can produce similar bone and cement strains in pre-clinical tests. *J Biomech* 2002;35:499–510, with permission.)

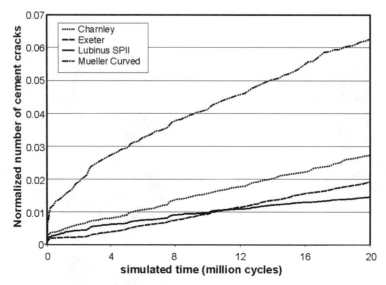

FIGURE 14-33. Damage accumulation in the cement mantle was simulated for the four stems shown in Fig. 14-3. The number of cement cracks versus simulated time is shown here. The number of cracks are normalized to the number of elements present in the cement mantle in the finiteelement models of the four reconstructions. (From Stolk J, Verdonschot N, Huiskes R. Can finite element based pre-clinical tests differentiate between cemented hip replacement stems according to clinical survival rates? In: 49th annual meeting of the Orthopaedic Research Society, Feb. 2–5, 2003, New Orleans, LA).

3.4.4 Strain-adaptive Bone Remodeling

The ability of bone to form optimal structures to support loads and to adapt structurally to changing loads was qualitatively described by Wolff's law (154,210). The ability implies that bone must have some internal sensors to detect stresses and strains. It also implies that bone must possess a mechano-chemical transduction mechanism to translate these mechanical signals to biochemical ones at the cellular level. A local change in mechanical signal must be sensed by the bone and translated by a transducer to a chemical remodeling potential. When this potential is integrated with genetic, hormonal, and metabolic factors, a remodeling signal is generated for modulating osteoblast and osteoclast activities, causing a net increase or decrease of bone mass. This entire process is known as the strain-adaptive remodeling paradigm (see also Chapter 4).

Over the years, a number of strain-adaptive bone-remodeling theories were formulated (15,23,57,81). The theories assume a relationship between local, strain-related variables and the net change of bone mass. Such variables are called remodeling signals, and the relationships are called remodeling rules. These rules are written as mathematical statements and are combined with FEA models of a bone or a bone–prosthesis structure. These models were used to explain the density patterns and trabecular architectures of bones as effects of their external loads (7,15,127,206, see also Chapter 4). Similar models were also applied to predict long-term bone remodeling around prostheses, to evaluate the consequences of stress shielding, and to preclinically test THA stem designs (84,89,187,205,209). The theories used for these computer-simulation analyses are briefly summarized in this section.

It is assumed for these theories that the bone cells react to a mechanical signal S, which is the local expression of bone deformation patterns caused by the external loads. The distribution of S is calculated in an FEA model of the bone with

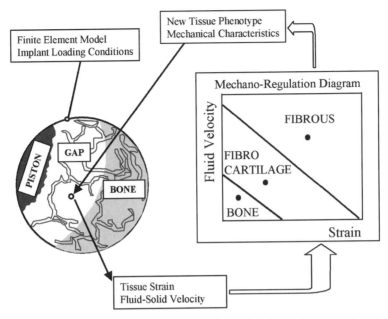

FIGURE 14-34. A proposed regulatory scheme for tissue differentiation at prosthetic bone interfaces. The strain and fluid-velocity distributions are calculated in an FEA model. Based on the transition criteria, illustrated in a phase diagram representing the differentiation rule, tissue phenotype characteristics are updated in every iteration. The simulation is continued until no more change occurs and homeostasis is reached. (From Huiskes R, van Driel WD, Prendergast PJ, et al. A biomechanical regulatory model for periprosthetic fibrous-tissue differentiation. *J Mater Sci Mater M* 1997;8:785–788, with permission.)

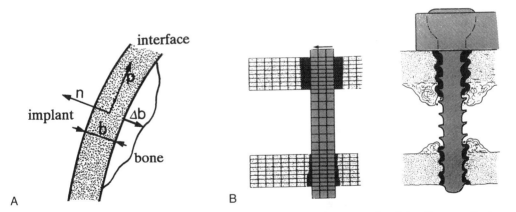

FIGURE 14-35. A: Interface layer with implant at the left and bone at the right. The coordinates n and p are taken parallel and normal to the interface. The thickness and growth of the interface are expressed by b and Δb, respectively. (From Weinans H, Huiskes R, Grootenboer HJ. Quantitative analysis of bone reactions at implant–bone interfaces. *J Biomech* 1993;26:1271–1281, with permission.) **B:** *(Left)* Simulation of the resorption process around a bone screw. The resorbed bone is indicated in black. (From Weinans H, Huiskes R, Grootenboer HJ. Quantitative analysis of bone reactions at implant–bone interfaces. *J Biomech* 1993;26:1271–1281, with permission.) *(Right)* The general resorption pattern around the bone screw fixations with fibrous tissue indicated in black. (Adapted from Perren SM. Induction der Knochenresorptio bei Prothesenlockerung. In: Morcher E, ed. *Die zementlose Fixation von Huftendoprothesen.* Berlin: Springer Verlag, 1983:38–40.)

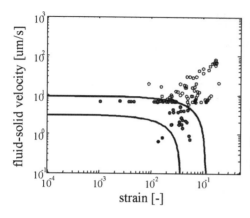

Element status after first iteration of both force-controlled and motion-controlled piston actuation

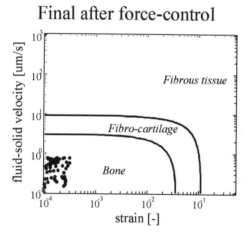

Final after force-control

Final after motion-control

FIGURE 14-36. Graphs illustrating phenotypic stages in gap tissue around a piston moving in bone (169) as evaluated in an FEA simulation; every dot represents an element. Initially all elements are fibrous. After the first iteration two elements were predicted to become bone, a large number to become fibrocartilaginous and the majority to be still fibrous, based on the strain and fluid velocity history computed. This first phase developed identical in both force and motion control of the piston. In the final homeostatic stage of the force-controlled simulation all elements turned to bone (90). In the motion-controlled simulation, however, the gap tissue was predicted as a final mixture of fibrous and fibrocartilaginous, with just a few islands of bone (184).

prosthesis. The signal value is compared with a target value S_{ref}, taking into account a threshold level s. Hence, the target signal value range is

$$(1 - s) S_{ref} \leq S \leq (1 + s) S_{ref} \qquad (19)$$

where s is expressed as a fraction. S_{ref} is the local signal value for normal bone under remodeling equilibrium. The distribution of S_{ref} is determined in an FEA model representing the natural bone without prosthesis, subject to identical loading conditions. If the signal exceeds the target range, then net bone mass M is added (dM/dt greater than 0); if it is below the target

range, bone is removed (dM/dt less than 0), as illustrated in Fig. 14-37. The adaptive process in the operated femur can then be expressed in the rate of net bone turnover

$$dM/dt = \tau A(\rho)[S - (1 - s) S_{ref}]$$
$$\text{if } S \leq (1 - s) S_{ref}$$
$$dM/dt = 0$$
$$\text{if } (1 - s) S_{ref} < S < (1 + s) S_{ref}$$
$$dM/dt = \tau A(\rho)[S - (1 + s) S_{ref}]$$
$$\text{if } S \geq (1 + s) S_{ref} \qquad (20)$$

with $0.01 \geq \rho \geq 1.73 \, \text{g/cm}^3$

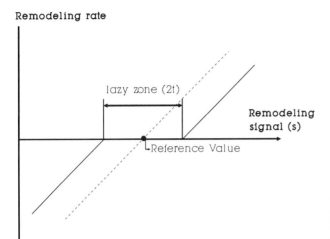

FIGURE 14-37. Relationship between remodeling rate and remodeling signal, with *(solid lines)* and without *(dotted lines)* a lazy zone (81).

where τ is a time constant expressed in grams per millimeters squared [joules/gram]/month, ρ is the apparent density of the bone (in g/cm^3), with a maximal value of 1.73, $A(\rho)$ is the free surface available for remodeling at the periosteum or in the internal bone structure, and s represents the threshold level. The time t is given in units of months.

During the simulation, remodeling takes place within the bone (internal remodeling, a change in apparent density ρ) and at its periosteal surface (external or surface remodeling, a change in shape). The rate of net bone turnover dM/dt can now be expressed as a rate of change in the external (periosteal) geometry, dx/dt, by

$$dM/dt = \rho A(dx/dt) \qquad (21)$$

with A the external surface area at which the rate of mass change dM/dt takes place (the external face of the element concerned) and x a characteristic surface coordinate, perpendicular to the periosteal surface. For the adaptation of the internal bone mass as a result of porosity changes we use

$$dM/dt = V(d\rho/dt) \qquad (22)$$

with V the volume in which the bone mass change takes place (the volume of the element concerned) and $d\rho/dt$ the rate of change in apparent density. Equation 20 can now be written in terms of dx/dt for surface remodeling and in terms of $d\rho/dt$ for internal remodeling. If we

substitute this in Eq. 20, the proportionality parameters τ/ρ and $\tau A/V$ appear, which regulate the rates of the remodeling processes at the surface and internally, respectively. In the latter location, $A(\rho)$ is the pore surface in the bone, which can be expressed in the apparent density ρ by using a theory of Martin (121).

For the mechanical signal S we take the average elastic energy per unit of mass (joules/gram) from a series of m external loading configurations, each consisting of joint and muscle forces; hence,

$$S = \frac{1}{m} \sum_{i=1}^{m} \frac{U_i}{\rho} \qquad (23)$$

where U_i is the strain-energy density (see appendix) for loading case i. The distribution of S_{ref} is determined accordingly in an FEA model of the intact (preoperative) bone. The distribution of the actual signal S in the THA model is updated iteratively. The external loading configurations are always assumed identical before and after the operation. Through forward Euler integration, the equations can be solved iteratively to find the new coordinates of the surface nodes and new apparent density values in the integration points after every iterative step. In the computer program, the integration is carried out in steps of $\tau \Delta t$, which represents the proceeding of the processes at an arbitrary computer-time scale. The time step in the integration process is variable and determined in each iterative step,

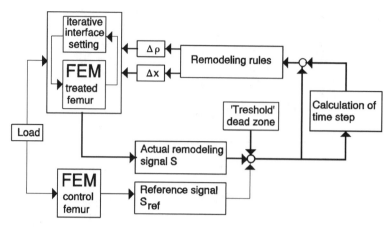

FIGURE 14-38. Schematic representation of the iterative computer-simulation model of bone remodeling around implants. (Adapted from Weinans H, Huiskes R, Van Rietbergen B, et al. Adaptive bone remodeling around bonded noncemented total hip arthroplasty: a comparison between animal experiments and computer simulation. *J Orthop Res* 1993;11:500–513.)

such that the maximal density change in the integration point where the maximal rate of density change occurs will not exceed $\frac{1}{2}\rho_{max}$ (= 0.865 g/cm^3) (186). The iterative simulation process is depicted in Fig. 14-38.

The value of the threshold s was determined experimentally for dogs as $s = 0.35$. The time constant τ was empirically determined in the same study as $\tau = 130$ g/[mm^2(J/g)month] to have the time t given in units of 1 month (208). For humans the threshold level is taken as $s = 0.75$ (87). A realistic time constant is not known for this case.

The simulation model just presented was validated with respect to six series of animal experiments with THA in dogs (186,208). In each series different stem materials and coating conditions were applied. The cortical bone areas and medullary bone densities were measured postmortem after 6 months and 2 years postoperatively and compared with the predictions of the simulation model. As shown in Fig. 14-39, the predictions of the model and the actual morphology found in the dogs were very similar, even in detail. When the predictions of overall bone remodeling were compared per series with the experimental averages and standard deviations, significant correspondence was obtained, as shown for one series in Fig. 14-40.

In regard to human configurations, we used internal remodeling only, studying cortical bone

as the main site for bone loss (74,77). Direct validation studies relative to individual patients were performed for the porous coated AML femoral stem (39–42). Four hip-replacement patients donated their postmortem femoral bones to the surgeon. They were used to measure periprosthetic bone density, using DEXA scanning (41). The postmortem contralateral femur was provided with the same prosthesis, and also evaluated with DEXA, as a model for the treated bone in the initial, directly postoperative situation. In this way the amount of periprosthetic bone lost per femoral region over time could be estimated (41). 3D FEA models for these cases were developed to "predict" the patterns of eventual bone resorption with the foregoing computative bone-remodeling schemes (102). The results of the simulations were very similar to those found from the postmortem measurements (Fig. 14-41). As evident from Fig. 14-41, in both the experimental and the computational studies we found a strong correlation between preoperative bone density and bone loss over time (102). On the one hand, this confirms the suitability of the computational method as a predictive tool for preclinical testing purposes. On the other hand, it indicates that estimates for postoperative bone loss can already be obtained for an individual patient at the time of treatment, simply by measuring preoperative bone density. If the bone is relatively dense, then extensive postoperative

Left Right

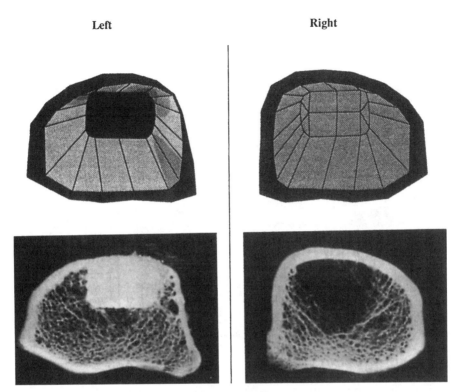

FIGURE 14-39. Animal experimental results (2 years' follow-up) of bone remodeling in canine femurs with fully bonded prostheses compared with the prediction using the remodeling simulation. The *left* femur is the treated case, and the *right* is the control. (Adapted from Van Rietbergen B, Huiskes R, Weinans H, et al. ESB Research Award 1992. The mechanism of bone remodeling and resorption around press-fitted THA stems. *J Biomech* 1993;26:369–382.)

bone loss is unlikely to occur. If it is relatively porous, the surgeon could better use a cemented prosthesis. The stems of those are relatively thin, hence producing much less stress shielding than the thick, canal-filling noncemented ones.

The computer-simulation method discussed here is now used routinely to test prosthetic designs preclinically relative to the stress-shielding failure scenario, on a relative basis, always comparing one configuration with another (87,89, 185,205,209).

4 INCOMPATIBLE DESIGN GOALS AND NUMERICAL DESIGN OPTIMIZATION

It is evident from the earlier discussion of failure scenarios that many design goals in THA are incompatible. In order to improve fit of non-cemented prostheses, modular components to be assembled at the operating table are useful. However, modularity implies more connections subject to wear. Hence, to prevent the "failed-bonding" failure scenario, components should be modular, but to prevent the "particulate-reaction" scenario, they should be monoblocs. They cannot be both at the same time, so sensible compromises will have to be found. There are many examples of incompatible design goals in THA (75). In an earlier section, we discussed the effects of femoral stem stiffness on bone and interface stresses. Basically, when the stiffness of the stem increases, the interface stresses decrease, but stress shielding increases. So a rigid stem promotes the stress-shielding scenario, and a flexible one promotes both the failed-bonding and the accumulated-damage scenarios. This is another notorious incompatibility in THA design goals, and again sensible compromises are

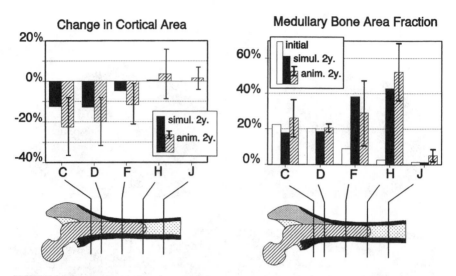

FIGURE 14-40. A comparison between 2-year experimental results in animals and those of the simulation for the uncoated-stem series. The predicted CBA and MBAF are within the 95% confidence interval of the experimental values. (Adapted from Van Rietbergen B, Huiskes R, Weinans H, et al. ESB Research Award 1992. The mechanism of bone remodeling and resorption around press-fitted THA stems. *J Biomech* 1993;26:369–382.)

indicated. To assist the designer in finding the best compromise available, numerical design optimization, using FEA models, can be a useful tool (30,35,82,83,104–106,189,190,212).

The usual approach to FEA is to consider a particular design (shape, material properties, etc.) and determine the stress patterns within the structure under specified loads. In numerical design optimization, this procedure is conceptually reversed in that a desired stress pattern in a THA structure is specified and the design characteristics by which it is to be realized are determined. As in the computer simulations discussed earlier, this is accomplished in an iterative procedure (Fig. 14-42). The process is started with an initial design for which the stresses, strains, or other mechanical variables (e.g., strain-energy density, SED) are determined from the initial FEA model. If the stress distributions deviate from the desired ones, the shape or material characteristics of the design are adapted in such a way that the stresses and strains are changed toward the specified values. This iterative process is repeated until the desired stress patterns are approximated as closely as possible or within a specified range of error. The way in

which the shape of the prosthesis is adapted in each iteration is determined by a search procedure that determines the search direction. Experience shows that it is an exception, rather than a rule, that the desired stress and strain distributions are realized precisely by the final design. One must be satisfied with a reasonable approximation of the desired stress and strain distributions.

An optimization process is conducted relative to particular criteria, for instance, minimal stress shielding, minimal interface tension, or minimal cement stress. These criteria are written in mathematical forms as *objective functions* to be minimized. In the optimization procedure, the values of these objective functions are minimized by the particular design characteristics evolving from the iterative process. Hence, these characteristics are "optimal" only relative to the particular objective function selected. This means the prosthetic designer must define the criteria very carefully. This optimization procedure must also include a check against unrealistic properties. For example, the stem of a femoral prosthesis cannot be bigger than the bone into which it is to be fixed. Or the elastic modulus

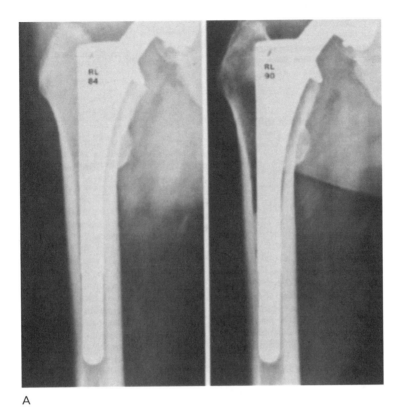

A

FIGURE 14-41A. Radiographs of a patient with an AML hip prosthesis (DePuy Inc., Warsaw, IN). *(Left)* immediate postoperatively and *(right)* after 6 years. (Adapted from Engh CA, McGovern TF, Bobyn JD, et al. A quantitative evaluation of periprosthetic bone-remodeling after cementless total hip arthroplasty. *J Bone Joint Surg Am* 1992;74:1009–1020.) Periprosthetic bone loss, ascribed to stress shielding is clearly visible.

of a material must fit within the range of what can actually be produced. For this reason, certain *boundary constraints* are required for use in the optimization procedure. Finally, the design variations considered in a particular prosthesis are limited to a particular, limited number of dimensional or material parameters. These are called *design variables*—for instance, parameters that define length or cross-sectional shape of a femoral stem or the parameters of a function that describe the allowable elastic modulus distribution field in a structure. The values of the selected design variables are varied in the process, but all other parameters remain fixed.

As an illustration (Fig. 14-43) we consider a procedure, applied to optimize the design of

a "metal-backed" acetabular cup (73,86). Previous FEA has shown that a metal-backed PE acetabular cup reduces some cement and cement–bone interface stresses (136). However, it was also found that this metal backing tends to increase interface shear stresses near the edges of the cup (34), as discussed in an earlier section of this chapter. Hence, the question posed was whether a metal-backing shape could be found that would minimize the cement and interface stresses over the whole cup. The solution procedure was based on a 2D FEA model with nonuniform bone properties (136). Other conditions simulated by the FEA model included the complete removal of the subchondral bone layer, a uniform cement-layer thickness of 3 mm, a femoral head diameter of 28 mm,

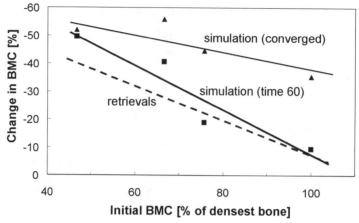

B

FIGURE 14-41B. Bone loss (%) over time versus initial bone mineral content (BMC) of four patients (% of densest bone; 41), compared with results of FEA strain-adaptive bone-remodeling simulations for the same patient group. (Adapted from Kerner J, Huiskes R, van Lenthe GH, et al. Correlation between pre-operative periprosthetic bone density and post-operative bone loss in THA can be explained by strain-adaptive remodeling. *J Biomech* 1999;32:695–703.) The simulation overestimates the percentages of bone lost when continued to full convergence (triangular dots), but matches the measurements after 60 iterations (square dots). Obviously, net resorption is overestimated in the simulations for the densest bone in particular. This can be an effect of the setting of the lazy zone (Fig. 14-37).

and a unit hip joint force in a direction corresponding to the maximal force during the stance phase of gait. The metal backing shell was assumed to be CoCrMd. A maximal shell thickness of 5 mm and a minimal thickness of zero were taken as boundary constraints in the optimization procedure. Three design variables were used: the thickness of the shell at the dome of

the cup, the thickness at the lateral edge, and the thickness at the medial edge. The objective function was the sum of the strain-energy density distribution for all nodal points in the cement elements. In this sense, the minimization procedure seeks a solution in which minimal load-transfer stresses would occur at the cement–bone interface. The mathematical formulation of the problem may be described as

Design variables:

$$\mathbf{v} = (t_l, t_d, t_m) \tag{24}$$

where t_l is the lateral shell thickness, t_d the shell thickness at the dome, and t_m the medial shell thickness (linear interpolation in between).

Boundary constraints:

$$0 < t_l \leq 5, 0 < t_d \leq 5, 0 < t_m \leq 5 \tag{25}$$

Objective function:

$$F(v) = \sum_{k=1}^{n} [U_k(v)]^p \tag{26}$$

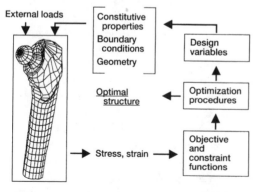

FIGURE 14-42. A general scheme for iterative optimization in combination with a FEA model.

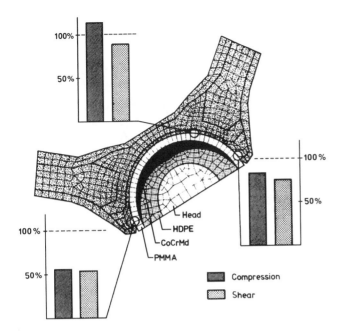

Head
HDPE
CoCrMd
PMMA

Compression
Shear

FIGURE 14-43. Compressive and shear-stress values at the cement–bone interface in an acetabular reconstruction for an "optimized" metal-backed shell normalized against the uniform-thickness case (100%) (73,86).

where U_k is the strain-energy density at nodal point k of the cement, n is the total number of nodal points, and p is an exponent.

Figure 14-43 shows the resulting optimal shape of the metal shell and the maximal cement–bone interface stress values (compression and shear) relative to those found for a shell of 2-mm uniform thickness. The optimal inner contour of the shell tends to make it as thick as possible at the cup dome (the maximal value of 5 mm) and as thin as possible at the cup edges. The reductions of stress compared with the case of the uniform shell thickness are on the order of about 15% at the medial and about 45% at the lateral side. At the cranial side, above the hip joint load, the compressive stress is slightly higher, and shear is slightly lower, than in the case of a uniformly thick metal backing.

For FEA of structures, parametric studies require selected design parameters that depend on the intuition and experience of the designer. For FEA optimization procedures the selection is automated, and the search for the optimal parameters is defined with respect to assumed physical and geometric constraints and criteria. Hence, FEA-integrated optimization can be a powerful tool in a prosthetic design process. These concepts are obviously not limited to shape optimization, but can also be applied to optimization of material properties and boundary conditions, taking conflicting design goals—such as adaptive bone resorption versus interface stress criteria—into account. For example, studies were conducted in which the probability of mechanical interface failure of a cemented stem was formulated mathematically as an objective criterion for optimization analysis. The integrated elastic energy in the bone was used for a constraint function, in the sense that the maximal amount of bone loss would be limited to a particular maximum value. To accomplish that, the elastic modulus distribution of the stem material was varied between zero and a maximum of 100 GPa. The parameters describing the potential modulus distribution were used as the design variables. Analyses were conducted in 2D and 3D models (104–106). Figure 14-44 shows an example of a configuration obtained in which the stem elastic modulus varies from high proximally to low distally. Compared to a full titanium stem (modulus 115 GPa), the amount of bone resorption predicted would decrease from 26% to 7.5%. This would also be realized by an "isoelastic" stem with a uniform modulus of 36 GPa, but for such a stem the peak interface stress would be a factor of three higher

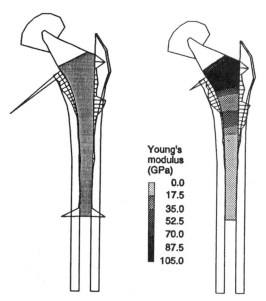

FIGURE 14-44. The stem stiffness distribution before *(left)* and after *(right)* an optimization procedure. Relative to a stem of homogenous elastic modulus, 18.5% reduced bone resorption in the bone, due to stress shielding, is predicted. At the same time, the peak interface stresses would be three times less. (Adapted from Kuiper JH, Huiskes R. Mathematical optimization of elastic properties—application to cementless hip stem design. *J Biomech Eng* 1997;119:166–174.)

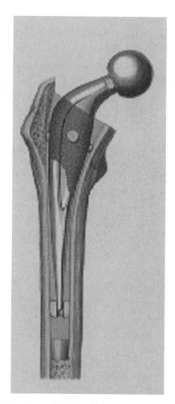

FIGURE 14-45. A longitudinal artist impression of the SHP hip stem. The fluted proximal part, evaluated in a numerical shape-optimization study significantly reduces cement and interface stress-transfer in that area (82,83,141). However, the lack of visual recognition points makes it hard for a surgeon to merge the placement of the stem correctly with the bone (182).

than for the optimized design. Evidently, it is questionable whether a material distribution like that in Fig. 14-44 could actually be produced, so the matter is rather academic at the moment. However, these results illustrate that in principle, solutions for incompatible design goals are to be found with numerical optimization methods.

It must be noted, however, that whether or not prostheses optimized in this way are successful also depends on other factors than just load transfer. For instance, an FEA procedure was applied to a cemented stem with the objective of minimizing cement and interface stresses by optimizing stem shape (82,83). This produced a typical shape, with a taper at the proximal/medial side, a belly-shaped middle region, and a strongly tapered distal end (Fig. 14-45). Relative to a conventional, straight femoral stem design, theoretical cement and interface stress reductions of 30% to 70% could be obtained with this optimized shape (83). These reductions were

also confirmed experimentally, albeit at a smaller scale (141). However, after clinical trials it turned out that the results with this femoral component were not really superior to those with conventional stems (182). One reason, it turned out, was that due to the unusual shape of the stem, an the lack of a collar, it was very difficult for the surgeon to place it correctly in the bone. The other was that a stem such as that relies on a firm bond between stem and cement. Because of cement-stem sliding and cement viscosity, this can not always be counted upon (91).

5 DISCUSSION

In this chapter, we treated the performance and endurance of THA and summarized what is known about failure mechanisms. It was argued that biomechanics is important in all activities of the innovation cycle. This is particularly so for design and design assessment of new prostheses, in which the engineering task is substantial. In order to rationalize the design process, five questions must always be addressed: (a) What clinical problem does a traditional design create? (b) How does this problem relate to the design characteristics? (c) What innovative feature would improve the design? (d) Does this feature indeed solve the clinical problem? (e) Will this innovative design cause another clinical problem, worse than the original one? To answer these questions is not an easy task, first because patient factors (both biological and functional ones) and surgical factors (technical feasibilities and skills) can hold many surprises in waiting. Second, although a clinical problem may be well documented, its cause in terms of precise failure mechanisms often remains obscure. Third, engineering design goals in THA tend to be incompatible; i.e., what prevents one failure mechanism often promotes another.

What will the future bring? Certainly, higher demands for hip replacements. People grow older now, compared with earlier generations, but their joints may be equally susceptible to OA. Although food quality is better than in the past, and the intensity of manual labor reduced, people tend to become heavier or put higher demands on their joints in sports. In addition, new "markets" are opening up in Africa and Asia. The question is whether there is still room for improving hip prosthetic quality, in terms of safety and efficacy. According to the Nordic registers, the hydroxylapatite-coated hip stem holds the record for prosthetic longevity—the stem, that is, not the cup! In the early days of hip replacement it was evident that cups were secure, on the average, for a longer time period than the stems. However, now it seems that femoral stem security and efficacy have been much improved, so that cup loosening is the earliest problem. So maybe that is what research should be concentrated upon now. Obviously, much more space in this chapter was devoted to stems than to cups. Also in the literature we find many more studies devoted to the former than to the latter. Finally,

a hip prosthesis is and remains an artificial joint, subject to wear and fatigue; so that is certainly an area for research and innovation. The best way to prevent hip-prosthetic failure, however, is not to have one at all. Instead, prevention or healing modalities might solve the problem in the future.

REFERENCES

1. Ahnfelt L, Herberts P, Malchau H, et al. Prognosis of total hip replacement. *Acta Orthop Scand [Suppl]* 1990;238.
2. American Academy of Orthopaedic Surgeons. *Musculoskeletal system research, current and future research needs.* AAOS Publication TFR-81, Chicago, 1981.
3. Amstutz HC, Campbell P, Kossovsky N, et al. Mechanism and clinical significance of wear debris-induced osteolysis. *Clin Orthop* 1992;276: 7–18.
4. Arroyo NA, Stark CF. The effect of textures, surface finish and precoating on the strength of bone cement/stem interfaces. *Proc Soc Biomat* 1987;13:218.
5. Barb W, Park JB, Kenner GH, et al. Intramedullary fixation of artificial hip joints with bone cement–precoated implants. Interfacial strengths. *J Biomed Mater Res* 1982;16:447–458.
6. Bartel DL, Bickness VL, Wright TJ. The effect of conformity, thickness, and material on stresses in ultra-high molecular weight components for total joint replacement. *J Bone Joint Surg* 1986;68-Am:1041–1051.
7. Beaupré GS, Orr TE, Carter DR. An approach for time-dependent bone modeling and remodeling-application: a preliminary remodeling simulation. *J Orthop Res* 1990;8:662–670.
8. Bergmann G, Graichen F, Rohlmann A. Is staircase walking a risk for the fixation of hip implants? *J Biomech* 1995;28:535–553.
9. Bergmann G, Deuretzbacher G, Heller M, et al. Hip contact forces and gait patterns from routine activities. *J Biomech* 2001;34:859–871.
10. Bobyn JD, Mortimer ES, Glassman AH, et al. Producing and avoiding stress shielding. Laboratory and clinical observations of noncemented total hip arthroplasty. *Clin Orthop* 1992;274:79–96.
11. Brunski JB, Aquilante FM, Pollack SR, et al. The influence of functional use of endosseous dental implants on tissue–implant interface. I. Histological aspects. *J Dent Res* 1979;10:1953–1969.
12. Burke DW, O'Connor DO, Zalenski EB, et al. Micromotion of cement and uncemented femoral components. *J Bone Joint Surg* 1991;73–13:22–37.

13. Carlsson L, Albrektsson B, Freeman MAR. Femoral neck retention in hip arthroplasty. *Acta Orthop Scand* 1988;59:6–8.

14. Carter DR, Vasu R, Harris WH. Stress distributions in the acetabular region—II: effects of cement thickness and metal backing of the total hip acetabular component. *J Biomech* 1982;15:165–170.

15. Carter DR, Fyhrie DP, Whalen RT. Trabecular bone density and loading history: regulation of connective tissue biology by mechanical energy. *J Biomech* 1987;20:785–794.

16. Chaboche JL. Continuum damage mechanics: part I—general concepts. *J Appl Mech* 1988;55:59–64.

17. Chaboche JL. Continuum damage mechanics: part II—damage growth, crack initiation, and crack growth. *J Appl Mech* 1988;55:65–72.

18. Charnley J. *Acrylic cement in orthopaedic surgery.* Edinburgh: E. and S. Livingstone, 1970.

19. Charnley J. *Low friction arthroplasty of the hip.* New York: Springer Verlag, 1978.

20. Chwirut DJ. Long-term compressive creep deformation and damage in acrylic bone cements. *J Biomed Mater Res* 1984;18:25–37.

21. Cohen B, Rushton N. Accuracy of DEXA measurement of bone mineral density after total hip arthroplasty. *J Bone Joint Surg* 1995;77-B:479–483.

22. Concensus Development Panel. *Total hip replacement in the United States.* Report of Consensus Conference, NIH, 1–3 March 1982, Bethesda, MD. *JAMA* 1982;248:1817–1821.

23. Cowin SC, Hegedus DH. Bone remodeling I: theory of adaptive elasticity. *J Elasticity* 1976;6:313–326.

24. Cristofolini L. A critical analysis of stress shielding evaluation of hip prostheses. *Crit Rev Biomed Eng* 1997;25:409–483.

25. Cristofolini L, Viceconti M, Toni et al. Influence of thigh muscles on the axial strains in a proximal femur during early stance in gait. *J Biomech* 1995;28:617–624.

26. Cristofolini, L, Viceconti M. Development and validation of a technique for strain measurement inside polymethyl methacrylate. *J Strain Anal* 2000;35:21–33.

27. Crowninshield RD, Tolbert JR. Cement strain measurement surrounding loose and well-fixed femoral component stems. *J Biomed Mater Res* 1983;17:819–828.

28. Crowninshield RD, Brand RA, Pedersen DR. A stress analysis of acetabular reconstruction in protrusio acetabulli. *J Bone Joint Surg* 1983;65-Am:495–499.

29. Dally JW, Riley WF. *Experimental stress analysis.* New York: McGraw-Hill, 1965.

30. Dalstra M. *Biomechanical aspects of the pelvic bone and design criteria for acetabular prostheses.* Ph.D.

thesis, Nijmegen University, The Netherlands, 1993.

31. Dalstra M, Huiskes R. Prestresses around the acetabulum generated by screwed cups. *Clin Mater* 1994;16:145–154.

32. Dalstra M, Huiskes R. Load transfer across the pelvic bone. *J Biomech* 1995;28:715–724.

33. Dalstra M, Huiskes R, Van Erning L. Development and validation of a three-dimensional finite element model of the pelvic bone. *J Biomech Eng* 1995;117:272–278.

34. Dalstra M, Huiskes R. The effects of total hip replacement on pelvic load transfer. Chapter IV *Biomechanical aspects of the pelvic bone and design criteria for acetabular prostheses.* Dalstra M, Doct. Diss. University of Nijmegen, Netherlands. 15 November 1993;ISBN 90-9006517-2.

35. Davy DT, Katoozian H. Three-dimensional shape optimization of femoral components of hip prostheses with frictional interfaces. *Trans ORS* 1994;40:223.

36. DiCarlo EF, Bullough PG. The biological responses to orthopaedic implants and their wear debris. *Clin Mater* 1992;9:235–260.

37. Diegel PD, Daniels AU, Dunn HK. Initial effect of collarless stem stiffness on femoral bone strain. *J Arthroplasty* 1989;4:173–179.

38. Eftekar MS, Doty SB, Johnston AD, et al. Prosthetic synovitis. In: Fitzgerald RH, ed. *The hip.* St. Louis: CV Mosby, 1985:169–183.

39. Engh CA, Bobyn JD. The influence of stem size and extent of porous coating on femoral bone resorption after primary cementless hip arthroplasty. *Clin Orthop* 1988;231:7–28.

40. Engh CA, Massin P. Cementless total hip replacement using the AML stem. 0–10 Year results using a survivorship analysis. *Nippon Seikeigeka Gakkai Zasshi* 1989;63:653–666.

41. Engh CA, McGovern TF, Bobyn JD, et al. A quantitative evaluation of periprosthetic bone-remodeling after cementless total hip arthroplasty. *J Bone Joint Surg Am* 1992;74:1009–1020.

42. Engh CA, Hooten JP Jr, Zettl-Schaffer KF, et al. Porous-coated total hip replacement. *Clin Orthop* 1994;298:89–96.

43. Faro LM, Huiskes R. Quality assurance of joint replacement. Legal regulation and medical judgement. *Acta Orthop Scand [Suppl]* 1992;250:1–33.

44. Felts, W, Yelin E. The economic impact of the rheumatic diseases in the United States. *J Rheumatol* 1989;16:867–884.

45. Finlay JB, Bourne RB, Landsberg RED, et al. Pelvic stresses *in vitro* —I. Malsizing of endoprostheses. *J Biomech* 1986;19:703–714.

46. Finlay JB, Bourne RB. Potential reinforcement-errors from the use of foil strain-gauges. *Trans Orthop Res Soc* 1989;14:491.

47. Finlay JB, Rorabeck CH, Bourne RB, et al. *In vitro* analysis of proximal femoral strains using

PCA femoral implants and a hip-abductor muscle simulator. *J Arthroplasty* 1989;4:335–345.

48. Furlong R. Six years use of the unmodified Furlong hydroxyapatite ceramic coated total hip replacement. *Acta Orthop Belg* 1993;59(Suppl 1):323–325.

49. Geesink RGT, Groot KDE, Klein CPAT. Chemical implant fixation using hydroxyl-apatite coatings. *Clin Orthop* 1987;225:147–170.

50. Geesink RG, Hoefnagels NH. Six-year results of hydroxyapatite-coated total hip replacement. *J Bone Joint Surg* 1995;77-Br:534–547.

51. Gilbert JL, Blommfield RS, Lautenschlager EP, et al. A computer-based biomechanical analysis of the three-dimensional motion of cementless hip prostheses. *J Biomech* 1992;25:329–340.

52. Goldring SR, Schiller AL, Roelke M, et al. The synovial-like membrane at the bone–cement interface in loose total hip replacements and its proposed role in bone lysis. *J Bone Joint Surg* 1983;65A:575–583.

53. Goodman SB, Aspenberg P, Song Y, et al. Effects of intermittent micromotion versus polymer particles on tissue ingrowth: experiment using a micromotion chamber implanted in rabbits. *J Appl Biomater* 1994;5:117–123.

54. Grazier KL, Holbrook TL, Kelsey JL, et al. *The frequency of occurence, impact and cost of musculoskeletal conditions in the United States.* Chicago: American Academy of Orthopaedic Surgeons, 1984.

55. Harrigan T, Harris WH. A three-dimensional nonlinear finite element study of the effect of cement-prosthesis debonding in cemented femoral total hip components. *J Biomech* 1991;24:1047–1058.

56. Harris WH. Is it advantageous to strengthen the cement–metal interface and use a collar for cemented femoral components of total hip replacement? *Clin Orthop* 1992;285:67–72.

57. Hart RT, Davy DT, Heiple KG. A computational method of stress analysis of adaptive elastic materials with a view toward application in strain induced remodeling. *J Biomech Eng* 1984;106:342–350.

58. Havelin LI, Espehaug B, Vollset SE, et al. The effect of the type of cement on early revision of Charnley total hip prostheses. A review of eight thousand five hundred and seventy-nine primary arthroplasties from the Norwegian Arthroplasty Register. *J Bone Joint Surg* 1995;77-Am:1543–1550.

59. Havelin LI, Espehaug B, Vollset SE, et al. Early aseptic loosening of uncemented femoral components in primary total hip replacement. A review based on the Norwegian Arthroplasty Register. *J Bone Joint Surg* 1995;77-Br:11–17.

60. Havelin LI, Engesaeter LB, Espehaug B, et al. The Norwegian Arthroplasty Register; 11 years and 73,000 arthroplasties. *Acta Orthop Scand* 2000;71:337–353.

61. Heller MO, Bergmann G, Deuretzbacher G, et al. Musculo-skeletal loading conditions at the hip during walking and stair climbing. *J Biomech* 2001;34:883–893.

62. Herberts P, Ahnfelt L, Malchau H, et al. Multi-center clinical trials and their value in assessing total joint arthroplasty. *Clin Orthop* 1989;249:48–55.

63. Herberts P, Malchau H. Long-term registration has improved the quality of hip replacement: a review of the Swedish THR Register comparing 160,000 cases. *Acta Orthop Scand* 2000;71:111–121.

64. Hinton E. *NAFEMS introduction to nonlinear finite element analysis.* Glasgow: Bell and Bain, 1992.

65. Hodge WA, Andriacchi TP, Galante JO. A relationship between stem orientation and function following total hip arthroplasty. *J Arthoplasty* 1991;6:229–235.

66. Hoffman O. The brittle strength of orthotropic materials. *J Comp Mater* 1967;1:200–206.

67. Hua J, Walker PS. Closeness of fit of uncemented stems improves the strain distribution in the femur. *J Orthop Res* 1995;13:339–346.

68. Huiskes R. Some fundamental aspects of human-joint replacement. *Acta Orthop Scand [Suppl]* 1980;185.

69. Huiskes R. Principles and methods of solid biomechanics. In: Ducheyne P, Hastings G, eds. *Functional behavior of orthopaedic materials. Vol. I: fundamentals.* Boca Raton, FL: CRC Press, 1984:51–98.

70. Huiskes R. Design, fixation, and stress analysis of permanent orthopedic implants: the hip joint. In: Ducheyne P, Hastings G, eds. *Functional behavior of biomaterials. Vol. II: applications.* Boca Raton, FL: CRC Press, 1984:121–162.

71. Huiskes R. Finite element analysis of acetabular reconstruction. *Acta Orthop Scand* 1987;58:620–625.

72. Huiskes R. The various stress patterns of press-fit, ingrown and cemented femoral stems. *Clin Orthop* 1990;261:27–38.

73. Huiskes R. New approaches to cemented hip-prosthetic design. In: Buchom G, Willert HG, eds. *Safety of implants.* Hans Huber Verlag, 1991:227–236.

74. Huiskes R. Stress shielding and bone resorption in THA: clinical versus computer-simulation studies. *Acta Orthop Belg* 1993;59(Suppl 1):118–129.

75. Huiskes R. Failed innovation in total hip replacement. *Acta Orthop Scand* 1993;64:699–716.

76. Huiskes R. Mechanical failure in total hip arthroplasty with cement. *Curr Orthop* 1993;7:239–247.

77. Huiskes R. Bone remodeling around implants can be explained as an effect of mechanical adaptation. In: Galante JO, Rosenberg AG, Gallaghan JJ, eds. *Total hip revision surgery.* New York: Raven Press, 1995:159–171.

78. Huiskes R. Biomechanics of noncemented total hip arthroplasty. *Curr Orthop* 1996;7:32–37.

79. Huiskes R, Janssen JD, Slooff TJ. A detailed comparison of experimental and theoretical stress-analyses of a human femur. In: Cowin SC, ed. *Mechanical properties of bone*. New York: The American Society of Mechanical Engineers, 1981:211–234.

80. Huiskes R, Strens PHGE, van Heck J, et al. Interface stresses in the resurfaced hip. *Acta Orthop Scand* 1985;56:474–478.

81. Huiskes R, Weinans H, Grootenboer HJ, et al. Adaptive bone-remodeling theory applied to prosthetic-design analysis. *J Biomech* 1987; 20(11/12):1135–1150.

82. Huiskes R, Boeklagen R. The application of numerical shape optimization to artificial joint design. In: Spilker RL, Simon BR, eds. *Computational methods in bioengineering*. New York: The American Society of Mechanical Engineers, 1988:185–198.

83. Huiskes R, Boeklagen R. Mathematical shape optimization of hip-prosthesis design. *J Biomech* 1989;22:793–804.

84. Huiskes R, Weinans H, Dalstra M. Adaptive bone remodeling and biomechanical design considerations for noncemented total hip arthroplasty. *Orthopedics* 1989;12:1255–1267.

85. Huiskes R, Strens P, Vroemen W, et al. Postloosening mechanical behavior of femoral resurfacing prostheses. *Clin Mater* 1990;6:37–55.

86. Huiskes R, van der Venne R, Spierings PTJ. Numeral shape optimization applied to cemented acetabular-cup design in THA. *Proc Ann Meet ORS* 1990;255.

87. Huiskes R, Weinans H, Van Rietbergen B. The relationship between stress shielding and bone resoption around total hip stems and the effects of flexible materials. *Clin Orthop* 1992;272:124–134.

88. Huiskes R, Hollister SJ. From structure to process, from organ to cell: recent developments of FE-analysis in orthopaedic biomechancics. *J Biomech Eng* 1993;115:520–527.

89. Huiskes R, Van Rietbergen B. Preclinical testing of total hip stems: the effects of coating placement. *Clin Orthop* 1995;319:64–76.

90. Huiskes R, van Driel WD, Prendergast PJ, et al. A biomechanical regulatory model for periprosthetic fibrous-tissue differentiation. *J Mater Sci Mater M* 1997;8:785–788.

91. Huiskes R, Verdonschot N, Nivbrant B. Migration, stem shape, and surface finish in cemented total hip arthroplasty. *Clin Orthop* 1998;355:103–112.

92. Huracek J, Spirig P. The effect of hydroxyapatite coating on the fixation of hip prostheses. A comparison of clinical and radiographic results of hip replacement in a matched-pair study. *Arch Orthop Trauma Surg* 1994;113:72–77.

93. Hwang W, Han KS. Cumulative damage models and multi-stress fatigue life prediction. *J Comp Mater* 1986;20:125–153.

94. Jacob HAC, Huggler AH. An investigation into biomechanical causes of prosthesis stem loosening within the proximal end of the human femur. *J Biomech* 1980;13:159–171.

95. Jasty M, Maloney WJ, Bragdon CR, et al. The initiation of failure in cemented femoral components of hip arthroplasties. *J Bone Joint Surg* 1991;73-Br:551–558.

96. Jasty M, Jiranek W, Harris WH. Acrylic fragmentation in total hip replacements and its biological consequences. *Clin Orthop* 1992;285:116–128.

97. Jasty M, O'Connor DO, Henshaw RM, et al. Fit of the uncemented femoral components and the use of cement influence the strain transfer to the femoral cortex. *J Orthop Res* 1994;12:648–656.

98. Kärrholm J. 1989; Roentgen stereophotogrammetry. Review of orthopaedic applications. *Acta Orthop Scand,* 60:491–503.

99. Kärrholm J, Borssén B, Löwenhielm G, et al. Does early micromotion of femoral stem prostheses matter? *J Bone Joint Surg Br* 1994;76:912–917.

100. Keaveny TM, Bartel DL. Effects of porous coating and collar support on early load transfer for a cementless hip prosthesis. *J Biomech* 1993;26:1205–1216.

101. Keller JC, Lautenschlager EP, Marshall GW, et al. Factors affecting surgical alloy/bone cement interface adhesion. *J Biomed Mater Res* 1980;14:1639–1651.

102. Kerner J, Huiskes R, van Lenthe GH, et al. Correlation between pre-operative periprosthetic bone density and post-operative bone loss in THA can be explained by strain-adaptive remodeling. *J Biomech* 1999;32:695–703.

103. Kohles SS, Vanderby R, Manley PM, et al. A comparison of strain gage analysis to differential infrared thermography in the proximal canine femur. *Trans Orthop Res Soc* 1989;14:490.

104. Kuiper JH, Huiskes R. Numerical optimization of hip-prosthetic material. In: Middleton J, Pande GN, Williams KR, eds. *Recent advances in computer methods in biomechanics and biomedical engineering*. Swansea, UK: Books & Journals Int, 1992:76–84.

105. Kuiper JH, Huiskes R. Mathematical optimization of elastic properties—application to cementless hip stem design. *J Biomech Eng* 1997;119:166–174.

106. Kuiper JH, Huiskes R. The predictive value of stress shielding for quantification of adaptive resorption around hip replacements. *J Biomech Eng* 1997;119:228–231.

107. Kuiper JH, Huiskes R. Friction and stem stiffness affect dynamic interface motion in total hip replacement. *J Orthop Res* 1996;14:36–43.

108. Landjerit B, Jacquard-Simon N, Thourot M, et al. Physiological loadings on human pelvis: a comparison between numerical and experimental simulations. *Proc Eur Soc Biomech* 1992;8:195.

109. Lanyon LE, Paul L, Rubin CT. *In vivo* strain measurements from bone and prosthesis following total hip replacements. *J Bone Joint Surg* 1981;63A:989–994.

110. Lemaitre J. How to use damage mechanics. *Nucl Eng Design* 1984;80:233–245.

111. Ling RSM. The use of a collar and precoating on cemented femoral stems is unnecessary and detrimental. *Clin Orthop* 1992;285:73–83.

112. Lionberger D, Walker PS, Granholm J. Effects of prosthetic acetabular replacement on strains in the pelvis. *J Orthop Res* 1985;3:372–379.

113. Maher SA, Prendergast PJ, Lyons CG. Measurement of the migration of a cemented hip prosthesis in an in vitro test. *Clin Biomech* 2001;16:307–314.

114. Maher SA, Prendergast PJ. Discriminating the loosening behaviour of cemented hip prostheses using measurements of migration and inducible displacement. *J Biomech* 2002;35:257–265.

115. Malchau H, Herberts P, Ahnfelt L. Prognosis of total hip replacement in Sweden. Followup of 92,675 operations performed 1978–1990. *Acta Orthop Scand* 1993;64:497–506.

116. Malchau M, Herberts P, Garelick G, et al. Prognosis of total hip replacement. Scientific Exhibit, 69th annual meeting of the Americal Academy of Orthopaedic Surgeons, February 13–17, 2002, Dallas, TX.

117. Maloney WJ, Jasty M, Burke DW, et al. Biomechanical and histologic investigation of cemented total hip arthroplasties. A study of autopsy-retrieved femurs after *in vivo* cycling. *Clin Orthop* 1989;249:129–140.

118. Maloney WJ, Smith RL, Schmalzried TP, et al. Isolation and characterization of wear particles generated in patients who have had failure of a hip arthroplasty, without cement. *J Bone Joint Surg* 1995;77-Am:1201–1210.

119. Mann KA, Bartel DL, Wright TM, et al. Coulomb frictional interfaces in modeling cemented total hip replacements: a more realistic model. *J Biomech* 1995;28:1067–1078.

120. Mann KA, Werner FW, Ayers DC. Modeling the tensile behavior of the cement–bone interface using nonlinear fracture mechanics. *J Biomech Eng* 1997;119:175–178.

121. Martin RB. The effects of geometric feedback in the development of osteoporosis. *J Biomech* 1972;5:447–455.

122. McKellop H, Campbeel P, Park SH, et al. The origin of submicron polyethylene wear debris in total hip arthroplasty. *Clin Orthop* 1995;311:3–20.

123. McNamara BP, Cristofolini L, Toni A, et al. Evaluation of experimental and finite element models of synthetic and cadaveric femora for pre-clinical design-analysis. *Clin Mater* 1995;17:131–140.

124. Mjöberg, B, Hanson LI, Selvik G. Instability, migration and laxity of total hip prostheses. A röntgen stereophotogrammetric study. *Acta Orthop Scand* 1984;55:504–506.

125. Morlock M, Schneider,E, Bluhm A, et al. Duration and frequency of every day activities in total hip patients. *J Biomech* 2001;34:873–881.

126. Mow VC, Ateshian GA, Spilker RL. Biomechanics of diathrodial joints: a review of twenty years of progress. *J Biomech Eng* 1993;115:460–467.

127. Mullender MG, Huiskes R. Proposal for the regulatory mechanism of Wolff's Law. *J Orthop Res* 1995;13:503–512.

128. Murphy BP, Prendergast PJ. Measurement of nonlinear microcrack accumulation rates in polymethylmethacrylate bone cement under cyclic loading. *J Mater Sci Mater M* 1999;10:779–781.

129. Murphy BP, Prendergast PJ. On the magnitude and variability of the fatigue strength of acrylic bone cement. *Int J Fatigue* 2000;22:855–864.

130. Murphy BP, Prendergast PJ. The relationship between stress, porosity, and nonlinear damage accumulation in acrylic bone cement. *J Biomed Mater Res* 2002;59:646–654.

131. Noble PC, Alexander JW, Lindahl LJ, et al. The anatomic basis of femoral component design. *Clin Orthop* 1988;235:148–165.

132. Oh I, Harris WH. Proximal strain distribution in the loaded femur. *J Bone Joint Surg* 1978;60A:75–85.

133. Olsson E. Gait analysis in hip and knee surgery. *Scand J Rehabil Med Suppl* 1986;15:1–55.

134. Osborn JF. The biological behavior of the hydroxyapatite ceramic coating on a titanium stem of a hip prosthesis. *Biomed Technol* 1987;32:177–183.

135. Pancanti A, Bernakiewicz M, Viceconti M. The primary stability of a cementless stem varies between subjects as much as between activities. *J Biomech* 2003;36:777–785.

136. Pedersen DR, Crowninshield RD, Brand RA, et al. An axial symmetric model of acetabular components in total hip arthroplasty. *J Biomech* 1982;15:305–315.

137. Perren SM. Induction der Knochenresorptio bei Prothesenlockerung. In: Morcher E, ed. *Die zementlose Fixation von Huftendoprothesen*. Berlin: Springer Verlag, 1983:38–40.

138. Perren SM, Ganz R, Rüter A. Oberflachliche Knochenresorption um Implantate. *Med Orthop Techn* 1975;95:6–10.

139. Perren SM, Rahn BA. Biomechanics of fracture healing. *Can J Surg* 1980;20:228–231.

140. Perrin T, Derr LD, Perry J, et al. Functional evaluation of total hip arthroplasty with five- to ten-year follow-up evaluation. *Clin Orthop* 1985;195:252–260.

141. Peters CL, Bachus KN, Craig, MA, et al. The effect of femoral prosthesis design on cement strain in cemented total hip arthroplasty. *J Arthroplasty* 2001;16:216–224.

142. Petty W, Miller GJ, Piotrowski G. *In vitro* evaluation of the effect of acetabular prosthesis implantation on human cadaver pelvis. *Bull Pros Res* 1980;17:80–89.

143. Pierson JL, Harris WH. Extensive osteolysis behind an acetabular component that was well fixed with cement—a case report. *J Bone Joint Surg* 1993;75-Am:305–315.

144. Pilliar RM, Lee JM, Maniatopoulos C. Observation on the effect of movement on bone ingrowth into porous-surfaced implants. *Clin Orthop Rel Res* 1986;208:108–113.

145. Prendergast PJ, Huiskes R, Søballe K. Biophysical stimuli during tissue differentiation at implant interfaces. *J Biomech* 1997;30:539–548.

146. Pritchett JW. Femoral bone loss following hip replacement. *Clin Orthop Rel Res,* 1995;314:156–161.

147. Puolakka TJS, Pajamaki KJJ, Halonen PJ, et al. The Finnish Arthroplasty Register: report of the hip register. *Acta Orthop Scand* 2001;72:433–441.

148. Raab S, Ahmed A, Provan JW. The quasistatic and fatigue performance of the implant/bone interface. *J Biomed Mater Res* 1981;15:159–182.

149. Radin EL, Rubin CT, Thrasher EL, et al. Changes in the bone–cement interface after total hip replacement. *J Bone Joint Surg* 1982;64A:1188–1194.

150. Rapperport DJ, Carter DR, Schurman DJ. Contact finite element stress analysis of the hip joint. *J Orthop Res* 1985;3:435–446.

151. Renaudin F, Lavst F, Skalli W, et al. A 3D finite element model of pelvis in side impact. *Proc Eur Soc Biomech* 1992;8:194.

152. Ries M, Pugh J, Au JC, et al. Cortical pelvic strains with varying size hemiarthroplasty in vitro. *J Biomech* 1989;22:775–780.

153. Ries MD, Gomez MA, Eckhoff DG, et al. An *in vitro* study of proximal femoral allograft strains in revision hip arthroplasty. *Med Eng Phys* 1994;16:292–296.

154. Roesler H. The history of some fundamental concepts in bone biomechanics. *J Biomech* 1987;20(11/12);1025–1034.

155. Rohlmann A, Cheal J, Hayes WC, et al. A nonlinear finite element analysis of interface condition in porous coated hip endoprostheses. *J Biomech* 1988;21:605–611

156. Ryd L. Micromotion in knee arthroplasty. *Acta Orthop Scand [Suppl]* 1986;220.

157. Saha S, Pal S. Mechanical properties of bone cement: a review. *J Biomed Mater Res* 1984;18:435–462.

158. Saikko VO, Pavolainen PO, Slätis P. Wear of the polyethylene acetabular cup. Metallic and ceramic heads compared in a hip simulator. *Acta Orthop Scand* 1993;64:391–402.

159. Sandborn PM, Cook, SD, Spires WP, et al. Tissue response to porous-coated implants lacking initial bone apposition. *J Arthroplasty* 1988;3:337–346.

160. Schimmel JW, Huiskes R. Primary fit of the Lord cementless total hip. *Acta Orthop Scand* 1988;59:638–642.

161. Schmalzried TP, Kwong LM, Jasty M, et al. The mechanism of loosening of cemented acetabular components in total hip arthroplasty. Analysis of specimens retrieved at autopsy. *Clin Orthop* 1992;274:60–78.

162. Schneider E, Kinast C, Eulenberger J, et al. A comparative study of the initial stability of cementless hip prostheses. *Clin Orthop* 1989;248:200–209.

163. Schneider E, Eulenberger J, Steiner W, et al. Experimental method for the *in vitro* testing of the initial stability of cementless hip prostheses. *J Biomech* 1989;22:735–744.

164. Schreurs BW, Buma P, Huiskes R, et al. Morsellized allografts for fixation of the hip prosthesis femoral component. A mechanical and histological study in the goat. *Acta Orthop Scand* 1994;65:267–275.

165. Schreurs BW, Huiskes R, Buma P, et al. Biomechanical and histological evaluation of a hydroxyapatite-coated titanium femoral stem fixed with an intramedullary morsellized bone grafting technique: an animal experiment on goats. *Biomaterials* 1996;17:1177–1186.

166. Selvik G. *A roentgen stereophotogrammetric method for the study of the kinematics of the skeletal system.* Thesis, Lund, 1974. Reprinted as *Acta Orthop Scand [Suppl],* 1989;232.

167. Shanbhag AS, Jacobs JJ, Glant TT, et al. Composition and morphology of wear debris in failed uncemented total hip replacement. *J Bone Joint Surg* 1994;76-Br:60–67.

168. Snorrason F, Kärrholm J. Primary stability of revision total hip arthroplasty: a roentgen stereophotogrammetric analysis. *J Arthroplasty* 1990;5:217–229.

169. Sballe K, Hansen ESB, Rasmussen H, et al. Tissue ingrowth into titanium and hydroxyapatite-coated implants during stable and unstable mechanical conditions. *J Orthop Res* 1992;10:285–299.

170. Södeqvist I, Wedin EA. Determining the movements of the skeleton using well-configured markers. Technical Note. *J Biomech* 1993;26:1473–1477.

171. Spears IR, Pfleiderer M, Schneider E, et al. The effect of interfacial parameters on cup–bone relative

micromotions. A finite element investigation. *J Biomech* 2001;34:113–120.

172. Stolk J, Verdonschot N, Huiskes R. Hip-joint and abductor-muscle forces adequately represent in vivo loading of a cemented total hip reconstruction. *J Biomech* 2001;34:917–926.

173. Stolk J, Verdonschot N, Cristofolini L, et al. Finite element and experimental models of cemented hip joint reconstructions can produce similar bone and cement strains in pre-clinical tests. *J Biomech* 2002;35:499–510.

174. Stolk J, Verdonschot N, Huiskes R. Stair climbing is more detrimental to the cement in hip replacement than walking. *Clin Orthop* 2002;405:294–305.

175. Stolk J, Maher SA, Verdonschot N, et al. Can finite element models detect clinically inferior cemented hip implants? *Clin Orthop* 2003;409:138–150.

176. Stolk J, Verdonschot N, Huiskes R. Can finite element based pre-clinical tests differentiate between cemented hip replacement stems according to clinical survival rates? In: 49th annual meeting of the Orthopaedic Research Society, Feb. 2–5, 2003, New Orleans, LA.

177. Stolk J, Verdonschot N, Mann KA, et al. Prevention of mesh-dependent damage growth in finite element simulations of crack formation in acrylic bone cement. *J Biomech* 2003;36:861–871.

178. Stolk J, Verdonschot N, Murphy BP, et al. Finite element simulation of anisotropic damage accumulation and creep in acrylic bone cement. *Eng Fract Mech* 2003;71:513–528.

179. Stolk J, Dormans KW, Sluimer J, et al. Is early bone resorption around non-cemented THA cups related to stress shielding? In: 50th annual meeting of the Orthopaedic Research Society, March 7–10, 2004, San Francisco, CA.

180. Stone MH, Wilkinson R, Stother IG. Some factors affecting the strength of the cement–metal interface. *J Bone Joint* Surg1989;71-Br:217–221.

181. Sugiyama H, Whiteside LA, Kaiser AD. Examination of rotational fixation of the femoral component in total hip arthroplasty. *Clin Orthop* 1989;249:122–128.

182. Sybesma T. *From laboratory to clinic: the study of a new cemented hip arthroplasty.* Ph.D. Thesis, University of Groningen, The Netherlands, 2002.

183. Tanner KE, Bonfield W, Nunn D, et al. Rotational movement of femoral components of total hip replacements in response to an anteriorly applied load. *Eng Med* 1988;17:127–129.

184. Van der Meulen MCH, Huiskes R. Why mechanobiology? *J Biomech* 2002;35:401–414.

185. Van Lenthe GH, de Waal Malefijt MC, Huiskes R. Stress shielding after total knee replacement may cause bone resorption in the distal femur. *J Bone Joint Surg* 1997;79-B:117–122.

186. Van Rietbergen B, Huiskes R, Weinans H, et al. ESB Research Award 1992. The mechanism of bone remodeling and resorption around press-fitted THA stems. *J Biomech* 1993;26:369–382.

187. Van Rietbergen B, Huiskes R. Load transfer and stress shielding of the hydroxyapatite-ABG hip. *J Arthroplasty (Suppl 1)* 2001;16:55–63.

188. Vasu R, Carter DR, Harris WH. Stress distributions in the acetabular region-I. Before and after total joint replacement. *J Biomech* 1982;15:155–164.

189. Vena P, Contro R, Huiskes R. Optimal design of interfaces in a femoral head surface replacement prosthesis considering nonlinear behavior. *Struct Optimization* 1999;18:162–172.

190. Vena P, Verdonschot N, Contro R, et al. Sensitivity analysis and optimal shape design for bone-prosthesis interface in a femoral head surface replacement. *Comp Meth Biomech Biomed Eng* 2000;3:245–256.

191. Verdonschot N, Huiskes R. The creep behavior of hand-mixed simplex P bone cement under cyclic tensile loading. *J Appl Biomater* 1994;5:235–243.

192. Verdonschot N, Huiskes R. Dynamic creep behavior of acrylic bone cement. *J Biomed Mater Res* 1995;29:575–5.81.

193. Verdonschot N, Huiskes R. A combination of continuum damage mechanics and the finite element method to analyze acrylic cement cracking around implants. In: Middleton J, Jones ML, Pande GN, eds. *Computer methods in biomechanics and biomedical engineering.* London: Gordon and Breach Science Publishers, 1995:25–33.

194. Verdonschot N, Huiskes R. Subsidence of THA stems due to acrylic cement creep is extremely sensitive to interface friction. *J Biomech* 1996;29:1569–1575.

195. Verdonschot N, Huiskes R. Mechanical effects of stem–cement interface characteristics in total hip replacement. *Clin Orthop* 1996;329:326–336.

196. Verdonschot N, Huiskes R. Cement debonding process of THA stems. *Clin Orthop* 1997;336:297–307.

197. Verdonschot N, Huiskes R. Acrylic cement creeps but does not allow much subsidence of femoral stems. *J Bone Joint Surg* 1997;79-B:665–669.

198. Verdonschot N, Huiskes R. The effects of cement-stem debonding in THA on the long-term failure probability of cement. *J Biomech* 1997;30:795–802.

199. Verdonschot N, Huiskes R. Surface roughness of debonded straight-tapered stems in cemented THA reduces subsidence but not cement damage. *Biomaterials* 1998;19:1773–1779.

200. Verdonschot N, Huiskes R. Creep properties of three low temperature–curing bone cements: a

preclinical assessment. *J Biomed Mater Res* 2000; 53:498–504.

201. Verdonschot N, Huiskes R, Freeman MAR. Preclinical testing of hip prosthetic designs: a comparison of finite element calculations and laboratory tests. *J Eng Med* 1993;207:149–154.

202. Verdonschot N, Tanck E, Huiskes R. Effects of prosthesis surface roughness on the failure process of cemented hip implants after stem–cement debonding. *J Biomed Mater Res* 1998;42:554–559.

203. Walker P, Mai SF, Cobb AG, et al. Prediction of clinical outcome of THR from migration measurements on standard radiographs. *J Bone Joint Surg* 1995;77-Br:705–714.

204. Weinans H, Huiskes R, Grootenboer HJ. Trends of mechanical consequences and modeling of a fibrous membrane around femoral hip prostheses. *J Biomech* 1990;23:991–1000.

205. Weinans H, Huiskes R, Grootenboer HJ. Effects of material properties of femoral hip components on bone remodeling. *J Orthop Res* 1992;10:845–853.

206. Weinans H, Huiskes R, Grootenboer HJ. The behavior of adaptive bone-remodeling simulation models. *J Biomech* 1992;25:1425–1441.

207. Weinans H, Huiskes R, Grootenboer HJ. Quantitative analysis of bone reactions at implant–bone interfaces. *J Biomech* 1993;26:1271–1281.

208. Weinans H, Huiskes R, Van Rietbergen B, et al. Adaptive bone remodeling around bonded noncemented total hip arthroplasty: a comparison between animal experiments and computer simulation. *J Orthop Res* 1993;11:500–513.

209. Weinans H, Huiskes R, Grootenboer HJ. Effects of fit and bonding characteristics of femoral stems on adaptive bone remodeling. *J Biomech Eng* 1994;116:393–400.

210. Wolff J. *Das Gesetz der Transformation der Knochen [The law of bone remodeling]*. Berlin: Springer-Verlag, 1892.

211. Yelin E. Arthritis. The cumulative impact of a common chronic condition. *Arthritis Rheum* 1992;35:489–497.

212. Yoon YS, Jang GH, Kim YY. Shape optimal design of the stem of a cement hip prosthesis to minimize stress concentration in the cement layer. *J Biomech* 1989;22:1279–1284.

213. Yuan X, Ryd L. Accuracy analysis for RSA: a computer simulation study on 3D marker reconstruction. *J Biomech* 2000;33:493–498.

214. Yuan R, Ryd L, Huiskes R. Wear particle diffusion and tissue differentiation in TKA–implant fibrous interface. *J Biomech* 2000;33:1279–1286.

215. Zhou XM, Walker PS, Robertson DD. Effect of press-fit femoral stems on strains in the femur. *J Arthroplasty* 1990;5:71–82.

APPENDIX: SOLID MECHANICS AND STRESS ANALYSIS

Some Principles of Solid Mechanics

Stress, Strain, and Hooke's Law

If a body is loaded, it deforms. Unless the body is regularly shaped (e.g., cube, bar, or beam) and the external load is evenly distributed and aligned with the geometry, these deformations produced in the body will not be uniform. The amount of deformation will vary throughout the body. To analyze the deformation, we select an infinitesimal cube of material inside the object and allow this cube to be stretched and compressed in the three edge directions. To quantify these deformations, we define a lineal strain along each edge, given as a change of length per original length (Fig. 14-A1a). These three lineal strains also define the dilatation (change of volume per original volume; this is equal to the algebraic sum of the three lineal strains) of the cube. The lineal strains and dilatation depend on the applied loading and on the material that constitutes the object. We also allow the shape of the cube to distort in its three planes (Fig. 14-A1b). These three angles are known as shear strains, and they also depend on the material properties and the external loads. These six variables completely describe the deformation of the tiny cube at any arbitrary point inside the body.

For a continuous body, load is transferred at every point inside the body. This implies that when we pass an imaginary plane through the

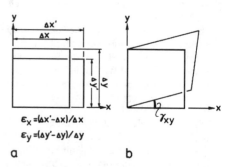

FIGURE 14-A1. Definitions of strain in the case of two-dimensional stress state. **a:** Direct strain; **b:** shear strain.

body, the material on one side of the plane will exert a force on the material at the other side. These are internal forces, transferred by chemical or physical bonds at the molecular level. Like the deformations, the magnitudes and orientations of these internal forces are not uniform but depend on the external loads, the shape of the object, and the intrinsic mechanical properties of the material making up the object. To describe these internal forces, we must first define the concept of stress. Simply stated, stress is defined as force per unit area. For convenience, the areas we choose are the faces of the tiny cube just described (Fig. 14-A2). On each face of the cube the force vector may be arbitrarily oriented. This means that on each face of the cube the stress vector will also be arbitrarily oriented. This stress vector may be decomposed into a component perpendicular to the face of the cube (normal stress) and a component parallel to the face of the cube (shear stress). In general, the shear stress component will have two components, each parallel to an axis of the chosen coordinate system. Thus, a total of nine stress components (three normal stresses and six shear stresses) must be known to define the state of stress acting on the cube (Fig. 14-A2). However, by conservation of angular momentum, the shear stresses are symmetric, i.e., $\tau_{xy} = \tau_{yx}$, $\tau_{yz} = \tau_{zy}$, $\tau_{zx} = \tau_{xz}$. Thus, only six independent stress components exist, three normal stress components (σ_x, σ_y, σ_z) and three shear stress components (τ_{xy}, τ_{yz}, τ_{zx}) (Fig. 14-A2). We note that the normal stresses can be either tensile (positive) or compressive (negative). We also note that these stress values vary with the orientation of the chosen cube (i.e., coordinate system) because the components of a vector vary with the orientation of the chosen coordinate system.

Central to solid mechanics theory is the relationship between stresses and strains for the body. This relationship is given by a constitutive equation. The stiffness of the material depends on the intrinsic mechanical properties of the material, i.e., the coefficients of the constitutive equation or material constants. If this material is linearly elastic, the generalized Hooke's law may be applied. In this case, the six strain components are linearly related to the six stress

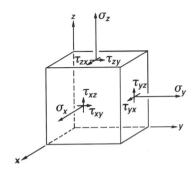

FIGURE 14-A2. Definition of the nine stress components relative to an infinitesimal cube in the material. Because $\tau_{zy} = \tau_{yz}$, $\tau_{xz} = \tau_{zx}$, and $\tau_{xy} = \tau_{yx}$, only six independent components remain to describe the three-dimensional stress state.

components by a matrix of 36 elastic constants (of which 21 are independent) given by

$$
\begin{bmatrix} \varepsilon_x \\ \varepsilon_y \\ \varepsilon_z \\ \gamma_{xy} \\ \gamma_{yz} \\ \gamma_{zx} \end{bmatrix} = \begin{bmatrix} S_{11} & S_{12} & S_{13} & S_{14} & S_{15} & S_{16} \\ S_{21} & S_{22} & S_{23} & S_{24} & S_{25} & S_{26} \\ S_{31} & S_{32} & S_{33} & S_{34} & S_{35} & S_{36} \\ S_{41} & S_{42} & S_{43} & S_{44} & S_{45} & S_{46} \\ S_{51} & S_{52} & S_{53} & S_{54} & S_{55} & S_{56} \\ S_{61} & S_{62} & S_{63} & S_{64} & S_{65} & S_{66} \end{bmatrix} \cdot \begin{bmatrix} \sigma_x \\ \sigma_y \\ \sigma_z \\ \tau_{xy} \\ \tau_{yz} \\ \tau_{zx} \end{bmatrix} \quad \text{(A1)}
$$

This is a coupled set of six equations, defined by matrix multiplication. For example, $\varepsilon_x = S_{11}\sigma_x + S_{12}\sigma_y + S_{13}\sigma_z + S_{14}\tau_{xy} + S_{15}\tau_{yz} + S_{16}\tau_{zx}$, etc. It shows that a particular strain value may depend on all six stress values and vice versa. Irrespective of the kind of material considered, this matrix is always symmetric (i.e., $S_{ij} = S_{ji}$), which implies a maximum of 21 independent components. This set of six equations defines a completely anisotropic material if all these 21 elastic constants in the matrix are different. For most materials, some form of symmetry of the microstructure exists. If the material is orthotropic, all but the constants S_{ii}, S_{12}, S_{13}, and S_{23} reduce to zero, which leaves nine independent constants in the matrix. If the material is transversely isotropic, which means that the properties are equal for two of the three principal directions, the number of independent constants reduces to five. For the isotropic case, the number reduces to only two independent elastic constants. Most often, these are expressed in terms of the Young's modulus (or elastic modulus) E and Poisson's ratio ν. Other constants are commonly used as well, such as the Lame constants (λ, μ), modulus of rigidity or shear modulus (μ), and the bulk modulus (κ). These constants may be expressed in terms of E and ν because only two constants are independent, and Eq. A1 may then be written as

$$
\begin{bmatrix} \varepsilon_x \\ \varepsilon_y \\ \varepsilon_z \\ \gamma_{xy} \\ \gamma_{yz} \\ \gamma_{zx} \end{bmatrix} = \begin{bmatrix} 1/E & -\nu/E & -\nu/E & 0 & 0 & 0 \\ -\nu/E & 1/E & -\nu/E & 0 & 0 & 0 \\ -\nu/E & -\nu/E & 1/E & 0 & 0 & 0 \\ 0 & 0 & 0 & (2+2\nu)/E & 0 & 0 \\ 0 & 0 & 0 & 0 & (2+2\nu)/E & 0 \\ 0 & 0 & 0 & 0 & 0 & (2+2\nu)/E \end{bmatrix} \cdot \begin{bmatrix} \sigma_x \\ \sigma_y \\ \sigma_z \\ \tau_{xy} \\ \tau_{yz} \\ \tau_{zx} \end{bmatrix} \quad \text{(A2)}
$$

When the material is transversely isotropic, a total of five elastic constants are required (A2, A30). For example, by approximation, cortical (haversian) bone is transversely isotropic. To describe cortical bone, a modulus is required for the longitudinal direction and another for the radial direction (the tangential direction has the same modulus as the radial one), along with two Poisson's ratios and a shear modulus.

We emphasize some important restrictions to linear elasticity theory and continuum mechanics. First, if a material is not linearly elastic, e.g., nonlinearly elastic, then Hooke's law does not apply. The material may also be plastic or viscoelastic in nature. For these types of material, the stress–strain laws are always much more complex. Biological materials cannot, in general, be described by infinitesimal linear elasticity theory, although bone can, by reasonable approximation. Second, the definitions of stress and strain presume that the material is continuous. This implies that no matter how small a cube we have chosen, the properties in the cube are supposed to be identical to those of the material at a larger scale. This assumes that there are no imperfections or voids (discontinuities) in the material. For real materials, this is hardly ever true. Even metals have imperfections in their lattice structure and at grain boundaries. Plastics usually possess a certain degree of porosity, although the pore sizes are extremely small. Bone is essentially discontinuous, particularly trabecular bone. Hence, stress–strain relationships and the calculated stresses and strains are always approximations. The quality of these approximations ranges from very good (e.g., metal) to very rough (e.g., trabecular bone). The approach to a discontinuous material such as bone is to designate a region in which dimensions are large relative to the characteristic size of the microstructure of imperfections and only consider the calculated stresses and strains in that region as averages.

Three- and Two-Dimensional and Uniaxial Stress States

If the characteristic features of a structure can be represented in a plane, and the external loads are also in that plane, then the stress state in the structure is 2D. A 2D problem may be described as a plane-stress or a plane-strain problem. In the *plane-stress* problem, the material is free to expand in the out-of-plane direction, and the normal stress in that direction is zero. This implies for Eqs. A1 and A2 that, when z is the out-of-plane direction, then $\gamma_{yz} = \gamma_{zx} = 0$ and $\sigma_z = \tau_{yz} = \tau_{zx} = 0$. For the *plane-strain* case, the material is constrained in the out-of-plane direction, and the lineal strain in that direction is zero. This implies for Eqs. A1 and A2 that $\varepsilon_z = \gamma_{yz} = \gamma_{zx} = 0$ and $\sigma_{yz} = \tau_{zx} = 0$. In both of these cases, the stress state within the plane can be characterized by three stress variables (e.g., σ_x, σ_y, and $\tau_{xy} = \tau_{yx} = \tau$).

In the *uniaxial stress* state, only one independent stress component exists. This implies for Eqs. 1 and 2 that, if x is the uniaxial direction, $\gamma_{xy} = \gamma_{yz} = \gamma_{zx} = 0$ and $\sigma_y = \sigma_z = \tau_{xy} = \tau_{yz} = \tau_{zx} = 0$. This state of stress occurs predominantly in long, slender bodies of regular prismatic shape (bars or columns), which are loaded externally at the end by axial tension or compression, transverse forces, or bending moments. This state of stress is most often used for tensile or compressive tests to determine the Young's modulus and Poisson's ratio of isotropic materials.

Principal Stresses and Stress Tensors

If we rotate the cube in Fig. 14-A2 relative to a fixed coordinate system external to the object, the values of the stress components will change even though the stress state within the material remains the same. Thus, different components may describe the same stress state inside

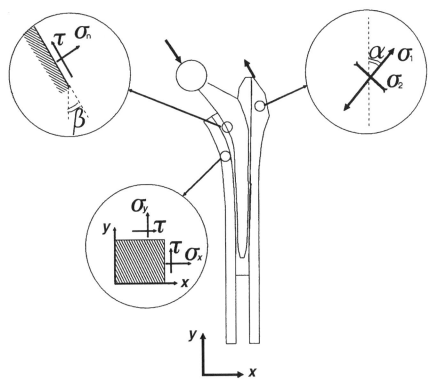

FIGURE 14-A3. The stress state in a point of a structure can be described in three ways: (i) principal stresses (σ_1, σ_2, and the principal-stress orientation α relative to the coordinate xy axes), (ii) coordinate stresses (σ_x, σ_y, and τ relative to a cube aligned with the coordinate axes), and (iii) interface stresses (compression/tension σ_n, normal to the interface, and shear τ, parallel to the interface, plus the orientation of the plane β). The principles of these representations are identical for three-dimensional stress states. One representation can directly and uniquely be converted to another by transformation of the coordinate system attitude.

the material. At one particular orientation of the cube, all shear-stress components acting on the face of the cube will vanish. This orientation defines the principal directions for the state of stress at the cube inside the material. The normal (perpendicular) stresses associated with this state are known as the *principal stresses*. For any arbitrary state of stress, the principal stresses are the maximal and minimal stresses at any point inside the object.

The state of stress is completely described by the six stress components. In its entirety, the state of stress is described as a stress tensor. Although the components may vary with the specific coordinate system chosen, the state of stress remains the same. In other words, the state of stress within an object does not depend on a specific

chosen coordinate system (i.e., observer). It depends solely on the loading, geometry, and material properties of the object. The simplest representations of a state of stress are either in the principal coordinate system or by the three principal normal stress components in an arbitrary coordinate system.

Bone–prosthesis structures often require stress information about *interfaces*, where different materials are connected. These interfaces do not always align with the external coordinate system, nor do they generally align with the principal stress directions. For that purpose, local coordinate systems at the point of interest can be introduced relative to which the interface normal and shear stresses are expressed. The three methods of stress representation (coordinate, principal, and interface stresses) are illustrated in Fig. 14-A3 for a 2D example.

Scalar Measures of Stress Intensity

The yield stress (or elastic limit) of a material is usually measured in uniaxial tensile and compressive or shear tests on material samples with simple geometric shapes. The question then is how to relate a 2D or 3D stress state, characterized by six stress components, to the yield stress data from uniaxial tests in order to estimate the probability of failure. For this purpose, an *equivalent* (or *effective*) *stress* is determined from a particular yield criterion. The von Mises yield criterion, for example, assumes that material will yield, i.e., deform plastically, when the distortion energy exceeds a certain value. The *von Mises stress* can be calculated from the equation

$$\sigma_{mi} = \left\{ \tfrac{1}{2} \left[(\sigma_1 - \sigma_2)^2 + (\sigma_1 - \sigma_3)^2 + (\sigma_2 - \sigma_3)^2 \right] \right\}^{1/2}$$

$$(A3)$$

where σ_1, σ_2, and σ_3 are the principal stress values in the material point of interest. This von Mises equivalent stress value can simply be compared with stress values obtained from samples of the material tested in the laboratory in uniaxial tension or compression to estimate the probability of failure. It gives reasonable predictions for isotropic materials. It works less satisfactorily for anisotropic elastic materials (such as bone) or viscoelastic materials. Still, it is often used for these materials as well to represent the six stress components in one generalized "stress intensity" factor, which greatly simplifies the interpretation and representation of results of stress analyses.

The *strain-energy density* (SED) also represents the stress state in a material but has not been directly related to a failure criterion. This quantity represents the elastic energy stored in the deformed material and can be calculated from the formula

$$U = \frac{1}{2}(\varepsilon_1 \sigma_1 + \varepsilon_2 \sigma_2 + \varepsilon_3 \sigma_3) \qquad (A4)$$

where ε_1, ε_2, and ε_3 and σ_1, σ_2, and σ_3 are the principal strains and stresses, respectively. This form of SED is valid only for isotropic materials, where the directions of principal strains and

principal stress are parallel. The SED function is commonly used to formulate nonlinearly elastic constitutive equations (hyperelastic materials). It is also used in strain-adaptive bone-remodeling theory.

Stress Analysis

Stress analysis in solid mechanics involves a particular structure with a given geometry made out of a particular material(s) with known elastic properties (i.e., Young's modulus and Poisson's ratio). The structure is loaded externally by forces and/or moments and is connected to the environment in a certain way. The objective of stress analysis may be to determine the stress and strain fields in the structure to see if the structure gives rise to excessive deformations or stresses that could cause mechanical failure.

Stress analysis may be conducted either numerically on a computer or with closed-form mathematical solutions. In the former case, a computer model is used, i.e., FEA. In the latter case, the solution is obtained in explicit mathematical formulas. These closed-form solutions are available only for particular, regularly shaped structures such as prismatic bars and beams. If applicable, closed-form solutions are always to be preferred over numerical ones because, in addition to the actual numerical results, they also render insight into the relationships among structural parameters, material properties, geometric factors, loads, and stress–strain patterns. As a rule, all calculated stresses and strains should be experimentally validated. Strains acting at the surface of a structure can be determined experimentally, either directly with measurements or indirectly using a laboratory model.

It is noted that the results of a stress analysis, whether experimental or analytical, depend on the model constructed to represent the structure. The accuracy of the stress and strain values obtained depends on the validity of the model used (i.e., geometry, constitutive equation for the material, material coefficients, loading conditions, and boundary conditions). Models are abstractions of reality, and they are used to simplify the actual problem. The essence of modeling is that

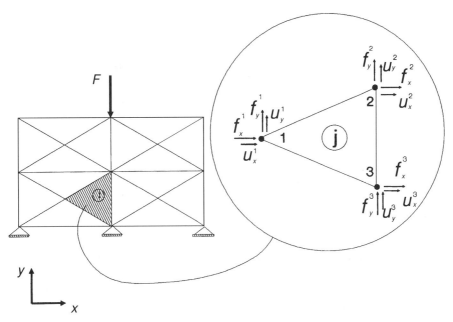

FIGURE 14-A4. A two-dimensional finite-element mesh and definition of nodal-point forces and nodal-point displacements.

each model must capture the salient characteristics of the problem appropriate to the needs of the situation. However, overly complex models are not necessarily better than simpler ones. There are no fixed rules for this modeling process. The question is never whether a model assumption is true in the real sense of the word (they almost never are) but whether a simplification is justified relative to the definition of the problem (A19).

Finite-element Analysis

FEA became a widely used method in orthopaedic biomechanics. It is a computer method suitable to determine stresses and strains at any given point inside a structure of arbitrary geometric and material complexity. A finite-element model relies on accurate constitutive representations of material characteristics (such as the elastic coefficients of generalized Hooke's law), geometric data, loading characteristics, and boundary and interfacial conditions. The principles of FEA are described in many textbooks (e.g., A16,A41). Attempts at more general introductions to FEA, particularly for orthopaedic biomechanics, have been published elsewhere (A19,A21,A26). Only the basic principles and a few pitfalls are reviewed here. To develop an FEA model, the shape of the structure to be analyzed is divided into small elements. For 3D analysis, elemental volumes of a particular shape (e.g., bricks) are used, and for a 2D analysis, elemental areas of a particular shape (e.g., triangles or quadrilaterals) are used. Each element has nodal points, usually at the corners of the element. At each nodal point three (or two in the case of 2D analysis) displacement components and three force components (two in a 2D analysis) are identified.

As an illustrative example, consider a 2D model with triangular elements, each with three nodal points (Fig. 14-A4). The displacement vector **u** and force vector **f** at each nodal point i can be written in terms of their components, as

$$\boldsymbol{u}^i = \begin{bmatrix} u_x^i \\ u_y^i \end{bmatrix} \boldsymbol{f}^i = \begin{bmatrix} f_x^i \\ f_x^i \end{bmatrix} (i = 1,2,3) \quad \text{(A5)}$$

For the entire structure with n elements, these

vectors at the *j*th element may be written as

$$\boldsymbol{u}^j = \begin{bmatrix} u^1 \\ u^2 \\ u^3 \end{bmatrix} = \begin{bmatrix} u_x^1 \\ u_y^1 \\ u_x^2 \\ u_y^2 \\ u_x^3 \\ u_y^3 \end{bmatrix} \quad \boldsymbol{f}^j = \begin{bmatrix} f_x^1 \\ f_y^1 \\ f_x^2 \\ f_y^2 \\ f_x^3 \\ f_y^3 \end{bmatrix} \quad (j=1,\ldots,n) \quad (A6)$$

where *n* is the total number of elements in the mesh. When the material of the element is linearly elastic, and the deformations are small relative to the dimensions of the element, there is a linear relationship between the nodal point force and the nodal point displacement components, which may be written in vector notation as

$$\mathbf{f}^j = \mathbf{Q}^j \mathbf{u}^j \qquad (A7)$$

Here $\mathbf{Q}^j$ is called the *stiffness matrix* of the *j*th element and consists of 6×6 components. Let us assume for a moment that the values of all these 36 components are known for every one of the elements. The structure is then numerically assembled, in the sense that all displacements and forces of the different elements belonging to the same nodal point are collected. Then one vector, **u**, is formed in which all displacement components in all the nodal points are collected, and one vector, **f**, is formed that contains all force components in all nodal points. Hence, we obtain an equation of the form

$$\mathbf{f} = \mathbf{Q}\mathbf{u} \qquad (A8)$$

where **Q** is the $m \times m$ stiffness matrix for the whole construction containing m^2 components, and *m* is the number of degrees of freedom in the model (usually $2n$ for a 2D model or $3n$ if the model is 3D). The value of each component is known from the assembling procedure. By Newton's third law of action and reaction, many of the force components at nodal points are zero. Hence, the components of the nodal-point force vector **f** are zero where no external force is applied, have a known value where external forces are applied, or are unknown where boundary constraints are applied. The components of the nodal point displacement vector **u** where the boundary conditions are applied are either unknown where the forces are prescribed or known where the displacements are prescribed. Hence, for each component (degree of freedom) at each nodal point, either the displacement is known or the force is known. In other words, Eq. A8 is a system of *m* linear, algebraic equations with *m* unknowns and hence can be solved to give the values of all displacements in all nodal points.

To determine the components of the stiffness matrices in Eq. A8, we must go back to the individual element and Eq. A7. We assume that the deformation in each element takes a specific form in such a way that the deformation within the element is determined by the relative displacements of the nodal points. For instance, the strain distribution in each element may be assumed to be uniform. This assumption makes possible the determination of the components of the element stiffness matrix from the volume of the element and its shape, elastic modulus, and Poisson's ratio. It also makes it possible to determine the strain in each element from the nodal point displacements and subsequently the stress in the element from Hooke's law.

In developing the FEA code as described earlier, we have made two important simplifications. First, we have limited the admissible deformation of each element to a uniform strain pattern (i.e., a linear displacement field) within the element. Second, we have assumed that all load transmission between elements is concentrated in the nodal points. Thus, all results obtained are approximate. In fact, the accuracy of the approximation depends on the kind of elements used and on the degree of mesh refinement. When the element density approaches infinity, the results converge to the exact solution.

Today, using the finite-element method is much simpler than suggested earlier because most of the work is done by readily available computer codes. The art of FEA now is really concerned with the development of the FEA model and the interpretation of its results rather than with the performance of the calculations. However, the development of an adequate FE model for a hip reconstruction is still not a trivial matter (A19). Of course, building a 3D anatomically realistic mesh is a lot more time consuming and complicated than building a 2D mesh. In the 3D case there could be significant restrictions on the maximal number of elements and nodal points used, depending on the capacity of the computer available. This is more problematic in prosthetic analysis because joint reconstructions are composite structures. For example, some parts of the composites have very small dimensions (e.g., acrylic cement layers) and require small elements. As a consequence of mesh continuity requirements, the adjacent material also needs relatively small elements, which increases the total number of elements in the structure. Potential solutions to this problem are limited by requirements for the minimal element aspect ratio; a brick element, for instance, that is relatively thin is said to be distorted and to produce errors.

When the mesh is constructed, the computer code needs external loading characteristics, elastic constants for each element, and specifications for the boundary and composite interface conditions. This again is not a trivial step in the process of modeling THR reconstructions because, as discussed above, these characteristics tend to vary greatly in a patient population and over time, and in general they are not known precisely. Hence, in order to analyze some of the problems, again, simplifying approximations must be used.

Geometry and FE Mesh

The FE mesh itself accounts for the geometry or shape of the arthroplasty components. Conceptually, every detail of the structures can be taken into account by using sufficiently small elements, but in practice this is hardly feasible; hence, the problem must be schematized to some degree. The refinement to which the structure is described by the mesh depends on the kind of information required (A19). A simplified alternative to a 3D model is a 2D one, representing the mid-frontal plane only. Such a model is quite easily assembled. However, it ignores the 3D elastic integrity of the bone.

In initiating an FE analysis, it is not advisable to immediately start developing the most expensive and complex model. As in all scientific endeavors, it is imperative to stop and think first what it is one wishes to accomplish and tune the model to those requirements. This, of course, requires an understanding of the relationships between model features and potential results.

Increasingly, FEA meshes of bones and THA structures are produced on the basis of geometric assessments from serial CT scanning. The CT delivers a 3D voxel mesh of density values from which the shape of the bone can be graphically reconstructed using contour detection algorithms. The graphic reconstruction then serves as a basis for the element mesh (A20,A23,A24). Advantages of this procedure are that mesh generation can be automated to some extent and that the apparent density of the bone material, by approximation related to its elastic modulus, is evaluated as well. Apart from this latter advantage and the convenience of the nondestructive geometric assessment, the problem of adequate mesh generation in a 3D volume remains. This problem can be solved with voxel-conversion methods (A15, A32).

In principle, each voxel from a CT scan can be converted directly into a cubic element. The cube corners provide the coordinates of the nodal points, and the voxel density its elastic modulus. In fact, the whole mesh is available by the time the CT scan is made, ready for FEA. An example of such a mesh of a THA structure is shown in Fig. 14-A5. There are, however, disadvantages to this efficient procedure: The number of elements may be excessive, and the boundaries of the model are ragged instead of smooth. As was shown in comparative tests, the ragged boundaries hardly affect the mechanical behavior of a model at large. This implies that although the stress values calculated at the boundary are not dependable, those within the material are precise (A14,A22). The problem of excessive numbers of elements can be solved with alternative FEA solution procedures that apply iterative optimization schemes. Examples are the element-by-element (EBE) procedure (A13,A17) and the row-by-row (RBR) procedure (A35,A36). The RBR procedure uses the fact that each element in the mesh has the same shape, dimension, and

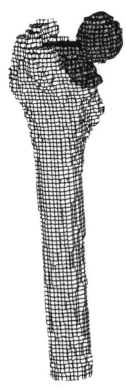

FIGURE 14-A5. Voxel model of an implanted femur. (Adapted from Skinner HB, Kilgus DJ, Keyak J, et al. Correlation of computed finite element stresses to bone density after remodeling around cementless femoral implants. *Clin Orthop* 1994;305:178–189.)

orientation, such that only a limited number of possible environments can exist. This makes the procedure much more efficient than EBE; hence, more elements can be used in the mesh. The RBR procedure does require each element to have the same elastic constants, which is not the case for EBE.

Global versus Local Mechanical Quantities

In many FE analyses of THA structures, local information about mechanical quantities is required. For example, one may need to evaluate the strength requirements of thin prosthetic coatings or study the stress environment of bone growing into pores. In such cases, the ratio between the typical volume to be studied and the dimensions of the whole THA structure may be

on the order of 10^3. An adequate FEA mesh for such a problem would imply too many elements for any computer. A traditional solution for this problem is to use FEA models for different levels, applying the local nodal-point forces of a global model as boundary conditions for a local one. The precision of this method is questionable, however, because the stiffness characteristics of the local model are usually not equal to those of the corresponding volume in the global model. As a result, equal nodal-point forces produce different deformation patterns (nodal-point displacements). This problem can be solved by the application of homogenization theory (A3,A12,A15). In homogenization theory, a representative volume element (RVE) is produced from the stiffness characteristics of a local volume of interest, evaluated with an FEA micromodel. The homogenized stiffness matrix of the RVE is substituted in the global mesh to determine its deformation characteristics, which then later serve as boundary conditions for an FEA of the local model, producing the local stresses and strains.

Loads

An FEA requires a numerical description of all external loads applied on the structure (point of application, magnitude, direction). These loads are usually variable and not always precisely known (A1,A7), so the question in FEA is often which approach to take in order to obtain useful information. A consideration always helpful is that FE analysis allows for easy parametric variation. Hence, the loads can be varied and the results studied in order to determine their relationships, and a "worst-case" situation can be defined. Often the worst-case (or typical-case) configuration is selected a priori from different possibilities. In such cases, it is advisable to investigate the sensitivity of the stress patterns to small deviations in the external loads. If different prosthetic designs are compared, different FEA meshes are needed. Consequently, it is not trivial that the 3D coordinates of the points where the external loads are applied are equal in all cases. Hence, the effects of different geometries on the stress and strain patterns are obscured by

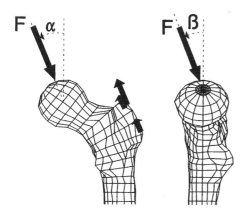

FIGURE 14-A6. The proximal part of a finite-element model of a femoral bone. A set of three joint forces and three muscle forces can be selected, which represent typical daily loading configurations. Orientation is shown; values are listed in Table 14-A1.

variations in load application location. Defining invariable points that are used to apply the external forces can repair this.

A set of three femoral loading cases can be considered that together represent average daily activities (Fig. 14-A6; Table 14-A1). Their magnitudes and directions have been chosen from telemetric measurements by Bergmann et al. (A1) and Kotzar et al. (A25) and are scaled for a person of 65 kg weight. The first two loading cases represent the peak joint forces that develop during the stance phase of normal walking (A1,A25), and the third loading case represents the maximal joint load during stair climb-

ing (A25). The first loading case has the largest joint force (2,132 N), whereas the third loading case has the largest out-of-plane component of this force. The insertions, orientations, and magnitudes of the corresponding forces in the three major muscles, the m. gluteus mimimus, the m. gluteus medius, and the m. gluteus maximus, have been taken from the work of Crowninshield and Brand (A4) and Dostal and Andrews (A8).

Hip joint and muscle loads working at the acetabulum reconstruction during gait have been specified for FEA analysis by Dalstra et al. (A6), based on data from the same authors as just mentioned for the femur.

Another approach to load selection is using representative loading cases. This approach is especially useful when the effects of particular design features of a prosthesis are to be studied in a comparative analysis, or when load-transfer mechanisms are to be studied. For instance, relative to femoral THA, the effects of the hip joint force may be separated into those resulting from the axial force, bending, and torsional components. The problem can then be analyzed for those three cases separately or for just the most important one. Finally, it is important to realize that most FEA models of implant structures use infinitesimal linear elastic theory and that their surfaces are perfectly bonded at the interfaces. In these models, the principle of superposition may be used. Hence, the stress patterns that result from the application of the hip joint force and the muscle forces together can be found from adding the results obtained from treating those forces separately. This is no longer possible when loose prosthetic components are analyzed, or when nonlinear (viscoelastic) tissues are included.

Material Properties

In the FEA model, each element must be assigned the appropriate elastic constants of the material. For an isotropic linearly elastic material, two material constants are required, e.g., Young's modulus and Poisson's ratio. This is the case for metallic implant materials. Acrylic cement and plastic components may be included in this category only by rough approximation

TABLE 14-A1. MAGNITUDES AND ORIENTATIONS OF HIP AND MUSCLE FORCES FOR THREE LOAD CASES (SEE FIG. 14-A6)

	Joint Force	M. Glut. Max.	M. Glut. Med.	M. Glut. Min.
F_1 (N)	2132	637	637	214.5
α_1 (°)	23.4	39.9	24.6	28.4
β_1 (°)	5.7	43.0	24.8	28.4
F_2 (N)	1586	45.5	739	143
α_2 (°)	21.9	28.2	20.8	25.1
β_2 (°)	−4.6	24.3	10.5	1.9
F_3 (N)	1690	637	637	214.5
α_3 (°)	25	63.8	42.5	42.0
β_3 (°)	−15	62.0	57.7	55.1

TABLE 14-A2. INDICATIVE VALUES OF YOUNG'S MODULI AND STATIC STRENGTHS FOR MOST MATERIALS AND INTERFACES USED IN THR RECONSTRUCTION

	Young's Modulus	Static Strength
CoCr alloy	200–200 GPa	800–1000 GPa under tension
Titanium	100–130 GPa	800–1500 GPa under tension
Acrylic cement (PMMA)	2–3 GPa	100 MPa under compression
		25–40 MPa under tension
UHMWPE	1 GPa	20–30 MPa under tension
Cortical bone	15–20 GPa	20–50 MPa under tension
		150–200 MPa under compression
Cancellous bone	500–1500 MPa	3–10 MPa under compression
Fibrous tissue	1 MPa	
Metal-acrylic–cement interface		5–8 MPa under shear
		5–10 MPa under tension
Hydroxylapatite–bone interface		30–50 MPa under shear
Acrylic cement–bone interface		2–4 MPa under shear
		7–10 MPa under tension

(A28). Cortical bone, by reasonable approximation, can be considered as linearly elastic and transversely isotropic, requiring five elastic constants for a complete description of its stress–strain relationship (A2,A30). The elastic relationship for cortical bone can also be simplified from transverse isotropy if the stresses and strains in the transverse and tangential directions are of lesser importance for the problem investigated.

Modeling cancellous bone is more complicated. To the first-order approximation, its elastic modulus can be expressed as a function of its porosity, measured by its apparent density. If a volume V (cm^3) weighs w (g) without the fatty marrow, then the apparent density is defined by $\rho = w/V$ (g/cm^3). The relationship between apparent density and the elastic modulus can be empirically defined by (A2a)

$$E = C\rho^\alpha \qquad (A9)$$

where C and α are constants; α is somewhere between 2 and 3, probably closer to 2 (A31). The elastic properties of cancellous bone also depend on the directionality of its structure, which can be the cause for anisotropic behavior (A10,A34). The elastic constants of trabecular bone can be determined fully from measurements of its volume fraction, fabric, and degree of tissue mineralization (A9,A31,A34,A35,A37). Of course, the elastic bone properties can be highly variable, depending on location and individual factors such as the degree of mineralization and osteoporosis (A5); see also Chapter 4.

To perform an FEA, information about strength of materials is not needed. However, this information is required for the interpretation of results. In Table 14-A2, indicative values for Young's moduli and the static strengths of the most important materials and interfaces used in THA are listed.

Nonlinear and Time-dependent Materials

A bone–prosthesis structure can behave in a nonlinear elastic manner when one or more of its materials have nonlinear elastic properties, when deformations are large relative to the characteristic dimensions of the structure, or when its interfaces are not rigidly bonded (A39,A40). Examples of essentially nonlinear materials are collageneous tissues such as fibrous tissue membranes, articular cartilage, and ligaments. Finite deformation nonlinearity is illustrated in Fig. 14-A7. Here a post consisting of two materials, a relatively stiff one with elastic modulus E' and length l_0 and a relatively soft and thin one with modulus E and thickness d_0, is considered. The cross-sectional area of the post is A, and the post is loaded by a uniformly distributed compressive force F over the thin layer.

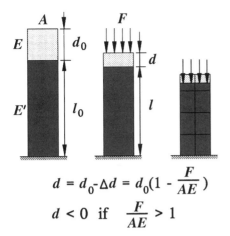

$$d = d_0 - \Delta d = d_0 \left(1 - \frac{F}{AE}\right)$$

$$d < 0 \quad \text{if} \quad \frac{F}{AE} > 1$$

FIGURE 14-A7. A post consisting of a relatively rigid material (E') and a flexible layer (E) is compressed by a force F. If the ratio $F/AE > 1$, a linear analysis of the problem will predict a negative thickness of the soft layer.

By simple linear elastic theory for uniaxial compression, it can easily be shown that in the deformed state, the length of the rigid post will reduce to

$$l = l_0 - l_0 F/AE' = l_0(1 - F/AE') \quad (A10)$$

and the thickness of the layer will reduce to

$$d = d_0 - d_0 F/AE = d_0(1 - F/AE) \quad (A11)$$

Let us now assume that $A = 100$ mm^2, $F = 1000$ N, $E' = 100$ MPa, and $E = 5$ MPa. It follows that $l = 0.9\ l_0$, indicating a reduction in length of 10%. It also follows that $d = d_0 - 2d_0 = -d_0$, which implies a negative thickness of the soft thin layer! The reason for this unrealistic result is that the problem was treated as if it were linear and that infinitesimal strain assumptions remained valid. For finite deformation problems, the simple infinitesimal strain tensor must be replaced by finite deformation tensors, and an appropriate elastic constitutive law must be used. Constitutive laws for soft materials such as rubber and cartilage have been developed. A general feature of these laws is that they allow for the stiffness of the thin layer to gradually increase with increasing compressive load.

Similar problems occur with linear FEA of bone–prosthesis structures where thin layers of a low modulus exist next to more rigid materials (A40). Thus, to analyze the fibrous tissue lining between bone and prostheses, a more complex FEA code is required. If a structure behaves nonlinearly, FEA must be performed in a stepwise fashion by increasing the external loads in small increments from zero until the desired end values are reached. The stiffness matrix in such an algorithm is updated with every increment of load. Hence, instead of solving Eq. A8, one must solve

$$\Delta \mathbf{f} = \mathbf{Q} \Delta \mathbf{u} \quad (A10)$$

for each increment of load (A11,A16,A41).

In a linear analysis, the external load is applied in one step because the deformations are always linearly related to the magnitude of the load. In a nonlinear analysis, one in fact simulates a process of structural deformation by gradually applied external loads, which introduces a time factor. If materials behave in a time-dependent way, the rate of the process becomes a factor of significance as well. Examples of such materials are viscoelastic ones (e.g., biphasic interface soft tissues) or plastics susceptible to creep or cold flow (e.g., PMMA and PE). The strategy for the solutions of these problems is similar to the above, in the sense that the process of deformation is simulated iteratively, updating the stiffness matrix in every iteration, depending on the time development of material constitutive parameters (A27,A29,A38).

Boundary and Interface Conditions

The boundary conditions for the FEA model are imposed on the exterior surfaces of the object. The boundaries can be divided into free, loaded, and fixed boundaries. At a free boundary, no stress (or load) is transferred, and it is not constrained by a connecting structure. At a loaded boundary, external loads are applied. At a fixed boundary, no motion is allowed, or the motion is constrained by some surrounding structure. The last ones are usually those where the FEA model is cut off from the environment with which it normally interacts. The

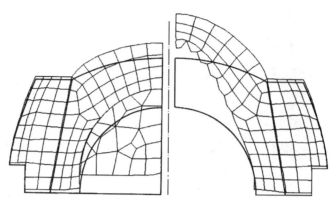

FIGURE 14-A8. Deformations determined by a finite-element model of an acetabular cup–bone composite structure (displacements are magnified to allow for visualization). When the femoral head is included in the model, the load transmission problem is a contact problem (*left*). In this case, the displacements at the surface of the cup are compatible. When the external force is applied directly on the inner surface of the cup with an assumed stress distribution, the resulting surface displacements may not be compatible with the form of the femoral head.

characteristics of this interaction must be accounted for by introducing prescribed displacements in the appropriate nodal points. This is not always easily realized, and as a result, artifacts can be introduced in the stress patterns near those boundaries. This is not a problem as long as the boundary region is remote from the region of interest.

Some problems that boundaries sometimes may present are illustrated in the example of Fig. 14-A8, where an FEA is applied to an acetabular THA component. The right side of Fig. 14-A8 represents the case in which the cup is assumed to be loaded internally by a distributed force, representing its interaction with an artificial metallic femoral head. The resulting surface deformation is shown (exaggerated to make it visible). Evidently, this is not a realistic representation because the inner cup boundary would in reality be forced to conform itself to the spherical contour of the stiff metallic femoral head. This problem can be solved by including the metal head in the FE model (left side of Fig. 14-A8) and allowing only compressive stress to be transferred at the head-cup connection as in a contact problem. To do this, the hip joint load is applied to the stem, and the femoral head then transfers the load to the cup in such a way that the head

is constrained to be in contact with the cup at all times.

At a connection (or interface) between two materials, which can be described as a surface, we can find stress transfer or relative motion, or a combination of both (Fig. 14-A9). The stress transferred across the connecting surface can be represented by a normal stress (σ_n) perpendicular to the plane (tension or compression) and two shear-stress components (τ_1 and τ_2). The relative motions can also be characterized by three relative displacement components, u_n in the normal direction and u_1 and u_2 in the tangential directions. Various conditions at the boundary may now be written as follows:

- Bonded interfaces:

$$\sigma_n \neq 0, \tau_1 \neq 0, \tau_2 \neq 0, \text{ and } u_n = u_1 = u_2 = 0$$
$$(A11)$$

- Loose interfaces without friction:

$$\tau_1 = \tau_2 = 0, \sigma_n \leq 0 \text{ (i.e., } \sigma_n \text{ can only be compressive)}$$
$$u_n \geq 0 \text{ (i.e., } u_n \text{ can only be separation), } u_n \neq 0, u_2 \neq 0$$
$$(A12)$$

- Loose interfaces with Coulomb friction:

$$\sigma_n \geq 0, \left(\tau_1^2 + \tau_2^2\right)^{1/2} \leq \mu|\sigma_n|, \text{ where } \mu \text{ is the Coulomb coefficient of friction,}$$
$$u_n \geq 0, u_1 \neq 0, u_2 \neq 0$$
$$(A13)$$

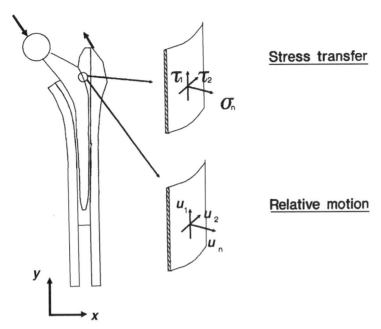

FIGURE 14-A9. Normal stress (σ_n) and shear stress (τ_1, τ_2) components transferred across a bonded interface. Normal (u_n) and tangential (u_1, u_2) displacement components are relative motions that may occur if the interface is unbonded.

When interfaces are unbonded and hence loose without friction (Eq. A12) or loose with friction (Eq. A13), the problem becomes nonlinear and must be solved iteratively, using load increments. For this purpose, most FE packages use the so-called gap elements to account for separation and sliding of the surfaces. The load transfer from intramedullary implants (e.g., hip stems) is affected more dramatically by interface conditions than by any other structural parameter, in particular when comparing a fully bonded with a fully unbonded case (A18).

REFERENCES

A1. Bergmann G, Graichen A, Rohlmann A. Hip joint loading during walking and running, measured in two patients. *J Biomech* 1993;26:969–990.

A2. Carter DR. Anisotropic analysis of strain rosette information from cortical bone. *J Biomech* 1978;11:199–202.

A2a. Carter DR, Hayes WC. The behavior of bone as a two-phase porous structure. *J Bone Joint Surg* 1977;59-A:954–962.

A3. Crolet JM, Aoubiza B, Meunier A. Compact bone: numerical simulation of mechanical characteristics. *J Biomech* 1993;26:677–689.

A4. Crowninshield RD, Brand RA. A physiologically based criterion of muscle force prediction in locomotion. *J Biomech* 1981;14:793–801.

A5. Currey JD. *Bones: structure and mechanics.* Princeton, NJ: Princeton University Press, 2002.

A6. Dalstra M, Huiskes R, Van Erning L. Development and validation of a three-dimensional finite-element model of the pelvic bone. *J Biomech Eng* 1995;117:272–278.

A7. Davy DT, Kotzar GM, Brown RH, et al. Telemetric force measurements across the hip after total arthroplasty. *J Bone Joint Surg* 1988;70-Am:45–50.

A8. Dostal WF, Andrews JF. A three dimensional biomechanical model of hip musculature. *J Biomech* 1981;14:802–881.

A9. Goulet RW, Goldstein SA, Ciarelli MJ, et al. The relationship between the structural and orthogonal compressive properties of trabecular bone. *J Biomech* 1994;27:375–389.

A10. Hayes WC, Snyder B. Toward a quantitative formulation of Wolff's law in trabecular bone. In: Cowin SC, ed. *Mechanical properties of bone.* New York: Am Soc Mech Engrs (ASME), 1981;45-AMD:43–69.

A11. Hinton E. *NAFEMS introduction to nonlinear finite element analysis.* Glasgow: Bell and Bain, 1992.

A12. Hollister SJ, Fyhrie DP, Jepsen KJ, et al. Application of homogenization theory to the study of trabecular bone mechanics. *J Biomech* 1991;24:825–839.

A13. Hollister SJ, Kikuchi N. Direct analysis of trabecular bone stiffness and tissue level mechanics using an element-by-element homogenization method. *Trans ORS* 1992;38:559.

A14. Hollister SJ, Brennan JM, Kikuchi N. Homogenization sampling analysis of trabecular bone microstructural mechanics. In: Middleton J, Pande GN, Williams KR, eds. *Recent advances in computer methods in biomechanics and biomedical engineering.* Swanswea, UK: Books & Journals Int. 1992:308–317.

A15. Hollister SJ, Brennan JM, Kikuchi N. A homogenization sampling prodedure for calculating trabecular bone effective stiffness and tissue level stress. *J Biomech* 1994;27:433–444.

A16. Hughes TJR. *The finite element method: linear static and dynamic finite element analysis.* Upper Saddle River, NJ: Prentice-Hall, 1987.

A17. Hughes JR, Ferencz RM, Hallquist JO. Large-scale vectorized implicit calculations in solid mechancs on a cray S-MP/48 utilizing EBE preconditioned conjugate gradients. *Comp Meth Appl Mech Eng* 1987;61:215–248.

A18. Huiskes R. The various stress patterns of press-fit, ingrown and cemented femoral stems. *Clin Orthop* 1990;261:27–38.

A19. Huiskes R, Chao EYS. A survey of finite element methods in orthopaedic biomechanics. *J Biomech* 1983;16:385–409.

A20. Huiskes R, Weinans H, Van Rietbergen B. The relationship between stress shielding and bone resoption around total hip stems and the effects of flexible materials. *Clin Orthop* 1992;272:124–134.

A21. Huiskes R, Hollister SJ. From structure to process, from organ to cell: recent developments of FE-analysis in orthopaedic biomechancics. *J Biomech Eng* 1993;115:520–527.

A22. Jacobs CR, Mandell JA, Beaupré GS. A comparative study of automatic finite element mesh generation techniques in orthopaedic biomechanics. *ASME* 1993;24:512–514.

A23. Kang YK, Park HC, Youm Y, et al. Three dimensional shape reconstruction and finite element analysis of femur before and after the cementless type of total hip replacement. *J Biomed Eng* 1993;15:497–504.

A24. Keyak JH, Meagher JM, Skinner HB, et al. Automated three-dimensional finite element modelling of bone: a new method. *J Biomed Eng* 1990;12:389–397.

A25. Kotzar GM, Davy DT, Goldberg VM, et al. Telemetrized *in vivo* hip joint force data: a report on two patients after total hip surgery. *J Orthop Res* 1991;9:621–633.

A26. Mackerle J. Finite and boundary element methods in biomechanics: a bibliography. *Eng Comput* 1992;9:403–435.

A27. Mow VC, Ateshian GA, Spilker RL. Biomechanics of diathrodial joints: a review of twenty years of progress. *J Biomech Eng* 1993;115:460–467.

A28. Pal S, Saha S. Stress relaxation and creep behaviour of normal and carbon fibre reinforced acrylic bone cement. *Biomaterials* 1982;3:93–95.

A29. Prendergast PJ, Huiskes R, Sballe K. Biophysical stimuli during tissue differentiation at implant interfaces. *J Biomech* 1997;30:539–548.

A30. Reilly DT, Burstein AH. The elastic and ultimate properties of compact bone tissue. *J Biomed Eng* 1975;8:393–405.

A31. Rice JC, Cowin SC, Bowman JA. On the dependence of the elasticity and strength of cancellous bone on apparent density. *J Biomech* 1988;21:155–168.

A32. Schneider E, Kinast C, Eulenberger J, et al. A comparative study of the initial stability of cementless hip prostheses. *Clin Orthop* 1989;248:200–209.

A33. Skinner HB, Kilgus DJ, Keyak J, et al. Correlation of computed finite element stresses to bone density after remodeling around cementless femoral implants. *Clin Orthop* 1994;305:178–189.

A34. Turner CH, Cowin SC, Rho JY, et al. The fabric dependence of the orthotropic elastic constants of cancellous bone. *J Biomech* 1990;23:549–561.

A35. Van Rietbergen B, Weinans H, Huiskes R, et al. A new method to determine trabecular bone elastic properties and loading using micromechanial finite element models. *J Biomech* 1995;28:69–81.

A36. Van Rietbergen B, Weinans H, Polman BJW, et al. Computational strategies for iterative solutions of large FEM applications employing voxel data. *Int J Num Meth Eng* 1996;39:2743–2767.

A37. Van Rietbergen B, Odgaard A, Kabel J, et al. Relationships between bone morphology and bone elastic properties can be accurately quantified using high-resolution computer reconstructions. *J Orthop Res* 1996;16:23–28.

A38. Verdonschot N, Huiskes R. Dynamic creep behavior of acrylic bone cement. *J Biomed Mater Res* 1995;29:575–581.

A39. Verdonschot N, Huiskes R. Mechanical effects of stem–cement interface characteristics in total hip replacement. *Clin Orthop* 1996;329:326–336.

A40. Weinans H, Huiskes R, Grootenboer HJ. Trends of mechanical consequences and modeling of a fibrous membrane around femoral hip prostheses. *J Biomech* 1990;23:991–1000.

A41. Zienkiewicz OC, Taylor RL. *The finite element method,* 5th ed. Oxford, UK: Butterworth-Heinemann, 2002.

BIOMECHANICS OF TOTAL KNEE REPLACEMENT DESIGNS

PETER S. WALKER

1 THE EVOLUTION OF TKR DESIGNS

Before the late 1960s, the treatments for arthritis of the knee were osteotomy, the interposition of metallic femoral condyles or tibial blocks, and uncemented metal hinges (192). In 1969, a cemented metal-plastic condylar replacement, the "polycentric," was developed by Gunston (76). This design, using the same cemented metal–plastic technology as that developed for the hip by Charnley, was the forerunner of the modern-day condylar replacements. Since that time, the term *total knee replacement* (TKR) has taken on a broad meaning encompassing the replacement of the femoral, tibial, and patello-femoral bearing surfaces, even including the complete mechanical replacement of the joint surfaces and ligaments with fixed and rotating hinges (Fig. 15-1). However, the large majority

of TKRs used today are condylar replacements, consisting of the following:

- A cobalt–chrome alloy femoral component of generally anatomical shape replacing the femoral condyles and the patella trochlea.
- A cobalt–chrome alloy or titanium alloy tibial tray to be affixed to the upper tibia.
- An ultrahigh-molecular-weight polyethylene (UHMWPE) tibial bearing component to be fixed into the tibial tray (in some variants, the entire tibial component is made from UHMWPE).
- An UHMWPE patella component (in some cases with a metal backing).

Within the category of condylar replacements are designs that preserve the posterior cruciate ligament (PCL) and that require resection, often substituting for its function by an intercondylar cam. Another notable condylar type is a meniscal

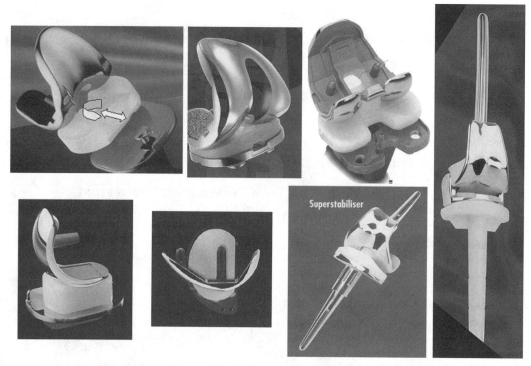

FIGURE 15-1. Examples of total knee replacements. (*Left*) Mobile bearing; (*left center*) condylar replacement, patella button, and Unicondylar; (*right center*) posterior stabilized and constrained condylar (superstabilized); (*right*) rotating hinge.

or mobile-bearing knee, where the plastic bearing component rotates and/or slides on the surface of the tibial tray. A compartmental replacement, or "uni," consists of components for only the medial or lateral side of the knee (167). In parallel with the design of TKRs (193) has been the development of instrumentation and techniques that have had as much influence on the clinical outcome as the TKR components themselves.

Starting in the 1970s, TKR development has been an evolutionary process, using intuitive design, empirical data, and laboratory studies (156). Paradoxically, some of the designs introduced in the 1970s have had successful long-term results, whereas some introduced more recently have exhibited serious problems. One might expect that a methodical design process would have been more routinely employed, leading to increasingly successful designs. However, there are a number of reasons why this has not been the case, or even possible. There has some-

times been too much reliance on introducing new design features on an intuitive basis, without adequate evaluation and testing. Even where design goals are rigorously specified, data on the mechanical conditions under which TKRs operate are incomplete. Finally, suitable testing methods have been insufficiently developed, or appropriate equipment has not been available.

The goals of TKR design include relief of pain, restoration of function, durability for the life of the patient, and reliability. However, in order to utilize such goals for design purposes, their biomechanical implications must be specified (Table 15-1). The criteria are targets against which a particular design can be measured. Any design solution can then be optimized to closely meet these ideal criteria.

The classical design approach is to identify a need, specify the objectives or goals, formulate different solutions, and select the solution most closely satisfying the objectives. Analysis and testing may be necessary to narrow down the

TABLE 15-1. FUNCTIONAL GOALS AND THE ASSOCIATED BIOMECHANICAL CRITERIA

Goals	Biomechanical Criteria
Relief of pain	Replacement of all articulating surfaces. Interface micromotion <50 μm between components and bone.
Restoration of function	Similar motion characteristics as in the normal knee. Soft tissue lengths within normal range. Similar laxity characteristics as in the normal knee. The same or larger muscle lever arms as normal.
Durability	Normal stresses at the interface and within the surrounding bone. Minimal wear of the articulating surfaces (<0.05 mm depth per year).
Reliability	Insensitive to misalignment or size mismatch. Function insensitive to different kinetics of patients.

selection process. Subsequently, further analysis and testing will be necessary to optimize and validate the final design. This process parallels the "Total Design" approach of Pugh (149), or the "Axiomatic Design" concepts of Suh (182). The process up to the point of surgical implantation is termed the "preclinical phase." Design tools may include computer modeling, kinematic studies, fixation evaluation, strength testing, and wear measurement. Evaluations during the "clinical phase" include functional assessment, radiographic evaluations, and kinematic studies including gait analysis. Hence, the complete design process includes both the preclinical and clinical phases.

There are several important limitations in the design process, however, which apply to most design problems in biomedical engineering. The forces and kinematics are not known with any certainty, and in any case vary from patient to patient. The properties of the structures into which the artificial joints are implanted and their subsequent remodeling are variable, while the remodeling rules for the biological materials are known only in general terms. The geometry of the bones and soft tissues is highly variable. Finally, there is a variability introduced by the surgical procedure and its implementation.

The development of validated preclinical design and evaluation methods has made steady progress. The most widely used numerical method has been finite-element analysis, applied to strength and contact stress analysis, as well as for the prediction of bone remodeling. Some models have included rules for bone remodeling and used iteration to predict the final stable situation. Cadaveric studies in various test machines have been used to study kinematics and ligament function. Cyclic load fatigue testing and long-term wear testing on joint simulators are essential parts of a TKR design project. All of these evaluation methods should be regarded as part of the design process as much as for final evaluation.

The degree to which clinical application constitutes "an experiment" depends on how many new features there are. In general, a clinical trial must be regarded as a necessary part of the experimental plan to test the design hypothesis and to determine whether design modification is necessary. The surgical technique should be included in this evaluation. The reason is that it is impossible to predict clinical outcomes with any certainty and even small design changes may have a negative effect. Herein lies an important difference between designing engineering components that can be tested under service conditions before being released generally, and developing implants for which there is invariably an element of risk in the first implantations. Predictive methods of clinical evaluation, where measurements taken in the short term predict a longer-term outcome, are particularly valuable.

2 BASIC DATA FOR DESIGN AND EVALUATION

2.1 Definitions of Motion

The knee has six degrees of freedom, namely:

Rotations: Flexion–extension (FE), varus–valgus (VV), internal–external (IE)

Displacements: Anterior–posterior (AP), medial–lateral (ML), proximal–distal (PD)

To quantify these motions during a range of flexion, Cartesian axis systems need to be defined in each bone with respect to well-defined bony landmarks. The motion from an initial reference position to a final position consists of sequence-dependent rotations called Eulerian or Cardan angles. A suitable order of rotation is flexion, varus, and internal rotation. In addition there is a displacement vector consisting of the x, y, and z coordinates of the origin of the femur with respect to the origin of the tibia, the coordinates being in the tibial reference frame. This system preserves the meaning of the degrees of freedom with respect to the commonly used orthopaedic terms stated above. Grood and Suntay (75) described a similar system for defining motions but where the rotations were sequence independent.

Many other methods have been used to describe three-dimensional (3D) motion. Blankevoort et al. (23) used the screw axis, but this is difficult to visualize and to relate to orthopaedic definitions. Churchill et al. (42) described motion by the femur rotating about a longitudinal axis centered on the medial side of the tibia in synchrony with flexion. Iwaki et al. (100) described the motion of an axis through the centers of the lateral and medial femoral condyles projected on to the upper tibial surface, progressively with flexion (Fig. 15-2). Such methods as these are not intended to be rigorous or complete definitions of motion, but rather to provide an easily visualized model of the important characteristics of the motion with respect to anatomical landmarks.

2.1.1 Motion as Described by Laxity Measurements

A fundamental way to characterize the motion of the knee is by the laxity and stability behavior.

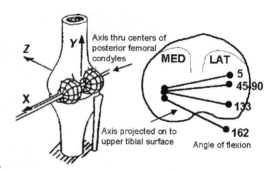

FIGURE 15-2. 3D motion described by the projection of a transverse femoral axis projected on to the tibial surface for different flexion angles. [Adapted from Iwaki et al. (100) and Nakagawa et al. (135).]

Laxity and stability are the opposite of each other, low laxity values implying high stability and vice versa. The value of this type of measurement is that it is an objective method of defining the constraints to motion in response to a specified set of external forces, which can be a combination of compression, shear, and torque, applied either in a single application or cyclically. Because of the difficulties of loading the knee in a clinical setting, most laxity measures of the natural knee have been carried out under no axial load, the Lachman test for AP displacement being the most well known. However, cadaveric specimens pose no problem with loading in many different ways.

Laxity is measured in millimeters per newton or degrees per newton-meter. In a TKR with flat or shallow tibial surfaces, the laxity is higher than for more dished surfaces. The rate of increase of laxity reduces with displacement or rotation from neutral. Laxity can also simply mean the total displacement or rotation away from the neutral position on the application of a defined force or a torque. Laxity can be measured in simple test equipment and is a useful indicator of the mechanical function of the knee.

In some of the earliest studies of laxity of the natural knee, the femur and the tibia were fixed at the required angle of flexion, and then the tibia was cyclically rotated IE about the axis of the tibia (212) and displaced cyclically in an AP direction (89). At a torque of 5 Nm (approximately what occurs in level walking) the average total rotational laxity at 25° flexion was 34°. This was increased after cutting various ligaments. The laxity was reduced by 80% when an axial load of 1,000 N was applied. In AP testing at 30° flexion, the average total AP laxity at 100 N shear force was 8 mm. This was reduced by 68% when an axial load of 1,500 N was applied. The reduction in laxity on load application was said to be due to "the uphill principle," notably the upward movement of the femur on the tibia due to the dishing of the tibia, especially on the medial side.

The methodologies for laxity measurement were subsequently improved for both *in vivo* (118) and *in vitro* situations (117,175). The IE laxity at a cyclic torque of 5 Nm was 35°. At 20° flexion for a cyclic AP force of 100 N, the average total AP laxity was 9 mm. These results agree with those given earlier. However, when axial loads were applied, the reductions in laxity were much less, only 15% for AP and only 25% for IE rotation. The authors ascribed the difference to whether the degrees of freedom other than that being tested were constrained or free, the concept of coupled motions described by Piziali and Rastegar (145). Magnitudes of coupled rotations and displacements were later measured by Gollehon et al. (72). Nevertheless, the authors concurred that joint congruency was the major factor contributing to the stabilizing effects of joint loading. Indeed, during *in vivo* testing, there was well over 50% reduction in AP laxity when the subjects tensed their muscles maximally.

Concerning the effect of flexion angle on laxity, in AP experiments with a cyclic force of 100 N, both Fukubayashi et al. (67) and Gollehon et al. (72) found that the maximum laxity occurred at 30° flexion (a total of 12 mm), with the minimum at 0° (9 mm) and a second minimum at 90° (10 mm). In rotation with a cyclic torque of 6 Nm, Blankevoort et al. (22) found a minimum total laxity of 20° at 0° of flexion, reaching 35° at 30° flexion, and increasing only slightly at higher angles. Blankevoort described this as an "envelope of passive motion."

All authors found that the resection of the cruciate ligaments resulted in large increases in AP displacements, increases by a factor of 2 to 3 being typical (Fig. 15-3). In IE rotation at 20° flexion, resection of the anterior cruciate ligament (ACL) increased total laxity by only 2° and resection of the lateral collateral ligament (LCL) increased laxity by 10°, while resection of both ligaments increased laxity by 15° (175). Gollehon et al. (72) found that isolated sectioning of the PCL produced no increase in rotational laxity. Isolated sectioning of the ACL produced no increase in internal rotation. It therefore appeared that the cruciates per se did not play a major role in controlling rotation, a situation of relevance to their role in TKR.

Laxity in the natural intact or cruciate-resected knee can be taken as a standard of comparison for knees with TKRs implanted. The ideal is that the knee with a TKR implanted should display the same laxity characteristics as the natural intact knee. At the same time, the

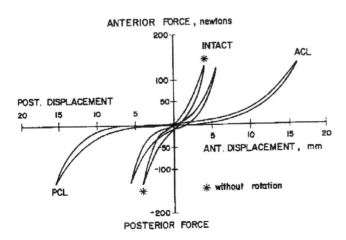

FIGURE 15-3. A typical dynamic recording of AP displacement with the knee at 30° of flexion. The displacement increased 30% when the tibia was allowed to rotate freely (uncoupled motion). Isolated section of either the ACL or the PCL produced almost three times the laxity of the intact knee (67).

effect of muscles as well as ligaments in controlling the position of the femur on the tibia, on the "effective laxity," is important (99,179).

2.1.2 Kinematics in Functional Activities

Knee kinematics in function can be approached at different levels. When studying the natural knee, the 3D motion can be measured for the neutral path of motion, or for specific activities such as walking, going up and down stairs, rising from a chair, and squatting. This is the realm of gait analysis that has been covered by many authors such as Inman et al. (97) and Andriacchi and Alexander (7). The segmental angles, especially those in the sagittal plane, are well documented and can be used as a comparison for knees after TKR. Other useful indicators are the ground-to-foot forces and pressures, and the electromyographic (EMG) signals from muscles.

When considering the relative femoral–tibial motion itself (153), the neutral path of motion is determined primarily by the ligaments and menisci and the shape of the joint surfaces, and is hence amenable to analysis using models in either two or three dimensions. The four-bar linkage was one of the first mechanical models of this type to explain the two-dimensional (2D) motion, primarily the femoral rollback on the tibial surface with flexion (223). More elaborate models have taken 3D motion and geometry into account (24,48,107,111,139).

Deviation from the neutral path of motion by the action of muscles has been shown to be due to the effect of shear forces acting in an anterior or posterior direction (115). For example, the quadriceps applies anterior shear to the tibia at low flexion angles and posterior shear at high flexion angles (57). Muscles such as the popliteus can also apply torque. In function, the ground-to-foot forces can apply shear and torque, whereas inertia forces come into play in faster activities. It is apparent that knee motion varies considerably as a function of the activity, and between individuals for the same activity.

Data on the relationship between IE rotation and AP displacement as a function of flexion angle were determined by Iwaki et al. (100), Hill et al. (84), and Nakagawa et al. (135). In these experiments, magnetic resonance imaging (MRI) sections were taken of cadaveric and living knees in unloaded and loaded situations (215), with the knee at angles from full extension to full flexion (Fig. 15-2). Under these conditions, from 45° to 120° flexion the femur externally rotated on the tibia ("internal tibial rotation") by 17°. From 90° to 162° flexion, there was 28° of rotation. The medial femoral condyle displaced posteriorly only a few millimeters in the higher flexion range, but the lateral condyle displaced progressively posteriorly, rolling off the back of the tibia at extreme flexion. This latter behavior had previously been observed in a radiographic study (83). Using fluoroscopy with image-matching based on CT models, active knee motion was studied for deep knee bend, rising from and sitting in a chair, and descending stairs (50). The mobility of the lateral condyle and relative immobility of the medial condyle were observed. This method has the potential for significant future development and is currently being used extensively to evaluate TKRs *in vivo*.

2.2 Forces in the Knee

Forces can be determined by an indirect method, solving the "total joint problem," where articular, muscle, and ligament forces are calculated, or by a direct method, where only the "articular surface problem" is solved (20,30,47). The forces acting in the knee during activity were calculated as long ago as the late 1960s using a knee model with the input of gait analysis, force plate data, EMG data, and geometric measurements of the limb (129,130,142) (Fig. 15-4). Since then, others have determined forces for different activities using a similar indirect method (8,81,129,130,136,172). A recent dynamic analysis in a young active subject calculated axial compressive forces of 1.7 to 2.3 bodyweight (BW) at 1 m/sec (104). At the other extreme, values of up to eight times BW were calculated for energetic downhill walking in young healthy subjects (106).

The forces in the shafts of two distal femoral replacements were determined by telemetry, the

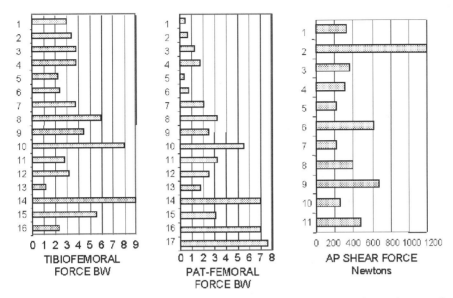

FIGURE 15-4. Forces in the knee for different activities. (*Left*) Tibio-femoral: *1*, Level walking (130); *2*, level walker (81); *3*, level walking (106); *5*, level walking (51); *7*, stair—descending (129); *8*, stair—descending (9); *9*, downhill (129); *10*, downhill (106); *11*, downstairs (187); *12*, rising from chair (59); *13*, cycling (62); *14*, isokinetic extension (137); *15*, squat descent (46); *16*, standing one leg (187). (*Center*) Patello-femoral. *1*, Level walking (152); *2*, level walking (120); *3*, level walking; *4*, level walking (106); *5*, level walking (51); *6*, level walking (187); *7*, stair—ascending (138); *8*, stair—ascending (152); *9*, stair—ascending (120); *10*, stair—descending (138); *11*, stair—descending (152); *12*, stair—descending (120); *13*, downhill (106); *14*, downhill (106); *15*, rising from chair (59); *16*, jogging (137); *17*, squat descent (46). (*Right*) The AP shear force in a direction to tense the PCL. *1*, Level walking (130); *2*, stair—ascending (129); *3*, level walking (187); *4*, level walking (9); *5* and *6*, dislocation forces for a range of TKRs; *7*, dislocation force for PCL-retaining knee under 500-N compression force (114); *8* and *9*, shear forces to reach dislocation point of Kinemax Condylar under 2,000-N and 1,000-N compression forces (161); *10* and *11*, as in *8* and *9*, but where the contact point reached 5 mm from edge of plastic.

first such measurement of its kind in the knee (185,186,187). Data were reported up to 2.5 years for the following activities: uni- and bilateral standing, walking, stair climbing and descending, treadmill walking, jogging, and jumping (Fig. 15-5). In the first subject the greatest averaged peak shaft forces found were jogging 3.6 BW, stair climbing 3.1 BW, walking 2.8 BW, treadmill walking 2.75 BW, and stair ascending 2.8 BW. It is notable that the first force peak occurring just on heel strike was much less than the subsequent large peak, which is at variance with the data of Morrison and makes the pattern of the knee force more like that of the hip, with only two major peaks during the stance phase. Bending moments about the AP axis (VV) and mediolateral axis (FE) peaked in the ranges 8.5 to 9.8 and 4.7 to 7.6 BW cm, respectively, over the

follow-up period. At most follow-up sessions, forces and moments during jogging were generally greater than those for other gait activities. In the second subject forces and moments were generally only 45% to 70% of those in the first subject, due to inadequate musculature around the knee.

There were significant axial torques occurring during walking and other activities. The torques act at the foot as a consequence of the twisting of the body as it swings over the planted foot. The direction of the torque was internal, such that the lateral tibial plateau would tend to move anteriorly. In walking, Taylor et al. (187) measured the peak torque at around 8 Nm.

Others have since determined force the patello-femoral forces, the results showing a wide range (Fig. 15-4). In walking activities, where the

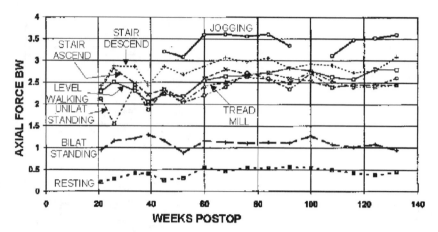

FIGURE 15-5. Axial compressive forces at the knee plotted over time, determined from a telemeterized distal femoral replacement. (Adapted from Taylor SJG, Walker PS. Forces and moments telemetered from two distal femoral replacements during various activities. *J Biomech* 2001;34:839–848, with permission.)

flexion angles in stance are about 20°, the patello-femoral forces are less than 2 BW, but in higher flexion, forces as high as 7 BW have been calculated. From several studies, the tibio-femoral shear forces were determined to be higher in a direction that would tense the PCL. In particular, in the telemetry study (187), the forces that would tense the ACL in walking were small.

Although calculated results (the indirect method) have the advantage that they can be applied to any number of subjects, the assumptions concerning relative muscle action and direction, joint contact points, and other factors, lead to uncertainty in the data (138). Telemetry studies produce direct and valid measurements of the forces in implants, although only a limited number of subjects can be studied for a variety of practical reasons. The validity of extrapolating the data to the intact joint depends on the extent to which the joint mechanics and surrounding musculature has been altered.

Knowledge of the force magnitudes is important for a number of reasons. In designing TKRs, the bearing surfaces should be designed to produce acceptable values of the contact areas and stresses, taking account of the forces that occur in the more strenuous activities, not only level walking. The varus or valgus moments redistribute the stresses over the tibial surface and in extreme cases can result in failure of trabecular bone or failure of fixation, or can cause an intramedullary stem to progressively resorb through a cortex. The shear forces and torques are of particular relevance to TKR because these forces are carried by the remaining cruciate ligaments, the condylar surfaces, plastic stabilizer posts, or linkages such as hinges. In addition, these forces act across the implant–bone interface and can affect fixation. In order to predict the long-term durability of TKRs, realistic force values are needed for input to various test machines and computer models.

2.3 Properties of Cancellous Bone

Any tests or analyses of the strength of TKR components or of the fixation require data of the mechanical properties of the trabecular bone. Most of the available data are for the tibia. The upper tibia consists of a shell of cortical bone with highly oriented cancellous bone within. Within 50 mm of the condylar surface, most of the trabecular structure has converged onto the cortices. For standard condylar replacements, the fixation is entirely within the cancellous structure. The regions of cancellous bone beneath the lateral and medial tibial plateaus are clearly more dense than the central region. This relation is maintained with depth, but with a widening of the less dense central region, until the trabeculae fuse into the cortices beneath the condylar flares.

The key mechanical properties are the elastic modulus and compressive strength, and their spatial variations in the upper tibia. These measurements were made by using an osteopenetrometer consisting of a probe that was gradually introduced into the cancellous bone, the force being continuously measured (91,93). The resisting force on the probe was calibrated to the local elastic modulus and compressive strength. They found that the properties varied considerably between knee specimens, but that the patterns were consistent. The medial condyle showed the highest stiffness and strength. The anterior part of the medial condyle and the posterior part of the lateral condyle were the strongest, consistent with the locations of the contact areas in function. However, there was no diminution of strength with depth below the resection level, as would be supposed from the radiographic appearance of the upper tibia. Goldstein et al. (71) tested cylinders of bone from the upper 10 mm of the upper tibia, and then from the 10-mm layer immediately below. They found very similar values for the modulus for the two layers, although slightly higher magnitudes than Hvid et al. (95). They determined a strong correlation between elastic modulus and compressive strength, as follows:

Elastic modulus = 37.7 × compressive strength

It was interesting that these and other studies found the stiffest and strongest bone was well within the boundaries of the tibia, rather than there being an increase in properties toward the boundary, until a hard cortical rim was reached. The densest bone corresponds with the femoral–tibial contact areas found in a number of studies (4), which is to be expected. The implications of the above studies to tibial fixation are that a resection level from just below the subchondral plate to around 10 mm below that will make little difference to the stiffness and strength of the support for the tibial component, and complete coverage of the upper tibia by the component is not necessary, because even if, say, 10% were not

covered, that might only represent a reduction of about 5% of the stiffness of support.

The foregoing data relate to the normal knee. However, data from knees that are arthritic and that are candidates for TKR are important. Studies have been carried out by Hvid (92) and by Wixson et al. (218). In the former study, strength measurements were made of the resected tibial surfaces of 150 consecutive total knee cases. Overall, the values for osteoarthritis (OA) and rheumatoid arthritis (RA) were similar, although Wixson et al. (218) found that rheumatoid bone was weaker and less stiff. In varus deformity, the bone on the medial side was much stronger than normal, while on the lateral side, the bone was weaker. When the knees were in neutral alignment, the medial side was still stronger than the lateral but not predominantly so, resembling the normal situation. In valgus, however, whereas it might be expected that the lateral bone would be stronger, the strengths of the medial and the lateral sides were similar. This is likely to be due to the finding that varus or valgus alignment alone does not predict the line of action of the ground-to-foot force, and that in many valgus knees, the force direction can still be central or even over the medial side of the knee (82).

An important consideration is the status of the bone during the ensuing years after TKR. The bone properties at the time of operation are most often abnormal because of the deformation. Furthermore, because of the relatively low activity level of most individuals prior to TKR, the overall bone density is found to be lower than normal. However, after realignment and restoration of more normal activity levels, changes in bone density are expected to occur over time, possibly to normal values. Hvid et al. (94) found that the dense bone on the medial side of a varus knee reduced in density over time, but the density on the lateral side did not increase. A similar phenomenon was noted in knees that were initially in valgus.

2.4 Patient Demographics

Fundamental data on patient age, weight, and frequency of everyday activities are required for the specification of mechanical testing.

TABLE 15-2. DEMOGRAPHICS

		Mean Height	Mean Weight
Men	(50–59 yr)	176.2 cm	85.6 kg
Men	(60–69 yr)	174.5 cm	82.2 kg
Women	(50–59 yr)	162.7 cm	75.2 kg
Women	(60–69 yr)	161.3 cm	70.6 kg

(Data from Centers for Disease Control. *Third national health and nutrition examination survey.* Maryland: CDC, 1988–94.)

Concerning patient height and weight, follow-up studies of TKR patients rarely report such data. Results from a 3-year U.S. health survey of the population-at-large produced the age–height–weight statistics shown in Table 15-2.

In a series of 9,200 TKR cases performed between 1971 and 1987 at the Mayo Clinic in Rochester, Minnesota, the average age of the patients was 67 years with a standard deviation of 11 years (150). This means that around 16% of the patients were younger than 56 years of age, with a life expectancy of at least 20 years.

In planning analyses or fatigue tests of TKR components, the frequency of different activities, and hence of the different force magnitudes and patterns, is important (32). McLeod et al. (121) instrumented nine subjects during activities of everyday living and recorded the angles of flexion of the knee, from which they were able to identify specific repetitive actions. Walking predominated, with undifferentiated motions also being substantial. In contrast, stair-ascending and -descending, where the forces may be higher, constituted only 2% of the total repetitive actions. Regarding the frequency of walking over an extended period, Seedhom and Wallbridge (173) carried out a study of 243 individuals. There were 144 female subjects and 99 male subjects of a range of ages and occupations. The total number of steps per day (for a given limb, the figures have to be divided by 2) were the following:

Males: mean 9,537   SD 4,761   range 1,600 to 35,500

Females: mean 9,839   SD 5,706   range 1,200 to 32,600

Translating these to annual figures for one limb gives 1,740,503 steps for males and 1,795,618

for females. This is far in excess of the frequently used assumption of 1 million steps per year.

Schmalzreid et al. (165) carried out a study using a similar method, but restricted their test subjects ($N = 111$) to those who had a hip or knee replacement. The overall average was 4,988 steps per day, translating to 910,310 steps per limb per year. The most active patient walked 3.5 times more than the average. Patients younger than 60 years old walked 30% more than those older than 60. Male patients walked 28% more than female patients.

These data need to be considered in analyses and testing. Statistical considerations are needed such that a given test would represent a stated percentage of the populations. In general, using an average value for patient weights, maximum forces, and number of cycles is probably not as useful as a test that takes values at, for example, 1 SD above the mean.

3 TYPES OF KNEE REPLACEMENT (206)

3.1 Fixed-bearing Condylar Replacements

The term "fixed-bearing" refers to the plastic bearing component being fixed securely into the metallic tibial tray. This type of design represents the major clinical usage today. Typical modern-day fixed-bearing condylar replacements were shown in Fig. 15-1. In this section, the main design features and the basic mechanical characteristics will be described.

3.1.1 Geometry of the Bearing Surfaces

A parametric description of the geometry of conventional condylar replacements is useful for modeling the knee, for predicting kinematics and ligament-length patterns, and for calculating the stresses on the bearing surfaces (Fig. 15-6) (161). In the sagittal view, most symmetric TKR designs take an average between the lateral and medial profiles of the natural knee (68), although some designs preserve a lateral–medial difference to obtain a differential

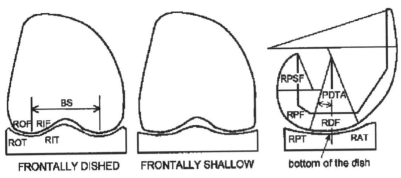

FIGURE 15-6. Geometric parameters of the bearing surfaces of a typical condylar replacement.

rollback in early flexion. If the distal-superior radius (RPSF) is reduced, this may increase the range of flexion slightly, but in reality there is only a small linear difference between the profiles whether a constant or decreasing radius is used. Likewise, the linear differences in the profile between using several arcs rather than two or three for the sagittal femoral profile is small. A computer model showed only small force differences on the bearing surfaces and in muscles for such differences in radii (221).

An important geometric parameter is the PDTA, or posterior-distal transition angle. If this is 20° or more, the large distal radius will contact the tibia during the entire stance phase of gait, reducing the contact stresses on the plastic. However, there are two possible disadvantages of this scheme. First, the distal-anterior trochlea can be too prominent, which can result in gait abnormalities due to the excessive forces required in the quadriceps and patellar ligament (8). Second, there can be a kinematic abnormality such that, in moving from extension to mid-flexion, the origin of the femur will displace anteriorly, which is opposite to the behavior in the natural knee. This is because, in the presence of axial compressive forces and relatively low shear forces, the femur locates at the bottom of the tibial dish. This phenomenon may be seen in fluoroscopy studies of deep knee bends or step ascending and descending, where the femur is found to slide anteriorly with flexion and posteriorly with extension, the so-called "paradoxical motion" (52,180).

Whereas the sagittal radii mainly affect the AP laxity, the frontal radii affect the rotational laxity.

The larger the frontal femoral and tibial radii, the greater will be the rotational laxity. However, there is a transition point in terms of the VV behavior. When the frontal radii are small, varus or valgus lift-off will pivot about the center of a frontal radius. For surfaces of larger radii, some ML skidding could occur.

There are two terms used to quantify the laxity behavior as a function of the radii:

Constraint is the resistance to a particular degree of freedom, such as AP, IE rotation, or VV, when there is a compressive force acting across the joint. This is measured in newtons of applied force/mm of AP displacement, or N mm of applied torque/degree of rotation. If the tibial surfaces are flat, the constraint is nominally zero, except for friction. For dished tibial surfaces, the relation is nonlinear with an increase in constraint with displacement from neutral. In a hinge the VV and AP constraint are infinite.

Conformity is a geometric measure of the closeness of fit of the contacting regions of the femoral and tibial bearing surfaces. An appropriate measure of conformity is relative radius of curvature. If the femoral convex radius is RF and the tibial concave radius is RT, the contact can be considered as a femoral radius RR on a flat tibial surface, where $1/RR = 1/RF - 1/RT$. An important application of RR is that it is directly related to the area of contact and the contact stresses.

It might be thought that constraint and conformity are synonymous. However, consider two knees, one with almost matching shallow profiles in the frontal view, and the other with almost matching dished profiles (Fig. 15-6). They are both equally conforming, but in rotation, the shallow surfaces are less constrained.

3.1.2 Replicating Normal Constraint

The constraint characteristics of the natural knee should ideally be replicated after insertion of a TKR (199). One solution was proposed in the geometry of the original Total Condylar design (194,208). For a geometry with two partially conforming radii in both the frontal and sagittal planes, when there is an axial compressive force acting, application of an AP shear force or a torque will result in a displacement or a rotation until an equilibrium position is reached. Even in the absence of the cruciate ligaments, radii can be found that produce reasonably normal laxity values. However, there is no mechanism for inducing the posterior femoral displacement and the internal tibial rotation as the knee flexes from zero to maximum.

Another approach to obtaining normal constraint in condylar TKRs was to closely repli-

cate the shapes of the anatomical surfaces. The general concept was introduced by Seedhom et al. (170,171) and Ewald (64), who molded a femoral shell to replicate the exact femoral surface anatomy, and then derived the shape of the tibial surface by a wax replica of the inside of the joint with the menisci removed and where the femur was put through a range of flexion. Walker (195,196) modified this concept by starting with a computer model of the femoral surface (68) writing equations to describe the laxity and stability characteristics of the natural knee, and then displacing and rotating the femoral component, according to the equations (Fig. 15-7). The downward locus of the multitude of points on the femoral surface accumulated at all of the flexion angles, displacements, and rotations described the tibial surface. It was assumed that the PCL would induce the posterior translation with flexion.

A factor that makes it difficult to exactly replicate the natural constraint is the friction between the metal and plastic surfaces (69,70). In the natural knee, the friction is so small as to have

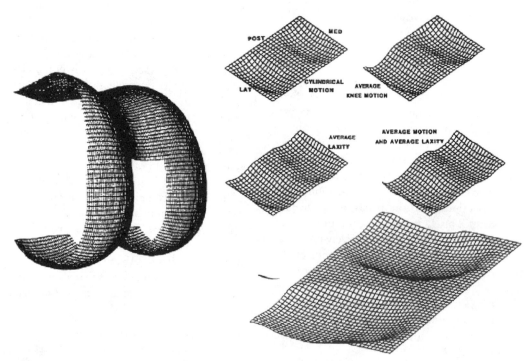

FIGURE 15-7. A femoral component determined from sectioning of anatomic knees. The tibial surfaces were generated using equations based on different motion and laxity criteria.

a minimal effect on the kinematics. In a TKR, however, the coefficient of friction is in the range of 0.05 to 0.1, the latter value applying when particles of debris become embedded in the plastic surface (195). The importance of friction can be appreciated in that, when a compressive force of 2,000 N is acting, the shear force required to overcome friction is up to 200 N, which is similar to the shear forces occurring in activity (Fig. 15-4). The effect is a reduction of laxity, an increase in stability, reduced forces on the cruciates, and periods of stick when the direction of the shear force is reversed. These phenomena were measured in a simulating machine under the application of shear forces and torques in a simulated walking cycle (159).

It is important to take into consideration the effect of muscle and gait patterns on the motion and laxity behavior of the natural and TKR knee *in vivo*. This places into perspective the studies of laxity and stability carried out on TKR components themselves, on cadaveric knees, or on the living knee in laboratory conditions. In addition, if a change occurs in the knee, such as a ruptured ligament, a resected ligament as part of a surgical procedure, or the presence of a TKR, muscle and gait patterns may well adapt to the altered mechanics. Examples of adaptation have been described for ACL-deficient knees and for stair climbing with different TKR designs (19,214).

3.1.3 Preservation of Both Cruciates

Potentially, the closest scheme for restoring normal constraint is to retain the cruciate ligaments, resurface the femoral condyles, and provide shallow tibial bearing surfaces. This scheme is based on preserving as many of the anatomical structures as possible, minimizing the shear forces on the plastic tibial surface and on the fixation, and maintaining the proprioceptive effects of the ligaments. Preservation of both cruciates was used in early unicompartmental designs (Marmor, Unicondylar), where one or both sides of the joint were replaced, and in designs with one-piece components (Townley, Duocondylar, Duopatella, Geomedic, Cloutier). Gait analysis of unicompartmentals has shown almost normal kinematic patterns (214) supporting the

principle of this scheme. The ideal indications for preserving both cruciates are in the younger and more active patients where the bone geometry and the surrounding ligaments are not severely compromised. However, certain factors have limited the application of cruciate-preserving TKRs: difficulty of precise profile matching and surgical placement, wear and deformation of thin low-conformity plastic, inadequate fixation, and limited exposure at surgery.

Efforts have been made to overcome these disadvantages, such as by improved surface designs, more accurate instrumentation and technique (6), more wear-resistant polyethylenes, better fixation design, and more rigorous selection of patients. The possibilities of using small incisions with more rapid recovery has also led to a resurgence of interest in unicompartmental replacement (133,188).

3.1.4 Preservation of the Posterior Cruciate

Today, almost two-thirds of the knees used worldwide are of the PCL-preserving type (168), although there is a gradual trend toward the posterior cruciate-substituting designs. Laboratory studies using cadaveric knees demonstrated the rationale for preserving the PCL (178). The femoral–tibial contact points in the sagittal plane were compared for flat versus dished tibial surfaces, and for PCL preservation versus PCL resection. Preserving the PCL prevented an excessively anterior contact point, and the shear force was shared between the ligament and the curved plastic surfaces. In the absence of the PCL, the contact points were too anterior for both flat and curved surfaces. The proportion of the AP shear force carried by the PCL was later shown to be very dependent on the radius of the tibial surfaces in the sagittal plane (RAT and RPT, Fig. 15-6).

In laboratory studies where compressive and shear forces were applied of magnitudes typical of those in activity, even a moderate sagittal radius of about 60 to 70 mm limited the AP displacement to only a few millimeters (198). The tests were extended to TKR patients by applying shear forces when the patients were standing on the knee. The AP displacements were inversely proportional to the weight of the patient and in a PCL-preserving design, the PCL was calculated to be carrying about one-third of the shear force. In a design without cruciates but with more dished tibial surfaces, the displacements were small and were limited almost entirely by the bearing surfaces rather than by the soft tissues.

A more detailed discussion of these issues is given in Section 4.3.

3.2 Guided Motion Knees

A Guided Motion Knee can be defined as a TKR where some characteristics of the motion, such as femoral rollback, are produced by mechanical interaction between the femoral and tibial components. The earliest examples of Guided Motion Knees were the Kinematic/Kinemax (KS) (204) and the Insall-Burstein Posterior Stabilized (PS) (98) designed in the late 1970s (Fig. 15-8). In the KS, the posterior displacement of the contact points was guided throughout the whole flexion range. In the PS design, posterior displacement was produced after about 70° of flexion. The magnitude of the posterior femoral displacement can be varied by the design of the cam surfaces. The contact point on the tibial post should be as low as possible to maximize the "hop height" before dislocation would occur. In order to accommodate IE rotation, suitable radii of the

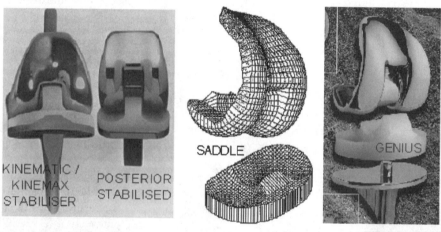

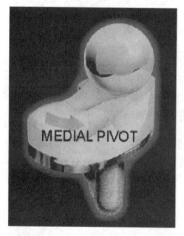

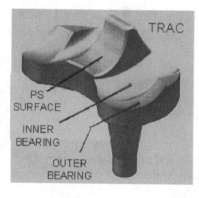

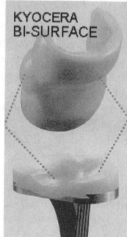

FIGURE 15-8. Examples of Guided Motion Knees where part or all the motions are guided by mechanical interactions between the femoral and tibial components.

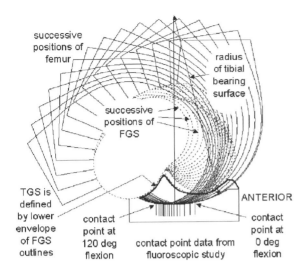

successive
positions of
femur

radius
of tibial
bearing
surface

successive
positions of
FGS

TGS is
defined
by lower
envelope
of FGS
outlines

contact
point at
120 deg
flexion

contact point data from
fluoroscopic study

ANTERIOR

contact
point at
0 deg
flexion

FIGURE 15-9. Method for synthesis of intercondylar guide surfaces. The femoral guide surface (FGS) is placed in successive flexion and posterior displacement positions. The tibial guide surface (TGS) is the lower envelope of the FGS profiles.

cam surfaces in horizontal sections are needed to avoid corner contacts.

Over the past two decades, there have been many variations of these posterior stabilized designs introduced by different manufacturers (169). In one study (204,205), software was produced where the shape of the femoral guide surface could be systematically varied, to determine combinations of femoral and tibial guide surfaces that closely reproduced a normal rollback pattern (Fig. 15-9) (51). One of the most effective configurations of guide surfaces was a convex femoral guide surface in a tibial saddle where there was continuous femoral rollback with flexion, with only a small AP laxity at the extremes. This guided motion satisfied the goals of providing rollback and controlling both anterior and posterior motion throughout the entire range of flexion. One manufacturer produced a design of this type, called the "Genius" (Astro Medical, Milano, Italy; not designed by the author), adding a mobile bearing to allow for IE rotation.

Recently two designs have been introduced where differential contact point locations between extension and flexion have been achieved. The TRAC knee, designed by Draganich and Pottenger (Biomet, Inc., Warsaw, Indiana) (56), used an inner pair of bearing surfaces that contacted from 5° hyperextension to 8° of flexion, and an outer pair of bearing surfaces that contacted more posteriorly throughout the remain-

ing flexion range. The Kyocera Bi-Surface knee (Kyocera Corp. Kyoto, Japan) (5) addressed the goal of achieving a very high range of flexion. For most of the flexion range, the knee behaves as a standard condylar replacement with moderately conforming bearing surfaces. Beyond 90° flexion, the load is transferred to a spherical surface protruding posteriorly from the femoral intercondylar region, contacting within a spherical depression at the posterior of the plastic tibial component. There is some similarity to the Variable Axis total knee (134). Because the surfaces are on the ML centerline, the resistance to rotational torque is minimized, which should further facilitate the maximum range of flexion possible for that joint. The Medial Pivot knee (Wright Mfg. Co, Memphis, TN) is a slightly different concept in that there are no guide surfaces or cams per se. Instead, the tibial bearing surfaces are shaped so that "normal knee motion" is possible, where the medial side remains in the same position during flexion but where the lateral femoral condyle can displace posteriorly with flexion. However, the design does not actively force this motion to occur.

These examples have shown that femoral–tibial motion can be guided by various designs of intercondylar guide surfaces or cams, or even by the bearing surfaces themselves (184,197). In addition, certain of the motions such as AP displacement and axial rotation are controlled, whereas in other cases motions are allowed.

3.3 Mobile-bearing or Meniscal Knees

Designs where a moving plastic bearing is interposed between the femoral condyle and the tibial plate, called meniscal knees or mobile-bearing knees, were first introduced in the late 1970s (34,73). These designs imitate the natural knee in that the plastic-bearing components resemble the menisci, the plastic accommodates AP translation as well as rotations, and a large contact area is maintained throughout all or much of the flexion range. The purpose of such designs is to minimize the wear and deformation of the plastic (158), to allow freedom of motion and position, and to allow for natural kinematics. There are a number of mechanical schemes that can be specified for a mobile-bearing knee (Fig. 15-10):

■ Allows IE rotation only. This has the advantage of allowing the knee to locate at a preferred rotational orientation, and to adjust to a new position without resistance (except friction) during activity.
■ Allows IE rotation about a medial axis. This allows more anatomical motion to occur where the centers of IE rotation in the horizontal plane of the upper tibia are located on the medial side (see Fig. 15-2).
■ Allows IE rotation and AP translation. This allows the knee to locate at a preferred rotational and translational orientation during

function. It can also allow natural knee kinematics where the location of the medial axis of rotation varies due to knee laxity and function.

■ Allows IE rotation and guides AP translation by a femoro-tibial cam, such as a posterior stabilizer or "saddle." This is preferable to a configuration with rotation only because it produces posterior translation in high flexion, but it requires partially conforming femoro-tibial bearing surfaces, at least in high flexion.
■ The same as the above, but where the tibial cam is fixed to the tibial plate. Because the plastic meniscus (or two menisci) slides AP, the femoral-plastic surfaces can be fully conforming.

In all of the above, rotation and AP translation can be unlimited, or limited by stops. Clinical experience has shown few problems with unlimited rotation for uncomplicated primary cases. However, in the absence of one or both cruciates, limits to AP translation seem advisable.

Referring now to specific designs (Fig. 15-11), the Oxford Knee was intended to be used as a unicompartmental replacement with preservation of both of the cruciates so that the AP pattern of motion could be achieved by a four-bar linkage mechanism. The lateral and medial bearings are independent and there is sufficient clearance to allow for IE rotation. By only providing for the femoro-tibial surfaces,

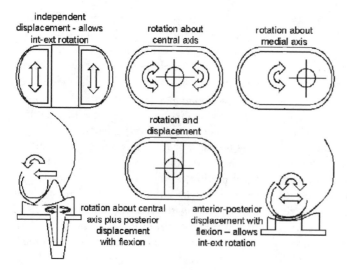

FIGURE 15-10. Mechanical schemes that can be used in mobile bearing knees.

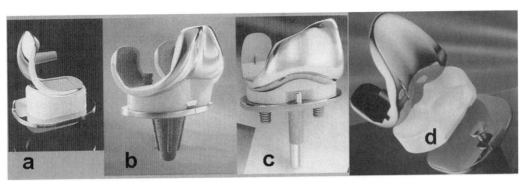

FIGURE 15-11. Examples of mobile bearing knees. **a:** The Oxford unicompartmental (Biomet). **b:** The LCS Rotating Platform (DePuy—J & J). **c:** The Polyzoides Rotaglide (Corin). **d:** The Zimmer MBK (Zimmer).

the sagittal radii could be made constant, thus producing complete area contact throughout the range of motion. Studies of passive motion in patients demonstrated that the menisci translated posteriorly with flexion, the lateral more than the medial (29). However, such passive studies do not replicate functional conditions where variable shear and torque forces will be present. The wear depth in retrievals has been much less than for total hips (148).

In the New Jersey Meniscal knee (LCS) (33,35,37), a one-piece metal tibial component was provided with tracks for sliding of two plastic menisci. In terms of freedom of motion, this was similar to the Oxford. When the LCS was used without the ACL, the menisci sometimes displaced too far posteriorly, causing problems including fracture of the menisci themselves (213). In terms of replicating natural knee mechanics, both the Oxford and the New Jersey were less constrained than the natural knee on the medial side.

A new version of the New Jersey knee was later introduced, the LCS Rotating Platform. The femoro-tibial contact was designed to be fully conforming up to about 20° of flexion, covering the stance phase of walking, but at higher flexion there was partial conformity. It is difficult to avoid this compromise in a femoral component design that includes a patellar flange and where the sagittal profile is similar to anatomical. This design has the advantage of simplicity and the long-term clinical results have been excellent with few mechanical problems. In terms of reproducing natural mechanics, although there

is freedom of IE rotation, there is no provision for AP translation and when the lateral condyle moves posteriorly, the medial condyle moves anteriorly, which is unphysiological. The consequence of this mechanism may be less than optimal muscle lever arms and a possible loss of some flexion. Recently, a new version of the LCS has been introduced, the AP Glide, where freedom of AP translation is superimposed on the rotation.

The Polyzoides Rotaglide (146) was probably the first to include both rotation and AP translation in a one-piece plastic design. This was achieved by locating the plastic on a smooth metal plate, with stops acting in slots and recesses to limit the motion. Limitation of motion was considered necessary because the design required the resection of both of the cruciates. Another feature of this design was complete conformity throughout the entire flexion range. This was achieved by a negative PDTA angle (see Fig. 15-6). The compromise was a patellar flange, which was recessed more than anatomical in the distal-anterior region.

The MBK (123) design solved the problem of obtaining complete femoro-tibial conformity throughout flexion, while maintaining an anatomically shaped patellar flange and sagittal profile. This was achieved by separating the lateral and medial, and patello-femoral bearing surfaces. This resulted in notches at the sides of the anterior femoral component, where the posterior-distal radius is carried forward. There is sufficient ML width to provide for all three bearing surfaces.

Although it might be considered that mobile-bearing knees are less constrained in certain degrees of freedom than most fixed-bearing designs, there are two factors which modify this view. First, in a fixed-bearing knee, relative femoral–tibial displacements can take place by rolling, which is not the case for a mobile-bearing knee (181). Second, friction between the plastic mobile bearing and the tibial plate can have a significant effect in a mobile-bearing design, as well as in a fixed-bearing design (159). The coefficient of friction with a large area of contact is larger than for small areas of contact for the same load (211). The result can be periods of stick and slip with reduced overall displacements and rotations in a mobile-bearing design (54,202).

3.4 Designs Providing Varus–valgus Stability

These designs can either be unlinked, as in the Superstabiliser-Constrained Condylar (CCK), or linked as in fixed or rotating hinges (203) (Fig. 15-12). The former can be regarded as an extension of designs with intercondylar guide surfaces described above, but where the plastic post is elevated (198). This arrangement provides for posterior displacement of the contact point in high flexion, some anterior displacement toward extension, and partial control of AP displacement in the mid-range. The main value of this design is in providing VV stability. An important design goal is to maximize the area of the plastic post for bending stiffness and strength. However, under extreme varus loading activities, a plastic post bends and deforms over time, making it unreliable in sustaining such loading in the long term (155). In most designs a metal reinforcing pin within the plastic post is provided, which improves the stiffness and strength. However, to provide more rigid and long-lasting support to VV moments, some type of linked device is needed. Over the years numerous different linked designs have been introduced. The characteristics of a linked design are:

- Stability is provided in all degrees of freedom, VV and hyperextension being particularly important, although there can be some laxity

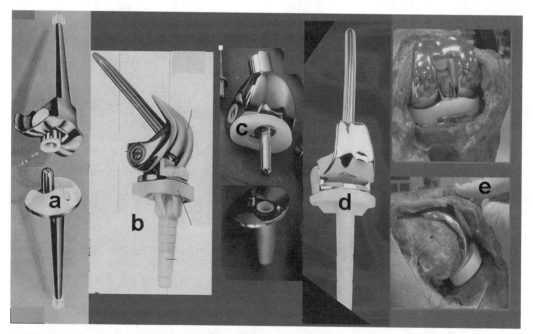

FIGURE 15-12. Linked types of TKR for serious instability and revision cases. **a:** Link endo Model (Waldemar-Link). **b:** Kinematic Rotating Hinge (Osteonics-Howmedica). **c:** Finn Knee (Biomet). **d:** Smiles Rotating Hinge (Stanmore Implants Worldwide). **e:** Zimmer Rotating Hinge (Zimmer).

(e.g., rotational) in one or more degrees of freedom.

- A linkage of some type, such as a hinge, provides the stability and prevents subluxation or dislocation.
- Intramedullary stems are required to provide adequate fixation.

The most conservative type of linked TKR is the intercondylar hinge. The linkage is housed in the intercondylar region, preserving the condyles on each side. Current variations of this type include the St George Endo Model (60) and the Zimmer Rotating Hinge. Advantages of an intercondylar design are preservation of bone and the fact that the axis of rotation can be placed in an anatomical location. Factors that need to be addressed in an intercondylar design are the restricted size of the bearing components, with an increased potential for wear and deformation; the possibility of fracture of the femoral condyles on either side of the intercondylar housing; the difficulty of linking the components at surgery; and the possibility of dislocation in extreme loading conditions (in some designs).

The least conservative type of linked TKR is the fixed hinge or rotating hinge. Surgery requires resection of about 25 mm from the distal femoral condyles, and 10 mm from the upper tibia. An axle is then used to connect the femoral and tibial components, usually with plastic bushings to act as the bearing. The total thickness of the implant is dictated by the required dimensions of the axle and bushings, and the ideal placement of the axle, which is close to the level of the epicondyles. A lower or more posterior axle location will reduce bone resection, but will result in abnormal tracking of the patella.

The fixed hinge is the simpler design, applicable to patients of low demand who require only a stable knee. Some of the long-term clinical follow-ups have shown survivorship similar to that of condylar knees (28). The rotating hinge, however, results in a more "natural feel" to the patient and is more durable in the long term (191). Examples are the Kinematic Rotating Hinge, the Finn, the Lacey, the PFC S-ROM, and the SMILES. More bone resection, however, is required to accommodate the

extra bearing surface compared with the fixed hinge. The rotation can be achieved by a flat polished metal surface pivoted on a flat plastic surface, or by a convex metal surface in a dished plastic surface. The latter is preferable because it provides a "soft" limit to rotation, reducing the possibility of instability or patello-femoral subluxation.

Cases with bone loss, including revision, need special consideration. Augments, such as spacers and wedges, are useful for filling bone defects and for accurately reproducing the joint line. The augments can be screwed or cemented to the main components. For larger defects, space-fillers made from metal or plastic are an alternative to bone grafting (31). Stems are useful for bypassing such larger defects or for protecting against fractures. When the TKR design carries VV moments, intramedullary stems are needed. In older patients, cemented stems are preferable. Uncemented fluted stems can be used if there is sufficient cortical thickness, in order to reduce the stress shielding of the cancellous bone near the joint. Empirically, suitable stem lengths for Superstabilizer types are 100 to 120 mm, while for rotating and fixed hinges 120 to 150 mm is needed. Revision of a failed cemented stem requires a new stem at least 50 mm longer (96). In all cases, stem centralizers are needed to prevent the stem tip from impacting the cortical wall, which frequently produces osteolysis, penetration, and even bone fracture. For cases with abnormal geometry, especially of very small size where bone preservation is a prerequisite, custom superstabilizers have been designed and made using CAD-CAM techniques (174).

3.5 Patello-femoral Joint

Unless the patella is normal in shape and has retained a viable cartilage layer, a patella resurfacing is most often used with a TKR (166). The resurfacing can be a dome, a rounded cone, or a Gaussian curve (Fig. 15-13). The dome has been widely used in condylar replacements but has several drawbacks:

- The plastic is thin at the sides, allowing overall deformation of the component and

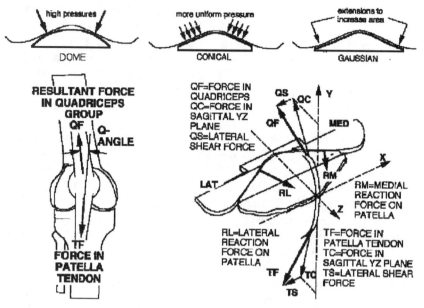

FIGURE 15-13. (*Top*) Three types of patella resurfacing designs shown in section. (*Bottom*) A generalized view of the patella with the knee in flexion, showing the various force vectors.

compressive failure of underlying trabecular bone, especially in activities with high flexion.

- If the femoral flange has an anatomic profile (to accept a retained patella), the dome has two local areas of high stress that are subject to wear and deformation.
- If the patellar flange has an arcuate profile to accept the dome, a retained anatomical patella is a poor fit.

The cone has increased plastic thickness at the sides, and larger contact areas in the form of two "lines" rather than "points." The Gaussian shape further increases both the thickness and the contact area. In all of the designs, a medial offset to the peak is an advantage and avoids the need to use a smaller size of symmetric design and medialize it. A rotating platform design produces the largest area of contact and potentially the least wear and deformation, at the expense of some extra thickness due to the metal backing.

Regarding stability, there is a perception that the dome is more forgiving in alignment and that the other types will tilt and load on the corners. In the front view, it can be seen that,

because of the angle between the lines of action of the patellar ligament and the quadriceps, the Q-angle, there will be a compressive force, tensile force, and lateral shear force on the patella itself (Fig. 15-13). The actual direction of the forces in the frontal plane will depend on the relative forces in the different parts of the quadriceps. The compressive force between the patella and the patellar flange increases with the flexion angle, reaching a maximum at about 90° flexion. A 3D force analysis can be carried out, based on the sectional view. If the resultant compressive force is central, equal resultants act on the lateral and medial facets. However, in general, the lateral reaction force will be larger than the medial, due to the laterally directed component of the quadriceps and patellar tendon forces. As the effective Q-angle increases (126), the lateral force will increase and the medial force will decrease. However, so long as both forces are positive, the patella will be stable. At the point where the medial force reaches zero, the patella will become unstable and will be subject to tilting and subluxation. This will occur at a Q-angle of approximately 12° (91). Except in cases of extreme valgus, this is unlikely, and hence, the cone and

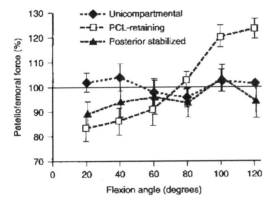

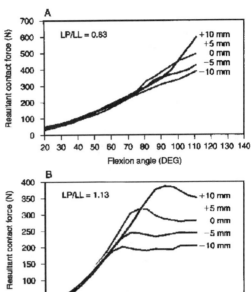

FIGURE 15-14. The mean change (±SEM) in the patello-femoral force with three designs of implant. The force after TKR is expressed as a percentage of the force in the intact knee specimens before TKR. (From Singerman R, Davy DT, Goldberg VM. Effects of patella alta and patella infera on patellofemoral contact forces. *J Biomech* 1994;27(8):1059–1065, with permission.)

Gaussian patellar components are likely to be stable.

After TKR, it is possible that the magnitude of the patello-femoral forces will change due to the type of TKR design, the placement of the components (177), ligament balancing, and other factors (41). In one study (125), it was found that the forces were unchanged after unicompartmental replacement and preservation of both cruciates (Fig. 15-14). For a PCL-retaining design, the patello-femoral force was 17% less than normal in extension and 25% more in full flexion. The explanation for the latter is that the PCL was not sufficiently tight to produce a sufficiently posterior contact point in high flexion. A PCL-substituting design gave 10% less force in extension, reverting to normal by about 80° flexion. The intercondylar cam produced a posterior contact point in high flexion, reducing the required force in the quadriceps.

In another study (176) the effect of the height of the patella relative to the joint line on the patello-femoral forces was investigated using a specially designed six-degree-of-freedom force transducer (Fig. 15-15). Whereas height had little effect up to about 60° flexion, a lower patella showed reduced forces after 60° due to off-loading from wraparound of the quadriceps on the anterior femur. The effect was even more

FIGURE 15-15. Values of the patello-femoral force in cadaveric knees using a modified Oxford-type knee Test Rig (see Fig. 15-16), with quadriceps loading, as a function of patella height. LP, height of the patella; LL, length of patella ligament. **A:** An initially high patella with LP/LL = 0.83. **B:** An initially low patella with LP/LL = 1.13. The values to the right of the curves are the shift in patella height from the reference position. (From Miller RK, Goodfellow JW, Murray DW, et al. *In vitro* measurement of patellofemoral force after three types of knee replacement. *J Bone Joint Surg* 80-B:900–906, with permission.)

pronounced for patellae that were tall relative to the length of the patellar ligament. There was also evidence that high-riding patellae were more liable to lateral subluxation.

4 EVALUATION AND TESTING OF TKR

4.1 Static or Quasi-static Tests

Numerous test rigs have been used for carrying out experiments on TKRs. If the goal is to measure the constraint of a TKR in the absence of surrounding muscles and soft tissues, a simple test rig can be used. With the TKR at the required flexion angle, any combination

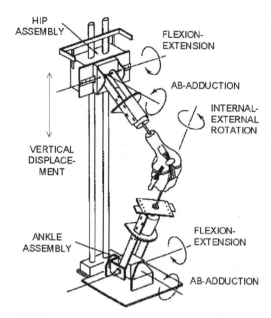

FIGURE 15-16. An Oxford Knee Test Rig designed for static or quasi-static testing of cadaveric knees in flexion. A downward force is applied at the "hip" and a balancing force is applied in the quadriceps. The angle of flexion is determined by the quadriceps length, which is adjustable. (From Zavatsky AB, O'Connor JJ. A model of the human knee ligaments in the sagittal plane. Part 1: response to passive flexion. *Proc Inst Mech Eng* 1992;206(H3):125–134, with permission.)

The forces have been measured by small turnbuckles, or by dissociation of bone blocks (119).

■ The force in the quadriceps and in the patellar tendon using force transducers (125).

■ The patello-femoral contact areas and pressures, and the effect of different relative forces in the components of the quadriceps (4).

■ The effect of different muscle forces on displacement and rotations at the knee (115).

The 3D motion of the knee under conditions of FE, where the quadriceps was continuously lengthened and shortened (157).

A sophisticated type of testing to study the kinematics of TKRs *in vitro* is to use a robot to control and monitor knee position (112,131) (Fig. 15-17). The principle of the method is that the robot positions the tibia on the femur at a succession of flexion angles. At each flexion angle, the angles (except flexion) and displacements are manipulated until the sum of the residual forces and moments as measured by a six-degree-of-freedom force transducer is minimized. This is then considered to be a neutral position. The succession of neutral positions is defined as the

of compressive force, VV moment, IE torque, and AP shear force can be applied and the resulting displacements measured. If it is required to study the patello-femoral joint also, an Oxford Knee Testing Rig is suitable (Fig. 15-16) (222). The advantage of the rig is that the external forces, balanced by forces in the quadriceps, give an approximation to the loading conditions in activity. Limitations of the method are the low force magnitude, the force may not simulate the direction of the external force at the knee in the frontal and sagittal planes, and only one muscle is represented. Such factors can be addressed in more sophisticated versions of the rig. Aspects that have been studied using an Oxford-type rig include:

■ The femoro-tibial contact point or area locations, determined radiographically or using pressure-sensitive film inside the knee (80,90).

■ The orientation of and forces in the ligaments.

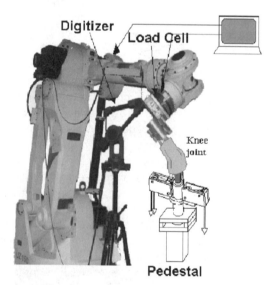

FIGURE 15-17. A robot used to position the knee precisely through a defined or measured motion path. The 3D kinematics is measured by the digitizer. The forces and moments across the knee are measured by the load cell. (Courtesy Guoam Li, Harvard Medical School, Boston. See Li et al., 2001).

neutral path of motion. Data have been obtained for the unloaded knee, and for when forces are applied in the quadriceps and hamstrings. The output has been expressed as projections of the epicondylar axis onto the top of the tibia. (Note that the studies by Iwaki et al. (100) cited previously show the projection of an axle through the centers of the circles of the posterior femoral condyles, which is angulated from the epicondylar axis—this produces different results.) A TKR is then implanted and the test is repeated. A comparison is then made between the neutral paths of motion. In addition to determining the neutral path, the robot equipment can be used to calculate ligament tensions. This is done by using the force data from the transducer with the ligament intact, and after resection. In a similar way, cam forces in a PS type of knee can be calculated.

4.2 Strength Testing

Each new knee component needs to be tested for strength prior to use in patients (Fig. 15-18). Strength requirements in general and the formulation of standards for testing were described by Paul (141,143). The test should replicate as far

as possible the physiological conditions, while maintaining mechanical simplicity. The rate of testing can be up to 5 Hz or even higher for metal components and up to 2 Hz where plastic is involved.

The strength of plastic posts in stabilized designs, the security of fixation of the plastic in the metal tray, and the security of mobile-bearing components can be tested using an applied cyclic shear force, preferably accompanied by a compressive force of around 1,000 N. From a compilation of available force data in the knee (Fig. 15-4), including that from a telemetrized distal femoral replacement (187), a suitable cyclic shear force in a direction that would tense the PCL is 750 N, interspersed with a force of 1,250 N applied for a total of 0.5 million cycles. The former represents vigorous walking, whereas the latter represents the extreme forces that could be applied in rapid ascending or descending. In the opposite direction (such that the ACL would be tensed), suitable values are 500 and 750 N. Again, a 10-million-cycle test is appropriate.

Designs such as Superstabilisers and Linked Hinges require testing in varus loading (Fig. 15-18). This can be accomplished using a cyclic force that is offset from the centerline

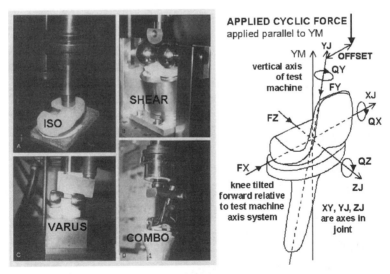

FIGURE 15-18. Various strength tests. *ISO*, testing the strength of tibial trays. *Shear*, applying a compressive force in combination with a shear component. *Varus*, a varus moment applied to a CCK type of TKR. *Combo* and *right*, the hinged TKR is set at an angle to the test machine axes so that a combination and forces of moments are applied by a single uniaxial force.

and medial to the medial femoro-tibial contact point. For comparative testing applicable to all designs, the offset distance from the center and the applied force should be the same. An extreme value of the external moment acting at the knee during activity is 6.5% BW times height, whereas a normal value is around 3.5% (8). To determine a suitable test force, consider a value of the external varus moment of 5% × BW × height = 67,500 N mm for a typical male. The moment carried by the reaction force of 3 BW on the medial condyle at 22 mm spacing is 44,550 N mm. Hence, the moment carried by the central post is 22,950 N mm. This can be applied by a force C of 1,000 N acting at 23 mm from the contact point or 45 mm from the center of the knee. Superstabilisers with plastic posts can show considerable progressive angular deformation, which is reduced but not eliminated by metal reinforcement. Fixed or rotating hinges show only small deformations.

To test the overall mechanical strength of a TKR, a complex Knee Simulator could be used. However, a uniaxial cyclic load machine can be used to apply multi-axial forces and moments. This is achieved by mounting the component at an angle and applying the force offset (Fig. 15-18). In this way, the following can be applied:

- Compressive force
- AP shear force
- Varus moment
- Hyperextension moment
- Axial torque

This test has the advantage of revealing weak points in a design not shown by simpler testing, as well as effectively applying several loading modes simultaneously.

The following data were obtained from Ahir et al. (2). Incidences of fatigue fracture of metallic tibial baseplates have been reported in the literature (1,124,128). The most commonly reported mechanism for fatigue fracture occurs where there is insufficient bone support, especially when combined with a distally well-fixed stem, increasing the load on the unsupported side of the tray (66). This situation can arise from a number of conditions. Tibial bone loss can occur due to severe varus or valgus defor-

mities (40) or as a result of stress shielding in response to a prostheses (66). The presence of a layer of fibrous tissue between the bone and cement may also produce inadequate support to the tray (Scott et al. 1986). Other clinical factors are axial malalignment, overloading due to patient weight and/or high activity level and poor fixation of the tibial component (1,124).

Tray design is an important factor, as fracture has occurred as a result of inadequate thickness, cruciate cut-outs with sharp corners and small radii between the tray and its rim (Fig. 15-19). (1,74,124). The choice of material and the manufacturing process are also significant. Cast CoCrMo alloy has a limited ductility and some trays made from this material have failed due to brittle fracture. There is little information on trays made from titanium alloy but Gradisar et al. (74) describe failure of one tray, which they attribute to the notch sensitivity of this material. Porous coating used on some materials, achieved by the sintering process, introduces microscopic notches on the surface of the implant, which reduces its strength and fatigue properties (128).

A test has been proposed by the International Standards Organization (ISO 14879-1, 1997) to determine the endurance properties of metallic tibial baseplates with respect to materials, manufacturing and design variables (Fig. 15-20). The test specimen is held as a cantilever:

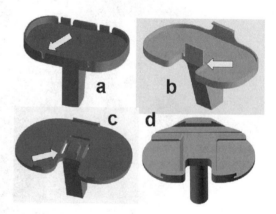

FIGURE 15-19. Designs of tibial trays that have had a clinical incidence of fracture (2). **a:** Total condylar. **b:** Kinematic. **c:** PCA. **d:** Kinemax A design, which has not shown any fracture in service. The arrows show locations of stress concentration.

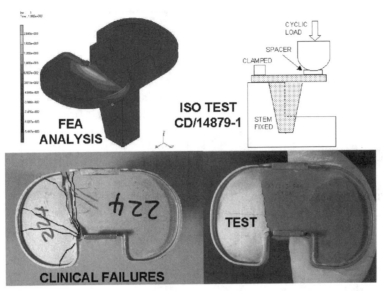

FIGURE 15-20. The ISO test for tibial tray strength. (*Top left*) FEA of a kinematic showing the weak area. (*Top right*) The ISO test. (*Bottom left*) Clinical failure of a kinematic, with lines showing other clinical failure directions. (*Bottom right*) Failure mode produced by the ISO test.

one-half is rigidly fixed, and the unsupported half is subjected to the loading. The unsupported condyle is loaded through a UHMWPE spacer using a metallic spherical indentor with a cyclic constant amplitude force perpendicular to the undeflected superior surface. The test specifies that the load is applied until the tibial baseplate exhibits failure or until 5 million cycles is achieved. In the ISO specification, the magnitude of the load was not specified. Experiments and analyses were carried out using tibial component designs, which had a documented clinical incidence of failure and designs that showed no such failure. The cyclic load which separated these two groups was originally found to be 500 N (2), but more recently 900 N was found to be represent a more suitable and stringent test load (3).

4.3 Laxity Measurement

In a typical *in vitro* laxity test on a TKR, a compressive load is applied, followed by a cyclic AP force or a cyclic torque. Wide variations are found in the displacement and rotational responses depending on the inherent constraint of the designs. However, in such tests the TKR is tested in isolation and not implanted in a knee joint, and hence, the results are representative only of the TKR surfaces and not of the combined effect of the surfaces plus the remaining soft tissues. Nevertheless, there is value in characterizing a TKR in this way, mainly to provide a measure of its inherent laxity and stability.

To determine the effect of soft tissue restraint on the laxity of a TKR, experiments were carried out by Luger et al. (114) in a knee simulator. Two designs of knee were tested, one of relatively "low constraint" intended to be used with retention of the PCL, the other of relatively "high constraint" to be used with resection of both cruciates. The knees were mounted in a simulator that could apply compressive forces down the axis of the tibia, and a cyclic AP shear force or a cyclic IE torque was applied (200). To simulate soft tissue restraint, rubber bumpers were used with stiffnesses to produce similar laxities to normal intact knees, or knees with ligaments resected (67).

Results were first obtained for cadaveric knees to act as a control. For the TKRs, laxity was measured at a modest axial compressive force of 500 N. With simulated soft tissue restraint, both designs were stable, the low-constraint knee giving slightly higher than physiological laxity

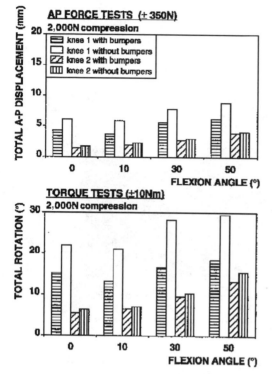

FIGURE 15-21. AP and rotational laxity values for two TKRs tested in a knee simulator. Knee 1 is of low constraint (PCL retention). Knee 2 is of high constraint (PCL resection). The "bumpers" represent soft tissue restraint.

levels, the high-constraint knee slightly less. Without the simulated soft tissue restraint, neither knee could sustain the high shear force pulling the tibia forward. When the axial force was increased to 2,000 N (3 BW), the AP laxity values were dramatically reduced (Fig. 15-21). For the low-constraint knee, the laxity values were 5 to 7 mm, soft tissue restraints reducing the laxity by about one-third. For the high-constraint knee, the total AP laxities were only 2 to 3 mm, soft tissue restraint making little difference.

For IE rotation, the pattern was very similar. There were physiological laxity values at 500 N compressive force with soft tissue restraint, but dislocation without soft tissue restraint. At the 2,000 N compressive force, the rotations were similar to physiological for the low-constraint knee, soft tissue restraint again reducing values by about one-third, but for the high-constraint knee, total rotations were only 4° to 13°, soft tissue restraint making almost no difference.

Several conclusions can be drawn from this study.

- For low-constraint TKRs (typically PCL retaining), in the absence of soft tissue restraint, the laxities were too high when the compressive forces were low. At higher compressive loads, the laxity values were in the normal range, with the soft tissues still playing a role at about a one-third level.
- For high-constraint TKRs (typically PCL substituting), the laxity levels were in the normal range at low compressive forces. However, at high compressive forces, there was overconstraint in both AP and IE rotation.
- In both types of knees, the curvatures of the bearing surfaces, primarily the dishing of the tibial surface, played a much more prominent role in controlling laxity, compared with normal intact knees. This was especially true for high-constraint TKRs.

For all types of TKR, surface friction between metal and polyethylene significantly contributes to the reduction in laxity at higher compressive loads, by about one-third below the level if the friction was zero (159). In contrast, the friction in a normal knee is close to zero. If small cement particles are embedded in the plastic surface, the increased friction reduces the laxity to very small levels (198).

The above results have implications to the laxity testing carried out on TKR components in isolation (Fig. 15-22). In all cases, an axial compressive force directed down the long axis of the tibia needs to applied; otherwise, it will be impossible to test the TKRs at all. For TKRs of low constraint, the laxity values measured in cyclic AP force or IE torque, when there is a modest (e.g., 500 N) compressive force acting, will be greatly in excess of those values when implanted in the knee. At high compressive forces, the laxity values will be approximately one-third higher than if the knee was implanted. For high-constraint knees, the laxity values will be reasonably representative of physiological at all loads. However, it should be pointed out that some TKR designs are of high constraint in one mode (e.g., AP) and of low constraint in another mode

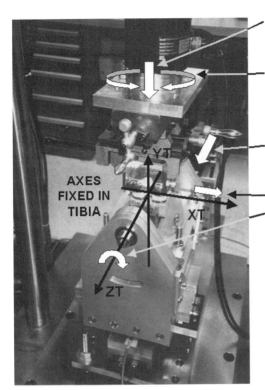

AXIAL FORCE APPLIED TO FEMUR

TORQUE APPLIED TO FEMUR
IN TORQUE TEST 3 OPTIONS:
1. AP DISPLACEMENT FREE
2. AP DISPLACEMENT FIXED
3. AP FORCE CONTROLLED TO ZERO

AP SHEAR FORCE APPLIED TO TIBIA
IN AP FORCE TEST 3 OPTIONS:
1. AXIAL ROTATION FREE
2. AXIAL ROTATION FIXED
3. AXIAL TORQUE CONTROLLED TO ZERO

ML DISPLACEMENT FREE IN ALL TESTS

VARUS-VALGUS ROTATION FREE IN ALL TESTS

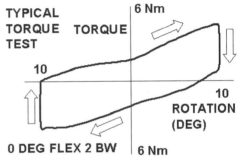

TYPICAL TORQUE TEST

0 DEG FLEX 2 BW

FIGURE 15-22. Equipment for measuring the laxity of TKRs in isolation, *in vitro*. In this particular machine, axial compression, AP force, axial torque, as well as the displacements and rotations, can all be controlled and measured. In addition, selected degrees of freedom can be uncoupled. This system allows for laxity testing for all types of TKR under a range of mechanical condition. (Courtesy Dr. Hani Haider, Department Orthopaedic Surgery, University of Nebraska, Omaha.)

(e.g., rotation). Typical rotating platform knees fit this category.

TKRs where either AP or rotation is unconstrained (except for friction) present a special problem in isolated laxity testing. In these cases, once friction is overcome, the laxity will be infinite. In reality, this does not occur. In this regard, interesting data was reported by Blunn et al. (25), who measured the wear tracks on retrieved unicompartmentals, some of which had been retrieved for instability, for which the plastic surfaces were close to being flat (Fig. 15-23). The average length of the wear tracks, presumably a composite of all motions of the patient, was 25 mm, most cases being within a few millimeters of this value. However, even allowing for "rollback" from extension to flexion, this value is higher than for the normal knee, certainly for the medial side, and hence, some dishing of the plastic surface may be indicated.

4.4 Functional Testing of TKRs in Knee Simulators

There are two basic types of knee simulator that have been used for kinematic studies of the knee. The first type is based on the original Oxford Rig (21,222), whereby a force is applied at the hip applying a flexing moment at the knee, and this is balanced by a force in the quadriceps (Fig. 15-16). A hamstrings muscle action can also be added (115). Typically, measurements are taken at a series of discrete angles, but continuous FE has been obtained (157) and dynamic computer-controlled motion to simulate walking and other activities has also been implemented (85). The Oxford type of rig has the advantage of being a reasonable simulation of the entire lower extremity in activities such as rising from a seated or crouching position, or even walking. 3D motion of the femoral and

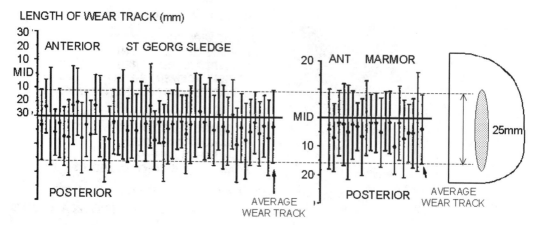

FIGURE 15-23. Position of the wear tracks on 52 retrieved St Georg Sledge unicompartmentals, and on 21 retrieved Marmor unicompartmentals. The average wear track is shown on the right (25).

tibial components can be measured by various means. For example, MacWilliams et al. (115) used a Flock-of-Birds Electromagnetic Tracking System (Ascension Technology, Colchester, VT). From their analytical model the shear force on the tibia due to the hamstrings progressively increased with flexion, affecting the shear displacements. This illustrates a limitation of simulator testing methods, that the ratio of the various muscle forces is not known. However, for the purposes of determining trends, or for comparative testing, an approximation of the muscle action may be sufficient.

The Oxford type of rig can be used in several ways to evaluate TKRs. In principle, a knee specimen can be implanted, a selected test carried out, and then the same test carried out after TKR implantation. For example, kinematics, muscle forces, and patello-femoral forces have all been measured in various studies. The general aim was to determine the effect of design parameters, or how a specific design compares with normal.

Knee simulating machines have been used for both kinematic and wear studies. For the latter purpose, the machines have typically been multichannel and constructed for durability for long-term wear testing. In some machines, flexion–extension, anterior–posterior displacement, and internal–external rotation, together with the compressive force, have been input. This is the so-called "displacement-input" ma-

chine (14,36). The displacements have to be chosen to be appropriate for the particular implant being tested. For example, the displacements for high-constraint designs will be less than for low-constraint designs. Values need to be obtained from calculations, or possibly from fluoroscopy if the particular implant is already in clinical use. Force data need to be obtained from computational methods or from direct measurements using telemetry (187).

The other type of Simulator is "force-input." Here, flexion–extension, AP shear force, internal–external torque, and compressive force are input (Fig. 15-24). The rationale behind this scheme is that the displacements and rotations will be a function of the design of the implant, notably its constraint in the different degrees of freedom (200). The basic assumptions of this scheme are:

- The external forces acting on the knee joint as a system are independent of the design of the TKR implanted.
- The kinematics of the joint, as described by the AP displacement and internal–external rotation, will be a function of the shape of the bearing surfaces the frictional characteristics of the articulating surfaces and the overall design of the TKR.
- For application to wear studies, the wear will be a direct function of the sliding, rolling, and tractive rolling conditions at the joint surfaces.

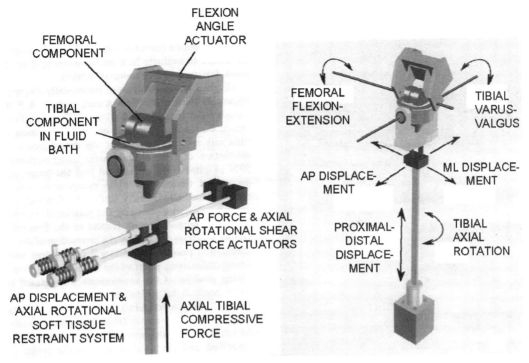

FIGURE 15-24. The mechanical scheme of a force-input knee simulator. Springs of appropriate strength simulate soft-tissue restraint.

One of the requirements for a simulator of this sort is that soft tissue restraint be accounted for. Using literature data (67), a set of springs was computed that would produce the same stiffnesses as the natural knee (53,78,79,200). For resected cruciates, the stiffnesses were reduced. In the initial tests to validate the Instron-Stanmore force-input Simulator, the kinematics were measured for two knee designs at the start of the test and after 5 million cycles (200). It was found that there was a reduction in the AP and rotary laxities. This was attributed to a gradually increasing conformity due to wear and deformation. Such a change in kinematics could not occur in a displacement-input simulator.

A further study was carried out to determine specifically the kinematics of different TKR designs, including fixed bearing and mobile bearing (53). Very large differences over at least a 2:1 range were found in the stance phase of walking, for both AP displacements and IE rotations. The authors then calculated the proportions of the applied forces that were carried by the

TKR surfaces and the soft tissue restraints, which highlighted the fundamentally different ways in which different designs functioned. Some relied primarily on the soft tissues for stability; some relied primarily on the bearing surfaces. Which is preferable is still an open question. However, it was noted that in order to achieve laxity values comparable with those of the natural knee, relatively low constraint was needed in the TKR itself, placing more reliance on the soft tissues. This places some additional requirements on the surgeon in correctly placing the components and balancing the soft tissues.

In a more recent study, four fixed-bearing and three mobile-bearing designs were tested for kinematics (77). The standard ISO test was applied, which showed large differences between designs, especially in IE rotation. An enhanced duty cycle was then applied, intended to simulate more vigorous activities. It was found that the differences in kinematics between designs was thereby increased, and in some cases, the relative values changed. Using the enhanced duty cycle,

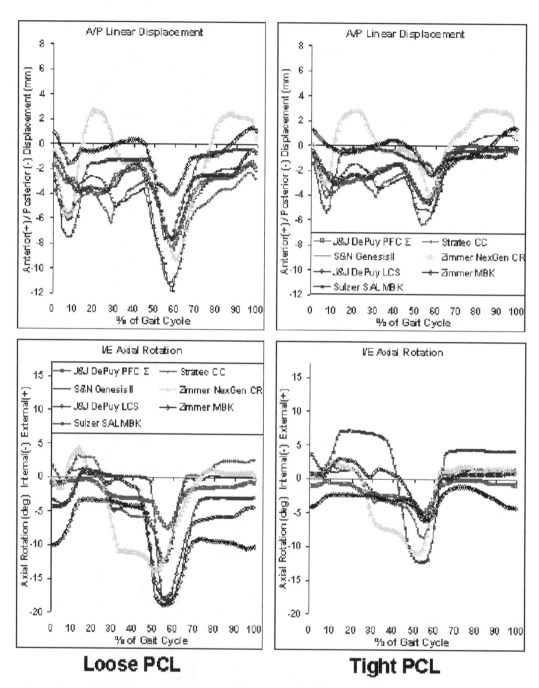

FIGURE 15-25. The differences in the AP and rotational motion patterns during an "enhanced" duty cycle (representing strenuous activities), comparing surgical insertion with a loose PCL with that of a tight PCL.

different setups were applied to simulate variations in surgical placement. Changing the line of action of the compressive force in the frontal plane, equivalent to a change in the frontal valgus angle, did not change the kinematics. Rotating the tibial component about a vertical axis shifted the IE rotational curves in the direction of misalignment. The largest effect on kinematics was changing the tightness of the PCL (Fig. 15-25). For a tight PCL, the displacements and rotations were greatly reduced; a loose PCL had the opposite effect. In all of the tests, the displacements and rotations of the mobile-bearing knees were in the same general range as for the fixed-bearing knees, or even less in some cases. This study provided insights into the relative kinematic behavior of TKRs in relation to patient factors and the alignment of the components at surgery.

4.5 Deformation and Wear of Plastic

The wear seen in retrieved TKRs is highly variable and depends on design, material properties, duration, and alignment (26,45,122,144,219). For partially conforming condylar replacements, on the application of load, a contact patch is produced on each condyle, the shape depending upon the geometry. Contacts approximating circular are called "point contacts," while for close frontal conformity, a cigar-shape called a "line contact" is formed. The contact area on each condyle varies considerably, from about 150 mm^2 for moderate- to high-conformity knees in early flexion, down to 30 mm^2 for low-conformity knees in flexion. The corresponding maximum compressive pressures in activity are 10 to 50 MPa, at the centers on the contact areas, the mean pressure being approximately maximum $\div$ 1.5. The compressive yield stress for polyethylene is in the region of 15 MPa. Hence, it can be seen that most condylar replacements overstress the plastic leading to deformation and residual stresses (63). In contrast, fully conforming mobile-bearing knees have contact areas (lateral and medial) of at least 300 mm^2 on each condyle, giving maximum contact pressures of only 5 MPa.

Within the contact area, at a microscopic level, there are a multitude of local contact points, depending on the microroughness of both the metal and plastic surfaces. There are several mechanisms whereby small plastic particles are released. Some of these mechanisms are fatigue processes requiring numerous cycles of sliding. Multidirectional sliding is more damaging than sliding in exactly the same direc-

tion. The wear processes are also dependent on whether the kinematics involve rolling, tractive rolling, or sliding. These wear processes are as follows:

- *Adhesive wear* occurs when the local shear force on transverse ripples or asperities causes shear deformation or stretching of a fibril, which is then released. The fibrils are typically 2 to 5 μm in length and 0.2 to 0.5 μm in diameter.
- Another form of *adhesive wear* occurs when a plastic asperity accumulates strain energy to the point where a crack develops and the surface particle is released. This typically produces granules of plastic 0.1 to 1.0 μm in size.
- A third form of *adhesive wear* is when a surface layer about 0.1 to 0.2 μm in thickness becomes sheared with respect to the underlying material, similar to the formation of a blister. Eventually, the layer fragments to form flakes, around 2 to 10 μm across.
- A small scratch on the metal surface with positive ridges will produce direct cutting or plowing into the plastic. Several passes across a groove in the plastic, especially at angles to previous passes, will release fibrils or granules. This is called *two-body abrasive wear*.
- If hard particles become drawn into in the contact area, they will also cut grooves in the plastic, causing *three-body abrasive wear*. Plastic particles themselves can produce this type of wear, but to a much lesser extent than hard particles such as metal, ceramic, or bone.
- *Pitting*, the release of small particles about 0.5 mm in size from the surface, is caused by cracks formed by repetitive tensile and compressive stresses at the surface as the contact areas slide over the surface. Around the periphery of the contact the stresses are tensile, whereas within the contact the stresses are compressive.
- *Delamination* is seen as gross disruption of the material to a depth of 0.5 mm or more and is due to the formation and propagation of subsurface cracks. These cracks are thought to be due to the subsurface shear stresses, which fluctuate in magnitude and direction.

Delamination (183) is the most destructive of all the wear mechanisms. This type of damage occurs when cracks form and propagate beneath the surface. A typical crack depth is 1 mm, and the initial area affected can be several millimeters across, seen initially as a white patch on the plastic surface. Once the cracks reach the surface, the consequent disruption of the surface leads to rapid delamination of adjacent areas, eventually covering the entire contact region. These cracks are associated with regions of maximum shear stress, which occur beneath the center of a contact area, at a depth of approximately 0.25 times the contact width, in general 1 to 2 mm. The direction of the shear stress is at 45° to the surface. Beneath the periphery of the contact area in the sectional plane, there are further peaks of shear stress, of lesser magnitude, oriented at 90° to the surface. The stress directions are opposite at the leading and trailing edges of the contact area. Hence, as the femoral component slides across the plastic, particular points beneath the plastic surface will experience shear stresses that change in direction, producing a fatigue situation. The

likelihood of a crack developing and the rate of crack propagation can be described by the strain energy input to an element of material during a complete activity cycle. A parameter to quantify this phenomenon, called a "damage function," was proposed by Sathasivam and Walker (160). The first steps in the calculation were to calculate a sequence of contact point locations during a gait cycle, then calculate the surface and subsurface stresses using FEA (Fig. 15-26). It was found that the regions with the highest damage function were at about 1 mm below the surface. The method was used to compare the damage function patterns for TKRs of different frontal and sagittal plane geometries. It was concluded that the TKR geometry that minimized delamination was a frontal conformity with only a small clearance, a large outer frontal radius, a large PDTA, and a medium (e.g., 60 mm) sagittal tibial radius (162). However, in order to reduce the constraint in rotation, a large tibial radius of, say, 80 mm could be used, for which there was only a small increase in the damage function. However, this might increase the surface wear due to sliding,

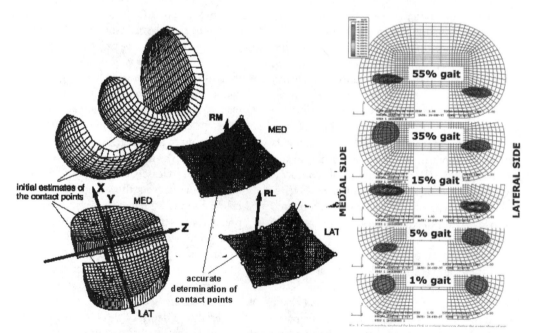

FIGURE 15-26. A computer model of a TKR, where an algorithm was developed to determine contact point locations for a sequence of intervals in a walking cycle. At each interval, contact areas were determined using FEA. A subsurface damage function was calculated for designs of different surface geometries (162).

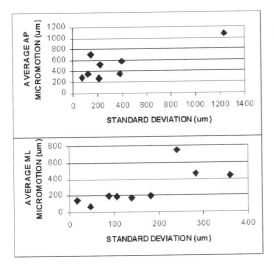

FIGURE 15-27. The total AP and ML motion between the plastic insert and the metal tibial tray when a cyclic load of ±100 N was applied. Each point represents a different design of component. (Data obtained from ref. 140.)

illustrating the trade-offs that are involved with TKR design.

Finally it should be noted that wear debris can originate from locations other than the bearing surfaces. "Back-side wear" between the plastic and the metal tray occurs due to micromotions at that interface (44,140) (Fig. 15-27). Snap-in capture mechanisms, combined with the manufacturing tolerances, can result in considerable motion under shear and torque, even up to 1 mm. If this is accompanied by a rough surface in the metal tray, severe wear can occur. The effects of such wear have been noted particularly in trays with holes for fixation screws, around which osteolytic lesions have developed.

4.6 Wear Testing Using Simulators

The most difficult, expensive, and time-consuming preclinical testing is measuring the long-term wear and deformation in TKRs (55,151,190). Physical tests, like computer models, are simplifications of reality that embody sufficient and appropriate characteristics of the actual situation, to address the question

being asked. In some cases, simple models suffice; in other cases, a complex model (including the human patient) is required.

- Any wear test should replicate as closely as possible the physiological situation, in terms of contact geometry, loads or pressures, crossover of wear tracks (e.g., produced by IE rotation superimposed on sliding), sliding velocity, lubricant, and temperature.
- Test duration should be sufficient to reach a steady-state wear rate, also considering that delamination (if it occurs) may require extended testing.
- Given that tests cannot exactly replicate physiological conditions (which vary in any case), tests should use a control of well-known clinical performance.
- Any wear test method, especially a simulating machine, should be validated by comparing its results with known clinical performance from retrievals and particle analysis.
- Testing under more stringent conditions than physiologic may be applicable for obtaining more rapid comparative results between materials on designs provided unrealistic situations (such as excess surface temperatures) are not obtained.

If the primary concern is to compare a new plastic or a new metal surface, a pin-on-plate test may be appropriate. A basic pin-on-plate test has been used to illustrate differences in wear between UHMWPE processed in different ways (113). A metal indentor with a spherical tip was reciprocated to and fro on UHMWPE plates under a constant load. In this test, shelf-aged material showed delamination and nonirradiated material showed mild surface wear, but the highly cross-linked material showed only a small amount of surface burnishing. Such a basic test was adequate for distinguishing between materials of widely different properties. However, with a spherical tip, the contact pressure will steadily decrease with time (up to a maximum), while the surface wear rate will probably be lower than physiologic because of the absence of wear tracks crossing at small angles from internal–external rotation.

One proposed test that attempted to replicate the sliding and contact conditions of TKRs was as follows (201):

- A metal pin with a spherical surface at the end (femoral) is slid to and fro on a flat plastic plate (tibial).
- The radius of the spherical end produces a similar relative radius of curvature to the TKR design envisaged.
- To account for IE rotation and the crossing over of sliding tracks, the pin is rotated cyclically about its own axis.
- The surrounding medium is 25% to 50% serum at 37°C.
- The fluid is changed every 2 days to minimize degradation.
- The sliding distance is a total of 10 mm.
- A static load of 1,000 N is applied, representing one condyle.
- Samples of fluid are collected every million cycles for particle analysis.
- The particles are characterized as granules, fibrils, and flakes, and the size ranges and the percentages of each are measured.
- The rate of testing is limited to 1 Hz (possibly 2 Hz maximum) to avoid overheating at the contact.

In such a test it is observed that, in the first few hundred thousand cycles, deformation of the plastic predominates over wear, whereas as the contact pressure thereby reduces, deformation reduces and wear predominates. If the objective of a test is to determine the effect of load, contact area, or contact pressure on wear, the above configuration can be reversed with a flat-ended plastic pin sliding on a flat metal plate. Such a test was used to determine the effect of contact area and pressure on the wear rate where plastic pins of different areas were tested under the same load (158). The objective of the test was to examine the rationale for using mobile-bearing knees or other designs with large contact areas. It was found that, for contact diameters of 17 mm and greater, the wear rates were substantially reduced when compared with diameters of 12 mm and less. This would, in general, support the use of TKRs of large contact areas from a wear and damage point of view. However, there may be an

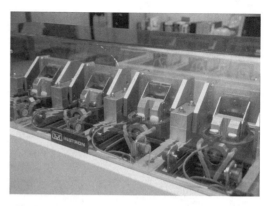

FIGURE 15-28. The four-channel Instron-Stanmore Force-Input knee simulator. Note that the mounting of the tibial components in the dish allows freedom of varus–valgus rotation about an AP axis.

upper limit to the area, after which "starved lubrication" with an increased wear rate may come into play.

To test a TKR for long-term durability where functional load and motion cycles are applied to an actual TKR, a knee simulator is required (Fig. 15-28). If the specified goals of a simulator are simplicity, low cost, reliability, and ease of use, a machine that applies a constant compression force and only FE is the result. However, such a machine is not likely to satisfy the criteria for a close simulation of reality, as show by Kawanabe et al. (103). They showed in a knee simulator that compared with a reference wear rate when only FE was applied, the subsequent superposition of internal rotation or AP displacement led to progressively higher wear rates. Based on the activities of typical patients, described in Section 2.4, a walking cycle is a suitable input, preferably with 5% to 10% of more rigorous cycles representing ascending and descending. The FE can be controlled by the machine, and the following forces cyclically applied: compressive force, varus moment, AP shear force, and IE torque. This is the force-input scheme described in Section 4.4 (Fig. 15-24).

In the test setup, the relative motions between the femur and tibia, except FE, are unconstrained, but to simulate soft tissue restraint, mechanical springs are mounted between the femoral and tibial holders. The assumption made with this type of simulating machine is that the forces which the knee experiences *in vivo* are independent of the type of TKR. This may not be strictly true because the contact point locations, or axis of rotation determined by the TKR, may affect the muscle forces needed to equilibrate the external forces on the knee. However, the major advantage of the scheme is that the laxities occurring during the activity cycles will be determined by the knee itself. This is important because the wear and damage will be in direct relation to the amount of rolling (58), tractive rolling, and sliding that takes place. In support of this, Blunn et al. (27) found that a cyclic load applied at the same location produced only light burnishing, rolling also produced light burnishing, but cyclic sliding produced surface wear and subsurface delamination. Wimmer et al. (217) showed wear pattern on retrievals which indicated that areas showing striated wear patterns were produced by cyclic tractive rolling.

Displacement-input machines have been used to compare wear of different TKR designs (10). The AP and IE rotation in the gait cycle were estimated based on the TKR constraint. In another study (49) representative motions of a TKR were determined from a fluoroscopy study. In this case, the machine differentiated between two types of UHMWPE, one irradiated and the other nonirradiated. Delamination occurred with the former but not with the latter. Also, the surface wear rates were higher for the irradiated material. Such a test, in that it duplicates the findings from retrievals, can be regarded as a validation of the test method, although this is not an absolute test. The input to a displacement-input simulator has been obtained from gait analysis using the point cluster technique (101). To validate any input to the test samples, it was proposed that the slip velocity profiles were the most important parameter. Such an approach is likely to yield wear rates that are representative of clinical cases, and also differentiate between the lateral and medial wear patterns.

It is evident that there are a number of alternate methods for predicting the wear of UHMWPE (or other materials) in TKR. Methods that have been used for quantifying the wear and deformation include:

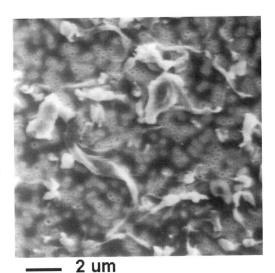

———   2 um

FIGURE 15-29. Wear particles filtered from the fluid using a Millipore filter system. The particles can be characterized as granules, fibrils, and flakes (38,39).

- *Surface profilometry.* Specified times after testing are required for complete recovery of the plastic from viscoelastic deformation. The method is precise but includes deformation as well as wear.
- *Gravimetric.* The major problem is the steady imbibing of fluid into the plastic samples. A soak control needs to be used so that weighings are taken at equivalent soak conditions. However, the soak control cannot be subjected to precisely the same mechanical conditions as the test samples (otherwise, the control would wear also), and hence, there will be some difference in fluid uptake.
- *Particle analysis* (Fig. 15-29). Methods have been developed for isolating, filtering, and analyzing the particles from the fluid used in tests, as well as from tissue around implants (38,39,86,87,108). Particles have been characterized as granules, fibrils, and sheets, shapes relevant to the tissue response. Ultimately the test results need to be compared alongside data obtained from clinical analyses.

Over the past decade there have been dramatic changes in an understanding of the factors leading to the surface wear and delamination of polyethylene. Retrieval studies showed a wide variety of wear severities as a function of design, type of polyethylene, and duration (18,26,43,45,61,88,102,164). In one study, autopsy retrievals were studied, more representative of well-functioning implants (110). Even for the same design, the severities and contact locations varied considerably. Some of the variations can be accounted for by surgical placement of components, soft tissue tensions, and activity patterns of the patient. All of this variation makes it difficult to specify reference wear behaviors for validating simulators.

Two major factors emerged as being responsible for the serious delamination type of wear (154). The hot-pressing procedure produced an interface about 1 mm below the surface in the flat-on-flat PCA design. Gamma-irradiation in air produced free radicals on the polyethylene chains, to which oxygen bonded shortly after the sterilization procedure, on the shelf (especially after long time periods such as 2 years or more), or in the patient (15,16,17). This oxidation resulted in a serious loss of mechanical properties, especially tensile strength and fatigue resistance (105). On the positive side, UHWPE which had been net-shape molded, as in the AGC MG1, and IB1 designs, showed only mild surface wear without delamination, even in long-term retrievals, which was confirmed by knee simulator wear testing (15). In about the mid- to late 1990s, most companies changed the processing method for UHMWPE, either gamma-irradiating in an inert atmosphere or using other sterilization methods such as gas plasma or ETO. This will undoubtedly reduce the incidence of delamination wear in TKRs inserted after that time.

More recently, the possibilities of reducing wear more dramatically have been proposed by using highly cross-linked polyethylene (132). Using an accelerated pin-on-plate test, Yao et al. (220) demonstrated that e-beam irradiated and melt-annealed highly cross-linked UHMWPE exhibited markedly improved delamination resistance and oxidation resistance, compared with a gamma-irradiated control. Using similar material in a knee simulator, a wear reduction of 80% was measured compared with the gamma-irradiated control (109). Data during the follow-ing decade will ascertain whether the potential for this new processed method will be realized.

4.7   Clinical Evaluation

The most commonly used method for evaluating the postoperative performance of a TKR is a clinical assessment such as the Knee Society or HSS scoring system. These methods provide an overall assessment of range of motion, the ability to perform various activities, and pain. It has been found that many total knee designs (with the exception of poor designs), even of different mechanical configuration such as PCL-preserving or -substituting, or even mobile-bearing knees, have very similar assessment scores. There are a number of possible explanations for this including the fact that a high proportion of the patients are older and have limited function in any case. The Knee Society has also specified a radiographic assessment (65,189) for documenting alignment (127) and interface radiolucencies (207). Survivorship analysis is commonly used to determine the failure rate over time based on different criteria, usually removal of at least one component for any cause such as pain, instability, wear, or fracture (150).

The most commonly used biomechanical assessment method in the past has been gait analysis (216). Important insights have been gained in the adaptation patterns adopted by patients due to abnormal contact points and patella tracking. Some studies have also been carried out using equipment such as the Cybex, which assesses muscular strength, although such results are not likely to relate specifically to the type of TKR in place.

In recent years, "fluoroscopic analysis" has been introduced as a method for determining the 3D orientation of the femoral and tibial components in an activity sequence (Fig. 15-30) (209). Originally, the method was derived from a 2D object recognition technique described by Wallace and Wintz (210) in their paper entitled "An efficient three-dimensional aircraft recognition algorithm using normalized Fourier descriptors." According to Banks and Hodge (11),

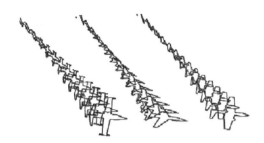

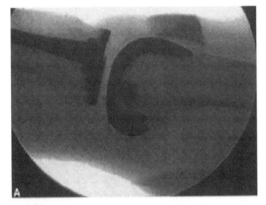

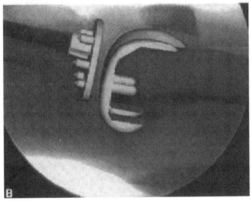

FIGURE 15-30. CAD models of the femoral and tibial components are profile-matched to fluoroscopic images. In this way the 3D orientation and position of the components relative to each other can be computed.

The kinematic measurement approach is based on imaging the knee joint as it moves, using x-ray fluoroscopy to obtain a sequence of images in which the prosthesis is projected as a 2-D perspective silhouette. These images are processed to extract the contours of the silhouette. The position and orientation of the TKR components are then estimated based on the position and orientation of the computer model (CAD) which generated the best matching contour.

Dennis et al. (51,52) similarly adapted the method to the study of knee movement *in vivo.* In recent publications, the accuracy is reported to be about 1° and 1 mm. Generally the results are stated to be shown as femoral–tibial contact positions, showing the lateral and medial contact point locations, joining the points with a line. It is noted that this does not exactly correspond to the "projection of the femoral axis on to the tibial surface" method used by Iwaki and others (see Fig. 15-2).

In some of the earlier studies (180), "paradoxical motion" was described for the deep knee bend activity where an anterior femoral translation was found with flexion in PCL preserving designs, due in part to a starting point at zero flexion posterior to the midline, because of the absence of the ACL. The motion patterns were variable between different patients, and were even variable for repeated trials by the same patient. PCL-substituting designs, on the other hand, showed less erratic patterns and showed posterior translation of the contact points with flexion. The differences between the two design types can be explained mainly by the geometry of the tibial-bearing surfaces. For the shallower surfaces of the PCL-preserving design, greater variation in contact position is possible because of the low constraint. This can be seen as an advantage in allowing such freedom of position without imposing high shear forces on the bearing components. For the more constrained PCL-substituting design, freedom of motion is reduced, especially in IE rotation (12).

An example of freedom of position was illustrated for the Mobile Bearing Knee (MBK) design using the fluoroscopic method (202). This MBK allows freedom of IE rotation as well as 4.5 mm of AP translation. This allows for a variable axis of IE rotation, rather than its being restricted to a single point as in the LCS design. Subjects with an MBK were asked to stand upright and then to twist the knee internally then externally. This was called the "twisting test."

A total of 15 patients successfully carried out this exercise. The average total rotation angle was 17.9°, with a range from 4.0° to 34.4° and a standard deviation of 8.8°. On average, the pivot point was within 1 mm of the centerline

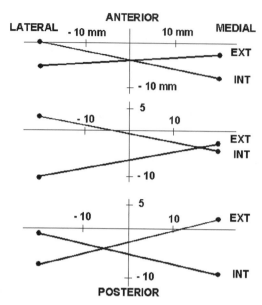

FIGURE 15-31. Three examples of the rotation of the femur on the tibial for the MBK in the twisting test. *(Top)* Central axis; *(center)* medial axis; *(bottom)* lateral axis.

of the tibia. Defining a central pivot point as within 5 mm of the centerline, there were three lateral pivots, seven central pivots, and five medial pivots. Particular examples of these three different locations of pivot points are shown in Fig. 15-31.

It was concluded that the particular design of MBK allowed freedom of position in rotation. This is one of the potential advantages of an MBK design, that there is freedom of the neutral rotational position and also freedom of motion during activities. The implication is that TKRs with high laxity, by allowing freedom of position, move in a variety of motion paths, which may not resemble normal knee motion. An extensive study of this subject has since been carried out by Banks and Hodge (13). However, the advantage of reproducing "normal knee motion" has yet to demonstrated, and considering the pathological condition of soft tissues in arthritic knees, it may not be possible in any case.

5 CONCLUDING REMARKS

Modern-day TKR systems usually consist of a group of designs for different indications. The designs can range from compartmental replacements (unis) to rotating hinges and even segmental replacements. The large majority of the usage is of the condylar replacement type, either PCL retaining or PCL substituting. Often there are several sets of instruments, depending on component placement specifications and surgeon preference.

Further advances in design and technique are being investigated on a number of fronts. An increase in the range of flexion achieved will be an advantage for many patients. Reduction in surface wear and delamination, using optimized molded or highly cross-linked UHMWPE, is likely to extend longevity. The improved materials, together with better plastic-tibial tray locking mechanisms, are likely to minimize backside wear also. More durable fixation may be achieved by revisiting bone ingrowth using enhanced porous materials and component designs. Improved accuracy and reproducibility of surgical technique (116) using navigation systems and robotics is already showing promise and may well become extensively used. Minimally invasive surgery, which provides reduced morbidity and more rapid recovery (147), especially for compartmental replacement, will become more frequently used.

All of the above require further advances in both research and technology, and an ongoing partnership including the biomechanician, the orthopaedic surgeon, and other specialists. The question is often raised as to whether tissue engineering or other biological approaches to treating osteoarthritis of the knee will supplant TKRs. Once the arthritis has reached an advanced stage, it is difficult to visualize a treatment more effective than a TKR, which even now has a high success rate of relieving pain and restoring function for at least 20 years. Both function and durability are likely to improve still further based on the advances under investigation today. Nevertheless, in early arthritis, tissue engineering is already finding applications, and this influence is likely to expand. Finally, the field of cause and prevention should not be overlooked. It may be possible to devise simple remedial measures which prevent or delay the onset of osteoarthritis.

ACKNOWLEDGMENTS

To the many collaborators with whom the author has worked over the years, to the granting agencies who have funded our research work, and to the manufacturing companies who have assisted in many ways. The manuscript was prepared by Ms. S. Lerner.

REFERENCES

1. Abernethy PJ, Robinson CM, Fowler RM. Fracture of the metal tibial tray after Kinematic total knee replacement. *J Bone Joint Surg* 1996;78-B (2):220–225.
2. Ahir AP, Blunn GW, Haider H, et al. Evaluation of a testing method for the fatigue performance of total knee tibial trays. *J Biomech* 1999;32:1049–1057.
3. Ahir AP, Blunn GW, Harrison M, et al. The fatigue performance of tibial trays using the International Standards Organization (ISO) test method. *J Biomech (in press)*.
4. Ahmed AM, Burke DL. In-vitro measurement of static pressure distribution in synovial joints—part 1: tibial surface of the knee. *J Biomech Eng* 1983;105:216–225.
5. Akagi M, Nakamura T. Matsusue Y, et al. The Bisurface total knee replacement: a unique design for flexion. *J Bone Joint Surg* 2000;82-A:1626–1633.
6. Altfield SF, Warren-Forward M, Wilton T, et al. Measurement of soft tissue in balance in total knee arthroplasty using electronic instrumentation. *Med Eng Phys* 1994;16:501–505.
7. Andriacchi TP, Alexander EJ. Studies of human locomotion: past, present, and future. *J Biomech* 2000;33:1217–1224.
8. Andriacchi TP, Yoder D, Conley A, et al. Patellofemoral design influences function following total knee arthroplasty. *J Arthroplasty* 1997; 12(3):243–249.
9. Andriacchi TP, Mikosz RP. Musculoskeletal dynamics, locomotion and clinical applications. In: Mow VC, Hayes WC, eds. *Basic orthopaedic biomechanics.* New York: Raven Press, 1991:51–92.
10. Ash HE, Burgess IC, Unsworth A. Long-term results for Kinemax and Kinematic knee bearings on a six-station knee simulator. *IMechE (Proc Inst Mech Eng)* 2000;214(5):437–447.
11. Banks SA, Hodge WA. Accurate measurement of three-dimensional knee replacement kinematics using single-plane fluoroscopy. *IEEE Trans Biomed Eng* 1996;43(6):638–649.
12. Banks SA, Markovich GD, Hodge WA. *In vivo* kinematics of cruciate-retaining and -substituting knee arthroplasties. *J Arthroplasty* 1997;12(3): 297–304.
13. Banks S, Hodge WA. Where's the pivot? Patterns of axial rotation in fixed and mobile bearing knee arthroplasties. *Trans Orthop Res Soc* 2002;27:0054.
14. Barnett PI, Mcwen HMJ, Auger DD, et al. Investigation of wear prostheses in a new displacement/force-controlled simulator. *J Eng Med* 2002; 216(H):51–61.
15. Bell CJ, Blunn GW, Walker PS, et al. Oxidation and wear resistance of directly moulded UHMWPE. In: 9th conference of the European Orthopaedic Research Society combined with the 4th EFFORT meeting. Abstract. Brussels, Belgium, June 3–4, 1999.
16. Bell C, Walker PS, Abeysundera M, et al. Effect of oxidation on delamination of ultra-high-molecular-weight polyethylene tibial components. *J Arthroplasty* 1998;13(3):280–290.
17. Bell CJ, Simmons J, King P, et al. Is oxidation of ultra high molecular weight polyethylene the main cause of delamination wear in total knee replacement? *Trans Orthop Res Soc* 1997;22(1):96.
18. Bell CJ, Walker PS, Sathasivam S, et al. Differences in wear between fixed bearing and mobile bearing knees. *Trans Orthop Res Soc* 1999;24:962.
19. Berchuck M, Andriacchi TP, et al. Gait adaptations by patients who have a deficient ACL. *J Bone Joint Surg* 1990;72-A:871–877.
20. Bergmann G, Graichen F, Rohlmann A. Hip joint loading during walking and running, measured in two patients. *J Biomech* 1993;26:969–990.
21. Biden E, O'Connor J. Experimental methods used to evaluate knee ligament function. In: Daniel DM, Akeson WH, O'Connor JJ, eds. *Knee ligaments, structure, function, injury and repair.* New York: Raven Press, 1990:135–151.
22. Blankevoort L, Huiskes R, de Lange A. The envelope of passive knee joint motion. *J Biomech* 1988;21(9):705–720.
23. Blankevoort L, Huiskes R, de Lange, A. Helical axes of passive knee joint motions. *J Biomech* 1990;23:1219–1229.
24. Blankevoort L, Huiskes R. Validation of a three-dimensional model of the knee. *J Biomech* 1996;29(7):955–961.
25. Blunn GW, Joshi AB, Lilley PA, et al. Polyethylene wear in unicondylar knee prostheses: 106 retrieved Marmor, PCA and St. Georg tibial components compared. *Acta Orthop Scand* 1992;63(3):247–255.
26. Blunn GW, Joshi AB, Minns RJ, et al. Wear in retrieved condylar knee arthroplasties. *J Arthroplasty* 1997;12(3):281–290.
27. Blunn GW, Walker PS, Joshi A, et al. The dominance of cyclic sliding in producing wear in total knee replacements. *Clin Orthop* 1991;273:253–260.

28. Böhm P, Holy T. Is there a future for hinged prostheses in primary total knee arthroplasty? *J Bone Joint Surg* 1998;80-B(2):302–309.

29. Bradley J, Goodfellow JW, O'Connor JJ. A radiographic study of bearing movement in unicompartmental Oxford knee replacements. *J Bone Joint Surg* 1987;69-B(4):598–601.

30. Brand RA, Pedersen DR, Davy DT, et al. Comparison of hip force calculations and measurements in the same patient. *J Arthroplasty* 1994;9:45–51.

31. Brooks PJ, Walker PS, Scott RD. Tibial component fixation in deficient tibial bone stock. *Clin Orthop* 1984;184:302–308.

32. Browne M, Langley RS, Gregson PJ. Reliability theory for load bearing biomedical implants. *Biomaterials* 1999;20:1285–1292.

33. Buechel FF, Keblish PA, Lee JM, et al. Low contact stress meniscal bearing unicompartmental knee replacement: long-term evaluation of cemented and cementless results. *J Orthop Rheumatol* 1994;7:31–41.

34. Buechel FF, Pappas MJ. New Jersey low contact stress knee replacement system. *Orthop Clin North Am* 1989;20(2):147–177.

35. Buechel FF, Pappas MJ. Long-term survivorship analysis of cruciate-sparing versus cruciate-sacrificing knee prostheses using meniscal bearings. *Clin Orthop* 1990;260:162–169.

36. Burgess IC, Kolar M, Cunningham JL, et al. Development of a six-station knee wear simulator and preliminary wear results. *Proc Inst Mech Eng* 1997;211(Part H):37–47.

37. Callaghan JJ, Squire MA, Goetz DD, et al. Cemented rotating-platform total knee replacement: a nine to twelve-year follow-up study. *J Bone Joint Surg* 2000;82-A(5):705–711.

38. Campbell P, Ma S, Schmalzried T, et al. Tissue digestion for wear debris particle isolation. *J Biomed Mater Res* 1994;28(4):523–526.

39. Campbell P, Ma S, Yeom B, et al. Isolation of predominantly submicron-sized UHMWPE wear particles from periprosthetic tissues. *J Biomed Mater Res* 1995;29:27–131.

40. Chen F, Krackow KA. Management of tibial defects in total knee arthroplasty. *Clin Orthop and Related Res* 1994;305:249–257.

41. Churchill D, Incavo SJ, Johnson CC, et al. The influence of femoral rollback on patellofemoral contact loads in total knee arthroplasty. *J Arthroplasty* 2001;16(7):909–918.

42. Churchill D, Incavo SJ, Johnson CC, et al. The transepicondylar axis approximates the optimal flexion axis of the knee. *Clin Orthop* 1998;356:111–118.

43. Collier JP, Mayor MB, McNamara JL, et al. Analysis of the failure of 122 polyethylene inserts from uncemented tibial knee components. *Clin Orthop* 1991;273:232–242.

44. Conditt M, Ismaily S, Pararic V, et al. Quantitative assessment of backside wear of polyethylene tibial inserts. *Trans Orthop Res Soc* 2002;27:0160.

45. Currier BH, Currier JH, Collier JP, et al. Shelf life and *in vivo* duration. Impacts on performance of tibial bearings. *Clin Orthop* 1997;342:111–122.

46. Dahlkvist NJ, Mayo P, Seedhom BB. Forces during squatting and rising from a deep squat. *Eng Med* 1982;11:69–76.

47. Davy DT, Kotzar G, Brown RH, et al. Telemetric force measurements across the hip after total arthroplasty. *J Bone Joint Surg* 1988;70A(1):45–50.

48. Delp SL, Loan PJ, Hoy MG, et al. An interactive graphics-based model of the lower extremity to study orthopaedic surgical procedures. *IEEE Trans Biomed Eng* 1990;37(8):757–767.

49. Deluzio KJ, O'Connor DO, Bragdon CR, et al. Development of an *in vitro* knee delamination model in a knee simulator with physiologic load and motion. Poster Session—Knee, 46th annual meeting, Orthop Res Soc, Orlando, FL, 2000.

50. Dennis D, Komistek RD, Scuderi G, et al. *In vivo* three-dimensional determination of kinematics for subjects with a normal knee or a unicompartmental or total knee replacement. *J Bone Joint Surg* 2001;83-A:104–115.

51. Dennis DA, Komistek RD, Hoff WA, et al. *In vivo* knee kinematics derived using an inverse perspective technique. *Clin Orthop* 1996;331:107–117.

52. Dennis DA, Komistek RD, Mahfouz MR, Haas BD, Stiehl JB. Multicenter determination of *in vivo* kinematics after total knee arthroplasty. *Clin Orthop* 2003;416:37–57.

53. DesJardins JD, Walker PS, Haider H, et al. The use of a force-controlled dynamic knee simulator to quantify the mechanical performance of total knee replacement designs. *J Biomech* 2000;33:1231–1242.

54. Des Jardins JD, Walker PS, Haider H, et al. An analysis of tibial component and soft tissue shear loads during a force controlled walking cycle for multiple TKR designs (Abstract). In: Ed. 9th conf Eur Orthop Res Soc, Brussels, 1999.

55. Dowson D, ed. *Advances in medical tribology.* London: Mechanical Engineering Publications, 1998.

56. Draganich L, Pottenger L. TRAC PS knee design and clinical outcome. In: Abstracts, ann symp Int Soc Technol Arthroplasty, Marseille, 1998;96–99.

57. Draganich LF, Andriacchi TP, Andersson GBJ. Interaction between intrinsic knee mechanics and the knee extensor mechanism. *J Orthop Res* 1987;5(4):539–547.

58. Elad D, Seliktar R, Mendes D. Synthesis of a knee joint endoprosthesis is based on pure rolling. *Eng Med* 1981;10(2):97–105.

59. Ellis MI, Seedhom BB, Wright V. Forces in the knee joint whilst rising from a seated position. *J Biomed Eng* 1984;6:113–120.

60. Engelbrecht E, Nieder E, Klüber D. Ten to twenty years of knee arthroplasty at the Endo-Klinik: a report on the long-term follow-up of the St. Georg Hinge and the medium-term follow-up of the Rotating Knee ENDO Model. Endo-Klinik, Holstenstrasse 2, D-22767 Hamburg, Germany.

61. Engh CA, Dwyer KA, Hanes CK. Polyethylene wear of metal backed tibial components in total and unicompartmental knee prostheses. *J Bone Joint Surg* 1992;74-B:9–17.

62. Ericson MO, Nisell R. Patellofemoral joint forces during ergometric cycling. *Phys Ther* 1987;67:1365–1369.

63. Estupinan JA, Bartel DL, Wright TM. Residual stresses in ultra-high molecular weight polyethylene loaded cyclically by a rigid moving indenter in nonconforming geometries. *J Orthop Res* 1998;16:80–88.

64. Ewald FC. Metal to plastic total knee replacement. *Orthop Clin North Am* 1975;6:811.

65. Ewald FC. The Knee Society Total Knee Arthroplasty roentgenographic evaluation and scoring system. *Clin Orthop* 1989;248:9–12.

66. Flivik G, Ljiung P, Rydholm U. Fracture of the tibial tray of the PCA knee. *Acta Orthop Scand* 1990;61:26–28.

67. Fukubayashi T, Torzilli PA, Sherman MF, et al. An *in vitro* biomechanical evaluation of anterior–posterior motion of the knee. Tibial displacement, rotation, and torque. *J Bone Joint Surg* 1982; 64-A:258–264.

68. Garg A, Walker PS. Prediction of total knee motion using a 3-dimensional computer-graphics model. *J Biomech* 1990;23:45–58.

69. Godest A-C, Beaugonin M, Haug E, et al. Simulation of a knee joint replacement during a gait cycle using explicit finite-element analysis. *J Biomech* 2002;35:267–275.

70. Godest A-C, Simonis de Cloke C, Taylor M, et al. A computational model for the prediction of total knee replacement kinematics in the sagittal plane. *J Biomech* 2000;33:435–442.

71. Goldstein SA, Wilson DL, Sonstegard DA, et al. The mechanical properties of human tibial trabecular bone as a function of metaphyseal location. *J Biomech* 1983;16(12):965–969.

72. Gollehon DL, Torzilli PA, Warren RF. The role of the posterolateral and cruciate ligaments in the stability of the human knee. *J Bone Joint Surg* 1987;69-A:233–242.

73. Goodfellow J, O'Connor J. The mechanics of the knee and prosthesis design. *J Bone Joint Surg* 1978;60-8:358–369.

74. Gradisar IA, Hoffmann ML, Askew MJ. Fracture of a fenestrated metal backing of a tibial knee component. *J Arthroplasty* 1989;4(1):27–30.

75. Grood ES, Suntay WJ. A joint co-ordinate system for the clinical description of three-dimensional motions: application to the knee. *J Biomech Eng* 1983;105:136.

76. Gunston FH. Polycentric knee arthroplasty prosthetic simulation of normal knee movement. *J Bone Joint Surg* 1971;53-B(2):272–277.

77. Haider H, Walker PS, Blunn GW. Are the kinematics of different TKR designs targeted for the same patient the same? *Trans Orthop Res Soc* 2002;27:0965.

78. Haider H, Walker PS. Matching spring stiffnesses to soft tissue restraint in knee simulator testing of total knee replacement under force control. In: Int Soc Technol Arthroplasty (ISTA), Hawaii, September 2001. Paper No. 276.

79. Haider H, Walker PS. Analysis and recommendations for the optimum spring configurations for soft tissue restraint in force-control knee simulator testing. In: Trans Orthop Res Soc, 48th annual meeting, Dallas, TX, February 2002.

80. Harris ML, Morberg P, Bruce WJM, et al. An improved method for measuring tibiofemoral contact areas in total knee arthroplasty: a comparison of K-Scan sensor and Fuji film. *J Biomech* 1999;32: 951–958.

81. Harrington IJ. A bioengineering analysis of force actions at the knee in normal and pathological gait. *Biomed Eng* 1976;11(1):167–172.

82. Harrington IJ. Static and dynamic loading patterns in knee joints with deformities. *J Bone Joint Surg* 1983;65-A(2):247–259.

83. Hefzy MS, Kelly BP, Cooke TDV. Kinematics of the knee joint in deep flexion: a radiographic assessment. *Med Eng Phys* 1983;20:302–307.

84. Hill PF, Vedi V, William A, et al. Tibiofemoral movement: the loaded and unloaded knee studies by MRI. *J Bone Joint Surg Br* 2000;82:1196.

85. Hillberry BM, Schaff JA, Cullom CD, et al. Laboratory knee simulation: a viable option. In: 10th annual meeting, Soc Biomater, Washington, DC, Apr 27–May 1, 1984:149.

86. Hirakawa K, Bauer TW, Stulberg BN, et al. Characterization of debris adjacent to failed knee implants of 3 different designs. *Clin Orthop* 1996; 331:151–158.

87. Hirakawa K, Bauer W, Yamaguchi M, et al. Relationship between wear debris particles and polyethylene surface damage in primary total knee arthroplasty. *J Arthroplasty* 1999;14(2):165–171.

88. Hood RW, Wright TM, Burstein AH. Retrieval analysis of total knee prostheses. *J Biomed Mater Res* 1983;17:829–842.

89. Hsieh HH, Walker PS. Stabilizing mechanisms of the loaded and unloaded knee joint. *J Bone Joint Surg* 1976;58-A(1):87–93.

90. Huberti HH, Hayes WC. Patellofemoral contact pressures. The influence of Q-angle and tendofemoral contact. *J Bone Joint Surg* 1984;66-A (5):715–724.

91. Hvid I. The stability of the human patello-femoral joint. *Eng Med* 1983;12(2):55–59.

92. Hvid I. Trabecular bone strength at the knee. *Clin Orthop* 1988;227:210–222.

93. Hvid I, Andersen K, Olesen S. Cancellous bone strength measurements with the osteopenetrometer. *Eng Med* 1984;13(2):73–78.

94. Hvid I, Bentzen SM, Jorgensen J. Remodelling of the tibial plateau after knee replacement. *Acta Orthop Scand* 1988;59(5):567–573.

95. Hvid I, Christensen P, Sondergard J, et al. Compressive strength of tibial cancellous bone. *Acta Orthop Scand* 1983;54:819–825.

96. Inglis AE, Walker PS. Revision of failed knee replacements using fixed-axis hinges. *J Bone Joint Surg* 1991;73-B(5):757–761.

97. Inman VT, Ralston HJ, Todd F. *Human walking*. Baltimore: Williams & Wilkins, 1981.

98. Insall JN, Lachiewicz PF, Burstein AH. The posterior stabilized condylar prosthesis: a modification of the total condylar design. *J Bone Joint Surg* 1982;64-A(9):1317–1323.

99. Iversen BF, Sturup J, Jacobsen K, et al. Implications of muscular defense in testing for the anterior drawer sign in the knee: a stress radiographic investigation. *Am J Sports Med* 1989;17(3):409–413.

100. Iwaki H, Pinskerova V, Freeman MAR. Tibiofemoral motion 1: the shapes and relative movements of the femur and tibia in the unloaded cadaver knee. *J Bone Joint Surg* 2000;82-B:1189–1195.

101. Johnson T, Andriacchi T, Laurent M. Development of a knee wear test method based on prosthetic *in vivo* slip velocity profiles. In: Session 5— Implant Wear I, 46th annual meeting, Orthop Res Soc, Orlando, FL, 2000.

102. Jones VC, Williams IR, Auger DD, et al. Quantification of third body damage to the tibial counterface in mobile bearing knees. *Proc Inst Mech Eng* 2001;215(H):171–179.

103. Kawanabe K, Clarke IC, Tamura J, et al. Effects of A-P translation and rotation on the wear of UHMWPE in a total knee joint simulator. In: Poster Session—Implant Wear, 47th annual meeting, Orthop Res Soc, San Francisco, CA, 2001.

104. Komisteck RD, Stiehl JB, Dennis DA, et al. Mathematical model of the lower extremity joint reaction forces using Kane's method of dynamics. *J Biomech* 1998;31:185–189.

105. Kurtz SM, Rimnac CM, Santner TJ, et al. Exponential model for the tensile true stress-strain behaviour of as-irradiated and oxidatively degraded ultra high molecular weight polyethylene. *J Orthop Res* 1996;14:755–761.

106. Kuster MS, Wood GA, Stachowiak GW, et al. Joint load considerations in total knee replacement. *J Bone Joint Surg* 1997;79-B:109–113.

107. Kwak SD, Blankevoort L, Ateshian GA. A mathematical formulation for 3D quasi-static multibody models of biarthrodial joints. *Comp Methods Biomech Biomed Eng* 2000;3:41–64.

108. Landry ME, Blanchard CR, Mabrey JD, et al. *Morphology of in vitro generated ultrahigh molecular weight polyethylene wear particles as a function of contact conditions and material parameters*. New York: John Wiley & Sons, *J Biomed Mater Res* 1999 Spring;48(1):61–69.

109. Laurent MP, Yao JQ, Bhamri S, et al. High cycle wear of highly crosslinked UHMWPE tibial articular surfaces evaluated in a knee wear simulator. In: 48th annual meeting, Orthop Res Soc, 2002.

110. Lavernia CJ, Sierra RJ, Hungerford DS, et al. Activity level and wear in total knee arthroplasty. *J Arthroplasty* 2001;16(4):446–453.

111. Li G, Gil J, Kanamori A, et al. A validated three-dimensional computational model of a human knee joint. *J Biomech Eng* 1999;121:657–662.

112. Li G, Zayontz S, Most E, et al. Cruciate-retaining and cruciate-substituting total knee arthroplasty. An *in vitro* comparison of the kinematics under muscle loads. *J Arthroplasty* 2001;16(8): (Suppl. 1).150–156.

113. Long M, Sauer W, Ries M, et al. Delamination wear study of crosslinked UHMWPE. In: Poster Session, 47th annual meeting, Orthop Res Soc, San Francisco, CA, 2001.

114. Luger E, Sathasivam S, Walker PS. Inherent differences in the laxity and stability between the intact knee and total knee replacements. *Knee* 1997;4: 7–14.

115. MacWilliams BA, Wilson DR, DesJardins JD, et al. Hamstrings cocontraction reduces internal rotation, anterior translation, and anterior cruciate ligament load in weight-bearing flexion. *J Orthop Res* 1999;17:817–822.

116. Mahaluxmivala MS, Bankes MJK, Nicolai P, et al. The effect of surgeon experience on component positioning in 673 press fit condylar posterior cruciate-sacrificing total knee arthroplasties. *J Arthroplasty* 2001;16(5):635–640.

117. Markolf KL, Bargar WL, Shoemaker SC, et al. The role of joint load in knee stability. *J Bone Joint Surg* 1981;63-A(4):570–585.

118. Markolf KL, Graff-Radford A, Amstutz HC. *In vivo* knee stability. *J Bone Joint Surg* 1978;60-A (5):664–674.

119. Markolf KL, Wascher DC, Finerman GAM. Direct *in vitro* measurement of forces in the cruciate ligaments. *J Bone Joint Surg Am* 1993;75-A(3):387–394.

120. Matthews LS, Sonstegard DA, Henke JA. Load bearing characteristics of the patello-femoral joint. *Acta Orthop Scand* 1977;48:511–516.

121. McLeod PC, Kettelkamp DB, Sprinivasan V, et al. Measurements of repetitive activities of the knee. *J Biomech* 1975;8:369–373.

122. McGloughlin TM, Kavanagh AG. Wear of ultra-high molecular weight polyethylene (UHMWPE) in total knee prostheses: a review of key influences. *Proc Inst Mech Eng* 2000;204(H):349–359.

123. Menchetti PPM, Walker PS. Mechanical evaluation of mobile bearing knees. *Am J Knee Surg* 1997;10:73–82.

124. Mendes DG, Brandon D, Galor L, et al. Breakage of the metal tray in total knee replacement. *Orthopaedics* 1984;7:860–862.

125. Miller RK, Goodfellow JW, Murray DW, et al. *In vitro* measurement of patellofemoral force after three types of knee replacement. *J Bone Joint Surg* 1998;80-B:900–906.

126. Mizuno Y, Kumagai M, Mattessich SM, et al. Q-angle influences tibiofemoral and patellofemoral kinematics. *J Orthop Res* 2001;19:834–840.

127. Moreland JR, Hanker GJ. Lower extremity axial alignment of normal males. In: Lawrence D. Dorr, ed. *The knee.* Baltimore: University Park Press, 1985:55–58.

128. Morrey BF, Chao EYS. Fracture of the porous-coated metal tray of a biologically fixed knee prosthesis. *Clin Orthop* 1988;228:182–189.

129. Morrison JB. Function of the knee joint in various activities. *Bio-Med Eng* 1969;4(12):573–580.

130. Morrison JB. The mechanics of the knee joint in relation to normal walking. *J Biomech* 1970;3(1):51–61.

131. Most ELIG, Otterberg E, Sabbag K, et al. The effect of posterior cruciate retention and substitution on tibial-femoral motion in total knee arthroplasty. *Trans Orthop Res Soc* 2001;26:1092.

132. Muratoglu OK, Bragdon CR, O'Connor DO, et al. A novel method of cross-linking ultra-high-molecular-weight polyethylene to improve wear, reduce oxidation, and retain mechanical properties. *J Arthroplasty* 2001;16(2):149–160.

133. Murray D, Webb J, Price A, et al. Minimally-invasive Oxford unicompartmental knee replacement. Proc Int Conf Knee Replacement 1974–2024, London, Institution of Mechanical Engineers, 1999.

134. Murray DG, Webster DA. The variable axis prosthesis: 2-year follow-up study. *J Bone Joint Surg* 1982;63-AL:687–694.

135. Nakagawa S, Kadoya Y, Todo S, et al. Tibiofemoral movement: full flexion in the living knee studied by MRI. *J Bone Joint Surg Br* 2000;82:1199.

136. Nisell R. Mechanics of the knee: a study of joint and muscle load with clinical applications. *Acta Orthop Scand* 1985;56(Suppl)216:7–47.

137. Nisell R, Ericson M. Patellar forces during isolinetic knee extension. *Clin Biomech* 1992;7:104–108.

138. Nissan M. Review of some basic assumptions in knee biomechanics. *J Biomech* 1980;13:(4):375–381.

139. Olanlokun KFT, Wills DPM. A spatial model of the knee for the preoperative planning of knee surgery. *Proc Inst Mech Eng J Eng Med* 2002;216(H):63–75.

140. Parks NL, Engh GA, Topoleski T, et al. Modular tibial insert micromotion: a concern with contemporary knee implants. The Coventry Award. *Clin Orthop Rel Res* 1998;356:10–15.

141. Paul JP. Development of standards for orthopaedic implants. *Proc Inst Mech Eng* 1997;211:119–126.

142. Paul JP. Forces transmitted by joints in the human body. *Proc Inst Mech Eng* 1967;181(3):8–15.

143. Paul JP. Strength requirements for internal and external prostheses. *J Biomech* 1999;32:381–393.

144. Peterson C, Benjamin JB, Szivek JA, et al. Polyethylene particle morphology in synovial fluid of failed knee arthroplasty. *Clin Orthop* 1999;359:167–175.

145. Piziali RL, Rastegar JC. Measurements of the nonlinear, coupled stiffness characteristics of the human knee. *J Biomech* 1977;10:45–55.

146. Polyzoides AJ, Dendrinos GK, Tsakonas H. The Rotaglide total knee arthroplasty. Prosthesis design and early results. *J Arthroplasty* 1996;11(4):453–459.

147. Price AJ, Webb J, Topf H, et al. Rapid recovery after Oxford unicompartmental arthroplasty through a short incision. *J Arthroplasty* 2001;16:970–976.

148. Psychoyios V, Crawford RW, O'Connor JJ, et al. Wear of congruent meniscal bearings in unicompartmental knee arthroplasty. *J Bone Joint Surg* 1998;80-B:976–982.

149. Pugh S. *Total design.* New York: Addison-Wesley, 1994.

150. Rand JA, Ilstrup DM. Survivorship analysis of total knee arthroplasty. *J Bone Joint Surg* 1991;73(39):397–409.

151. Rawlinson J, Furman B, Li S, et al. Kinematics, stresses, and damage from a TKR simulator and a finite-element model. In: Session 36—Knee Arthroplasty, 47th annual meeting, Orthop Res Soc, San Francisco, CA, 2001.

152. Reilly DT, Martens M. Experimental analysis of the quadriceps muscle force and patello-femoral joint reaction force for various activities. *Acta Orthop Scand* 1972;43:126–137.

153. Reinschmidt C, van den Bogert AJ, Nigg BM, et al. Effect of skin movement on the analysis of skeletal knee joint motion during running. *J Biomech* 1997;30:729–732.

154. Rimnac CM, Klein RW, Betts F, et al. Post-irradiation aging of ultra-high molecular weight polyethylene. *J Bone Joint Surg* 1994;76-A(7): 1052–1056.

155. Robie BH, Daellenbach KK, Bolanos A, et al. Retrieval analysis of constrained condylar tibial components. *Trans Orthop Res Soc* 1997;22:644.

156. Robinson R. Evolution of condylar knee replacement. *J Arthroplasty (in press)*.

157. Rovick JS, Reuben JD, Schrager RJ, et al. Relation between knee motion and ligament length patterns. *Clin Biomech* 1991;6(4):213–220.

158. Sathasivam S, Walker PS, Campbell PA, et al. The effect of contact area on wear in relation to fixed bearing and mobile bearing knee replacements. *J Biomed Mater Res* 2001;58(3):382–390.

159. Sathasivam S, Walker PS. A computer model with surface friction for the prediction of total knee kinematics. *J Biomech* 1997;30(2):177–184.

160. Sathasivam S, Walker PS. A computer model to predict subsurface damage in tibial inserts of total knees. *J Orthop Res* 1998;16:564–571.

161. Sathasivam S, Walker PS. Optimisation of the bearing surface geometry of total knees. *J Biomech* 1994;27(3):255–264.

162. Sathasivam S, Walker PS. The conflicting requirements of laxity and conformity in total knee replacement. *J Biomech* 1999;32:239–247.

163. Sathasivam S, Walker PS, Pinder I, et al. Custom constrained condylar total knees using CAD-CAM. *Knee* 1999;6:49–53.

164. Schmalzried TP. Current concepts review. Wear in total hip and knee replacements. *J Bone Joint Surg* 1999;81-A(1):115–136.

165. Schmalzried TP, Szuszczewicz ES, Northfield MR, et al. Quantitative assessment of walking activity after total hip or knee replacement. *J Bone Joint Surg* 1998;80-A:54–59.

166. Scott RD. Prosthetic replacement of the patellofemoral joint. *Orthop Clin North Am* 1979;10(1):129–137.

167. Scott RD, Santore RF. Unicondylar unicompartmental replacement for osteoarthritis of the knee. *J Bone Joint Surg* 1981;63-A(4):536–544.

168. Scott RD, Volatile TB. Twelve years' experience with posterior cruciate-retaining total knee arthroplasty. *Clin Orthop* 1986;205:100–107.

169. Scott WN, Rubinstein M. Posterior stabilized knee arthroplasty. *Clin Orthop* 1986;205:138–145.

170. Seedhom BB, Longton EB, Dowson D, et al. The Leeds Knee. In: Proc Total Knee Replacement Conf, London, 1974. London: Mechanical Engineering Publications, 1975:108–114.

171. Seedhom BB. Conformity and the patella surface. In: Proc Total Knee Replacement Conf, London, 1974. London: Mechanical Engineering Publications, 1975:175–177.

172. Seedhom BB, Terayama K. Knee forces during the activity of getting out of a chair with and without the aid of arms. *Biomed Eng* 1976;11:278–282.

173. Seedhom BB, Wallbridge NC. Walking activities and wear of prostheses. *Ann Rheum Dis* 1985;44:838.

174. Sathasivam S, Walker PS, Pinder I, et al. Custom constrained condylar total knees using CAD-CAM. *Knee* 1999;6:49–53.

175. Shoemaker SC, Markolf KL. Effects of joint load on the stiffness and laxity of ligament-deficient knees. *J Bone Joint Surg* 1985;67-A(1):136–146.

176. Singerman R, Davy DT, Goldberg VM. Effects of patella alta and patella infera on patello-femoral contact forces. *J Biomech* 1994;27(8): 1059–1065.

177. Singerman R, Pagan HD, Peyser AB, et al. Effect of femoral component rotation and patellar design on patellar forces. *Clin Orthop* 1997;334:345–353.

178. Soudry M, Walker PS, Reilly DT, et al. Effects of total knee replacement design on femoral–tibial contact conditions. *J Arthroplasty* 1986;1(1): 35–45.

179. Steele JR, Roger GJ, Milburn PD. Tibial translation and hamstring activity during active and passive arthrometric assessment of knee laxity. *Knee* 1995;1(4):217–223.

180. Stiehl JB, Komistek RD, Dennis DA, et al. Fluoroscopic analysis of kinematics after posterior-cruciate-retaining knee arthroplasty. *J Bone Joint Surg* 1995;77-B(6):884–889.

181. Stukenborg-Colsman C, Ostermeier S, Wenger KH, et al. Relative motion of a mobile bearing inlay after total knee arthroplasty—dynamic *in vitro* study. *Clin Biomech* 2002;17:49–55.

182. Suh NP. *Axiomatic design.* Oxford, UK: Oxford University, 2001.

183. Suh NP. *Tribophysics.* Englewood Cliffs, NJ: Prentice Hall, 1986:114–122.

184. Takei T. A posterior stabilised TKR based on converging condyles. In: Annual meeting of the Japanese Knee Society, Ohita, Japan, 2002;20–22.

185. Taylor SJG, Perry JS, Meswania JM, et al. Telemetry of forces from proximal femoral replacements and relevance to fixation. *J Biomech* 1997;30(3):225–234.

186. Taylor SJG, Walker PS. Forces and moments telemetered from two distal femoral replacements during various activities. *J Biomech* 2001;34:839–848.

187. Taylor S, Walker PS, Perry J, et al. The forces in the distal femur and the knee during walking and other activities measured by telemetry. *J Arthroplasty* 1998;13(4):428–437.

188. Toksvig-Larsen S. Minimally-invasive surgery for the next decade? In: Proc Int Conf Knee Replacement 1974–2024, London, 1999. London:

Professional Engineering Publishing, Institution of Mechanical Engineers, 1999:261–263.

189. Uematsu O, Hsu HP, Kelley KM, et al. Radiographic study of kinematic total knee arthroplasty. *J Arthroplasty* 1987;2:317–326.

190. Unsworth A. Tribology of human and artificial joints. *Part H: J Eng Med Proc IME* 1991;205:163–172.

191. Unwin PS, Walker PS, Blunn GW. Rotating hinge, hydroxyapatite coated versus fixed hinged, uncoated distal femoral replacement. A study of 402 cases. In: 10th Int Symp, Int Soc Limb Salvage (ISOLS). Cairns, Australia, 1999.

192. Walker PS. Human joints and their artificial replacements, Chapter 6. Springfield, IL: Charles C Thomas, 1977;253–275.

193. Walker PS. Design of a knee prosthesis system. *Acta Orthop Belgica* 1980;46(6):766–775.

194. Walker PS. The total-condylar knee and its evolution. In: Ranawat CS, ed. *Total condylar arthroplasty. Techniques, results and complications.* New York: Springer-Verlag, 1985:7–23.

195. Walker PS. Bearing surface design in total knee replacement. *Eng Med* 1988;17(4):149–156.

196. Walker PS. Design of Kinemax total knee replacement bearing surfaces. *Acta Orthop. Belgica* 1991;57(Suppl. II):108–113.

197. Walker PS. A new concept in guided knee motion total knee arthroplasty. *J Arthroplasty* 2001; 16:157–163.

198. Walker PS, Ambarek MS, Morris JR, et al. Anterior–posterior stability in partially conforming condylar knee replacement. *Clin Orthop* 1995;310:87–97.

199. Walker PS, Blunn GW. Biomechanical principles of total knee replacement design. In: Mow VC, Hayes WC, eds. *Basic orthopaedic biomechanics,* 2nd ed. Philadelphia: Lippincott-Raven, 1997:461–493.

200. Walker PS, Blunn GW, Broome DR, et al. A knee simulating machine for performance evaluation of total knee replacements. *J Biomech* 1997;30(1):83–89.

201. Walker PS, Blunn GW, Lilley PA. Wear testing of materials and surface for total knee replacement. *J Biomed Mater Res (Appl Biomater)* 1996;33:159–175.

202. Walker PS, Komistek RD, Barrett DS, et al. Motion of a mobile bearing knee allowing translation and rotation. *J Arthroplasty* 2002;17:(1):11–19.

203. Walker PS, Manktelow ARJ. Comparison between a constrained condylar and a rotating hinge in revision knee surgery. *Knee* 2001;8:269–279.

204. Walker PS, Sathasivam S. Controlling the motion of total knee replacements using intercondylar guide surfaces. *J Orthop Res* 2000;18(1):48–55.

205. Walker PS, Sathasivam S. The design of guide surfaces for fixed-bearing and mobile-bearing knee replacements. *J Biomech* 1999;32:27–34.

206. Walker PS, Sathasivam S. Design forms of total replacement. *Proc Inst Mech Eng* 2000;214(H):101–119.

207. Walker PS, Sathasivam S, Cobb A, et al. A comparison between cemented, press-fit, and HA-coated interfaces in Kinemax total knee replacement. *Knee* 2000;9:71–78.

208. Walker PS, Wang C-J, Masse Y. Joint laxity as a criterion for the design of condylar knee prostheses. Proc Total Knee Replacement Conf. London: Mechanical Engineering Publications for The Institution of Mechanical Engineers, 1975:22–29.

209. Walker SA, Komistek R, Hoff W, et al. "*In vivo*" pose estimation of artificial knee implants using computer vision. *Biomed Sci Instrum* 1996;32:143–150.

210. Wallace TP, Wintz PA. An efficient three-dimensional aircraft recognition algorithm using normalized fourier descriptors. *Comput Graphics Image Processing* 1980;13:99–126.

211. Wang A, Essner A, Klein R. Effect of contact stress on friction and wear of ultra-high molecular weight polyethylene in total hip replacement. *Proc Inst Mech Eng* 2001;215:133–139.

212. Wang C-J, Walker PS. Rotatory laxity of the human knee joint. *J Bone Joint Surg* 1974;56-A(1):161–170.

213. Weaver JK, Derkash RS, Greenwald AS. Difficulties with bearing dislocation and breakage using a movable bearing total knee replacement system. *Clin Orthop* 1993;290:244–252.

214. Weinstein JN, Andriacchi TP, Galante J. Factors influencing walking and stair-climbing following unicompartmental knee arthroplasty. *J Arthroplasty* 1986;1:109–115.

215. Williams A, Vedi V, Gedroyc W, et al. "Dynamic" M.R.I. scanning of the weight-bearing asymptomatic knee-tibio-femoral motion during flexion. In: Proc EFORT Congress, Brussels, 1999:44.

216. Wilson SA, McCann PD, Gotlin RS, et al. Comprehensive gait analysis in posterior-stabilized knee arthroplasty. *J Arthroplasty* 1996;11(4):359–367.

217. Wimmer MA, Andriacchi TP, Loos RN, et al. A striated pattern of wear in ultrahigh-molecular-weight polyethylene components of Miller-Galante total knee arthroplasty. *J Arthroplasty* 1998;13(1):8–16.

218. Wixson RL, Elasky N, Lewis J. Cancellous bone material properties in osteoarthritic and rheumatoid total knee patients. *J Orthop Res* 1989;7:885–892.

219. Wrona M, Mayor MB, Colliers JP, et al. The correlation between fusion defects and damage in

tibial bearings. *Clin Orthop Rel Res* 1994;229:92–103.

220. Yao JQ, Gsell R, Laurent MP, et al. Improved delamination resistance of melt-annealed electron-beam irradiated highly crosslinked UHMWPE knee inserts. In: Soc Biomater 28th annual meeting, 2002.

221. Yu CH, Walker PS, Dewar ME. The effect of design variables of condylar total knees on the joint forces in step climbing based on a computer model. *J Biomech* 2001;34:1011–1021.

222. Zavatsky AB. A kinematic-freedom analysis of a flexed-knee-stance testing rig. *J Biomech* 1997;30(3):277–280.

223. Zavatsky AB, O'Connor JJ. A model of the human knee ligaments in the sagittal plane. Part 1: response to passive flexion. *Proc Inst Mech Eng* 1992;206(H3):125–134.

INDEX

Note: Page numbers followed by f indicate figures; page numbers followed by t indicate tables.